A Pattern Based Approach

Atlas of Genitourinary Pathology

SARA E. WOBKER, MD, MPH
Department of Pathology and Laboratory Medicine
University of North Carolina at Chapel Hill
Chapel Hill, North Carolina

SEAN R. WILLIAMSON, MD, FASCP
Department of Pathology
Robert J. Tomsich Pathology and Laboratory Medicine Institute
Cleveland Clinic
Cleveland, Ohio

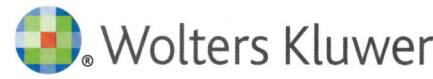 Wolters Kluwer

Philadelphia • Baltimore • New York • London
Buenos Aires • Hong Kong • Sydney • Tokyo

Acquisitions Editor: Nicole Dernoski
Development Editor: Ariel Winter
Editorial Coordinator: Tim Rinehart
Marketing Manager: Phyllis Hitner
Production Project Manager: Sadie Buckallew
Design Coordinator: Stephen Druding
Manufacturing Coordinator: Beth Welsh
Prepress Vendor: TNQ Technologies

Library of Congress Cataloging-in-Publication Data is available upon request from the publisher.

ISBN-13: 978-1-4963-9766-9

To all of my teachers, especially the patients.
To my partner Ben, ready with encouragement or baked goods when times were tough.
Sara E. Wobker, MD, MPH

To my wife, Alexandra, who makes me a better person.
In memory of my mentor, Dr. David J. Grignon, who lived each day as if practicing genitourinary pathology were an absolute treat.
Sean R. Williamson, MD

Considering the broad and expanding knowledge base in diagnostic pathology, a conceptual framework is necessary for learners, especially those at the beginning of their training. Whereas other textbooks may be encyclopedic, with detailed information regarding each diagnostic entity, this book provides a broad conceptual approach based on morphologic patterns that can be recognized by both new learners and those aiming to explore differential diagnostic possibilities. Our goal is to provide the framework for approaching diagnosis of common genitourinary diseases, with numerous images for the entities highlighting their most useful diagnostic features. To that end, more than 1350 images are provided covering the full range of genitourinary pathology, including prostate, bladder, kidney, testis, and external genitalia. For each organ, we begin with an overview of normal and "near normal" before discussing abnormal findings. Disease processes are grouped by broad morphologic pattern, usually a "low-power" assessment that will help guide the reader to the appropriate section of the book. Within each section, disease processes are described based on additional helpful patterns and diagnostic features unique to that entity.

We are fortunate to be "standing on the shoulders of giants"— series editors Dr. Christina Arnold, Dr. Dora Lam-Himlin, and Dr. Elizabeth Montgomery—as we developed this book. Following the success of the editions that came before the genitourinary atlas, this book is structured in a similar manner, reflecting a belief that grouping disease processes by morphologic patterns can facilitate learning and increase diagnostic efficiency. As such, we have included numerous checklists, key features, diagnostic pearls and pitfalls, frequently asked questions, and sample notes in the text. The goal is to make the text approachable for new learners while also serving as a practical reference during sign-out for practicing pathologists.

- Each chapter begins with the "Unremarkable and Nonneoplastic" to orient the reader to the organ and point out variations of normal which may be confusing to learners.

- "Pearls and Pitfalls" are provided throughout the book to highlight things commonly discussed in real time at the microscope during teaching sessions, focusing on real-life conundrums.

- The "Frequently Asked Questions" section reflects both testable and practical questions heard from consulting pathologists and trainees.

- "Key Features" are provided as succinct lists to summarize topics for easy reference.

- In select entities where specific diagnostic challenges are common, "Sample Notes" are provided as a template for how the authors relay complex information in a concise manner, often with important references that are useful for clinical decision-making.

- "Near Misses" are included to alert the reader to close calls and tips for avoiding pitfalls in difficult diagnoses.

- The "Quiz" questions for each chapter serve to emphasize the most important points of the chapter and solidify the reader's knowledge. Topics are selected to reflect both diagnostic challenges and board-testable facts to serve as board preparation.

ACKNOWLEDGMENTS

We extend our gratitude to the diverse group of supporters who helped us throughout the inception and completion of this book. Dr. Wobker is especially grateful for Dr. Elizabeth Montgomery's sponsorship that led to the opportunity to work on this book. We thank Dr. Steven Billings for helpful review of dermatologic aspects of the external genitalia section, and Drs. Khaleel I. Al-Obaidy, Giovanna Giannico, Ondrej Hes, Chia-Sui "Sunny" Kao, Andres Matoso, Ankur R. Sangoi, Steven C. Smith, and Matthew J. Wasco for providing figures. We thank our editorial team for their encouragement throughout the process.

CONTENTS

CHAPTER OUTLINE

THE UNREMARKABLE AND NONNEOPLASTIC PROSTATE

ANATOMY AND HISTOLOGY

Since both resection specimens and needle biopsy samples from the prostate are common in surgical pathology practice, some knowledge of anatomy and the zonal architecture of the normal prostate can be helpful to orient samples as viewed under the microscope and avoid a few specific diagnostic pitfalls. This chapter will include some discussion of the most relevant aspects of anatomy and prostate zones with implications for diagnostic practice; however, for more detailed discussion, other thorough reviews are available.[1] The modern understanding of prostatic zonal anatomy was heavily influenced by the pioneering work from McNeal et al.,[2-5] which established the main prostatic zones.

KEY FEATURES: Zones of the Prostate

The main prostate zones[1] are as follows:

1. The peripheral zone (where most cancers are thought to originate), a crescent-shaped area that rims the lateral and posterior areas of the prostate
2. The transition zone (the epicenter of benign prostatic hyperplasia), typically manifesting as bilateral periurethral circumscribed nodules, although sometimes asymmetrical
3. The central zone (relatively infrequently involved by cancer), a cone-shaped area that becomes more prominent toward the base of the prostate, adjacent to the ejaculatory ducts
4. The anterior fibromuscular stroma, an anterior area that often lacks glandular structures, although not always

Most core needle biopsies collected via transrectal ultrasound-guided approach are intentionally targeted toward the posterolateral aspects of the gland (particularly the peripheral zone), attempting to have the highest diagnostic yield for cancer while minimizing sampling of benign nodular hyperplasia. However, with the evolution of multiple novel biopsy techniques more recently, other approaches are sometimes taken, including magnetic resonance imaging (MRI)–targeted biopsies of specific lesions, as well as transperineal saturation biopsies that attempt to "map" the prostate for location and extent of any potential cancers.[6,7] The histology of these biopsies is generally similar, with the possible exceptions that transperineal biopsies can contain fragments of skin in place of colorectal tissue, and that some may be predominantly fibromuscular stroma, if not targeted at the peripheral zone.

Awareness of these anatomic zones can assist with orienting the prostatic tissue on the slide. In general, whole-mount processing of radical prostatectomy specimens makes orientation easy[8]; however, since this technique can be challenging for routine adoption in pathology practices, its use is in the minority, with only 16% of participants in an International Society of Urological Pathology (ISUP) consensus using the whole-mount technique.[8] Therefore, in conventional sections, several subtle clues may be helpful to distinguish different anatomic regions of the prostate if sections are not clearly labeled or if there is a concern they have been mislabeled.

KEY FEATURES: Orienting Prostatic Tissue on the Microscopic Slide

- Skeletal muscle is admixed with the prostate stroma in the anterior and apex.[1,9] If there is a concern that apex and base margins are not correctly labeled, the presence of skeletal muscle usually favors apical location (Figure 1.1)
- Since skeletal muscle intermingles with the prostate in the apex and anterior, glands within skeletal muscle are not necessarily malignant (Figure 1.2)
- Malignant glands within skeletal muscle do not necessarily constitute extraprostatic extension, but this often indicates close proximity to the prostatic apex (see Sample Note)[10] (Figure 1.3)
- The verumontanum usually forms a triangular protuberance in the urethra at mid-prostate.[1] This "arrow" consistently points toward the anterior (Figure 1.4)
- The paired ejaculatory ducts are located posterior to the urethra on each side of midline, usually visualized in sections from mid-gland or the base of the prostate (Figure 1.5). In conventional cassettes, one ejaculatory duct may be present in each (left/right) posterior section. A rich vascular network is often visible in the posterior midline surrounding the ejaculatory ducts (Figure 1.6)

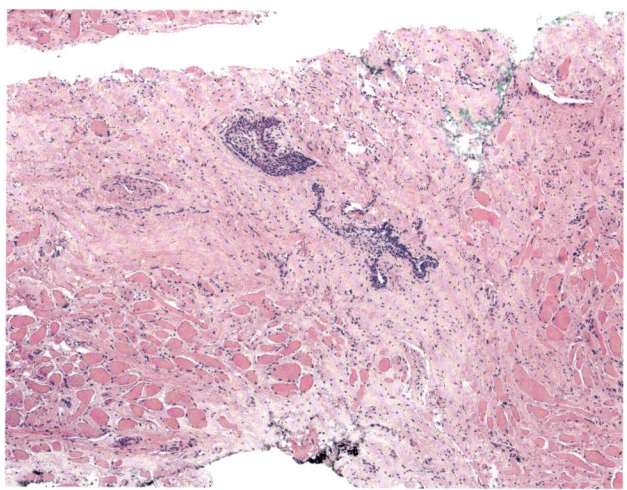

Figure 1.1. Skeletal muscle is admixed with the prostate in the apex (shown here) and anterior, which may assist in orientation of tissue sections.

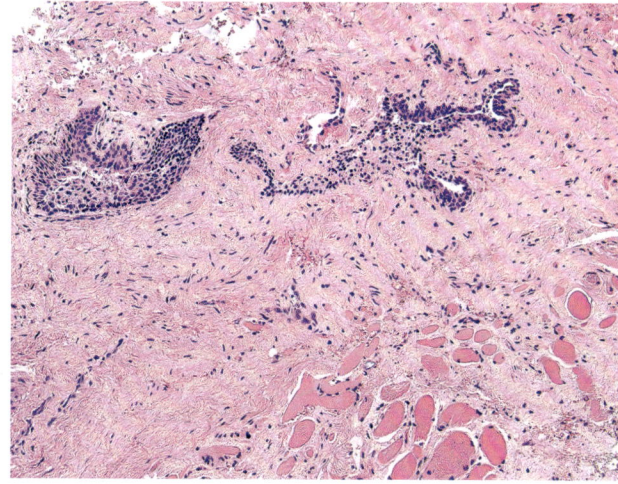

Figure 1.2. Benign glands can be admixed with skeletal muscle. This is not necessarily an indicator of malignancy.

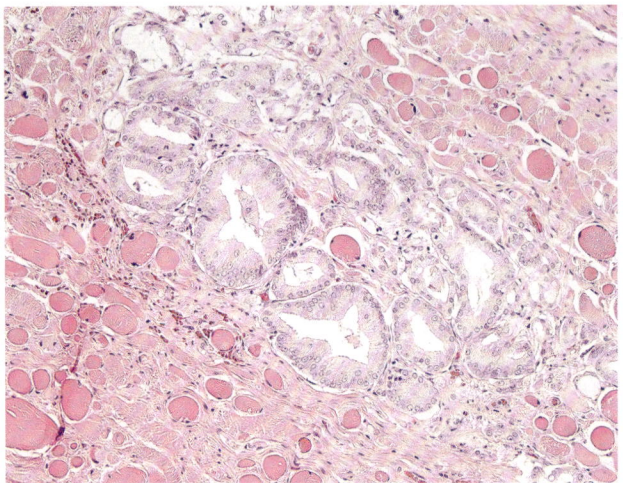

Figure 1.3. Malignant glands within skeletal muscle do not necessarily constitute extraprostatic extension, but this often indicates proximity to the prostatic apex.

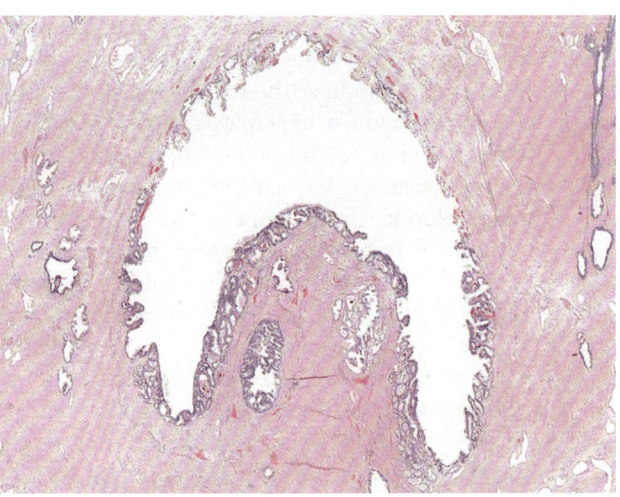

Figure 1.4. The verumontanum is a protuberance in the prostatic urethra that points toward the anterior, which can be helpful for orientation.

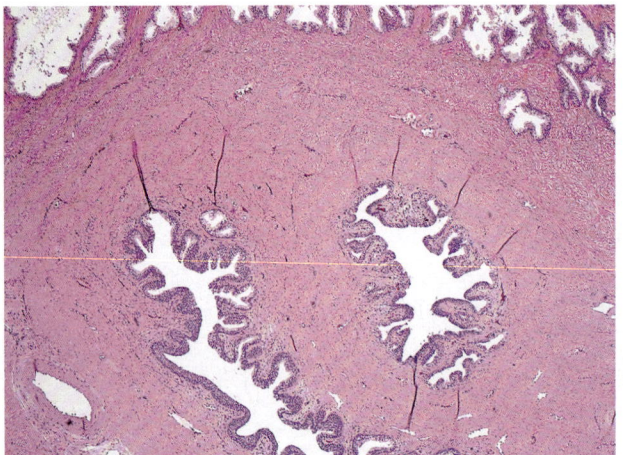

Figure 1.5. The ejaculatory ducts are located posterior to the urethra at the base of the prostate, just left and right of midline.

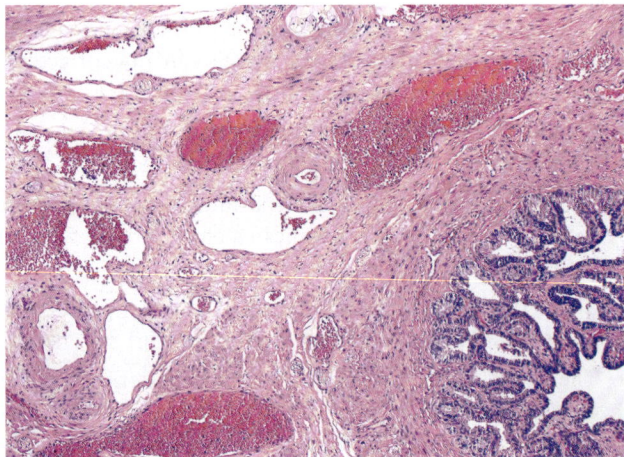

Figure 1.6. There is often a rich vascular network (left) surrounding the ejaculatory ducts (right).

- Depending on the extent of dissection, sections from the base of the prostate may contain larger muscle bundles, consistent with bladder muscularis propria, that contrast to the confluent fibromuscular stroma of the prostate (Figure 1.7). Involvement of these larger bundles microscopically constitutes pT3a prostate cancer (bladder neck invasion)[9] (Figure 1.8)

- The anterior fibromuscular stroma is often devoid of glandular tissue, which can serve to distinguish it from posterior peripheral zone in tissue sections

- The central zone is located in the midline of the prostate posteriorly, predominantly toward the base of the prostate, and has unique histologic features, often including dense fibromuscular stroma, slightly larger and more haphazardly arranged nuclei, and "Roman arch" bridging[1,11] (Figures 1.9 and 1.10). This can be mistaken for high-grade prostatic intraepithelial neoplasia (PIN), but does not have the hyperchromatic nuclei or prominent nucleoli of true PIN. Nonetheless, it is possible for true PIN to involve the central zone (Figure 1.11)

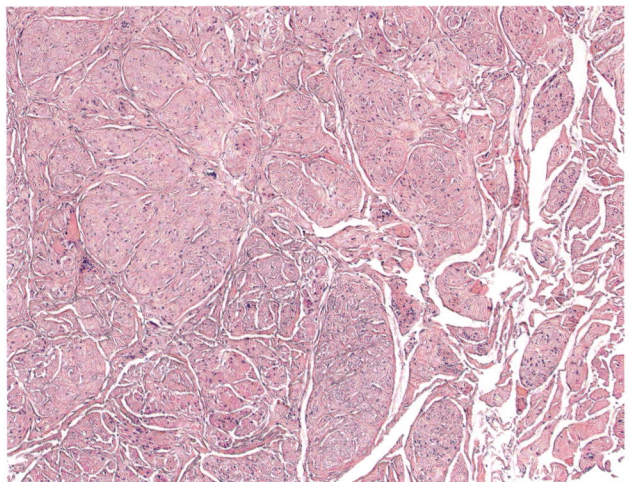

Figure 1.7. The bladder neck can be discerned microscopically based on larger discrete muscle bundles, in contrast to the confluent smooth muscle of the prostatic stroma.

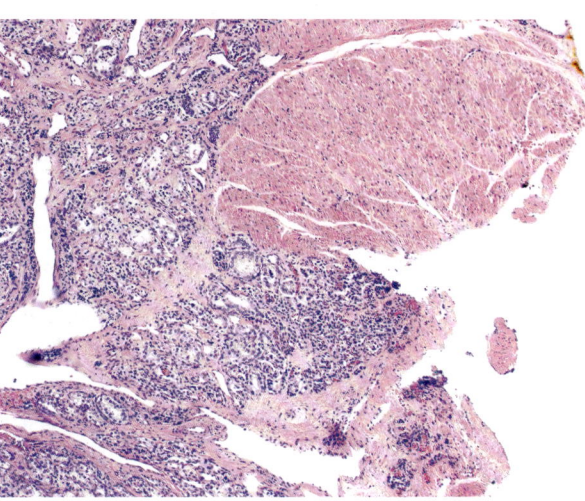

Figure 1.8. Invasion of the bladder neck muscle by prostatic adenocarcinoma constitutes pT3a.

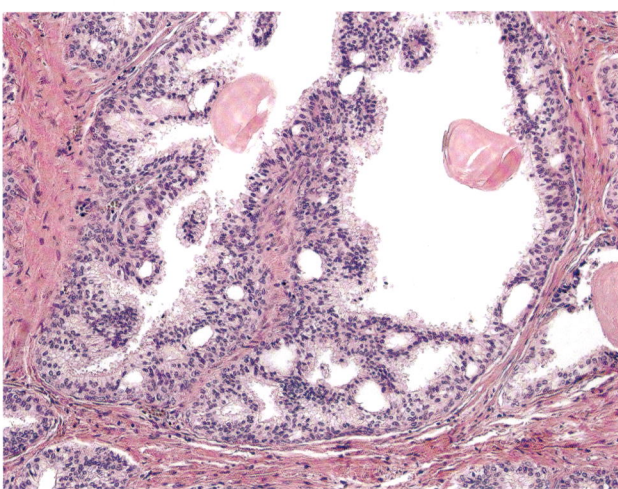

Figure 1.9. The normal central zone of the prostate has a cribriform-like morphology that may be confused for prostatic intraepithelial neoplasia (PIN) or cancer.

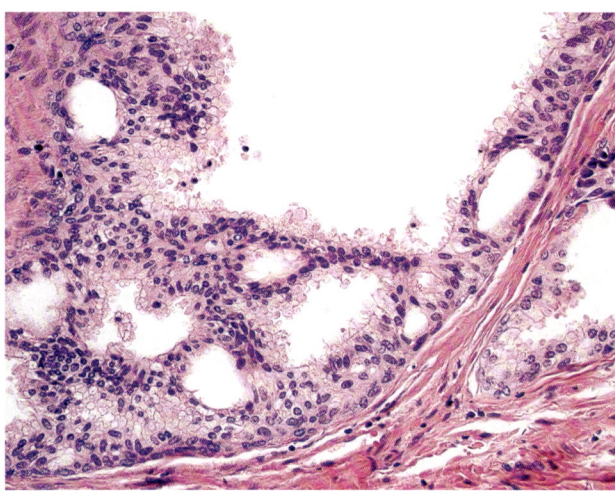

Figure 1.10. The central zone contains frequent "Roman arch" bridging structures.

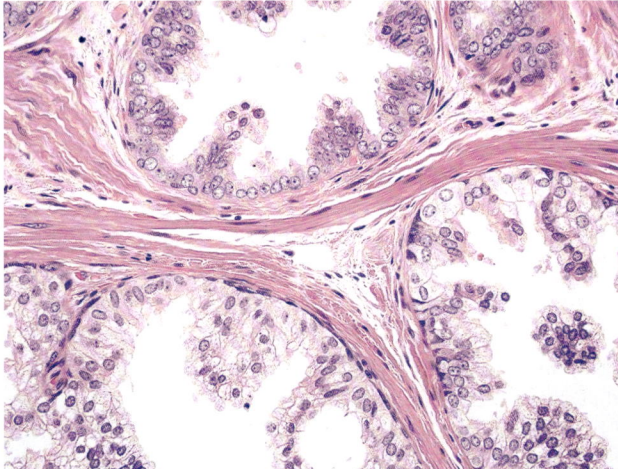

Figure 1.11. Despite that the central zone morphology (bottom) can be confused for prostatic intraepithelial neoplasia (PIN), it is possible for the central zone to be involved by PIN (top).

SAMPLE NOTE: Carcinoma Involving Skeletal Muscle in Needle Biopsy

Prostate, left lateral mid, core needle biopsy:

- Prostatic adenocarcinoma, Gleason score 3 + 3 = 6 (Grade Group 1), involving 40% of the length of one core (4 mm tumor focus)
- Carcinoma involves skeletal muscle—see Comment

Comment: In specimen #, the prostatic adenocarcinoma involves skeletal muscle. This does not necessarily indicate extraprostatic extension; however, it may indicate close proximity to the apex of the prostate (see reference).

Sadimin ET, Ye H, Epstein JI. Should the involvement of skeletal muscle by prostatic adenocarcinoma be reported on biopsies? *Hum Pathol.* 2016;49:10-14.

THE PROSTATE "CAPSULE" AND BOUNDARIES

Although it is common in clinical language to refer to the prostate "capsule," the prostate does not have a true capsule anatomically speaking.[11] Generally, in the posterolateral regions of the prostate (the areas where assessment for extraprostatic extension is usually most critical), the plane of adipose tissue is typically regarded as the most definitive boundary for organ-confined vs non–organ-confined cancer.[9] Another problem with the term "capsule" is that this can also be used by urologists to refer to the plane between the transition zone and the peripheral zone, in which dissections for nodular hyperplasia are carried out. As such, terms such as capsular invasion or penetration should largely be avoided, instead terminologies such as extraprostatic extension or organ-confined could be used.

PEARLS AND PITFALLS: Extraprostatic Extension in Needle Biopsy Samples

- Extraprostatic extension can be identified in needle biopsies when malignant cells are identified in adipose tissue
- Carcinoma cells closely approaching adipose tissue on one side only does not necessarily constitute extraprostatic extension

THE PROSTATIC GLANDULAR EPITHELIUM

The prostatic glandular epithelium itself is composed of two cell populations: the secretory and basal cells. The prototypical benign secretory cell layer has pale cytoplasm, an undulating contour, and ovoid nuclei without prominent nucleoli[12] (Figure 1.12). Common normal variations within the benign glandular epithelium can include lipofuscin pigment, which can have various colorations in stained tissue sections (brown, golden, but also gray or blue; Figures 1.13-1.15).[13,14] The basal cell layer, when well visualized, and depending on the laboratory preparation, is typically composed of cells with ovoid nuclei, often appearing perpendicular to those of the secretory layer with little to no cytoplasm.[15] The basal cells often have a blue-gray or slate staining color (Figures 1.16-1.18), compared to the darker purple or violet staining of the secretory cell nuclei.[16] An unusual finding that can be encountered occasionally in benign (as well as malignant) tissue is so-called Paneth-like neuroendocrine cells. These are scattered interspersed cells within the prostatic glandular epithelium that have brightly eosinophilic granules (Figure 1.19).[17,18] Despite being termed "Paneth-like," this terminology is probably a misnomer, as these are more akin to the gastrointestinal neuroendocrine cells rather than true Paneth cells, with positive immunohistochemical staining for neuroendocrine markers (Figure 1.20).[17] This is currently not considered to have any clinical significance, as scattered neuroendocrine cells can be present in both normal prostate tissue and conventional adenocarcinomas.[17]

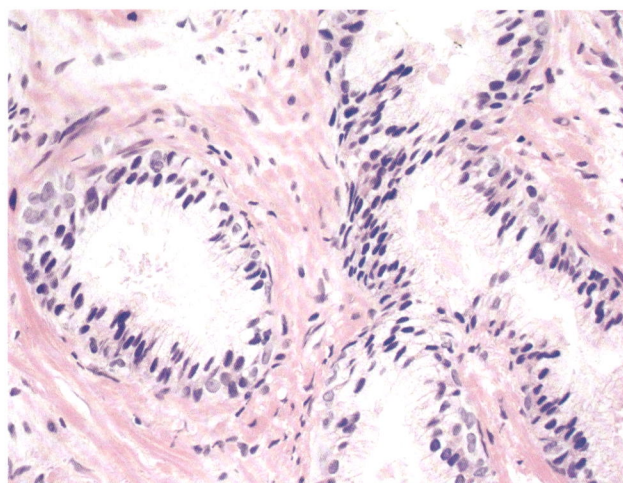

Figure 1.12. The normal prostatic glandular epithelium contains secretory cells with pale cytoplasm and oval, purple-staining nuclei.

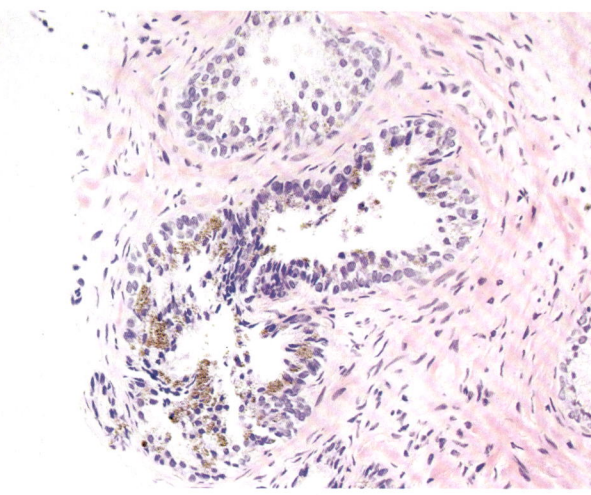

Figure 1.13. Pigment in benign prostatic glandular epithelium can vary in color. This example is brown.

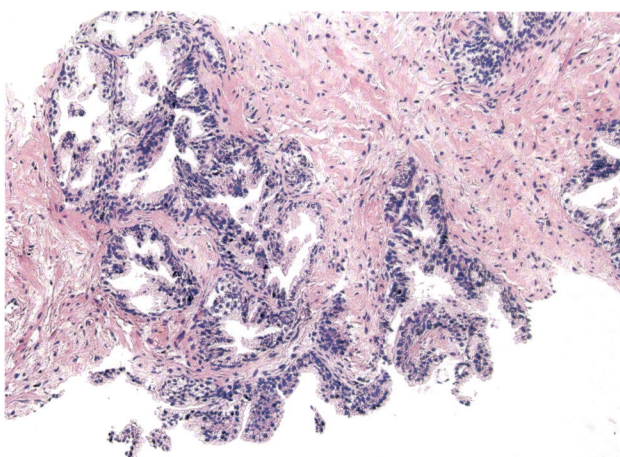

Figure 1.14. This focus of benign prostatic glands appears dark at low magnification due to cytoplasmic pigment.

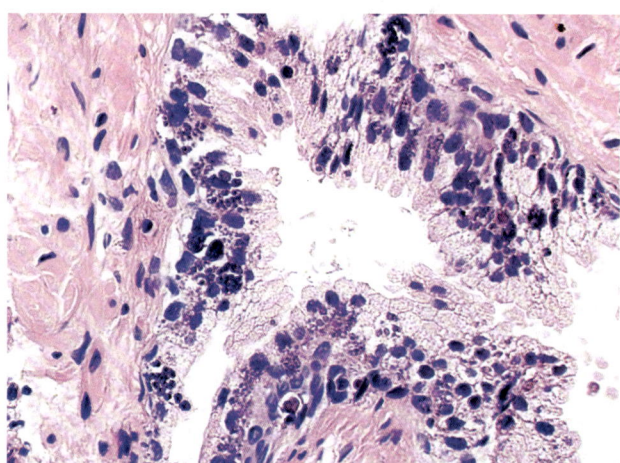

Figure 1.15. At high magnification, the same focus from Figure 1.14 shows a dark blue or purple pigment.

PEARLS AND PITFALLS: Distinguishing Basal Cells From Secretory Cells by Morphology

- In optimal tissue sections with benign glands, basal cells can be readily distinguished from secretory cell nuclei by their slightly different staining qualities (blue-gray or slate color rather than purple or violet) (Figures 1.16-1.18)
- In lesions suspicious for cancer, compressed nuclei at the base of the glandular epithelium are not necessarily basal cells, especially if they do not have a strikingly different staining quality than the suspicious nuclei (Figures 1.21 and 1.22)
- Immunohistochemistry for basal cell markers should always be undertaken for morphologically suspicious lesions, even if they have compressed nuclei at the base of the gland that might be basal cells
- Basal cells can have relatively prominent nucleoli, which can mimic cancer, especially with basal cell hyperplasia that narrows the lumen or obscures the secretory cell layer (Figure 1.23). Comparison to basal cells of adjacent obviously benign glands can be helpful, along with immunohistochemistry for basal cell markers

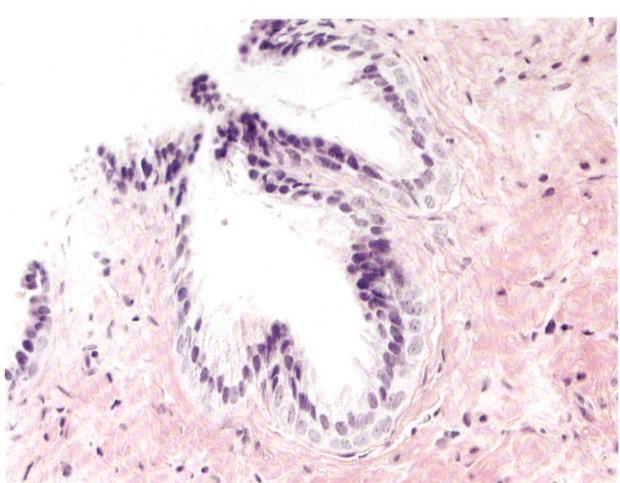

Figure 1.16. In well-visualized benign glands, the basal cell layer will contain nuclei with a blue-gray color, distinct from the purple color of the secretory cell nuclei.

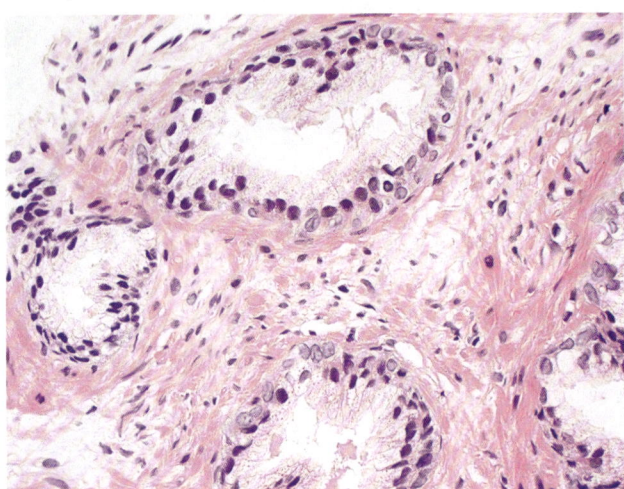

Figure 1.17. The basal layer may also have small nucleoli.

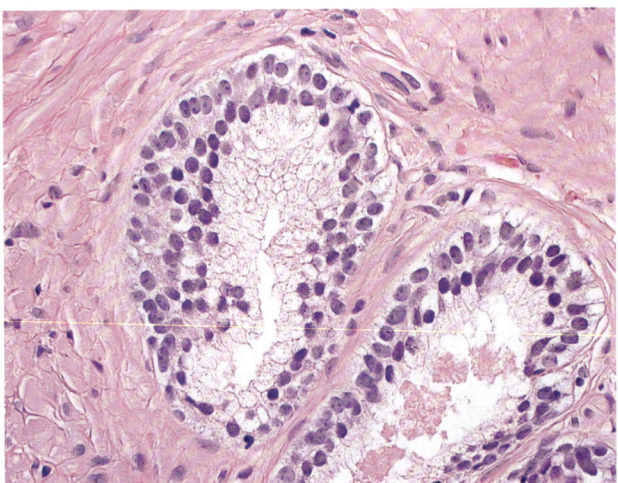

Figure 1.18. In some benign glands, prominent nucleoli in the basal cell layer may lead to confusion with prostatic intraepithelial neoplasia (PIN) or cancer.

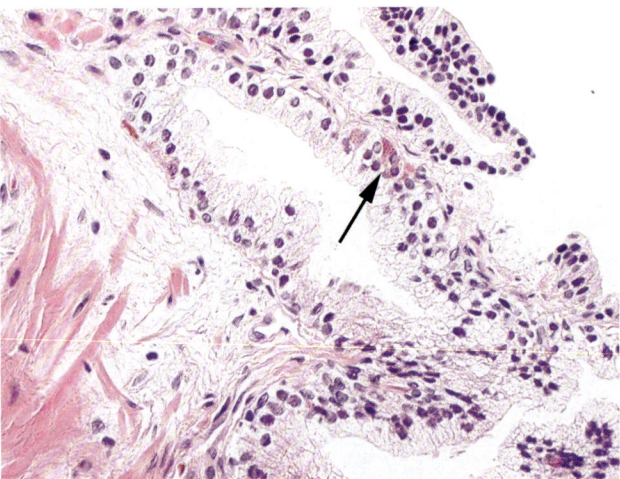

Figure 1.19. So-called Paneth-like neuroendocrine cells (arrow) can be found in benign prostatic tissue. These are occasional cells with eosinophilic cytoplasmic granules, usually at the base of the glandular epithelium.

SIMPLE ATROPHY

Simple atrophy is so common in prostatic tissue that it may debatably be considered a relatively normal finding. In general, it is postulated to be aging-related and potentially a sequela of an inflammatory insult; however, it is possible to encounter atrophy in prostatic specimens even from men at age 30 to 40 years.[11,19] Simple atrophy is composed of glands with scant cytoplasm, typically arranged into angulated structures with pointed corners (Figure 1.24), which usually makes it unlikely to mimic malignancy. In contrast to prostate cancer, which often elicits no stromal changes, atrophic glands can be variably rimmed by stromal fibrosis (Figures 1.25 and 1.26).[19] Other, more deceptive patterns of atrophy, such as partial atrophy, are discussed later in the sections discussing small gland lesions.

PROSTATIC NODULAR HYPERPLASIA

Prostatic nodular hyperplasia is composed of variable proportions of glands and stroma, arranged into circumscribed nodules. This is usually easier to appreciate in larger surgical pathology specimens, such as transurethral resections or radical or simple prostatectomy specimens. In needle biopsy samples, it is for the most part not possible to recognize glandular hyperplasia, since the glandular component of nodular hyperplasia is essentially identical to normal glandular tissue, other than its arrangement into nodules. Therefore,

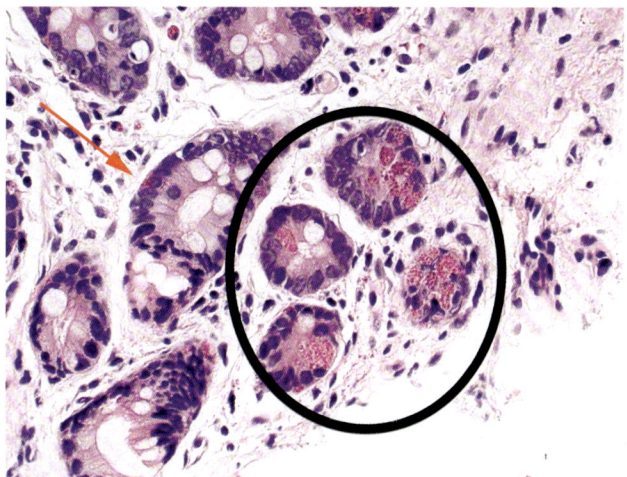

Figure 1.20. Paneth-like cells in the prostate are likely misnamed, as they are more analogous to the basally located neuroendocrine cells (arrow) that have granules beneath the nucleus in this image of the small intestine, in contrast to true Paneth cells (circle), which have larger granules above the nucleus.

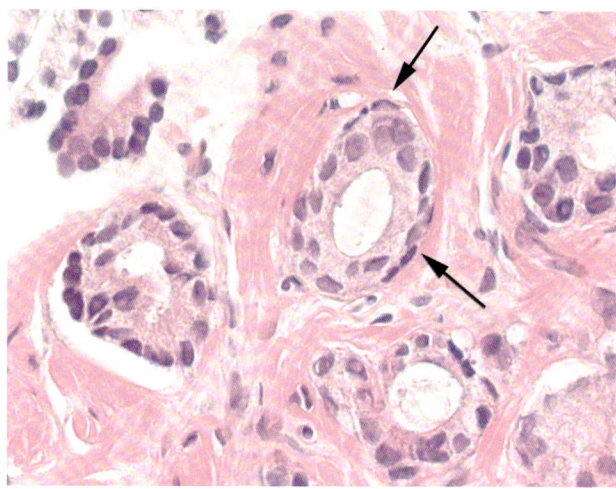

Figure 1.21. Some prostate cancers can contain compressed nuclei at the base of the glands, resembling basal cells (arrows).

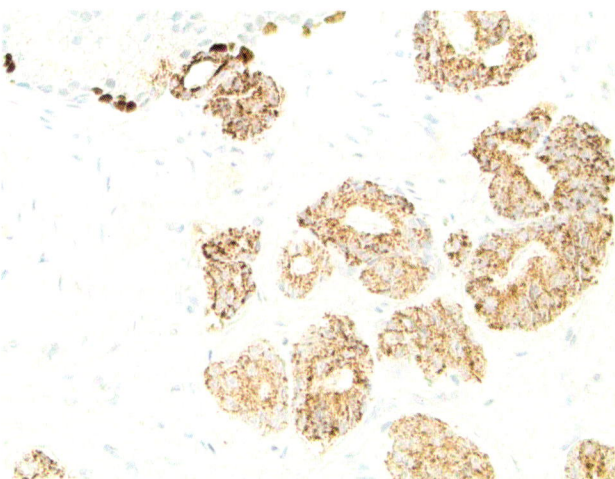

Figure 1.22. The same case from Figure 1.21 evaluated with double immunohistochemical staining for alpha-methylacyl-CoA racemase (AMACR) and p63 shows positivity for AMACR but no basal cells.

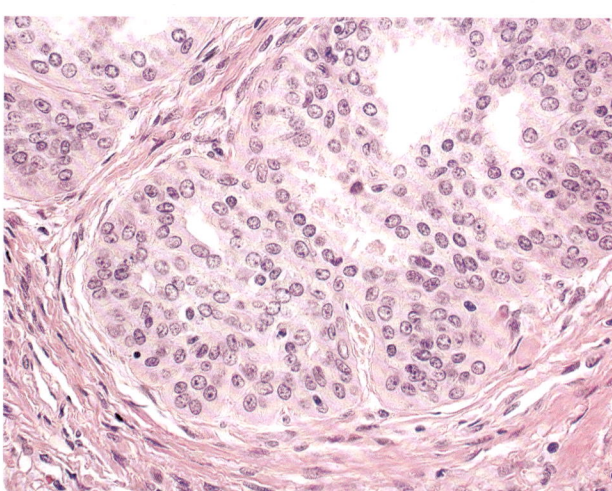

Figure 1.23. Basal cell hyperplasia can narrow the lumen of involved glands. With prominent nucleoli, this may be confused for carcinoma.

diagnosis of glandular hyperplasia in needle biopsy samples should typically be avoided[20]; however, stromal-predominant hyperplastic nodules can sometimes be recognized in needle biopsy samples by a few morphologic clues.

KEY FEATURES: Prostatic Nodular Hyperplasia in Needle Biopsy Specimens

- Histologic features that are helpful in identifying stromal hyperplastic nodules (Figures 1.27-1.31) include the following:
  - Increased stromal cellularity
  - Scattered blood vessels with slight thickening/hyalinization
  - A scattered population of lymphocytes

It is generally optional to comment on the presence of stromal nodules in needle biopsy samples; however, with the increasing usage of specialized biopsy techniques, such as MRI-targeted biopsy,[6,7] it may sometimes be relevant to mention the presence of stromal nodules, when they might account for the clinical "lesion" in a negative biopsy.

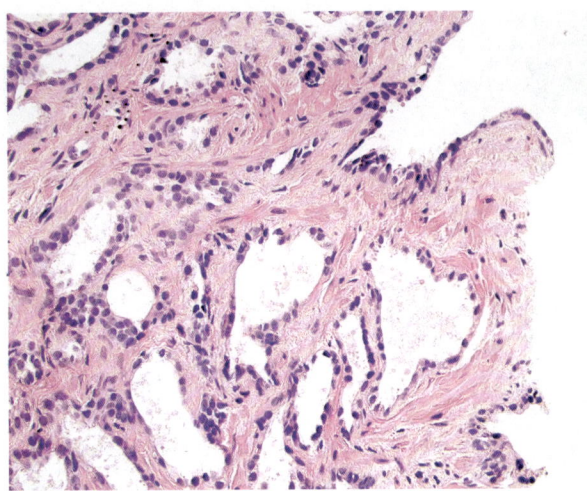

Figure 1.24. Simple atrophy is composed of glands with scant cytoplasm, often arranged into jagged glandular shapes with some pointed tips.

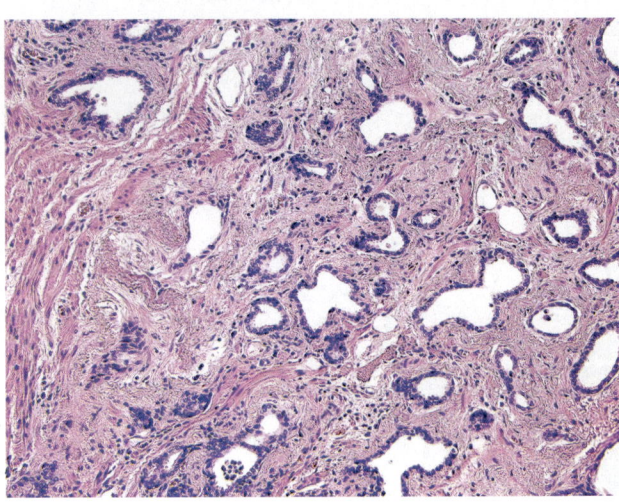

Figure 1.25. In contrast to prostate cancer, atrophy often is surrounded by stromal fibrosis or inflammation.

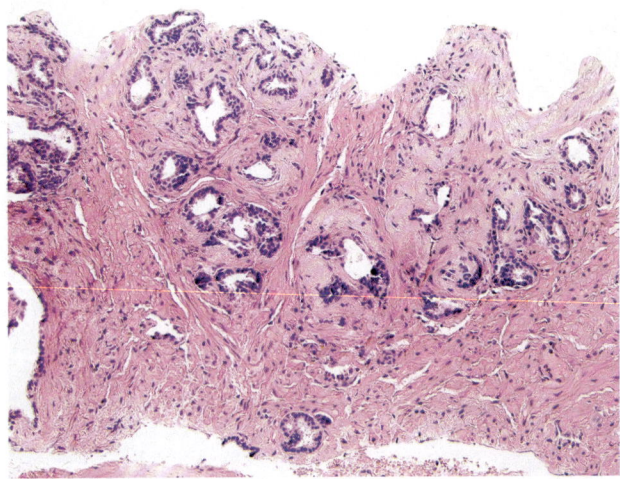

Figure 1.26. This needle biopsy example shows prominent hyalinization around atrophic glands.

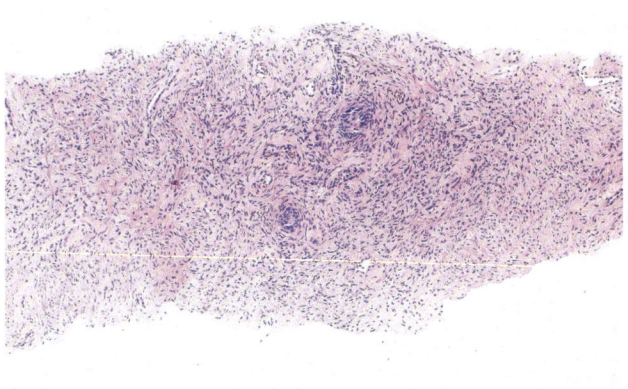

Figure 1.27. Occasionally stromal nodules can be detected in prostate needle biopsies. This example shows hypercellular stroma with only a few glands.

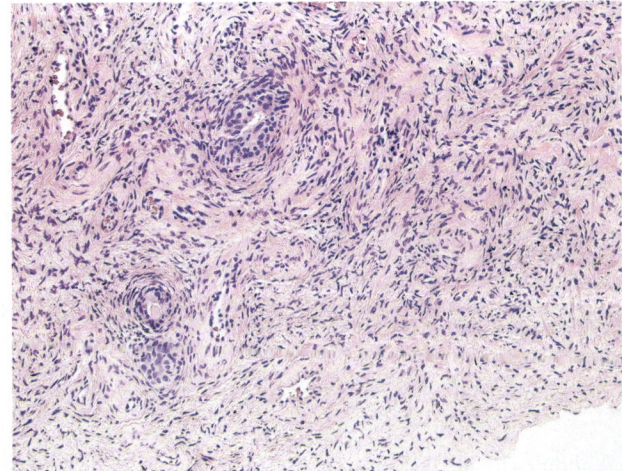

Figure 1.28. At higher magnification, the same case from Figure 1.27 shows rare glands and hypercellular stroma with scattered lymphocytes.

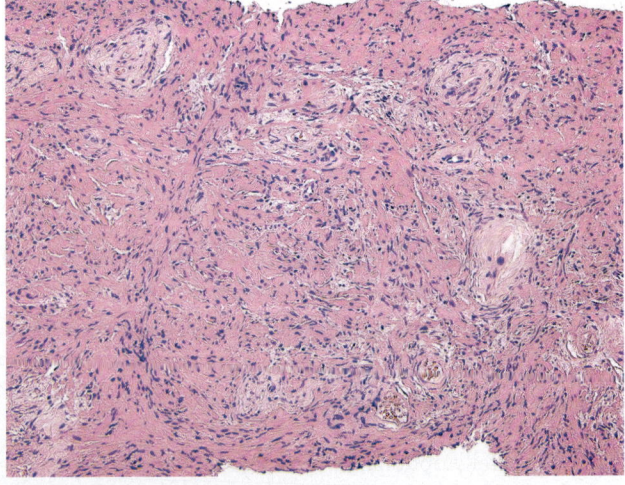

Figure 1.29. This example of a prostatic stromal nodule shows eosinophilic fibromuscular stroma with scattered blood vessels showing slightly hyalinized walls.

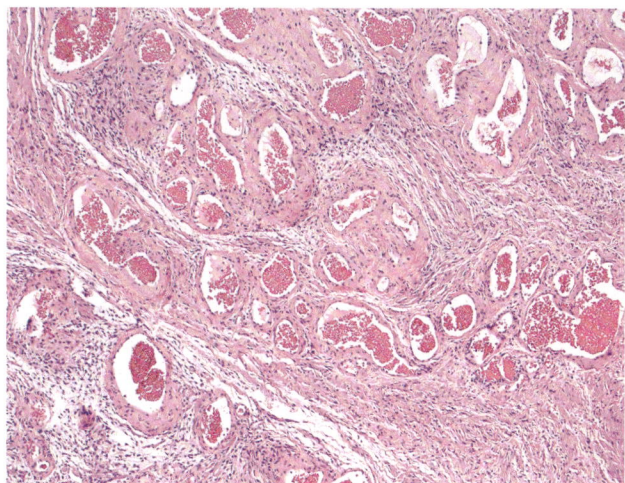

Figure 1.30. Rarely, prostatic stromal nodules can have such prominent vasculature that they resemble a vascular lesion.

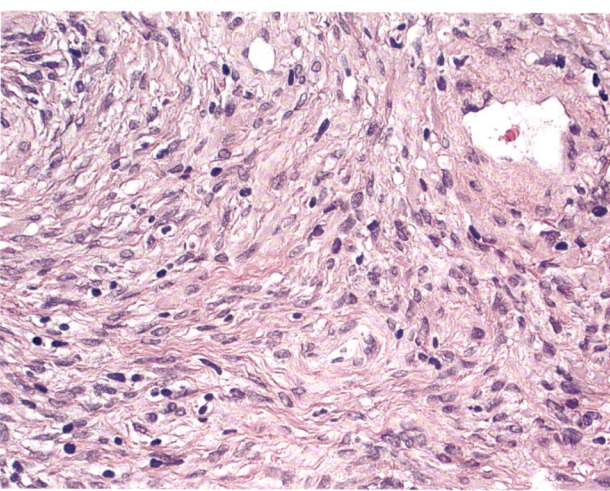

Figure 1.31. At high magnification, prostatic stromal nodules often have occasional scattered lymphocytes.

BENIGN SEMINAL VESICLE AND EJACULATORY DUCT TISSUE

Encountering seminal vesicle or ejaculatory duct in needle biopsy can occasionally be a source of diagnostic confusion, due to the inherent cytologic atypia and sometimes crowded glandular architecture of these structures.[21]

PEARLS AND PITFALLS: Clues to the Presence of Benign Seminal Vesicle/Ejaculatory Duct Tissue in Biopsy Samples

- Benign seminal vesicle and ejaculatory duct tissue often show a striking degree of nuclear size variation (Figures 1.32 and 1.33), much greater than that of prostate cancer, which is paradoxically monotonous
- Large globules of yellow-brown pigment are often present within the cytoplasm of the cells (Figure 1.34)
- Nuclei of benign seminal vesicle/ejaculatory duct tissue may contain intranuclear cytoplasmic invaginations (nuclear pseudoinclusions), which is conversely rare in prostate cancer (Figure 1.35)
- In biopsy samples, seminal vesicle tissue is often located at the tip or edge of the biopsy core, presumably because the biopsy needle punches into the main lumen and no longer can capture tissue (Figure 1.36)
- Nucleoli can be present, mimicking prostate cancer (Figures 1.37 and 1.38)

An interesting feature of benign seminal vesicle and ejaculatory duct tissue is that amyloid deposition is sometimes present in the stroma surrounding the epithelium, which is thought to be aging-related (Figures 1.39-1.42). This amyloid appears to have no relation to systemic amyloidosis and is thought to be composed of semenogelin I.[22] Given the lack of apparent clinical significance of this phenomenon, it is debatable whether it should be documented in surgical pathology reports. On the one hand, it is typically clinically insignificant; however, it is possible that it can be noted clinically, such as on imaging studies, mimicking invasion by cancer[23-25] (see Sample Note).

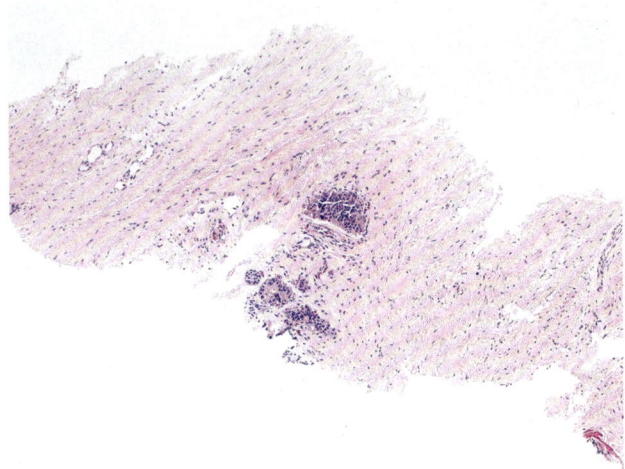

Figure 1.32. Seminal vesicle tissue can be deceptive in needle biopsy samples. This example demonstrates a few crowded glands at the edge of the core.

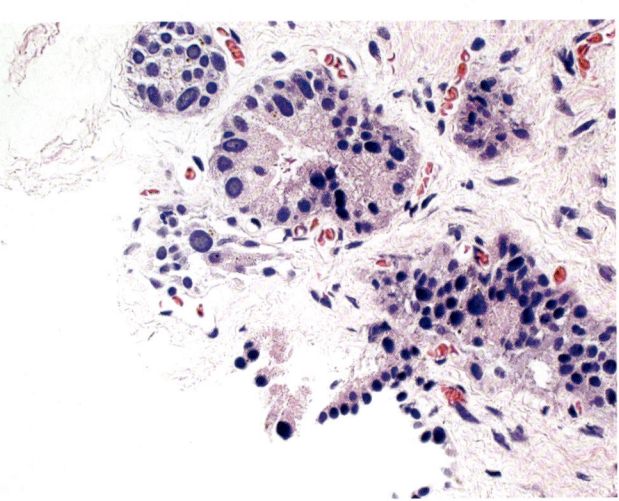

Figure 1.33. At higher magnification, the same case from Figure 1.32 shows more variation in nuclear size than typically expected of prostate cancer.

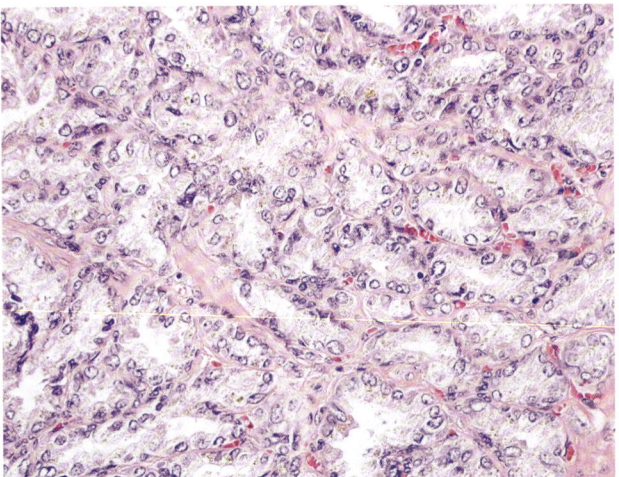

Figure 1.34. Seminal vesicle tissue often has granules of yellow-brown pigment, facilitating recognition.

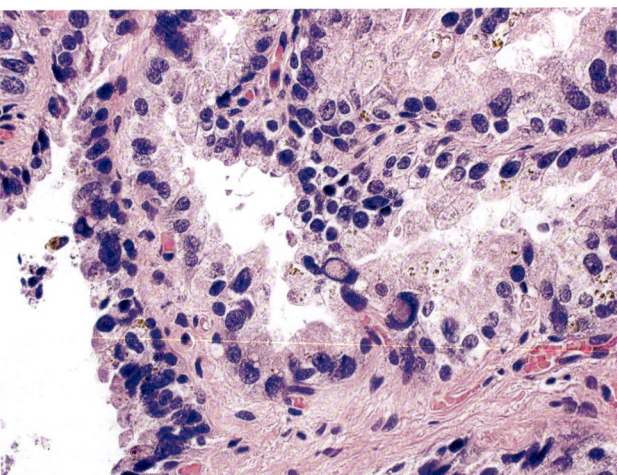

Figure 1.35. Another clue to the recognition of seminal vesicle tissue is the presence of intranuclear cytoplasmic invaginations or pseudoinclusions, which are rare in prostate cancer.

SAMPLE NOTE: Amyloid in Benign Seminal Vesicle/Ejaculatory Duct Tissue

Amyloid deposition of seminal vesicle—see Comment

Comment: Amyloid deposition in the seminal vesicle and ejaculatory duct is thought to be a localized phenomenon related to ejaculatory proteins (likely semenogelin) and unrelated to systemic amyloid. In this case, no definite amyloid is identified in other locations (perivascular, etc.) to raise concern for systemic deposition.

Conversely, the presence of amyloid in other locations, such as throughout the prostate stroma, or especially in a perivascular location in small prostatic or soft tissue blood vessels, should likely trigger a clinical evaluation for the possibility of systemic amyloidosis (Figures 1.43 and 1.44). Immunohistochemistry can be used to attempt to subtype the amyloid, as antibodies are available to kappa and lambda light chains (AL type) or amyloid A (AA type), among others; however, such evaluation is not always conclusive. When tissue material is limited, a practical approach is to refer paraffin-embedded tissue samples to a laboratory that offers mass spectroscopy for amyloid subtyping, if clinically indicated.

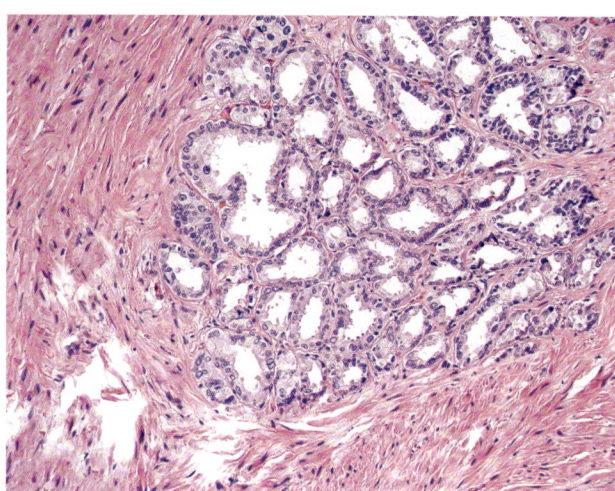

Figure 1.36. Seminal vesicle tissue in needle biopsy samples is often at the end or edge of the core, since the biopsy likely punches into the large lumen.

Figure 1.37. This focus of seminal vesicle glands could be confused for prostatic adenocarcinoma due to crowded round glands.

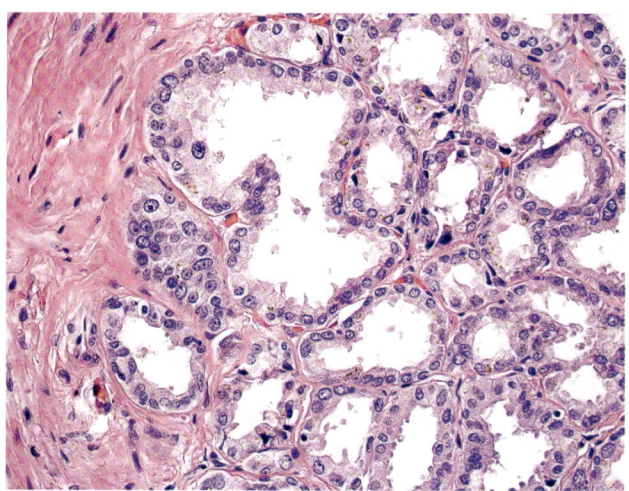

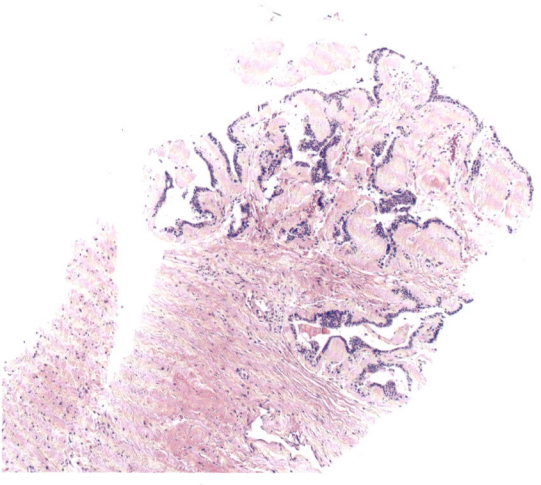

Figure 1.38. The same case from Figure 1.37 contains some prominent nucleoli. However, clues to the recognition of seminal vesicle tissue include scattered yellow-brown pigment and varied nuclear size.

Figure 1.39. Amyloid deposition is occasionally present in the seminal vesicle or ejaculatory duct, which is thought to have no clinical significance.

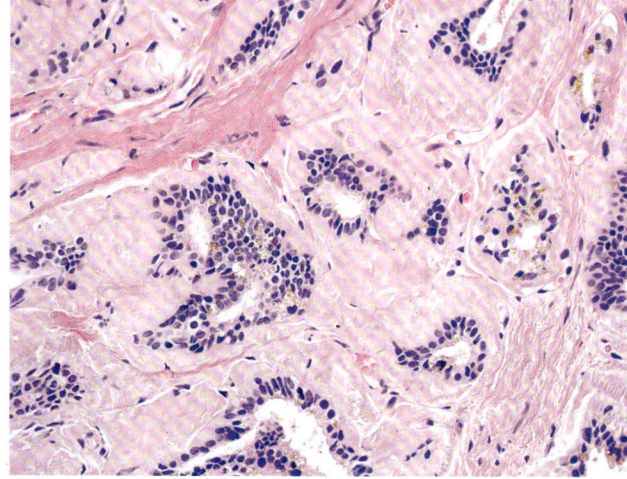

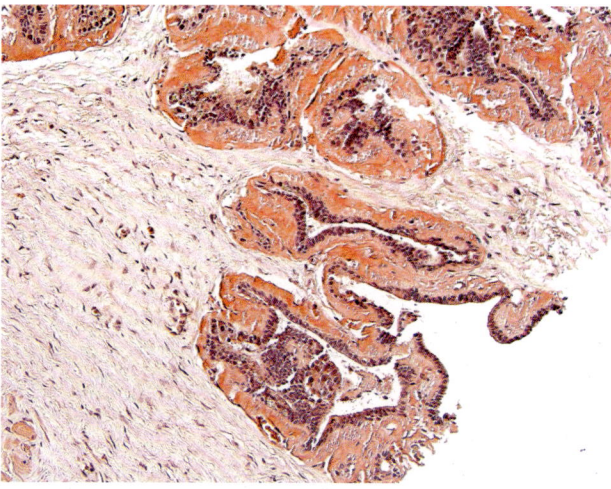

Figure 1.40. Amyloid rims benign seminal vesicle glands, which contain some yellow-brown pigment.

Figure 1.41. Congo red staining highlights seminal vesicle amyloid, similar to other forms of amyloid.

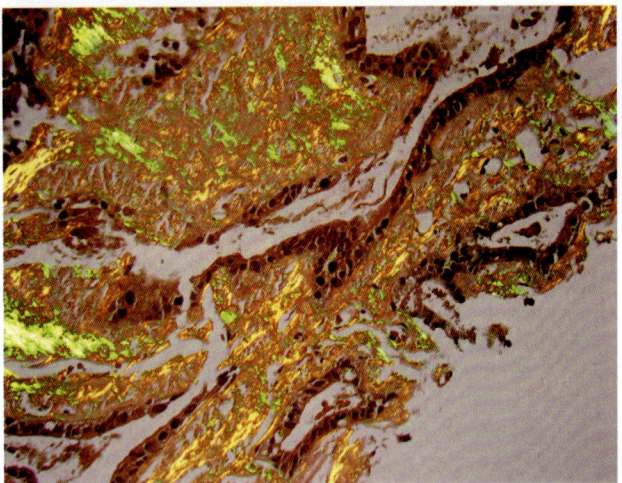

Figure 1.42. With polarization, this seminal vesicle with amyloid shows the classic green birefringence.

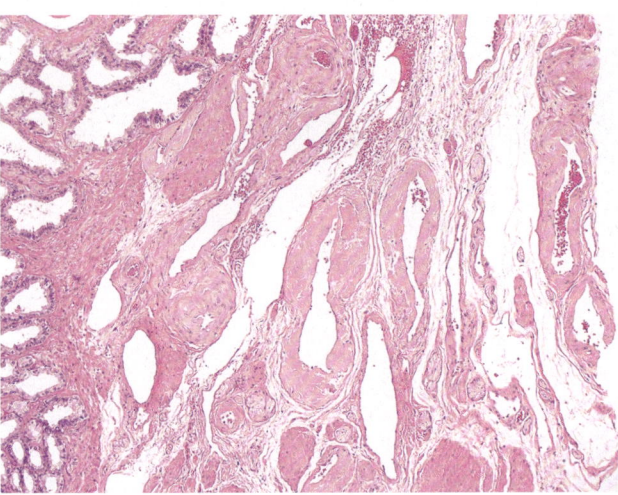

Figure 1.43. In contrast to seminal vesicle amyloid, which is likely not clinically significant, amyloid in prostatic blood vessels may be a sign of systemic deposition. This case shows large thickened blood vessels at right with benign prostatic tissue at left.

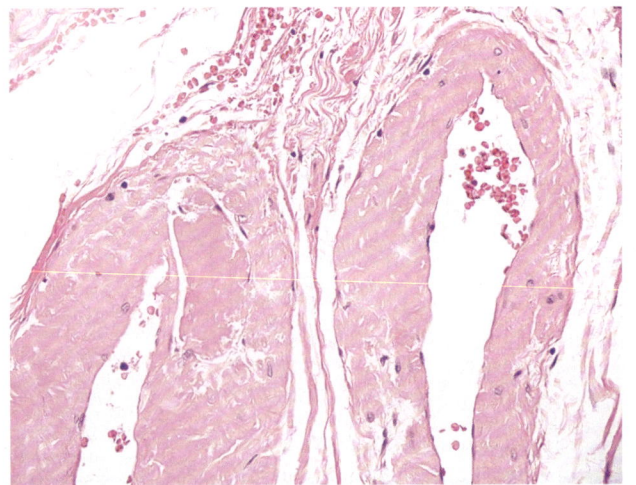

Figure 1.44. At high magnification, the same case from Figure 1.43 shows a waxy, cracked consistency of the vascular amyloid.

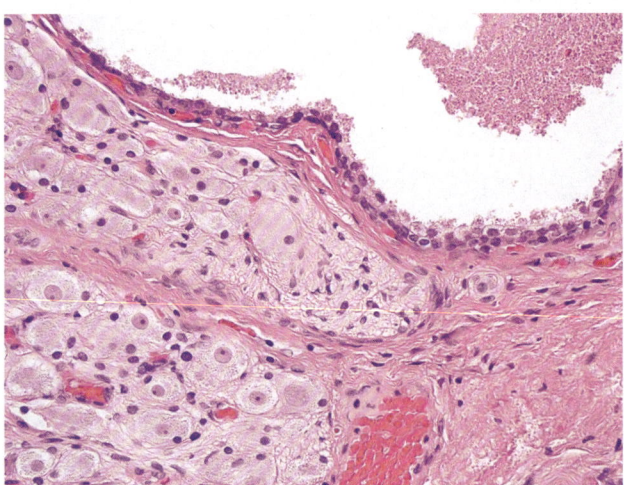

Figure 1.45. Ganglia can be found in the periprostatic tissue and occasionally in close juxtaposition to benign prostatic glands.

GANGLIA AND PARAGANGLIA

Ganglia are encountered relatively commonly in prostate specimens and usually pose little diagnostic confusion due to their apparent composition by nerve fibers and large ganglion cells (Figure 1.45). However, paraganglia are rarer and may be a source of diagnostic difficulty due to their similarity to poorly formed gland or solid adenocarcinoma (Figures 1.46 and 1.47).[26-29] Contrasting to prostate cancer, paraganglia are positive for neuroendocrine markers, such as chromogranin, whereas they are negative for prostate-specific markers, such as prostate-specific antigen (PSA).[26-29] Of note, it has been recently recognized that paragangliomas and pheochromocytomas are often positive for GATA3, which may complicate distinction from urothelial carcinoma.[30,31] To our knowledge, this has not been studied in normal paraganglia; however, it may be reasonable to suspect that positive staining can also be found in this context.

IMMUNOHISTOCHEMISTRY

Immunohistochemistry plays an important role in diagnosis of prostatic specimens, particularly biopsies; however, use of immunohistochemistry should be judicious.

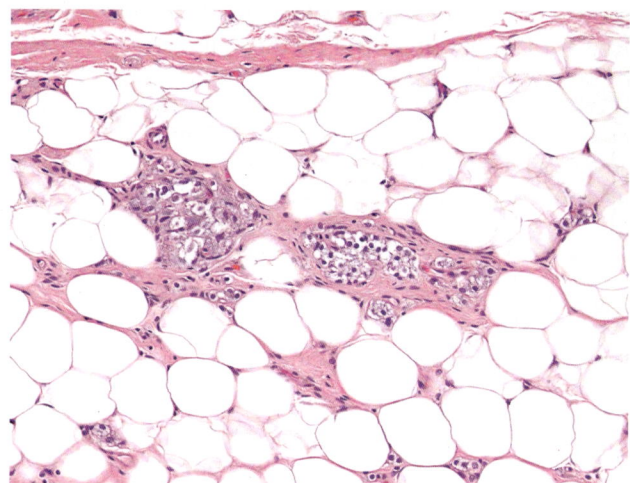

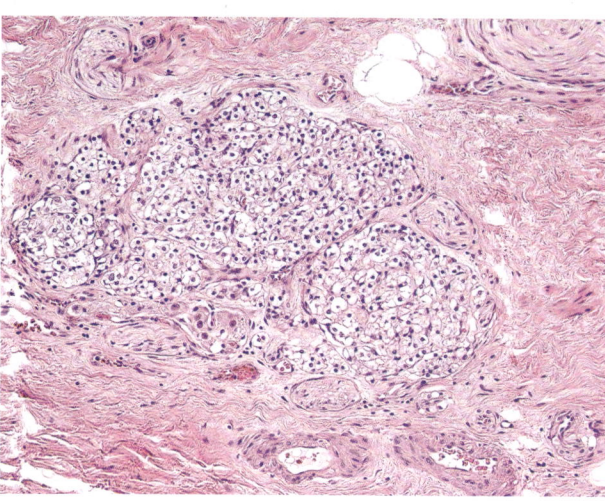

Figure 1.46. Paraganglia in and around the prostate can be more deceptive, as the mononuclear cell pattern can be confused for carcinoma or extraprostatic extension of carcinoma, as the small nests of cells in this case intermingle with adipose tissue.

Figure 1.47. This example of periprostatic paraganglion could be confused for pattern 4 or 5 prostatic adenocarcinoma due to formation of solid nests of cells with pale to clear cytoplasm.

Routine immunohistochemistry in all benign biopsies, or in biopsies with unequivocal cancer, is not appropriate.[32] It is typically helpful to use more than one antibody in a multiplex assay or "cocktail" that contains alpha-methylacyl-CoA racemase (AMACR) and one or more basal cell markers. However, there are several possible formulations for this (Table 1.1).

Some noteworthy exceptions to the usual staining patterns of prostate cancer do exist. For example, although prostate cancer inherently lacks basal cells, rare cases of prostatic adenocarcinoma with aberrant p63 positivity in the cancer cells have been described.[33-38] In contrast to the basal cell distribution shown by p63 staining in lesions with true basal cells, this staining result is typically nonbasal (Figures 1.48 and 1.49) and labels much or all the cancer cells themselves. Prostate cancers with aberrant p63 staining are often atrophic in appearance. Similarly, a minority of prostate cancers can have aberrant positivity for high-molecular-weight cytokeratin in the cancer glands. These are often higher-grade cancers (Figure 1.50).[39-42] Fortunately, these are also typically not the same tumors that have aberrant p63 staining, so that if the two markers are used complementarily, the true absence of basal cells should be detected.

Scenarios Potentially Warranting Immunohistochemical Staining

Of course, the decision to utilize immunohistochemistry in prostate biopsy samples requires the clinical judgment of the reporting pathologist and may be influenced by specific criteria at a given institution regarding surveillance or treatment eligibility. However, some more common scenarios in which there is a stronger or lesser need for immunohistochemistry are shown in Table 1.2 (Figures 1.51 and 1.52).

ARTIFACTS AND CONTAMINANTS IN PROSTATE SPECIMENS

The most common nonprostatic tissue found in prostate specimens is colorectal tissue captured via the transrectal nature of ultrasound-guided biopsies (Figure 1.53). In most cases, this is readily recognizable as rectal tissue and it poses no diagnostic challenge. However, in exceptional cases, there may be either (1) abnormal findings, such as polyps or inflammatory processes,[43] or (2) rectal tissue closely juxtaposed to prostate tissue, mimicking atypical glands or cancer.[44] This latter situation can be compounded by the lack of basal cells in colorectal tissue if immunohistochemistry is used, as well as occasional positivity for AMACR in rectal glands.

TABLE 1.1: Immunohistochemical Antibody Combinations for Confirmation of Prostate Cancer

Antibody	Chromogen	Pro	Con
Alpha-methylacyl-CoA racemase (AMACR) + p63	Single color (cytoplasmic vs nuclear)	Technically simpler than dual-color assays, conserves tissue compared with individual antibodies on separate slides	Strong AMACR may mimic or obscure basal cells, lacks additional basal cell detection of high-molecular-weight cytokeratin
AMACR + p63 + high-molecular-weight cytokeratin (cytokeratin 5/6, 14, 34βE12, others)	Dual color	Basal cells appear in a different color than AMACR, conserves tissue compared with individual antibodies on separate slides	Technically more difficult to perform than single-color methods
p63 alone	Single color		More difficult to assess without a concurrent positive marker
High-molecular-weight cytokeratin alone	Single color		More difficult to assess without a concurrent positive marker
ERG	Single color or in combination with others	Positive strongly favors adenocarcinoma or occasionally prostatic intraepithelial neoplasia (PIN)	Only positive in approximately 40% of prostate cancer
PTEN	Single color or in combination with others	Abnormal negative ("loss") favors malignancy and higher-grade/aggressive cancer	Interpretation of absence of staining can be challenging

Adapted from Epstein JI, Egevad L, Humphrey PA, Montironi R. Members of the ISUP Immunohistochemistry in Diagnostic Urologic Pathology Group. Best practices recommendations in the application of immunohistochemistry in the prostate: report from the International Society of Urologic Pathology consensus conference. *Am J Surg Pathol.* 2014;38(8):e6-e19.

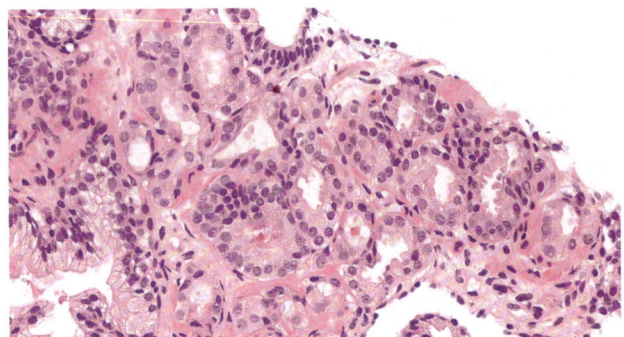

Figure 1.48. Rare prostate cancers can be p63-positive. This example shows a proliferation of small glands with prominent nucleoli. (Courtesy Ankur R. Sangoi, MD, El Camino Hospital.)

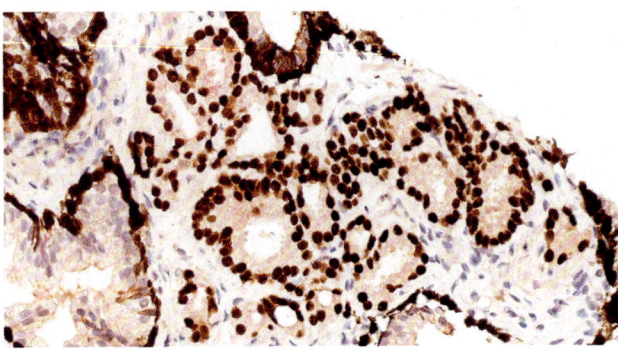

Figure 1.49. The same prostatic adenocarcinoma from Figure 1.48 shows nuclear staining of the cancer glands for p63. Although the adjacent basal cells show both cytoplasmic (high-molecular-weight cytokeratin) and nuclear (p63) staining in a basal distribution, the cancer glands show only nuclear staining for p63, supporting their distinction from a true benign basal cell population. (Courtesy Ankur R. Sangoi, MD, El Camino Hospital.)

PEARLS AND PITFALLS: Recognizing Distorted Rectal Tissue in Prostate Biopsies

- Features that can mimic cancer when rectal tissue is juxtaposed to or interdigitated with prostate tissue include luminal blue mucin, elongated nuclei, nucleoli, mitotic figures, absence of basal cells detected with immunohistochemistry, and AMACR positivity[44] (Figures 1.54-1.57)
- Clues to recognizing rectal tissue in this setting include presence of lamina propria (Figure 1.58), detached location of the fragment, inflammatory cells (of the normal lamina propria), goblet cells, or presence of muscularis propria[44]

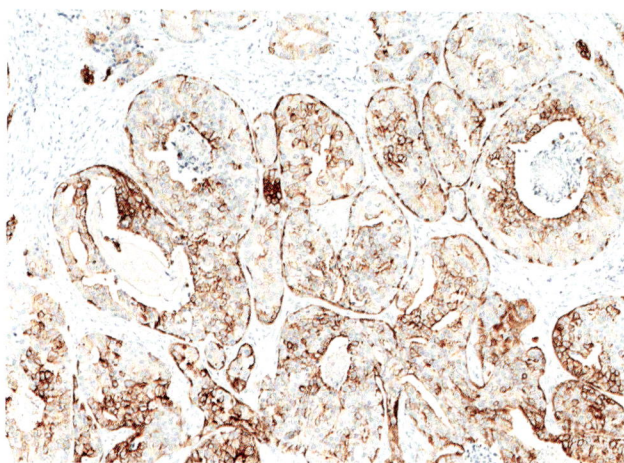

Figure 1.50. Rare prostate cancers can be positive for high-molecular-weight cytokeratin, especially high-grade cancers. This example shows intraductal carcinoma with high-molecular-weight cytokeratin staining of the basal cells; however, there is also substantial staining of the cancer cells as well.

TABLE 1.2: Scenarios for Immunohistochemistry Use in Prostate Biopsy

Scenario	Necessity	Notes
Atypical glands in a single core biopsy	Usually	Diagnosis may range from benign (if the presence of basal cells would allow confident classification as a benign mimic such as partial atrophy, Figures 1.51 and 1.52) to atypical or malignant
Atypical glands in additional biopsies with one or more showing Gleason score 3 + 3 = 6 (Grade Group 1) cancer	Maybe	Some active surveillance criteria use the number of positive biopsies (two or three sites) and percentage (50%) involvement of biopsies to determine eligibility, although this is changing and often depends on the institution and practitioner
Atypical glands in additional biopsies with one or more showing Gleason score 3 + 4 = 7 (Grade Group 2) cancer	Maybe	In general, prostate cancer management is driven by the highest-grade biopsy, so the need for confirming additional foci of Gleason score 3 + 3 = 6 (Grade Group 1) in a case with overall Gleason score 3 + 4 = 7 (Grade Group 2) may depend on the institutional criteria for treatment. In most cases, there would not be a significant management difference with additional small foci of Gleason score 3 + 3 = 6 (Grade Group 1) cancer
Atypical glands in additional biopsies with one or more showing Gleason score Gleason score 4 + 3 = 7 (Grade Group 3) or higher cancer	Unlikely	With high-grade cancer, additional small foci of Gleason score 3 + 3 = 6 (Grade Group 1) or Gleason score 3 + 4 = 7 (Grade Group 2) are unlikely to change the clinical management plan
Large cribriform cancer that may be entirely intraductal carcinoma	Usually	If there is a possibility that a large cribriform proliferation is entirely intraductal carcinoma, it is often reasonable to confirm with immunohistochemistry. Although some would consider pure intraductal carcinoma to be indication for treatment alone, cases with minimal or no invasion may not be as aggressive as those with associated high-grade invasive cancer. This is an emerging area of interest
High-grade invasive cancer + possible intraductal carcinoma	Unlikely	Although intraductal carcinoma is generally excluded from grading, in the setting of high-grade (pattern 4 or higher) invasive cancer, it is not clear at present that subtracting an intraductal component from the grade improves prognostication
Routine immunohistochemistry of all biopsies	Never	Routine immunohistochemistry of all biopsies prior to morphologic review or for all benign biopsies is not warranted. This has the potential to cause more confusion than clarity, as some benign lesions may have a patchy basal cell layer, in which occasionally glands show none in the plane of section

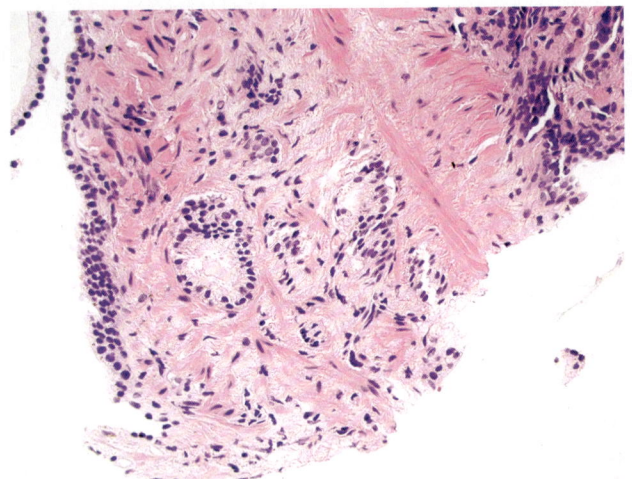

Figure 1.51. When a small focus of atypical glands is present in a prostate needle biopsy with no definite cancer in other specimens, it is usually worthwhile to perform immunohistochemistry. This case shows a focus of a few crowded round glands adjacent to a benign gland.

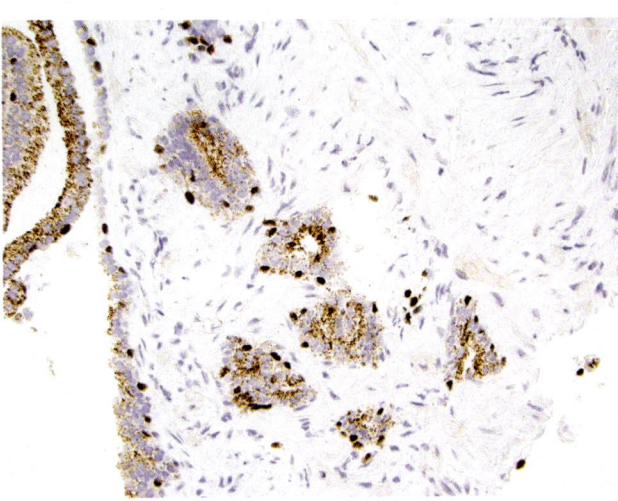

Figure 1.52. Using a single-color p63 and alpha-methylacyl-CoA racemase (AMACR) immunohistochemical stain, the same case from Figure 1.51 shows an intact, patchy basal cell layer with moderate staining for AMACR, supporting a benign diagnosis. Despite the AMACR staining, the focus does not show features of prostatic intraepithelial neoplasia (PIN) morphologically.

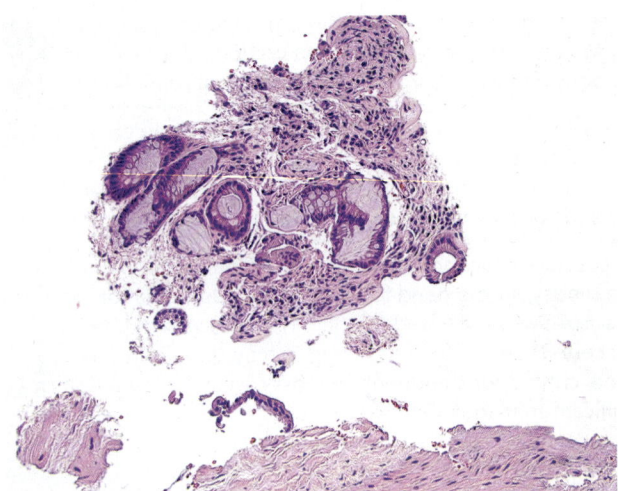

Figure 1.53. Colorectal tissue is a common contaminant in prostatic needle biopsies. When the fragment is detached and contains apparent blue mucin, lamina propria, and goblet cells, it is usually straightforward to disregard as colorectal tissue.

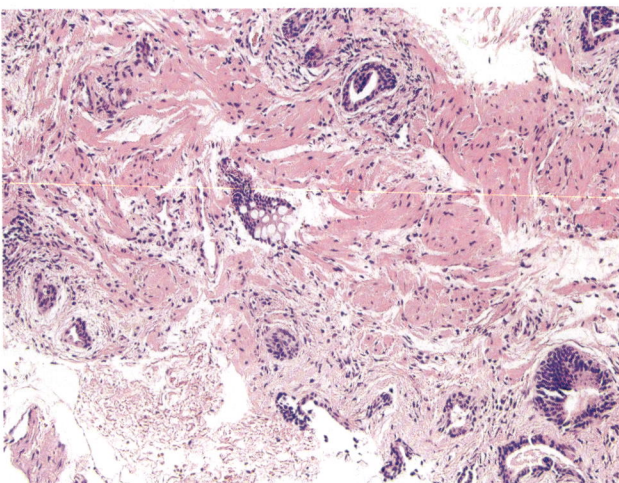

Figure 1.54. Scenarios in which colorectal tissue can cause challenges in prostatic biopsy specimens include implantation of the colorectal glands into the prostatic tissue. This example shows a single colorectal gland in the middle of the biopsy core, which could be confused for prostatic adenocarcinoma or prostatic intraepithelial neoplasia (PIN) with cytoplasmic vacuoles.

Abnormalities in the squamous tissue from the anal or perineal areas that may be captured in transrectal or transperineal biopsies have been less frequently reported but can be potentially encountered as well. In general, the presence of detached fragments of atypical or malignant cells that are not part of the tissue core should raise consideration of a specimen contaminant before being diagnosed as prostatic malignancy. Some laboratories offer molecular techniques of tissue identity testing to confirm whether a component of the tissue belongs to the same patient or represents a specimen contaminant.

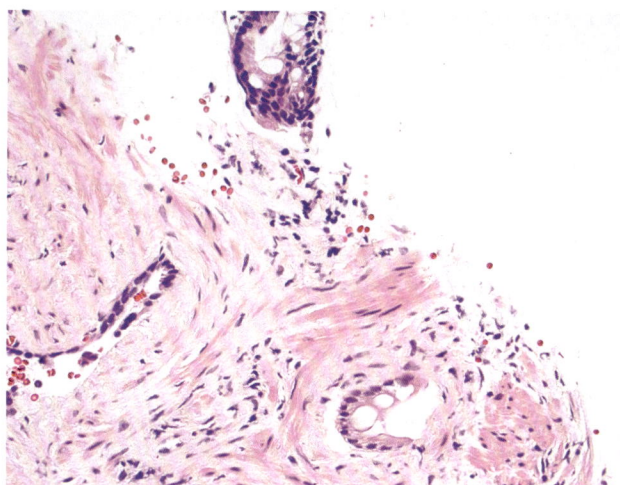

Figure 1.55. This example of colorectal tissue in a prostate biopsy shows a detached colorectal gland (top) in addition to one implanted in the biopsy core (bottom right).

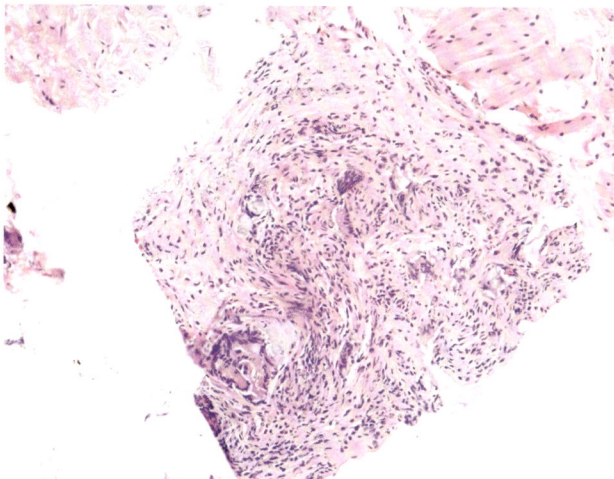

Figure 1.56. This example of colorectal tissue was misdiagnosed in a prostate biopsy as atypical glands suspicious for cancer. The morphology is somewhat distorted, but there is a suggestion of lamina propria.

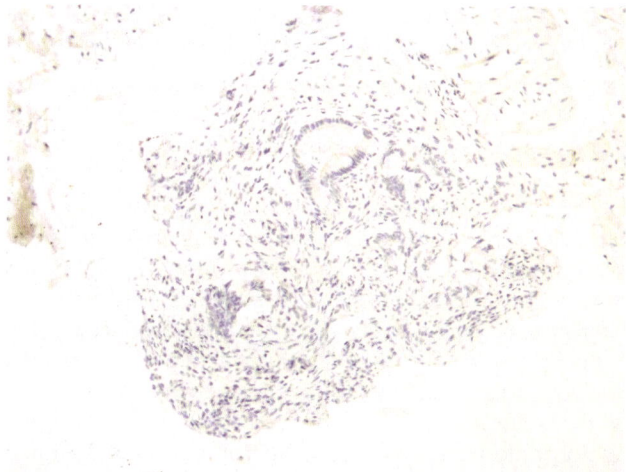

Figure 1.57. Absence of staining for basal cell markers in this fragment of colorectal tissue may have compounded the confusion with prostatic adenocarcinoma. This example also has no significant alpha-methylacyl-CoA racemase (AMACR) staining in the cocktail stain; however, this does not necessary help resolve the diagnosis, as some prostate cancers are negative and some colorectal tissue can be positive.

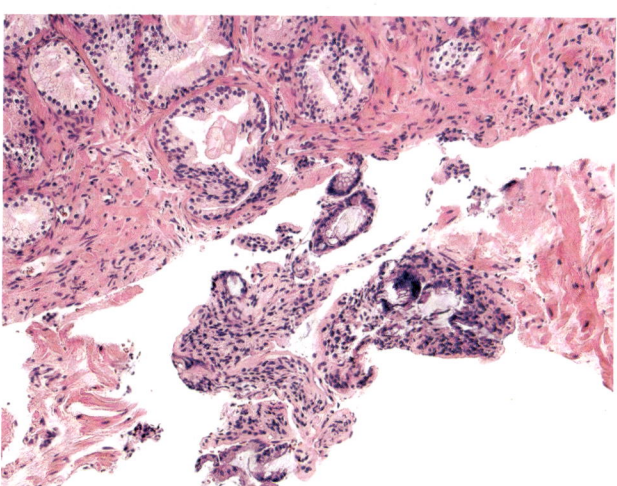

Figure 1.58. Although colorectal glands in prostate biopsy may appear hyperchromatic, detached configuration and the presence of lamina propria are helpful to discriminate from prostatic adenocarcinoma.

SMALL ROUND GLAND EPITHELIAL LESIONS

The most common diagnostic challenge in prostate cancer pathology is a lesion with a histologic appearance of small, round glandular structures, since the most common pattern of low-grade prostate cancer is that of small, ring-shaped glands with a monolayered appearance. This section in the pattern-based approach discusses small gland lesions, including low-grade cancer and its mimics.

BENIGN MIMICS OF CANCER

Adenosis (Atypical Adenomatous Hyperplasia)

Adenosis or atypical adenomatous hyperplasia are synonymous names that can be used interchangeably.[21] Some authors have argued that the designation adenosis has less potential for confusion, since it does not contain the word "atypical," which may be confused with a suspicious diagnosis (atypical glands or atypical small acinar proliferation)[45]; however, both names are sufficiently well established in the scientific literature to be used.

PEARLS AND PITFALLS: Adenosis/Atypical Adenomatous Hyperplasia

- Occurs in the transition zone of the prostate as a part of hyperplastic nodules, typically manifesting as a circumscribed hyperplastic nodule (Figure 1.59)
- Composed predominantly of usual benign, branched glands
- At the outer edge, the glands are small and round, imparting resemblance to low-grade prostatic adenocarcinoma (Figures 1.60 and 1.61)[21,46,47]
- May also have a patchy or discontinuous basal layer using immunohistochemical staining (Figures 1.62-1.65) and some degree of AMACR positivity, compounding the mimicry of prostate cancer[21,46,47]
- May have identifiable nucleoli or luminal crystalloids (Figure 1.62), brightly eosinophilic structures typically forming geometric shapes[47]
- However, no significant cytologic difference between the small round glands that lack basal cells (or appear to) and those that do contain basal cells

FAQ: How Do I Evaluate a Focus of Prostatic Glands in Which a Subset of the Glands Lacks Basal Cells?

When evaluating morphologically or immunohistochemically for basal cells, foci of prostatic glands should always be evaluated as a whole. Several entities in prostate pathology can have a discontinuous or patchy basal cell layer, such that a subset of the glandular structures may appear to lack basal cells entirely. Most common examples include adenosis (atypical adenomatous hyperplasia), sclerosing adenosis, partial atrophy, and PIN. However, when evaluating such foci as a whole, if the cytology is essentially identical in the small glands that appear to lack basal cells and other glands that appear benign and contain unequivocal basal cells, then a benign (or at most atypical) diagnosis should usually be rendered. In contrast, if there is a stark difference in cytology between the glands that lack basal cells and those that contain them (such as nuclear enlargement, hyperchromasia, or presence of prominent nucleoli), this would favor a diagnosis of malignancy (or least atypical, depending on the other features). In other words, absence of basal cells in a few glands that are morphologically not distinctive from adjacent benign glands should not automatically yield an atypical or malignant diagnosis.

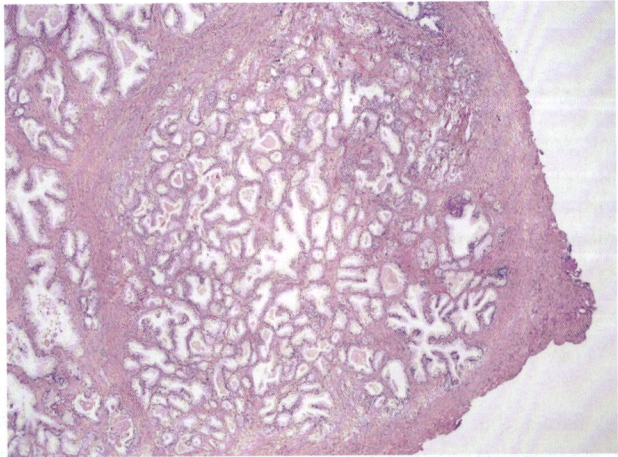

Figure 1.59. Adenosis or atypical adenomatous hyperplasia usually manifests as a well-circumscribed nodule, resembling nodular hyperplasia.

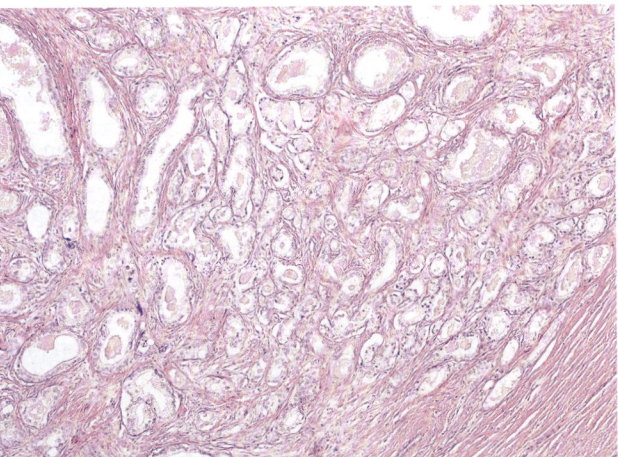

Figure 1.60. In adenosis, there is a transition from large benign-appearing glands to small, crowded round glands.

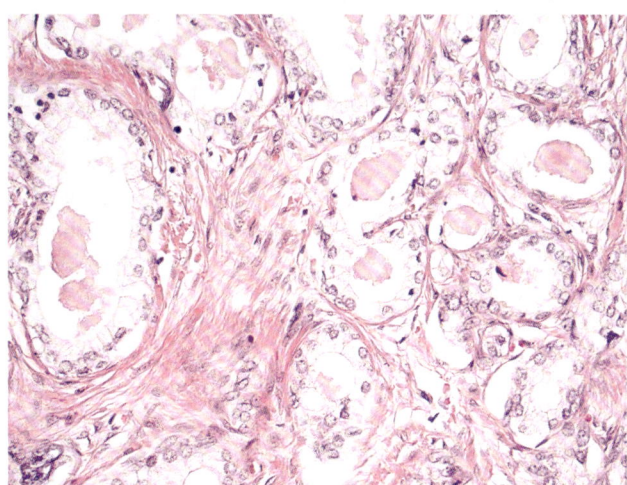

Figure 1.61. At high magnification, the small round glands of adenosis/atypical adenomatous hyperplasia (adenosis) are morphologically similar to typical benign glands.

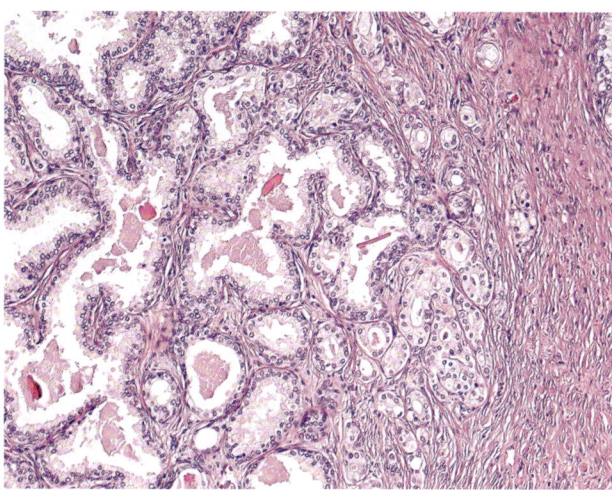

Figure 1.62. This example of adenosis/atypical adenomatous hyperplasia is particularly deceptive, due to numerous small crowded glands at the edge of the lesion. Crystalloids are present in some of the lumens, further resembling cancer.

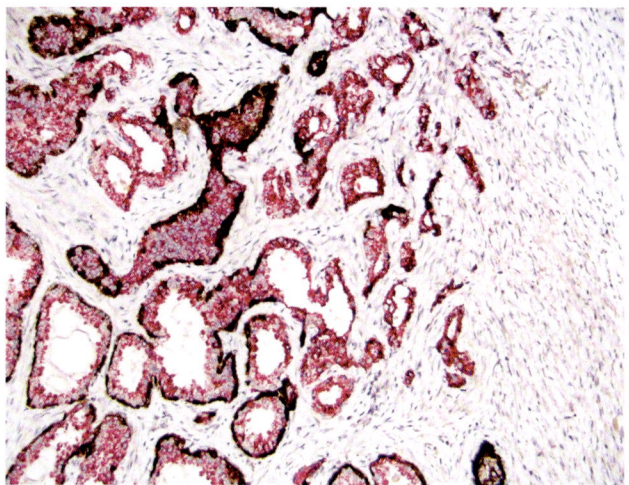

Figure 1.63. In this dual-color alpha-methylacyl-CoA racemase (AMACR) and basal cell immunohistochemical stain, the same case from Figure 1.62 shows several of the small glands to lack basal cells and the entire lesion is positive for AMACR. However, several of the small glands have a patchy basal cell layer, arguing against diagnosis of carcinoma.

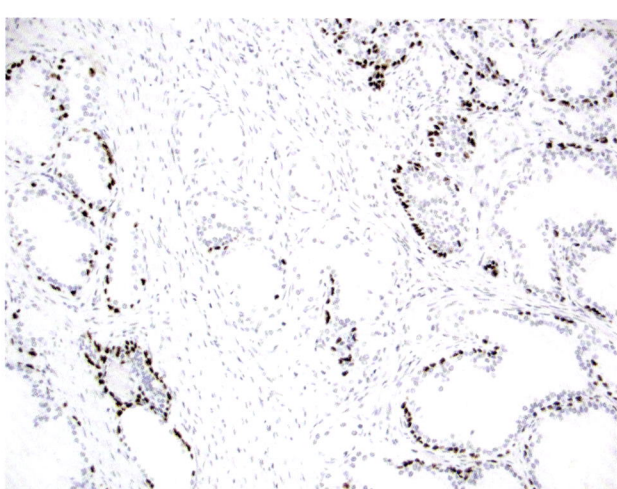

Figure 1.64. In this example of adenosis, p63 staining shows decreased density of the basal layer in the small glands; however, several basal cells are present and there is not a striking cytologic difference between the glands with basal cells and those without.

Since adenosis has some features that overlap with those of prostatic adenocarcinoma, such as the proliferation of small glands, presence of crystalloids, and a partial lack of basal cells, it has been postulated that it might be a precursor lesion,[48] particularly for transition zone cancers. Using molecular techniques, a few studies have found that these lesions are typically lacking the *ERG* gene rearrangements that are present in approximately 40% of prostate cancers.[49,50] However, since *ERG* rearrangements appear to be less common in transition zone cancers,[51-54] it is unclear if this would be the optimal evidence for refuting the status of adenosis as a precursor. Nonetheless, there is currently no evidence that adenosis carries an increased risk for development of cancer, and thus, no clinical action is currently recommended.[21,46] It is also debatable whether it is necessary to document the presence of adenosis in reports. For smaller lesions that are easily recognized as part of a hyperplastic nodule in transurethral resection specimens, it is likely reasonable that they not be specifically mentioned; however, for lesions encountered in needle biopsy or more florid examples in transurethral resection, it is reasonable to document that the focus was evaluated and judged to be adenosis/atypical adenomatous hyperplasia and not cancer.

Sclerosing Adenosis

Sclerosing adenosis is similar in many ways to adenosis/atypical adenomatous hyperplasia. For example, it shares the composition by large, branched (classically benign) glands and smaller, crowded glands. It may also have a discontinuous basal layer, with some of the small crowded glands appearing to lack basal cells.[21,46,47] However, the main differences between sclerosing adenosis and usual adenosis are that sclerosing adenosis also contains hypercellular stroma, which may compress some glands into small clusters of cells that could mimic even higher-grade cancer (Figures 1.66-1.71).[55-58] In normal benign prostate tissue, the basal cells are not myoepithelial (differing from the breast). However, sclerosing adenosis is unique in the prostate, in that the basal cells do have a myoepithelial phenotype, including positive staining for immunohistochemical markers such as S100 or muscle-specific actin (Figures 1.68 and 1.71),[55-58] in addition to the usual p63 or high-molecular-weight cytokeratin positivity of basal cells. Rarely sclerosing adenosis can have a greater degree of nuclear atypia, increasing the mimicry of prostatic adenocarcinoma; however, these cases have been found to still contain a myoepithelial cell layer and have no clear evidence of more aggressive behavior, favoring their similarity to conventional sclerosing adenosis.[55]

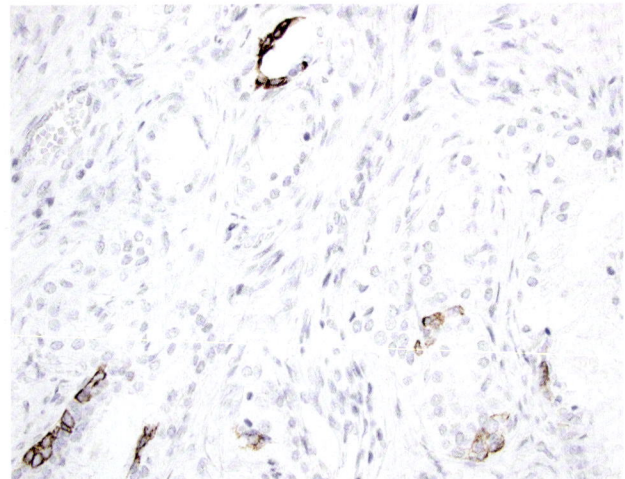

Figure 1.65. Using high-molecular-weight cytokeratin staining in the same lesion from 1-64, similarly several of the small glands appear to lack basal cells, but they are morphologically similar to other small glands with basal cells.

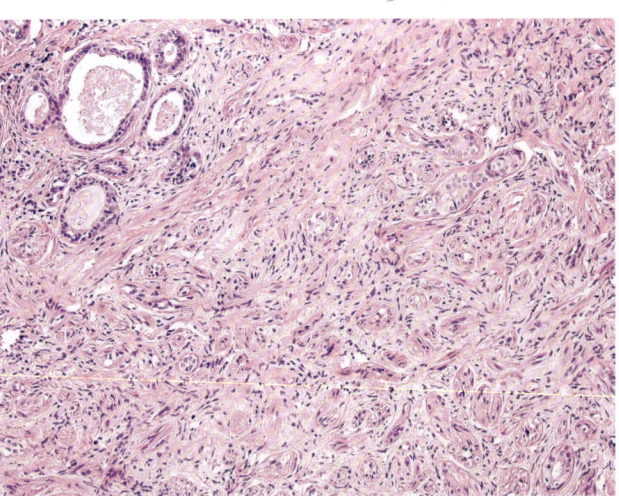

Figure 1.66. Sclerosing adenosis is composed of small benign glands in a cellular stroma that may mimic cancer, including pattern 4 or higher cancer. This example shows a transition from benign glands at upper left to cellular stroma at lower right.

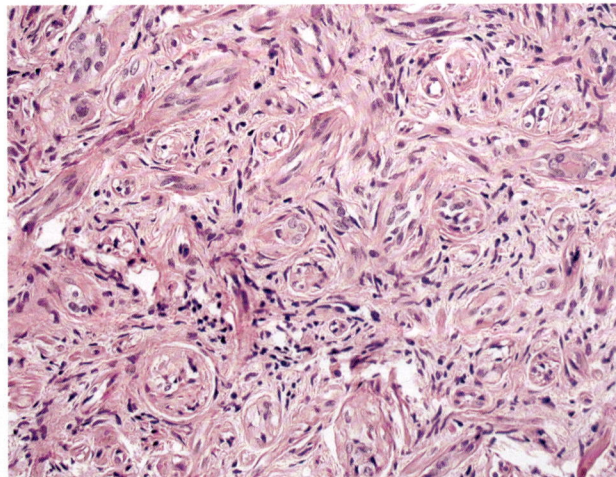

Figure 1.67. At higher magnification, the same case as Figure 1.66 shows numerous compressed glands that may be difficult to distinguish from blood vessels or stromal cells. However, some small clusters of epithelial cells may raise a differential diagnosis of poorly formed glands of prostatic adenocarcinoma.

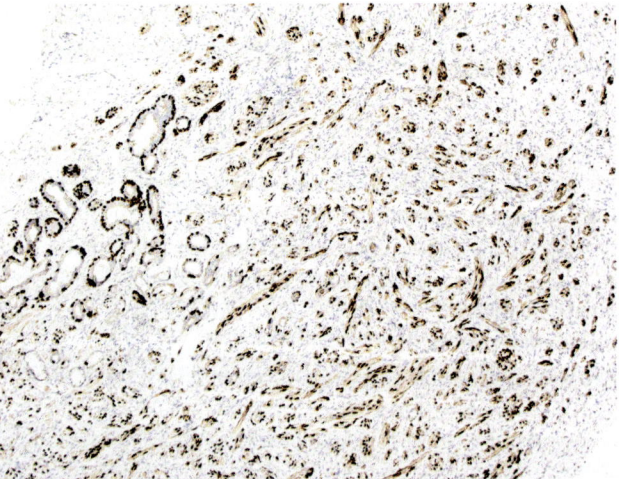

Figure 1.68. The same case from Figures 1.66 and 1.67 shows numerous glandular structures with basal cells on this single-color p63 and alpha-methylacyl-CoA racemase (AMACR) stain, even more numerous than appreciable by morphology.

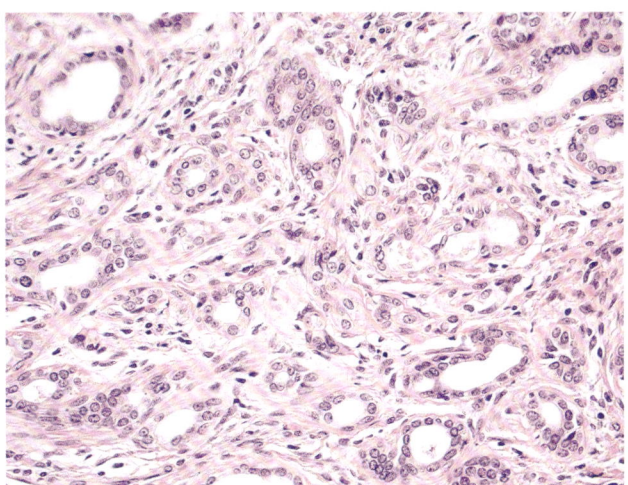

Figure 1.69. In other examples of sclerosing adenosis, glands may be more obvious but crowded, leading to concern of fused or poorly formed glands of prostatic adenocarcinoma.

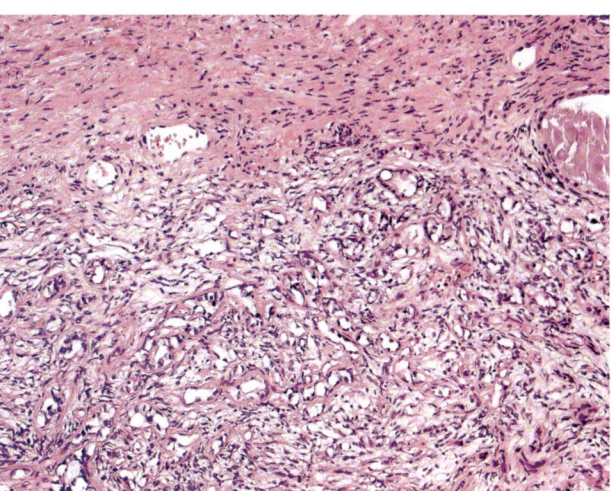

Figure 1.70. This example of sclerosing adenosis shows very cellular stroma with glands that are difficult to recognize.

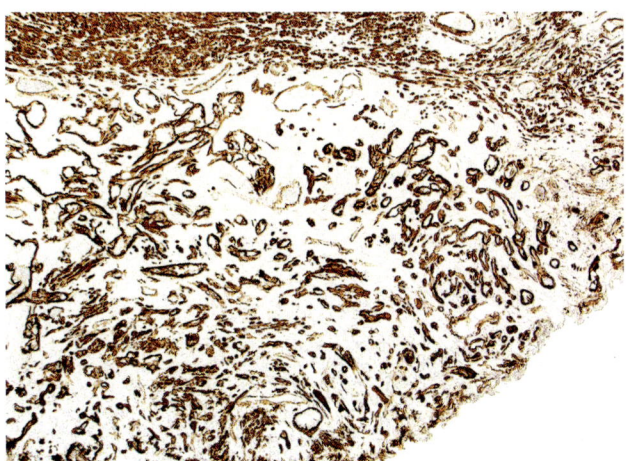

Figure 1.71. Immunohistochemistry shows a smooth muscle actin–positive cell layer around the glands in this example of sclerosing adenosis, supporting myoepithelial differentiation and contrasting to usual basal cells, which are not myoepithelial.

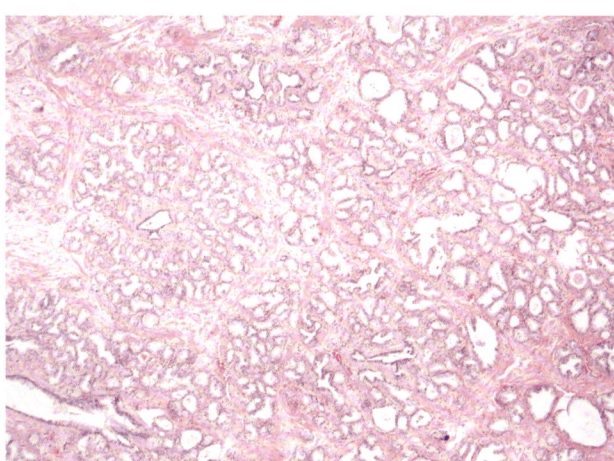

Figure 1.72. Diffuse adenosis of the peripheral zone is a rare proliferation of benign-appearing but crowded glands, often occurring in younger patients. This specimen from a 45-year-old man shows areas of lobular crowded glands (left) and other areas with less obvious lobular configuration (right).

Diffuse Adenosis of Peripheral Zone

Diffuse adenosis of the peripheral zone is a rare lesion that has been described in only one study to date.[59] In contrast to conventional adenosis, which forms a circumscribed nodule in the transition zone, rare examples under this name have been noted to exhibit crowded, nonlobular, but benign-appearing acini in the peripheral zone (Figures 1.72 and 1.73), often in younger patients (average age 49 years).[59] These were noted to typically contain an intact, although often patchy, layer of basal cells in the 55% of cases that were evaluated with immunohistochemistry.[59] Despite the apparent benign nature of diffuse adenosis itself, the authors noted an association with cancer, suggesting that it be considered a potential risk factor for prostatic adenocarcinoma.[59]

Atrophy

As noted previously in the Section The Unremarkable and Nonneoplastic Prostate, atrophy is potentially so common in prostate pathology to be considered a relatively normal finding. In particular, simple atrophy (discussed previously) rarely causes diagnostic difficulty. However, several other patterns of atrophy have been described, including simple atrophy with cysts, sclerotic atrophy, postatrophic hyperplasia (also known as hyperplastic or lobular atrophy), and partial atrophy.[19,60] Postatrophic hyperplasia refers to essentially a lobular configuration of atrophic but crowded glands, which are often hyperchromatic (Figures 1.74 and 1.75). This name implies a putative mechanism of proliferation of the atrophic glands; however, whether it instead represents a crowded lobule that has subsequently undergone atrophy remains open to debate. Most of the discussion here will focus on partial atrophy, which has the most potential to mimic prostatic adenocarcinoma.

Partial Atrophy

Partial atrophy is so named because the cells have decreased cytoplasm compared to normal glands, although cytoplasm is not as attenuated as in other types of atrophy. This means that the glandular structures are not necessarily basophilic, leading to potential confusion with prostatic adenocarcinoma.[19] In addition, the cytoplasmic height is typically not much greater than the height of the nucleus (Figure 1.76), whereas there may be an abundant amount of lateral cytoplasm before the next nucleus is encountered in a histologic section (Figures 1.77-1.83). Nucleoli can also be identifiable, and luminal border is often at least partially straight,

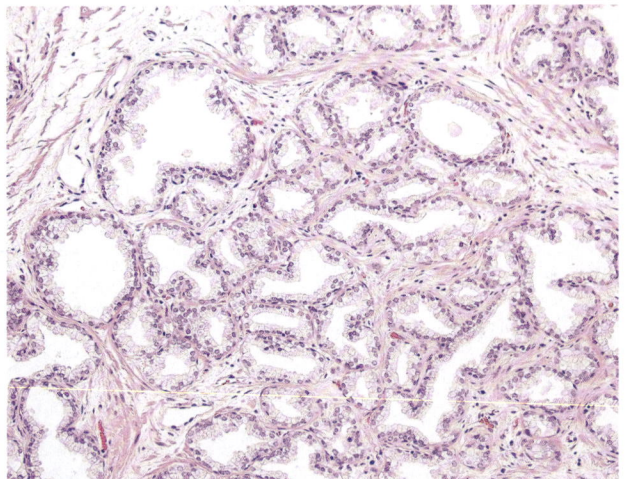

Figure 1.73. In diffuse adenosis of the peripheral zone, small round glands are morphologically benign but crowded, often with a less lobular configuration.

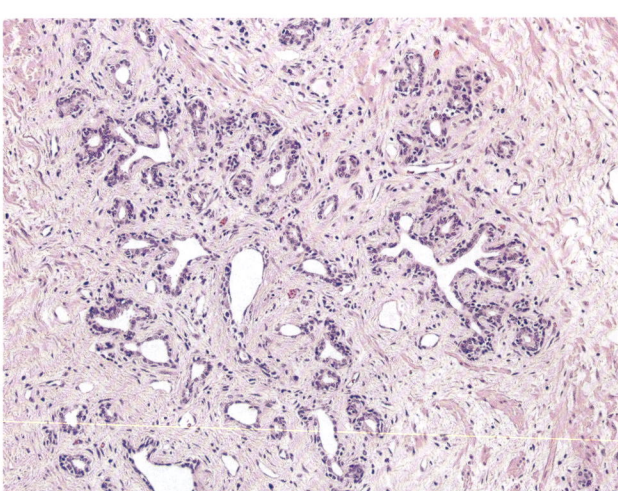

Figure 1.74. Postatrophic hyperplasia is typically composed of a lobular configuration of glands with an atrophic appearance. Although the glands may appear morphologically crowded and small, the lobular orientation is a clue to the benign diagnosis.

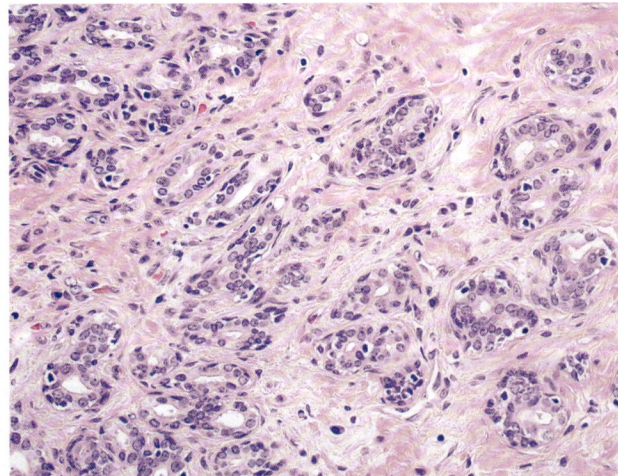

Figure 1.75. At high magnification, this example of postatrophic hyperplasia may mimic cancer due to the small clusters of glands with a hyperchromatic appearance; however, a normal basal cell layer is present.

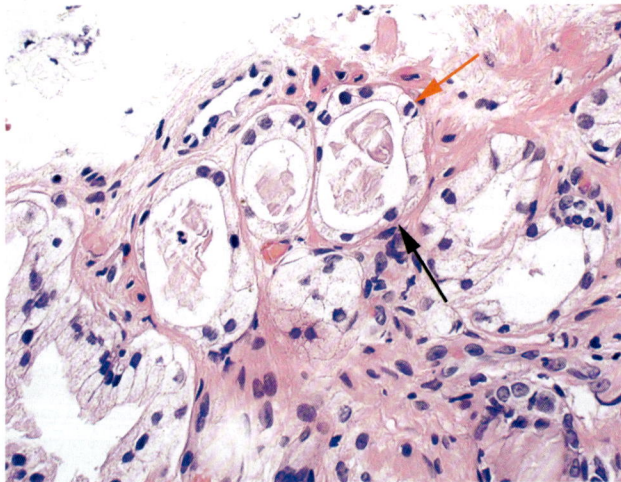

Figure 1.76. In partial atrophy, glands are small and crowded. Some nuclei are very small and compressed, as if they have been "pinched" (red arrow). The cytoplasm is not much taller than the nuclei (black arrow), and there is abundant lateral cytoplasm before the next nucleus.

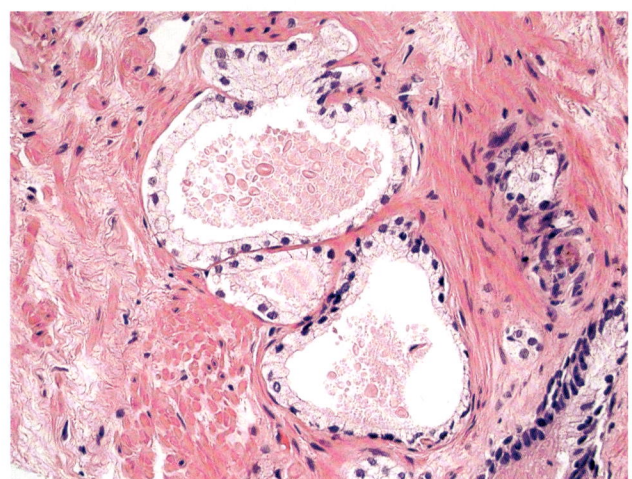

Figure 1.77. This example of partial atrophy is composed of larger, dilated glands. Although basal cells are not morphologically obvious, the cytoplasm is not much taller than the nuclei in several areas and the nuclei are not atypical.

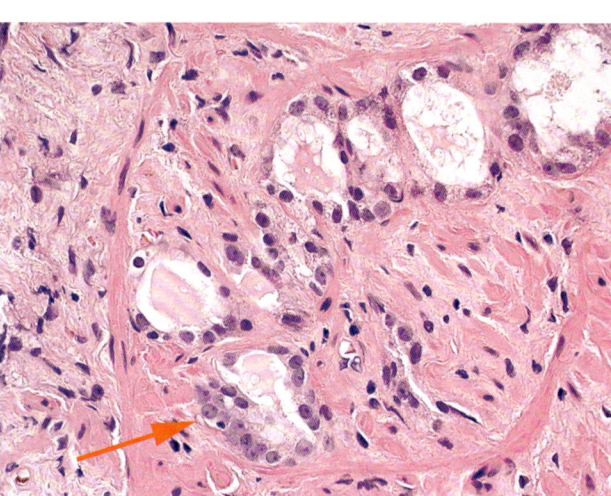

Figure 1.78. Occasional prostate cancers can have atrophy-like features. This example shows glands with short and wide cytoplasm resembling partial atrophy; however, areas with prominent nucleoli similar to usual cancer are also present (arrow).

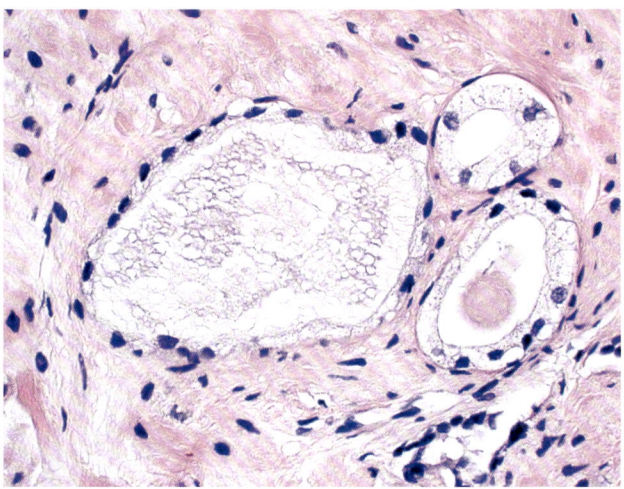

Figure 1.79. In this example of partial atrophy, there is one gland with attenuated cytoplasm and two round glands with a sharp luminal border.

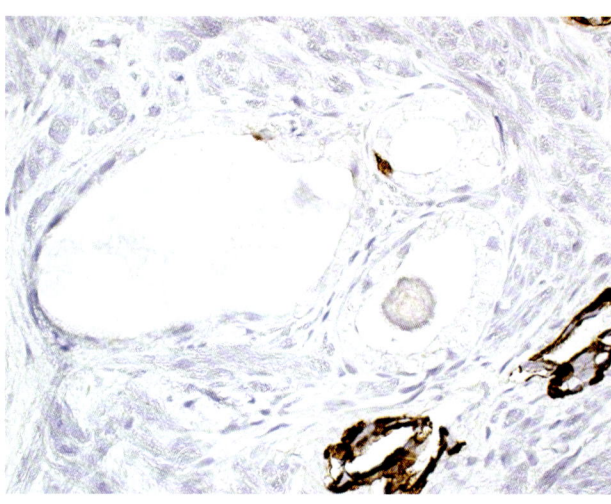

Figure 1.80. Using immunohistochemistry with a dual-color basal cell and alpha-methylacyl-CoA racemase (AMACR) cocktail, the same focus from Figure 1.79 shows extremely rare basal cells and no significant staining for AMACR. Despite the paucity of basal cells, the lesion can be interpreted as benign.

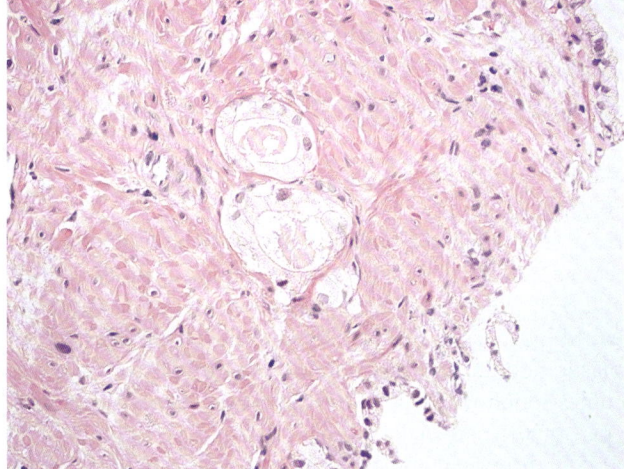

Figure 1.81. This focus of partial atrophy closely mimics cancer, composed of three small round glands.

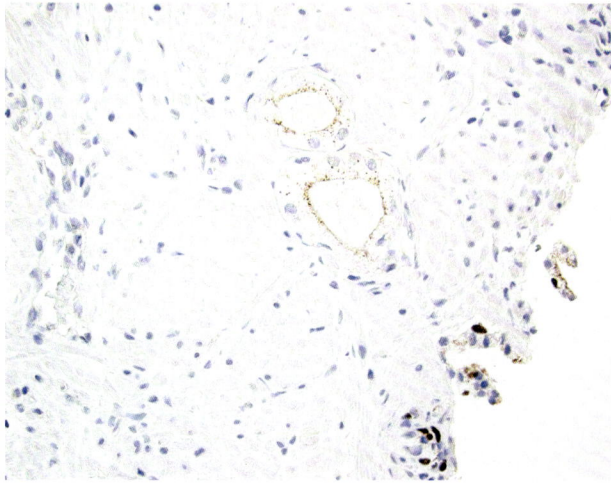

Figure 1.82. On a single-color p63 and alpha-methylacyl-CoA racemase (AMACR) stain, no basal cells are visualized in the same focus from Figure 1.81. There is no significant AMACR staining.

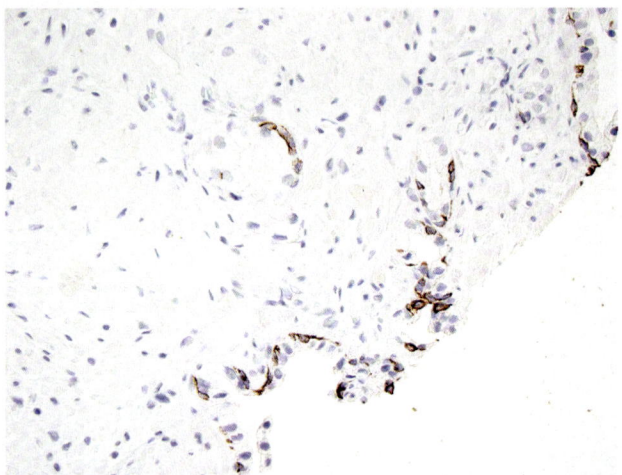
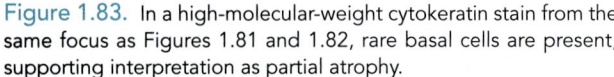

Figure 1.83. In a high-molecular-weight cytokeratin stain from the same focus as Figures 1.81 and 1.82, rare basal cells are present, supporting interpretation as partial atrophy.

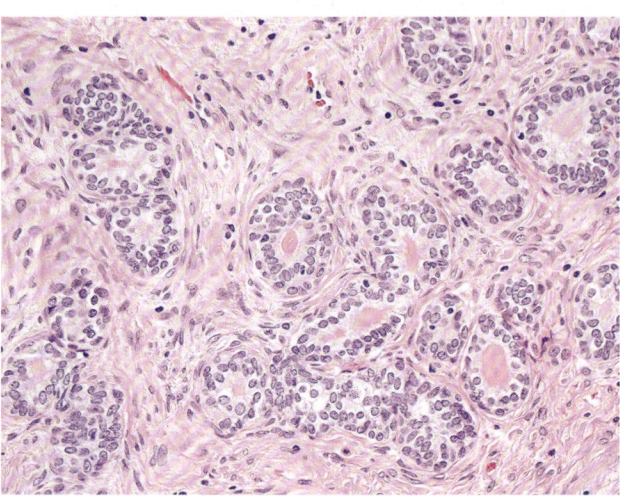

Figure 1.84. Basal cell hyperplasia can manifest as small round glands. This example is relatively evident as having two cell populations.

leading to the mimicry of prostatic adenocarcinoma encountered for this entity.[61-63] Basal cells are often not apparent using morphology alone; however, immunohistochemistry usually reveals a patchy but intact basal cell layer. Nonetheless, some cases may show no definite basal cells by immunohistochemistry, which should not necessarily preclude confident interpretation as partial atrophy in the appropriate context. Although AMACR may be occasionally positive in partial atrophy,[61] it is often of limited or weak intensity.[62]

PEARLS AND PITFALLS: Diagnosis of Partial Atrophy

Potential pitfalls:

- Basal cells inapparent by morphology
- Small, crowded, round glands with pale cytoplasm
- Often straight luminal border
- Some nucleoli visible

Helpful diagnostic clues:

- Decreased basal apical cell dimension (cytoplasm barely taller than the nucleus)
- Large lateral cytoplasm dimension (abundant lateral cytoplasm before the next nucleus)
- Occasional small, dark, "pinched" nuclei
- Basal cells often present in patchy distribution using immunohistochemistry (may be completely absent in some of the glands)
- AMACR often minimal or negative (but sometimes positive)

Basal Cell Hyperplasia (Small Gland Pattern)

Basal cell hyperplasia can exhibit several different histologic patterns, which are discussed in each of the pattern-based sections. Occasionally, basal cell hyperplasia can form small, round glands (Figures 1.84 and 1.85), which may be confused with the usual pattern of prostatic acinar adenocarcinoma. In most cases, this proliferation makes up the majority of, or the entirety of, a hyperplastic nodule, and therefore, the nature of the lesion can be recognized based on its circumscription within a nodule. However, rare cases of basal cell hyperplasia can form only part of a hyperplastic nodule, yielding a pseudoinfiltrative appearance (Figures 1.86-1.90).[64] Both normal and hyperplastic basal cells can contain appreciable nucleoli, which can add to the diagnostic difficulty (Figure 1.88). Additionally, basal cell hyperplasia can contain mitotic figures and crystalloids.[64]

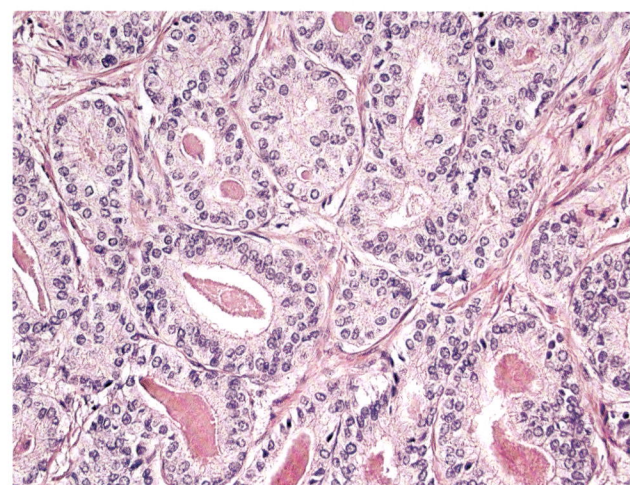

Figure 1.85. This example of basal cell hyperplasia mimicked a low-grade prostatic adenocarcinoma due to extremely crowded arrangement of round glands.

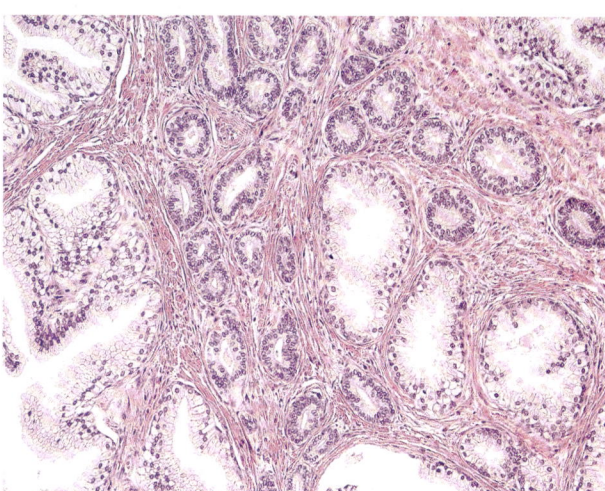

Figure 1.86. Occasionally, basal cell hyperplasia can have a pseudoinfiltrative appearance due to the glands making up only a part of a hyperplastic nodule, raising the possibility that they are cancer glands infiltrating between benign glands.

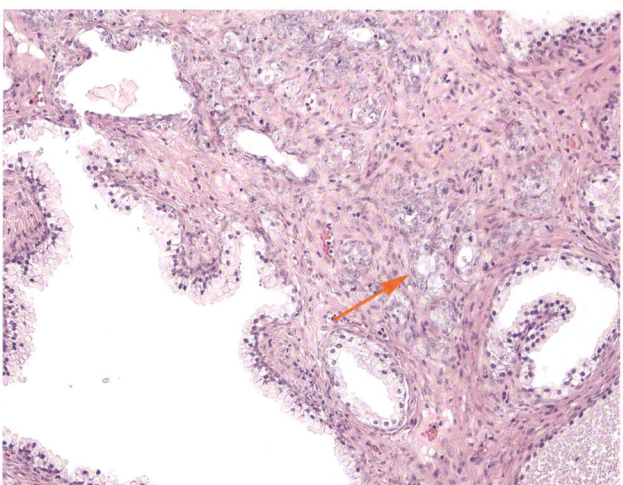

Figure 1.87. This example of basal cell hyperplasia was extremely deceptive due to its partial composition of a hyperplastic nodule. Some of the basal cell hyperplasia glands contain blue mucin (red arrow), and they appear to infiltrate between benign glands.

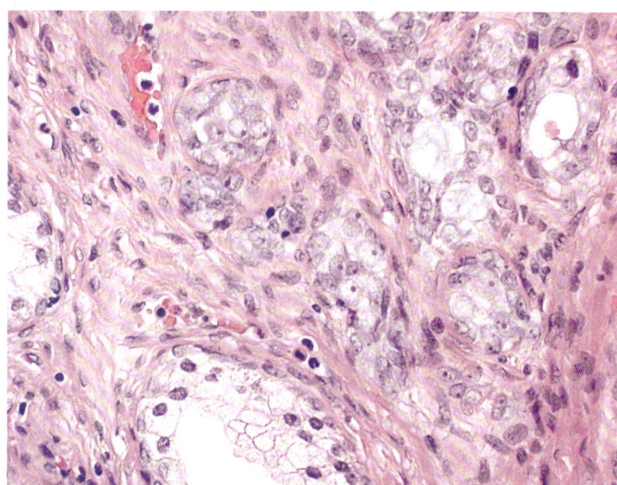

Figure 1.88. High magnification of the same case from Figure 1.87 shows prominent nucleoli and blue mucin. See also Figures 1.89 and 1.90.

PEARLS AND PITFALLS: Recognizing Basal Cell Hyperplasia

- Similarity of nuclei with nucleoli to the basal cells of adjacent benign glands (Figure 1.91)

- Recognition of an apparent dual cell population despite nucleoli or atypia

- Immunohistochemistry: Although glands appear to be filled with basal cells, sometimes labeling for basal markers will appear as predominantly a single layer or a few layers at the periphery of the glands,[65] or in a checkerboard pattern (Figures 1.92 and 1.93)

It is relevant to keep in mind that rare prostate cancers can be p63-positive[33-35,37] and others, especially high-grade cancers, can be high-molecular-weight cytokeratin positive.[39-42,66] However, fortunately, positivity for both markers typically does not occur in the same case and the staining distribution of staining in such cases is not basally located, instead typically labeling the cancer diffusely in a nonbasal distribution.

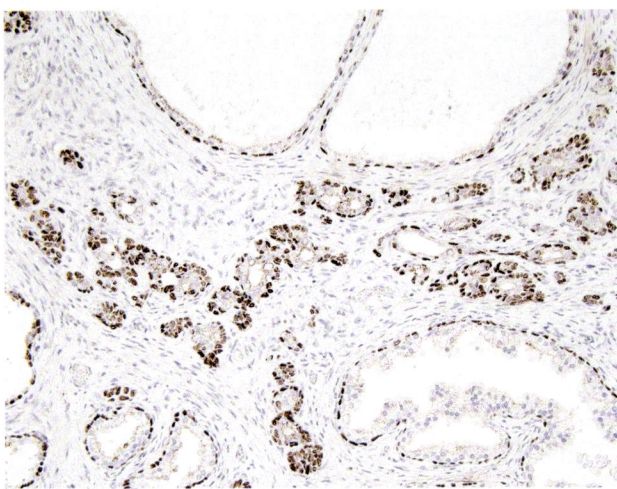

Figure 1.89. Immunohistochemistry with a single-color p63 and alpha-methylacyl-CoA racemase (AMACR) stain shows a robust layer of basal cells in all of the pseudoinfiltrative glands from Figures 1.87 and 1.88.

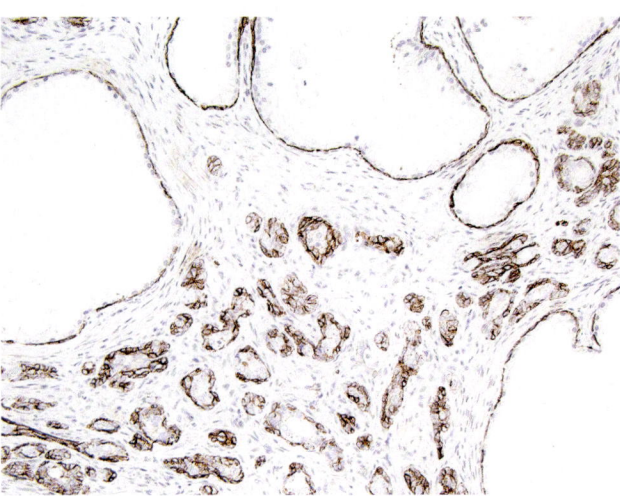

Figure 1.90. The same case from Figures 1.87-1.89 shows a robust basal cell layer with high-molecular-weight cytokeratin staining.

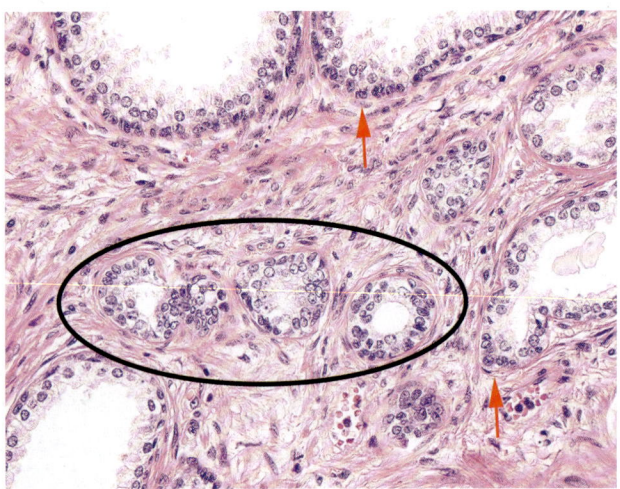

Figure 1.91. When considering a differential diagnosis between basal cell hyperplasia and prostatic adenocarcinoma, it is helpful to compare the suspicious glands (circle) to the basal cells of obviously benign glands (red arrows).

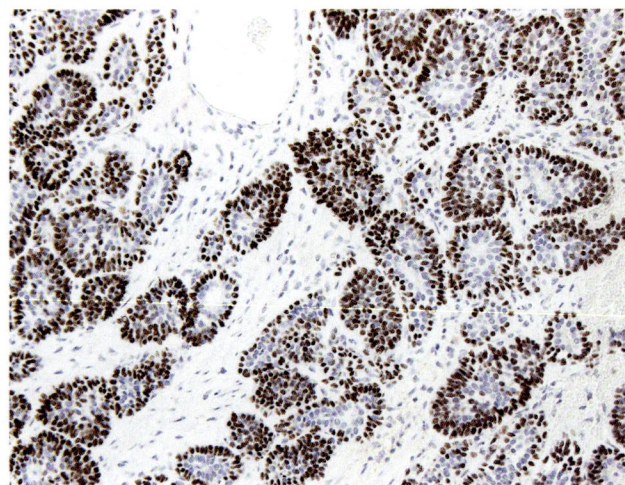

Figure 1.92. When using immunohistochemistry in basal cell hyperplasia, although the glands appear to be filled with basal cells morphologically, the staining may be more peripheral, as in this example of p63 staining, or in a checkerboard pattern with some morphologically similar cells being negative.

FAQ: Can Prostate Cancer Be Positive for Basal Cell Markers?

Yes, rare cancers can be positive for p63 (Figures 1.48 and 1.49) or high-molecular-weight cytokeratin. However, positivity for both markers is rarely, if ever, found in the same tumor. Prostate cancer with unexpected p63 positivity typically shows diffuse labeling of the cancer cells in a nonbasal distribution (luminal).[33-35,37] Of note, some distinctive morphologic findings have been reported in these cases, including infiltrative glands, nests, and cords with an atrophic appearance of the cytoplasm (scant cytoplasm) or basaloid appearance.[33,40] Although the significance of this finding is not totally understood, some data suggest that the behavior of these cancers may not be totally reflected by conventional grading, in which case it may be appropriate to defer using conventional grading.[33]

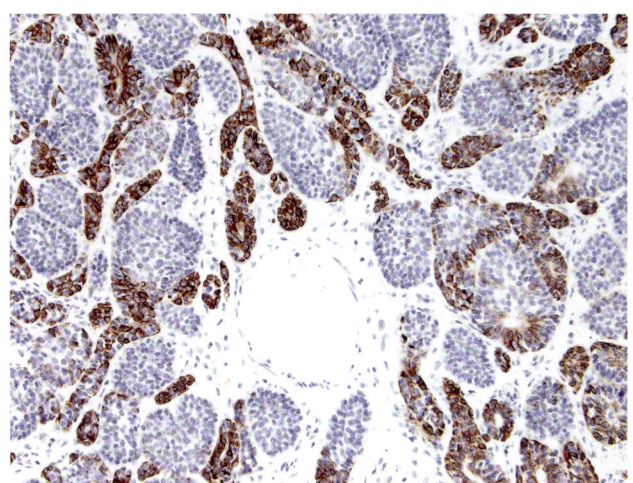

Figure 1.93. The same case of basal cell hyperplasia from Figure 1.92 shows high-molecular-weight cytokeratin only partially in most of the glands, despite their morphologic appearance of being filled by basal cells.

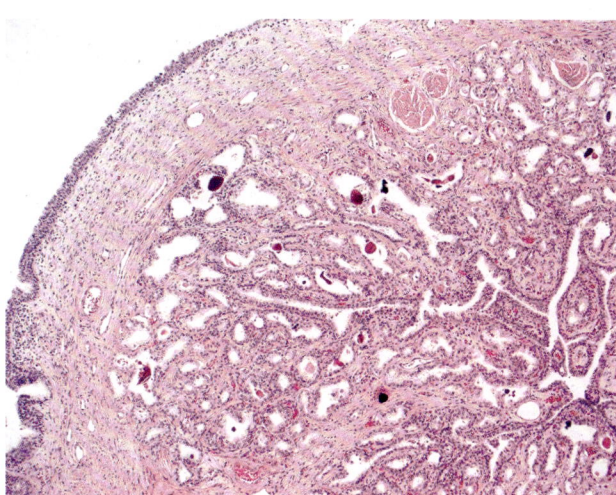

Figure 1.94. The verumontanum sometimes contains a crowded architecture of small round glands, although usually with a normal lobular architecture.

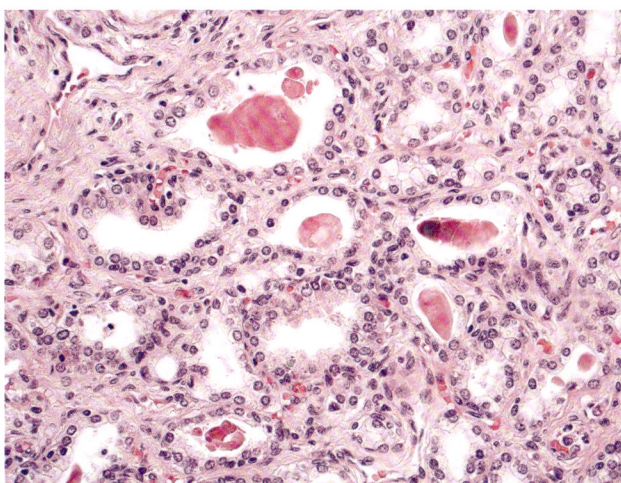

Figure 1.95. At high magnification, the verumontanum glands have benign cytology and often dark-colored luminal concretions.

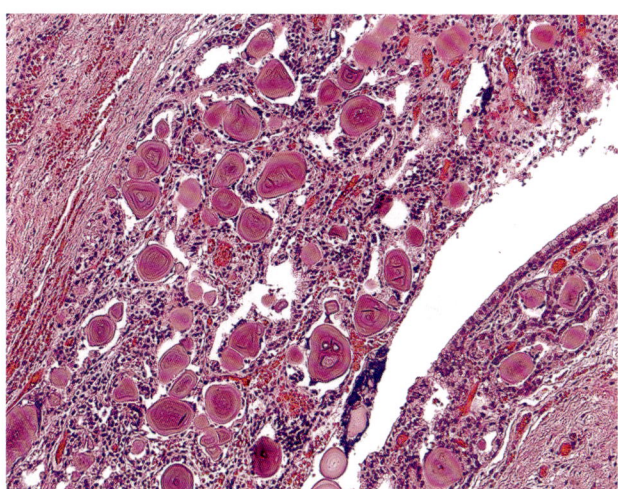

Figure 1.96. In some examples of verumontanum mucosal glands (or hyperplasia), the dark concretions may be extremely numerous, which can be used as a diagnostic clue if found in a biopsy specimen.

Verumontanum Mucosal Glands, Normal and Hyperplastic

The verumontanum or seminal colliculus is a landmark within the prostatic urethra near the insertion of the ejaculatory ducts that typically forms a rounded or triangular hump in tissue sections, pointed toward the anterior aspect of the prostate gland.[1,11,67,68] This can contain small, rounded, crowded glands, which may appear on first examination to be suspicious for adenocarcinoma (Figures 1.94 and 1.95).[67] In radical prostatectomy specimens, this is typically not a diagnostic problem, as the restriction of this proliferation to the specific anatomic region of the verumontanum is apparent. However, when especially florid or encountered in a biopsy specimen, this pattern may be deceptive.[68] These glands often have concretions similar to corpora amylacea that are more numerous than conventional benign tissue, and frequently, these have a red-orange, bronze, or deep purple color (Figures 1.96-1.98), different from the typical pink appearance of corpora amylacea.[68] Despite the crowded acinar appearance of this lesion, basal cells are appreciable by morphology or immunohistochemistry, and cytologic features are typically bland, contrasting to true adenocarcinomas, which may sometimes extend to the urethra.[67,68]

> **PEARLS AND PITFALLS: Clues to Diagnosis of Verumontanum Mucosal Gland Hyperplasia**[68]
> - Predominantly lobular architecture
> - Often immediately beneath urothelium
> - Corpora amylacea/orange-red concretions often numerous
> - Basal cells identifiable by morphology or immunohistochemistry

Nephrogenic Adenoma

Nephrogenic adenoma is a relatively well-known entity with a proliferation of cells with a renal tubular phenotype, particularly in the urinary bladder; however, it also may cause a diagnostic challenge in the prostatic urethra. Patterns of nephrogenic adenoma include tubular, papillary, and flat.[16,46,47,69-71] Primarily the tubular pattern is discussed here for its potential to be confused with prostate cancer (Figures 1.99-1.102).[71] Nephrogenic adenoma was originally considered a metaplastic process, considering its frequent association with inflammation or irritation of the urinary tract, which suggests that it may be a

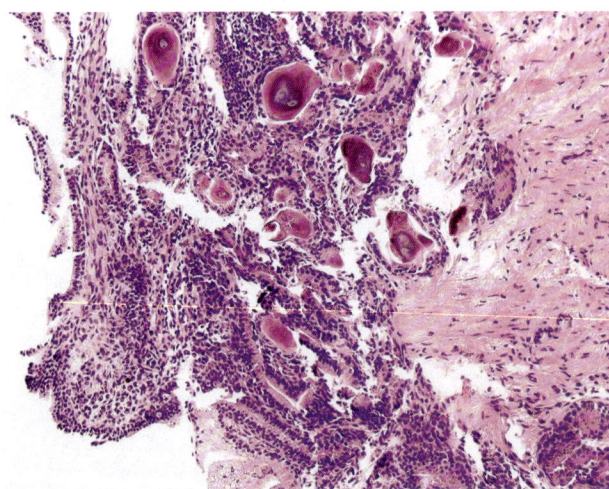

Figure 1.97. In this example, verumontanum glands were captured in a needle biopsy appearing as a complex glandular proliferation but with prominent dark concretions.

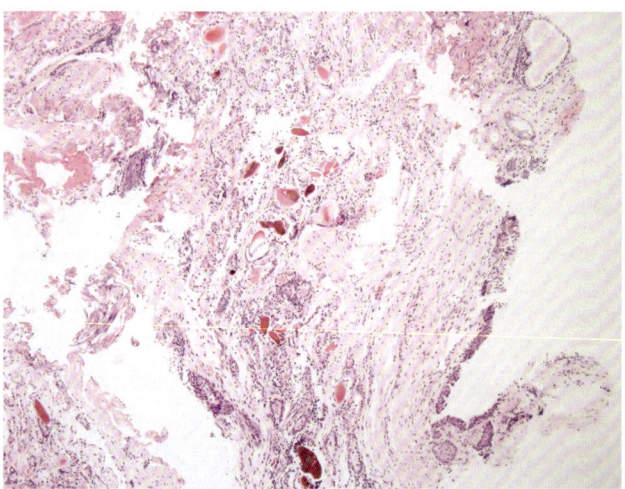

Figure 1.98. In this case, verumontanum glands appear distorted in a transurethral resection specimen; however, the dark concretions are a clue that may help to avoid concern for cancer.

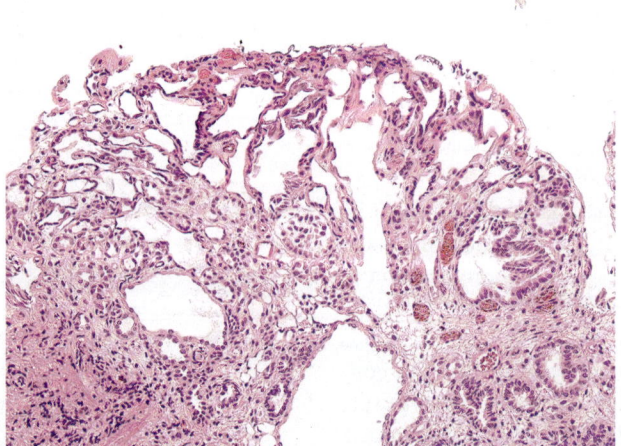

Figure 1.99. Nephrogenic adenoma involving the prostatic urethra usually manifests as crowded glands or tubular structures just under the urethral mucosa.

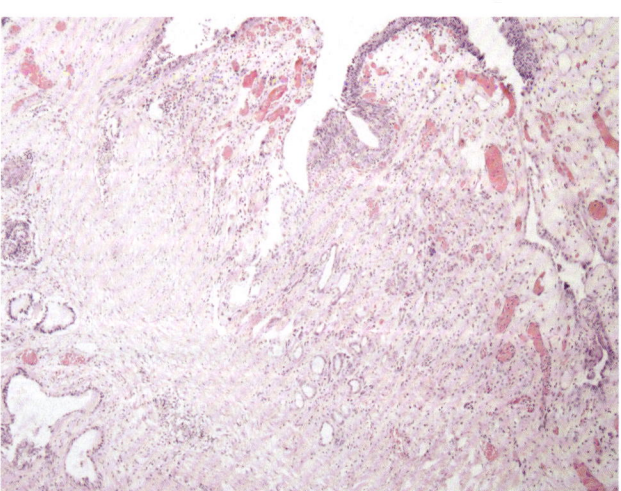

Figure 1.100. In this case of nephrogenic adenoma found in transurethral resection, several tubular structures are present just below the urethral mucosa.

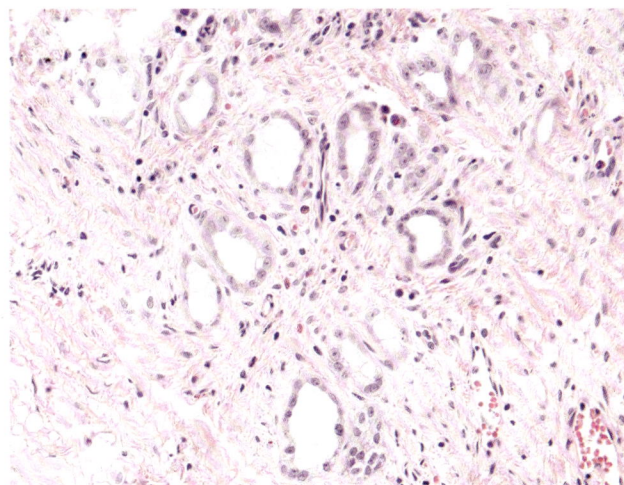

Figure 1.101. The classic pattern of nephrogenic adenoma forms small tubules or glands, which could be confused for prostate cancer.

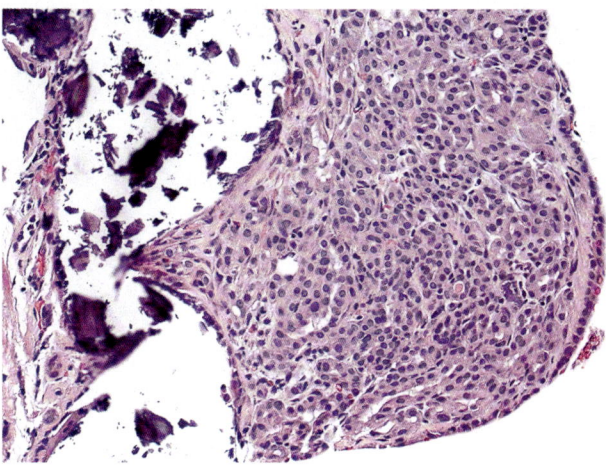

Figure 1.102. This example of nephrogenic adenoma encountered in a needle biopsy shows an extremely crowded proliferation of tubular structures at the tip of the core, which likely represents the urethral lumen.

metaplastic response to injury. However, an interesting study found that in renal transplant recipients, the lesion has the sex chromosomes of the kidney donor rather than the recipient, suggesting that it likely represents implantation and growth of shed renal tubular cells into a site of urinary mucosal injury.[72] As such, it seems that nephrogenic adenomas are most consistently positive for renal tubular marker PAX8 (Figure 1.103),[73,74] whereas they can have a few different phenotypes resembling perhaps different sites of renal tubular cells, with variable positivity for other markers such as AMACR and GATA3 (Figure 1.104).[75]

PEARLS AND PITFALLS: Nephrogenic Adenoma in Prostatic Specimens

- Can have a prostate cancer–like staining pattern with typical prostate immunohistochemical cocktails (absence of basal cells and AMACR positivity) (Figure 1.104)
- Positivity for high-molecular-weight cytokeratin in the tubules in a nonbasal distribution[75] and positivity for PAX8 can be used to confirm the diagnosis
- Other morphologic clues include the following:
  - Prominent basement membrane layer around many of the tubules/glands (Figure 1.105)
  - Frequent localization near the mucosa of the urethra
  - Association with inflammation (Figure 1.105), and sometimes a hobnail-shaped configuration of the cells or prominent nucleoli (Figure 1.106)[71]

Mesonephric Remnant and Hyperplasia

Mesonephric remnants are rare benign inclusions sometimes found in the prostatic or periprostatic tissue, analogous to the counterpart in the gynecologic tract.[21,76-78] Locations noted have included bladder neck smooth muscle, soft tissue around the seminal vesicle at the prostatic base, within anterior fibromuscular stroma of the prostate, and within the prostatic tissue among acini.[76] This lesion may be underrecognized, as some cases likely overlap substantially with lobules of atrophic prostatic glands; however, the more florid and hyperplastic cases may have the potential for diagnostic confusion, being mistaken for prostatic adenocarcinoma or extraprostatic extension of cancer (when in the periprostatic tissue).[76] Several features of mesonephric remnant resemble those of nephrogenic adenoma, including positivity for PAX8 immunohistochemistry, as well as formation of small glandular structures with cuboidal cell lining. In contrast to nephrogenic adenoma, which by its nature occurs near urothelial mucosa (eg, the prostatic urethra), mesonephric remnants tend to be found in locations distant from the urethral mucosa. Other features of

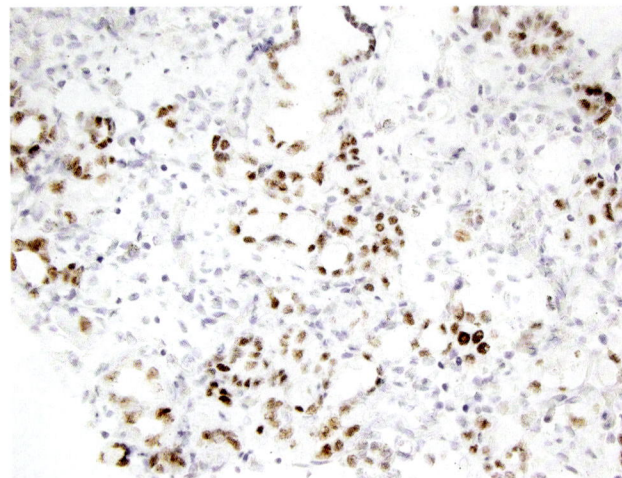

Figure 1.103. Consistent positive immunohistochemistry for PAX8 is helpful in confirming nephrogenic adenoma, which is rarely, if ever, positive in prostatic adenocarcinoma.

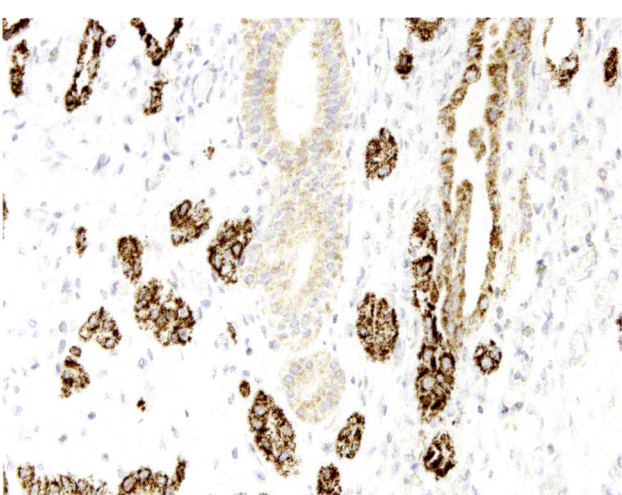

Figure 1.104. If a prostate immunohistochemical "cocktail" is used, such as this p63 and alpha-methylacyl-CoA racemase (AMACR) single-color assay, it may led to confusion with prostatic adenocarcinoma, as nephrogenic adenoma will have no basal cell layer and often cytoplasmic positivity for AMACR.

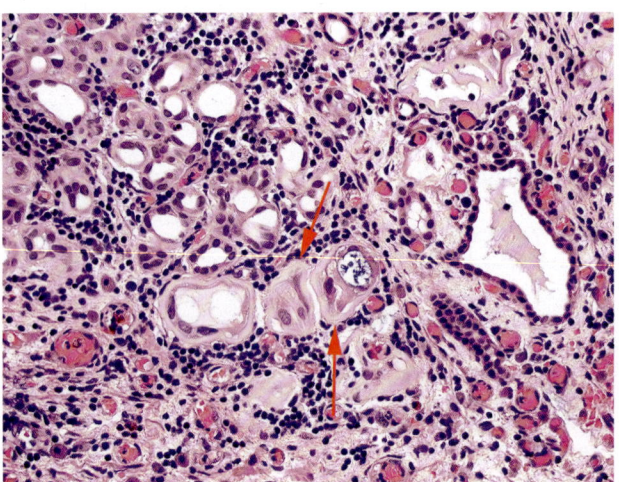

Figure 1.105. Other features of nephrogenic adenoma include a frequent background of chronic inflammation and a prominent basement membrane layer around the glands (red arrows).

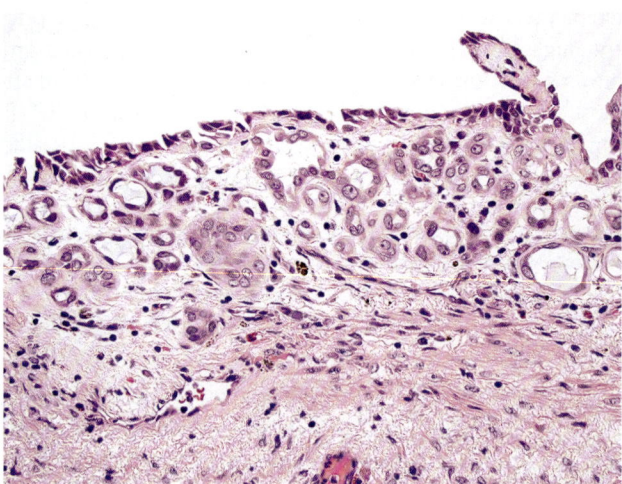

Figure 1.106. This example of nephrogenic adenoma of the prostatic urethra has prominent nucleoli, which could lead to confusion with prostatic adenocarcinoma. The location just under the mucosa of the urethra is a clue.

mesonephric remnant include a lobular architecture, colloid-like luminal material (Figure 1.107), dilated tubules or cysts, and micropapillary tufts.[76] When mesonephric remnants are found within benign prostatic tissue, it is of no clinical significance if they are disregarded as atrophic glands; however, when potentially confused for prostate cancer or extraprostatic extension of cancer, their negative staining for prostatic markers (PSA and others) and positive staining for PAX8 (Figure 1.108) are diagnostically useful.[76,78]

Benign Glands With Radiation Atypia

A general rule for histopathology of prostate specimens is that marked nuclear pleomorphism tends to argue against prostatic adenocarcinoma and favor another diagnosis, whether it be benign seminal vesicle or ejaculatory duct tissue, benign glands with radiation change, or urothelial carcinoma. As such, apparently random variation in nuclear size within prostatic glandular tissue should often raise suspicion for previous radiation change. Additionally, a patient history of radiation is often not conveyed upon submission of specimens for examination, frequently requiring the pathologist to verify such a

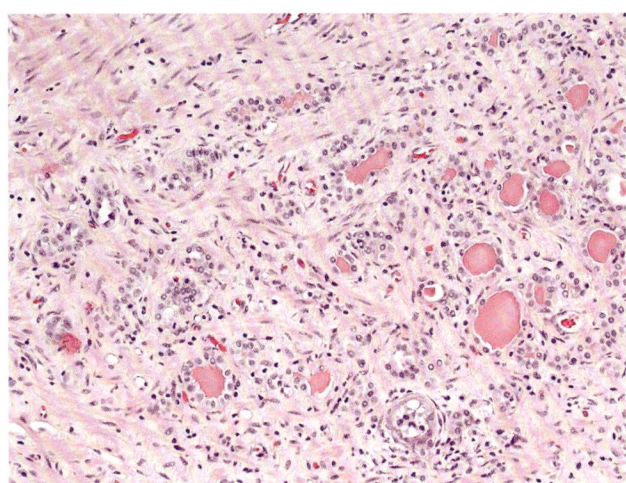

Figure 1.107. Mesonephric remnants are rare lesions in and around the prostate. This example would likely be disregarded as a benign process such as atrophy; however, when found in periprostatic tissue, this entity may lead to uncertainty. This example is composed of small tubules with eosinophilic colloid-like material.

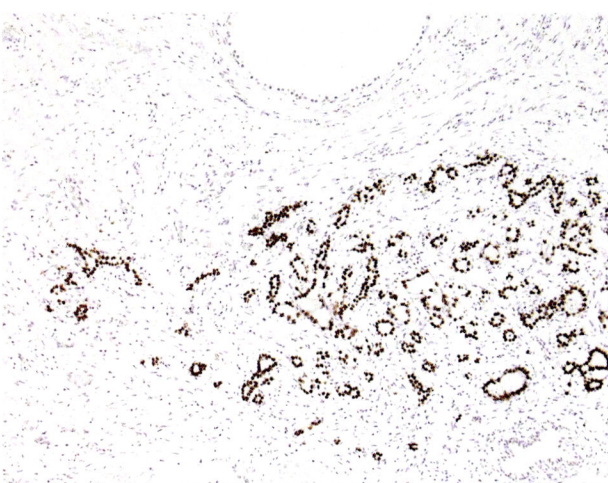

Figure 1.108. PAX8 positivity can help confirm the diagnosis of mesonephric remnant, which also highlights a lobular architecture in this case.

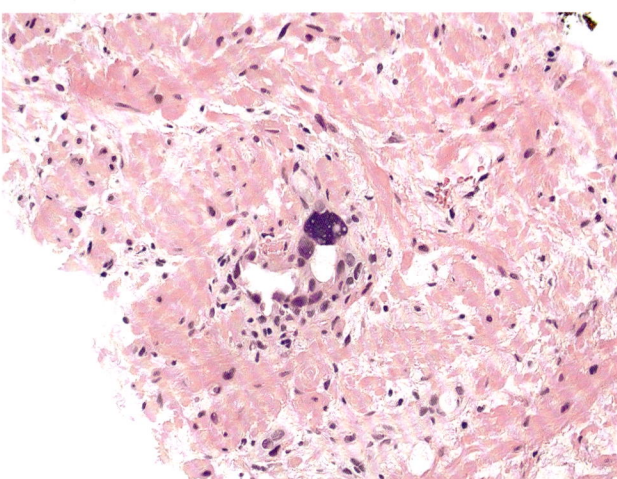

Figure 1.109. Benign prostatic tissue with radiation effect can display marked nuclear atypia in the basal cells, which may be disconcerting. However, pleomorphism is unusual in prostate cancer and should raise consideration of radiation change.

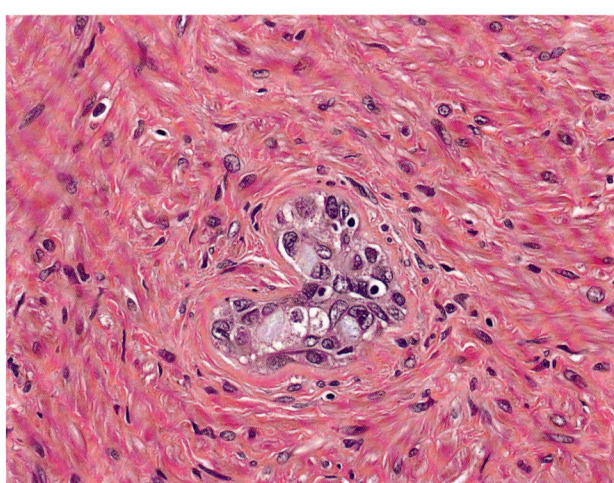

Figure 1.110. This example of benign prostatic tissue with radiation change demonstrates a lesser degree of nuclear atypia, but this may be a clue to the posttreatment nature of the specimen if not communicated.

history within available medical records. In benign tissue with radiation change, glands often appear atrophic with scant cytoplasm of the luminal or secretory cells. However, the basal cells are enlarged and sometimes quite atypical and hyperchromatic with prominent nucleoli (Figures 1.109 and 1.110).[79,80] Despite this potentially worrisome appearance, lobular architecture can often still be recognized. Radiation change of soft tissues, such as marked vascular damage (Figure 1.111), obliteration of small blood vessels, or atypical cells within nerves can also be a clue to the posttreatment nature of a specimen when not communicated. A recently reported interesting finding that could cause diagnostic confusion is that these basal cells may also be positive for GATA3 immunohistochemistry (Figures 1.112-1.114),[81,82] which could lead to confusion with urothelial carcinoma. Despite the recognition of this phenomenon in prostates with radiation treatment, GATA3 positivity can also be found in benign prostate tissue without a radiation history, although perhaps at a lesser level.[81,83] Prostate cancer, in contrast, is consistently negative for GATA3 with extremely rare reported exceptions.[81,83-87] If prostatic adenocarcinoma is a diagnostic concern, immunohistochemistry in these glands will show the atypical cells to be positive for basal cell markers.

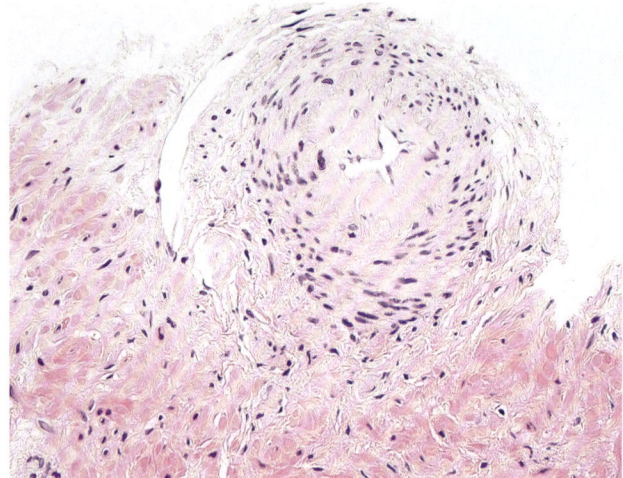

Figure 1.111. This blood vessel from a postradiation prostate biopsy shows intimal thickening and enlarged nuclei in the wall, which are clues that the prostate has been previously treated with radiation.

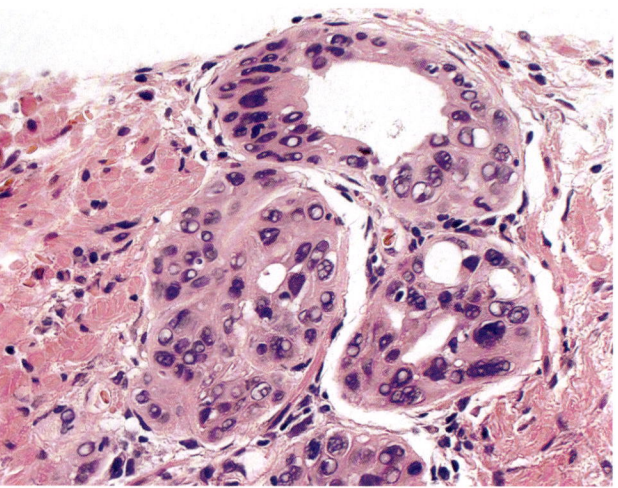

Figure 1.112. This example of radiation atypia in benign prostatic glands demonstrates numerous basal cell nuclei with enlarged nuclei of varying size.

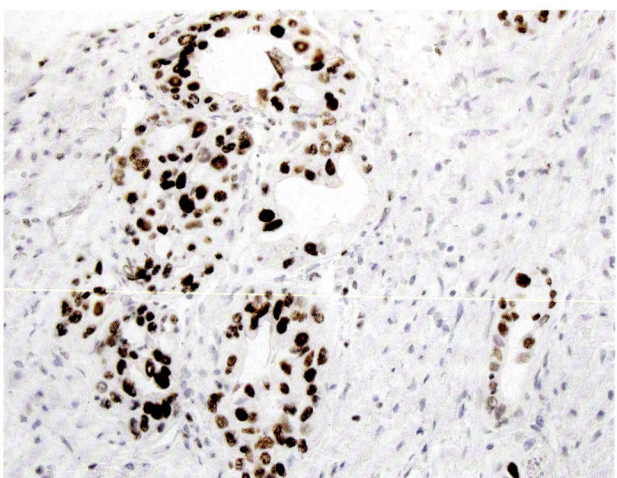

Figure 1.113. Immunohistochemistry in the same case from Figure 1.112 shows substantial GATA3 positivity, which has been recently described in postradiation benign glands.

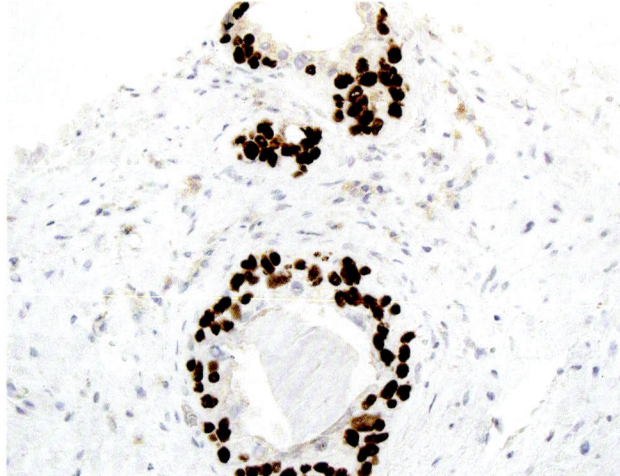

Figure 1.114. Immunohistochemistry for p63 in the case from Figures 1.112 and 1.113 shows most of the cells to be basal cells, arguing against prostate cancer.

Cowper Glands

Benign Cowper glands (bulbourethral glands) are a rare finding in prostatic samples, as these are located beyond the apex of the prostate around the internal base of the penis; however, they can occasionally be captured in biopsies, especially those from the prostatic apex.[16,46,47,88] The small, crowded, foamy gland appearance (Figure 1.115) may lead to confusion with prostatic adenocarcinoma, such as foamy gland variant cancer. However, clues to the nonneoplastic nature of these structures include a lobular or circumscribed configuration surrounding a central duct, with a background of skeletal muscle. Occasional associated benign-appearing glands often transition into the mucinous glands (Figure 1.116). If in doubt, immunohistochemistry can aid in the recognition of Cowper glands, as they typically have positive staining for high-molecular-weight cytokeratin in ductal cells and in a basal-like distribution in some of the lobules. Likewise, p63 often shows at least a patchy positive cell layer (Figure 1.117).

PROSTATIC ACINAR ADENOCARCINOMA

Prostatic acinar adenocarcinoma is, of course, the main concern within the spectrum of "small gland" lesions that has led to the recognition of the numerous benign mimics

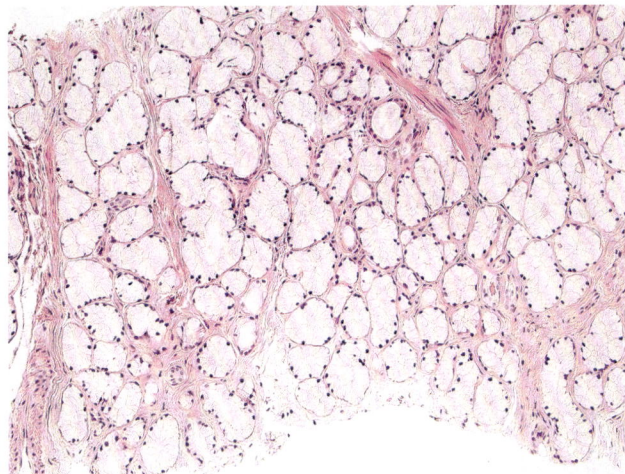

Figure 1.115. Cowper or bulbourethral glands can appear as crowded small round glands with mucinous features in a needle biopsy, especially from the apex of the prostate.

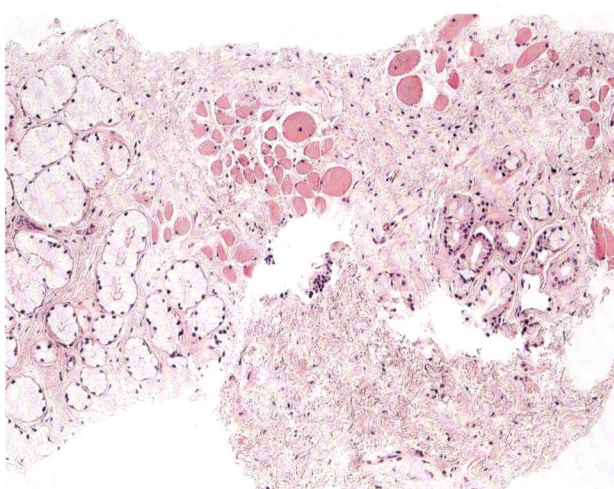

Figure 1.116. Clues to the recognition of Cowper glands in prostate biopsies include the intimate association with skeletal muscle and associated benign ducts (right).

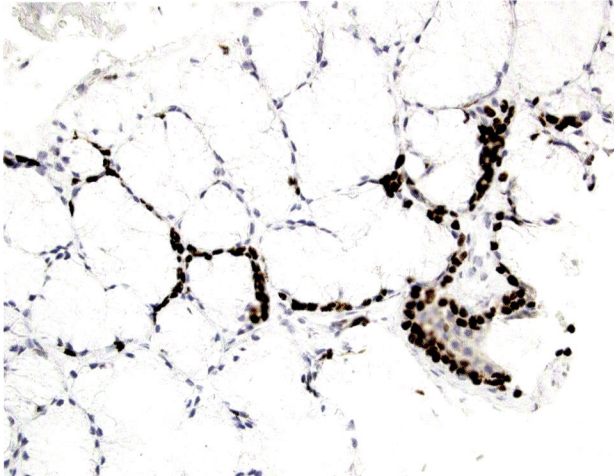

Figure 1.117. This example of Cowper glands on prostate needle biopsy shows no significant alpha-methylacyl-CoA racemase (AMACR) staining and a patchy p63-positive cell layer on a single-color dual stain for both markers.

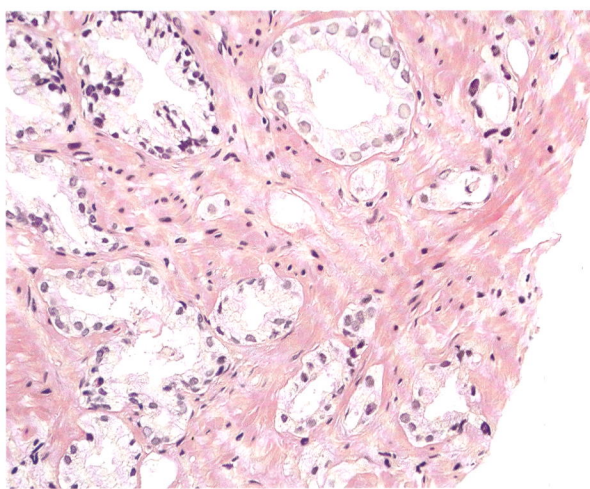

Figure 1.118. One of the strongest features for histologic diagnosis of prostatic adenocarcinoma is the presence of prominent nucleoli, as shown in this case with relatively pale round glands, some containing prominent nucleoli.

discussed here. The classic prostatic adenocarcinoma is composed of crowded, small, ring-shaped glandular structures with a monolayered appearance. Nuclei are enlarged and sometimes hyperchromatic, often with at least focally prominent nucleoli (Figure 1.118). Cytoplasm is also dark or amphophilic compared with reference benign epithelium (Figures 1.119 and 1.120).[89] However, prostate cancer differs from many other cancers in that the tumor cells are classically monotonous (not pleomorphic), the glandular shapes are round/regular, and the tumor does not usually elicit a stromal/desmoplastic response.

Diagnostic Criteria for Minimal Prostate Cancer

Although large foci of prostatic adenocarcinoma are usually readily recognizable due to their crowded small gland pattern, cytologic atypia, and infiltrative growth pattern, a common challenge in surgical pathology practice is to determine whether a limited focus of atypical glands in a biopsy sample is sufficient to render the diagnosis of malignancy, overwhelmingly in regard to Gleason score 3 + 3 = 6 (Grade Group 1) cancer.[89,90] A commonly used system for evaluating such atypical foci is to tally the histologic features in favor of and against cancer to arrive at an overall assessment (listed in Table 1.3 and illustrated in Figures 1.121-1.144).[89] With numerous features in favor of a diagnosis of cancer and few

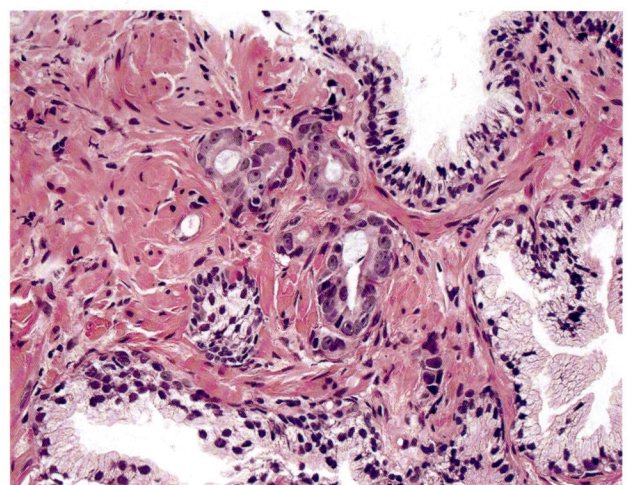

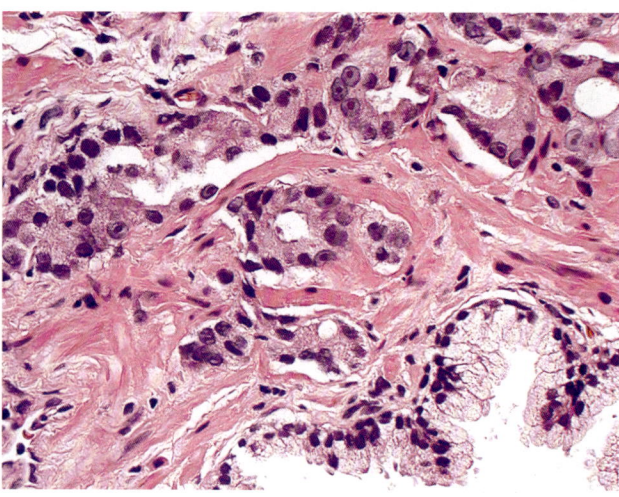

Figure 1.119. This small focus of prostatic adenocarcinoma is dark or amphophilic compared with the adjacent benign glands.

Figure 1.120. High magnification of this prostatic adenocarcinoma shows prominent nucleoli, overall dark or amphophilic color, and a contrasting color to the adjacent benign glands (bottom).

TABLE 1.3: Features in Favor of and Against Prostatic Adenocarcinoma in Biopsy Samples

	Favors Cancer	Favors Benign	Mimics, Exceptions, Notes
Small round glands	X		**Mimics:** Partial atrophy, atypical adenomatous hyperplasia (adenosis), nephrogenic adenoma (usually near urethra), mesonephric remnant (rare, PAX8+, prostate markers negative)
Tufted glandular epithelium		X	**Exceptions:** PIN-like cancer, pseudohyperplastic cancer
Prominent nucleoli	X		**Mimics:** Prominent basal cells, basal cell hyperplasia, PIN, partial atrophy (sometimes)
Crowded glands (Figure 1.121)	X		**Mimics:** Nodular hyperplasia, atypical adenomatous hyperplasia (adenosis), peripheral zone adenosis, verumontanum mucosal gland hyperplasia, seminal vesicle, or ejaculatory duct tissue
Mitotic figures (Figures 1.122 and 1.123)	X	Less common	**Note:** More often in cancer but can be found in PIN, benign glands
Dark or amphophilic cytoplasm (Figure 1.124)	X		**Note:** Particularly helpful if contrast to nearby benign glands
Nuclear hyperchromasia and enlargement	X		**Mimics:** PIN, radiation atypia of benign basal cells
Infiltrative growth pattern (Figures 1.125 and 1.126)	X		
Stromal hyalinization (Figure 1.127)		X	**Notes:** Prostate cancer usually lacks stromal response or desmoplasia of other organ cancers; stromal hyalinization often present around atrophic glands; recent evidence suggests true desmoplasia (stromogenic cancer) is a more aggressive feature
Blue mucin (Figures 1.128-1.130)	X		**Mimics:** Basal cell hyperplasia, colorectal epithelium (depends on staining technique)
Luminal crystalloids (Figures 1.131 and 1.132)	X	Less common	**Note:** Common in cancer but can also be found in benign glands and PIN

TABLE 1.3: Features in Favor of and Against Prostatic Adenocarcinoma in Biopsy Samples   (Continued)

	Favors Cancer	Favors Benign	Mimics, Exceptions, Notes
Corpora amylacea/concretions/calcifications (Figures 1.133 and 1.134)		X	**Note:** Rare in cancer, but not impossible
Sharp luminal border	X		**Mimic:** Partial atrophy
Absence of basal cells	X		**Mimics:** Basal cell layer often attenuated in PIN, partial atrophy, atypical adenomatous hyperplasia (adenosis) **Notes:** Some glands in these mimics may entirely lack basal cells, but few basal cells usually present in others
Presence of basal cells (Figures 1.135 and 1.136)		X	**Notes:** Smaller, compressed-appearing nuclei sometimes present in cancer glands but do not stain for basal cell markers. Rare prostate cancers have aberrant p63 staining in the cancer cells (nonbasal location) **Exception:** Intraductal cancer appears high grade (usually cribriform) but intact basal cell layer
Glomeruloid structures (glomerulations) (Figure 1.137)	X		**Notes:** Pathognomonic of cancer (never found in benign prostate) **Mimic:** Telescoping of benign epithelium into lumen (not cribriform) (Figure 1.138)
Perineural invasion (Figure 1.139)	X		**Notes:** Specific for cancer if true wrapping around nerve, but rarely benign glands may abut nerve (Figure 1.140)
Collagenous micronodules (mucinous fibroplasia) (Figures 1.141 and 1.142)	X		**Notes:** Pathognomonic of cancer
AMACR positive	X	Less common	**Notes:** Characteristic of cancer but also found in PIN, sometimes atypical adenomatous hyperplasia (adenosis), partial atrophy
AMACR negative or weak (Figure 1.143)	Subset	X	**Exceptions:** Strong AMACR characteristic of cancer but a considerable minority of cancers are negative or weak (up to 20%)
ERG positive (Figure 1.144)	X		**Notes:** Probably highly specific for cancer, rare cases of PIN
ERG negative	X	X	**Notes:** Only 40-50% of cancers have ERG rearrangements

AMACR, alpha-methylacyl-CoA racemase; PIN, prostatic intraepithelial neoplasia.

or none against, diagnosis of prostatic adenocarcinoma can usually be made. With a mixture of features in favor of and against cancer, diagnostic options typically include benign mimics of cancer, if the findings can be confidently classified with the use of immunohistochemistry. Alternatively, a report of atypical glands/atypical small acinar proliferation may be necessary when a satisfactory explanation for the atypical glands cannot be reached with confidence. Similarly, if there are multiple features against a diagnosis of cancer, but a smaller number of suspicious features, diagnostic options would again include benign mimics or an atypical diagnosis.

CHECKLIST: Diagnosis of small foci of prostatic adenocarcinoma[a]

☐ Multiple concerning cytologic or architectural features (see Table 1.3)

☐ Complete absence of basal cells using immunohistochemistry in all morphologically atypical glands

☐ No established benign mimic that could account for all features

☐ Typically, not less than three atypical glands (but number varies based on other findings)

☐ If practice setting allows, second pathologist agreement

[a]If criteria are not met, a diagnosis of atypical glands (atypical small acinar proliferation) is usually reasonable.

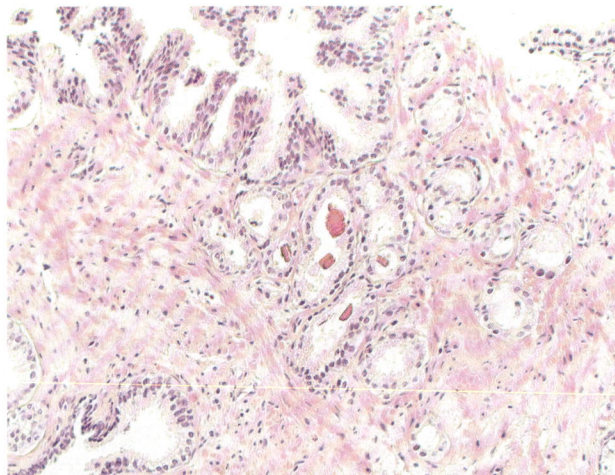

Figure 1.121. Glandular crowding is a clue to diagnosis of prostatic adenocarcinoma, such as in this case with relatively pale cytoplasm. Crystalloids are also present in the lumens.

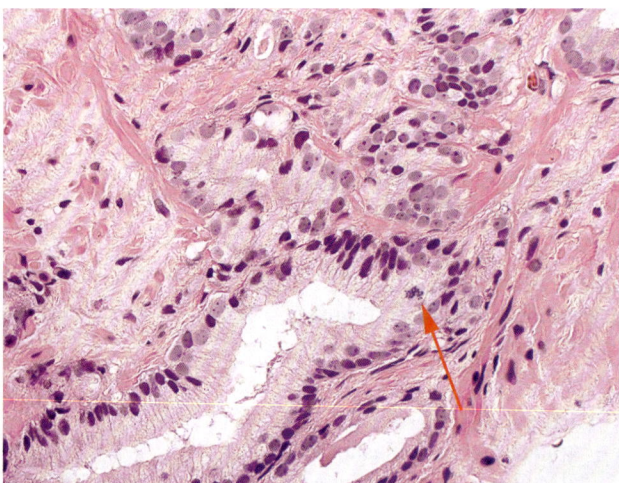

Figure 1.122. Mitotic figures are more common in prostate cancer (arrow), but their presence is not specific for cancer.

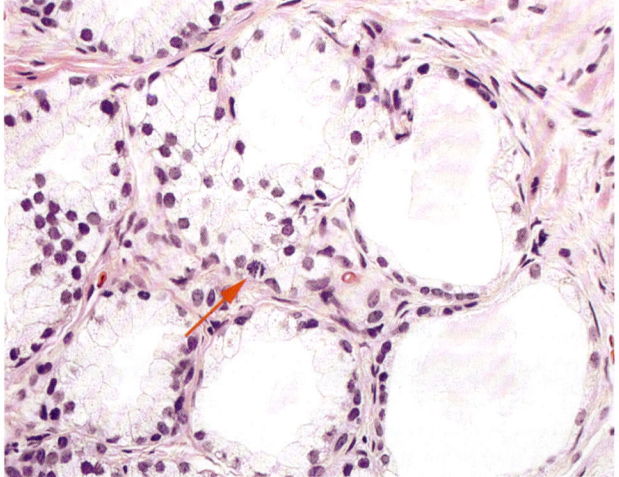

Figure 1.123. Mitotic figures can also be observed in benign glands (arrow).

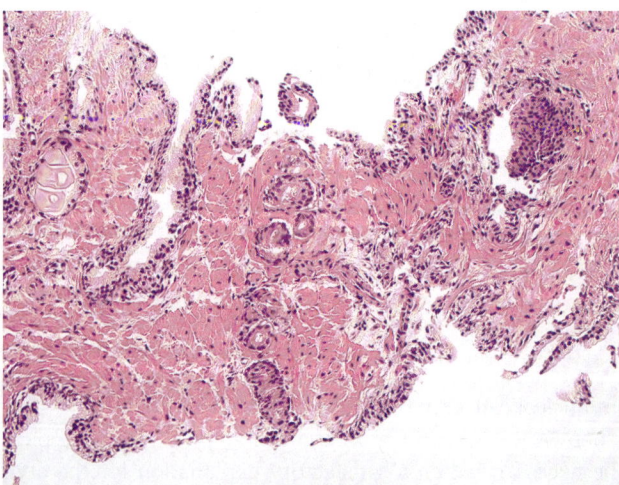

Figure 1.124. Infiltrative architecture is a helpful clue to diagnosis of prostatic adenocarcinoma in needle biopsy samples. This case demonstrates a linear configuration of glands across the biopsy core, which can be considered a form of infiltrative pattern. The cancer glands are also darker than adjacent benign glands in this case.

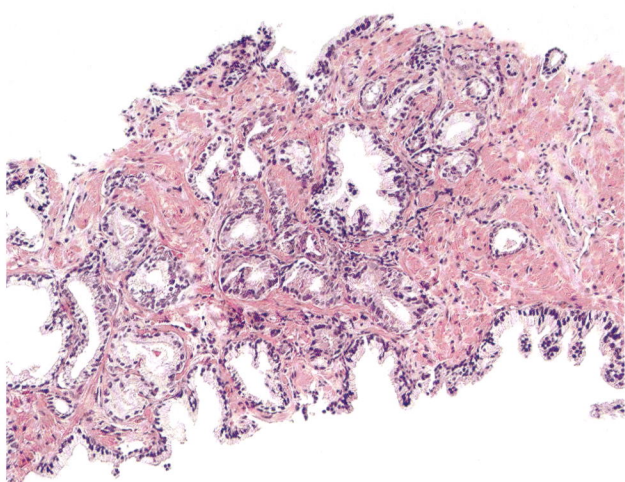

Figure 1.125. In this case of prostatic adenocarcinoma in a needle biopsy, infiltration is well visualized by multiple atypical glands on both sides of benign glands.

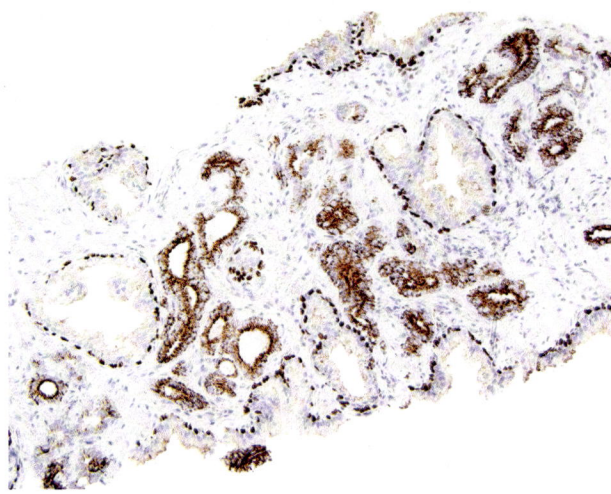

Figure 1.126. Immunohistochemistry for alpha-methylacyl-CoA racemase (AMACR) and p63 (single color) in the same case from Figure 1.125 highlights the cancer glands infiltrating around benign glands.

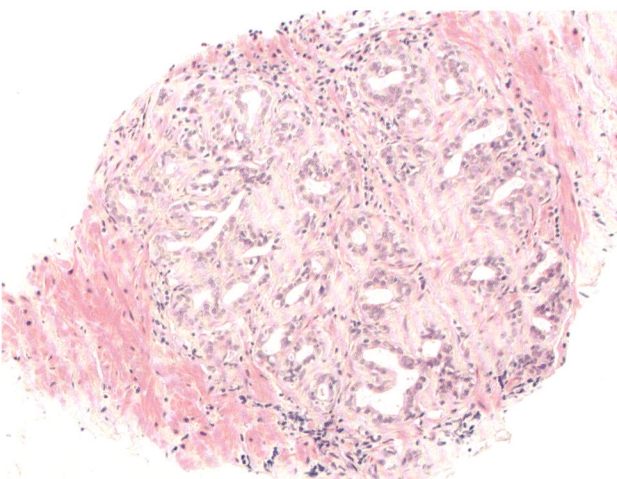

Figure 1.127. Sclerotic stroma is more common with benign processes, such as atrophy, shown here, although rare cancers can have reactive stroma.

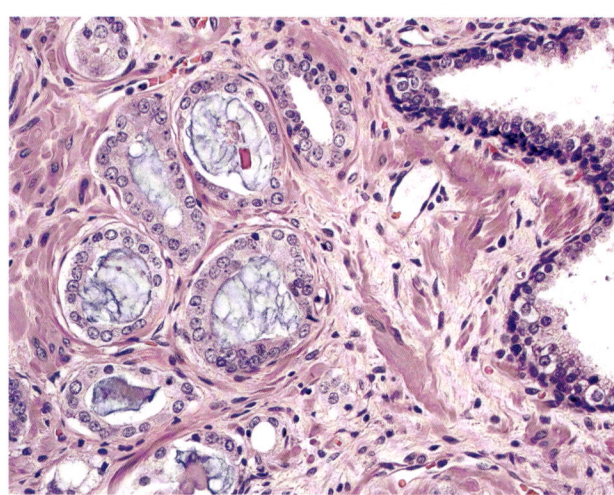

Figure 1.128. Blue mucin is a helpful diagnostic clue for prostatic adenocarcinoma, which may vary in prominence depending on laboratory staining procedures. This case shows extremely prominent blue mucin in the cancer glands (left), compared with a benign gland (right).

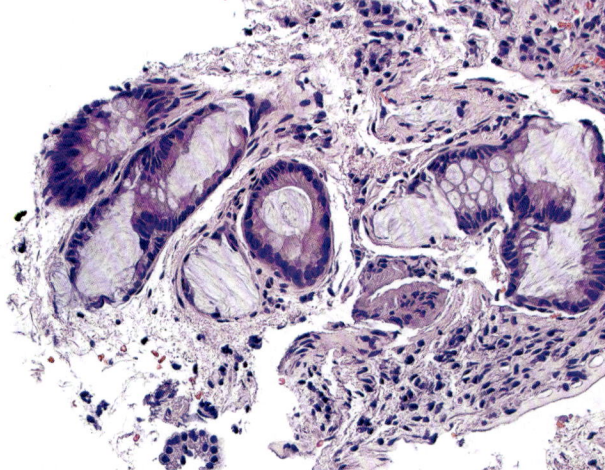

Figure 1.129. Other mimics can have prominent blue mucin, including colorectal tissue sampled in prostatic needle biopsy, as shown here.

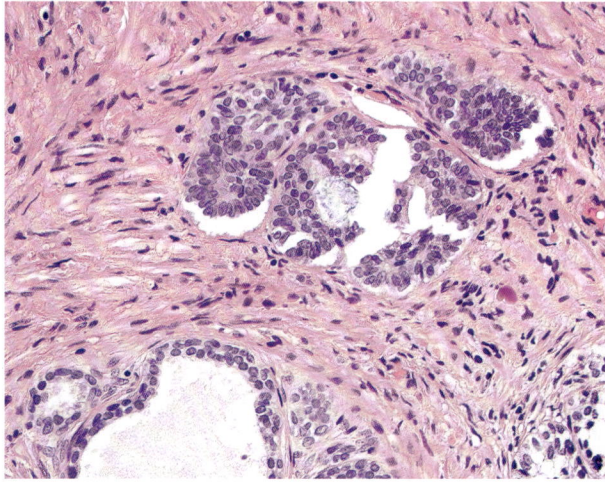

Figure 1.130. Basal cell hyperplasia can also contain luminal blue mucin, so this is not specific for cancer.

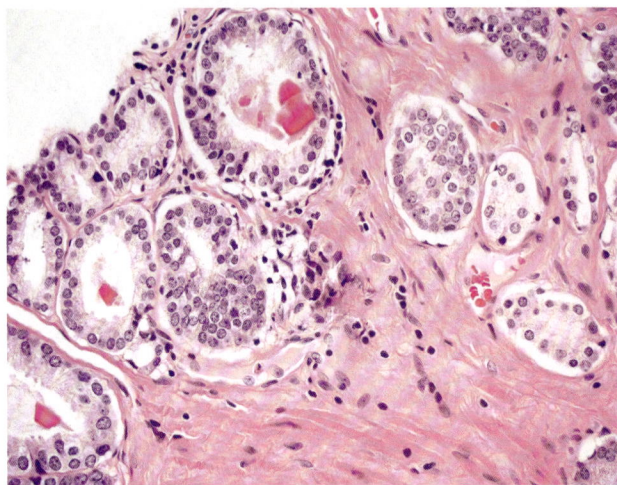

Figure 1.131. Crystalloids are brightly eosinophilic structures in glandular lumens with varied geometric shapes. These are more commonly found in cancer glands, but they are not specific for malignancy.

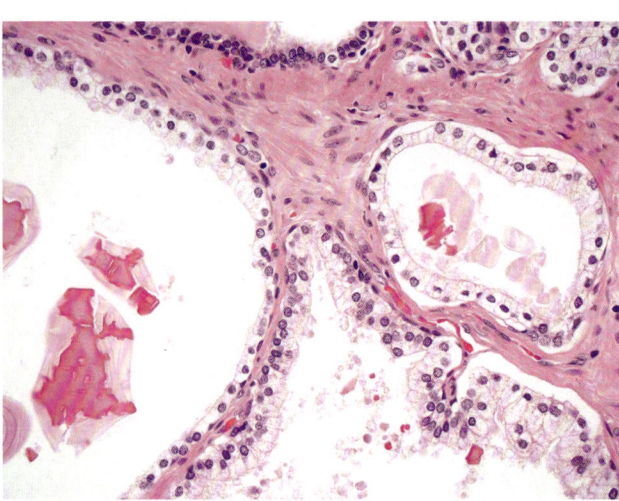

Figure 1.132. This case shows crystalloids within benign glands, highlighting the lack of specificity of this finding for prostatic adenocarcinoma.

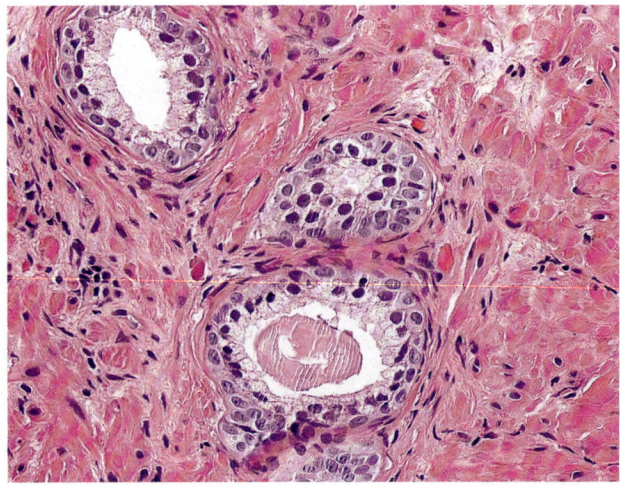

Figure 1.133. Corpora amylacea are more commonly found in benign glands, as shown here, and rarely in cancer.

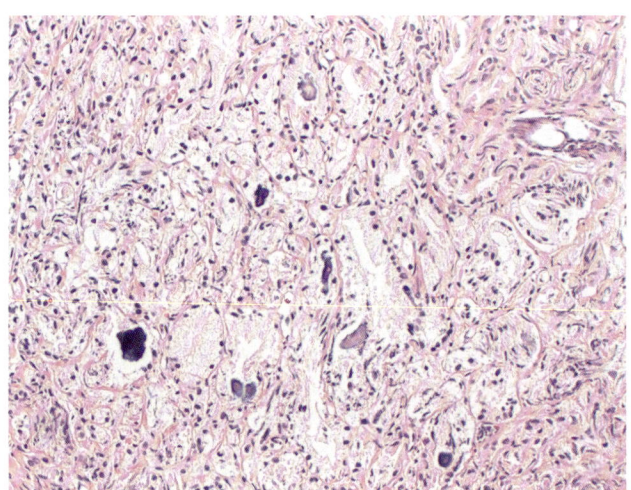

Figure 1.134. Very rare prostate cancers contain corpora or calcifications, as shown here.

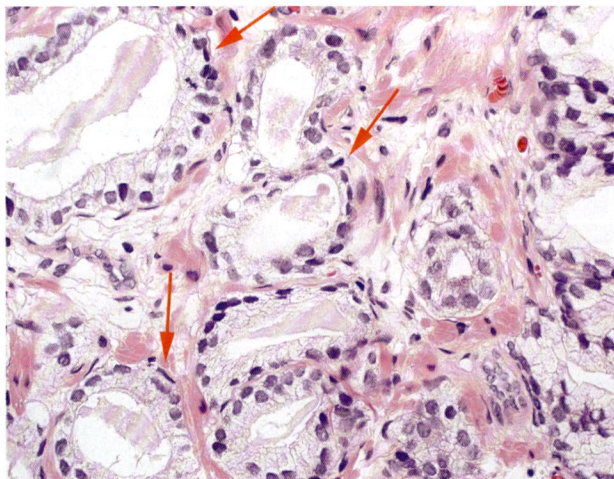

Figure 1.135. Although the presence of basal cells argues against a diagnosis of malignancy, prostate cancers can have compressed nuclei at the edges of the glands (arrows), mimicking basal cells.

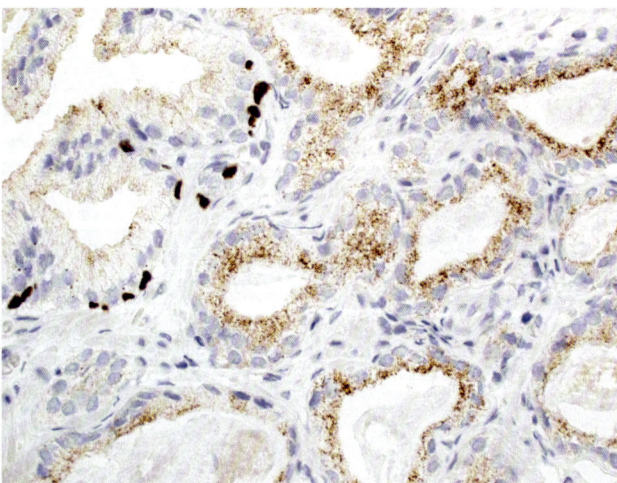

Figure 1.136. The same case from Figure 1.135 shows no basal cells using p63 and alpha-methylacyl-CoA racemase (AMACR) single-color immunohistochemistry.

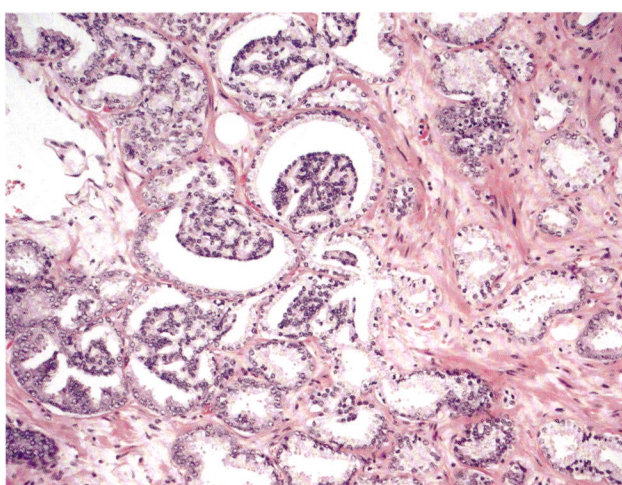

Figure 1.137. Glomeruloid structures or glomerulations are formations that mimic the architecture of a glomerulus, with a central cribriform tuft, often attached at only one site to a peripheral round gland. These are considered highly specific for prostate cancer, and this component is graded as pattern 4.

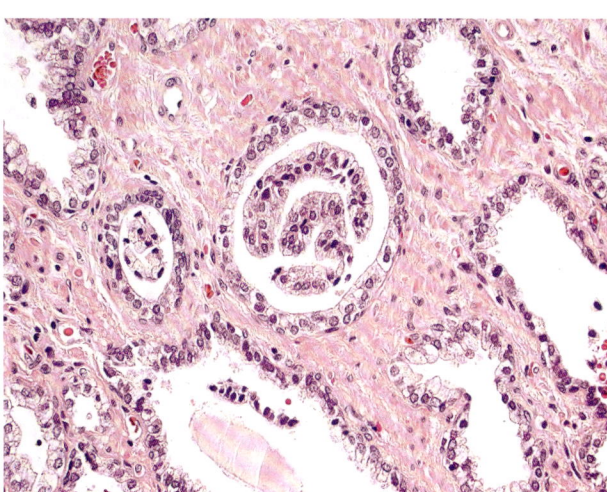

Figure 1.138. Telescoping of epithelium into the glandular lumen is essentially the only scenario where a benign gland could mimic glomerulation.

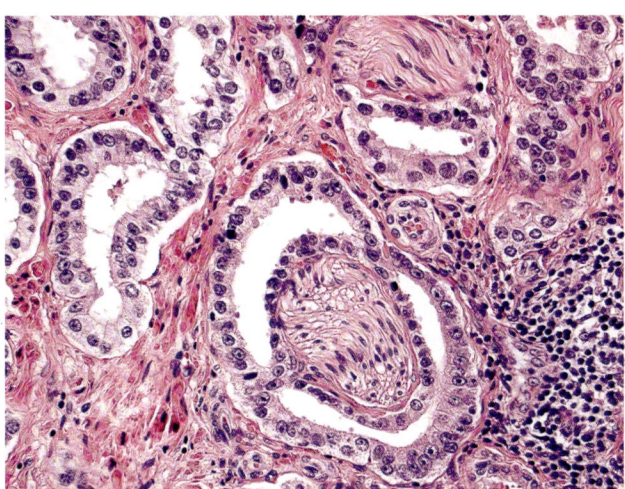

Figure 1.139. Perineural invasion is highly specific for prostatic adenocarcinoma in the appropriate context, when atypical glands circumferentially wrap around a nerve in the perineural space.

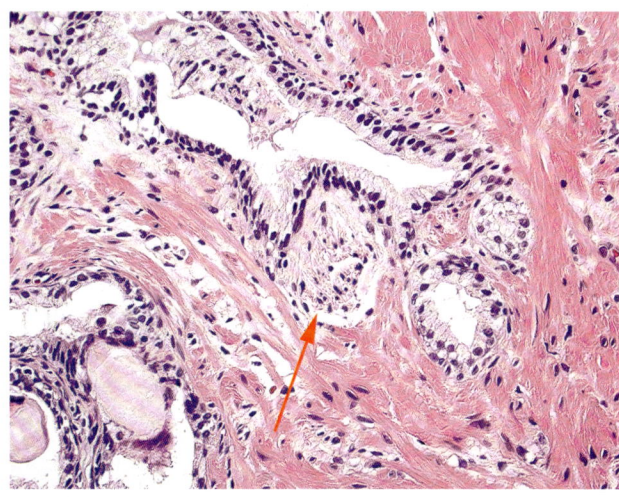

Figure 1.140. Benign glands can abut nerves (arrow), so the juxtaposition of a gland and a nerve is not sufficient for diagnosis of malignancy.

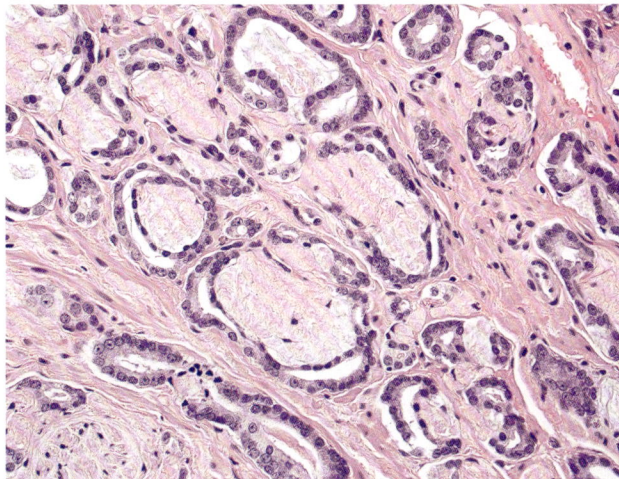

Figure 1.141. Collagenous micronodules or mucinous fibroplasia are considered diagnostic of prostate cancer. These structures are pale eosinophilic deposits of collagen thought to occur from mucin rupturing out of the glands.

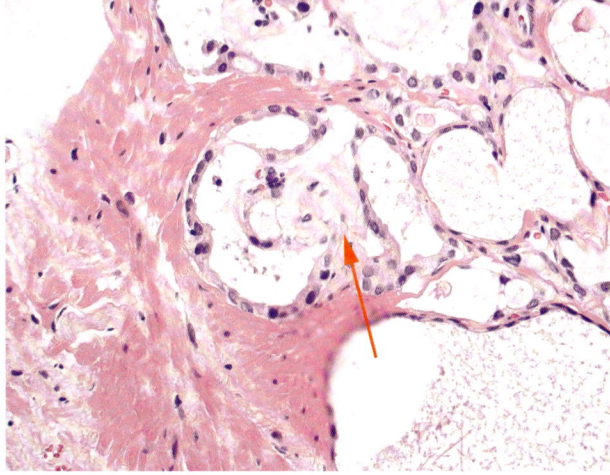

Figure 1.142. This example shows early formation of collagenous micronodules/mucinous fibroplasia (arrow) in a background of mucin rupturing from a gland.

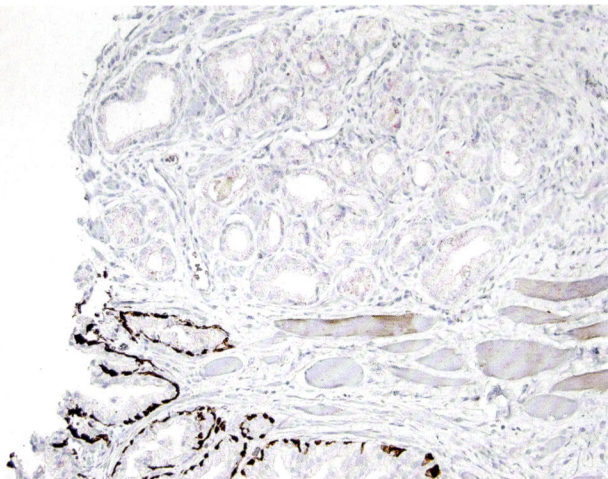

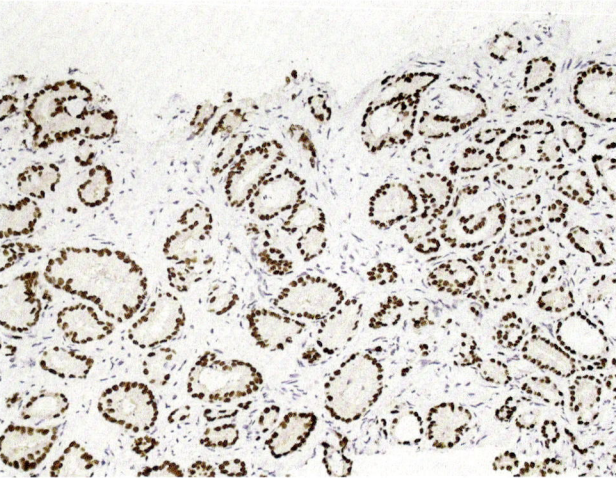

Figure 1.143. Although alpha-methylacyl-CoA racemase (AMACR) positivity is helpful for diagnosis of prostatic adenocarcinoma, this example shows absence of basal cells with minimal to no AMACR staining in a dual-color AMACR (red), high-molecular-weight cytokeratin, and p63 (both brown) preparation.

Figure 1.144. Positive nuclear staining for ERG is supportive of a diagnosis of prostatic adenocarcinoma; however, this is found in only 40%-50% of prostate cancers.

FAQ: Which Features are Highly Specific for Prostate Cancer?

Prominent nucleoli are generally considered one of the best features for diagnosis of prostatic adenocarcinoma; however, this is not entirely specific, being found in several benign mimics. Only a few features are considered highly specific for prostatic adenocarcinoma:

1. Mucinous fibroplasia or collagenous micronodules (Figures 1.141 and 1.142) are cancer glands associated with pale nodules of extracellular collagenous material.[91] It is hypothesized that this collagen deposition results from mucin spillage and organization into the nodules.[92]

    a. This also has relevance for grading, as it can markedly distort the shape of the glands, which is discussed in the next section on grading.

2. Glomeruloid structures or glomerulations[92] manifest as round glandular structures that contain a luminal cribriform nodule, often attached at one side, imparting resemblance to a glomerulus (Figure 1.137). When fully developed, this is considered diagnostic of cancer; however, a potential mimic is sloughing or "telescoping" of the glandular epithelium into the lumen (Figure 1.138). When the luminal proliferation is not truly cribriform, it is not considered specific for cancer.

3. Perineural invasion is considered specific for diagnosis of prostate cancer in a biopsy sample. If used for diagnostic purposes, the perineural invasion should ideally circumferentially wrap the nerve within the perineural space (Figure 1.139), as it is possible for benign glands to abut nerves (Figures 1.140).[89,90,92]

FAQ: What is the Meaning of Atypical Glands or Atypical Small Acinar Proliferation?

Atypical glands and atypical small acinar proliferation are synonymous terms that refer to a focus of prostatic glands that is suspicious for adenocarcinoma but insufficient to make the diagnosis with certainty. This is often either due to a small number of glands or incompletely developed features of carcinoma. There is no specific number of glands that is sufficient to make a diagnosis of malignancy; however, it is rare for less than three glands to meet criteria for malignancy, especially as the only focus for a given patient.

Apart from the features that are highly specific for prostate cancer (see FAQ), numerous other features are associated with cancer but not totally specific for the diagnosis. Prominent nucleoli are generally considered the strongest feature (Figures 1.118 and 1.120)[93]; however, nucleoli alone are not entirely specific, as they can be present in benign mimics.[89] Prominent nucleoli are also not perfectly sensitive. Although they are almost invariably found in large areas of cancer, they can be absent, particularly in small areas of cancer in biopsy samples, or with small foci of foamy gland variant cancer (Figure 1.145).[94,95] Other helpful features include an infiltrative growth pattern, manifesting as atypical glands on both sides of benign glands, or linear growth across the entire width of the needle core (Figures 1.124 and 1.125). Small, round, crowded glands make up the prototypical prostate cancer; however, infrequent cancers can have a tufted, undulating configuration, resembling PIN (Figures 1.146 and 1.147). Hyalinization around glands typically favors a benign or atrophic process (Figure 1.127), whereas only a subset of prostate cancers generate a stromal response or desmoplasia like cancers of other organs.

Grading

The grading system for prostate cancer has undergone several revisions since the initial scheme reported by Gleason.[96-98] The current scheme endorsed by ISUP and the World Health Organization (WHO) now utilizes five Grade Groups that add a new face to the previous

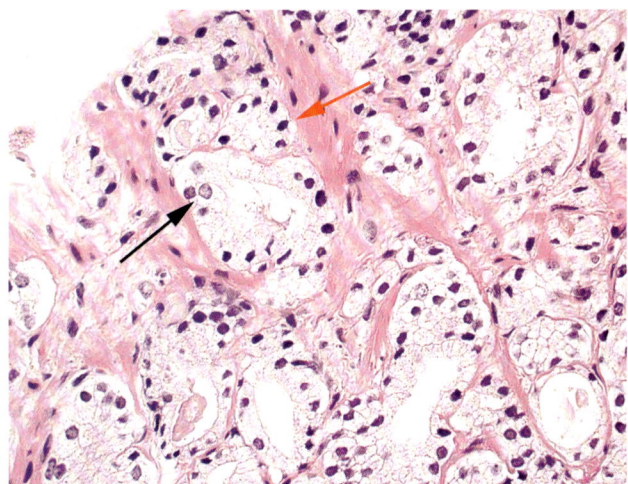

Figure 1.145. In some cases, especially foamy gland variant of prostatic adenocarcinoma, the cancer nuclei may be small and condensed (red arrow); however, other areas often have larger nuclei, more closely resembling those of conventional cancer (black arrow).

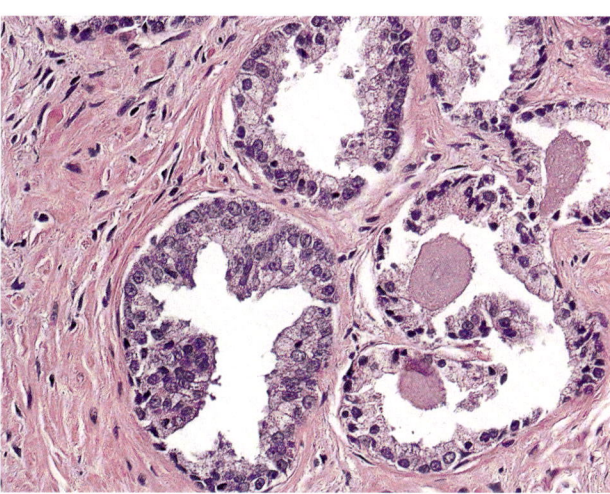

Figure 1.146. Some prostate cancers have a tufted glandular configuration, resembling prostatic intraepithelial neoplasia (PIN) or benign glands.

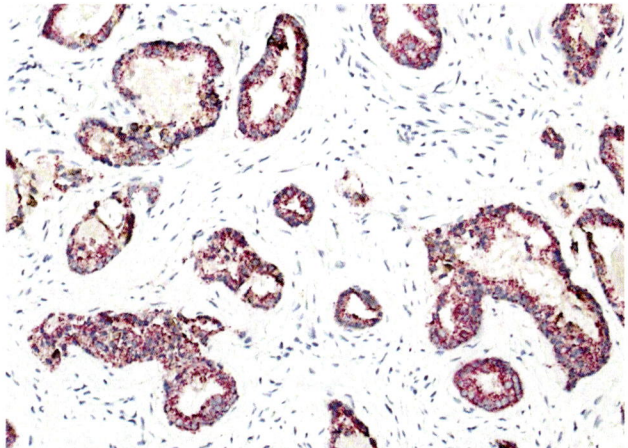

Figure 1.147. The same case from Figure 1.146 shows absence of basal cells (brown) and alpha-methylacyl-CoA racemase (AMACR) positivity (red) in a dual-color immunohistochemistry preparation.

TABLE 1.4: The Prostate Cancer Grade Group System, Endorsed by ISUP and WHO

Grade Group 1	Gleason score 3 + 3 = 6 or less
Grade Group 2	Gleason score 3 + 4 = 7
Grade Group 3	Gleason score 4 + 3 = 7
Grade Group 4	Gleason score 4 + 4 = 8 Gleason score 3 + 5 = 8 Gleason score 5 + 3 = 8 (rare)
Grade Group 5	Gleason score 4 + 5 = 9 Gleason score 5 + 4 = 9 Gleason score 5 + 5 = 10

ISUP, International Society of Urological Pathology; WHO, World Health Organization.

Gleason scores (Table 1.4).[99] This has some advantages over the historical use of Gleason score only. Firstly, it simplifies the understanding for patients, as a score of 3 + 3 = 6 has the potential to be misconstrued as a high grade (6 of 10), whereas Grade Group 1 clearly indicates the lowest grade. Secondly, it requires separation of Gleason score 3 + 4 = 7 (Grade Group 2) and Gleason score 4 + 3 = 7 (Grade Group 3), which have significantly different prognoses, yet which had been historically not discriminated as both score 7.[99]

The underlying histologic patterns responsible for each grade pattern have mostly remained similar with a few changes, foremost being that cribriform growth is now considered pattern 4 inherently (ie, there is no cribriform pattern 3).[96] Other changes include classification of glomeruloid structures as pattern 4 and a retirement of the term "hypernephroid," which is likely quite rare and lacks interobserver agreement. A summary of the various grade patterns is shown in Table 1.5 and Figures 1.148-1.163.

BASAL CELL CARCINOMA (SMALL GLAND PATTERN)

Although the overwhelming majority of small gland proliferations with prominent basal cells represent basal cell hyperplasia, rare basal cell carcinomas do occur and can be difficult to distinguish from basal cell hyperplasia. The most helpful findings that would favor basal cell carcinoma over basal cell hyperplasia for a small gland proliferation include perineural

TABLE 1.5: Histologic Patterns Making Up Each Grade Pattern

Histology	Grade Pattern	Exceptions
Separate, well-formed glands (Figures 1.148 and 1.149)	Pattern 3	
Poorly formed glands (Figures 1.150-1.153)	Pattern 4	
Fused glands (Figures 1.154 and 1.155)	Pattern 4	
Cribriform glands (Figures 1.156-1.158)	Pattern 4	
Ductal variant (Figure 1.159)	Pattern 4	PIN-like cancer considered a variant of ductal by some authors, which can be pattern 3
Single cells (Figures 1.160 and 1.161)	Pattern 5	
Solid (Figure 1.162)	Pattern 5	
Comedonecrosis (Figure 1.163)	Pattern 5	Currently debated whether intraductal carcinoma with comedonecrosis must be verified with immunohistochemistry and excluded from the grade. A majority of foci of comedonecrosis are within intraductal carcinoma

PIN, prostatic intraepithelial neoplasia.

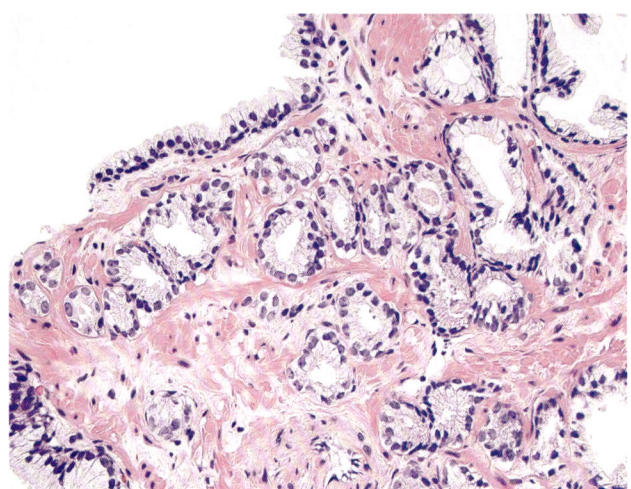

Figure 1.148. Pattern 3 adenocarcinoma is composed of discrete, well-formed glands in a ring-shaped configuration, as shown in this biopsy sample.

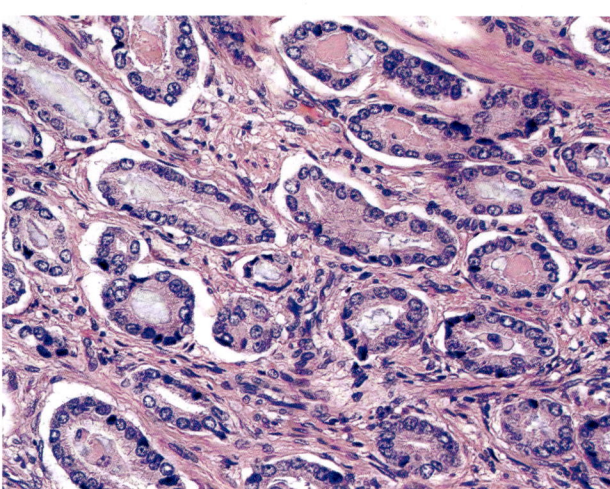

Figure 1.149. This example of pattern 3 prostatic adenocarcinoma shows crowded small round glands with nucleoli and luminal blue mucin.

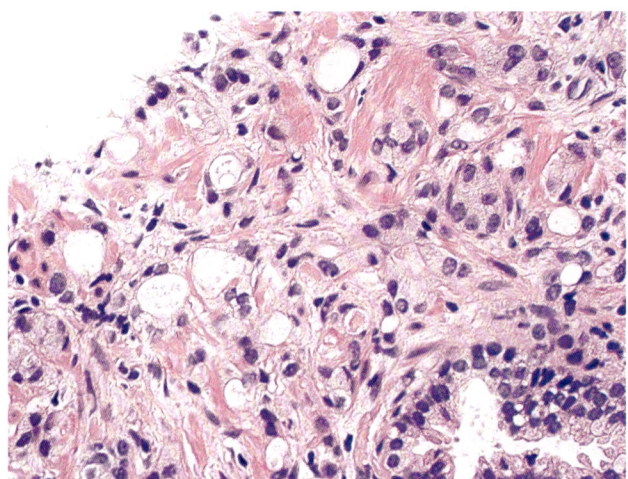

Figure 1.150. Poorly formed glands, composed of clusters of cells with variable glandular lumens, are classified as pattern 4. This morphology should make up multiple glands in the same area before being interpreted as pattern 4, to avoid overinterpretation of the edge of pattern 3 glands.

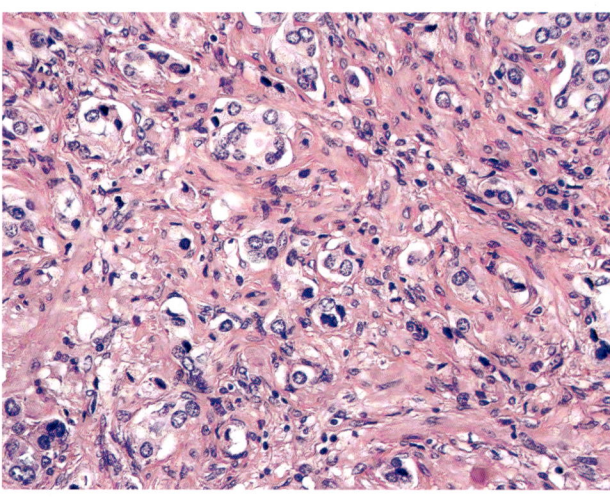

Figure 1.151. In this example of pattern 4 poorly formed glands, there are many clusters of only a few cells with variable lumen formation, although debatable whether there are enough single cells to regard as pattern 5.

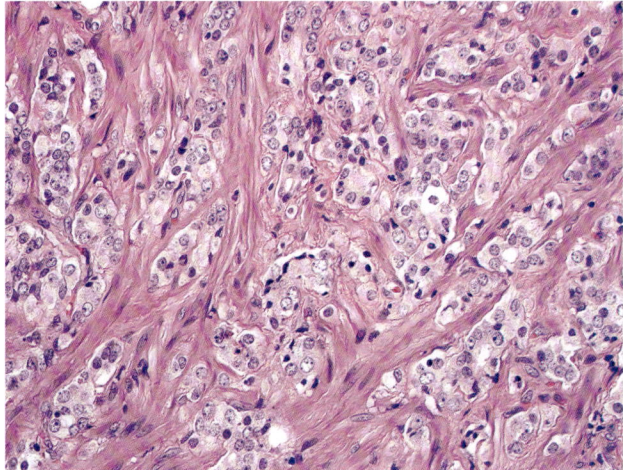

Figure 1.152. In this example of pattern 4 poorly formed glands, there are clusters of cells and cord-like structures, suggesting gland formation, with most lacking discrete lumens.

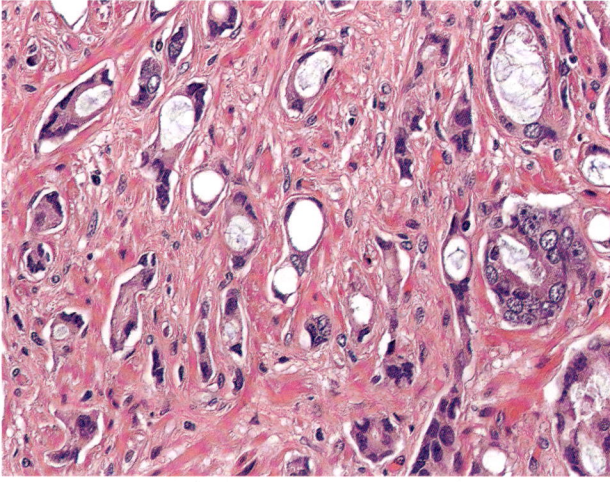

Figure 1.153. This field shows a mixture of patterns 3 and 4. There are poorly formed glands, some of which have only two to three nuclei and an eccentric glandular lumen.

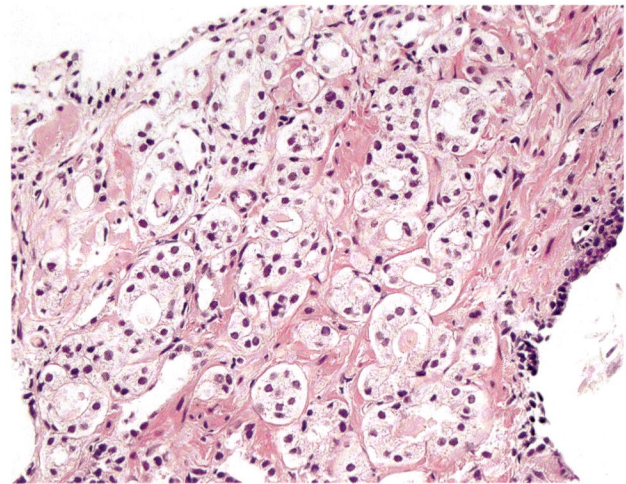

Figure 1.154. Glandular fusion, resulting from ring-shaped glands abutting one another without intervening stroma is graded as pattern 4. This field would likely be graded as Gleason score 3 + 4 = 7 (Grade Group 2).

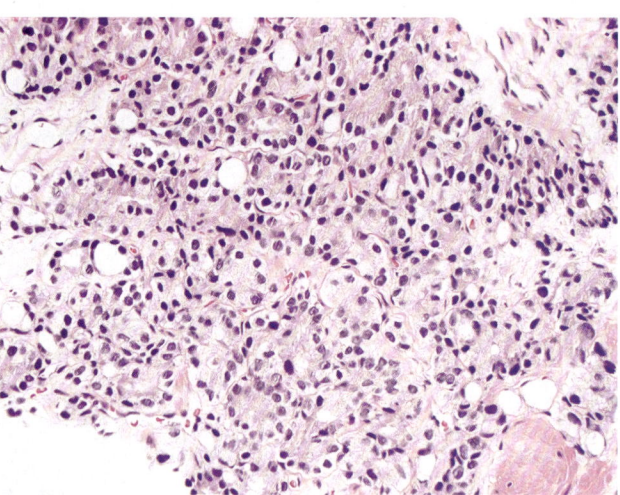

Figure 1.155. This field shows prominent glandular fusion in a crowded focus of small glands.

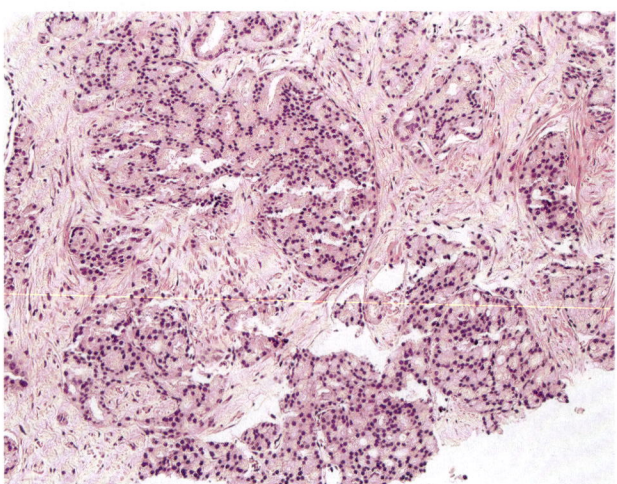

Figure 1.156. Cribriform growth of prostatic adenocarcinoma is composed of large areas of cancer cells with multiple "punched out" lumens, which is considered pattern 4.

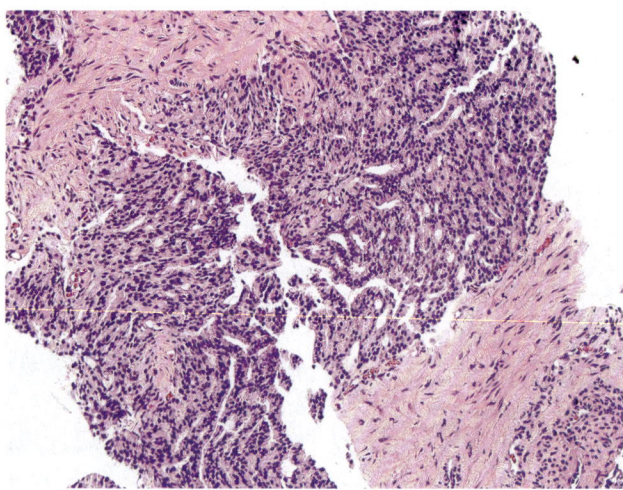

Figure 1.157. This biopsy core shows a large area of cribriform cancer (pattern 4) stretching across the entire width of the core. This often results in biopsy fragmentation.

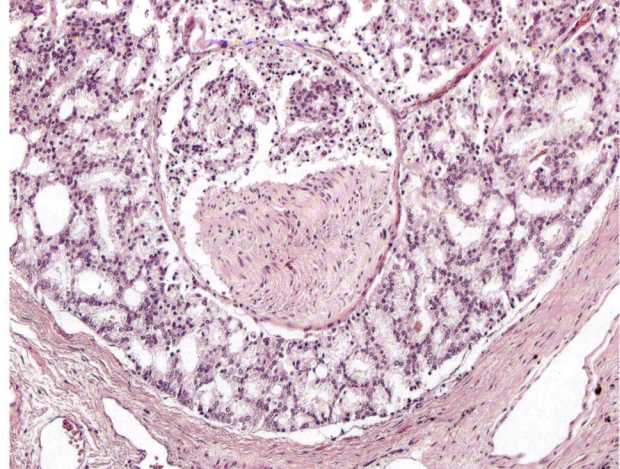

Figure 1.158. This cribriform invasive prostatic adenocarcinoma engulfs a nerve, supporting invasive pattern 4 carcinoma rather than intraductal carcinoma.

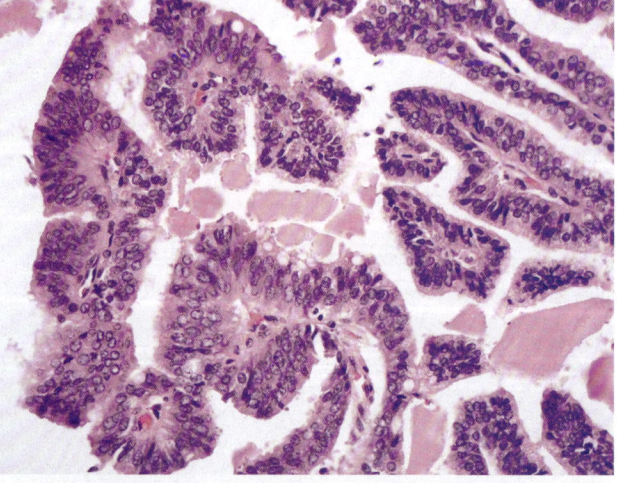

Figure 1.159. Ductal variant prostatic adenocarcinoma is composed of columnar cells with pseudostratified nuclei, resembling an adenomatous colon polyp, graded as pattern 4.

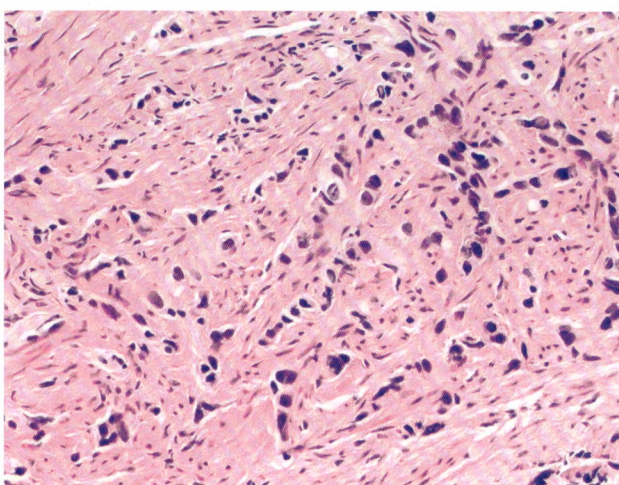

Figure 1.160. Single cells infiltrating in linear rows or cords are graded as pattern 5.

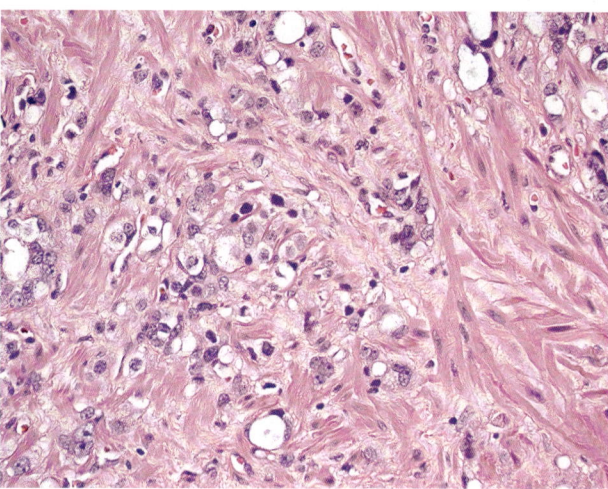

Figure 1.161. Clusters of single cells without gland formation are graded as pattern 5.

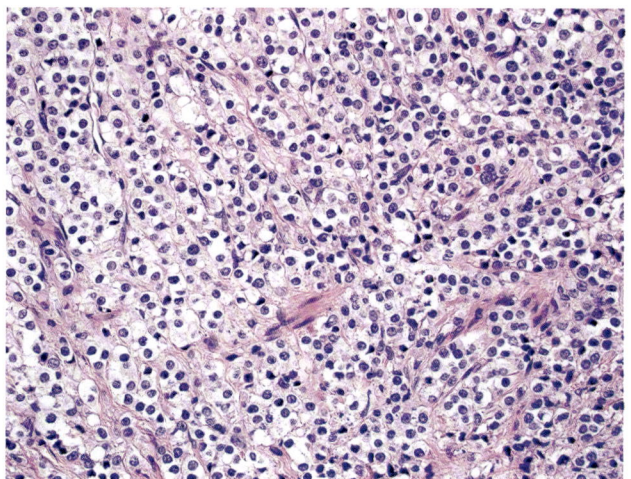

Figure 1.162. Solid growth without gland formation is also graded as pattern 5.

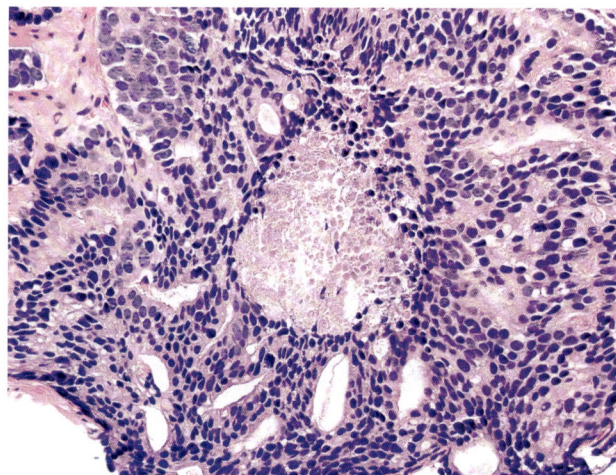

Figure 1.163. Prostatic adenocarcinoma with comedonecrosis is considered pattern 5. However, it has been recently recognized that these foci are often intraductal carcinoma. As current thinking is that intraductal carcinoma should not be graded, it is controversial how to approach these cases. We would avoid using immunohistochemistry for the sole purpose of excluding such foci from the grade and primarily grade based on the morphology , unless there is concern that all of the cancer is intraductal.

invasion, extraprostatic extension (Figures 1.164 and 1.165), and peripheral zone location or extension into the peripheral zone.[100] In the absence of these findings, extreme caution should be exercised before diagnosing basal cell carcinoma of the prostate, especially in a small sample.

POORLY FORMED GLAND LESIONS AND MIMICS

PARAGANGLION

Paraganglion tissue can be encountered in prostatic resection specimens and rarely needle biopsy samples.[21,26-29] Owing to formation of nests of cells without overt glandular lumens (Figures 1.166 and 1.167), paraganglia can be confused for prostate cancer with poorly formed gland pattern (Gleason pattern 4). Awareness of this occurrence and judicious use of immunohistochemistry (such as neuroendocrine markers and prostate-specific markers)

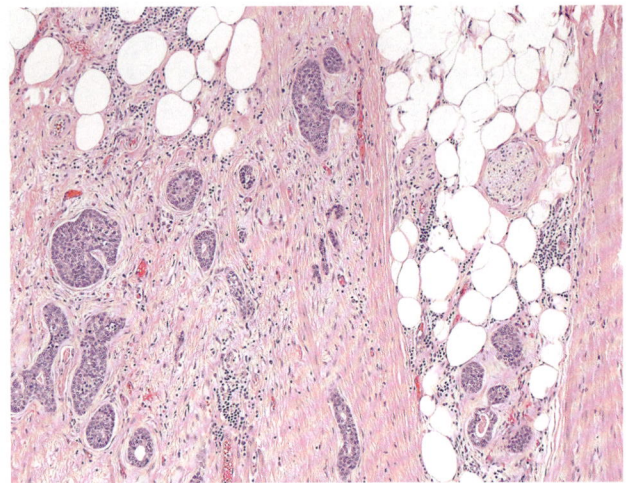

Figure 1.164. Basal cell carcinoma is a rare form of prostate cancer. This example is composed of small glands resembling those of basal cell hyperplasia; however, they extend outside of the prostate into adipose tissue, supporting malignancy.

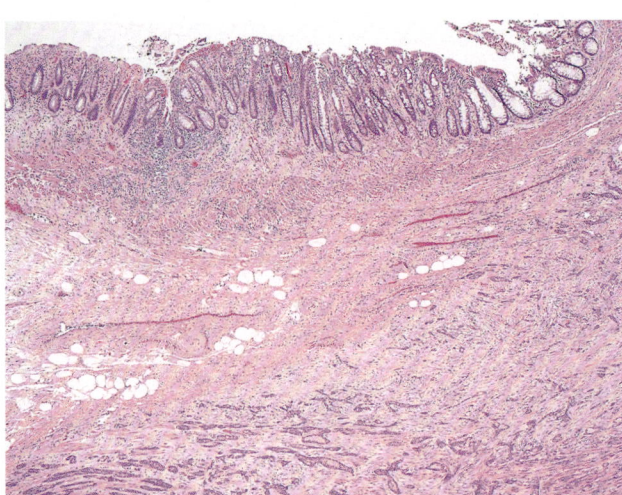

Figure 1.165. The same case of basal cell carcinoma from Figure 1.164 also showed invasion to the rectal wall.

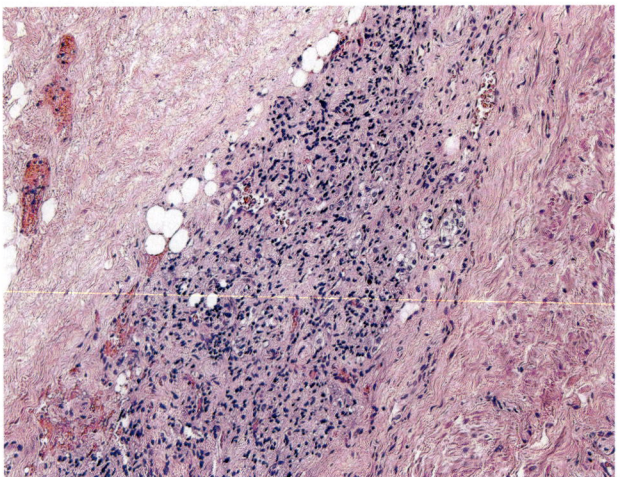

Figure 1.166. Paraganglion tissue can be deceptive in prostatic specimens, mimicking pattern 4 or 5 prostatic adenocarcinoma or extraprostatic extension. In difficult cases, immunohistochemistry for prostatic and neuroendocrine markers can be helpful to confirm paraganglion tissue.

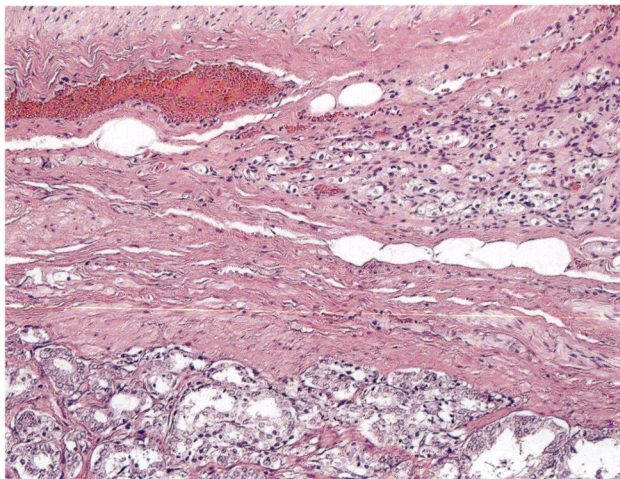

Figure 1.167. In this case, paraganglion tissue is present in the extraprostatic tissue (top) adjacent to prostatic adenocarcinoma (bottom), which may lead to confusion with extraprostatic extension.

in challenging cases can help avoid the pitfall of misdiagnosis as pattern 4 prostatic adenocarcinoma. In general, it is helpful to use both positive and negative markers for the suspected diagnosis, as, for example, weak nonspecific staining for a prostate marker may lead to confusion if used in isolation. Conversely, conventional prostate cancer can also have positivity for neuroendocrine markers, although usually in a patchy distribution.

XANTHOMA

Prostatic xanthoma (Figures 1.168-1.170) is a rare benign lesion that can be misdiagnosed as pattern 4 or 5 adenocarcinoma, as individual cells or solid nests of cells with foamy cytoplasm can be encountered in high-grade cancers.[101] Awareness of this entity, particularly when there is no conventional associated gland-forming carcinoma, can help to avoid this pitfall. Xanthoma cells are positive for histiocytic markers, such as CD68 (or likely CD163, although this has not been studied), and negative for cytokeratin immunohistochemistry. The xanthoma cells are usually negative for prostatic markers such as PSA or prostate-specific acid phosphatase (PSAP), but some positivity has been occasionally reported, possibly representing phagocytosis by the histiocytes or in some cases perhaps weak nonspecific staining.[101] Of course, xanthoma will show lack of staining with high-molecular-weight cytokeratin or p63 antibodies, which should not be taken as support for diagnosis of prostatic adenocarcinoma. Weak AMACR positivity has also been noted.[101]

POORLY FORMED GLAND PROSTATIC ADENOCARCINOMA

Poorly formed gland prostate cancer has gained increased interest recently with the updated grading systems.[97,102,103] Introduced as a category of pattern 4 cancer in the 2005 ISUP Consensus, poorly formed glands were referred to as a cluster of glands with poorly formed glandular lumens in sufficient number that a tangential section of pattern 3 could be argued against.[97] Usually this is straightforward for diagnosis as adenocarcinoma; however, mimics of poorly formed gland cancer could include sclerosing adenosis (discussed previously) and a tangential section of the edge of benign glandular epithelium. In the latter circumstance, this can often be distinguished from cancer by examining additional tissue levels, in which the ill-defined glands will be found to be part of a larger benign gland. Poorly formed gland cancer is typically made up of small clusters of cells that may form a lumen, but without the architecture of a conventional glandular structure. For example, this can consist of two to three eccentrically located nuclei with cytoplasm forming a glandular lumen (Figure 1.171).

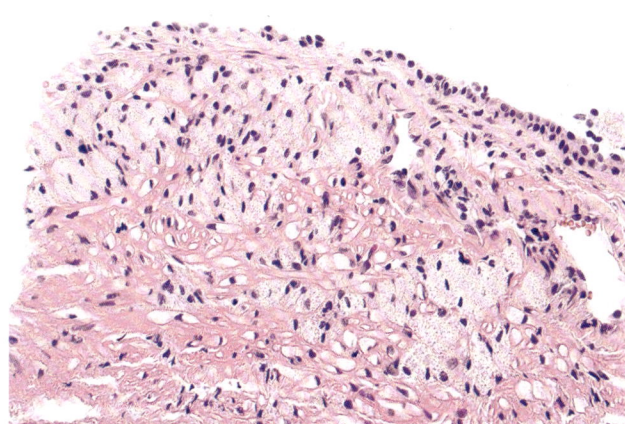

Figure 1.168. Prostatic xanthoma should be distinguished from high-grade prostatic adenocarcinoma.

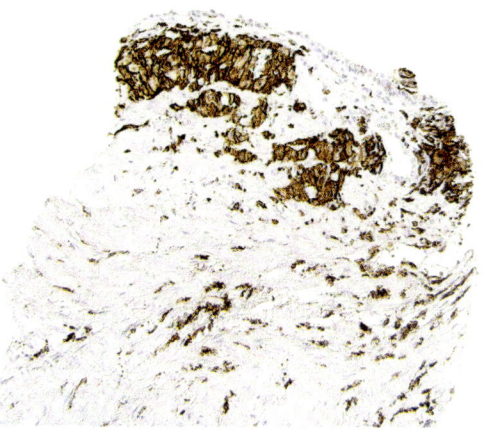

Figure 1.169. In the case from Figure 1.169, immunohistochemistry showed positivity for macrophage marker CD163, arguing against adenocarcinoma.

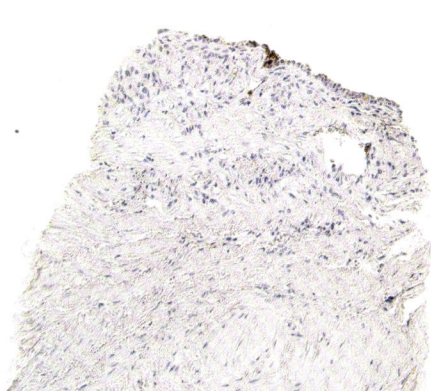

Figure 1.170. In the same case from Figures 1.168 and 1.169, prostate-specific antigen (PSA) staining is negative in the foamy cells, arguing against carcinoma.

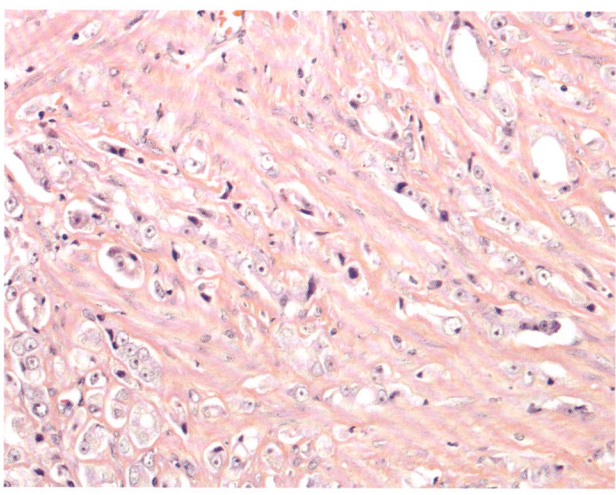

Figure 1.171. Poorly formed gland prostatic adenocarcinoma is composed of glands and clusters of cells. This case shows prominent nucleoli, making recognition as malignant straightforward.

Sometimes there may be only a suggestion of a lumen or none at all, yet there do not appear to be sufficient numbers of single cells or solid growth to warrant a diagnosis of pattern 5. One study recommended that this not be used as justification for pattern 4 if there are five or less such glandular structures, or if they are interspersed with well-formed glands, such that they could be tangential sectioning of the well-formed glands. It was recommended that more than 10 poorly formed glands could be diagnosed with greater certainty as pattern 4.[102]

CANCER WITH TREATMENT EFFECT

Prostatic adenocarcinoma with radiation or androgen deprivation therapy effect typically manifests as small clusters of cells or individual cells with a poorly formed gland pattern (Figures 1.172-1.176).[79,80] For grading purposes, the current recommendation is that such cancers not be graded, as they have had at least partly the desired response to treatment, yet poorly formed glands or single cells would be graded as patterns 4-5, which may falsely

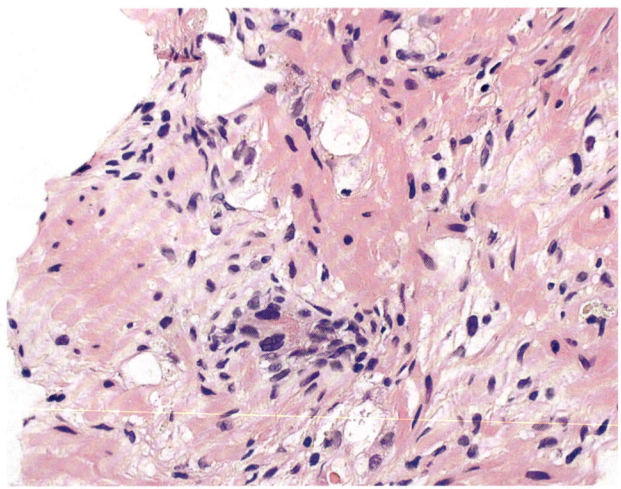

Figure 1.172. Prostatic adenocarcinoma with radiation effect is often markedly distorted, appearing as foamy vacuolated "holes" in the tissue with often relatively small condensed nuclei. A benign gland with atypia of the basal cells is present at bottom center.

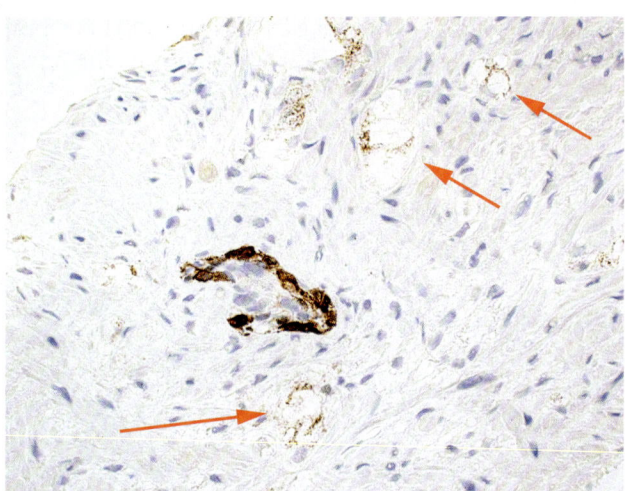

Figure 1.173. The same case from Figure 1.172 shows basal cells in the benign gland. The adenocarcinoma with treatment effect (arrows) shows no basal cells and weak staining for alpha-methy-lacyl-CoA racemase (AMACR) in this p63 and AMACR single-color immunohistochemical stain.

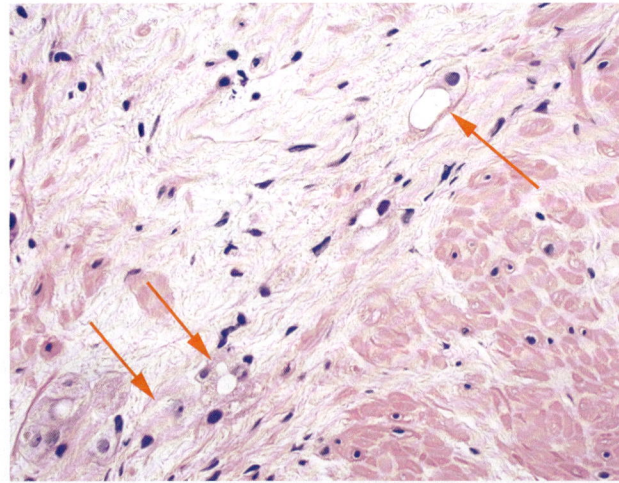

Figure 1.174. In this example of prostatic adenocarcinoma with radiation effect, there are poorly formed glands with only a few nuclei (arrows) and eccentrically oriented cytoplasmic lumens. Focally prominent nucleoli are visible at bottom left.

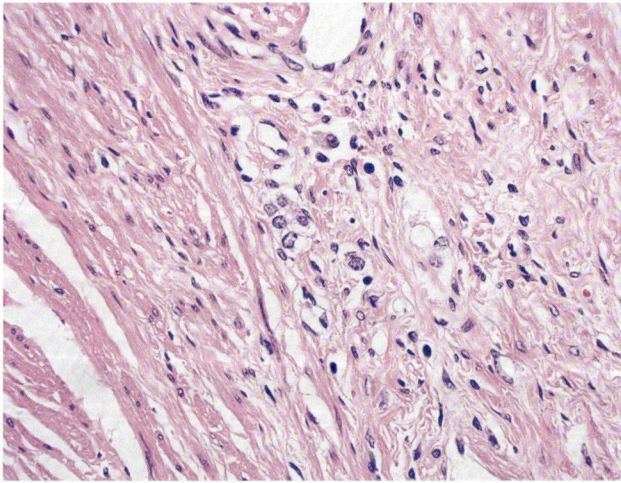

Figure 1.175. This example of prostatic adenocarcinoma with androgen deprivation therapy effect shows single cells and clusters of cells that would normally be graded as pattern 4 or pattern 5. However, this appearance would not be graded, as it is showing at least a partial therapy response.

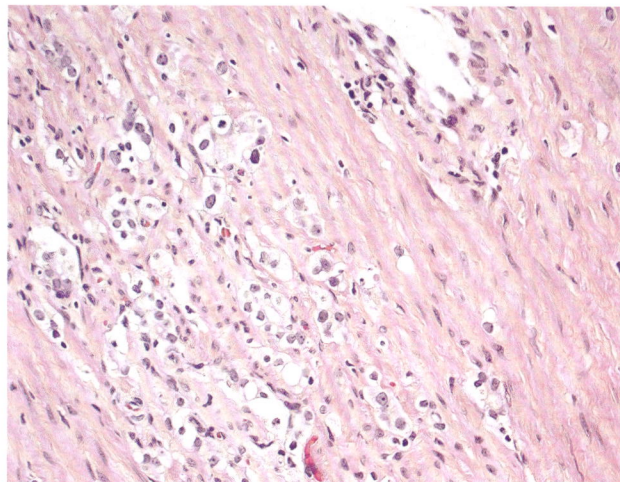

Figure 1.176. Another example of prostatic adenocarcinoma with androgen deprivation therapy effect shows bland nests and clusters of cells with small nuclei and minimal gland formation.

inflate the grade.[80] However, some cancers after treatment show conventional cancer histology, in which case it is reasonable to assign a grade with a comment noting that despite the history of treatment, no morphologic changes are appreciable and the cancer can be graded normally.[79] There is evidence that cancers with marked radiation effect found on surveillance biopsies do not have an outcome different from that of patients with negative biopsies, whereas cancers without appreciable treatment effect have a significantly higher rate of local failure.[104-106] So, it is important for pathologists to be aware of treatment effect on prostate cancer to avoid potentially triggering unnecessary salvage therapy. However, in many institutions, posttreatment biopsies are not performed routinely, rather only when biochemical failure (PSA increase) or other recurrence has already been identified, so this population is likely biased toward patients who are indeed experiencing recurrent cancer. 5α-Reductase inhibitors such as finasteride and dutasteride are in general a milder form of androgen deprivation therapy, and they may have some effects on prostate cancer morphology. However, one major study found that urologic pathologists were not able to reliably discriminate cancers that were treated from those that were not.[107] Therefore, the current recommendation is that prostate cancer should be graded normally in the setting of 5α-reductase inhibitor therapy. Other therapies predominantly ablate the prostatic tissue, such as high-intensity focused ultrasound (HIFU), cryoablation, laser therapies, and others. Currently, it is thought that the morphology in the viable areas is not necessarily distorted by these treatments, and therefore, grading as usual is recommended for any viable cancer.

FAQ: **When Can Prostate Cancer With Treatment Effect Be Graded?**

- In general, prostatic adenocarcinoma after radiation or androgen deprivation therapy with poorly formed glands and single cells showing at least partly bland nuclei should not be graded, as this often represents shrinkage of the cancer glands in response to the therapy

- Discrete glands (pattern 3) and cribriform structures (pattern 4) are unlikely to be mimicked by therapy effect and can usually be graded (with a note indicating that despite the history of treatment, no treatment-related changes are appreciable)

- A mixture of cancer glands with and without features of treatment effect usually should not be graded, but may be described in a note, indicating approximate grades of the evaluable areas

- Viable prostate cancer after other destructive/ablative therapies, such as HIFU or cryoablation (Figure 1.177) can usually be graded normally, as these are not thought to distort the morphology of the viable areas that are not ablated by the treatment

FAQ: What are Clues to Recognize That Prostatic Adenocarcinoma May Have Been Previously Treated?

Androgen deprivation therapy:

- Basal cell layer may be unusually prominent in benign glands (Figure 1.178)
- Benign nodular hyperplasia tissue may contain abrupt squamous metaplasia (Figure 1.179)
- Cancer is predominantly poorly formed glands, atrophic-appearing cancer, or single cells, at least partly with bland nuclei

Radiation therapy:

- Basal cell layer in benign tissue may contain enlarged, atypical nuclei, with more size variation than a typical prostate cancer (Figure 1.180)
- Stromal fibrosis may be present
- Blood vessels and nerves may show chronic damage/fibrosis or atypical nuclei
- Cancer is predominantly poorly formed glands, atrophic-appearing cancer, or single cells, at least partly with bland nuclei

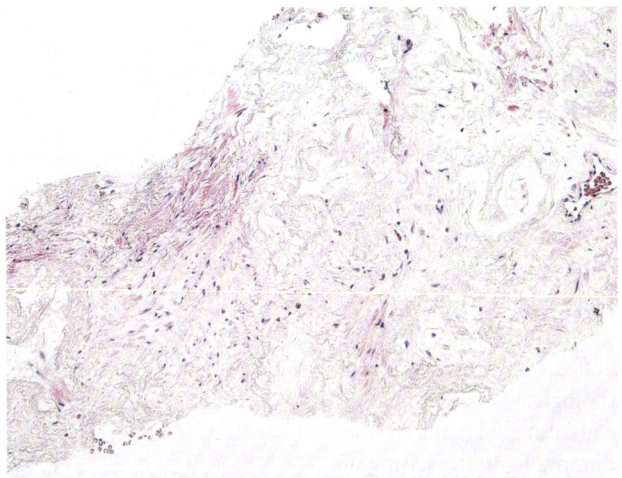

Figure 1.177. Cryotherapy is an ablative therapy that can show fibrosis or hyalinization in posttreatment prostate samples. If residual cancer is viable, current thinking is that it can be graded as usual.

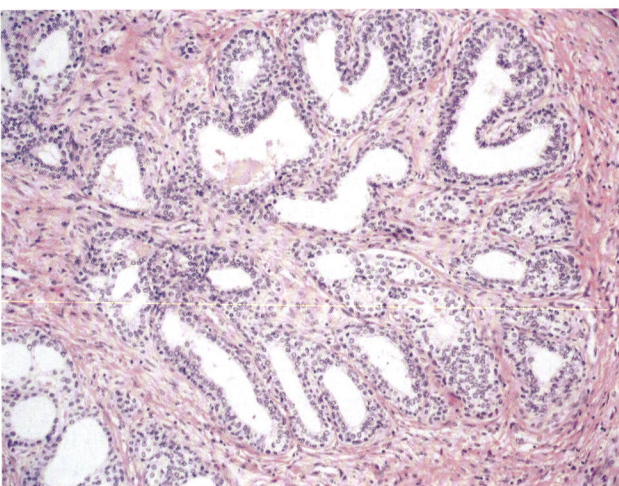

Figure 1.178. If a history of prior treatment is not provided, very prominent basal cells in the benign tissue can be a clue to prior androgen deprivation therapy.

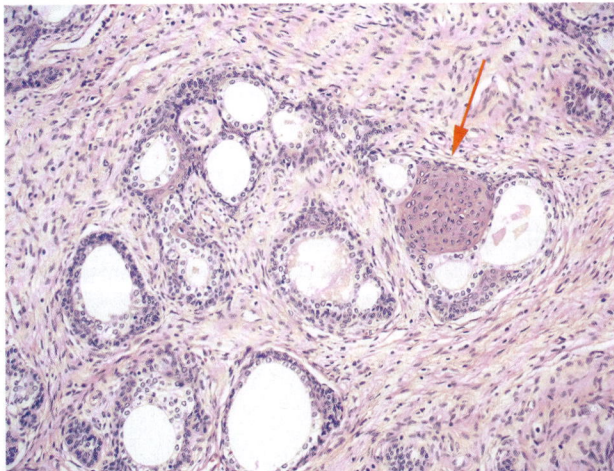

Figure 1.179. Abrupt squamous metaplasia (arrow) within the benign tissue in nodular hyperplasia is a strong clue to prior androgen deprivation therapy.

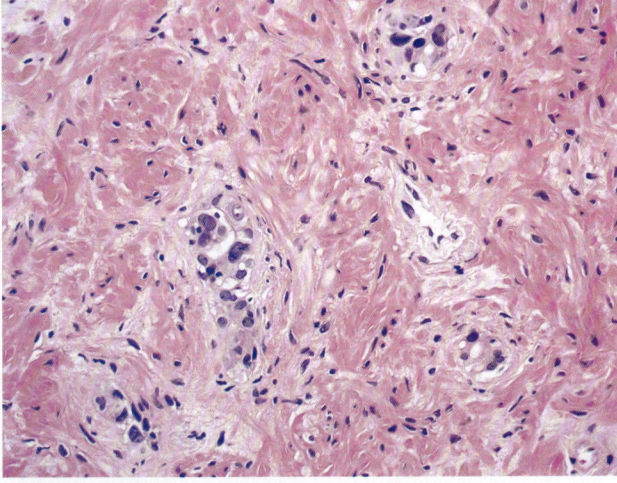

Figure 1.180. Prominent variation in nuclear size of the basal cells in benign glands is a clue to prior radiation therapy.

SAMPLE NOTE: Prostatic Adenocarcinoma With Therapy Effect

Note: The cancer and benign prostatic tissue show changes suggestive of (modality) effect. Review of the patient's medical records confirms prior treatment with (agent). In this context, Gleason grading is generally not applicable, as cancer cells with treatment effect typically shrink and coalesce, which would mimic higher grade patterns (pattern 4 or 5), despite having at least partially the desired response to treatment. The tumor cells in this specimen show (mild to marked) treatment effect.

LARGE/COMPLEX GLAND EPITHELIAL LESIONS

BENIGN MIMICS OF "LARGE GLAND" LESIONS

Basal Cell Hyperplasia (Large Gland Pattern)

Basal cell hyperplasia with a small gland pattern was previously discussed. However, basal cell hyperplasia can also form large glands that sometimes appear cribriform (Figures 1.181-1.183).[65] Usually this can be readily discriminated from adenocarcinoma, as the large cribriform glands are made up of cells that are similar to the basal cells of nearby normal glands; however, some florid examples may be deceptive. In particular, some unique lesions have been described as florid basal cell hyperplasia, basal cell adenoma, adenoid basal tumor, and adenoid cystic–like tumor.[64,100] The main features that help in discriminating such lesions from the rare occurrence of basal cell carcinoma and adenoid cystic carcinoma (discussed later in this section) include somewhat older age, a predominant transition zone location, circumscription (lack of infiltration), and lack of perineural invasion in basal cell hyperplasia.[100] Of note, rare cases with these benign adenoid cystic–like proliferations can contain cribriform structures with collagenous spherules, closely mimicking salivary adenoid cystic carcinoma, yet current thinking is to regard them as part of the spectrum of nodular hyperplasia so long as they appear confined within hyperplastic nodules and not infiltrative (Figures 1.184 and 1.185).[100] As noted previously, high-molecular-weight cytokeratin and p63 consistently show positive staining in basal cell hyperplasia, often with a multilayered pattern but lacking in the luminal-most layer.

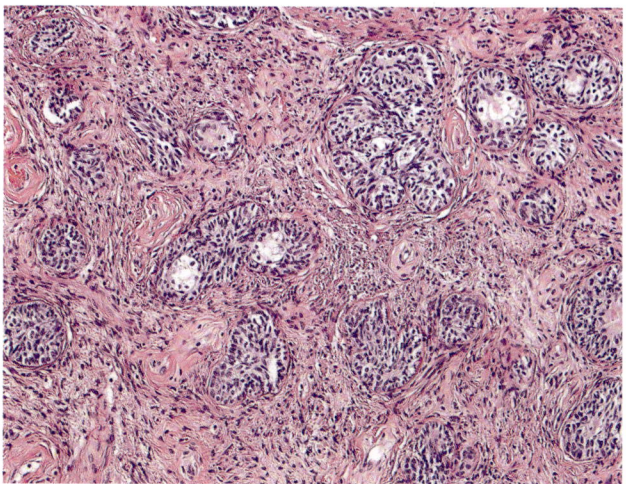

Figure 1.181. Basal cell hyperplasia can sometimes form large glandular structures that may raise a differential diagnosis with malignant large gland processes.

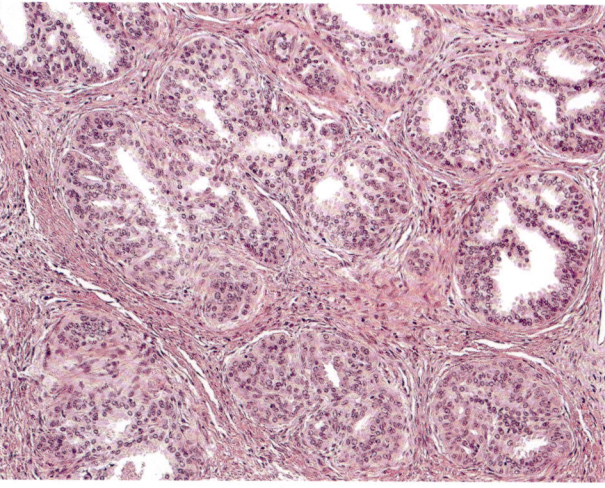

Figure 1.182. This example of basal cell hyperplasia shows cribriform structures; however, the increased basal cells have similar cytologic features to those of normal benign glands.

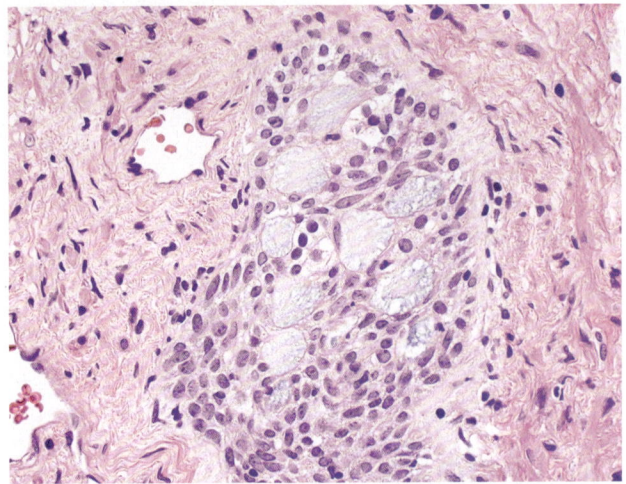

Figure 1.183. This basal cell hyperplasia gland shows cribriform formation and blue mucin; however, the elongated shape of the nuclei is a clue to distinguish from prostatic adenocarcinoma.

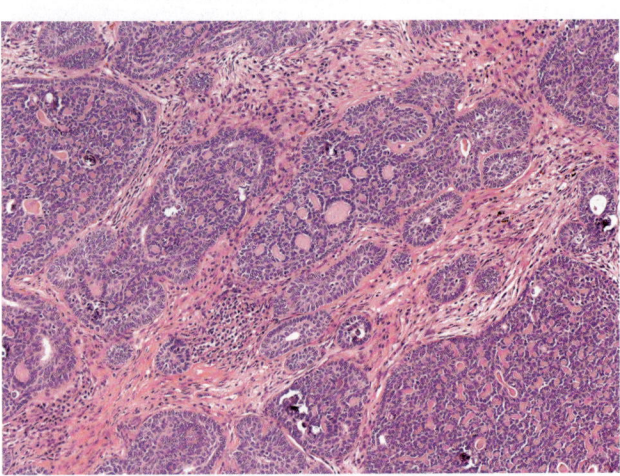

Figure 1.184. Very rarely basal cell hyperplasia can form large cribriform structures mimicking adenoid cystic carcinoma of the salivary gland.

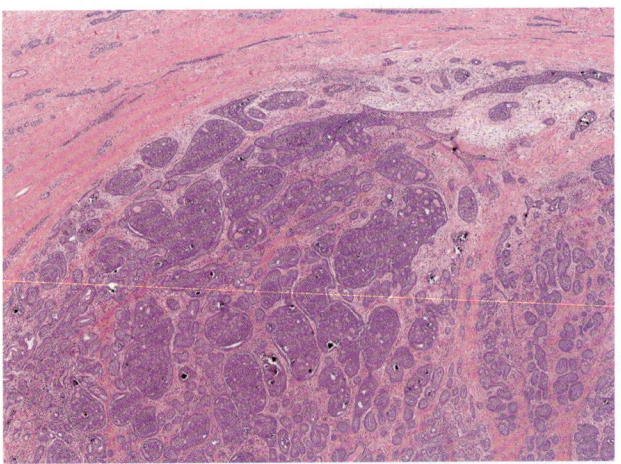

Figure 1.185. If adenoid cystic-like areas of basal cell hyperplasia remain well circumscribed within hyperplastic nodules, as illustrated by the well-defined border of this lesion, it support classification as basal cell hyperplasia rather than basal cell carcinoma.

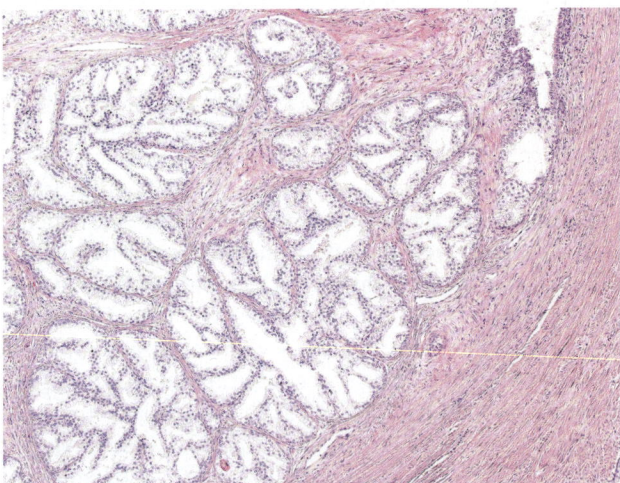

Figure 1.186. Clear cell cribriform hyperplasia is part of the spectrum of prostatic nodular hyperplasia, manifesting as complex or cribriform glands within hyperplastic nodules.

Clear Cell Cribriform Hyperplasia

Clear cell cribriform hyperplasia is a rare lesion typically encountered in the transition zone of the prostate as a part of nodular hyperplasia.[21,47,108,109] Despite the cribriform architecture, which might be concerning for pattern 4 cancer or intraductal carcinoma, cytologic features are more in keeping with benign prostatic tissue (Figures 1.186-1.189), including pale foamy/clear cytoplasm and bland nuclei with inconspicuous nucleoli. If needed to confirm the diagnosis, immunohistochemistry shows a normal basal cell layer. Although this has an unusual appearance, it is thought to be part of the spectrum of benign nodular hyperplasia.

Central Zone

As noted in the Unremarkable and Nonneoplastic Prostate section, central zone tissue has a few features that differ from those of typical benign prostatic tissue. Relevant to the discussion of "large gland lesions," it can contain Roman bridge–like structures that impart a cribriform appearance (Figures 1.190-1.192), potentially mimicking PIN, intraductal carcinoma, or perhaps invasive cancer. In contrast to PIN and cancer, central zone should have relatively inconspicuous nucleoli, although it is possible to have central zone involvement by true PIN. Awareness of the location from which the sample is taken can also be helpful in recognizing central zone, as it is present predominantly at the base, in the midline posteriorly.

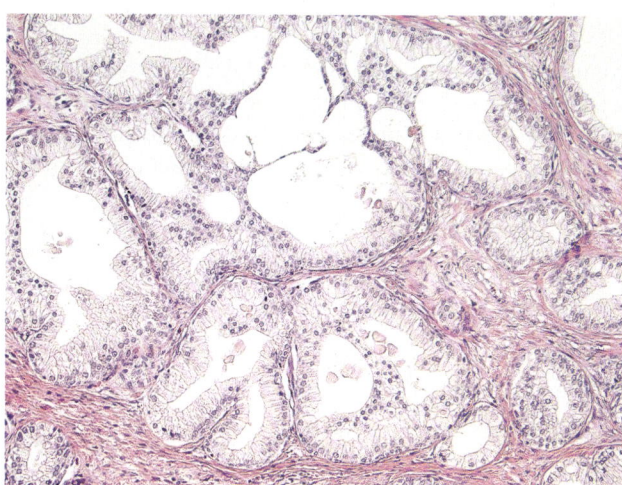

Figure 1.187. This case of cribriform hyperplasia shows bridging structures of the epithelium, although the glandular cytology is similar to that of benign glands.

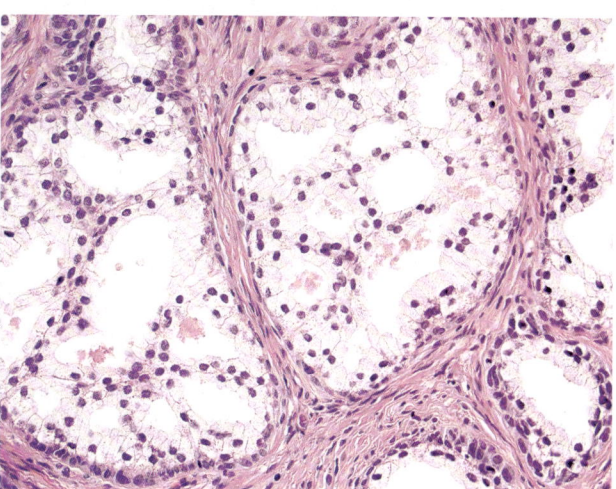

Figure 1.188. At high magnification, this case of cribriform hyperplasia has multiple lumens that appear "punched-out"; however, there is no nuclear atypia and a basal layer is apparent.

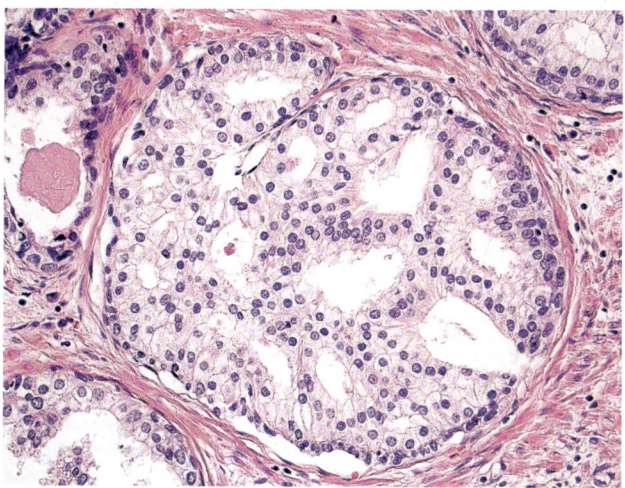

Figure 1.189. This case of cribriform hyperplasia is relatively cellular; however, the basal layer is appreciable and nucleoli are not conspicuous.

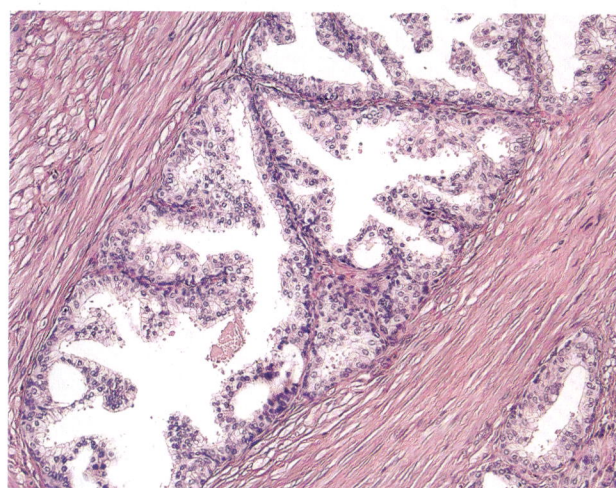

Figure 1.190. The normal central zone can contain "Roman bridge" structures, which should not be confused for prostatic intraepithelial neoplasia (PIN) or intraductal carcinoma.

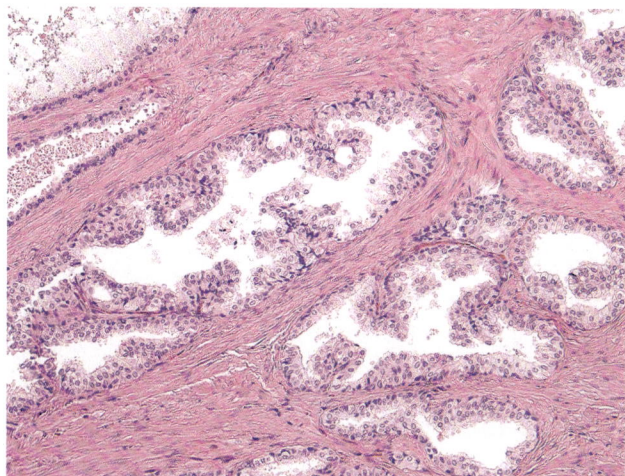

Figure 1.191. This example of benign central zone tissue shows dense eosinophilic stroma and tufted glands with a few "Roman bridges."

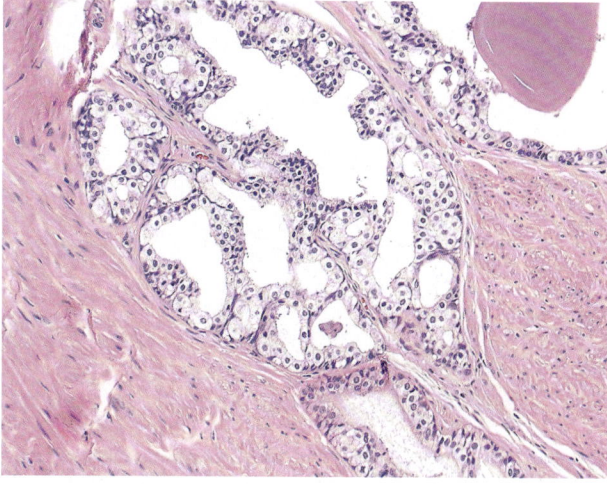

Figure 1.192. Occasionally, central zone tissue appears almost cribriform, resembling cribriform hyperplasia.

Prostatic Infarct

Prostatic infarct is a relatively common finding particularly in nodular hyperplasia specimens (transurethral resection or simple prostatectomy), rarely in prostatic biopsy. Relevant to the discussion of "large gland" lesions, it can contain reactive glands or squamous metaplasia, which can be confused for malignancy, such as urothelial carcinoma or squamous cell carcinoma involving the prostate.[110,111]

KEY FEATURES: Prostatic Infarct

- Zonal pattern:
  - Central necrosis or hyalinization
  - Rim of reactive glands with squamous metaplasia (Figures 1.193-1.196)
  - Surrounded by normal prostatic tissue

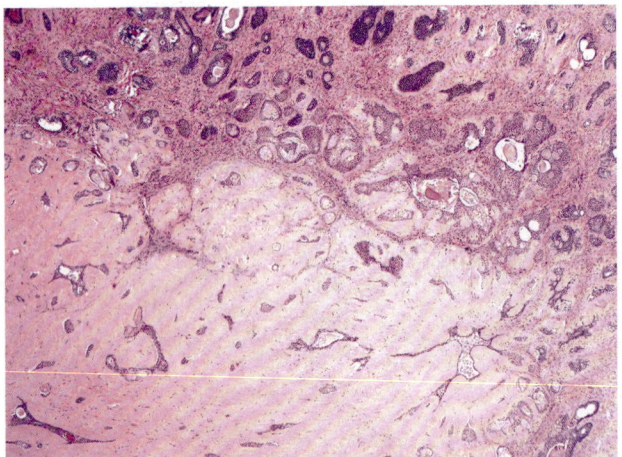

Figure 1.193. Prostatic infarct is composed of a zone of infarct or fibrosis, typically surrounded by a zone of squamous metaplasia, followed by a zone of normal prostatic tissue, in a "bull's-eye" pattern.

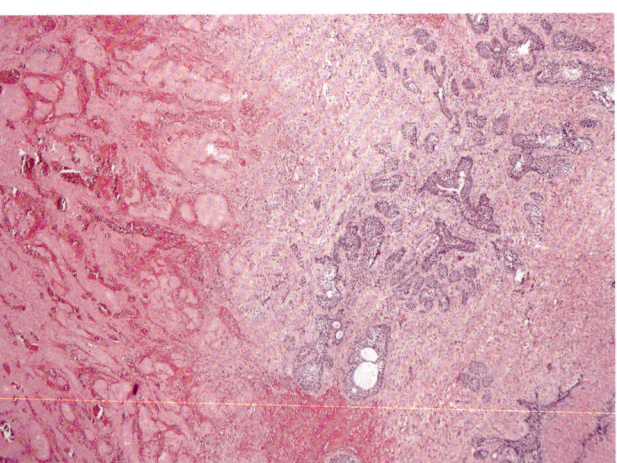

Figure 1.194. This prostatic infarct shows a more hemorrhagic area of necrosis, surrounded by glands with squamous metaplasia.

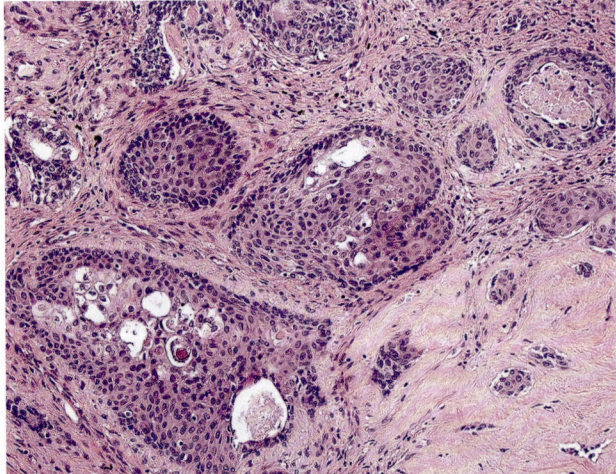

Figure 1.195. The squamous metaplasia of prostatic infarcts may appear concerning for squamous cell carcinoma or urothelial carcinoma involving prostatic ducts; however, atypia should be relatively minimal. The fibrotic zone at bottom right is a clue to the zonation pattern of infarct.

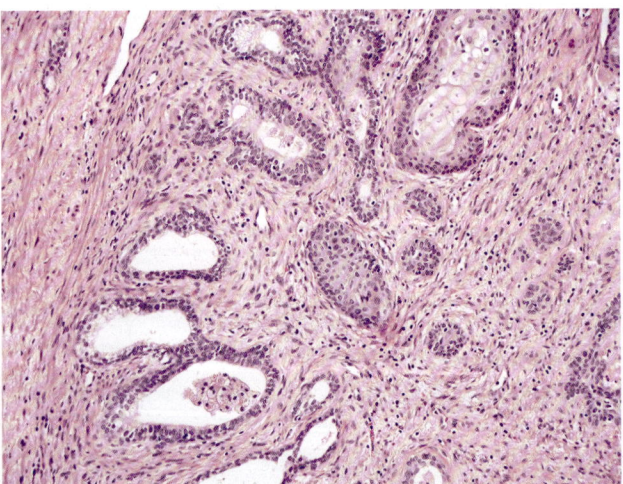

Figure 1.196. Outside the infarct, the glands around a prostatic infarct will transition from squamous to normal.

The etiology of this phenomenon is not totally clear. Although it has been postulated that it might be related to vascular disease in general,[112] other studies have found no significant association with vascular disease,[110] suggesting that it may be primarily a function of prostate size. Perhaps as large prostates reach a critical size, the interplay of the gland enlargement and confined anatomic space of the pelvis compromises the blood supply to certain areas. Of note, the serum PSA can rapidly reach a high level with prostatic infarct, with some patients having sudden elevation of more than 200 ng/mL over their baseline level.[110]

Benign Glands With Androgen Deprivation Therapy Effect (Squamous Metaplasia)

As noted in the FAQ on treatment effect (page 52), an unusual large gland lesion can occur with androgen deprivation therapy in which benign glands have abrupt squamous metaplasia partially filling the gland (Figure 1.197). This phenomenon has been previously associated with estrogen-related therapies[79,80,113]; however, we have continued to encounter it occasionally even with modern antiandrogen treatments. Awareness of this phenomenon facilitates discrimination from squamous or urothelial carcinoma spreading in preexisting spaces and may be a clue to the posttreatment nature of the specimen, if such history is not provided.

HIGH-GRADE PROSTATIC INTRAEPITHELIAL NEOPLASIA

Prostatic intraepithelial neoplasia (PIN) is considered the foremost putative precursor lesion of prostate cancer (Figure 1.198). Notably though its significance is relatively minimal when found in isolation. In the biopsy setting, the risk of finding cancer in a repeat biopsy after a PIN diagnosis has been estimated at 22%. As this compares to a risk of cancer of about 15% to 19% following a benign diagnosis on initial biopsy, PIN usually does not elicit any management changes on its own.[114] Extensive PIN found in multiple biopsies has been suggested to have a higher risk of cancer. In one study, a threshold of four or more sites was used for the definition of "widespread" PIN.[115]

Regarding morphology, PIN can have several patterns, including flat (Figures 1.199 and 1.200), tufted (most common, Figures 1.201-1.203), micropapillary (Figures 1.204 and 1.205), and inverted or hobnail PIN (with nuclei aligned at the cell apex, Figures 1.206-1.208).[116] Other rare patterns include PIN with vacuoles, among others.[114] Although cribriform PIN has historically been considered one of the main patterns of PIN, thinking is

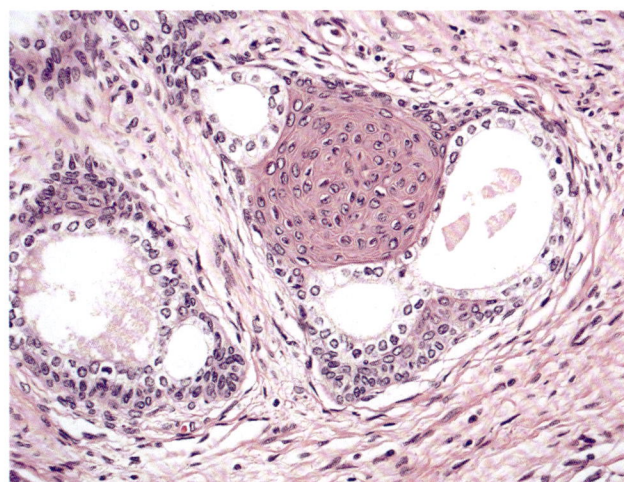

Figure 1.197. Abrupt squamous metaplasia within a benign gland is a clue to prior androgen deprivation therapy.

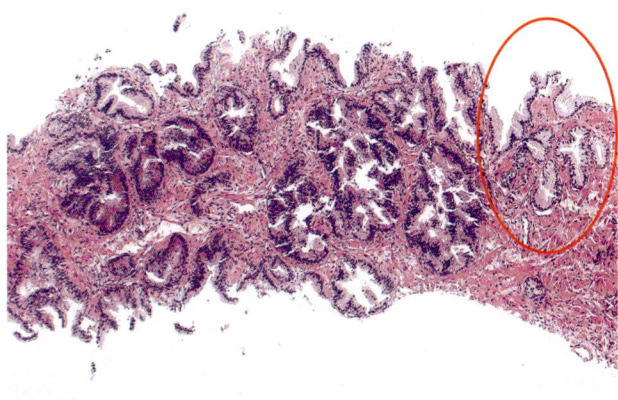

Figure 1.198. Prostatic intraepithelial neoplasia (PIN) is the main putative precursor of prostate cancer. In this needle biopsy, it is evident that a large area of glands has darker cytoplasm and nuclei than the adjacent normal glands (circle), which should prompt confirmation at higher magnification for features of PIN, especially prominent nucleoli.

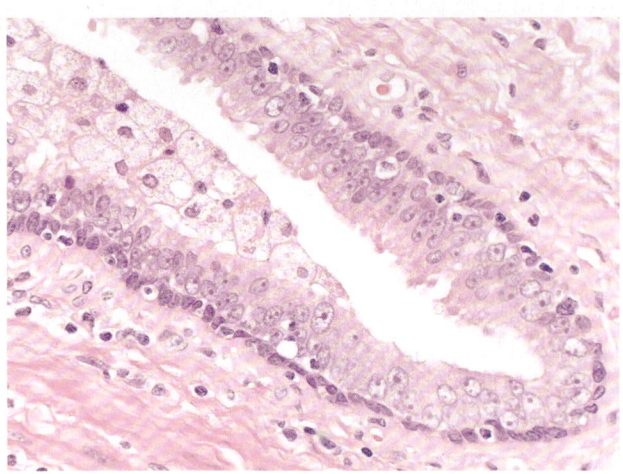

Figure 1.199. Occasionally, prostatic intraepithelial neoplasia (PIN) can show a flat architectural pattern with enlarged nuclei containing prominent nucleoli, without significant tufting or papillary structures.

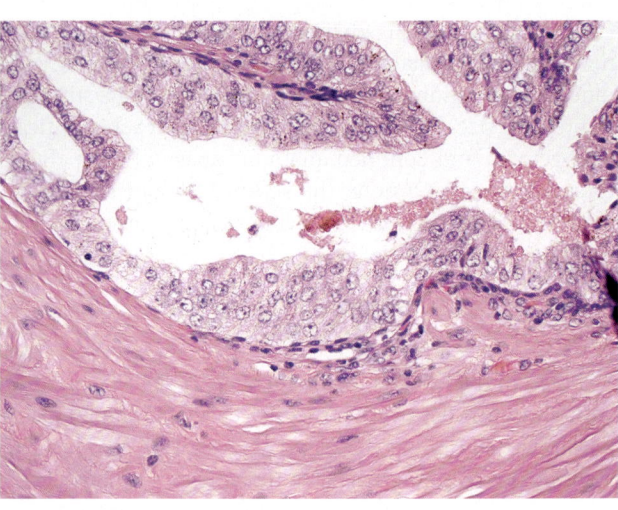

Figure 1.200. This focus of prostatic intraepithelial neoplasia (PIN) is partially flat.

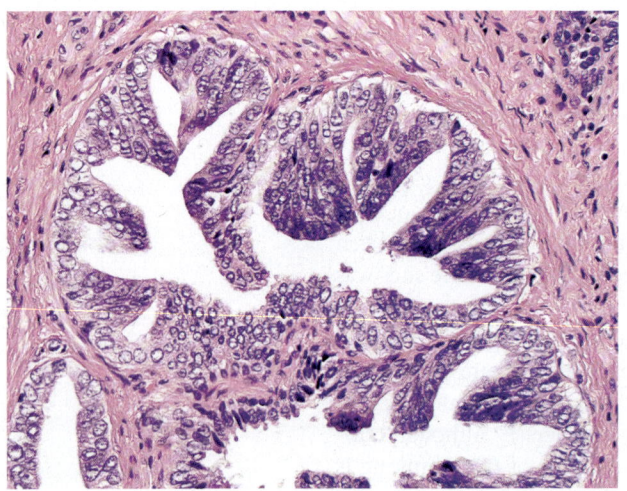

Figure 1.201. Tufted pattern is the most common pattern of prostatic intraepithelial neoplasia (PIN), with an undulating luminal contour.

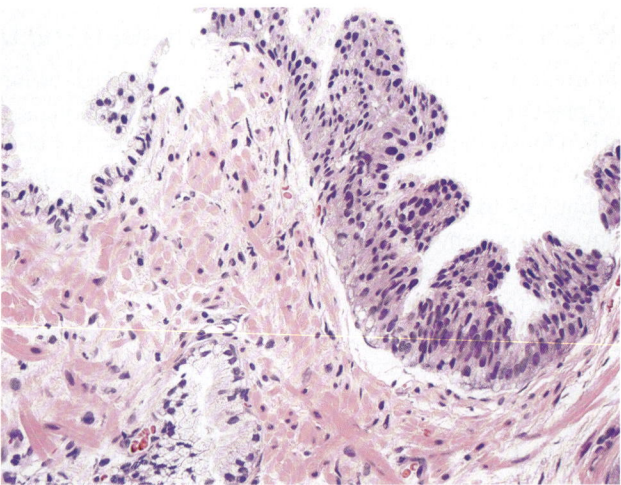

Figure 1.202. In this focus of tufted prostatic intraepithelial neoplasia (PIN), the abnormal glands (right) have obviously darker cytoplasm and nuclei than the adjacent normal glands (left).

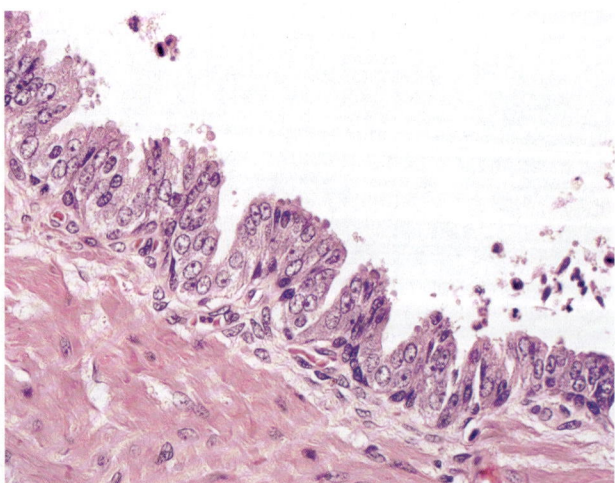

Figure 1.203. At high magnification, this focus of tufted prostatic intraepithelial neoplasia (PIN) has prominent nucleoli.

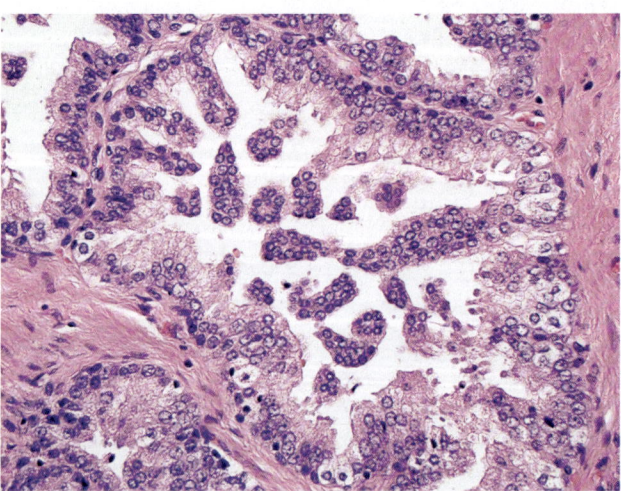

Figure 1.204. Micropapillary prostatic intraepithelial neoplasia (PIN) is composed of budding structures that have no fibrovascular cores, some of which appear detached in the lumen.

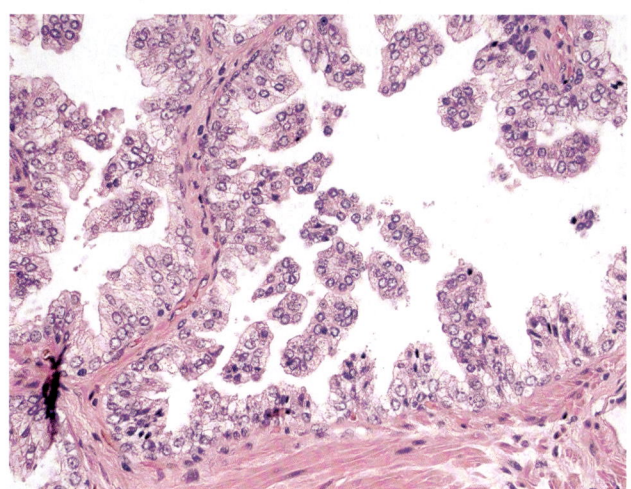

Figure 1.205. This example of micropapillary prostatic intraepithelial neoplasia (PIN) shows multiple small clusters of epithelial cells with nuclear atypia in the lumen.

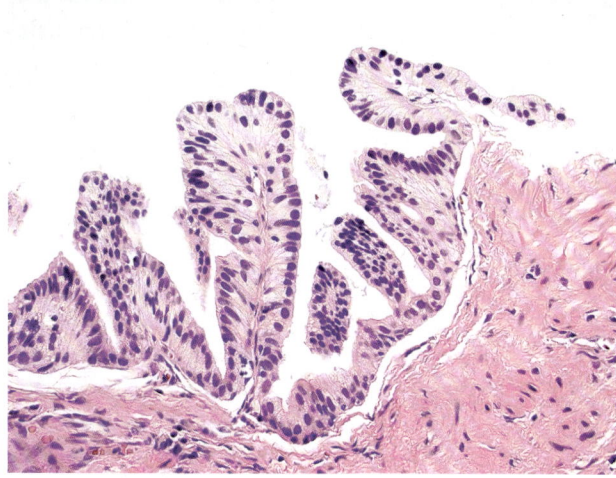

Figure 1.206. A relatively uncommon pattern of prostatic intraepithelial neoplasia (PIN) is so-called inverted or hobnail PIN, in which the nuclei are aligned toward the apex of the cell. In some of these cases, the nuclei are less atypical than those of usual PIN; however, this odd architectural pattern should prompt consideration of inverted PIN.

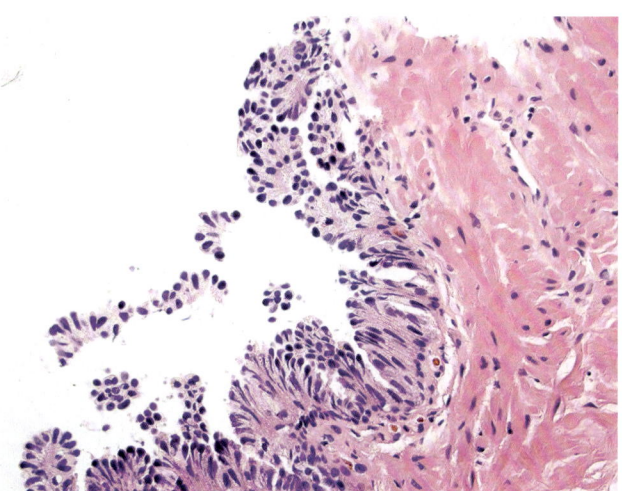

Figure 1.207. In this case of inverted or hobnail pattern prostatic intraepithelial neoplasia (PIN), the nuclei are aligned at the cell apex with a hobnail-shaped configuration.

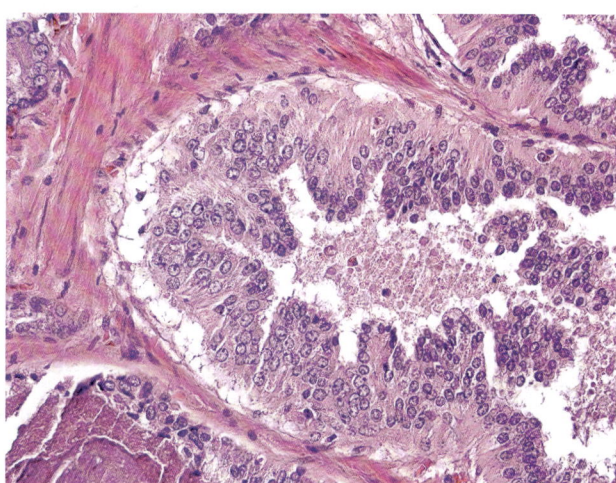

Figure 1.208. This inverted prostatic intraepithelial neoplasia (PIN) is similar to the more common tufted PIN; however, the nuclei are predominantly aligned away from the basement membrane.

increasingly shifting to raise concern for intraductal carcinoma (which is considerably higher risk) whenever a cribriform intraductal proliferation is encountered. As discussed later with intraductal carcinoma, a term "atypical intraductal proliferation" can be used for lesions that are worrisome for being beyond the spectrum of PIN, yet not definitive for intraductal carcinoma.[117,118] This should usually be accompanied by a comment indicating that repeat sampling is likely warranted. In current practice, only lesions with high-grade nuclear features (enlarged, hyperchromatic nuclei with nucleoli, similar to those of adenocarcinoma) should be diagnosed as PIN. Historical categories of low-grade or intermediate-grade PIN should no longer be diagnosed, due to lack of reproducibility and because even high-grade PIN has only a minimally increased risk of cancer itself. Some authors use a general rule that nucleoli should be visible at 20× objective magnification to diagnose PIN.[114]

CHECKLIST: Diagnosis of high-grade prostatic intraepithelial neoplasia (PIN)

☐ Hyperchromatic cells within a preexisting glandular space (tufted, flat, or micro-papillary configuration)

☐ Nucleoli usually conspicuous (evident at 20 × magnification) and/or nuclei enlarged compared with adjacent benign

☐ No associated small round glands lacking basal cells (may warrant diagnosis of PIN with atypical glands or small focus of adenocarcinoma)

☐ No significant cribriform proliferation (usually warrants diagnosis of intraductal carcinoma or atypical intraductal proliferation)

☐ Absence of marked nuclear pleomorphism (usually warrants diagnosis of intra-ductal carcinoma or atypical intraductal proliferation)

☐ Absence of comedonecrosis (usually warrants diagnosis of intraductal carci-noma or atypical intraductal proliferation)

MALIGNANT LARGE GLAND AND GLAND-LIKE LESIONS

Cribriform Cancer

Despite a recent explosion of interest in cribriform intraductal carcinoma,[117,118] cribriform growth does exist as a pattern of invasive cancer. In fact, it is increasingly thought that cribriform growth connotes one of the most aggressive variations of pattern 4, perhaps warranting specific documentation in pathology reports.[119-125] Cribriform invasive cancer manifests as large areas of glandular proliferation with numerous "punched out" lumens (Figures 1.209 and 1.210). Cribriform cancer can include areas of perineural invasion or comedonecrosis, although more than half of foci of prostate cancer with comedonecrosis are actually intraductal carcinoma.[126]

Intraductal Carcinoma

It is now increasingly recognized that many cribriform proliferations in the prostate that were previously assumed to be invasive cancer are in fact intraductal carcinoma.[117,118] Intraductal carcinoma is almost always associated with high-grade invasive prostate can-cer, so misinterpretation as invasive cancer is usually not a significant error. However, a notable minority of cases have intraductal carcinoma in the absence of invasive cancer or only with low-grade invasive cancer,[127] sometimes referred to as "precursor-like" intraductal

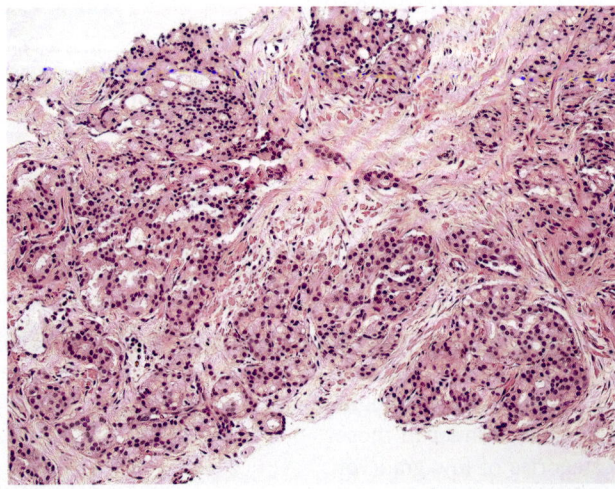

Figure 1.209. This needle biopsy shows large areas of cribriform growth, representing cribriform invasive prostatic adenocarcinoma.

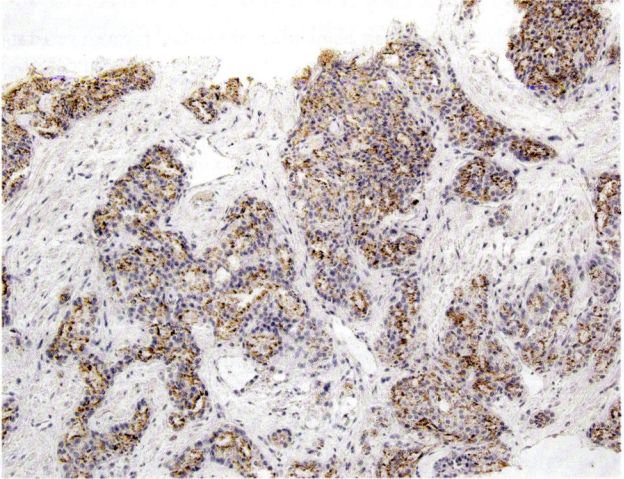

Figure 1.210. Immunohistochemistry in the same case from Figure 1.209 shows increased cytoplasmic staining for alpha-methyla-cyl-CoA racemase (AMACR) and absence of basal cells (single-color p63 and AMACR stain).

carcinoma.[128] Such exceptions have led to the current recommendation that intraductal carcinoma be distinguished from invasive cancer and not graded, as patients with intraductal carcinoma in the absence of invasion likely have a more favorable prognosis than a predominant pattern 4 would imply. However, it is uncertain at present whether subtracting an intraductal carcinoma component before assigning a grade provides superior prognostication to providing a grade overall, when there is obvious invasive cancer. As such, how carefully one must exclude intraductal carcinoma from the differential diagnosis is an area of controversy. In general, most experts would agree that it is not necessary to perform immunohistochemistry solely for the purpose of excluding intraductal carcinoma from the grade, when there is overt high-grade (pattern 4 or higher) invasive cancer.[117,118]

In larger specimens, it is often possible to recognize intraductal carcinoma based on morphology alone, as it often has an especially prominent basal cell layer (Figure 1.211) and sometimes the cribriform proliferation partially involves benign glands (Figures 1.212-1.214). In the biopsy setting, however, it can be more difficult to determine whether a cribriform proliferation is invasive cancer or intraductal carcinoma. Likewise, discriminating PIN from intraductal carcinoma is critically important, as PIN has minimal, if any, management implications, whereas intraductal carcinoma is at minimum an indication for repeat biopsy and perhaps an indication for definitive treatment.

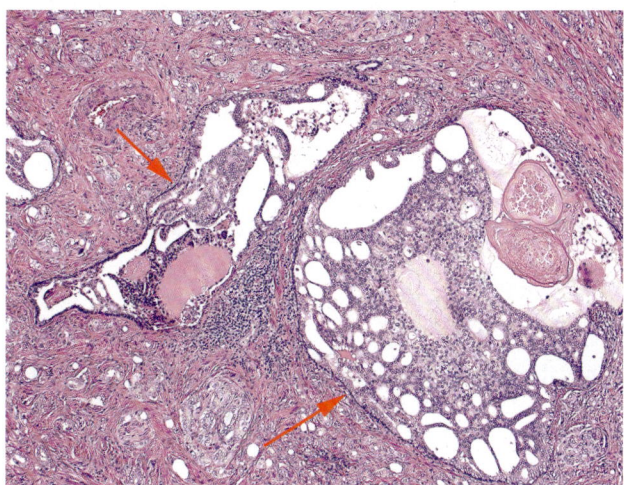

Figure 1.211. Intraductal carcinoma often has an extremely prominent basal cell layer (arrows) that contrasts to the marked atypia of the cancer cells.

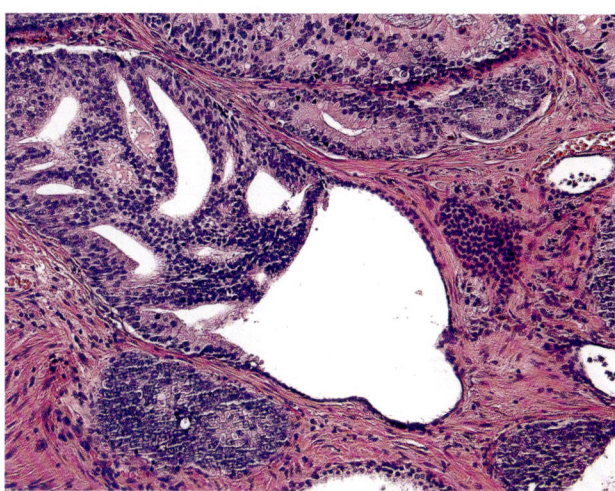

Figure 1.212. In some fields, intraductal carcinoma can be visualized partially involving benign glands.

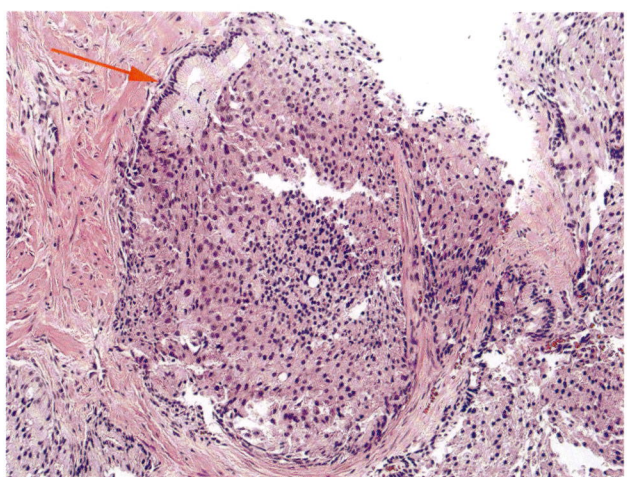

Figure 1.213. This focus is intraductal carcinoma with a predominantly solid growth pattern. A small rim of benign uninvolved gland can be visualized at one edge (arrow).

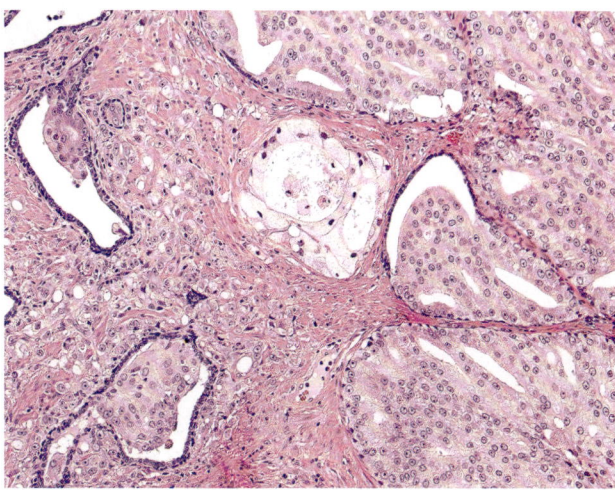

Figure 1.214. In this example of intraductal carcinoma, the intraductal component has very similar cytology to the adjacent invasive cancer, and it can be seen partially filling benign glands with a residual basal cell layer.

KEY FEATURES: Discriminating intraductal carcinoma from PIN

- Proposed diagnostic features for intraductal carcinoma include the following:
  - Solid or dense cribriform proliferation (with cells making up at least 50% to 70% of the lumen)
  - Loose cribriform or micropapillary proliferation with either marked nuclear atypia or nonfocal comedonecrosis[117,129]
    - **Note:** The original proposal for marked nuclear atypia used the criterion of nuclei 6× normal size[129]; however, this can be the subject of debate (nuclear diameter, which is rare, vs area, which is more common).[130] We would interpret this criterion more flexibly as nuclear atypia that is markedly beyond that normally expected of PIN (Figure 1.215)

FAQ: What Is "Atypical Intraductal Proliferation"?

"Atypical intraductal proliferation" or "atypical cribriform lesion" is not a specific entity itself but rather a diagnostic term for lesions encountered in biopsy samples that are debatably stretching the limits of PIN (Figures 1.216-1.220) but not yet fulfilling definitive criteria for intraductal carcinoma. As such, this term may be used to convey to clinicians that the patient requires further investigation, such as with prostate imaging or additional biopsies to further evaluate for intraductal or invasive cancer.

SAMPLE NOTE: Atypical Intraductal Proliferation

Prostate, left lateral base, core needle biopsy:

- Atypical intraductal proliferation—see Comment

Comment: The biopsy shows atypical cells growing within a retained basal cell layer. The differential diagnosis is between high-grade PIN and intraductal carcinoma. Repeat biopsy with or without MRI guidance is recommended.

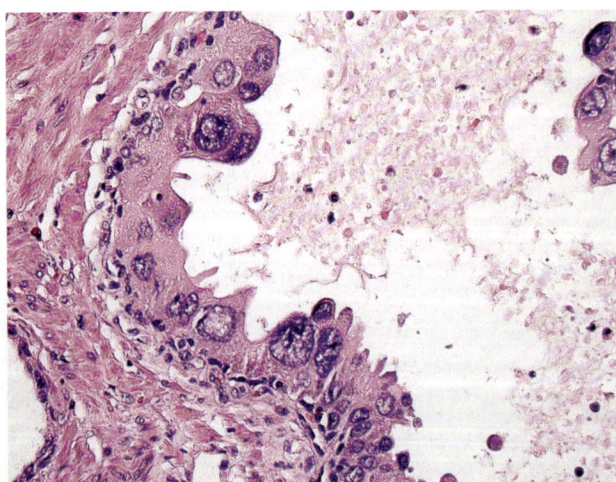

Figure 1.215. The proposed criterion for marked cytologic atypia to diagnose intraductal carcinoma used nuclei 6× larger than normal. We would interpret this as marked nuclear atypia that is well beyond what is normally expected of prostatic intraepithelial neoplasia (PIN).

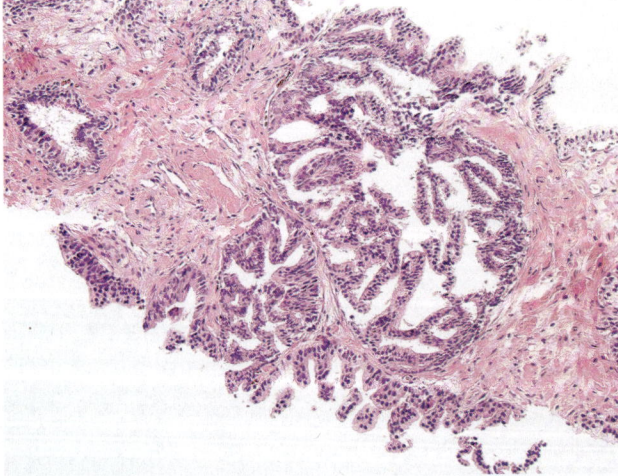

Figure 1.216. For lesions that do not entirely fulfill the criteria for intraductal carcinoma, such as this biopsy showing a loose cribriform proliferation, the terminology of atypical intraductal proliferation or atypical cribriform lesion has been proposed. This connotes a lesion potentially more worrisome than prostatic intraepithelial neoplasia (PIN), yet not fulfilling definite features of intraductal carcinoma.

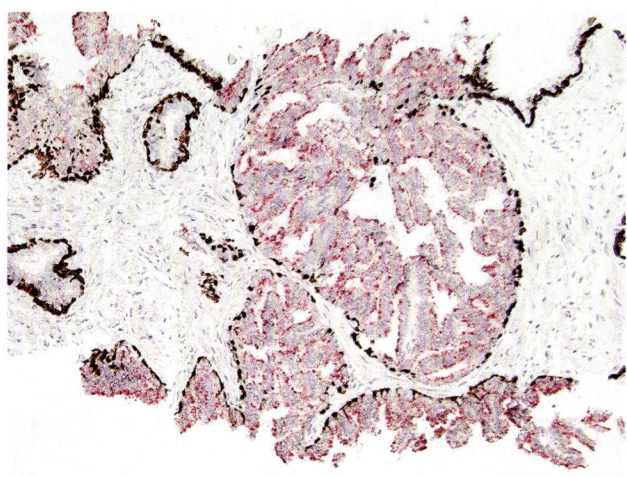

Figure 1.217. The same focus from Figure 1.216 shows a basal cell layer (brown) and increased staining for alpha-methylacyl-CoA racemase (AMACR) (red) in this dual-color cocktail stain.

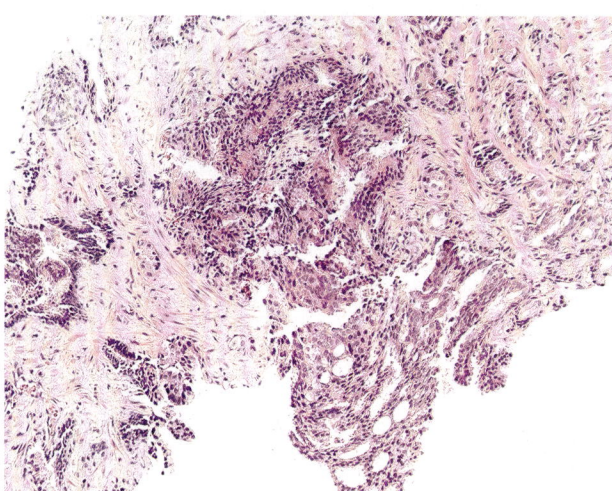

Figure 1.218. This focus was an isolated lesion in a patient's entire prostate biopsy set, showing a single cribriform gland with several small round glands adjacent to it.

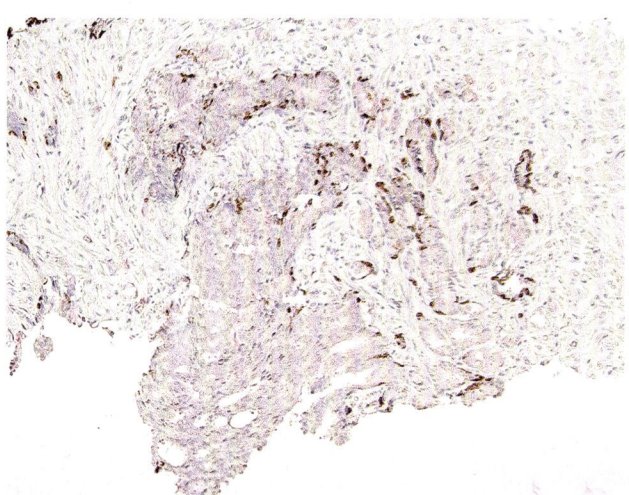

Figure 1.219. The same focus from Figure 1.218 shows a patchy basal cell layer in the cribriform gland (brown) and weak staining for alpha-methylacyl-CoA racemase (AMACR) (red). Most of the small round glands have at least focal basal cells, arguing against associated adenocarcinoma. This was diagnosed as atypical intraductal proliferation and further studies (imaging or repeat biopsy) were recommended.

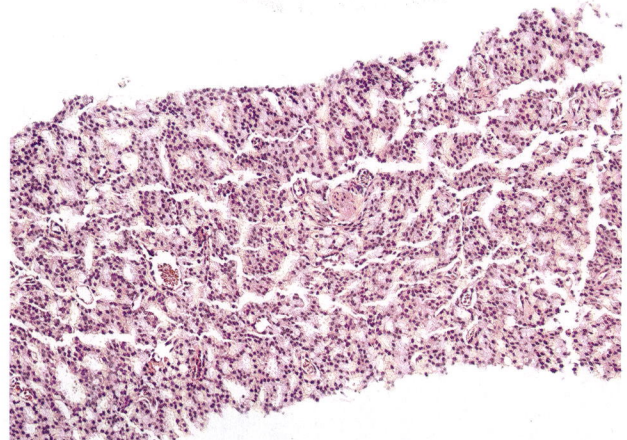

Figure 1.220. The same patient from Figures 1.218 and 1.219 had a first repeat biopsy showing only a small focus of Gleason score 3 + 3 = 6 (Grade Group 1) cancer (not pictured). His third biopsy under magnetic resonance imaging (MRI) guidance finally identified a large area of Gleason score 4 + 4 = 8 (Grade Group 4) cribriform cancer, shown here.

Ductal Adenocarcinoma

Originally described as "endometrioid," ductal prostatic adenocarcinoma is a specific variant of prostate cancer that is primarily characterized by columnar cytology, with pseudostratified nuclei resembling those of an adenomatous colonic polyp (Figures 1.221 and 1.222).[117,118,131,132] Ductal prostatic adenocarcinoma is inherently graded as pattern 4, or Gleason score 4 + 4 = 8 (Grade Group 4) if pure. Areas of solid growth or necrosis would be graded as pattern 5.

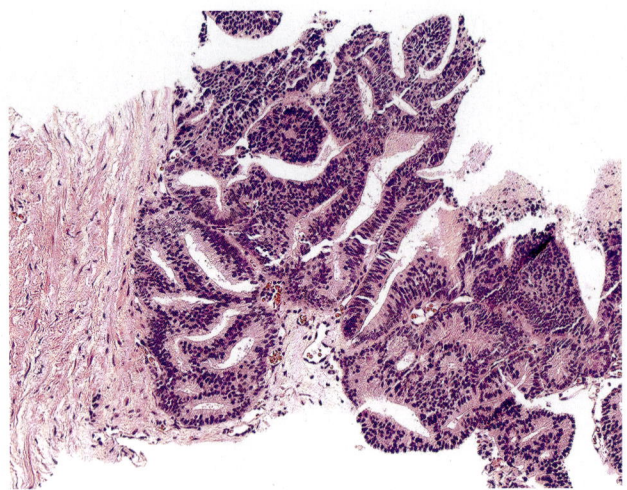

Figure 1.221. Ductal variant prostatic adenocarcinoma, when present in needle biopsy samples, may result in fragmentation of the cores due to large areas of cribriform growth with little stroma to hold the tissue together. This field shows ductal carcinoma making up the tip of the biopsy core.

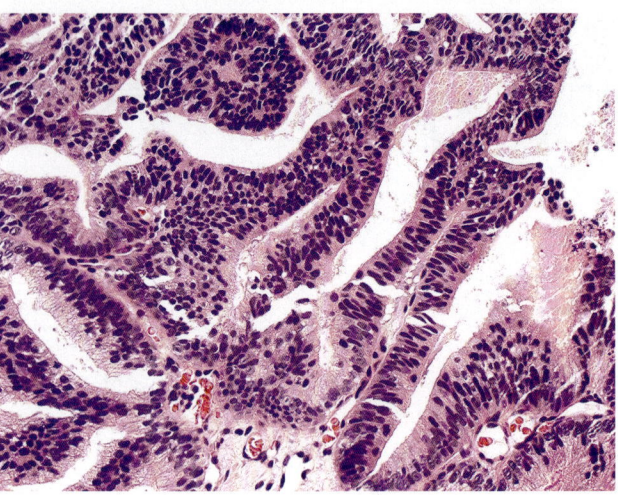

Figure 1.222. At higher magnification, the same case from Figure 1.221 shows columnar cytology, resembling an adenomatous colon polyp.

FAQ: What are the Criteria for Diagnosing Prostatic Ductal Adenocarcinoma?

The most universal criterion for ductal variant prostate cancer is that cells should have a columnar configuration, resembling that of an adenomatous colon polyp, with elongated, pseudostratified nuclei.[117] However, there is some debate regarding the precise boundaries of the diagnostic spectrum for ductal cancer. Some pathologists would consider papillary architecture to be a highly supportive feature (Figures 1.223 and 1.224).[133] Although cribriform architecture is common, it is nonspecific,[133] and we would usually reserve the designation of ductal variant for only cancers with the columnar cytology and nuclear pseudostratification.

PEARLS AND PITFALLS: Unique Clinicopathologic Features of Ductal Prostate Cancer

- May present as a prostatic urethral or urinary bladder mass, mimicking a urothelial neoplasm clinically (Figure 1.225) and causing obstruction or hematuria
- In a subset of cases, may occur in the central prostate, involving large periurethral ducts or the verumontanum
- Peripheral zone involvement also occurs, like conventional prostate cancer
- Graded inherently as pattern 4, and if pure, Gleason score 4 + 4 = 8 (Grade Group 4)
- Often associated with higher clinicopathologic stage

Immunohistochemistry of ductal cancer may show some unusual patterns, including cytokeratin 20 or CDX2 positivity, which could lead to potential confusion with colorectal or other adenocarcinomas. However, staining for prostatic markers, such as PSA and NKX3.1, is consistently positive.[134,135] Ductal cancer can also occasionally grow within preexisting spaces, like intraductal prostate cancer, with a focally intact basal cell layer. In contrast to acinar intraductal carcinoma, it is generally considered that ductal variant cancer can be diagnosed as malignant and graded, even if there is a focally intact basal cell layer, as ductal cancer rarely, if ever, occurs without invasion.[117]

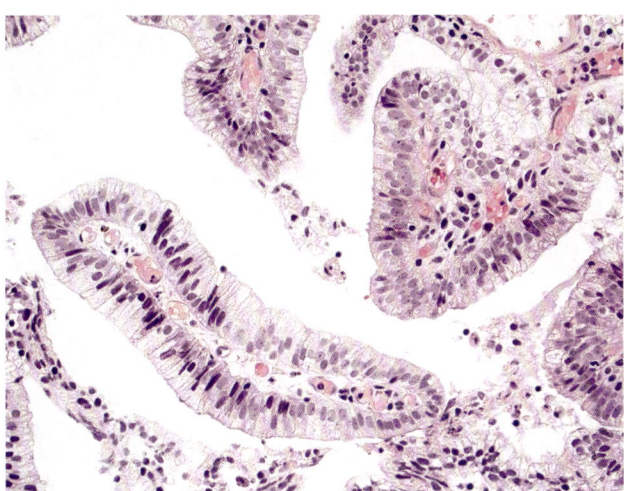

Figure 1.223. Ductal carcinomas also often have papillary archi-tecture. This case shows more clear to pale cytoplasm, yet still with elongated nuclei.

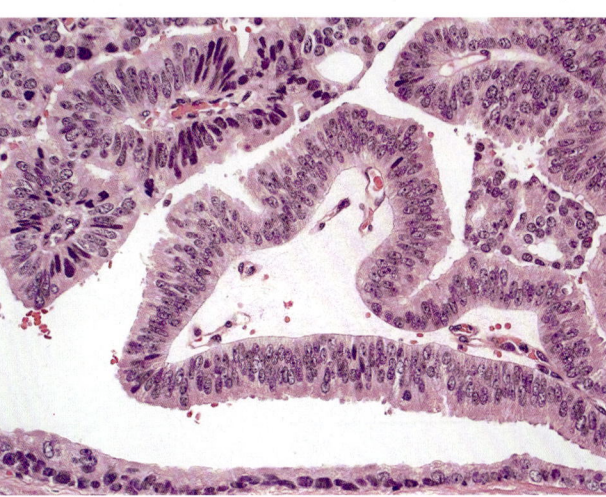

Figure 1.224. This papillary ductal carcinoma shows columnar cells with eosinophilic cytoplasm.

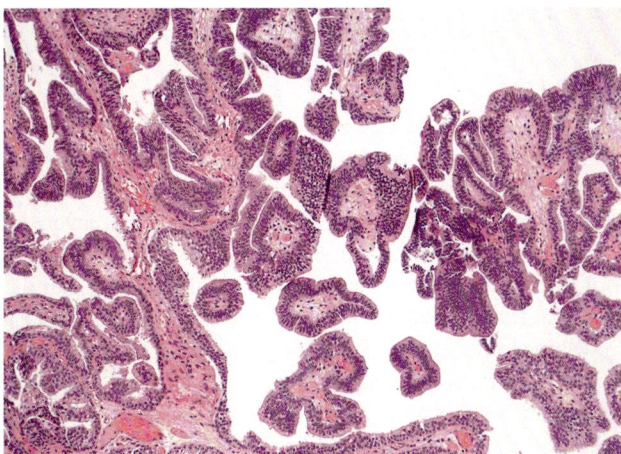

Figure 1.225. This ductal prostatic adenocarcinoma presented as a prostatic urethral lesion and was referred as a consultation case for the possibility of a benign prostatic urethral polyp. However, atten-tion to the elongated atypical nuclei will help to avoid this diagnos-tic pitfall.

FAQ: What is the Difference Between Ductal and Intraductal Carcinoma?

The nomenclature for ductal and intraductal carcinoma can be confusing. In duc-tal variant cancer, the word "ductal" refers to the cytology of columnar cells with pseudostratified nuclei. This is considered inherently malignant and Gleason pat-tern 4 if unequivocal features are present. In contrast, in intraductal carcinoma, it refers to the growth within preexisting ducts, typically with acinar (cuboidal) cytology. The vast majority of intraductal carcinoma is associated with extensive high-grade invasive cancer; however, the current paradigm is that intraductal car-cinoma is not graded, in view of rare cases where there is only intraductal carci-noma without invasion.[117] Nonetheless, this is a current area of debate.

PIN-like (Ductal) Carcinoma

A special form of prostate cancer that is debatably related to ductal carcinoma is so-called PIN-like ductal carcinoma or PIN-like carcinoma.[136,137] This form has columnar cytology like typical ductal cancer; however, it is arranged in smaller glands with flat or undulating

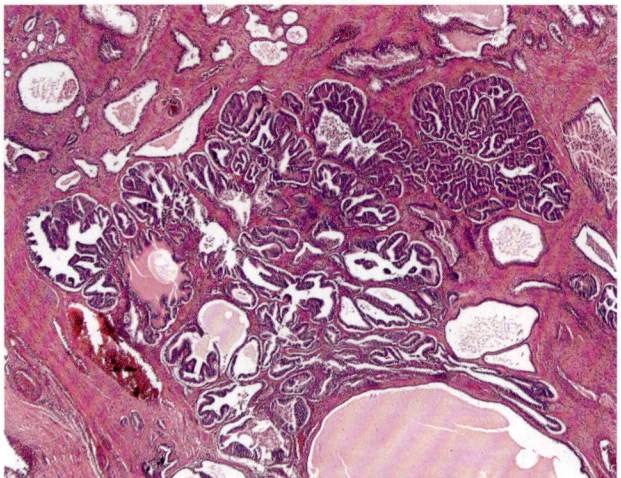

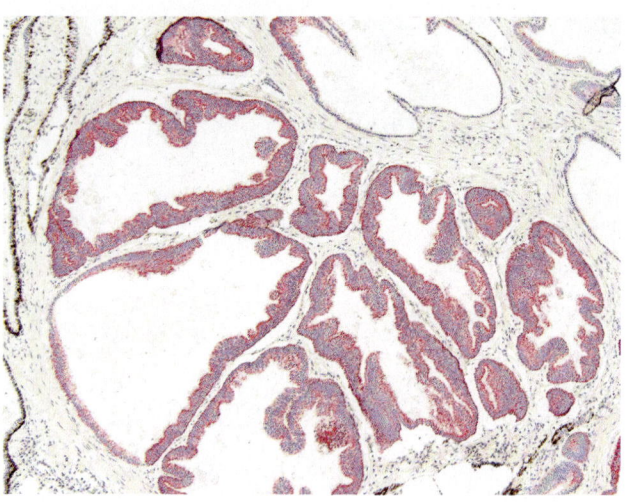

Figure 1.226. Rare invasive prostatic adenocarcinoma can closely resemble prostatic intraepithelial neoplasia (PIN), referred to as PIN-like carcinomas or PIN-like ductal carcinomas. This example shows a sizable focus of glands with undulating contours, resembling PIN. (Courtesy of Giovanna Giannico, MD, Vanderbilt University Medical Center.)

Figure 1.227. The same case from Figure 1.226 shows absence of basal cells (brown) and increased staining for alpha-methylacyl-CoA racemase (AMACR) (red), supporting invasive carcinoma. (Courtesy of Giovanna Giannico, MD, Vanderbilt University Medical Center.)

lining, morphologically resembling PIN. (Figures 1.226 and 1.227) In biopsy specimens, this variant is often identified as strips of atypical epithelium on the edges of the core, indicating large glands which have been cut across. When immunohistochemistry is applied, PIN-like ductal carcinoma shows multiple PIN-like glands without a basal cell layer. As PIN often has a patchy basal layer, and rare glands may appear to have no basal cells, diagnosis of PIN-like carcinoma should be reserved for specimens with multiple such glands, in which it would be difficult to accept that a basal layer was missed due to patchy distribution. It is a subject of debate whether this should be considered part of the spectrum of ductal prostatic adenocarcinoma or more in keeping with acinar carcinoma; however, current thinking is that this pattern can be graded as pattern 3 (not inherently pattern 4 like typical ductal cancer).[137] A recent study found that PIN-like cancers with thin papillary projections into the cystic spaces more often were associated with extraprostatic extension of the PIN-like cancer, leading the authors to suggest that this specific morphology should be an exception to grading PIN-like cancer as pattern 3, instead being graded as pattern 4 like typical ductal cancer.[136]

Basal Cell Carcinoma (Large Gland Pattern)

As noted previously for small gland lesions, occasional basal cell carcinomas of the prostate do occur, despite being considerably rare compared with basal cell hyperplasia.[138] In the large gland spectrum of morphology, some basal cell carcinomas are composed of large cribriform glands, resembling adenoid cystic carcinoma of the salivary gland, and others show more solid growth (Figure 1.228). In fact, a subset of basal cell carcinomas (half or less) have been shown to have *MYB* gene rearrangement, akin to adenoid cystic carcinoma of the salivary gland, especially those with adenoid cystic–like morphology.[139,140] Immunohistochemistry of basal cell carcinoma typically shows multiple layers of cells positive for basal cell markers such as high-molecular-weight cytokeratin and p63 (Figure 1.229), with negative staining of the innermost layer.[138] As basal cell hyperplasia can sometimes have large cribriform glands, the most helpful features for distinguishing basal cell carcinoma from hyperplasia include the presence of perineural invasion or extraprostatic extension and involvement of the peripheral zone or extension into the peripheral zone.[100] As noted previously, rare cases of basal cell hyperplasia can have adenoid cystic-like morphology, so an adenoid cystic pattern alone should not be considered inherently indicative of malignancy.

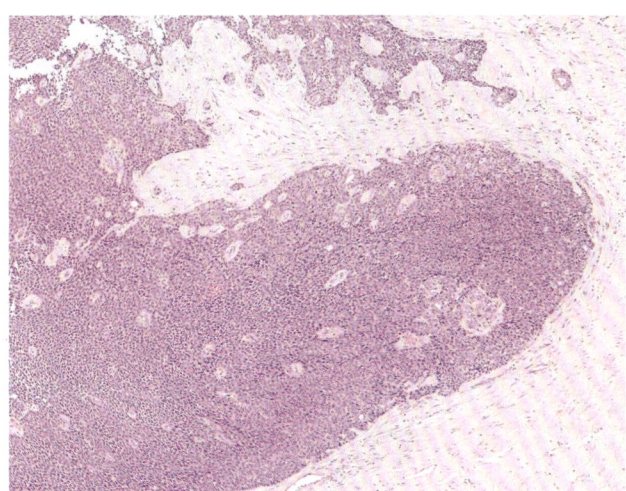

Figure 1.228. Basal cell carcinoma of the prostate is rare and can include tumors resembling adenoid cystic carcinoma or solid invasive tumors as shown here.

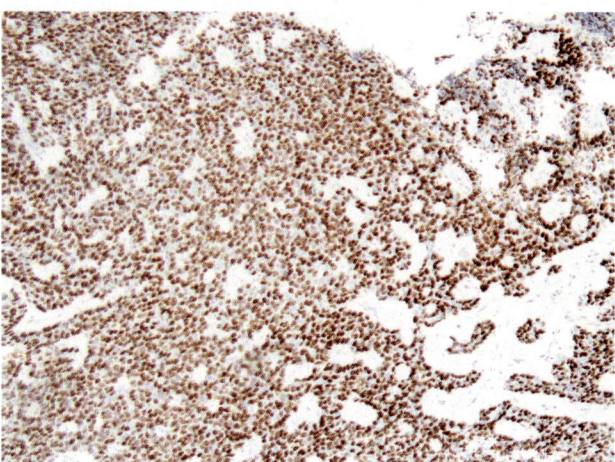

Figure 1.229. The same tumor from Figure 1.228 shows substantial staining for p63 although the luminal-most cells are negative, which is a frequent pattern in basal cell carcinoma. The same case was negative for GATA3 (not pictured), arguing against urothelial carcinoma.

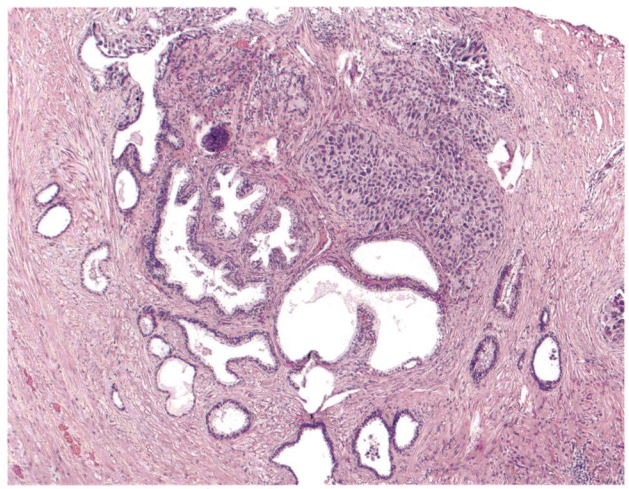

Figure 1.230. Urothelial carcinoma involving the prostate can grow within prostatic ducts, mimicking an intraductal component of prostate cancer.

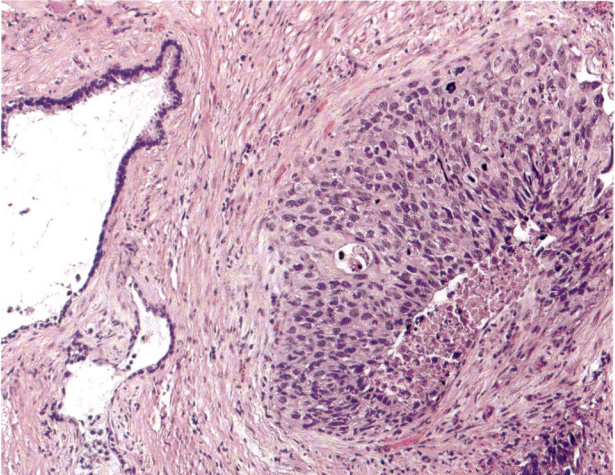

Figure 1.231. A clue to the diagnosis of urothelial carcinoma in the prostate is the greater cytologic atypia and variation of nuclear size as compared with prostate cancer.

Urothelial Carcinoma Involving the Prostate

Although most neoplasms of the prostate are primary prostatic adenocarcinomas, occasionally other malignancies can involve the prostate, the most common being urothelial carcinoma. As urothelial carcinoma can involve prostatic ducts, it has the potential to be confused for intraductal carcinoma or high-grade prostatic adenocarcinoma (Figures 1.230-233). Helpful clues to recognize urothelial carcinoma involving the prostate include a greater degree of nuclear size variation or atypia than in prostatic adenocarcinoma, and the presence of an in situ component in the urethra. Immunohistochemistry is extremely helpful in challenging cases, with positivity for p63 and GATA3 in urothelial carcinoma, contrasting to PSA, NKX3.1, or prostein positivity in prostatic adenocarcinoma.[84,141-144] This distinction is critically important, as the treatments for urothelial carcinoma and prostatic adenocarcinoma are drastically different, even when prostate cancer is of high grade or stage. Rarely prostatic adenocarcinoma can even have features suggesting papillary formation (Figures 1.234-1.236), further causing difficulty with urothelial carcinoma vs prostatic adenocarcinoma.[145] Therefore, a relatively low threshold should be used for performing immunohistochemistry in any tumor with equivocal features.

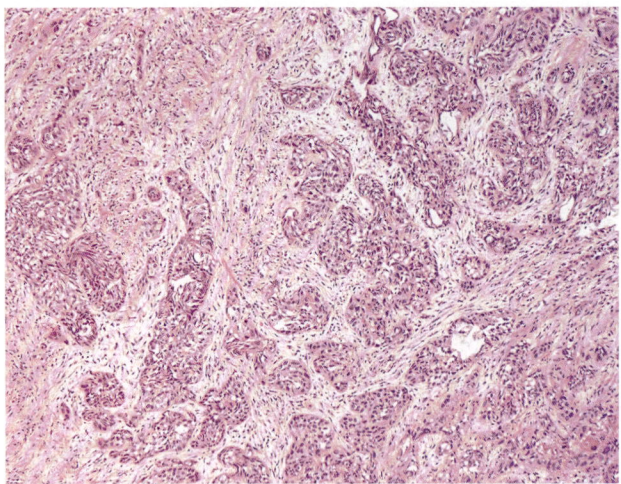

Figure 1.232. This example of urothelial carcinoma involving the prostate exhibits desmoplastic reaction, supporting stromal invasion.

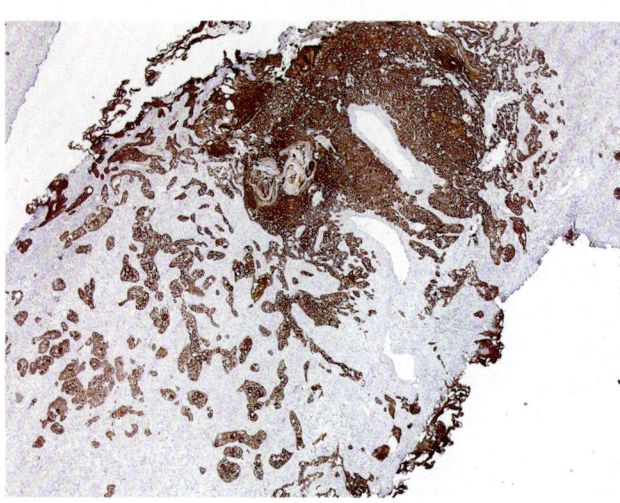

Figure 1.233. Diffuse high-molecular-weight cytokeratin staining in this case supports the diagnosis of urothelial carcinoma involving the prostate.

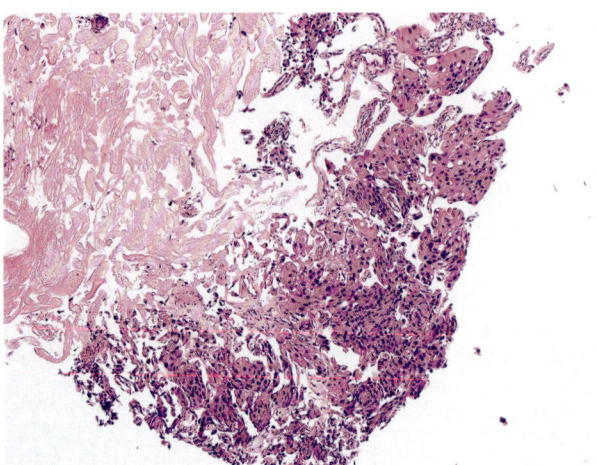

Figure 1.234. Rare prostate cancer can be exceedingly pleomorphic or papillary, mimicking urothelial carcinoma. Therefore, a high index of suspicion should be maintained for tumors with atypical features for urothelial carcinoma or with a prior history of prostate cancer.

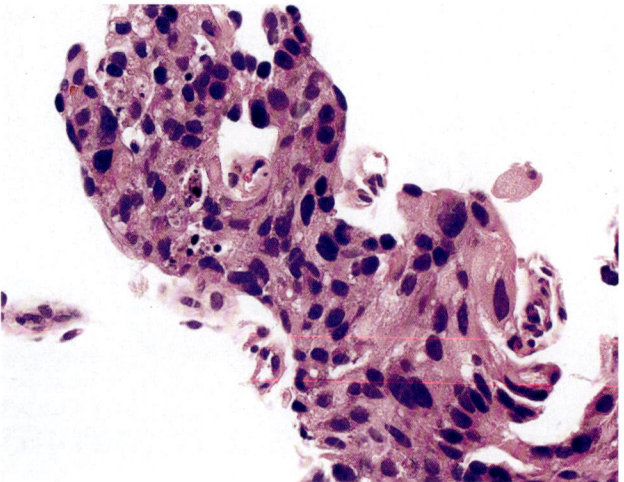

Figure 1.235. The same case from Figure 1.234 shows prostatic adenocarcinoma shows more prominent nuclear size variation than is typical.

Other Malignancies Involving the Prostate

Other malignancies secondarily involving the prostate are quite rare, but unusual patterns should always prompt consideration of secondary involvement, like other surgical pathology specimens. Usually the diagnosis of a high-stage malignancy of another organ is well known; however, in rare cases, secondary involvement, such as by colorectal cancer or rare other malignancies (Figures 1.237 and 1.238), can be deceptive.[146]

PLEOMORPHIC TUMORS

As discussed in the previous section, urothelial carcinoma is characteristically more pleomorphic than prostatic adenocarcinoma, and thus, urothelial carcinoma involving the prostate should be a differential diagnostic consideration for high-grade malignancy with marked pleomorphism in prostatic specimens.

CHECKLIST: Poorly differentiated prostatic adenocarcinoma

☐ Absence of urothelial carcinoma or urothelial carcinoma in situ in the urethra (except rare collision tumor, usually requires immunohistochemistry)

☐ Positive prostatic markers (one or more of PSA, NKX3.1, prostein, PSAP)

☐ Lacking urothelial immunohistochemical phenotype[a] (GATA3, p63, high-molecular-weight cytokeratin)

☐ Lacking neuroendocrine morphology/immunohistochemical phenotype

☐ Optional: well-differentiated prostatic glandular component (acinar or cribriform) is helpful but not always identifiable

[a]Exceptions exist for individual markers.

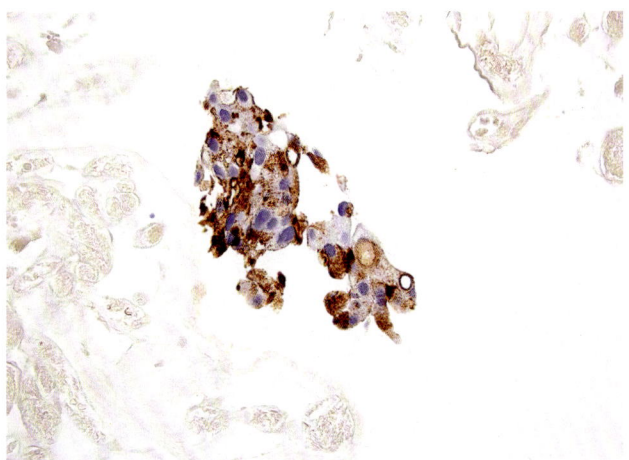

Figure 1.236. Immunohistochemistry for prostate-specific antigen (PSA) in the case from Figures 1.234 and 1.235 shows positive staining, supporting recurrent prostate cancer. This tumor was also negative for GATA3 and focally positive for prostein (p501s, not pictured).

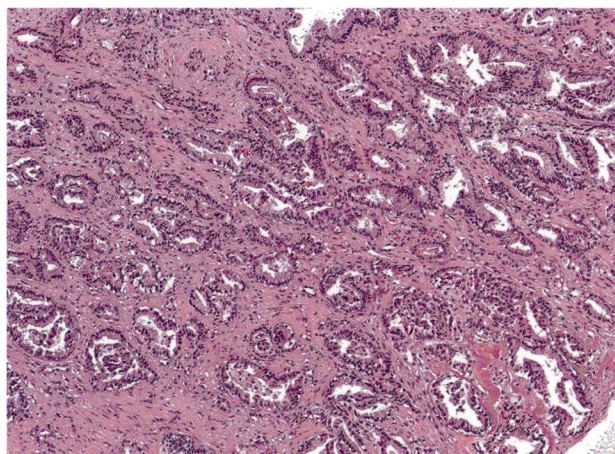

Figure 1.237. Extremely rarely, other nonprostatic tumors can involve the prostate. This is an example of lung adenocarcinoma metastatic to the prostate, which could closely mimic a primary prostate cancer without knowledge of the clinical history of lung cancer. (Courtesy of Matthew J. Wasco, MD, St. Joseph Mercy Health System.)

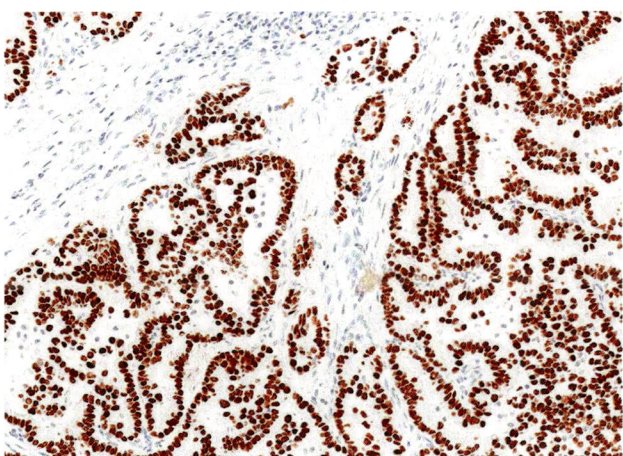

Figure 1.238. The same case from Figure 1.237 shows positive staining for TTF1. (Courtesy of Matthew J. Wasco, MD, St. Joseph Mercy Health System.)

Prostatic Adenocarcinoma With Increased Pleomorphism

Although most prostatic adenocarcinomas have quite uniform cytology (despite nuclear enlargement and prominent nucleoli), rare examples may show increased pleomorphism without forming a recognized variant (Figure 1.239). Therefore, differential diagnosis between prostatic adenocarcinoma and other types of carcinoma should usually be considered, especially urothelial carcinoma involving the prostate. At the same time, awareness that some cases of prostatic adenocarcinoma can have a greater degree of pleomorphism is important.

Prostatic Adenocarcinoma With Pleomorphic Giant Cell Features

A specific variant of prostate cancer known as carcinoma with pleomorphic giant cells has been rarely encountered and is highly aggressive.[147-149] A recent study found that even when this finding is very focal (<5%), the behavior still appears to be quite aggressive.[147] These tumors typically show transition from conventional prostatic adenocarcinoma to markedly atypical forms with giant cells (Figure 1.240). A diagnostic problem for such cases is that positivity for prostatic markers, such as PSA and prostein (Figure 1.241) may be decreased or absent in the giant cell component. NKX3.1 is the most sensitive marker at present (Figure 1.242), although it likewise can be decreased or occasionally negative in the giant cell component.[147]

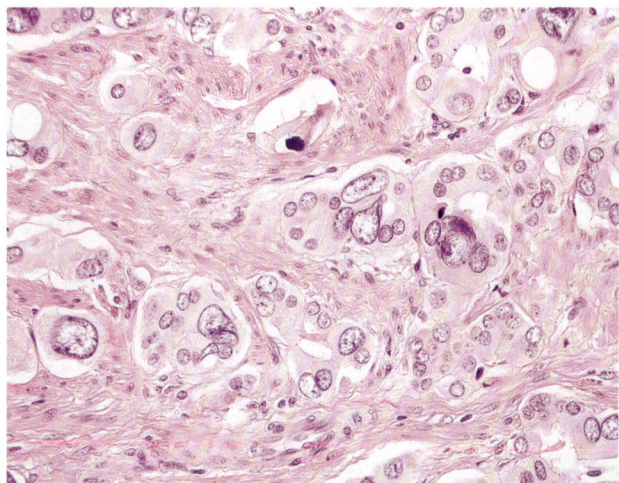

Figure 1.239. Rare prostate cancers can exhibit more marked atypia. This example shows typical gland forming morphology; however, some nuclei are much more enlarged than usual for prostatic adenocarcinoma.

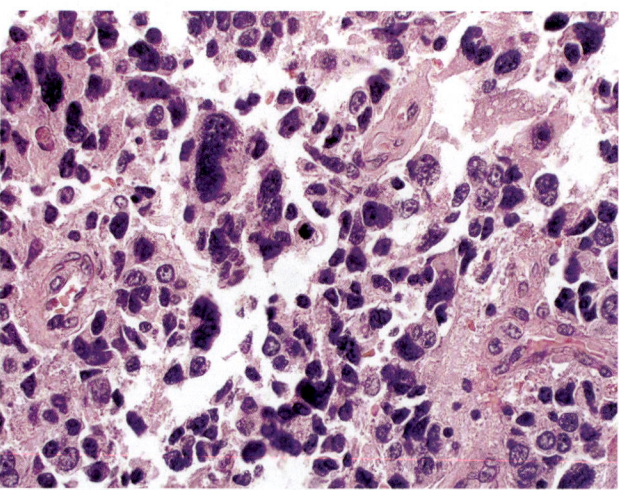

Figure 1.240. Pleomorphic giant cell variant of prostatic adenocarcinoma is a specifically named variant with very poor prognosis, composed of poorly differentiated tumor cells with giant bizarre tumor cells, very different from those of conventional adenocarcinoma.

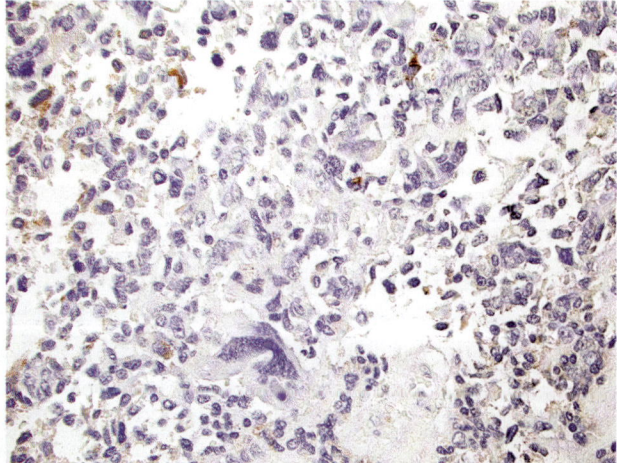

Figure 1.241. The same case from Figure 1.240 shows negative staining for prostate-specific antigen (PSA) in the pleomorphic giant cells and minimal staining in the adjacent mononuclear cells.

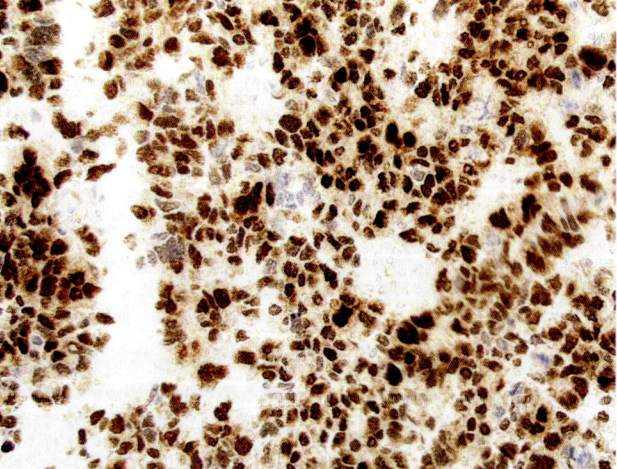

Figure 1.242. NKX3.1 immunohistochemical staining appears to be one of the most helpful markers for confirming the prostatic origin of pleomorphic giant cell prostate cancer (same case from Figures 1.240 and 241).

Prostatic Adenosquamous Carcinoma

When encountering a neoplasm with mixed features of prostatic adenocarcinoma and squamous or urothelial carcinoma, it is important to ensure that this does not represent coincidence of both prostate cancer and urothelial carcinoma. However, rare prostate cancers do transition from adenocarcinoma to squamous differentiation (Figures 1.243 and 1.244), sometimes in the posttreatment setting.[150,151] Helpful clues to support this occurrence would include 1) absence of urothelial carcinoma by history or in adjacent areas of the urothelium and 2) intimate admixture of prostatic adenocarcinoma (with positive prostatic immunohistochemical markers) and squamous carcinoma. We have occasionally used molecular techniques in this setting, to show the same gene fusion (such as *ERG* rearrangement) in both components.[151] However, *ERG* fusions are only present in 40% to 50% of prostate cancers, so a negative result does not exclude prostate origin. Although *ERG* fusion may be present genetically, ERG immunohistochemical staining is not always present in poorly differentiated or neuroendocrine tumors, as the protein expression depends on androgen signaling.[152,153] As such, fluorescence in situ hybridization (FISH) or other molecular techniques may detect the fusion despite negative immunohistochemistry.

TUMORS WITH A NEUROENDOCRINE APPEARANCE

Prostatic Adenocarcinoma With Neuroendocrine Marker Staining

Prostate cancer histology inherently can resemble a neuroendocrine neoplasm, due to its relatively uniform cytology and occasional formation of rosette-like structures. It is important to note that even conventional prostate cancer can contain cells with neuroendocrine marker immunohistochemical staining, in as much as 30% to 100% of cases.[17] This is usually in a patchy distribution and in cells that otherwise resemble conventional prostate cancer cells and at present should not be interpreted as evidence of transformation from prostate cancer to a neuroendocrine neoplasm in the absence of suspicious morphology.

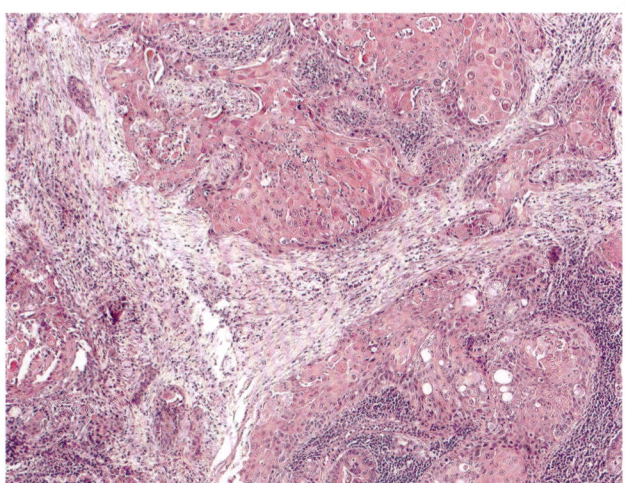

Figure 1.243. Rare prostate cancers can transition to squamous differentiation. This lymph node metastasis from a patient with prostatic adenocarcinoma showed abrupt transition to squamous differentiation in the metastatic lesion in lymph nodes only.

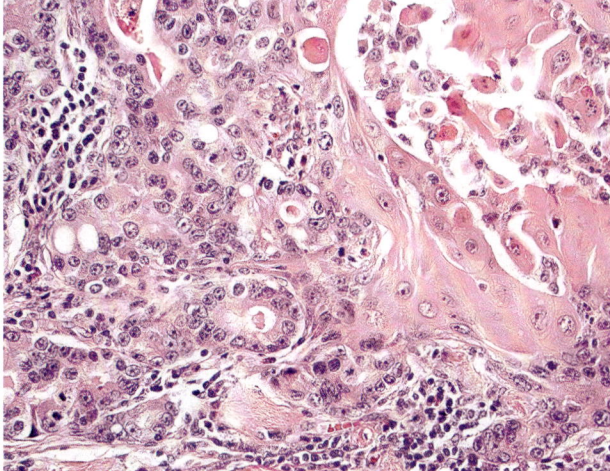

Figure 1.244. The same lesion from Figure 1.243 shows transition from prostatic adenocarcinoma (left) to squamous carcinoma (right). Immunohistochemistry (not pictured) showed intermingling of cells positive for prostatic and squamous markers.

FAQ: What Do I Do If a Clinician Asks to Test a Prostate Cancer for Neuroendocrine Differentiation (Small Cell Carcinoma)?

Clinicians may sometimes ask the pathologist if there is evidence of neuroendocrine differentiation (such as small cell carcinoma) in a tumor that was otherwise reported as a conventional prostate cancer, especially in patients with an atypical pattern of metastatic disease or with a lack of response to therapy. If immunohistochemistry is then applied, showing some patchy neuroendocrine marker staining, it may lead to confusion as to whether the tumor has developed a neuroendocrine phenotype. In this scenario, we typically recommend against using neuroendocrine marker immunohistochemistry unless there is a morphologic suspicion of small cell carcinoma or another specific neuroendocrine variant, as the significance of even moderate amounts of neuroendocrine marker staining in an otherwise conventional prostate cancer is not clearly established at present.[17] If immunohistochemical staining has already been done, showing patchy positive cells, but the features still do not appear to be those of small cell or neuroendocrine carcinoma, it can be reported that there is focal or patchy positive staining but that overall the features do not meet criteria for small cell carcinoma or another variant. In this scenario, the clinical significance is uncertain at present.

Prostatic Adenocarcinoma With Paneth Cell–Like Neuroendocrine Cells

A specific variant of prostatic adenocarcinoma contains tumor cells with prominent eosinophilic cytoplasmic granules.[18,154,155] This has been termed Paneth-like neuroendocrine cells for its resemblance to Paneth cells of the gastrointestinal tract; however, this is likely a misnomer, as true Paneth cells are not neuroendocrine cells. Rather, these cells are probably more akin to the eosinophilic neuroendocrine cells in the gastrointestinal tract (Figure 1.245).[17] At present, this pattern is not thought to have any clinical significance when it is identified in usual prostatic adenocarcinoma (Figures 1.246 and 1.247). The only relevance for the pathologist is that occasionally tumors may have solid-appearing nests composed of such cells, in which case usual grading would suggest pattern 4 or 5 (Figure 1.248). However, some data on these rare tumors suggest that they are not as aggressive as conventional cancers with pattern 4/5.[155] As such, the current recommendation is that such a solid component be excluded from grading, whereas gland-forming cancer with scattered Paneth-like cells can be graded as usual (pattern 3-4).[155]

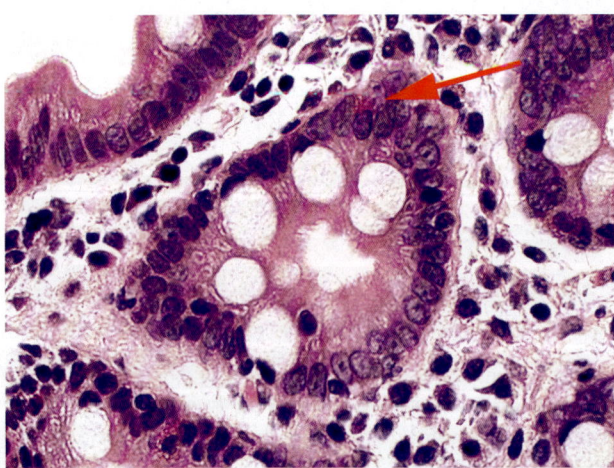

Figure 1.245. So-called "Paneth-like" neuroendocrine cells of the prostate are probably more akin to the neuroendocrine cells of the gastrointestinal tract (arrow) rather than true Paneth cells, which instead have larger granules above the nucleus.

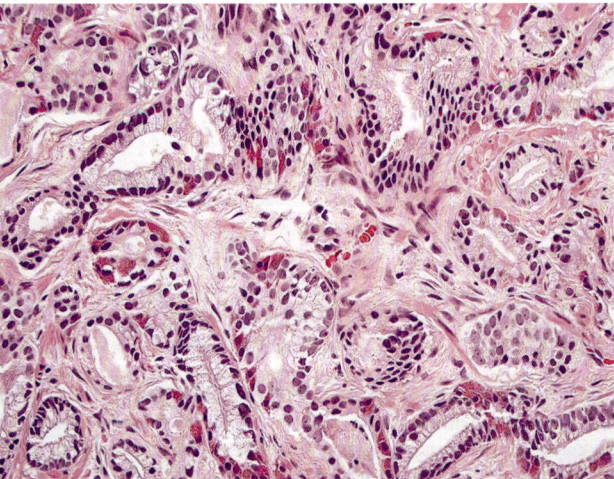

Figure 1.246. Occasional prostate cancers contain scattered cells with brightly eosinophilic granules, so-called Paneth-like neuroendocrine cells. In a case such as this with conventional architecture and only scattered eosinophilic cells, current thinking is that the tumor can be graded as usual.

In addition to tumors with these brightly eosinophilic granules, it has been recently recognized that a similar pattern of neuroendocrine cells with basophilic or amphophilic cytoplasm (without granules) also occurs (Figure 1.249).[156] This pattern would be even more prone to interpretation as Gleason pattern 5, as the eosinophilic granules are not present to identify the cells as neuroendocrine. A helpful clue, however, is that eosinophilic granular cells are often focally admixed with the nongranular cells (Figure 1.250). Like the eosinophilic counterpart, the current limited data on these rare variants suggest they not be graded, as the behavior seems to be more favorable than that of typical pattern 5 cancer.[155,156] Both the granular and nongranular forms of these neuroendocrine cells typically label for synaptophysin and chromogranin, and the proliferation rate assessed by Ki67 is low, in line with the hypothesis that these are not aggressive cancers.[155,156]

Carcinoid Tumor (Well-Differentiated Neuroendocrine Tumor)

Carcinoid tumor (well-differentiated neuroendocrine tumor) of the prostate has been reported; however, in modern classification, it is likely that most of these represent prostatic

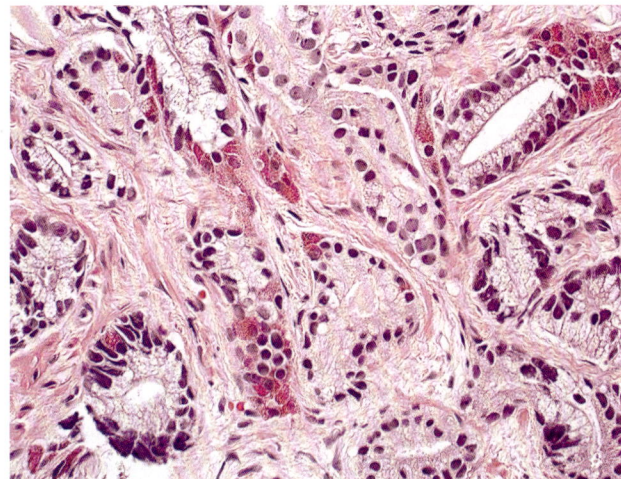

Figure 1.247. Higher magnification of the case from Figure 1.246 shows scattered cells with brightly eosinophilic granules. The prominence of these cells may vary based on laboratory staining techniques.

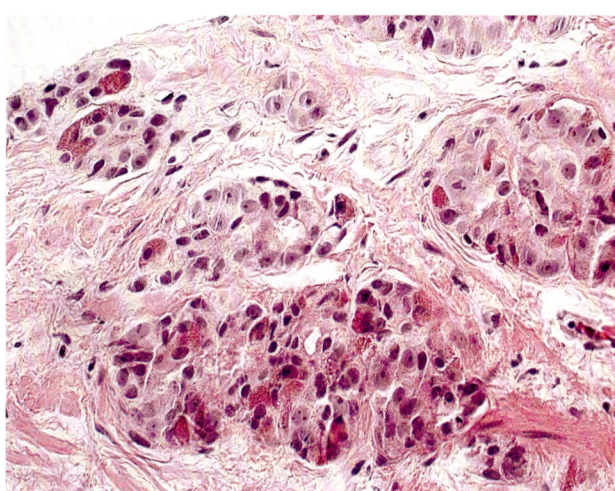

Figure 1.248. When Paneth-like neuroendocrine cells form solid nests in prostate cancer, current thinking is that they should not be graded, as this does not necessarily appear to be as aggressive as pattern 4 or 5 cancer based on the limited outcome data that are available.

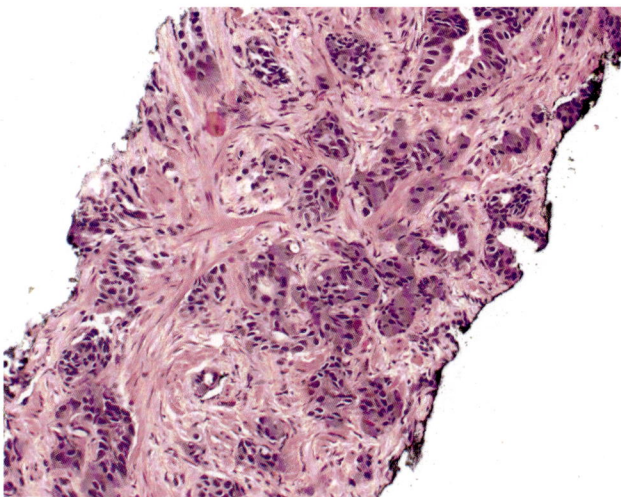

Figure 1.249. Rarely, a variant of prostate cancer with Paneth-like neuroendocrine cells lacking granules but with deeply amphophilic cytoplasm has been reported.

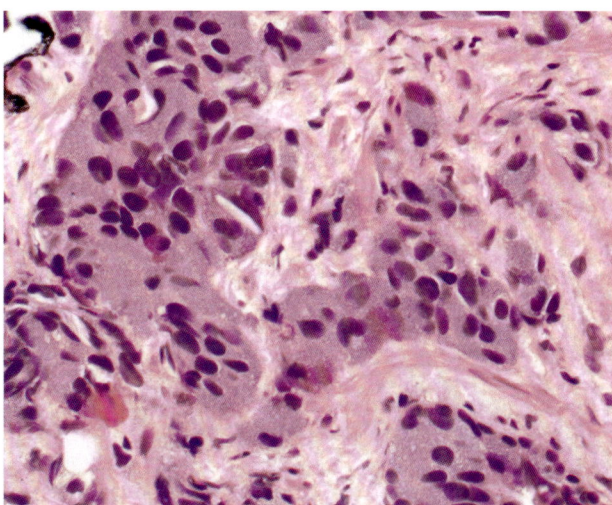

Figure 1.250. A clue to recognition of the rare prostate cancers with Paneth-like neuroendocrine cells showing amphophilic cytoplasm is that there is often a small component of eosinophilic cells admixed.

adenocarcinoma with neuroendocrine marker staining or a Paneth cell–like component.[17] As such, extremely restrictive criteria should be used before making a diagnosis of prostatic carcinoid, if ever. Associated prostatic adenocarcinoma should be absent, coupled with typical carcinoid morphology and negative PSA staining before rendering this diagnosis.

Prostate Cancer With Diffuse Neuroendocrine Marker Positivity

An emerging category of uncertain significance at present in prostatic adenocarcinoma that does not have definite neuroendocrine or small cell morphology, yet which has substantial neuroendocrine marker staining.[17,157] These tumors typically have both prostatic marker positivity (PSA, NKX3.1) and neuroendocrine marker positivity, and they are usually high grade, often occurring in patients with prior androgen deprivation therapy.[17] The histologic features of these tumors are somewhat variable, not corresponding well to a specific entity, like small cell carcinoma. Therefore, the precise role of this occurrence in diagnostic practice and clinical treatment remains to be better established.

SMALL BLUE CELL PATTERN TUMORS

SMALL CELL CARCINOMA

Prostate cancer can progress from typical adenocarcinoma to small cell neuroendocrine carcinoma (Figures 1.251 and 1.252), especially in the setting of long-standing treatment, such as androgen deprivation therapy. However, small cell carcinoma can also occur without prior treatment.[17] The features of these small cell carcinomas are similar to those of other organs, with neuroendocrine marker staining (synaptophysin Figure 1.253, chromogranin, CD56), and often TTF1 positivity (Figure 1.254). Frequently staining for PSA (Figure 1.255) or NKX3.1 is negative, and there is usually high proliferative activity (Ki67 >50%, often approaching 90% to 100%, Figure 1.256).[17] Therefore, the immunohistochemical phenotype is typically not helpful in determining whether the small cell carcinoma is arising from the prostate or another origin. The presence of *ERG* gene rearrangement in a small cell carcinoma would lend support to prostatic origin (although only present in 40%-50% of prostate cancers); however, it is noteworthy that in these tumors, ERG immunohistochemistry is typically negative, even with genetically confirmed fusion, due to the requirement of androgen signaling for protein expression.[17,153] Difficulty discriminating prostatic from another origin, such as the urinary bladder, may not be a major problem, since as the clinical paradigm generally shifts to a small cell carcinoma–like treatment plan without regard for the organ of origin.

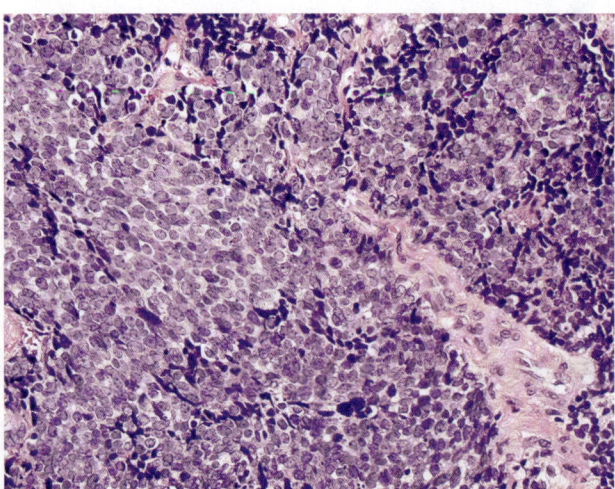

Figure 1.251. Occasional prostatic adenocarcinomas can progress to small cell neuroendocrine carcinoma, which shows similar features to small cell carcinoma of other organs, including a small blue cell pattern, crush artifact, nuclear molding, and stippled chromatin.

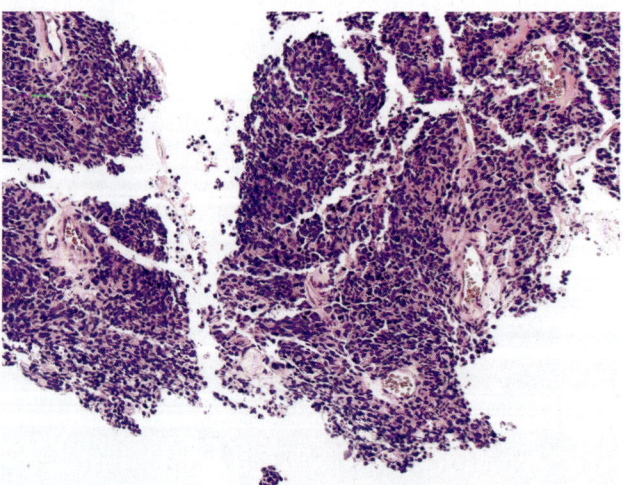

Figure 1.252. This small cell carcinoma of apparent prostatic origin demonstrates a cellular small blue cell pattern with tissue fragmentation.

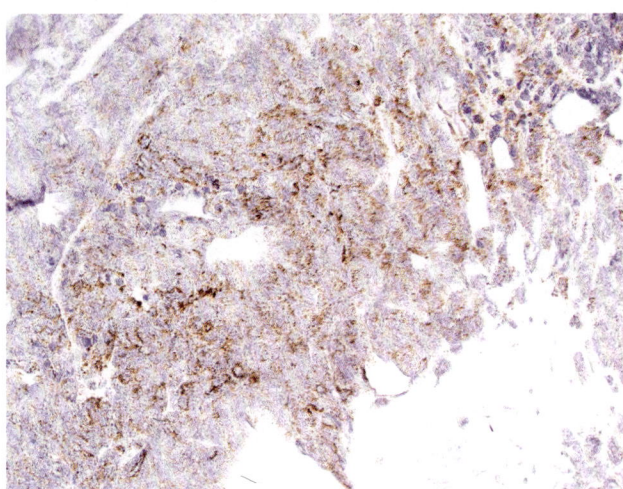

Figure 1.253. Prostatic small cell carcinomas usually show positivity for synaptophysin (pictured) and other neuroendocrine markers.

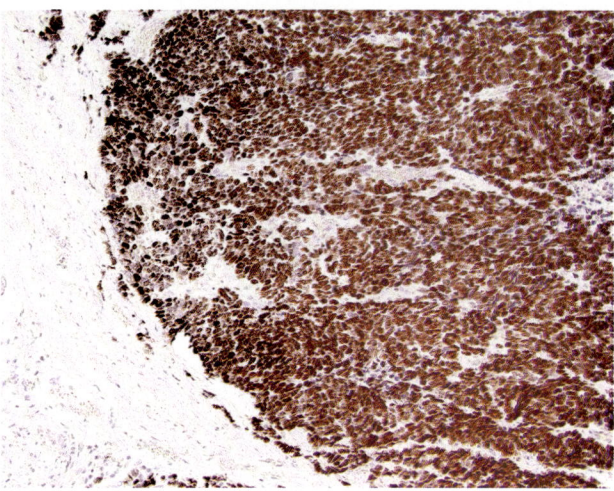

Figure 1.254. Prostatic small cell carcinoma can be positive for TTF1. Therefore, this should not be interpreted as suggesting lung origin.

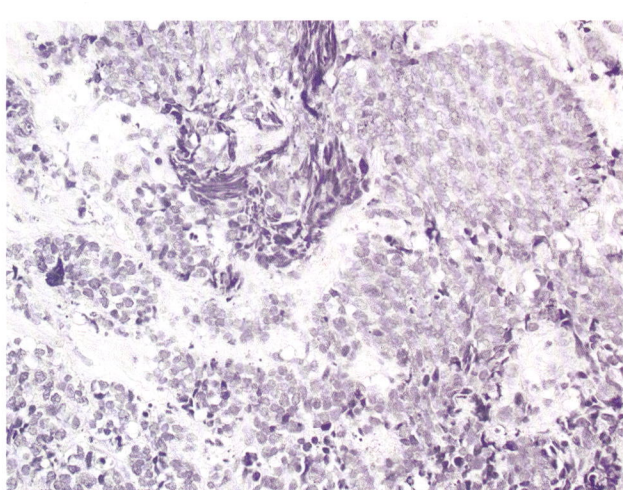

Figure 1.255. Immunohistochemical staining for prostate markers, like prostate-specific antigen (PSA) (pictured) and NKX3.1 is often absent in small cell carcinoma of prostate origin.

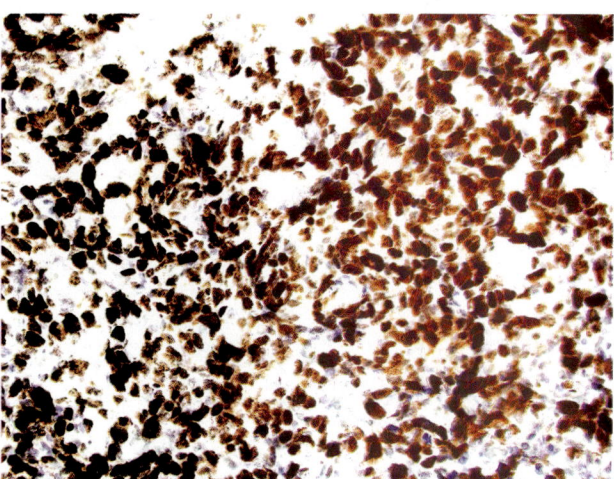

Figure 1.256. The Ki67 or MIB-1 proliferative rate is usually extremely high in small cell carcinoma of the prostate, which may aid in distinguishing it from high-grade conventional prostatic adenocarcinoma.

SMALL CELL–LIKE CHANGE IN PROSTATIC NEOPLASMS

An unusual morphologic pattern has been described in prostatic neoplasms including PIN and invasive and intraductal carcinoma, referred to as small cell–like change.[158,159] In this morphologic pattern, large glands, often with cribriform architecture, show a peripheral layer of cells with typical prostate cancer cytology, surrounding a central area of basophilic cells with scant cytoplasm, resembling small cell carcinoma (Figures 1.257 and 1.258). Although it is tempting to hypothesize that this might represent an early form of transformation to neuroendocrine differentiation, these structures are largely lacking evidence of neuroendocrine differentiation, with negative synaptophysin and chromogranin staining and low Ki67 proliferation indices. Interestingly, they may nonetheless have some positivity for TTF1.[158,159] It is currently unclear if this represents a phenomenon of degenerative changes of the luminal cells or maturation of the luminal cells compared with the peripheral cells; however, a less prominent degree of cytologic changes can be seen more commonly in cribriform structures (Figures 1.259 and 1.260), suggesting that this represents the extreme end of the morphologic spectrum of this change.

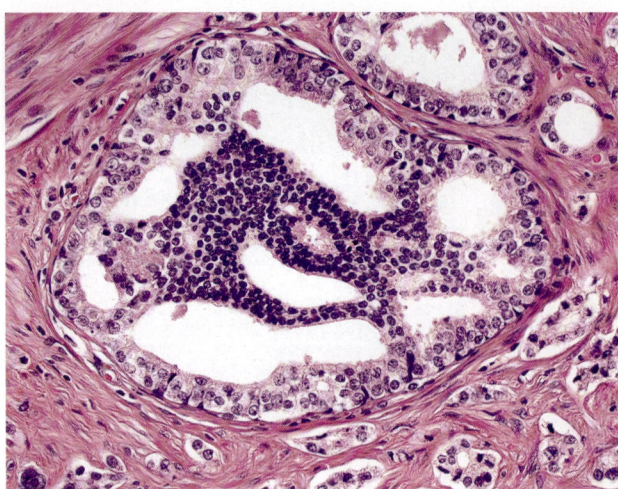

Figure 1.257. An unusual phenomenon referred to as "small cell–like change" within prostatic neoplasms shows a component of small blue cells that does not seem to be related to true neuroendocrine differentiation, based on lack of neuroendocrine marker staining and low proliferative activity.

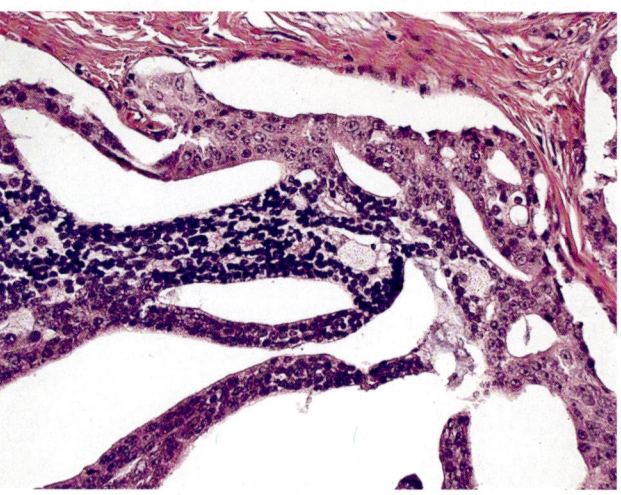

Figure 1.258. In small cell–like change, the peripheral tumor cells have typical features of prostatic adenocarcinoma with prominent nucleoli, whereas the central cells have much smaller, blue, crowded nuclei.

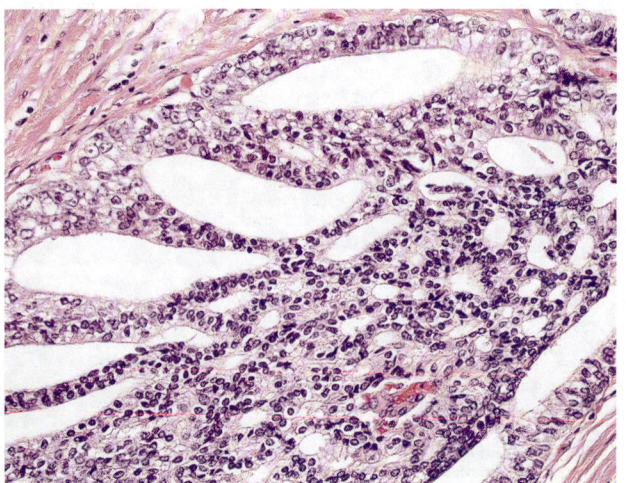

Figure 1.259. Small cell–like change may represent the extreme end of a more common morphologic pattern. This cribriform structure in a prostatic adenocarcinoma shows typical cancer nuclei peripherally and smaller, more condensed nuclei centrally.

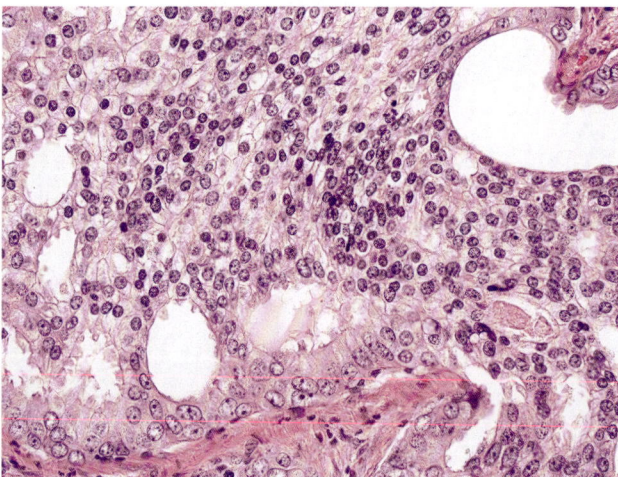

Figure 1.260. In this cribriform structure in prostate cancer, the peripheral nuclei have prominent nucleoli, whereas the central nuclei are smaller with less conspicuous nucleoli. This may be the early end of the spectrum of the same phenomenon as small cell–like change.

POORLY DIFFERENTIATED PROSTATIC ADENOCARCINOMA

In some cases, including metastatic and primary prostatic samples, poorly differentiated prostatic adenocarcinoma of Gleason score 5 + 5 = 10 (Grade Group 5) or similar grade can raise a differential diagnosis of small cell carcinoma (Figure 1.261). In this setting, it may be helpful to test for neuroendocrine markers, prostatic markers (PSA, NKX3.1), Ki67 proliferative activity, and TTF1. Small cell carcinomas usually will have a paucity of prostate marker positivity, positive neuroendocrine marker staining, and occasionally TTF1 positivity. The Ki67 index will usually be extremely high in small cell carcinoma (>50% and often approaching 90%), whereas this is not typical of even high-grade prostatic adenocarcinoma.[17]

OTHER SMALL BLUE CELL PATTERN TUMORS

Other small blue cell patterns tumors are relatively rare in the prostate. The prostate can be involved by various types of lymphoma.[160,161] In children, the prostate and bladder are established sites for the development of embryonal rhabdomyosarcoma.[162,163]

STROMAL LESIONS

INFLAMMATORY PROCESSES

Some degree of acute or chronic inflammation is not unusual in the prostate (Figure 1.262), and typically, diagnoses of acute prostatitis and chronic prostatitis should be avoided based solely on pathology specimens, as these are primarily clinical diagnoses. It is generally optional to report the presence of focal inflammation in prostatic specimens. When present, acute and chronic inflammation often are associated with prostatic glands, possibly representing inflammatory reaction to duct obstruction. Extensive, monotonous chronic inflammation that does not follow a periglandular distribution (Figure 1.263) should raise concern for prostatic involvement by lymphoma, which is not unthinkable given the frequency of diseases such as chronic lymphocytic leukemia/small lymphocytic lymphoma in the older population in whom prostate diseases are more common.[161] Conversely, some prostatic adenocarcinomas can be deceptively infiltrative with single cells such that they can mimic inflammation (Figures 1.264 and 1.265).

Nonspecific Granulomatous Prostatitis

One pattern of inflammation encountered frequently in the prostate is so-called nonspecific granulomatous prostatitis.[16,164] This is thought to occur from idiopathic duct obstruction and rupture, often forming an impressive nodule of histiocytic cells and chronic inflammation, sometimes with a spindle-shaped or epithelioid appearance of the histiocytic cells that may mimic a neoplasm (Figures 1.266-1.269). This may also form a clinical lesion on the digital rectal examination. The association with ducts and presence of scattered giant cells are helpful in recognizing this as an inflammatory and not a neoplastic process; however, if necessary, epithelial or prostatic immunohistochemical markers such as cytokeratin, PSA, or NKX3.1 may be used to argue against an epithelial neoplasm.

Other Patterns of Granulomatous Prostatitis

Other than nonspecific granulomatous prostatitis, other recognizable patterns of granulomas in the prostate include those from bacillus Calmette-Guérin (BCG) therapy for urothelial carcinoma. This often manifests as large necrotizing granulomas (Figure 1.270), in which case the clinical history of either BCG therapy or bladder cancer in general is usually sufficient to conclude that the necrotizing granulomas are related to this treatment. Secondly, previous transurethral resection can form granulomas with a pattern reminiscent

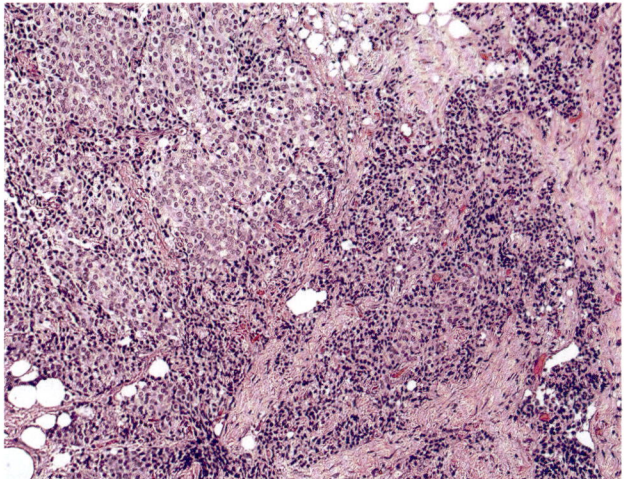

Figure 1.261. This high-grade prostatic adenocarcinoma transitions from areas of solid pattern 5 morphology to crushed cells with indistinct cytoplasm, raising the question of small cell or neuroendocrine differentiation. However, neuroendocrine markers were negative in this case and the immunohistochemical phenotype was similar to the adjacent adenocarcinoma, arguing against small cell carcinoma.

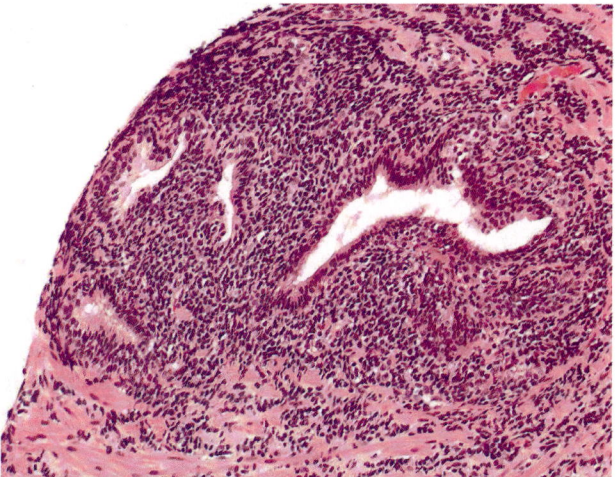

Figure 1.262. It is not unusual for prostatic specimens to have some degree of chronic, or less frequently, acute inflammation, especially in a periglandular distribution. It is typically not advisable to use the terminology acute/chronic prostatitis, as these are clinical diagnoses; however, descriptive terms acute and chronic inflammation can be used.

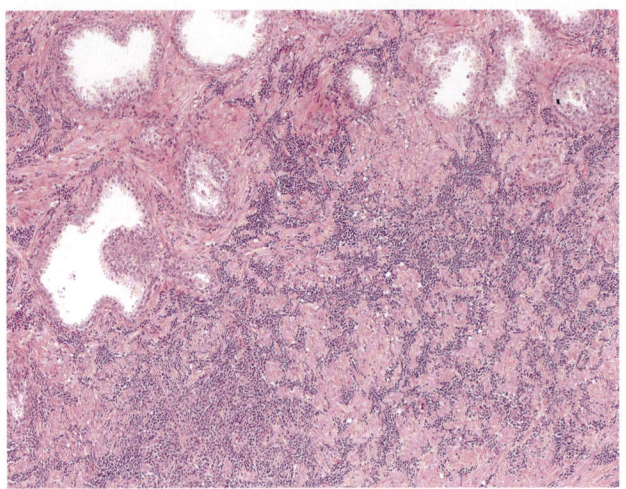

Figure 1.263. When there is extensive chronic inflammation in prostatic specimens, especially when it is not in a periglandular distribution, it is worth considering the possibility of prostate involvement by lymphoma, such as chronic lymphocytic leukemia/small lymphocytic lymphoma in this case. This is also relatively common in the older patient demographic in whom prostate cancer is most common.

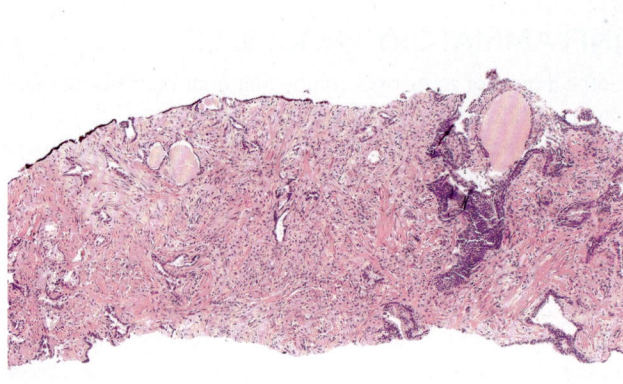

Figure 1.264. Occasionally infiltrative prostate cancers with single cells can mimic an inflammatory process. This example shows an area of atrophy with infiltrating single cells of prostatic adenocarcinoma that could be mistaken for inflammatory cells at low magnification.

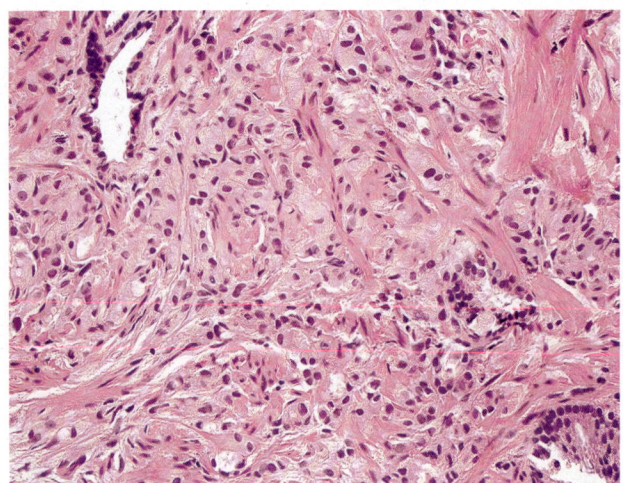

Figure 1.265. At high magnification, the same case from Figure 1.264 shows the mononuclear cells to be cancer cells.

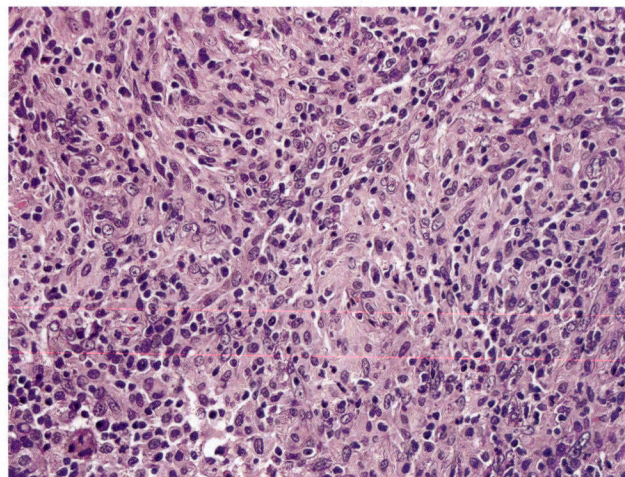

Figure 1.266. Nonspecific granulomatous prostatitis manifests as sheets of histiocytes, which may be spindle-shaped, and associated chronic inflammation. This may form a palpable nodule on the digital rectal examination.

of a rheumatoid nodule, showing central fibrinous debris, surrounded by a palisading rim of histiocytic cells (Figures 1.271 and 1.272).[164] Again, confirming a history of prior transurethral resection is usually sufficient to verify this etiology, making special stains for microorganisms typically unnecessary. In the absence of one of these recurring patterns, it may be reasonable to investigate for specific infectious organisms, such as fungi or mycobacteria.

Malakoplakia

Malakoplakia sometimes occurs in the prostate, similar to its involvement of other organs. As in other sites, it is associated with long-standing urinary tract infections, such as with *Escherichia coli* in most cases, followed by *Klebsiella pneumoniae*, among others. Some cases are associated with concomitant prostate cancer (Figure 1.273).[165] As in other sites, malakoplakia can be recognized by the sheets of epithelioid histiocytes (von Hansemann cells) containing targetoid structures (Michaelis-Gutmann bodies) that are positive for von Kossa (calcium) and periodic acid–Schiff (PAS) stains.

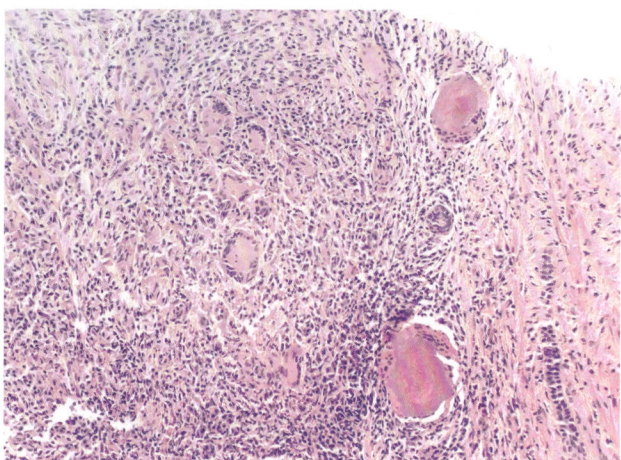

Figure 1.267. Histiocytic giant cells can be a clue to the nature of the process in nonspecific granulomatous prostatitis.

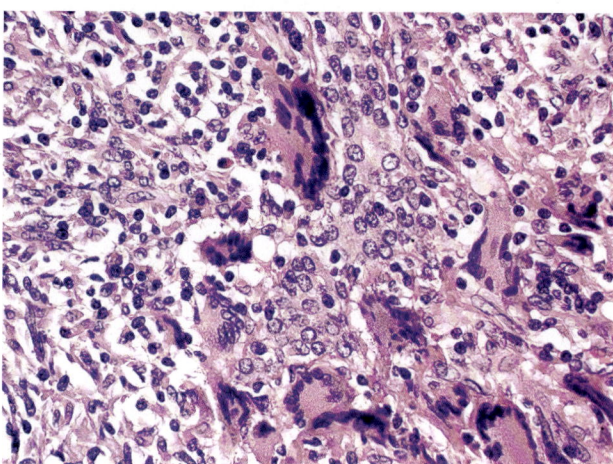

Figure 1.268. Care should be taken to avoid misdiagnosis of nonspecific granulomatous prostatitis as a neoplasm, particularly when the histiocytic cells are epithelioid or if they may mimic giant tumor cells.

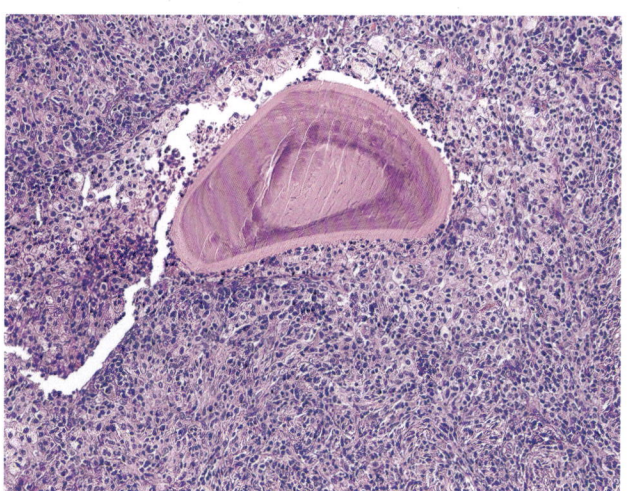

Figure 1.269. In this case of nonspecific granulomatous prostatitis, entrapment of corpora amylacea lends support to the hypothesis that this results from duct rupture.

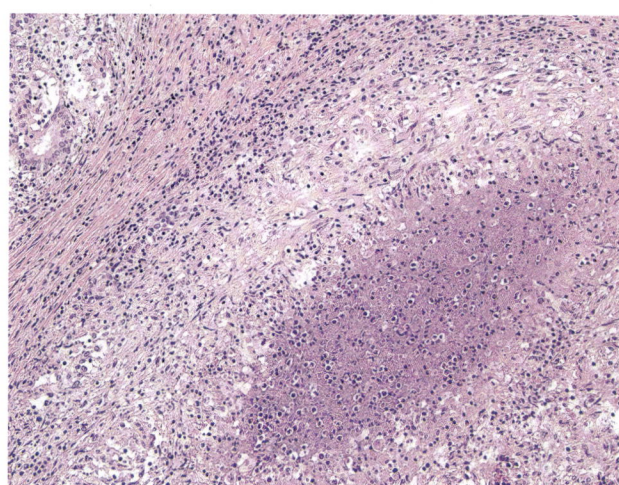

Figure 1.270. The typical etiology for large necrotizing granulomas in the prostate is prior bacillus Calmette-Guérin (BCG) therapy. If there is a clinical history of BCG treatment or bladder cancer, this is usually sufficient to conclude that the granulomas are the result of BCG treatment.

NONNEOPLASTIC PROCESSES

Benign Prostatic Hyperplasia (Stromal)

Nodular hyperplasia of the prostate ranges from nodules resembling normal glandular tissue to a mixture of hypercellular stroma and glands to nodules entirely composed of stroma. The latter is usually readily recognizable as a stromal nodule in the typical context; however, stromal nodules rarely can cause diagnostic challenges when extensive or in unusual contexts, such as presenting as a bladder mass or lesion (see Chapter 2). When extensive stromal predominant nodular hyperplasia is present in prostatic specimens, especially transurethral resections, the differential diagnosis of prostatic stromal or mesenchymal neoplasms may be considered. The three most helpful histologic findings of stromal nodules are hypercellular stroma, prominent blood vessels with thickened walls, and a sprinkling of lymphocytes (Figures 1.274-1.277). If there is extensive stromal hyperplasia making up multiple slides, the best tool for distinguishing from a prostatic stromal tumor (discussed later) is to identify discrete nodules. Whereas hyalinized vessels are typical of stromal nodules, some authors note these to be less conspicuous in prostatic stromal tumors, with a more diffuse growth pattern.[163,166]

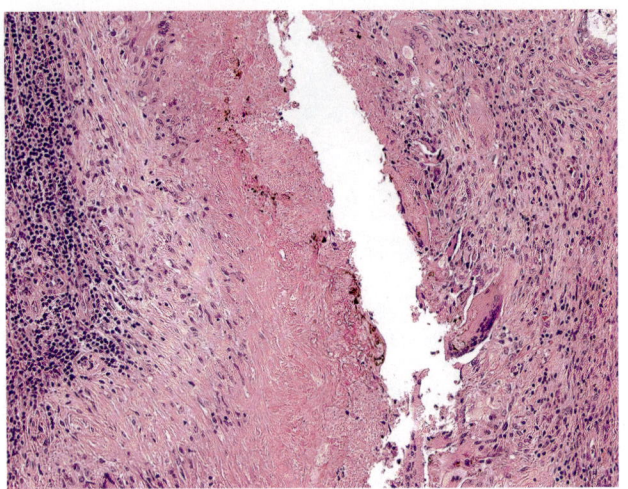

Figure 1.271. Previous transurethral resection granulomas in the prostate often manifest as necrobiotic debris surrounded by a rim of palisaded histiocytes, resembling a rheumatoid nodule.

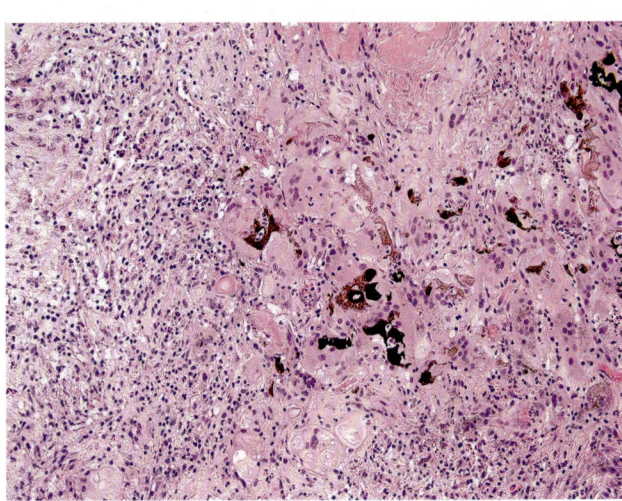

Figure 1.272. Previous transurethral resection granulomas may also contain histiocytes engulfing red-brown material, likely representing the cauterized tissue from the prior resection.

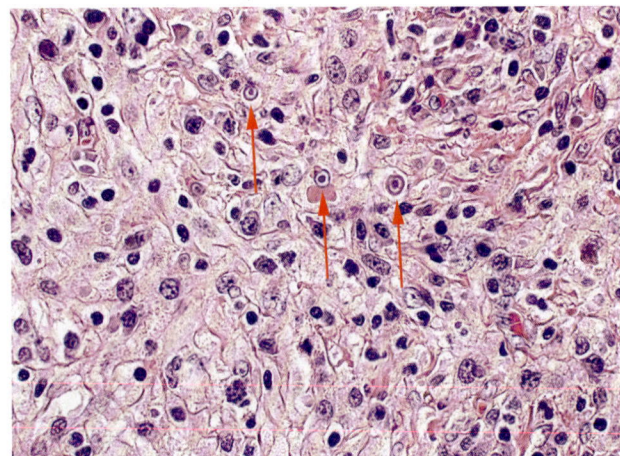

Figure 1.273. Malakoplakia can occasionally involve the prostate, with similar features to its involvement of other sites. Michaelis-Gutmann bodies are noted with arrows.

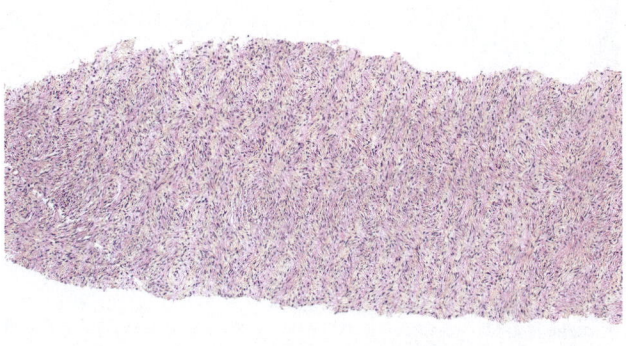

Figure 1.274. Prostatic stromal nodules are composed of cellular spindle-shaped cells and can occasionally be captured in needle biopsy samples.

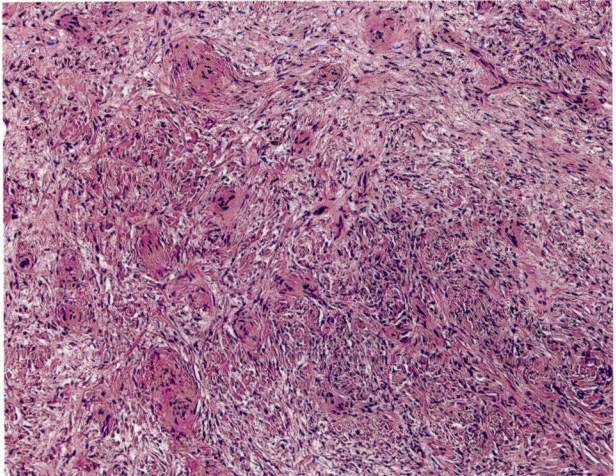

Figure 1.275. Characteristic features of prostatic stromal nodules include cellular stroma and blood vessels with slightly hyalinized, thickened walls.

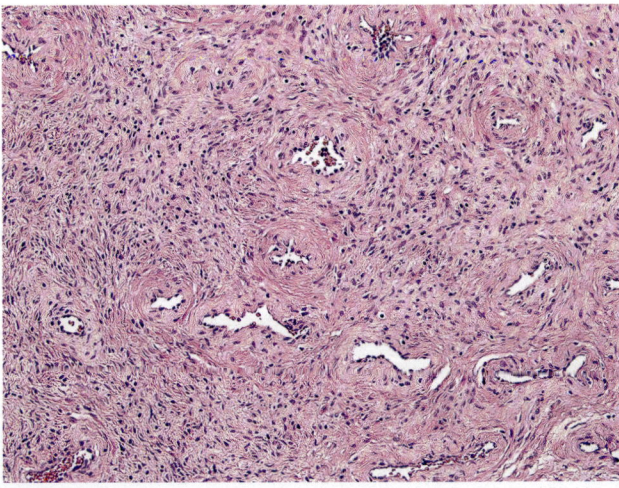

Figure 1.276. In this prostatic stromal nodule, the prominent blood vessels and loose cellular stroma are appreciable. There are scattered lymphocytes in the stroma.

NEOPLASTIC PROCESSES

Stromal Tumor of Uncertain Malignant Potential

The most common mesenchymal neoplasm of the prostate is the so-called stromal tumor of uncertain malignant potential (STUMP), which has been variably known by other names, including atypical stromal hyperplasia, prostatic stromal hyperplasia with bizarre nuclei, and phyllodes tumor, among others.[163,166] In the absence of frank sarcoma, prostatic STUMP typically behaves in an indolent manner, typically cured by complete surgical resection. Several main histologic patterns have been described. The most common resembles nodular hyperplasia but contains abnormal stromal cells with degenerative, smudged-appearing nuclear chromatin (Figures 1.278 and 1.279). Other patterns include hypercellular stromal overgrowth (without the large atypical cells, Figures 1.280-1.282), a myxoid pattern (Figure 1.283), a phyllodes-like pattern with leaf-like structures invaginating into the epithelium (Figure 1.284), and a round cell pattern.[167,168] Associated epithelial proliferations have also been described in association with STUMP, including crowded glands, prominent basal cells (Figures 1.283 and 1.284), papillary projections, basal cell hyperplasia, cribriform hyperplasia, or urothelial or squamous metaplasia.[169]

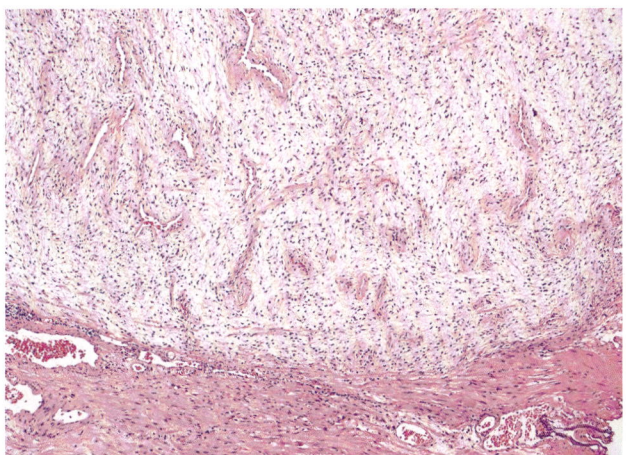

Figure 1.277. Occasional prostatic stromal nodules have a more myxoid appearance.

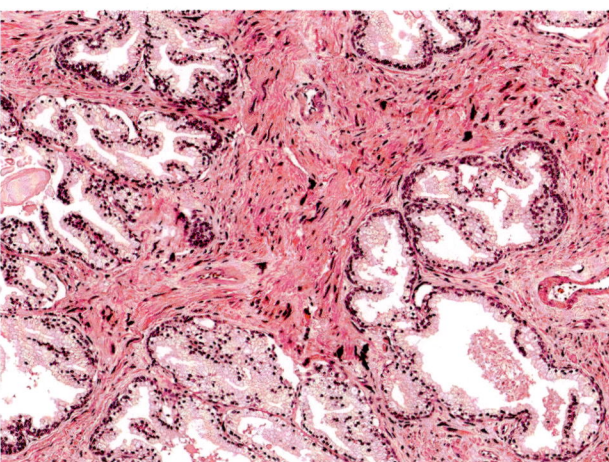

Figure 1.278. The most common pattern of prostatic stromal tumor of uncertain malignant potential (STUMP) is composed of nodular hyperplasia–like tissue, with large atypical hyperchromatic stromal cells.

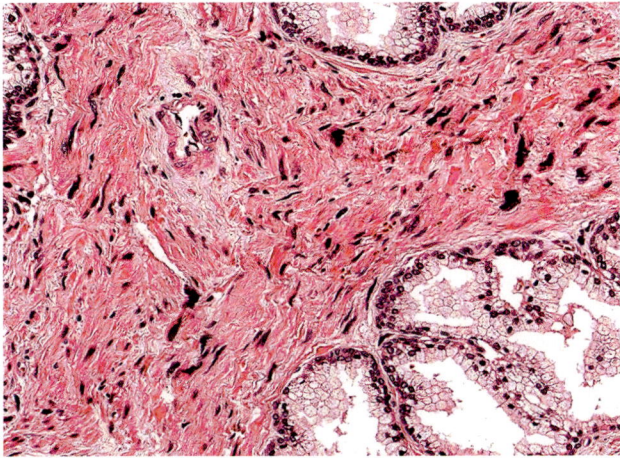

Figure 1.279. The stromal cells in stromal tumor of uncertain malignant potential (STUMP) often have a smudged, degenerative-appearing chromatin pattern.

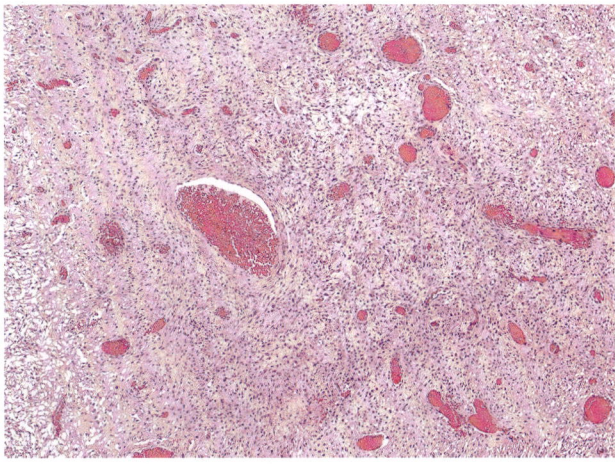

Figure 1.280. An alternate pattern of stromal tumor of uncertain malignant potential (STUMP) is diffuse growth of stroma without large atypical cells but lacking the nodular architecture of nodular hyperplasia. This example includes some prominent vessels, reminiscent of nodular hyperplasia.

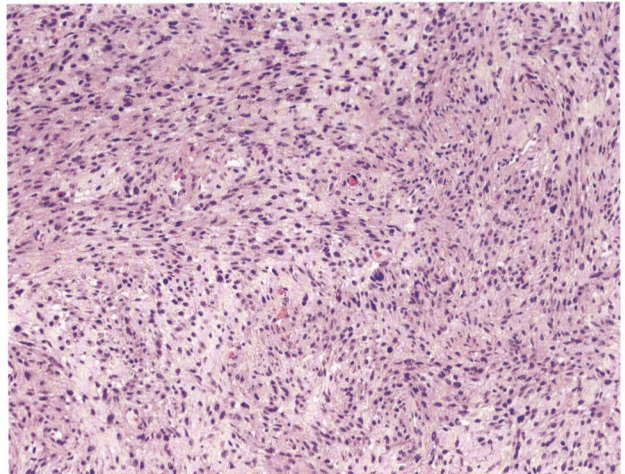

Figure 1.281. At higher magnification, the case from Figure 1.280 shows monotonous proliferation of prostatic stromal cells without distinct nodular architecture.

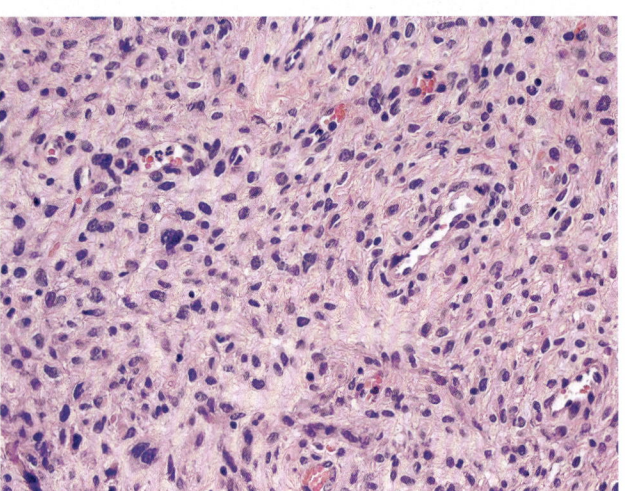

Figure 1.282. At high magnification, this stromal tumor of uncertain malignant potential (STUMP) has very mild cytologic atypia, which would be unusual for nodular hyperplasia.

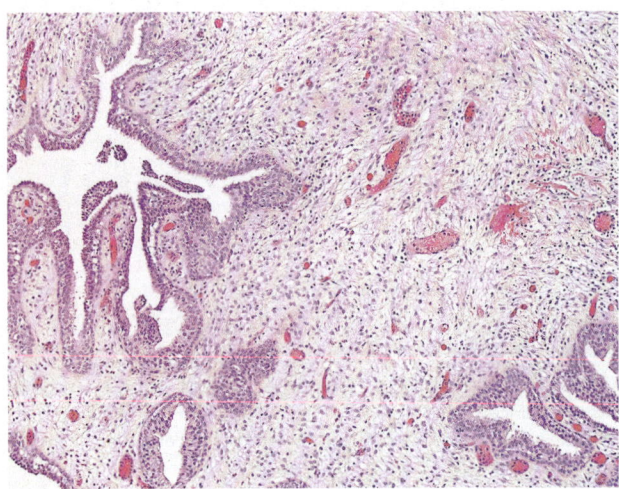

Figure 1.283. Other patterns of stromal tumor of uncertain malignant potential (STUMP) include more myxoid stroma. This example also includes prominent basal cells in the glandular epithelium, which is one of the recognized epithelial proliferations in STUMP.

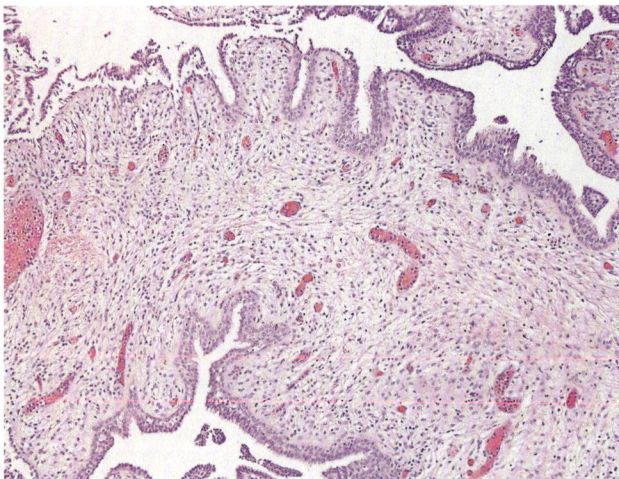

Figure 1.284. This prostatic stromal tumor of uncertain malignant potential (STUMP) has slightly myxoid stroma and a suggestion of phyllodes-like invagination into the epithelium. There are prominent basal cells in the glandular epithelium.

Recognizing nodular hyperplasia–like tissue with markedly enlarged, degenerative stromal cells essentially clinches the diagnosis. However, for the other patterns, the most helpful discriminator from conventional nodular hyperplasia is the presence of discrete nodules in nodular hyperplasia vs sheet-like overgrowth of one element in STUMP. Immunohistochemistry is not necessarily of great help in this differential. STUMP is commonly positive for CD34 and progesterone receptor, variably for estrogen receptor and smooth muscle markers, such as smooth muscle actin and desmin.[163,166] However, these findings overlap significantly with other mesenchymal tumors that may be in the differential diagnosis, such as gastrointestinal stromal tumor (GIST), leiomyoma, leiomyosarcoma, or solitary fibrous tumor. The histologic pattern resembling nodular hyperplasia is overall the most helpful feature in discrimination from other mesenchymal tumors, supplemented by occasional selective immunohistochemical markers, such as STAT6 to discriminate solitary fibrous tumor (positive) from STUMP (negative or focal positive),[170] or DOG1 for GIST (positive).

Stromal Sarcoma

Even rarer than STUMP is its unequivocally malignant counterpart, prostatic stromal sarcoma, which may occur as a transition or dedifferentiation from STUMP.[167] Features discriminating stromal sarcoma from STUMP include increased cellularity, cytologic atypia, mitotic activity (or atypical mitotic figures), and necrosis (Figures 1.285-1.287).[163,166,167,171] In contrast to STUMP, stromal sarcoma is aggressive and requires multidisciplinary management, similar to other sarcomas.

Sarcomatoid Carcinoma

In contrast to the bladder, in which sarcomatoid carcinoma should be near the top of the differential diagnosis list for most spindle cell proliferations, sarcomatoid carcinoma is extremely rare but not impossible in the prostate.[172] It should usually be considered carefully among a differential diagnosis that includes sarcomatoid urothelial carcinoma involving the prostate, STUMP, sarcoma, and other mesenchymal tumors. Features that can assist in confirming a diagnosis of sarcomatoid prostate cancer include coexistent high-grade prostatic adenocarcinoma (Figure 1.288) or positivity for prostate markers in an epithelial component, with transition to the sarcomatous malignancy. Also, a history of urothelial carcinoma or nearby urothelial neoplasm should typically be absent, unless there is exceptional evidence to support two collision neoplasms. We have occasionally used molecular techniques to support that a sarcomatous malignancy is of prostatic origin, such as by demonstrating *TMPRSS2-ERG* fusion,[151] in challenging cases.

Solitary Fibrous Tumor

Solitary fibrous tumor is worth particular discussion, as the genitourinary tract is a known site of occurrence[166,171,173-175] and there can be substantial overlap between the morphology of STUMP (predominantly the stromal hyperplasia–like pattern without atypical cells) and solitary fibrous tumor (Figures 1.289-1.291). CD34 immunohistochemistry is of little help, as both can be positive. However, with the recent recognition of *STAT6* gene fusion in solitary fibrous tumor, immunohistochemistry for STAT6 has emerged as a helpful marker. Although focal staining for STAT6 has been reported in STUMP, labeling is much more consistent and diffuse in true solitary fibrous tumor.[170] Other clues can include the hemangiopericytoma-like vascular pattern of solitary fibrous tumor, contrasting to the occasional hyalinized round vessels of nodular hyperplasia or STUMP.

Other Spindle Cell Lesions

Although specialized stromal tumors of the prostate are the most common spindle cell lesions of this organ, other neoplasms can arise in the prostate, including leiomyosarcoma,

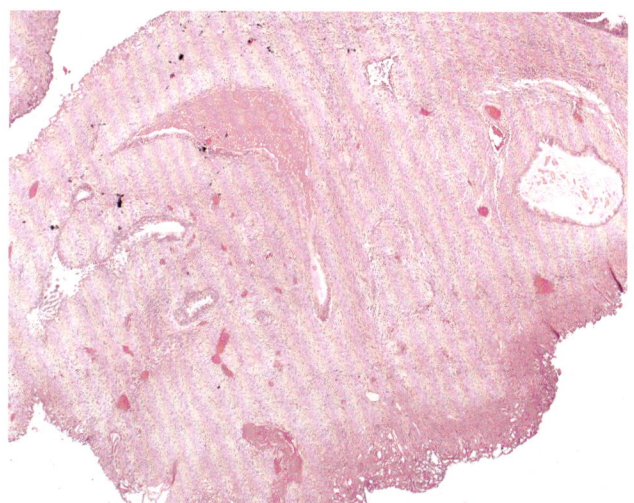

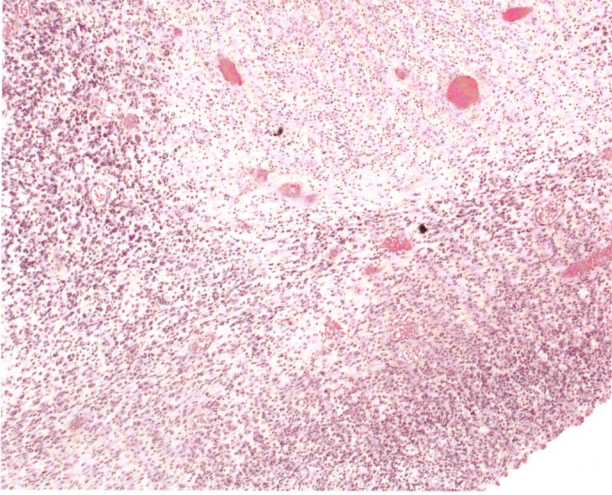

Figure 1.285. In this patient with prostatic stromal sarcoma, there is a background of stromal tumor of uncertain malignant potential (STUMP) with hypercellular stroma.

Figure 1.286. Other areas from the same patient from Figure 1.285 show a progression to a more cellular neoplasm with cytologic atypia.

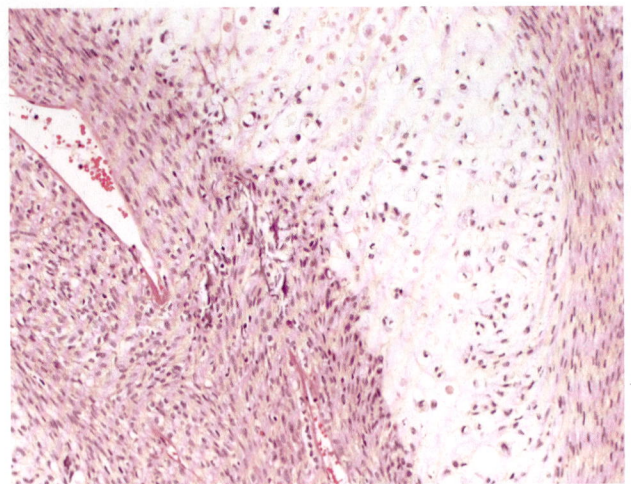

Figure 1.287. This prostatic stromal sarcoma includes areas of cartilaginous differentiation.

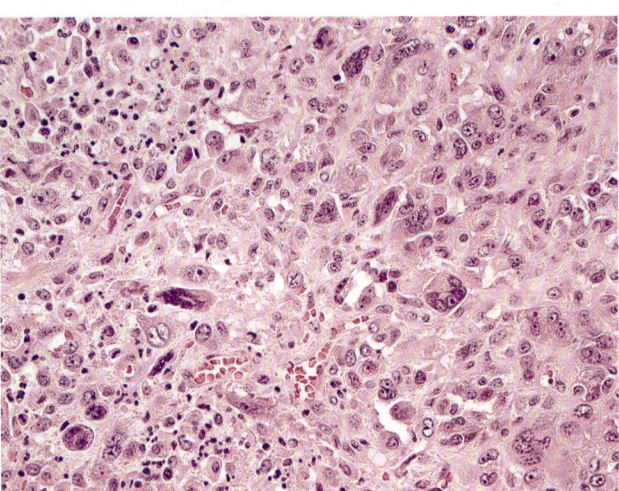

Figure 1.288. Although much rarer than sarcomatoid urothelial carcinoma, occasional prostatic adenocarcinomas can become sarcomatoid. This patient had a prior resection of high-grade prostatic adenocarcinoma and later developed a recurrent perirectal tumor with sarcomatoid morphology and minimal immunohistochemical positivity for epithelial markers.

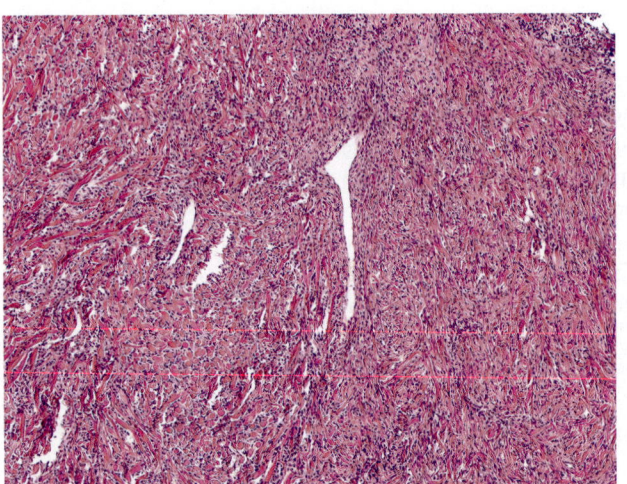

Figure 1.289. Solitary fibrous tumor can occur in the prostate and can have morphologic overlap with stromal tumor of uncertain malignant potential (STUMP). This case demonstrates a spindle cell solitary fibrous tumor with a suggestion of staghorn or hemangiopericytoma-like vasculature.

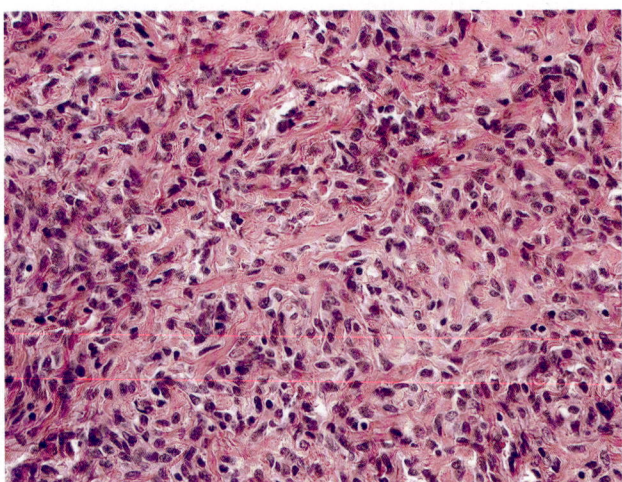

Figure 1.290. At higher magnification, this prostatic solitary fibrous tumor shows spindle-shaped cells with intervening collagen. This tumor was positive for STAT6 immunohistochemistry (not pictured), supporting solitary fibrous tumor over stromal tumor of uncertain malignant potential (STUMP).

rhabdomyosarcoma, solitary fibrous tumor, and myofibroblastic proliferations. Rarely GIST can be sampled in prostatic biopsy, likely typically representing rectal GIST mimicking a prostatic mass or being inadvertently sampled via the transrectal approach.[176] Leiomyoma occurs extremely rarely in the prostate, with many of the historical reports probably representing STUMP. As such, this diagnosis should be made with great caution and only with ample resection specimens (transurethral resection or surgical resection) rather than biopsy.[163] In contrast, leiomyosarcoma does occur at this location and has similar features to leiomyosarcoma of other sites, including evidence of smooth muscle differentiation (either as evidenced by classic smooth muscle morphology or ideally at least two immunohistochemical markers positive, of which we typically use smooth muscle actin, caldesmon, and desmin). This would be coupled with cytologic atypia or mitotic activity to indicate malignancy and without the features of STUMP discussed previously. Rhabdomyosarcoma also occurs in the bladder or prostate, primarily in childhood, almost all of which are embryonal subtype. Other soft tissue–type tumors that have been reported include angiosarcoma and rare others.

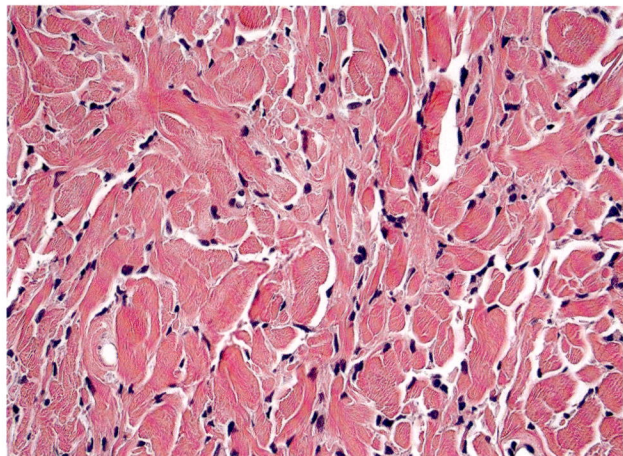

Figure 1.291. Solitary fibrous tumor can also have more prominent intercellular collagen.

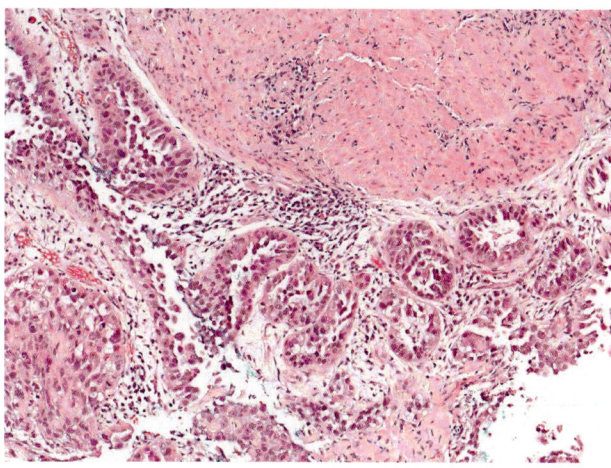

Figure 1.292. Primary seminal vesicle adenocarcinoma is extremely rare. This tumor detected in a prostatic needle biopsy was positive for PAX8 and cytokeratin 7 and negative for GATA3, cytokeratin 5, p63, prostate-specific antigen (PSA), and prostate-specific membrane antigen (PSMA), supporting a primary seminal vesicle carcinoma. (Courtesy of Matthew J. Wasco, MD, St. Joseph Mercy Health System.)

TUMORS OF THE SEMINAL VESICLE

SEMINAL VESICLE CARCINOMA

Primary seminal vesicle carcinoma has been reported, but it is vanishingly rare and should be diagnosed only when there is clear evidence of a tumor primarily originating from the seminal vesicle and not the prostate, bladder, rectum, or other organs.[177] These tumors may be large and solid or cystic. They often show papillary or glandular patterns (Figure 1.292), and immunohistochemistry may show positivity for cytokeratin 7, sometimes cytokeratin 20, and typically not PSA.[177,178] Exceedingly rare squamous cell carcinomas of the seminal vesicle have been reported.

MIXED EPITHELIAL AND STROMAL TUMOR

Mixed epithelial and stromal tumor of the seminal vesicle, also known as cystadenoma, fibroadenoma, phyllodes tumor, among numerous other names, is a rare benign neoplasm of the seminal vesicle formed by spindle cell stroma and benign glandular epithelium.[177,179]

MESENCHYMAL TUMORS OF THE SEMINAL VESICLE

Various mesenchymal tumors of the seminal vesicle have been reported, generally with similar features to those of soft tissue sites, including leiomyoma (some of which might actually represent mixed epithelial and stromal tumor), schwannoma, mammary-type myofibroblastoma, and solitary fibrous tumor, among others.[177]

REPORTING ELEMENTS FOR PROSTATIC SPECIMENS

Other works have described recommended reporting for prostatic specimens in detail.[180-183] This chapter will emphasize some pragmatic aspects in prostate cancer reporting, including most recent updates and areas of controversy and continued debate.

BIOPSY REPORTING

In prostate biopsy samples, the most agreed upon parameters considered necessary for reporting include the grade and extent of cancer per specimen (per jar/bottle). There is no universal agreement for how to report extent (i.e., either percentage or millimeter length), but it is recommended that some form of quantification be given for needle biopsy specimens (see Sample Note). At present, it remains reasonable to give both the Gleason score and Grade Group (see Sample Note), although it may be possible in the future to report only Grade Groups, as the comfort with this system increases, possibly eventually replacing the Gleason score completely.

SAMPLE NOTE: Documenting Prostatic Adenocarcinoma in Needle Biopsy

Prostate, left lateral mid, core needle biopsy:

- Prostatic adenocarcinoma, Gleason score 3 + 3 = 6 (Grade Group 1), involving 40% of the length of one core (4 mm tumor focus)

FAQ: Should I Report Separate Grades and Extents of Multiple Cores in the Same Slide?

It is debated whether it is necessary to report separate grades and quantification per biopsy core when there are multiple readily identifiable cores in the same specimen container. On the one hand, the clinician submitting multiple biopsies in the same container would imply that he or she does not need separate diagnoses. However, if the cancer in such separate cores is significantly different, such as one core showing Gleason score 3 + 4 = 7 (Grade Group 2) and another showing Gleason score 4 + 4 = 8 (Grade Group 4), it would be reasonable to convey this information, as it could potentially represent two separate tumors in the prostate. Our approach is to give separate diagnoses if it would make a significant difference to the overall grade. Otherwise, the cancer can be lumped into a single diagnosis (see Sample Notes). In some samples, if either numerous cores are submitted together or if there is extensive fragmentation, or both, it is impossible to determine how many cores are involved.[182] In these cases, it is reasonable to report simply an overall percentage of involvement (i.e., 20% of the tissue from multiple fragmented cores, or similar wording).

SAMPLE NOTE: Documenting Prostatic Adenocarcinoma in Multiple Cores With the Same Grade

Prostate, left lateral mid, core needle biopsy:

- Prostatic adenocarcinoma, Gleason score 3 + 3 = 6 (Grade Group 1), involving 40% of the tissue, 2 of 2 cores (up to 5 mm tumor focus)

SAMPLE NOTE: Documenting Prostatic Adenocarcinoma in Multiple Cores With Different Grades

Prostate, left lateral mid, core needle biopsy:

- Prostatic adenocarcinoma, Gleason score 4 + 4 = 8 (Grade Group 4), involving 20% of the length of one core (3 mm tumor focus)
- Prostatic adenocarcinoma, Gleason score 3 + 4 = 7 (Grade Group 2), involving 30% of the length of a separate core (4 mm tumor focus); percentage of Gleason pattern 4 = 30%

KEY FEATURES: Prostate Biopsy reporting

- Perineural invasion is currently an optional reporting parameter, as it has not consistently been found to have prognostic relevance in multivariable analyses.[182] We currently document it when easily recognized in biopsy samples but not in radical prostatectomy samples, in which it is almost ubiquitous

- If benign seminal vesicle/ejaculatory duct tissue is present in a needle biopsy, it is reasonable to note it for documentation purposes. It is largely not possible to distinguish seminal vesicle from ejaculatory duct in a biopsy sample. Therefore, if cancer invades this tissue, it should be reported with a comment explaining that it may not necessarily represent pT3b disease if from the intraprostatic ejaculatory duct

- If carcinoma involves adipose tissue in a needle biopsy, especially when tumor cells are found on both sides of adipocytes (Figures 1.293 and 1.294), it can be reported that extraprostatic extension is present (at least pT3a)

FAQ: What Is a Global or Composite Grade for Prostate Biopsy?

There is good agreement that each separately submitted specimen should receive its own grade and cancer quantification. In addition to this, some pathologists have proposed that a global or composite grade, considering all the positive biopsies and giving an estimated overall grade, may be helpful to the clinician.[184-186] For example, when multiple biopsies show Gleason score 3 + 4 = 7 (Grade Group 2) and one biopsy shows a minute focus of Gleason score 4 + 4 = 8 (Grade Group 4), the typical clinical paradigm would be to label the patient as having Grade Group 4 cancer. However, this is often an overestimate,[184] if the tumor is Grade Group 2 and a small pattern 4 area has been captured fortuitously at the edge of the tumor in one biopsy. Conversely, other authors would argue that this is best left to the clinician, who might incorporate other factors into decision-making, such as imaging findings.[96] At present, it is optional to give a composite or global grade, in addition to separate grades per specimen.

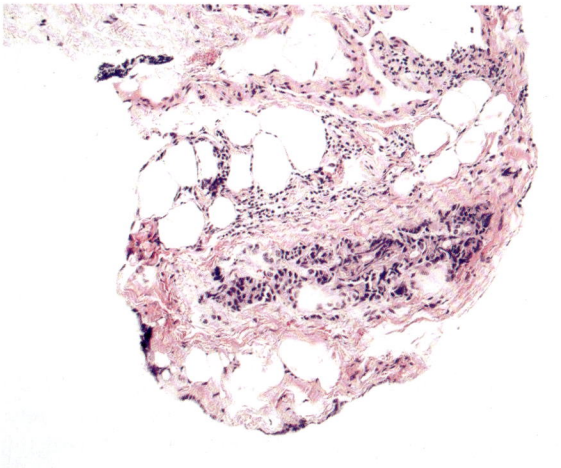

Figure 1.293. If prostatic adenocarcinoma is clearly within adipose tissue, extraprostatic extension can be diagnosed in a needle biopsy sample, such as in this case which shows adipocytes on both sides of the carcinoma cells.

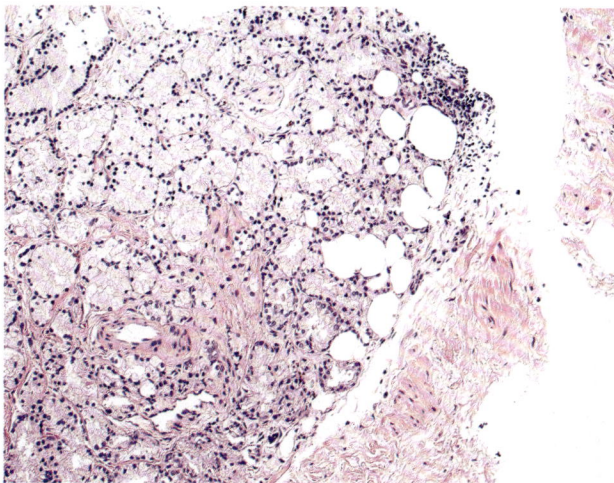

Figure 1.294. In this needle biopsy of prostatic adenocarcinoma, extraprostatic extension can be diagnosed due to intermingling of the carcinoma with adipocytes.

FAQ: Which Biopsy Parameters are Most Important for Active Surveillance Eligibility?

Historically, some of the most common pathology criteria for enrollment in active surveillance[187-189] included

- Gleason score 6 or less
- Maximum two positive biopsy sites (cores)
- Less than 50% involvement of the most involved core

However, various institutions have utilized other schemes for active surveillance eligibility, such as increasing the limit of positive cores to three cores or 33% to 50% of cores/sites. Gleason score 3 + 4 = 7 (Grade Group 2) is also increasingly being allowed in some schemes.[187-189] Since we may not be aware which criteria a given urologist will use for surveillance eligibility, we recommend considering each inflection point carefully, especially making a first diagnosis of pattern 4 in a patient who would otherwise have Grade Group 1 cancer.

FAQ: How Do I Report Prostate Cancer With a Gap of Benign Intervening Tissue Within the Cancer?

As less than 50% involvement of a single core is one of the more common requirements for active surveillance eligibility, the way the pathologist measures the cancer may affect surveillance eligibility. If there is a sizable gap of benign tissue intervening and it is included in the measurement (Figures 1.295 and 1.296), the involvement could be measured at greater than 50%, making the patient ineligible for surveillance. Several studies have investigated this problem.[190-194] In general, there remains incomplete agreement as to whether it is preferable to include the intervening benign tissue or mentally subtract it. Some data suggest that this is more likely to represent one large tumor rather than multiple incidental minute tumors.[190,191] Our approach, which is also endorsed by a recent expert consensus,[189] is to report the inclusive percentage with an explanatory comment (see Sample Note).

SAMPLE NOTE: Documenting Discontinuous Prostatic Adenocarcinoma in a Biopsy Core

Prostate, left lateral mid, core needle biopsy:

- Prostatic adenocarcinoma, Gleason score 3 + 3 = 6 (Grade Group 1), discontinuously involving 70% of the length of one core (two foci of 1 mm each, spanning 8 mm)—see Comment

Comment: Specimen A contains two foci of adenocarcinoma measuring 1 mm each but spanning an area of 8 mm of the biopsy core. The optimal method for quantification of tumor in such biopsies remains controversial (20% vs 70%). Two studies[192,193] have found that measuring such foci as if they were continuous correlated better with risk of extraprostatic extension and positive surgical margins than subtracting the intervening tissue, whereas another found neither method of measurement to be clearly superior in predicting biochemical recurrence.[194] Other data[190] indicate that this finding in approximately 75% of cases corresponds to a single tumor focus in same region of the radical prostatectomy specimen rather than multiple small tumors. Molecular biomarkers have shown a matching pattern in approximately the same percentage (75%) of cases,[191] with only 25% showing discordant biomarker patterns in the separate foci.

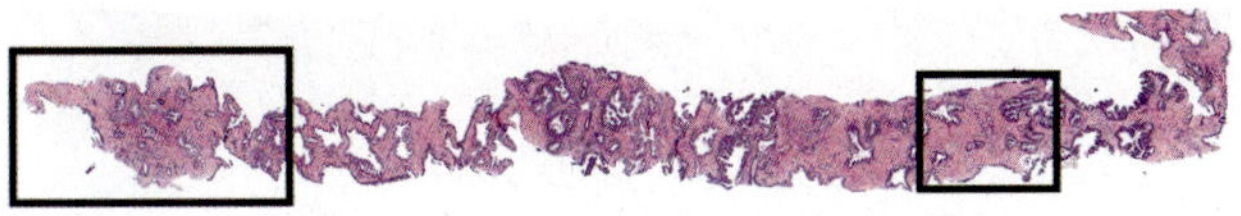

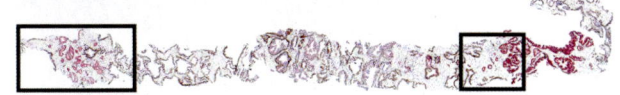

Figure 1.295. It is debatable how to quantify discontinuous involvement of prostate biopsies by cancer. This example shows two foci of prostatic adenocarcinoma (boxes) separated by a large gap of benign intervening tissue.

Figure 1.296. Immunohistochemistry with a dual-color basal cell and alpha-methylacyl-CoA racemase (AMACR) stain in the case from Figure 1.295 highlights the two foci of adenocarcinoma (boxes), with the right-sided focus arising associated with prostatic intraepithelial neoplasia (PIN). This cocktail stain also includes ERG protein staining, which showed that only the right focus was positive, suggesting two different unrelated clones of cancer.

Another parameter that is now recommended for reporting in prostate biopsy and radical prostatectomy specimens is the percentage of Gleason grade patterns, particularly percentage of pattern 4.[98] Coupled with the new Grade Group system which discriminates Gleason score 3 + 4 = 7 (Grade Group 2) from Gleason score 4 + 3 = 7 (Grade Group 3), documenting the percentage of pattern 4 will illustrate to the clinician whether the grade is closer to Grade Group 1 (with a low percentage of pattern 4) or approaching Grade Group 3 (with a high percentage of pattern 4). The latter patient would less likely be considered for active surveillance.

SAMPLE NOTE: Reporting Percentage of Gleason Pattern 4

Prostate, left lateral mid, core needle biopsy:

- Prostatic adenocarcinoma, Gleason score 3 + 4 = 7 (Grade Group 2), involving 30% of the length of one core (3 mm tumor focus); percentage of Gleason pattern 4 = 10%

RADICAL PROSTATECTOMY REPORTING AND STAGING

Other resources include frequently updated lists of relevant reporting parameters[195]; however, this chapter will address some select topics in pathologic staging and reporting of radical prostatectomy specimens that are diagnostically challenging or controversial.

Extraprostatic Extension

The simplest criterion for diagnosis of extraprostatic extension is when cancer extends into adipose tissue or breaks the plane of adjacent adipose tissue (Figures 1.297 and 1.298). This is relatively straightforward, as there is usually no adipose tissue within the prostate.[196] In the rare case when adipose tissue is abnormally within the prostate, it often has an unusual appearance with variable adipocytes, ranging from very small to usual size, intimately admixed with benign glands or nerves (Figures 1.299 and 1.300).[197] A more controversial criterion for diagnosing extraprostatic extension is when cancer bulges significantly beyond the contour of the prostate but does not involve adipose tissue (Figure 1.301).[9] It has been suggested that this can be diagnosed as extraprostatic extension in the posterolateral areas when it protrudes in this way and lacks a condensed band of smooth muscle stroma around the tumor. It is recommended that extraprostatic extension be quantified as either focal or nonfocal. The two most prevalent criteria for quantifying extraprostatic extension as focal include only a few glands outside the prostate[198] or less than one high-power field of extraprostatic extension in only one to two sections.[199]

Tertiary (or Minor High-Grade) Pattern

An area that remains somewhat controversial in prostate pathology reporting is documentation of a tertiary or minor high-grade pattern. Some pathologists would advocate that a third most prevalent pattern greater than 5% be moved to the secondary pattern, such that a tumor with 60% pattern 4, 30% pattern 3, and 10% pattern 5 would be diagnosed as Gleason score 4 + 5 = 9 (Grade Group 5).[200,201] Conversely, others would advocate that the

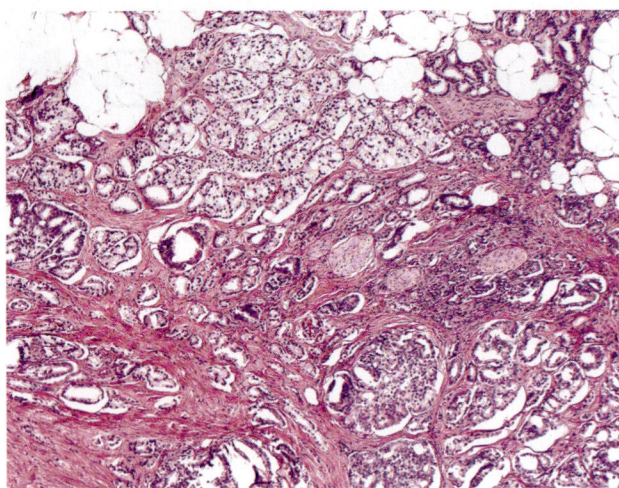

Figure 1.297. Extraprostatic extension can be diagnosed when prostate cancer breaks the plane into adipose tissue or directly involves adipose tissue.

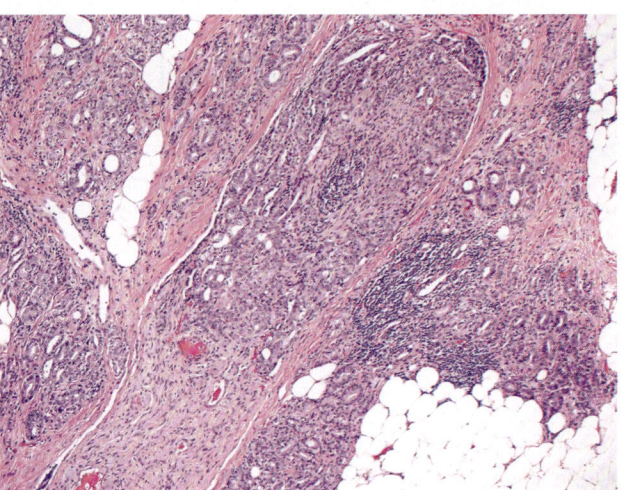

Figure 1.298. In this example of extraprostatic extension of prostatic adenocarcinoma, there are cancer glands at multiple planes within adipose tissue and intermingled with a large nerve.

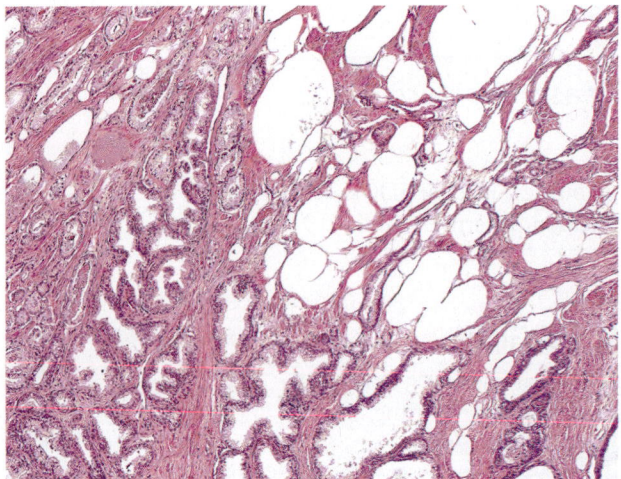

Figure 1.299. Very rarely adipose tissue can be intermingled with the prostate. In such cases, the adipose tissue often has unusual architecture with variable size adipocytes abnormally abutting glands or nerves. This field has adenocarcinoma at the left edge; however, adipose tissue is also present among benign glands (center and right).

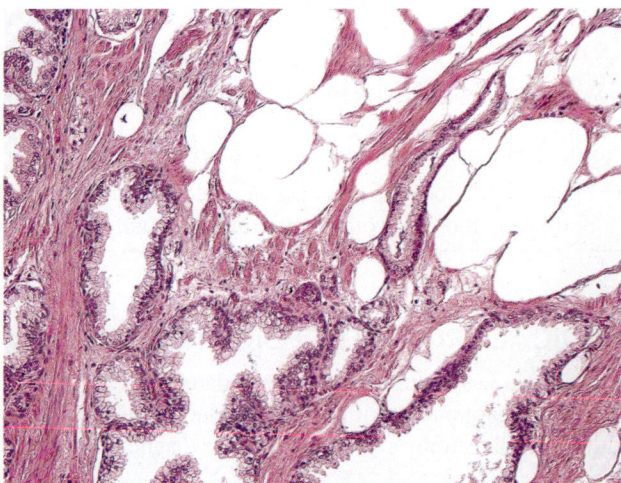

Figure 1.300. This rare example of intraprostatic fat shows abnormal small adipocytes abutting a benign gland at bottom and other adipocytes of varying sizes.

same tumor should be reported as Gleason score 4 + 3 = 7 (Grade Group 3) with tertiary pattern 5 (or with a minor high-grade pattern). At present, a larger fraction of experienced urologic pathologists are using the former method,[201] which is also endorsed by an expert consensus recommendation.[200] Some data presented in abstract form do support a cutoff between 5% and 10% as associated with biochemical recurrence.[202] As such, we are currently using the 5% cutoff with the caveat that this is debated.

Intraductal Carcinoma and Cribriform Cancer

There is considerable controversy over the reporting of intraductal carcinoma at present. In general, the current recommendation is that intraductal carcinoma is not graded, to account for the rare cases where the neoplastic proliferation is entirely intraductal or associated with only minimal invasive cancer. However, most experts currently agree that it is not necessary to perform immunohistochemistry solely for the purpose of excluding intraductal carcinoma from the grade, when there is overt and extensive high-grade (pattern 4 or higher) invasive cancer.[117,118] To our knowledge, there is no evidence at present that subtracting the intraductal component from the grade in this setting provides superior prognostication, and indeed this would be contrary to the many large controlled trials correlating Gleason grade with outcome that predated widespread recognition of intraductal carcinoma and routine use of immunohistochemistry. Therefore, our approach is to use immunohistochemistry only when there is suspicion that the entire tumor is intraductal, in which case the behavior may be more favorable than that of a Gleason score 4 + 4 = 8 (Grade Group 4) or similar tumor.

In addition to intraductal carcinoma, there is growing evidence that cribriform cancer is among the more aggressive patterns of prostate cancer.[119-125] Although this is not specifically required as a reporting parameter at present,[195] some pathologists are beginning to consider it as a potentially important parameter in future schemes.[122]

NEAR MISSES

ADENOSIS (ATYPICAL ADENOMATOUS HYPERPLASIA)

Adenosis or atypical adenomatous hyperplasia can be deceptive in prostatic specimens due to its composition of small crowded round glands. These may have several overlapping features with prostatic adenocarcinoma, including partial absence of basal cells, luminal crystalloids, and a small round gland architecture. Figure 1.302 illustrates an especially challenging case in a transurethral resection of the prostate which closely resembles low-grade adenocarcinoma by morphology. There is variable staining for AMACR (red). However, many of the glands have patchy basal cells (Figure 1.303). At high magnification, there is a small subset of glands with absence of basal cells and increased AMACR staining (Figure 1.304); however, interpreting this lesion as a whole would favor atypical adenomatous hyperplasia (adenosis).

DUCTAL PROSTATIC ADENOCARCINOMA INVOLVING URETHRA

When it occurs in prostatic biopsy specimens or radical prostatectomy specimens, ductal adenocarcinoma is generally readily recognizable due to its complex cribriform and papillary architecture. However, a deceptive scenario can manifest when ductal adenocarcinoma involves the urethra and presents to the urologist as potentially a urothelial neoplasm

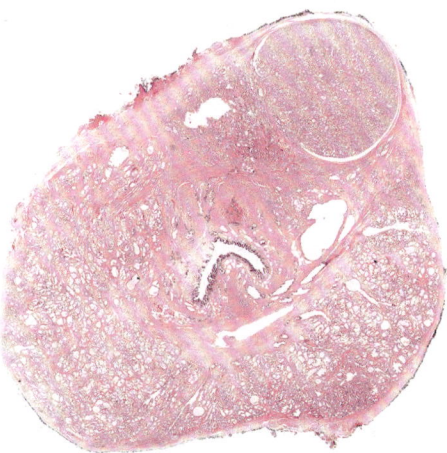

Figure 1.301. It is debatable whether prostate cancer that bulges well beyond the prostate without intermingling with adipose tissue should be considered extraprostatic extension. This example has a large, circumscribed nodule of low-grade adenocarcinoma in the anterior that markedly distorts the configuration of the prostate; however, it remains circumscribed with a thin layer of fibromuscular stroma.

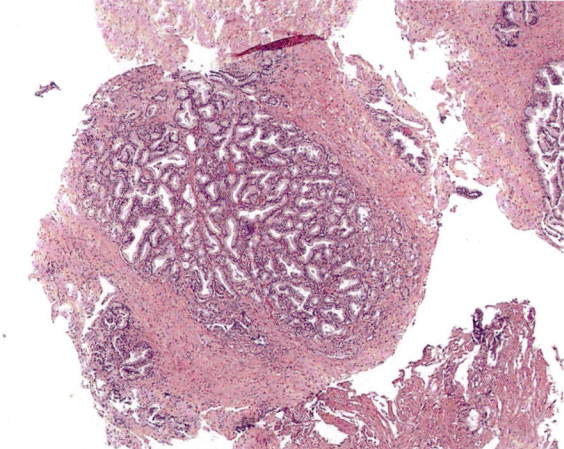

Figure 1.302. Adenosis (or atypical adenomatous hyperplasia) can sometimes be very deceptive in prostatic specimens, such as transurethral resection. This focus of crowded glands is suspicious for a low-grade adenocarcinoma.

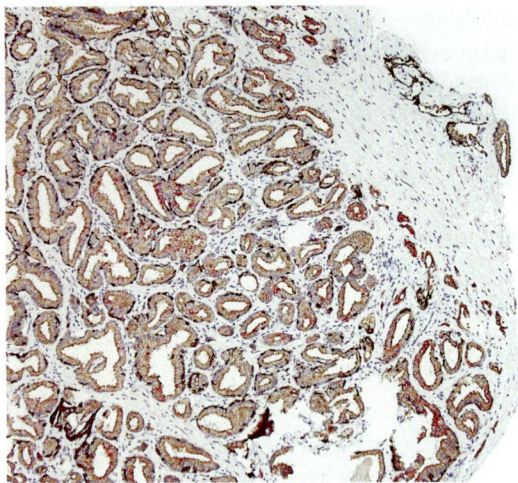

Figure 1.303. The same focus from Figure 1.302 using a basal cell (brown) and alpha-methylacyl-CoA racemase (AMACR) (red) dual-color stain shows that most of the glands have at least a patchy basal cell layer with variable positivity for AMACR.

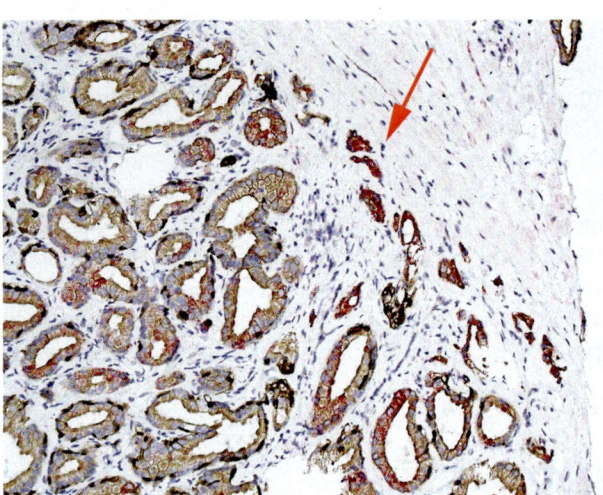

Figure 1.304. At higher magnification, the case from Figures 1.301 and 1.302 shows several glands with alpha-methylacyl-CoA racemase (AMACR) staining and absence of basal cells (arrow); however, this should not be interpreted as adenocarcinoma in the context of the entire lesion, which suggests adenosis.

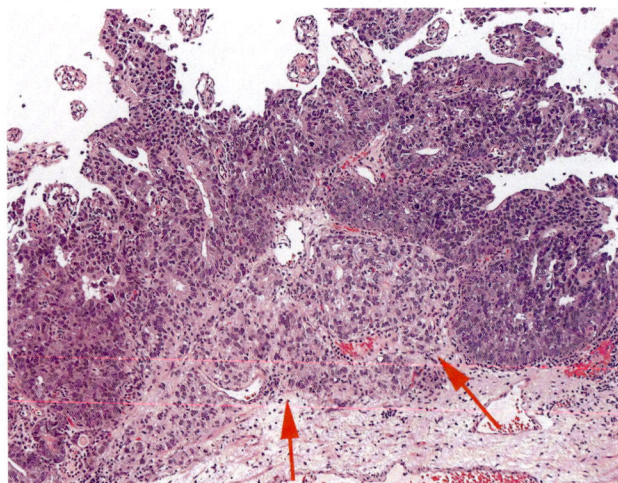

Figure 1.305. Occasionally ductal variant prostatic adenocarcinoma may lead to confusion with urothelial carcinoma, particularly when it involves the urethra or bladder. This case has a papillary surface component in the urethra, resembling a urothelial neoplasm; however, there is an underlying suggestion of cribriform glands (arrows), which is a clue to the diagnosis of prostatic adenocarcinoma.

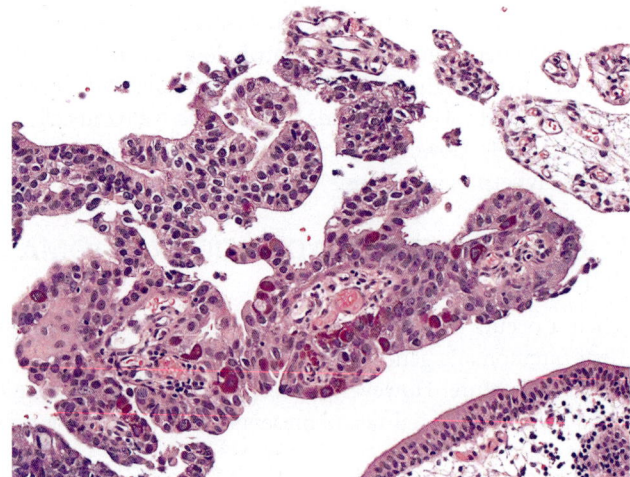

Figure 1.306. The papillary component of the same lesion from Figure 1.305 could also be confused for a papillary urothelial carcinoma; however, this field is notable for Paneth-like neuroendocrine with bright red granules, which is also a clue to the prostatic origin of this tumor.

(Figures 1.305 and 1.306). Although the classic appearance of papillary ductal carcinoma is relatively straightforward due to columnar cells with pseudostratified hyperchromatic nuclei, some areas of papillary ductal carcinoma can have low-grade atypia, mimicking a prostatic urethral polyp.

PARAGANGLION TISSUE

Ganglia are much more common in prostatic specimens than paraganglia. However, paraganglia can be much more deceptive due to their composition by a primarily solid architecture of pale cells (Figures 1.307-1.310), mimicking pattern 4 or 5 prostatic adenocarcinoma. Clues to this diagnosis include a spatially separate location from adenocarcinoma, if any is present, and sometimes adjacent ganglia with nerves and ganglion cells. If difficult cases, immunohistochemistry can be used, showing positive neuroendocrine markers and negative prostatic markers (Figures 1.309 and 1.310).

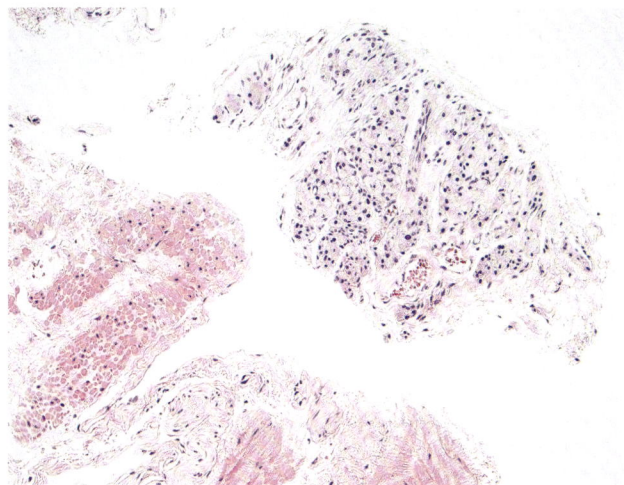

Figure 1.307. Paraganglion tissue may be deceptive in prostate biopsies. This field shows a solid nest of epithelioid cells with pale cytoplasm. A clue helping to identify it as paraganglion is that it is located at the edge of the core without associated glands.

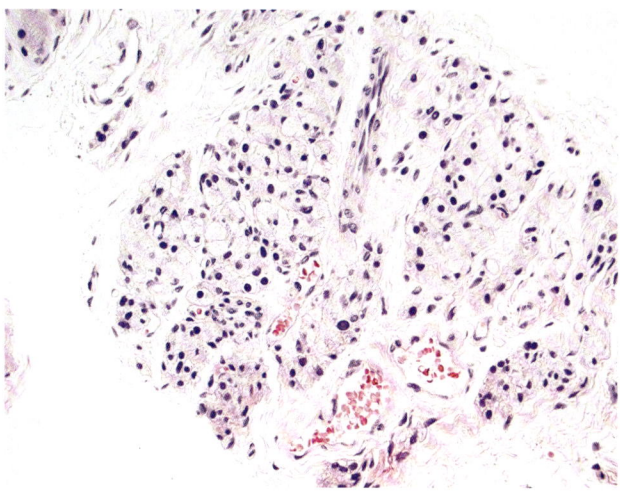

Figure 1.308. Higher magnification of the paraganglion from Figure 1.307 shows pale solid nests of cells, which could be confused for pattern 4 or 5 prostatic adenocarcinoma.

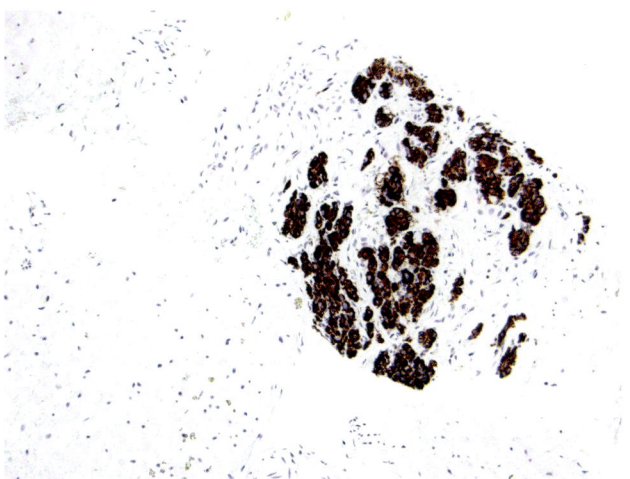

Figure 1.309. This paraganglion shows strong staining for chromogranin.

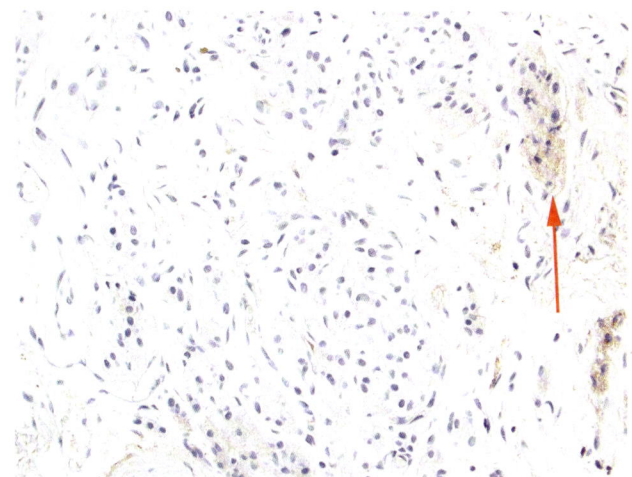

Figure 1.310. The paraganglion from Figures 1.307-1.309 is largely negative for prostate-specific antigen (PSA) immunohistochemical staining; however, there is focal weak staining at the edge (arrow), which could lead to misinterpretation as carcinoma if used in isolation.

UROTHELIAL CARCINOMA VS HIGH-GRADE PROSTATIC ADENOCARCINOMA

Although there are some general guides that discriminate urothelial carcinoma from prostatic adenocarcinoma, such as papillary architecture and increased pleomorphism in the former and cellular monotony and cribriform formation or rosette-like structures in the latter, a given case can be potentially deceptive. Figures 1.311 and 1.312 show a case of prostatic adenocarcinoma recurrent in a urinary bladder biopsy with areas mimicking urothelial carcinoma. When any unusual findings are present, a low threshold should be used for requesting immunohistochemistry (Figures 1.313-1.315) to confirm this distinction. Figures 1.316-1.319 show the opposite, an unusual case of a urothelial neoplasm with gland-like formation, mimicking prostatic adenocarcinoma.

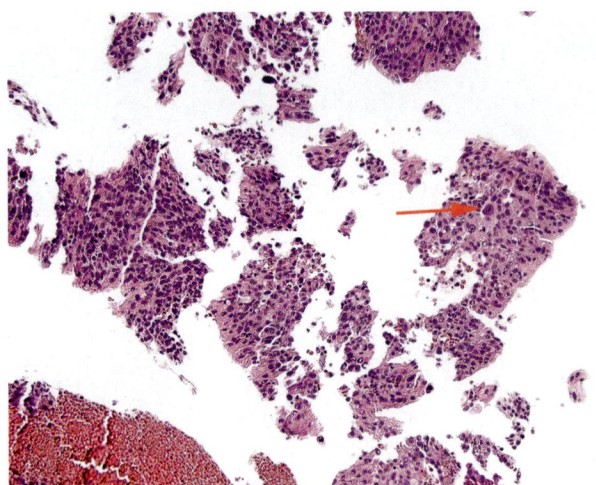

Figure 1.311. This case of prostatic adenocarcinoma shows detached strips of malignant epithelial cells, which could be confused with urothelial carcinoma; however, even the more pleomorphic cells have very prominent nucleoli (arrow), which may be a clue to the prostatic origin.

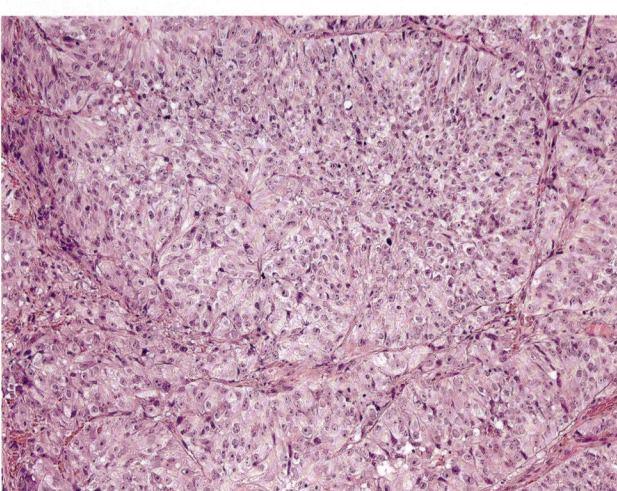

Figure 1.312. Other areas from the same tumor in Figure 1.311 show invasive solid nests of cells. Although there is somewhat greater pleomorphism than a typical prostatic adenocarcinoma, the consistent prominent nucleoli are a clue to the diagnosis.

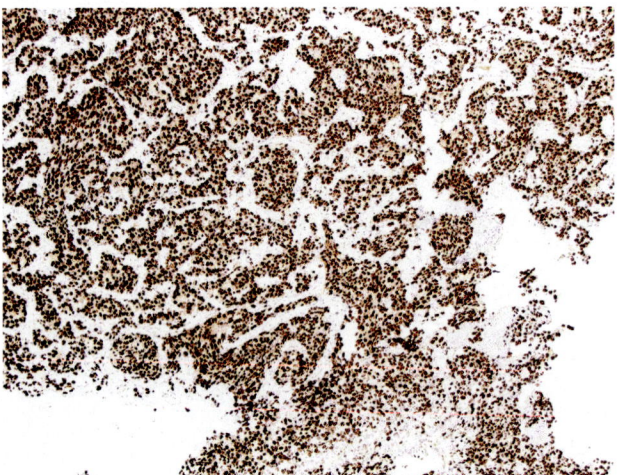

Figure 1.313. The tumor from Figures 1.311 and 1.312 shows diffuse staining for NKX3.1, supporting prostatic origin.

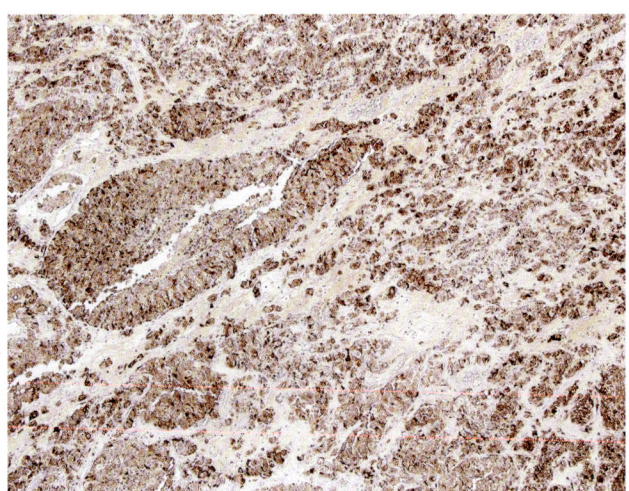

Figure 1.314. Prostate-specific antigen (PSA) is also positive in the tumor from Figures 1.311-1.313.

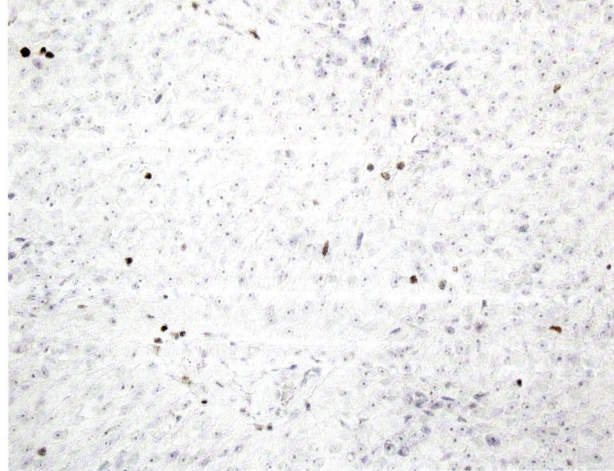

Figure 1.315. GATA3 staining in the same tumor from Figures 1.311-1.314 shows a negative result in the tumor cells. Scattered small positive nuclei represent intermingled lymphocytes, which are often positive for this marker.

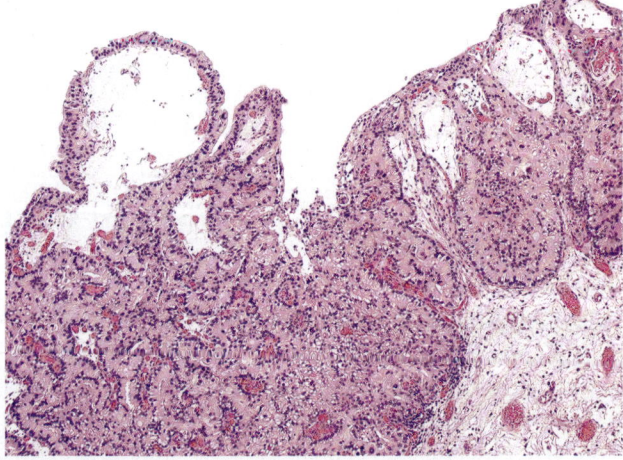

Figure 1.316. This case of urothelial carcinoma shows an unusual pattern of surface growth with nuclear alignment, resembling the cribriform or rosette-like architecture of prostatic adenocarcinoma.

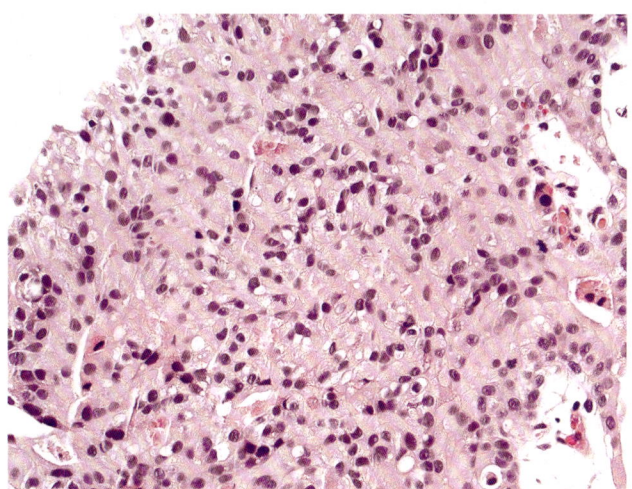

Figure 1.317. At higher magnification, the tumor from Figure 1.316 shows monomorphic nuclei and rosette-like structures, resembling prostatic adenocarcinoma.

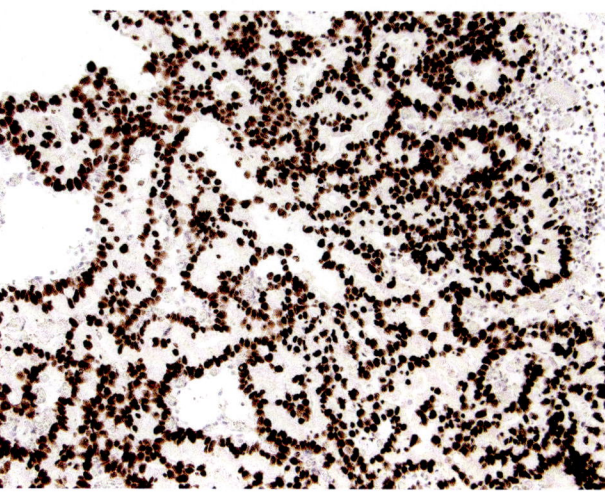

Figure 1.318. Immunohistochemistry shows the tumor from Figures 1.316 and 1.317 to be positive for GATA3.

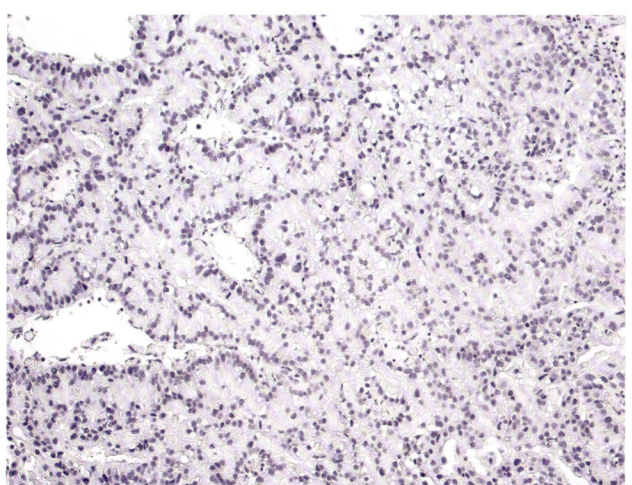

Figure 1.319. The same tumor from Figures 1.316-1.318 is negative for prostate-specific antigen (PSA).

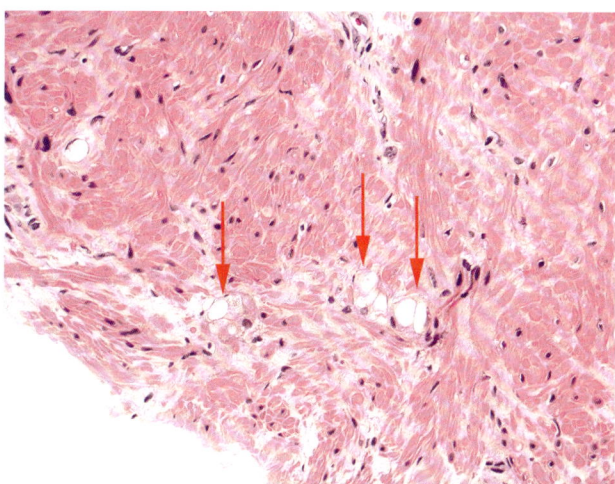

Figure 1.320. Prostatic adenocarcinoma with radiation therapy effect often appears as histiocyte-like cells or poorly formed glands with rings of cytoplasm forming small lumens and only rare small nuclei (arrows).

PROSTATIC ADENOCARCINOMA WITH TREATMENT EFFECT

Prostatic adenocarcinoma with either androgen deprivation therapy or radiation therapy effect can be quite deceptive in surgical pathology specimens. Fortunately, the most deceptive patterns with severe treatment effect largely show nonaggressive behavior; however, in modern practice, biopsies and resections of posttreatment patients are usually performed preferentially when the primary treatment has failed. Figures 1.320 and 1.321 show a case of prostatic adenocarcinoma with marked radiation therapy effect, manifesting as single cells and poorly formed glands with histiocyte-like cytoplasm and nuclei. Immunohistochemistry is helpful in this context, as cancer glands with treatment effect still show a generally similar pattern to that of adenocarcinoma (Figures 1.322 and 1.323).

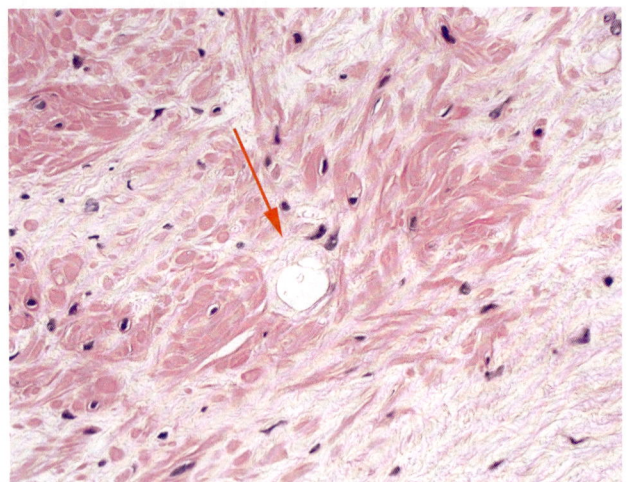

Figure 1.321. This rare gland of prostatic adenocarcinoma with radiation effect appears as essentially a ring of cytoplasm with no nucleus (arrow).

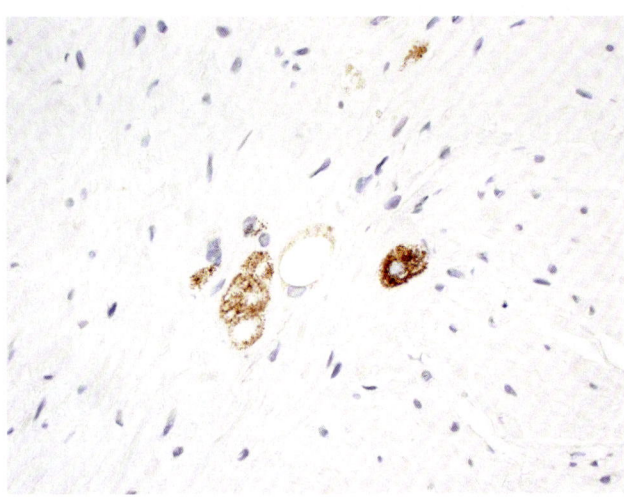

Figure 1.322. Immunohistochemistry with a single-color p63 and alpha-methylacyl-CoA racemase (AMACR) cocktail stain shows no basal cells and AMACR positivity, as typical of adenocarcinoma in general, in this case of prostatic adenocarcinoma with radiation effect.

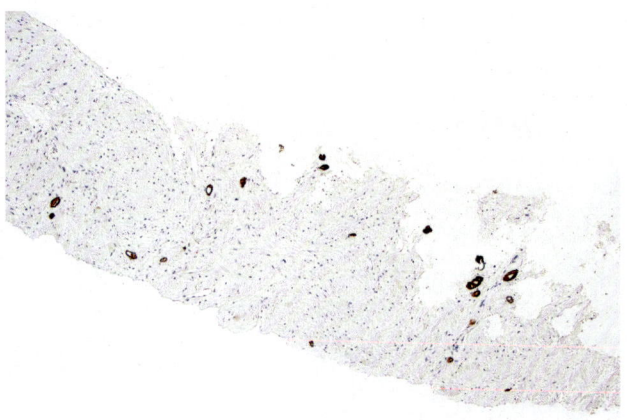

Figure 1.323. The same case from Figures 1.320-1.322 using a cytokeratin immunohistochemical stain highlights the poorly formed glands and confirms them to be of epithelial origin.

References

1. Fine SW, Reuter VE. Anatomy of the prostate revisited: implications for prostate biopsy and zonal origins of prostate cancer. *Histopathology*. 2012;60(1):142-152.

2. McNeal JE. Regional morphology and pathology of the prostate. *Am J Clin Pathol*. 1968;49(3):347-357.

3. McNeal JE. Origin and evolution of benign prostatic enlargement. *Invest Urol*. 1978;15(4):340-345.

4. McNeal JE. The zonal anatomy of the prostate. *Prostate*. 1981;2(1):35-49.

5. McNeal JE. Anatomy of the prostate and morphogenesis of BPH. *Prog Clin Biol Res*. 1984;145:27-53.

6. Grummet J. How to biopsy: transperineal versus transrectal, saturation versus targeted, what's the evidence? *Urol Clin North Am*. 2017;44(4):525-534.

7. Scattoni V, Maccagnano C, Capitanio U, Gallina A, Briganti A, Montorsi F. Random biopsy: when, how many and where to take the cores? *World J Urol*. 2014;32(4):859-869.

8. Samaratunga H, Montironi R, True L, et al. International Society of Urological Pathology (ISUP) consensus conference on handling and staging of radical prostatectomy specimens. Working group 1: specimen handling. *Mod Pathol*. 2011;24(1):6-15.

9. Magi-Galluzzi C, Evans AJ, Delahunt B, et al. International Society of Urological Pathology (ISUP) consensus conference on handling and staging of radical prostatectomy specimens. Working group 3: extraprostatic extension, lymphovascular invasion and locally advanced disease. *Mod Pathol*. 2011;24(1):26-38.

10. Sadimin ET, Ye H, Epstein JI. Should the involvement of skeletal muscle by prostatic adenocarcinoma be reported on biopsies? *Hum Pathol*. 2016;49:10-14.

11. Fine SW, McKenney JK. Prostate. In: Mills SE, ed. *Histology for pathologists*. 4th ed. Philadelphia: Wolters Kluwer Health/Lippincott Williams & Wilkins; 2012:987-1002.

12. deVries CR, McNeal JE, Bensch K. The prostatic epithelial cell in dysplasia: an ultrastructural perspective. *Prostate*. 1992;21(3):209-221.

13. Amin MB, Bostwick DG. Pigment in prostatic epithelium and adenocarcinoma: a potential source of diagnostic confusion with seminal vesicular epithelium. *Mod Pathol*. 1996;9(7):791-795.

14. Brennick JB, O'Connell JX, Dickersin GR, Pilch BZ, Young RH. Lipofuscin pigmentation (so-called "melanosis") of the prostate. *Am J Surg Pathol*. 1994;18(5):446-454.

15. Mao P, Angrist A. The fine structure of the basal cell of human prostate. *Lab Invest*. 1966;15(11):1768-1782.

16. Hameed O, Humphrey PA. Pseudoneoplastic mimics of prostate and bladder carcinomas. *Arch Pathol Lab Med*. 2010;134(3):427-443.

17. Fine SW. Neuroendocrine tumors of the prostate. *Mod Pathol*. 2018;31(S1):S122-S132.

18. Weaver MG, Abdul-Karim FW, Srigley J, Bostwick DG, Ro JY, Ayala AG. Paneth cell-like change of the prostate gland. A histological, immunohistochemical, and electron microscopic study. *Am J Surg Pathol*. 1992;16(1):62-68.

19. De Marzo AM, Platz EA, Epstein JI, et al. A working group classification of focal prostate atrophy lesions. *Am J Surg Pathol*. 2006;30(10):1281-1291.

20. Benign prostatic hyperplasia. In: Epstein JI, Cubilla AL, Humphrey PA, eds. *Tumors of the Prostate Gland, Seminal Vesicles, Penis, and Scrotum*. Washington, DC: American Registry of Pathology in collaboration with the Armed Forces Institute of Pathology; 2011:23-47.

21. Srigley JR. Benign mimickers of prostatic adenocarcinoma. *Mod Pathol*. 2004;17(3):328-348.

22. Linke RP, Joswig R, Murphy CL, et al. Senile seminal vesicle amyloid is derived from semenogelin I. *J Lab Clin Med*. 2005;145(4):187-193.

23. Jager GJ, Ruijter ET, de la Rosette JJ, van de Kaa CA. Amyloidosis of the seminal vesicles simulating tumor invasion of prostatic carcinoma on endorectal MR images. *Eur Radiol*. 1997;7(4):552-554.

24. Kaji Y, Sugimura K, Nagaoka S, Ishida T. Amyloid deposition in seminal vesicles mimicking tumor invasion from bladder cancer: MR findings. *J Comput Assist Tomogr*. 1992;16(6):989-991.

25. Ramchandani P, Schnall MD, LiVolsi VA, Tomaszewski JE, Pollack HM. Senile amyloidosis of the seminal vesicles mimicking metastatic spread of prostatic carcinoma on MR images. *AJR Am J Roentgenol*. 1993;161(1):99-100.

26. Freedman SR, Goldman RL. Normal paraganglia in the human prostate. *J Urol*. 1975;113(6):874-875.

27. Howarth SM, Griffiths DF, Varma M. Paraganglion of the prostate gland: an uncommon mimic of prostate cancer in needle biopsies. *Histopathology*. 2005;47(1):114-115.

28. Kawabata K. Paraganglion of the prostate in a needle biopsy: a potential diagnostic pitfall. *Arch Pathol Lab Med*. 1997;121(5):515-516.

29. Ostrowski ML, Wheeler TM. Paraganglia of the prostate. Location, frequency, and differentiation from prostatic adenocarcinoma. *Am J Surg Pathol*. 1994;18(4):412-420.

30. So JS, Epstein JI. GATA3 expression in paragangliomas: a pitfall potentially leading to misdiagnosis of urothelial carcinoma. *Mod Pathol*. 2013;26(10):1365-1370.

31. Perrino CM, Ho A, Dall CP, Zynger DL. Utility of GATA3 in the differential diagnosis of pheochromocytoma. *Histopathology*. 2017;71(3):475-479.

32. Epstein JI, Egevad L, Humphrey PA, Montironi R. Members of the ISUP Immunohistochemistry in Diagnostic Urologic Pathology Group. Best practices recommendations in the application of immunohistochemistry in the prostate: report from the International Society of Urologic Pathology consensus conference. *Am J Surg Pathol*. 2014;38(8):e6-e19.

33. Giannico GA, Ross HM, Lotan T, Epstein JI. Aberrant expression of p63 in adenocarcinoma of the prostate: a radical prostatectomy study. *Am J Surg Pathol*. 2013;37(9):1401-1406.

34. Osunkoya AO, Hansel DE, Sun X, Netto GJ, Epstein JI. Aberrant diffuse expression of p63 in adenocarcinoma of the prostate on needle biopsy and radical prostatectomy: report of 21 cases. *Am J Surg Pathol*. 2008;32(3):461-467.

35. Tan HL, Haffner MC, Esopi DM, et al. Prostate adenocarcinomas aberrantly expressing p63 are molecularly distinct from usual-type prostatic adenocarcinomas. *Mod Pathol*. 2015;28(3):446-456.

36. Uchida K, Ross H, Lotan T, et al. DeltaNp63 (p40) expression in prostatic adenocarcinoma with diffuse p63 positivity. *Hum Pathol*. 2015;46(3):384-389.

37. Wu A, Kunju LP. Prostate cancer with aberrant diffuse p63 expression: report of a case and review of the literature and morphologic mimics. *Arch Pathol Lab Med*. 2013;137(9):1179-1184.

38. Baydar DE, Kulac I, Gurel B, De Marzo A. A case of prostatic adenocarcinoma with aberrant p63 expression: presentation with detailed immunohistochemical study and FISH analysis. *Int J Surg Pathol*. 2011;19(1):131-136.

39. Oliai BR, Kahane H, Epstein JI. Can basal cells be seen in adenocarcinoma of the prostate? an immunohistochemical study using high molecular weight cytokeratin (clone 34betaE12) antibody. *Am J Surg Pathol*. 2002;26(9):1151-1160.

40. Brimo F, Epstein JI. Immunohistochemical pitfalls in prostate pathology. *Hum Pathol*. 2012;43(3):313-324.

41. Ali TZ, Epstein JI. False positive labeling of prostate cancer with high molecular weight cytokeratin: p63 a more specific immunomarker for basal cells. *Am J Surg Pathol*. 2008;32(12):1890-1895.

42. Shah RB, Zhou M, LeBlanc M, Snyder M, Rubin MA. Comparison of the basal cell-specific markers, 34betaE12 and p63, in the diagnosis of prostate cancer. *Am J Surg Pathol*. 2002;26(9):1161-1168.

43. Ye H, Montgomery E, Epstein JI. Incidental anorectal pathologic findings in prostatic needle core biopsies: a 13-year experience from a genitourinary pathology consult service. *Hum Pathol*. 2010;41(12):1674-1681.

44. Schowinsky JT, Epstein JI. Distorted rectal tissue on prostate needle biopsy: a mimicker of prostate cancer. *Am J Surg Pathol*. 2006;30(7):866-870.

45. Epstein JI. Adenosis vs. atypical adenomatous hyperplasia of the prostate. *Am J Surg Pathol*. 1994;18(10):1070-1071.

46. Trpkov K. Benign mimics of prostatic adenocarcinoma. *Mod Pathol*. 2018;31(S1):S22-S46.

47. Netto GJ, Epstein JI. Benign mimickers of prostate adenocarcinoma on needle biopsy and transurethral resection. *Surg Pathol Clin*. 2008;1(1):1-41.

48. Cheng L, Shan A, Cheville JC, Qian J, Bostwick DG. Atypical adenomatous hyperplasia of the prostate: a premalignant lesion? *Cancer Res*. 1998;58(3):389-391.

49. Cheng L, Davidson DD, Maclennan GT, et al. Atypical adenomatous hyperplasia of prostate lacks TMPRSS2-ERG gene fusion. *Am J Surg Pathol*. 2013;37(10):1550-1554.

50. Green WM, Hicks JL, De Marzo A, Illei PP, Epstein JI. Immunohistochemical evaluation of TMPRSS2-ERG gene fusion in adenosis of the prostate. *Hum Pathol*. 2013;44(9):1895-1901.

51. Liu S, Yoshimoto M, Trpkov K, et al. Detection of ERG gene rearrangements and PTEN deletions in unsuspected prostate cancer of the transition zone. *Cancer Biol Ther*. 2011;11(6):562-566.

52. Falzarano SM, Navas M, Simmerman K, et al. ERG rearrangement is present in a subset of transition zone prostatic tumors. *Mod Pathol*. 2010;23(11):1499-1506.

53. Bismar TA, Trpkov K. TMPRSS2-ERG gene fusion in transition zone prostate cancer. *Mod Pathol*. 2010;23(7):1040-1041; author reply 1–2.

54. Guo CC, Zuo G, Cao D, Troncoso P, Czerniak BA. Prostate cancer of transition zone origin lacks TMPRSS2-ERG gene fusion. *Mod Pathol*. 2009;22(7):866-871.

55. Cheng L, Bostwick DG. Atypical sclerosing adenosis of the prostate: a rare mimic of adenocarcinoma. *Histopathology*. 2010;56(5):627-631.

56. Grignon DJ, Ro JY, Srigley JR, Troncoso P, Raymond AK, Ayala AG. Sclerosing adenosis of the prostate gland. A lesion showing myoepithelial differentiation. *Am J Surg Pathol*. 1992;16(4):383-391.

57. Jones EC, Clement PB, Young RH. Sclerosing adenosis of the prostate gland. A clinicopathological and immunohistochemical study of 11 cases. *Am J Surg Pathol*. 1991;15(12):1171-1180.

58. Sakamoto N, Tsuneyoshi M, Enjoji M. Sclerosing adenosis of the prostate. Histopathologic and immunohistochemical analysis. *Am J Surg Pathol*. 1991;15(7):660-667.

59. Lotan TL, Epstein JI. Diffuse adenosis of the peripheral zone in prostate needle biopsy and prostatectomy specimens. *Am J Surg Pathol*. 2008;32(9):1360-1366.

60. Billis A. Prostatic atrophy. Clinicopathological significance. *Int Braz J Urol*. 2010;36(4):401-409.

61. Wang W, Sun X, Epstein JI. Partial atrophy on prostate needle biopsy cores: a morphologic and immunohistochemical study. *Am J Surg Pathol*. 2008;32(6):851-857.

62. Przybycin CG, Kunju LP, Wu AJ, Shah RB. Partial atrophy in prostate needle biopsies: a detailed analysis of its morphology, immunophenotype, and cellular kinetics. *Am J Surg Pathol*. 2008;32(1):58-64.

63. Oppenheimer JR, Wills ML, Epstein JI. Partial atrophy in prostate needle cores: another diagnostic pitfall for the surgical pathologist. *Am J Surg Pathol*. 1998;22(4):440-445.

64. Hosler GA, Epstein JI. Basal cell hyperplasia: an unusual diagnostic dilemma on prostate needle biopsies. *Hum Pathol*. 2005;36(5):480-485.

65. Rioux-Leclercq NC, Epstein JI. Unusual morphologic patterns of basal cell hyperplasia of the prostate. *Am J Surg Pathol*. 2002;26(2):237-243.

66. Sharma M, Miyamoto H. Prostatic adenocarcinoma with aberrant diffuse expression of high molecular weight cytokeratin. *Pathology*. 2018;50(7):787-789.

67. Gagucas RJ, Brown RW, Wheeler TM. Verumontanum mucosal gland hyperplasia. *Am J Surg Pathol*. 1995;19(1):30-36.

68. Gaudin PB, Wheeler TM, Epstein JI. Verumontanum mucosal gland hyperplasia in prostatic needle biopsy specimens. A mimic of low grade prostatic adenocarcinoma. *Am J Clin Pathol*. 1995;104(6):620-626.

69. Williamson SR, Lopez-Beltran A, Montironi R, Cheng L. Glandular lesions of the urinary bladder: clinical significance and differential diagnosis. *Histopathology*. 2011;58(6):811-834.

70. Pina-Oviedo S, Shen SS, Truong LD, Ayala AG, Ro JY. Flat pattern of nephrogenic adenoma: previously unrecognized pattern unveiled using PAX2 and PAX8 immunohistochemistry. *Mod Pathol*. 2013;26(6):792-798.

71. Allan CH, Epstein JI. Nephrogenic adenoma of the prostatic urethra: a mimicker of prostate adenocarcinoma. *Am J Surg Pathol*. 2001;25(6):802-808.

72. Mazal PR, Schaufler R, Altenhuber-Muller R, et al. Derivation of nephrogenic adenomas from renal tubular cells in kidney-transplant recipients. *N Engl J Med*. 2002;347(9):653-659.

73. Tong GX, Melamed J, Mansukhani M, et al. PAX2: a reliable marker for nephrogenic adenoma. *Mod Pathol*. 2006;19(3):356-363.

74. Tong GX, Weeden EM, Hamele-Bena D, et al. Expression of PAX8 in nephrogenic adenoma and clear cell adenocarcinoma of the lower urinary tract: evidence of related histogenesis? *Am J Surg Pathol*. 2008;32(9):1380-1387.

75. McDaniel AS, Chinnaiyan AM, Siddiqui J, McKenney JK, Mehra R. Immunohistochemical staining characteristics of nephrogenic adenoma using the PIN-4 cocktail (p63, AMACR, and CK903) and GATA-3. *Am J Surg Pathol*. 2014;38(12):1664-1671.

76. Chen YB, Fine SW, Epstein JI. Mesonephric remnant hyperplasia involving prostate and periprostatic tissue: findings at radical prostatectomy. *Am J Surg Pathol*. 2011;35(7):1054-1061.

77. Gikas PW, Del Buono EA, Epstein JI. Florid hyperplasia of mesonephric remnants involving prostate and periprostatic tissue. Possible confusion with adenocarcinoma. *Am J Surg Pathol*. 1993;17(5):454-460.

78. Bostwick DG, Qian J, Ma J, Muir TE. Mesonephric remnants of the prostate: incidence and histologic spectrum. *Mod Pathol*. 2003;16(7):630-635.

79. Evans AJ. Treatment effects in prostate cancer. *Mod Pathol*. 2018;31(S1):S110-S121.

80. Evans AJ, Ryan P, Van derKwast T. Treatment effects in the prostate including those associated with traditional and emerging therapies. *Adv Anat Pathol*. 2011;18(4):281-293.

81. Tian W, Dorn D, Wei S, et al. GATA3 expression in benign prostate glands with radiation atypia: a diagnostic pitfall. *Histopathology*. 2017;71(1):150-155.

82. Wobker SE, Khararjian A, Epstein JI. GATA3 positivity in benign radiated prostate glands: a potential diagnostic pitfall. *Am J Surg Pathol*. 2017;41(4):557-563.

83. Miettinen M, McCue PA, Sarlomo-Rikala M, et al. GATA3: a multispecific but potentially useful marker in surgical pathology: a systematic analysis of 2500 epithelial and nonepithelial tumors. *Am J Surg Pathol*. 2014;38(1):13-22.

84. Chang A, Amin A, Gabrielson E, et al. Utility of GATA3 immunohistochemistry in differentiating urothelial carcinoma from prostate adenocarcinoma and squamous cell carcinomas of the uterine cervix, anus, and lung. *Am J Surg Pathol*. 2012;36(10):1472-1476.

85. Higgins JP, Kaygusuz G, Wang L, et al. Placental S100 (S100P) and GATA3: markers for transitional epithelium and urothelial carcinoma discovered by complementary DNA microarray. *Am J Surg Pathol*. 2007;31(5):673-680.

86. Hoang LL, Tacha D, Bremer RE, Haas TS, Cheng L. Uroplakin II (UPII), GATA3, and p40 are highly sensitive markers for the differential diagnosis of invasive urothelial carcinoma. *Appl Immunohistochem Mol Morphol*. 2015;23(10):711-716.

87. Ordonez NG. Value of GATA3 immunostaining in tumor diagnosis: a review. *Adv Anat Pathol*. 2013;20(5):352-360.

88. Cina SJ, Silberman MA, Kahane H, Epstein JI. Diagnosis of Cowper's glands on prostate needle biopsy. *Am J Surg Pathol*. 1997;21(5):550-555.

89. Epstein JI. Diagnosis of limited adenocarcinoma of the prostate. *Histopathology*. 2012;60(1):28-40.

90. Magi-Galluzzi C. Prostate cancer: diagnostic criteria and role of immunohistochemistry. *Mod Pathol*. 2018;31(S1):S12-S21.

91. Bostwick DG, Wollan P, Adlakha K. Collagenous micronodules in prostate cancer. A specific but infrequent diagnostic finding. *Arch Pathol Lab Med*. 1995;119(5):444-447.

92. Baisden BL, Kahane H, Epstein JI. Perineural invasion, mucinous fibroplasia, and glomerulations: diagnostic features of limited cancer on prostate needle biopsy. *Am J Surg Pathol*. 1999;23(8):918-924.

93. Bostwick DG, Srigley J, Grignon D, et al. Atypical adenomatous hyperplasia of the prostate: morphologic criteria for its distinction from well-differentiated carcinoma. *Hum Pathol*. 1993;24(8):819-832.

94. Hudson J, Cao D, Vollmer R, Kibel AS, Grewal S, Humphrey PA. Foamy gland adenocarcinoma of the prostate: incidence, Gleason grade, and early clinical outcome. *Hum Pathol*. 2012;43(7):974-979.

95. Nelson RS, Epstein JI. Prostatic carcinoma with abundant xanthomatous cytoplasm. Foamy gland carcinoma. *Am J Surg Pathol*. 1996;20(4):419-426.

96. Kryvenko ON, Epstein JI. Prostate cancer grading: a decade after the 2005 modified gleason grading system. *Arch Pathol Lab Med*. 2016;140(10):1140-1152.

97. Epstein JI, Allsbrook WC Jr, Amin MB, Egevad LL. The 2005 International Society of Urological Pathology (ISUP) consensus conference on gleason grading of prostatic carcinoma. *Am J Surg Pathol*. 2005;29(9):1228-1242.

98. Epstein JI, Egevad L, Amin MB, et al. The 2014 International Society of Urological Pathology (ISUP) consensus conference on gleason grading of prostatic carcinoma: definition of grading patterns and proposal for a new grading system. *Am J Surg Pathol*. 2016;40(2):244-252.

99. Epstein JI, Zelefsky MJ, Sjoberg DD, et al. A contemporary prostate cancer grading system: a validated alternative to the gleason score. *Eur Urol*. 2016;69(3):428-435.

100. McKenney JK, Amin MB, Srigley JR, et al. Basal cell proliferations of the prostate other than usual basal cell hyperplasia: a clinicopathologic study of 23 cases, including four carcinomas, with a proposed classification. *Am J Surg Pathol*. 2004;28(10):1289-1298.

101. Chuang AY, Epstein JI. Xanthoma of the prostate: a mimicker of high-grade prostate adenocarcinoma. *Am J Surg Pathol*. 2007;31(8):1225-1230.

102. Zhou M, Li J, Cheng L, et al. Diagnosis of "poorly formed glands" gleason pattern 4 prostatic adenocarcinoma on needle biopsy: an interobserver reproducibility study among urologic pathologists with recommendations. *Am J Surg Pathol*. 2015;39(10):1331-1339.

103. Gottipati S, Warncke J, Vollmer R, Humphrey PA. Usual and unusual histologic patterns of high Gleason score 8 to 10 adenocarcinoma of the prostate in needle biopsy tissue. *Am J Surg Pathol*. 2012;36(6):900-907.

104. Crook JM, Bahadur YA, Bociek RG, Perry GA, Robertson SJ, Esche BA. Radiotherapy for localized prostate carcinoma. The correlation of pretreatment prostate specific antigen and nadir prostate specific antigen with outcome as assessed by systematic biopsy and serum prostate specific antigen. *Cancer*. 1997;79(2):328-336.

105. Crook JM, Bahadur YA, Robertson SJ, Perry GA, Esche BA. Evaluation of radiation effect, tumor differentiation, and prostate specific antigen staining in sequential prostate biopsies after external beam radiotherapy for patients with prostate carcinoma. *Cancer*. 1997;79(1):81-89.

106. Crook JM, Malone S, Perry G, et al. Twenty-four-month postradiation prostate biopsies are strongly predictive of 7-year disease-free survival: results from a Canadian randomized trial. *Cancer.* 2009;115(3):673-679.

107. Lucia MS, Epstein JI, Goodman PJ, et al. Finasteride and high-grade prostate cancer in the Prostate Cancer Prevention Trial. *J Natl Cancer Inst.* 2007;99(18):1375-1383.

108. Frauenhoffer EE, Ro JY, el-Naggar AK, Ordonez NG, Ayala AG. Clear cell cribriform hyperplasia of the prostate. Immunohistochemical and DNA flow cytometric study. *Am J Clin Pathol.* 1991;95(4):446-453.

109. Ayala AG, Srigley JR, Ro JY, Abdul-Karim FW, Johnson DE. Clear cell cribriform hyperplasia of prostate. Report of 10 cases. *Am J Surg Pathol.* 1986;10(10):665-671.

110. Milord RA, Kahane H, Epstein JI. Infarct of the prostate gland: experience on needle biopsy specimens. *Am J Surg Pathol.* 2000;24(10):1378-1384.

111. Mostofi FK, Morse WH. Epithelial metaplasia in "prostatic infarction". *AMA Arch Pathol.* 1951;51(3):340-345.

112. Strachan JR, Corbishley CM, Shearer RJ. Post-operative retention associated with acute prostatic infarction. *Br J Urol.* 1993;72(3):311-313.

113. Grignon D, Troster M. Changes in immunohistochemical staining in prostatic adenocarcinoma following diethylstilbestrol therapy. *Prostate.* 1985;7(2):195-202.

114. Epstein JI. Precursor lesions to prostatic adenocarcinoma. *Virchows Arch.* 2009;454(1):1-16.

115. Netto GJ, Epstein JI. Widespread high-grade prostatic intraepithelial neoplasia on prostatic needle biopsy: a significant likelihood of subsequently diagnosed adenocarcinoma. *Am J Surg Pathol.* 2006;30(9):1184-1188.

116. Argani P, Epstein JI. Inverted (Hobnail) high-grade prostatic intraepithelial neoplasia (PIN): report of 15 cases of a previously undescribed pattern of high-grade PIN. *Am J Surg Pathol.* 2001;25(12):1534-1539.

117. Wobker SE, Epstein JI. Differential diagnosis of intraductal lesions of the prostate. *Am J Surg Pathol.* 2016;40(6):e67-e82.

118. Magers M, Kunju LP, Wu A. Intraductal carcinoma of the prostate: morphologic features, differential diagnoses, significance, and reporting practices. *Arch Pathol Lab Med.* 2015;139(10):1234-1241.

119. Choy B, Pearce SM, Anderson BB, et al. Prognostic significance of percentage and architectural types of contemporary gleason pattern 4 prostate cancer in radical prostatectomy. *Am J Surg Pathol.* 2016;40(10):1400-1406.

120. Dong F, Yang P, Wang C, et al. Architectural heterogeneity and cribriform pattern predict adverse clinical outcome for Gleason grade 4 prostatic adenocarcinoma. *Am J Surg Pathol.* 2013;37(12):1855-1861.

121. Hollemans E, Verhoef EI, Bangma CH, et al. Large cribriform growth pattern identifies ISUP grade 2 prostate cancer at high risk for recurrence and metastasis. *Mod Pathol.* 2019;32(1):139-146.

122. Iczkowski KA, Paner GP, Van der Kwast T. The new realization about cribriform prostate cancer. *Adv Anat Pathol.* 2018;25(1):31-37.

123. Keefe DT, Schieda N, El Hallani S, et al. Cribriform morphology predicts upstaging after radical prostatectomy in patients with Gleason score 3 + 4 = 7 prostate cancer at transrectal ultrasound (TRUS)-guided needle biopsy. *Virchows Arch.* 2015;467(4):437-442.

124. Lee TK, Ro JY. Spectrum of cribriform proliferations of the prostate: from benign to malignant. *Arch Pathol Lab Med.* 2018;142(8):938-946.

125. Siadat F, Sykes J, Zlotta AR, et al. Not all gleason pattern 4 prostate cancers are created equal: a study of latent prostatic carcinomas in a cystoprostatectomy and autopsy series. *Prostate.* 2015;75(12):1277-1284.

126. Madan R, Deebajah M, Alanee S, et al. Prostate cancer with comedonecrosis is frequently, but not exclusively, intraductal carcinoma: a need for reappraisal of grading criteria. *Histopathology.* 2019;74(7):1081-1087.

127. Khani F, Epstein JI. Prostate biopsy specimens with gleason 3+3=6 and intraductal carcinoma: radical prostatectomy findings and clinical outcomes. *Am J Surg Pathol.* 2015;39(10):1383-1389.

128. Miyai K, Divatia MK, Shen SS, Miles BJ, Ayala AG, Ro JY. Heterogeneous clinicopathological features of intraductal carcinoma of the prostate: a comparison between "precursor-like" and "regular type" lesions. *Int J Clin Exp Pathol.* 2014;7(5):2518-2526.

129. Guo CC, Epstein JI. Intraductal carcinoma of the prostate on needle biopsy: histologic features and clinical significance. *Mod Pathol.* 2006;19(12):1528-1535.

130. Varma M, Egevad L, Delahunt B, Kristiansen G. Reporting intraductal carcinoma of the prostate: a plea for greater standardization. *Histopathology.* 2017;70(3):504-507.

131. Seipel AH, Delahunt B, Samaratunga H, Egevad L. Ductal adenocarcinoma of the prostate: histogenesis, biology and clinicopathological features. *Pathology.* 2016;48(5):398-405.

132. Amin A. Prostate ductal adenocarcinoma. *Appl Immunohistochem Mol Morphol.* 2018;26(7):514-521.

133. Seipel AH, Delahunt B, Samaratunga H, et al. Diagnostic criteria for ductal adenocarcinoma of the prostate: interobserver variability among 20 expert uropathologists. *Histopathology.* 2014;65(2):216-227.

134. Seipel AH, Samaratunga H, Delahunt B, et al. Immunohistochemical profile of ductal adenocarcinoma of the prostate. *Virchows Arch.* 2014;465(5):559-565.

135. Seipel AH, Samaratunga H, Delahunt B, Wiklund P, Clements M, Egevad L. Immunohistochemistry of ductal adenocarcinoma of the prostate and adenocarcinomas of non-prostatic origin: a comparative study. *APMIS.* 2016;124(4):263-270.

136. Paulk A, Giannico G, Epstein JI. PIN-like (ductal) adenocarcinoma of the prostate. *Am J Surg Pathol.* 2018;42(12):1693-1700.

137. Tavora F, Epstein JI. High-grade prostatic intraepithelial neoplasialike ductal adenocarcinoma of the prostate: a clinicopathologic study of 28 cases. *Am J Surg Pathol.* 2008;32(7):1060-1067.

138. Ali TZ, Epstein JI. Basal cell carcinoma of the prostate: a clinicopathologic study of 29 cases. *Am J Surg Pathol.* 2007;31(5):697-705.

139. Bishop JA, Yonescu R, Epstein JI, Westra WH. A subset of prostatic basal cell carcinomas harbor the MYB rearrangement of adenoid cystic carcinoma. *Hum Pathol.* 2015;46(8):1204-1208.

140. Magers MJ, Iczkowski KA, Montironi R, et al. MYB-NFIB gene fusion in prostatic basal cell carcinoma: clinicopathologic correlates and comparison with basal cell adenoma and florid basal cell hyperplasia. *Mod Pathol.* 2019;32(11):1666-1674.

141. Chuang AY, DeMarzo AM, Veltri RW, Sharma RB, Bieberich CJ, Epstein JI. Immunohistochemical differentiation of high-grade prostate carcinoma from urothelial carcinoma. *Am J Surg Pathol.* 2007;31(8):1246-1255.

142. Oliai BR, Kahane H, Epstein JI. A clinicopathologic analysis of urothelial carcinomas diagnosed on prostate needle biopsy. *Am J Surg Pathol.* 2001;25(6):794-801.

143. Gurel B, Ali TZ, Montgomery EA, et al. NKX3.1 as a marker of prostatic origin in metastatic tumors. *Am J Surg Pathol.* 2010;34(8):1097-1105.

144. Sheridan T, Herawi M, Epstein JI, Illei PB. The role of P501S and PSA in the diagnosis of metastatic adenocarcinoma of the prostate. *Am J Surg Pathol.* 2007;31(9):1351-1355.

145. Gordetsky J, Epstein JI. Pseudopapillary features in prostatic adenocarcinoma mimicking urothelial carcinoma: a diagnostic pitfall. *Am J Surg Pathol.* 2014;38(7):941-945.

146. Osunkoya AO, Netto GJ, Epstein JI. Colorectal adenocarcinoma involving the prostate: report of 9 cases. *Hum Pathol.* 2007;38(12):1836-1841.

147. Alharbi AM, De Marzo AM, Hicks JL, Lotan TL, Epstein JI. Prostatic adenocarcinoma with focal pleomorphic giant cell features: a series of 30 cases. *Am J Surg Pathol.* 2018;42(10):1286-1296.

148. Lotan TL, Kaur HB, Alharbi AM, Pritchard CC, Epstein JI. DNA damage repair alterations are frequent in prostatic adenocarcinomas with focal pleomorphic giant cell features. *Histopathology.* 2019;74(6):836-843.

149. Parwani AV, Herawi M, Epstein JI. Pleomorphic giant cell adenocarcinoma of the prostate: report of 6 cases. *Am J Surg Pathol.* 2006;30(10):1254-1259.

150. Parwani AV, Kronz JD, Genega EM, Gaudin P, Chang S, Epstein JI. Prostate carcinoma with squamous differentiation: an analysis of 33 cases. *Am J Surg Pathol.* 2004;28(5):651-657.

151. Alhamar M, Vladislav T, Smith SC, et al. Gene fusion characterization of rare aggressive prostate cancer variants - adenosquamous carcinoma, pleomorphic giant cell carcinoma, and sarcomatoid carcinoma: an analysis of 19 cases. *Histopathology.* 2020. doi:10.1111/his.14205.

152. Hermans KG, van Marion R, van Dekken H, Jenster G, van Weerden WM, Trapman J. TMPRSS2:ERG fusion by translocation or interstitial deletion is highly relevant in androgen-dependent prostate cancer, but is bypassed in late-stage androgen receptor-negative prostate cancer. *Cancer Res.* 2006;66(22):10658-10663.

153. Schelling LA, Williamson SR, Zhang S, et al. Frequent TMPRSS2-ERG rearrangement in prostatic small cell carcinoma detected by fluorescence in situ hybridization: the superiority of fluorescence in situ hybridization over ERG immunohistochemistry. *Hum Pathol.* 2013;44(10):2227-2233.

154. Adlakha H, Bostwick DG. Paneth cell-like change in prostatic adenocarcinoma represents neuroendocrine differentiation: report of 30 cases. *Hum Pathol.* 1994;25(2):135-139.

155. Tamas EF, Epstein JI. Prognostic significance of paneth cell-like neuroendocrine differentiation in adenocarcinoma of the prostate. *Am J Surg Pathol.* 2006;30(8):980-985.

156. So JS, Gordetsky J, Epstein JI. Variant of prostatic adenocarcinoma with Paneth cell-like neuroendocrine differentiation readily misdiagnosed as Gleason pattern 5. *Hum Pathol.* 2014;45(12):2388-2393.

157. Prendeville S, Al-Bozom I, Comperat E, et al. Prostate carcinoma with amphicrine features: further refining the spectrum of neuroendocrine differentiation in tumours of primary prostatic origin? *Histopathology.* 2017;71(6):926-933.

158. Kryvenko ON, Williamson SR, Trpkov K, et al. Small cell-like glandular proliferation of prostate: a rare lesion not related to small cell prostate cancer. *Virchows Arch.* 2017;470(1):47-54.

159. Lee S, Han JS, Chang A, et al. Small cell-like change in prostatic intraepithelial neoplasia, intraductal carcinoma, and invasive prostatic carcinoma: a study of 7 cases. *Hum Pathol.* 2013;44(3):427-431.

160. Bostwick DG, Iczkowski KA, Amin MB, Discigil G, Osborne B. Malignant lymphoma involving the prostate: report of 62 cases. *Cancer.* 1998;83(4):732-738.

161. Chu PG, Huang Q, Weiss LM. Incidental and concurrent malignant lymphomas discovered at the time of prostatectomy and prostate biopsy: a study of 29 cases. *Am J Surg Pathol.* 2005;29(5):693-699.

162. Hansel DE, Netto GJ, Montgomery EA, Epstein JI. Mesenchymal tumors of the prostate. *Surg Pathol Clin.* 2008;1(1):105-128.

163. Tavora F, Kryvenko ON, Epstein JI. Mesenchymal tumours of the bladder and prostate: an update. *Pathology.* 2013;45(2):104-115.

164. Epstein JI, Hutchins GM. Granulomatous prostatitis: distinction among allergic, nonspecific, and post-transurethral resection lesions. *Hum Pathol.* 1984;15(9):818-825.

165. Medlicott S, Magi-Galluzzi C, Jimenez RE, Trpkov K. Malakoplakia associated with prostatic adenocarcinoma: report of 4 cases and literature review. *Ann Diagn Pathol.* 2016;22:33-37.

166. McKenney JK. Mesenchymal tumors of the prostate. *Mod Pathol.* 2018;31(S1):S133-S142.

167. Herawi M, Epstein JI. Specialized stromal tumors of the prostate: a clinicopathologic study of 50 cases. *Am J Surg Pathol.* 2006;30(6):694-704.

168. Sadimin ET, Epstein JI. Round cell pattern of prostatic stromal tumor of uncertain malignant potential: a subtle newly recognized variant. *Hum Pathol.* 2016;52:68-73.

169. Nagar M, Epstein JI. Epithelial proliferations in prostatic stromal tumors of uncertain malignant potential (STUMP). *Am J Surg Pathol.* 2011;35(6):898-903.

170. Guner G, Bishop JA, Bezerra SM, et al. The utility of STAT6 and ALDH1 expression in the differential diagnosis of solitary fibrous tumor versus prostate-specific stromal neoplasms. *Hum Pathol.* 2016;54:184-188.

171. Hansel DE, Herawi M, Montgomery E, Epstein JI. Spindle cell lesions of the adult prostate. *Mod Pathol.* 2007;20(1):148-158.

172. Hansel DE, Epstein JI. Sarcomatoid carcinoma of the prostate: a study of 42 cases. *Am J Surg Pathol.* 2006;30(10):1316-1321.

173. Herawi M, Epstein JI. Solitary fibrous tumor on needle biopsy and transurethral resection of the prostate: a clinicopathologic study of 13 cases. *Am J Surg Pathol.* 2007;31(6):870-876.

174. Westra WH, Grenko RT, Epstein J. Solitary fibrous tumor of the lower urogenital tract: a report of five cases involving the seminal vesicles, urinary bladder, and prostate. *Hum Pathol.* 2000;31(1):63-68.

175. Kouba E, Simper NB, Chen S, et al. Solitary fibrous tumour of the genitourinary tract: a clinicopathological study of 11 cases and their association with the NAB2-STAT6 fusion gene. *J Clin Pathol.* 2017;70(6):508-514.

176. Herawi M, Montgomery EA, Epstein JI. Gastrointestinal stromal tumors (GISTs) on prostate needle biopsy: a clinicopathologic study of 8 cases. *Am J Surg Pathol.* 2006;30(11):1389-1395.

177. Cheng L, Billis A, Bostwick DG, Iczkowski KA. Seminal vesicle tumors. In: Moch H, Humphrey PA, Ulbright TM, Reuter VE, eds. *WHO Classification of Tumours of the Urinary System and Male Genital Organs*. Vol 8. 4th ed. Lyon: International Agency for Research on Cancer; 2016:181-183.

178. Ormsby AH, Haskell R, Jones D, Goldblum JR. Primary seminal vesicle carcinoma: an immunohistochemical analysis of four cases. *Mod Pathol*. 2000;13(1):46-51.

179. Reikie BA, Yilmaz A, Medlicott S, Trpkov K. Mixed epithelial-stromal tumor (MEST) of seminal vesicle: a proposal for unified nomenclature. *Adv Anat Pathol*. 2015;22(2):113-120.

180. Egevad L, Judge M, Delahunt B, et al. Dataset for the reporting of prostate carcinoma in core needle biopsy and transurethral resection and enucleation specimens: recommendations from the International Collaboration on Cancer Reporting (ICCR). *Pathology*. 2019;51(1):11-20.

181. Fine SW, Amin MB, Berney DM, et al. A contemporary update on pathology reporting for prostate cancer: biopsy and radical prostatectomy specimens. *Eur Urol*. 2012;62(1):20-39.

182. Grignon DJ. Prostate cancer reporting and staging: needle biopsy and radical prostatectomy specimens. *Mod Pathol*. 2018;31(S1):S96-S109.

183. Kench JG, Judge M, Delahunt B, et al. Dataset for the reporting of prostate carcinoma in radical prostatectomy specimens: updated recommendations from the International Collaboration on Cancer Reporting. *Virchows Arch*. 2019;475(3):263-277.

184. Arias-Stella JA III, Shah AB, Montoya-Cerrillo D, Williamson SR, Gupta NS. Prostate biopsy and radical prostatectomy Gleason score correlation in heterogenous tumors: proposal for a composite Gleason score. *Am J Surg Pathol*. 2015;39(9):1213-1218.

185. Athanazio D, Gotto G, Shea-Budgell M, Yilmaz A, Trpkov K. Global Gleason grade groups in prostate cancer: concordance of biopsy and radical prostatectomy grades and predictors of upgrade and downgrade. *Histopathology*. 2017;70(7):1098-1106.

186. Varma M, Berney D, Oxley J, Trpkov K. Gleason score assignment is the sole responsibility of the pathologist. *Histopathology*. 2018;73(1):5-7.

187. Briganti A, Fossati N, Catto JWF, et al. Active surveillance for low-risk prostate cancer: the European Association of Urology position in 2018. *Eur Urol*. 2018;74(3):357-368.

188. Matoso A, Epstein JI. Defining clinically significant prostate cancer on the basis of pathological findings. *Histopathology*. 2019;74(1):135-145.

189. Amin MB, Lin DW, Gore JL, et al. The critical role of the pathologist in determining eligibility for active surveillance as a management option in patients with prostate cancer: consensus statement with recommendations supported by the College of American Pathologists, International Society of Urological Pathology, Association of Directors of Anatomic and Surgical Pathology, the New Zealand Society of Pathologists, and the Prostate Cancer Foundation. *Arch Pathol Lab Med*. 2014;138(10):1387-1405.

190. Arias-Stella JA III, Varma KR, Montoya-Cerrillo D, Gupta NS, Williamson SR. Does discontinuous involvement of a prostatic needle biopsy core by adenocarcinoma correlate with a large tumor focus at radical prostatectomy? *Am J Surg Pathol*. 2015;39(2):281-286.

191. Fontugne J, Davis K, Palanisamy N, et al. Clonal evaluation of prostate cancer foci in biopsies with discontinuous tumor involvement by dual ERG/SPINK1 immunohistochemistry. *Mod Pathol*. 2016;29(2):157-165.

192. Karram S, Trock BJ, Netto GJ, Epstein JI. Should intervening benign tissue be included in the measurement of discontinuous foci of cancer on prostate needle biopsy? Correlation with radical prostatectomy findings. *Am J Surg Pathol*. 2011;35(9):1351-1355.

193. Schultz L, Maluf CE, da Silva RC, Falashi Rde H, da Costa MV, Schultz MI. Discontinuous foci of cancer in a single core of prostatic biopsy: when it occurs and performance of quantification methods in a private-practice setting. *Am J Surg Pathol*. 2013;37(12):1831-1836.

194. Brimo F, Vollmer RT, Corcos J, et al. Prognostic value of various morphometric measurements of tumour extent in prostate needle core tissue. *Histopathology*. 2008;53(2):177-183.

195. Paner GP, Srigley JR, Zhou M, et al. Protocol for the Examination of Radical Prostatectomy Specimens From Patients With Carcinoma of the Prostate Gland 2019. Available at https://documents.cap.org/protocols/cp-malegenital-prostate-radicalprostatectomy-19-4041.pdf.

196. Sung MT, Eble JN, Cheng L. Invasion of fat justifies assignment of stage pT3a in prostatic adenocarcinoma. *Pathology*. 2006;38(4):309-311.

197. Nazeer T, Kee KH, Ro JY, et al. Intraprostatic adipose tissue: a study of 427 whole mount radical prostatectomy specimens. *Hum Pathol*. 2009;40(4):538-541.

198. Epstein JI, Carmichael MJ, Pizov G, Walsh PC. Influence of capsular penetration on progression following radical prostatectomy: a study of 196 cases with long-term followup. *J Urol.* 1993;150(1):135-141.

199. Wheeler TM, Dillioglugil O, Kattan MW, et al. Clinical and pathological significance of the level and extent of capsular invasion in clinical stage T1-2 prostate cancer. *Hum Pathol.* 1998;29(8):856-862.

200. Epstein JI, Amin MB, Reuter VE, Humphrey PA. Contemporary gleason grading of prostatic carcinoma: an update with discussion on practical issues to implement the 2014 International Society of Urological Pathology (ISUP) Consensus Conference on Gleason Grading of Prostatic Carcinoma. *Am J Surg Pathol.* 2017;41(4):e1-e7.

201. Fine SW, Meisels DL, Vickers AJ, et al. Practice patterns in reporting tertiary grades at radical prostatectomy: survey of a large group of experienced urologic pathologists. *Arch Pathol Lab Med.* 2020;144(3):356-360.

202. Jamal M, Schultz D, Williamson SR, et al. Clinical significance of percentage of gleason pattern 5 as a tertiary pattern in prostate cancer at radical prostatectomy. *Mod Pathol.* 2018;31:352 (abstract).

CHAPTER OUTLINE

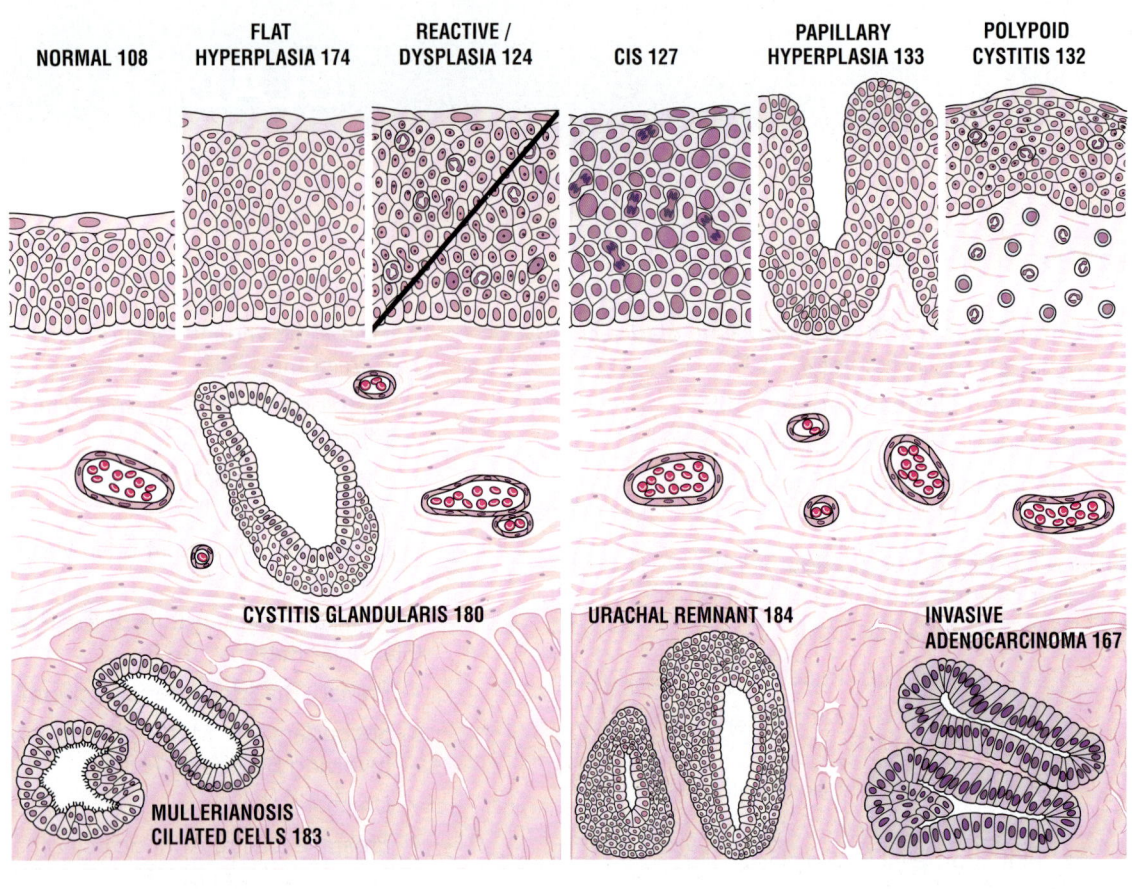

NORMAL 108

FLAT
HYPERPLASIA 174

REACTIVE /
DYSPLASIA 124

CIS 127

PAPILLARY
HYPERPLASIA 133

POLYPOID
CYSTITIS 132

CYSTITIS GLANDULARIS 180

URACHAL REMNANT 184

INVASIVE
ADENOCARCINOMA 167

MULLERIANOSIS
CILIATED CELLS 183

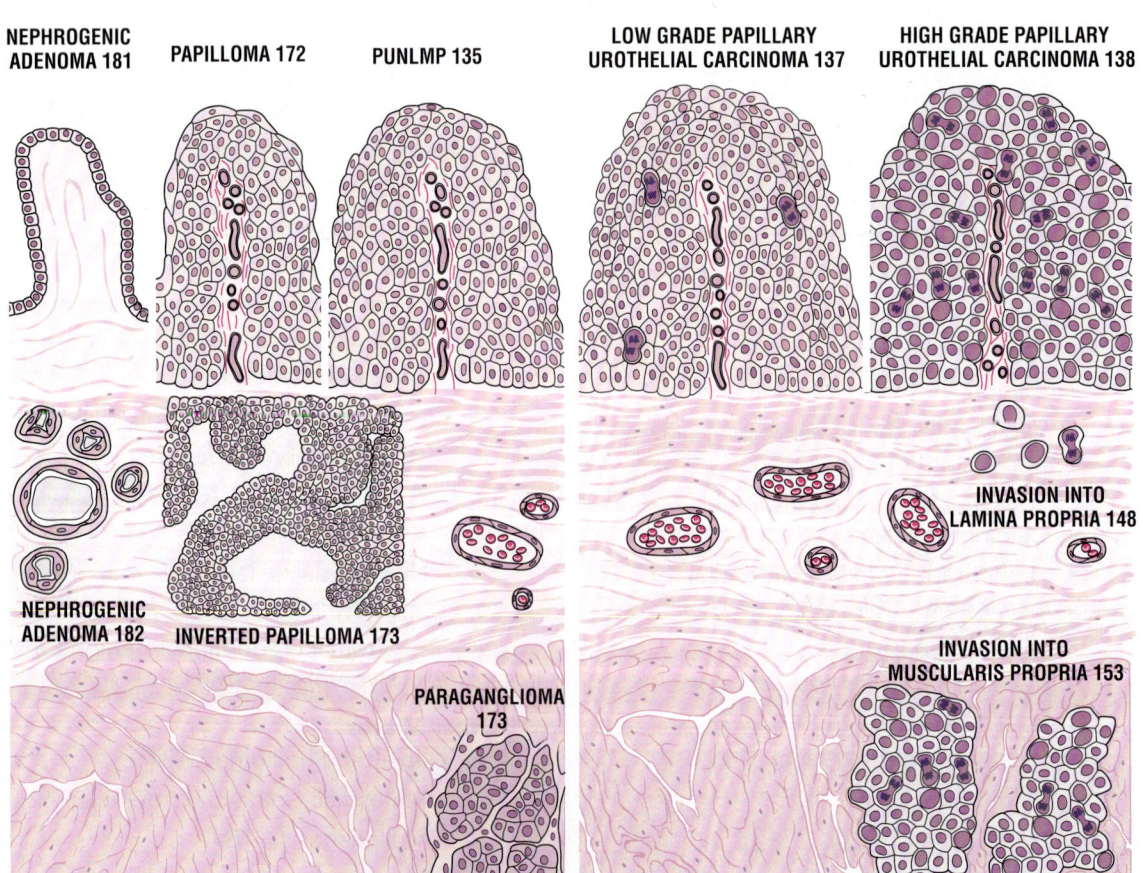

NEPHROGENIC
ADENOMA 181

PAPILLOMA 172

PUNLMP 135

LOW GRADE PAPILLARY
UROTHELIAL CARCINOMA 137

HIGH GRADE PAPILLARY
UROTHELIAL CARCINOMA 138

NEPHROGENIC
ADENOMA 182

INVERTED PAPILLOMA 173

PARAGANGLIOMA
173

INVASION INTO
LAMINA PROPRIA 148

INVASION INTO
MUSCULARIS PROPRIA 153

THE UNREMARKABLE AND NONNEOPLASTIC BLADDER

ANATOMY AND HISTOLOGY

The urinary bladder is a hollow viscus situated in the deep pelvis, which can expand to hold up to 500 mL of urine. Expansion of the bladder is permitted by interlacing bundles of smooth muscle and its multilayered urothelial lining which can fold into the bladder when empty. Urothelium is present throughout the urinary tract, starting from the renal pelvis, extending to the ureters, bladder, and terminating in the urethra, where it transitions to squamous epithelium. The general histology of these anatomic areas is similar, with a 5 to 7 cell layer–thick urothelium lined by umbrella cells. Beneath the urothelium lies the lamina propria, loose connective tissue containing numerous small lymphatics, and the wispy muscle fibers of the muscularis mucosae (Figures 2.1-2.4). Of note, the trigone muscle layer is derived from the bladder detrusor muscle and the ureter muscle and, therefore, lacks muscularis mucosae. The detrusor muscle, or muscularis propria, of the bladder is the deepest layer, containing thick fascicles of smooth muscle that interdigitate to allow for expansion and contraction of the bladder. The bladder is loosely encased in a layer of adipose tissue, the perivesical fat, which permits expansion as the bladder fills.[1]

The bladder is a roughly pyramid-shaped organ, with the point of the pyramid aligned inferiorly toward the urethra and the flat "dome" situated superiorly. The other anatomic regions of the bladder include the trigone, a flattened triangular area of urothelium located between the ureteral orifices and urethra on the posterior wall. The ureteral orifices, also denoted as the ureterovesical junctions, are located on the right and left sidewalls of the bladder, and the ureter courses through the muscularis propria within the bladder for some distance before emerging into the retroperitoneum and terminating in the renal pelvis.

> **PEARLS AND PITFALLS: Normal Elements of Bladder Wall**
>
> - Fat can be identified at any level within the bladder wall (Figure 2.5)
> - Presence of fat in a TURBT (transurethral resection of bladder tumor) specimen should not prompt concern for perforation or involvement of perivesical tissue
> - Ganglia and paraganglia are a normal component of bladder and may be identified in the muscularis propria (Figure 2.6)

THE NEAR-NORMAL BLADDER

von Brunn Nests

von Brunn nests (VBN) are rounded clusters of normal urothelium located within the lamina propria. They occur in both ureter and bladder. VBN represent downward invagination and budding of the urothelial surface and as such are a normal part of the urothelial mucosa. They are usually well circumscribed with focal attachment to the surface urothelium, depending on the plane of section. They tend to appear at roughly the same horizontal depth in the lamina propria, without irregular extension beyond that level.[2] VBN proliferations are common in the ureter and should not be confused for a neoplasm in a small biopsy specimen (Figure 2.7). However, there is morphologic overlap with proliferation of VBN and superficial sampling of nested variant of urothelial carcinoma, which will be discussed later in the chapter (Figure 2.8). One should be especially cautious of diagnosing nested variant of urothelial carcinoma in the ureter because of the frequency of proliferation of VBN in this location.

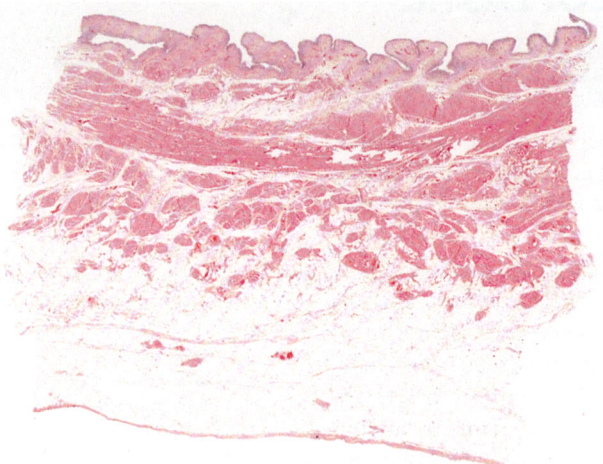

Figure 2.1. Whole slide image of the bladder wall showing the different compartments of the bladder. The surface urothelium shows slight infolding in its empty, decompressed state. Immediately below the urothelium is the lamina propria, with loose edematous stroma and thin muscle bundles. The thick, intersecting muscles of the muscularis propria are located beneath the lamina propria. The perivesical fat is located at the deepest aspect of the bladder.

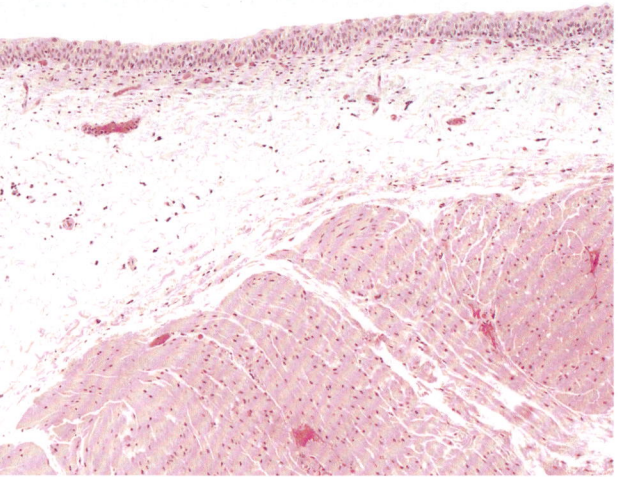

Figure 2.2. Low-power image of bladder wall showing benign urothelium, lamina propria, and muscularis propria. The lamina propria is comprised of loose, edematous stroma and vessels. In the lower right corner of the image, the muscularis propria shows thick muscle bundles, some of which are oriented perpendicular to the plane and others parallel.

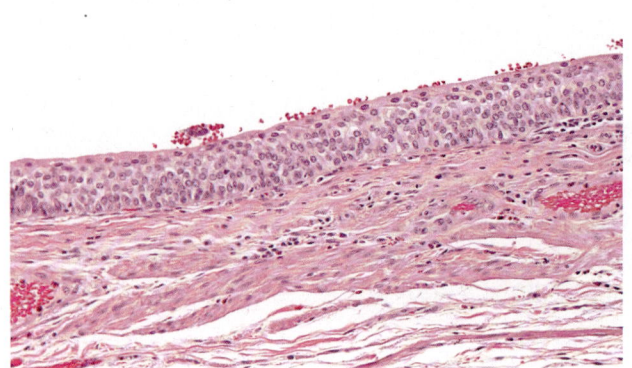

Figure 2.3. Benign urothelium at high power shows the usual 5 to 7 cell thickness of the epithelial layer. The cytology of the urothelial cells shows open, pale chromatin with pinpoint nucleoli. The higher power image of the lamina propria shows large vessels and thin, wispy muscles characteristic of this compartment.

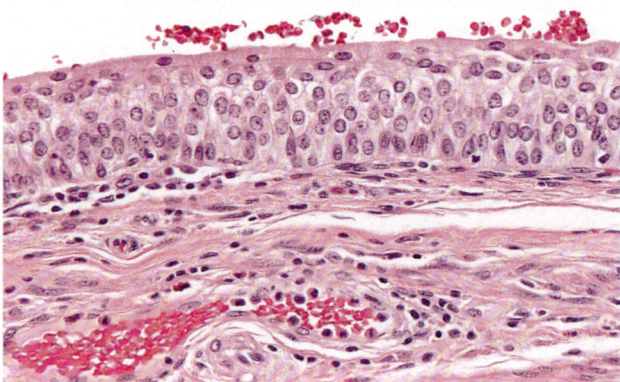

Figure 2.4. At high magnification, the urothelium shows a well-oriented 5 to 7 cell thick epithelial layer. Cytologically, rare nuclear grooves are present, a common finding in benign urothelium. Umbrella cells are located on the luminal surface and cover 2 to 3 cells each. These cells allow for expansion of the bladder while protecting the underlying lamina propria from urine. A large, gaping vessel is present in the lamina propria. These vessels are a useful landmark when deciding if small muscle bundles are in the lamina propria or the muscularis propria.

SAMPLE NOTE: Superficial Sampling of Atypical Urothelial Proliferation (See Note)

Note: The specimen is composed of a superficial sampling of urothelium with rounded nests of urothelial cells present in the lamina propria. The differential diagnosis includes proliferation of VBN and nested variant of urothelial carcinoma. Recommend clinical correlation and repeat sampling if warranted.

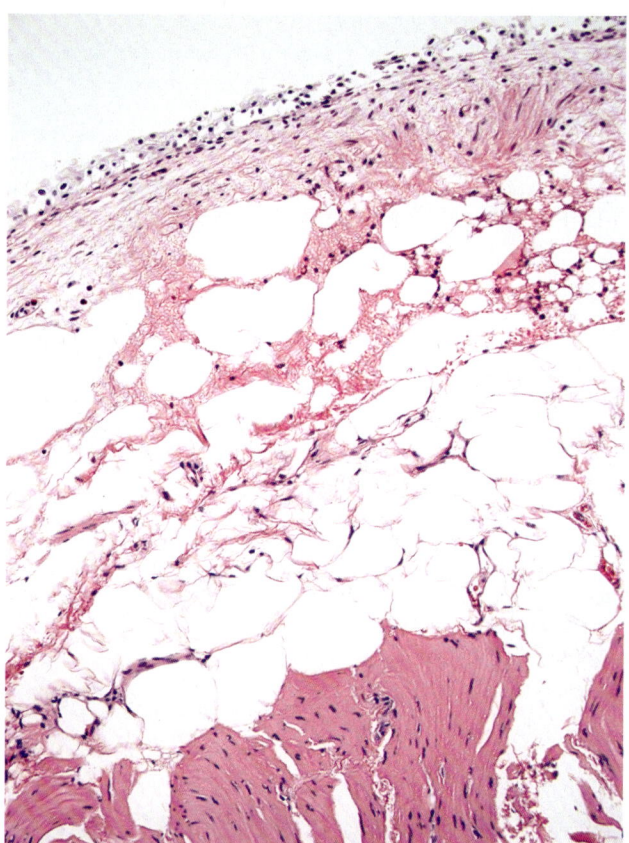

Figure 2.5. In the bladder wall, fat can be identified at any level. In this example, fat is present at multiple levels, including the lamina propria above the muscularis propria. Due to this possibility, it is not possible to definitively diagnose extravesical extension in a TURBT (transurethral resection of bladder tumor) specimen.

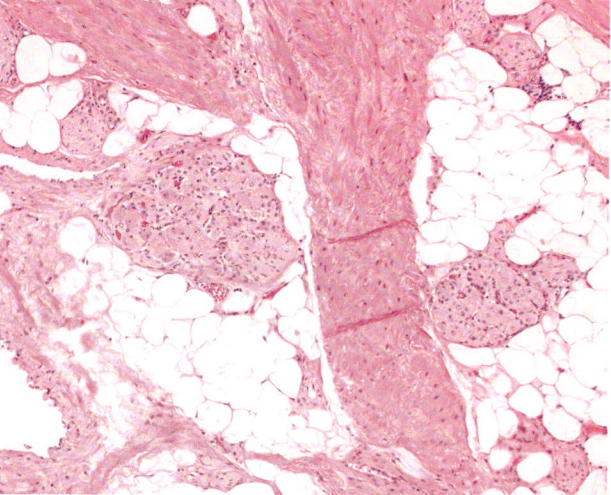

Figure 2.6. Visceral paraganglia are a normal finding in the bladder at the level of the muscularis propria. Paraganglia are composed of neuroendocrine and sustentacular cells and are arranged in small nodules. They are the origin of bladder paragangliomas when they arise as larger masses.

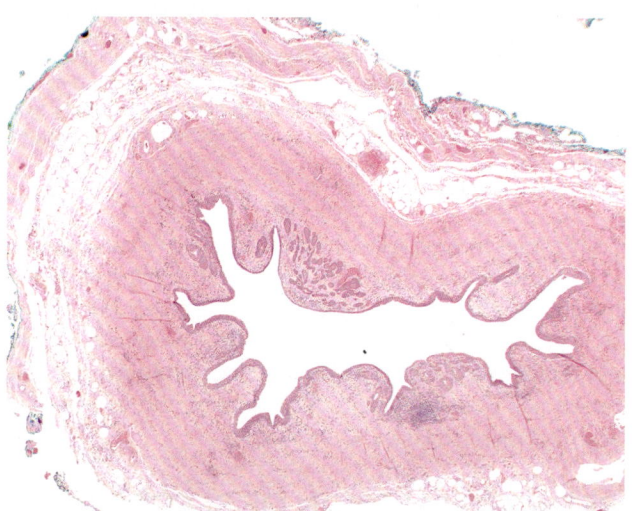

Figure 2.7. von Brunn nests are a common finding in both the bladder and ureter. These small bland nests of urothelium are located just beneath the urothelial surface and usually extend to the same depth and lack irregular downward growth.

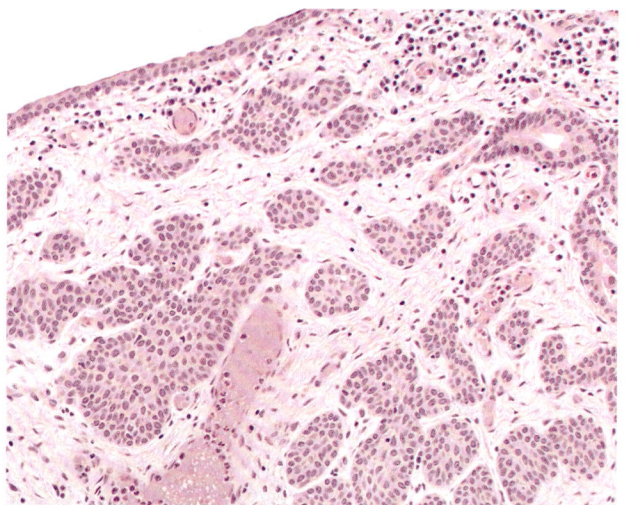

Figure 2.8. Higher power image of von Brunn nests (VBN) from Figure 2.7 showing bland cytology, focal cystic change (top right of image). In small and superficial biopsy specimens, a proliferation of small urothelial nests such as this raises the differential diagnosis of VBN and small nested urothelial carcinoma. A diagnosis of "atypical urothelial proliferation" is warranted for these types of cases.

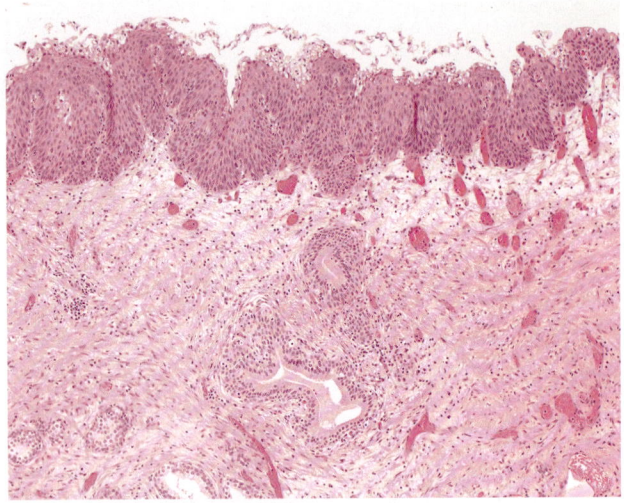

Figure 2.9. Squamous metaplasia is a reactive process often associated with chronic irritation from a catheter or infection. It manifests as a transformation from the usual urothelial lining to a squamous epithelium, which may or may not keratinize. In this case, it is nonkeratinizing.

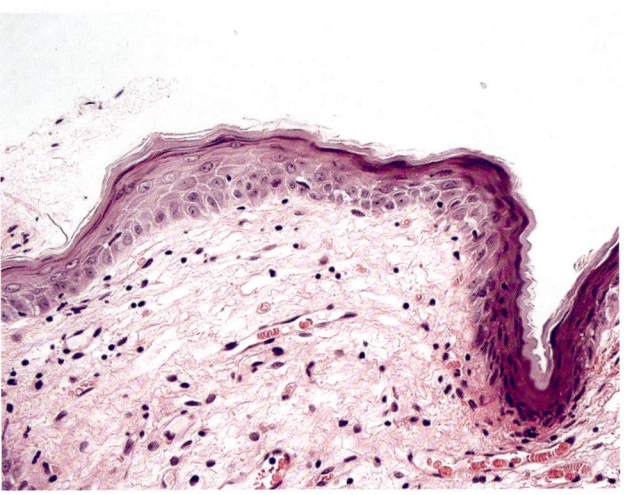

Figure 2.10. Keratinizing squamous metaplasia is pictured here, with the superficial layer showing flaky keratin. These lesions are often white on cystoscopy, and the keratin debris may be apparent in urine cytology if collected.

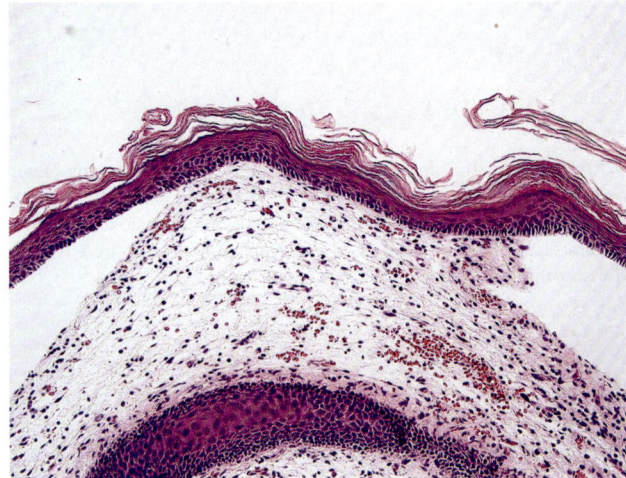

Figure 2.11. Additional image of keratinizing squamous metaplasia showing detached keratin debris. Keratinizing squamous metaplasia carries an increased risk of development of carcinoma and should be specifically commented on when identified in a bladder biopsy.

Chronic irritation may lead to squamous metaplasia of the urothelium. The usual transitional type epithelium is replaced with squamous epithelium (Figure 2.9). Common causes include chronic urinary tract infections, chronic catheterization, and some specialized infections such as schistosomiasis. The metaplastic epithelium may be glycogenated (most commonly found in the trigone of the female bladder) or keratinizing. Keratinizing squamous metaplasia carries an increased risk of development of carcinoma, and its presence should be included in the final report (Figures 2.10 and 2.11).

BIOPSY AND TRANSURETHRAL RESECTION OF BLADDER TUMORS

Cystoscopically, the unremarkable bladder reveals a pink-tan smooth to mildly trabeculated surface without exophytic growths or marked erythema. Using ureteroscopy, the upper urothelial tract demonstrates similar white-tan flattened urothelium lining the ureters and renal pelvis.

Histologic evaluation of the bladder is achieved by the use of cold cup biopsy or TURBT. Cystoscopy is a procedure that fills the bladder with clear fluid and evaluates the mucosa using white- or blue-light flexible scopes, looking for mucosal irregularities or tumors.

Cystoscopy can be performed in the urologist's office, without anesthesia, for surveillance of bladder cancer recurrence, initial workup of hematuria, or other lower urinary symptoms. During office-based flexible cystoscopy, cold cup biopsies may be obtained for evaluation of mucosal abnormalities. Specific cystoscopic findings include erythema, which may represent cystitis or urothelial carcinoma in situ (CIS), papillary neoplasms, or obvious invasive tumors. Some cystoscopic findings may suggest a high-grade tumor, such as necrosis or sessile growth pattern; however, histologic confirmation is necessary for final diagnosis. Blue-light cystoscopy is a recent technological advance where a light-sensitive substance (hexaminolevulinate) is instilled in the bladder prior to cystoscopy. Blue-light outperforms white-light cystoscopy in the detection of CIS and other high-risk lesions.[3,4]

Cold cup biopsies are subject to a number of artifactual distortions. When a large bite of tissue is present, you may have all layers of the bladder represented even in a small biopsy (Figure 2.12). However, these small biopsies often show significant crush artifact given the pincher-type forceps that are used. This can lead to difficulty assessing nuclear atypia for grading and displacing urothelial cells into the lamina propria, mimicking invasion. When possible, attempts should be made to identify intact, unperturbed urothelium for evaluation (Figure 2.13). Chronic inflammation, especially when crushed, can also mimic invasive disease (Figure 2.14). A simple pan-keratin stain can be used in this instance to rule out invasive carcinoma. With increased inflammation comes other changes in both the urothelium and the possibility of nonurothelial diagnoses; disrupted urothelial surfaces may harbor nephrogenic adenomas (Figure 2.15).

PEARLS AND PITFALLS: Cystoscopy and Ureteroscopy

- Cystoscopy notes can provide guidance for the pathologist and should be reviewed with each bladder biopsy or TURBT specimen
- If you are uncertain if a lesion represents a true papillary neoplasm, check the cystoscopic appearance in the procedure note. Papillary tumors are usually quite evident by cystoscopy; beware making a diagnosis of a papillary neoplasm if none was seen on cystoscopy
- Ureteroscopy involves a very small scope and, therefore, results in very small biopsies. Beware over diagnosing a neoplasm or invasion on a small, crushed biopsy, as the clinical ramifications are very significant in the upper urinary tract

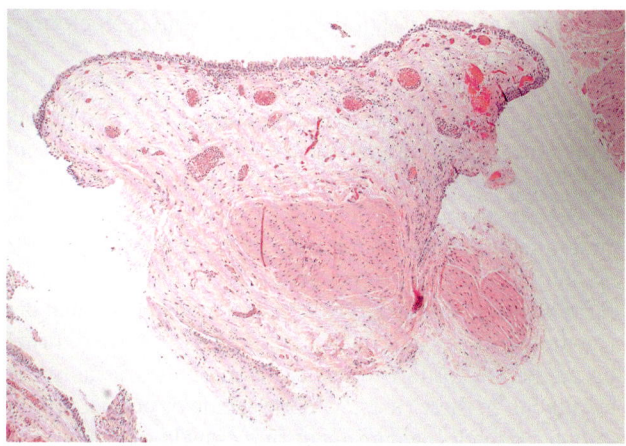

Figure 2.12. Cold cup biopsies can be obtained during office-based cystoscopy and may be used for initial screening of mucosal abnormalities. In this image, the biopsy is well oriented with a full urothelial surface represented and underlying lamina propria with a small amount of muscularis propria sampled.

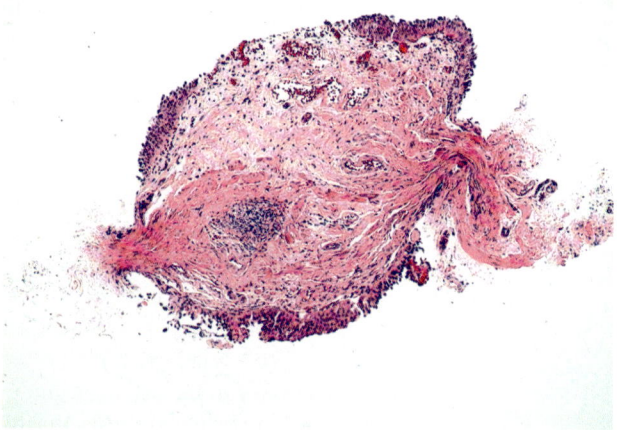

Figure 2.13. A more representative example of cold cup biopsy with crush artifact at either end of the specimen. This biopsy shows mostly intact urothelium, which is satisfactory for evaluation. Focal areas of denudation may be procedure related or part of the pathologic process and should be interpreted with both possibilities in mind.

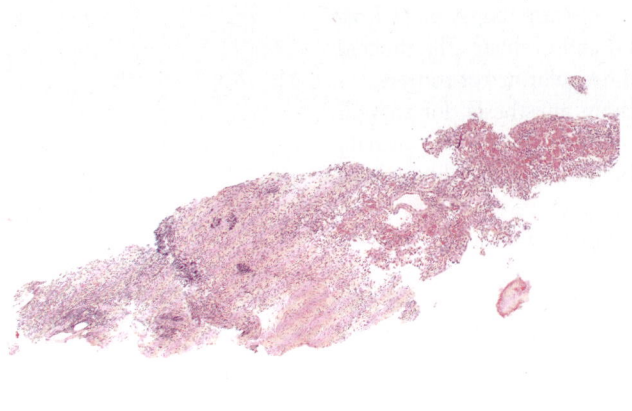

Figure 2.14. Cold cup biopsy with crush artifact and minimal urothelium present for evaluation. At low power, the left side of the specimen is predominantly lamina propria with chronic inflammation, which can mimic invasive disease. The finding of inflammation and urothelial disruption is a soft clue for the finding on the right side of the specimen—a nephrogenic adenoma.

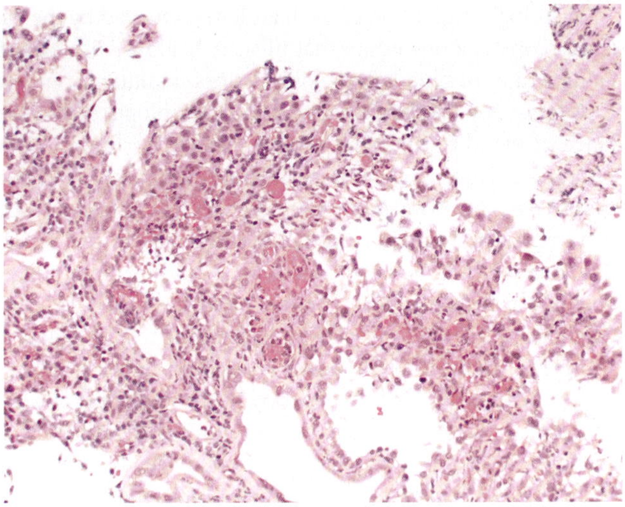

Figure 2.15. Higher power image of the nephrogenic adenoma present in Figure 2.14. Multiple tubules are present in lamina propria and lining of both tubules and surface shows hobnail cytology. The tubules are lined with an amorphous pink basement membrane-like material.

FAQ: What is the Clinical Approach to Workup of a Suspicious Bladder Mass?[5]

- Suspicious bladder lesions are first evaluated with office cystoscopy, urine cytology, and biopsy or TURBT
- Once tumor is identified, secondary evaluation includes complete TURBT
- Noninvasive low-grade tumors may be observed or treated with intravesical therapy
- Lamina propria involvement by low-grade tumors should be followed up with repeat TURBT; if residual disease, cystectomy may be considered
- If high grade is suspected based on sessile appearance, complete TURBT with sampling of muscularis propria is necessary; possible mapping biopsies with sampling of prostatic urethra
- Non–muscle-invasive high-grade tumors may be observed or treated with intravesical therapy
- Muscle-invasive high-grade tumors require definitive treatment with cystectomy and possible neoadjuvant chemotherapy

---

Once a tumor is detected with cystoscopy and cold cup biopsy, a larger resection may be necessary for accurate staging of the tumor. A TURBT can be performed during cystoscopy under spinal or general anesthesia, as it requires longer procedure time and removal of deeper layers of the bladder wall. The general purpose of a TURBT is to remove all possible tumor burden, with sufficient sampling of muscle wall for accurate staging. The most critical element for staging is evaluation of muscularis propria invasion.

TURBT is performed using electrocautery, and therefore, a major artifact is thermal distortion of tissue (Figure 2.16). The urologist may start the resection with the current turned to a relatively high level, causing marked distortion and destruction of superficial tumor. Assigning histologic grade can be difficult in these cases, with low-grade or normal urothelium showing artifactual hyperchromasia, nuclear enlargement, and crowding (Figures 2.17 and 2.18). Ideally, the current is lower as the urologist performs the deeper part of the resection involving detrusor muscle; however, cautery at the deep aspect of tumors may lead to an inability to determine if a muscle bundle is detrusor or if tumor is present. In some cases, a cytokeratin stain may be useful to highlight cauterized tumor, and in some cases, adding desmin staining can highlight obscured large muscle bundles.

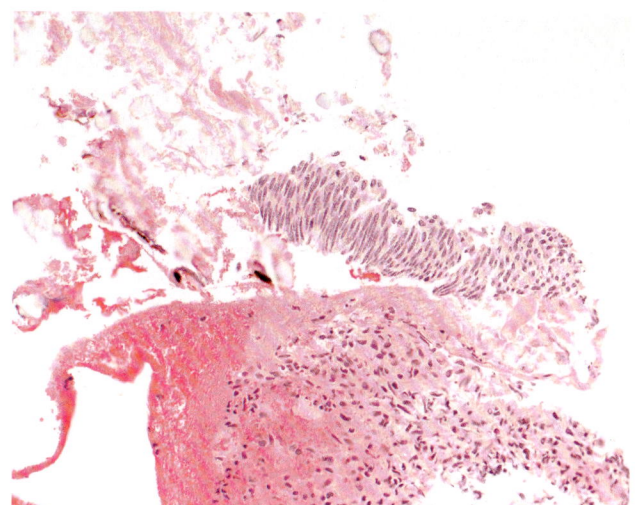

Figure 2.16. Unlike cold cup biopsies, TURBT (transurethral resection of bladder tumor) specimens are collected using electrocautery. As a result, thermal changes are evident in both the urothelium and surrounding tissue. In the urothelium, thermal artifact results in elongated cells with smudged cytoplasm and loss of distinct nuclear features. Caution is warranted when interpreting specimens with marked thermal artifact.

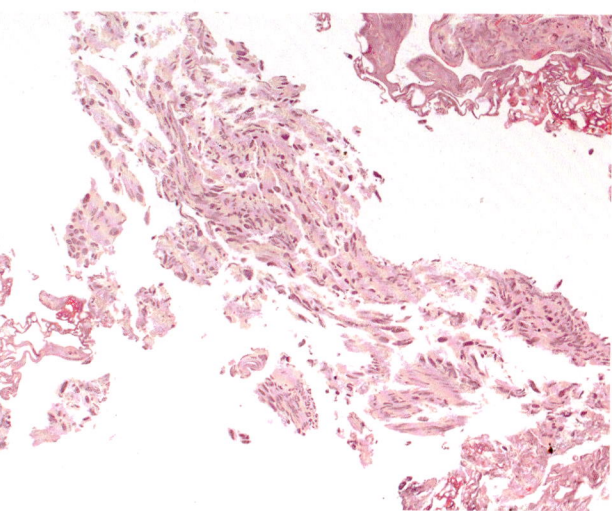

Figure 2.17. Another example of thermal artifact distorting urothelial tissue. In the top right corner, the tissue is almost unrecognizable and appears homogenized with no distinct nuclei remaining. The middle of the specimen shows some intact cells; however, the nuclear features are obscured by thermal artifact.

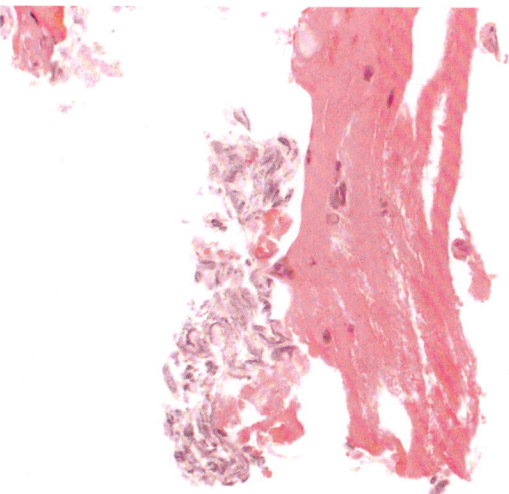

Figure 2.18. Thermal artifact has completely obscured this small fragment of urothelium. No definitive diagnosis can be rendered in cases with this degree of cautery.

A TURBT produces irregularly sized chips of tumor and bladder, which may be embedded tangentially and lead to artifacts. When a flat lesion is sectioned in a nonperpendicular plane, it may appear artifactually thickened (Figures 2.19-2.22). This could lead to an overdiagnosis of urothelial hyperplasia or potential confusion for CIS if through the basal layers. For papillary lesions, tangential sectioning can obscure the papillae entirely by obliquely sectioning one side of the fibrovascular core (Figures 2.23 and 2.24). In these cases, identifying other sectioned cores may help confirm the diagnosis of a papillary lesion. Tangential sectioning of an obvious papillary lesion may lead to confusion over assignment of histologic grade. Similar to the flat lesion that is sectioned through the basal layer, tangential sectioning of a papillary lesion may also result in the appearance of a higher-grade lesion. A pseudopapillary appearance can also occur in small biopsy specimens when the urothelial surface becomes detached and folds over on itself (Figures 2.25 and 2.26). A thorough search for definitive fibrovascular cores is critical before diagnosis of a papillary neoplasm.

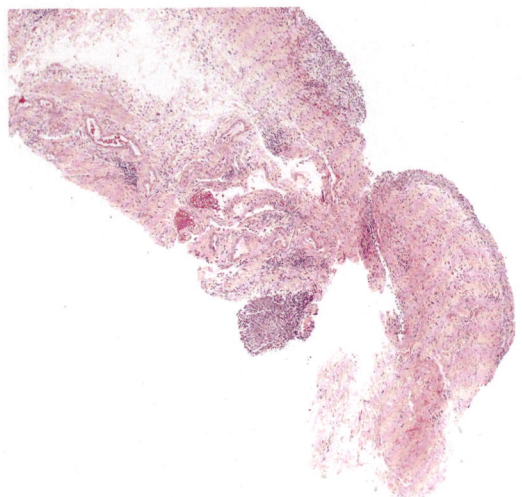

Figure 2.19. Tangential sectioning can cause interpretive errors in small biopsies. In this cold cup biopsy, a small area of apparently thickened urothelium is present in the middle of the biopsy. At first glance, this may prompt a diagnosis of hyperplasia or atypia in a flat lesion.

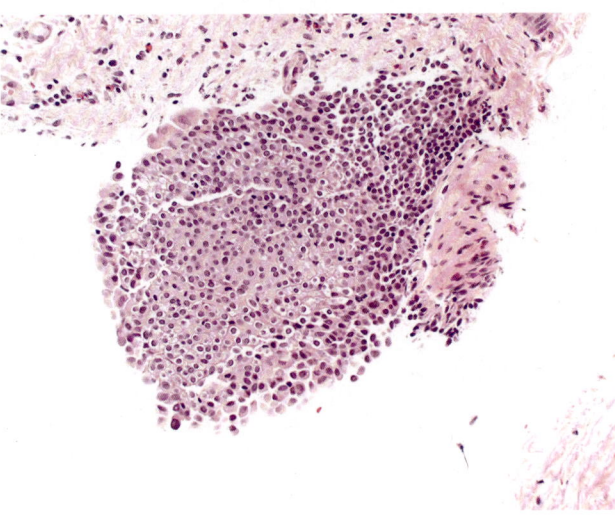

Figure 2.20. At higher power, the thickened area of urothelium shows some minimal atypia with occasional larger cells present, particularly at the periphery of the lesion. Before considering a diagnosis of atypia, one may consider obtaining deeper levels to identify proper tissue orientation.

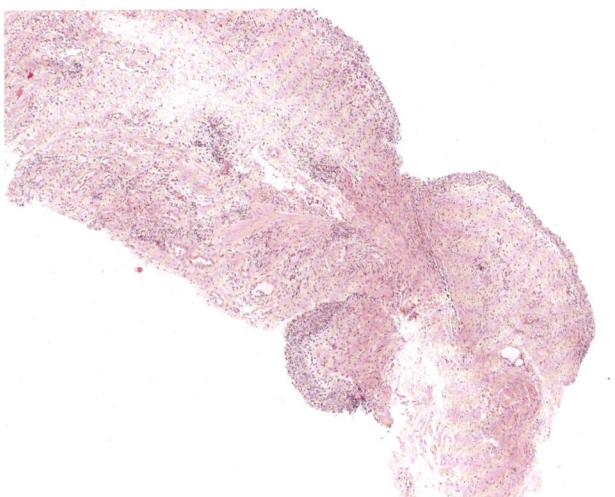

Figure 2.21. Deeper level of same specimen as Figure 2.19 showing the area of thickened urothelium now much thinner with better orientation of urothelial surface.

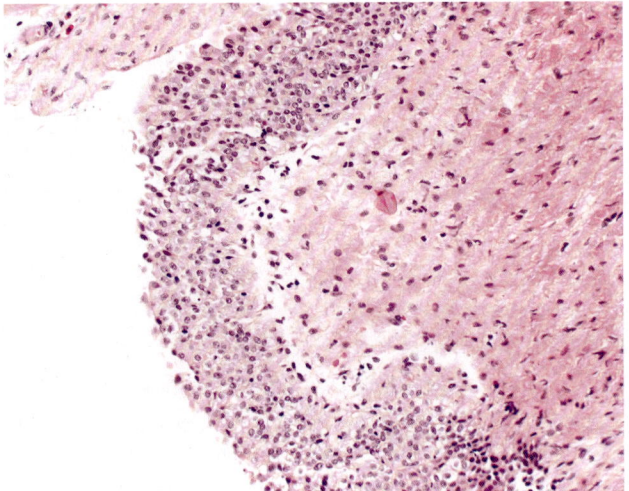

Figure 2.22. Higher power image of same area as Figure 2.20. Urothelium is thinner, and the few darker cells appear to be predominantly umbrella cells. Polarity is minimally altered, as compared with the artifactually jumbled in Figure 2.20. When possible, interpret the most well-oriented level of tissue available on the slide, or order recut levels if you have any suspicion that tangential sectioning is confounding interpretation.

KEY FEATURES: Necessary elements for pathology report for a bladder biopsy or TURBT:

- Histologic grade
- Presence/absence of invasion
- Depth of invasion
- Presence/absence of muscularis propria in the specimen
- Presence/absence of CIS
- Presence/absence of lymphovascular space invasion

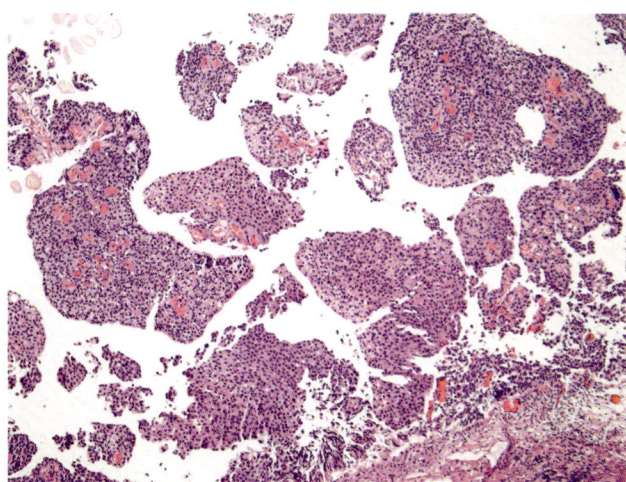

Figure 2.23. Tangential sectioning is especially common in papillary lesions, where the fragmented nature of the lesion leads to embedding of papillary fronds both perpendicular and parallel to the plane of sectioning. In this image, the papillary nature of the lesion is evident from the numerous vessels present in the center of free-floating urothelial tissue, indicating fronds cut perpendicular to the long fibrovascular core.

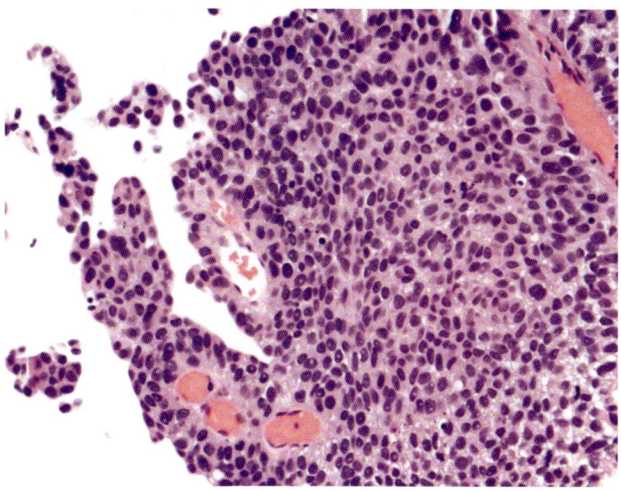

Figure 2.24. Atypical urothelial cells surround numerous vessels in the lower left-hand area of the specimen, consistent with fibrovascular cores. A vessel cut in longitudinal/parallel orientation is present in the upper right corner of the specimen.

The American Joint Committee on Cancer (AJCC) staging for urothelial cancer differs slightly depending on whether or not the lesion is flat or papillary.[6] For flat lesions, a noninvasive in situ component is represented by CIS and is staged as pTis. A noninvasive papillary lesion, regardless of its cytologic grade, is staged as pTa. For tumors that invade the lamina propria, the staging is the same regardless of the architectural pattern of the tumor.

CHECKLIST: Systematic Approach to Bladder Biopsy or TURBT Specimen

☐ Assess urothelial surface
- o Thickness
    - ■ Normal thickness, consider benign urothelial tissue, papilloma
    - ■ Thickened, consider hyperplasia, CIS or papillary neoplasm
- o Architecture
    - ■ Flat
    - ■ Papillary
- o Atypia
    - ■ None—benign, papilloma
    - ■ Mild—reactive changes, PUNLMP
    - ■ Moderate—dysplasia, low-grade papillary
    - ■ Severe—CIS, high-grade papillary

☐ Assess lamina propria
- o Invasion—scan for irregular nests, small nests or single cells, paradoxical maturation (round and pink)
- o Evidence of treatment effect—BCG (bacillus Calmette-Guerin) granulomas, radiation changes

☐ Assess muscularis propria
- o Presence/absence of muscularis propria—adequacy of TURBT resection
- o Invasion—must involve thick, round muscle bundles for definitive muscularis propria invasion

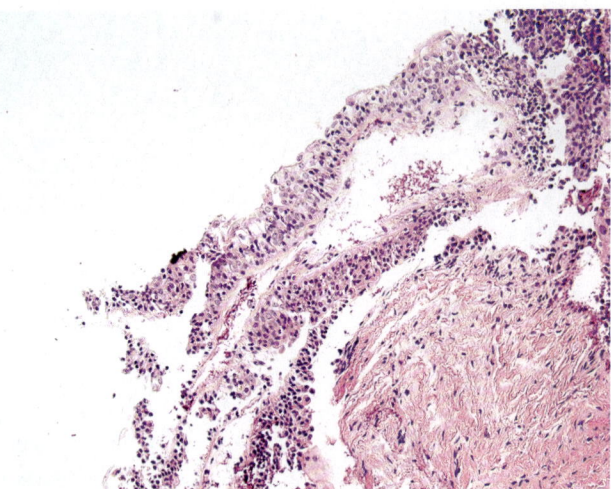

Figure 2.25. Unusual folding of the urothelium creates the illusion of a papillary fragment of tissue. In this image, the urothelial surface is detached and has folded over on itself to create the impression of a papillary frond. While there are red blood cells in the middle of the folded tissue, no definitive fibrovascular cores are identified. A papillary neoplasm should not be diagnosed without intact fibrovascular cores surrounded by urothelium.

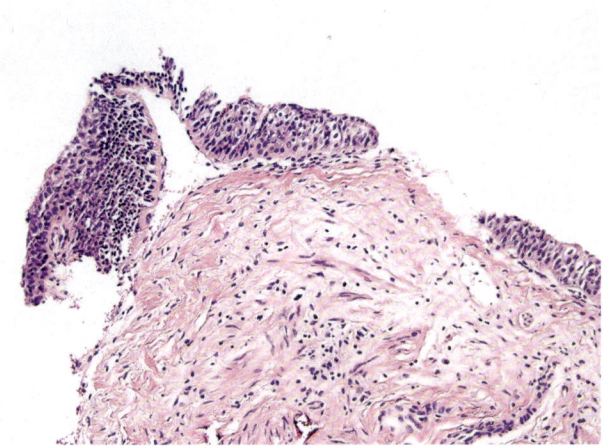

Figure 2.26. Another example of pseudopapillary structure in a specimen where the urothelium is partly detached and tented above the lamina propria. The empty space below the urothelium lacks fibrovascular cores and is not a true papillary frond.

SURFACE LESIONS OF THE BLADDER

Surface lesions of the urothelium generally correspond to mucosal surface irregularities seen on cystoscopy, including erythema or a velvety, irregular mucosa. Urologists sample these mucosal changes by cold cup biopsy. Cold cup biopsies are ideal for initial evaluation of mucosal findings, because they can be done in the office without general anesthesia, unlike a TURBT. A downside to cold cup biopsy is the relatively small sample size, which is prone to tangential sectioning and potentially tissue exhaustion if the block is not leveled carefully during sectioning. Clinical findings that may prompt an office biopsy include hematuria, lower urinary tract symptoms, or recurrent urinary tract infections. Each of these clinical scenarios may contribute valuable information to your interpretation of the bladder biopsy, so a review of the cystoscopy procedure notes and clinic notes is critical to accurate diagnosis.

FLAT LESIONS OF THE BLADDER

Using the "Checklist: Approach to Bladder Biopsy or TURBT Specimen," the first step is to scan the surface epithelium to detect changes in the thickness of the urothelium, overall architectural pattern, and assess for presence of atypia. If the urothelium is of normal thickness (5-7 cells), is predominantly flat, and lacks atypia at medium magnification (10×), this most likely represents a benign process (Figure 2.27). The cells are aligned in an orderly manner, with the long axis of nuclei oriented perpendicular to the interface with the lamina propria. An intact umbrella cell layer is useful, but can be seen in atypical and malignant processes as well. Cytologic findings in benign urothelium include dispersed chromatin and longitudinal grooves within the nucleus (Figure 2.28). Benign urothelial mucosa may be sampled due to equivocal cystoscopic findings or in an effort to map out areas of CIS in the bladder. Areas of increased vascularity or dense chronic inflammation may also contribute to an unusual cystoscopic appearance, leading the urologist to biopsy the area (Figure 2.29).

Chronic Cystitis

Chronic cystitis is a general clinical term to describe inflammation within the bladder manifested by lower urinary tract symptoms, including urinary frequency, painful urination, or hematuria. There is not always a direct correlation between the clinical impression of cystitis and the histologic appearance. However, histologic descriptive diagnoses in this category include follicular cystitis, interstitial cystitis, and polypoid cystitis.

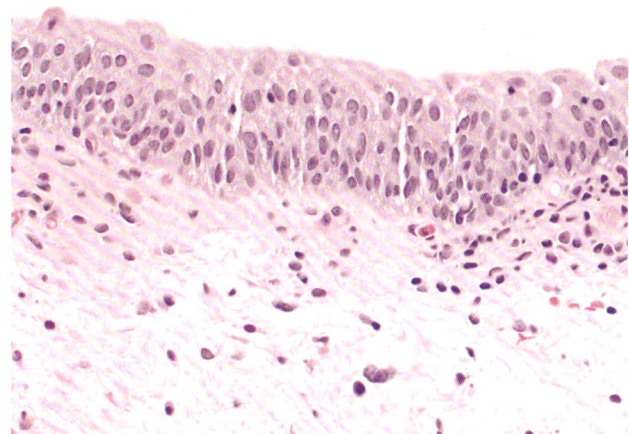

Figure 2.27. This image of benign urothelium is useful as a reference demonstrating the usual 5 to 7 layer thickness, maintained cell polarity and intact umbrella layer. At scanning (10×) magnification, no atypical cells are evident.

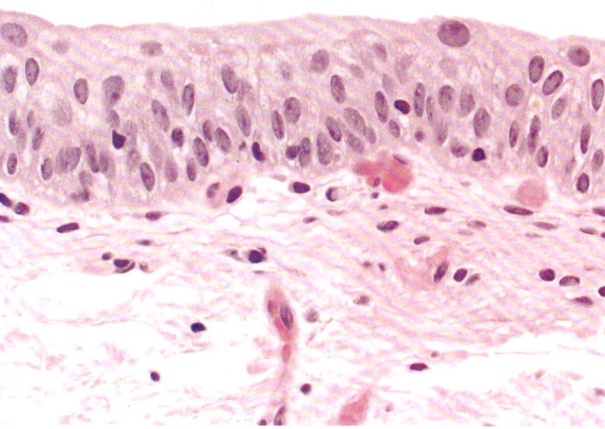

Figure 2.28. The cytologic features of benign urothelium include abundant eosinophilic cytoplasm and nuclei with open chromatin with occasional nuclear grooves.

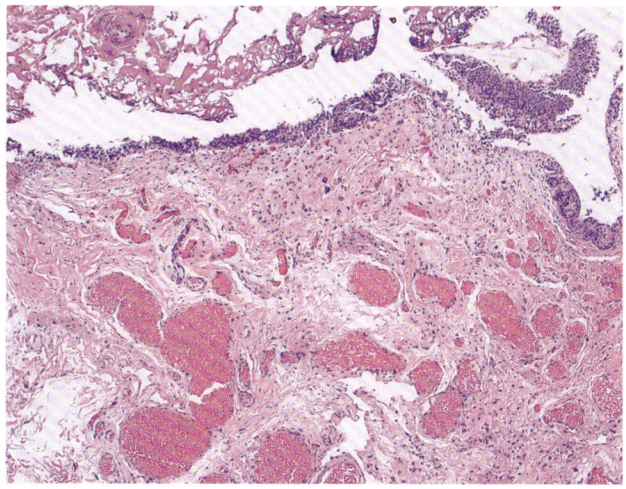

Figure 2.29. Prominent vessels within the lamina propria are evident cystoscopically and may prompt the urologist to target a biopsy in that area. The overlying urothelium appears reactive, which may also have contributed to a roughened or erythematous appearance to the lesion.

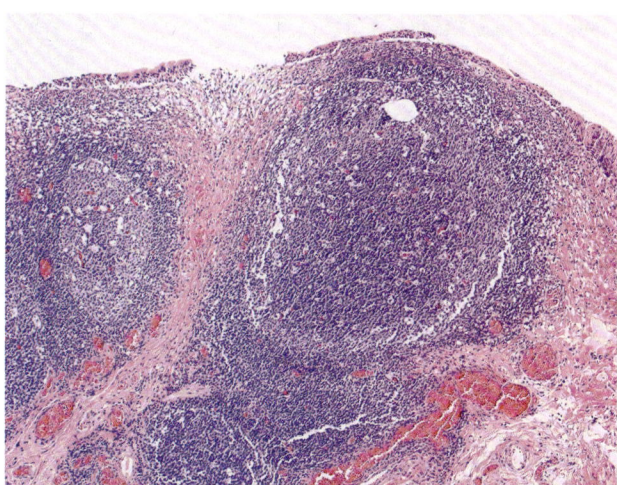

Figure 2.30. Follicular cystitis shows well-formed lymphoid follicles in the lamina propria, leading to mucosal nodularity which can be seen cystoscopically. It is a nonspecific finding and can be caused by multiple inflammatory conditions.

Follicular cystitis is a form of chronic inflammation in which germinal centers have formed within the lamina propria (Figure 2.30). The histologic appearance is nonspecific, but may be related to chronic urinary tract infection or other inflammatory reaction to BCG or intravesical chemotherapy. Cystoscopically, a small mucosal bump may be seen representing the bulging of the urothelium over the well-formed germinal centers.

Interstitial cystitis is a clinical diagnosis often made in older women with painful bladder symptoms. These symptoms may prompt cystoscopic evaluation, which can show erythematous, friable bladder mucosa. Unfortunately, there are no specific pathologic diagnostic criteria for interstitial cystitis, though clinicians often ask for a specific diagnosis in this entity (Figures 2.31 and 2.32). The histopathologic findings in these biopsies are not predictive of severity of disease.[7,8] The "Hunner ulcer" is often ascribed to this entity, though it is not specific for interstitial cystitis. Cystoscopically, Hunner ulcer shows a heaped up nodule with small vessels radiating outward. When biopsied, the Hunner ulcer is usually wedge shaped, with punctate hemorrhage and surrounding granulation tissue. No topline diagnosis of interstitial cystitis should be rendered; rather, excluding a more serious condition of dysplasia, CIS, or malignancy and a description of the findings is appropriate.

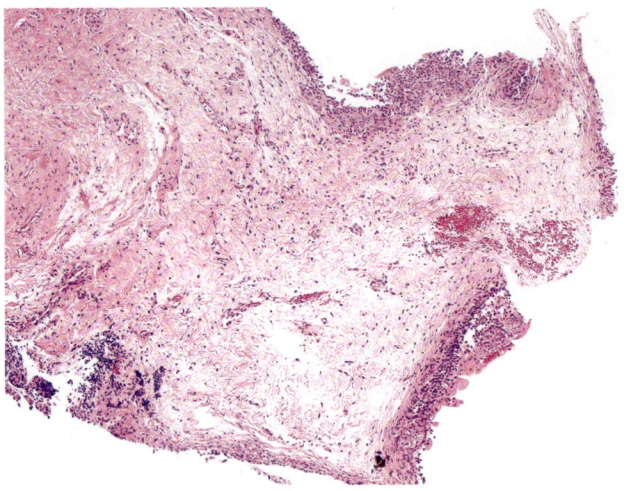

Figure 2.31. Interstitial cystitis is a clinical diagnosis with nonspecific histopathologic appearance. The urothelium may show reactive atypia, and the lamina propria contain numerous vessels with surrounding edema and inflammatory cell infiltrate.

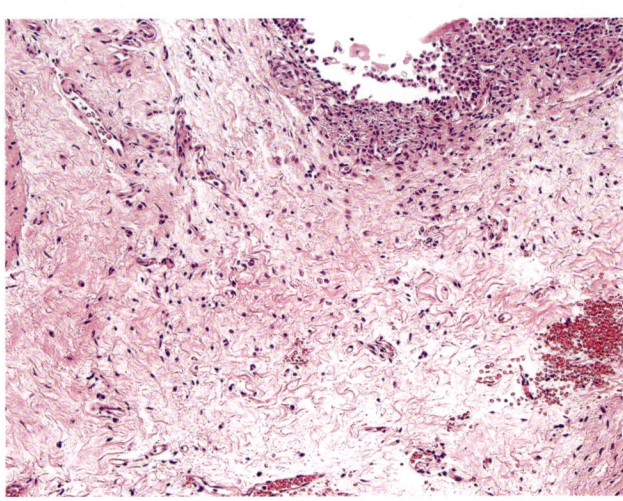

Figure 2.32. Medium-power image of Figure 2.31 showing increased chronic inflammatory cell infiltrate and vessels with overlying urothelium with reactive atypia.

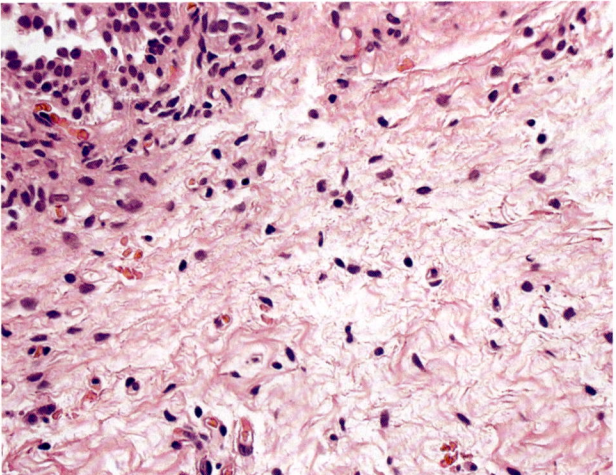

Figure 2.33. At higher power, the chronic inflammatory cells are a mix of lymphocytes, plasma cells, and occasional mast cells.

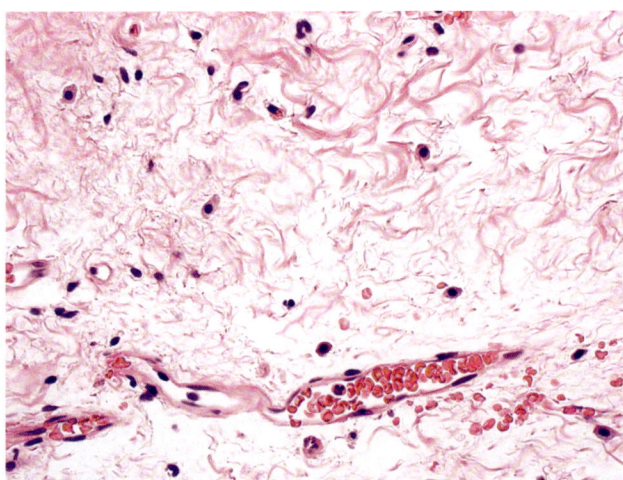

Figure 2.34. Clinicians may ask for a count of mast cells as part of their diagnostic workup for interstitial cystitis; however, no diagnostic cutoff for mast cell count exists and their significance is uncertain.

Occasionally, clinicians may ask for a mast cell count as part of their workup for interstitial cystitis; however, no diagnostic cutoff for mast cell count exists, and their significance is uncertain (Figures 2.33 and 2.34).

KEY FEATURES: Spectrum of atypia and dysplasia
- Atypia is defined as the presence of one or more cellular or architectural features that deviate from that of an otherwise normal appearing cell or group of cells[9]
  - Cytologic atypia is manifest by nuclear enlargement, change in nuclear shape, chromatin clumping, prominent nucleoli, or irregular nuclear outlines
  - Architectural atypia includes denudation, thickening, or changes in cell polarity
  - Reactive changes are included in atypia
- Dysplasia is defined as a preneoplastic or neoplastic process
  - Cytologic and architectural dysplasia are evidenced by more severe alterations in the cells than expected in atypia
  - Changes worrisome for dysplasia or CIS should be included in the dysplastic category

Urothelium With Reactive Changes

Urothelium that either is thickened or demonstrates atypia at medium magnification should be closely examined for a more specific finding. First, reactive changes should be considered and the patient's clinical history should be examined for potential causes, including urinary tract infection, stones, instrumentation or catheterization, and history of intravesical therapy or radiation. Clinical presentation includes lower urinary tract symptoms such as frequency, urgency, or dysuria. Cystoscopic findings demonstrate patches of erythema or roughened urothelium.

PEARLS AND PITFALLS: Reactive Urothelial Changes

- No change or mild thickening of the urothelium
- Obvious inflammation, often in the form of lymphocytes or neutrophils in the lamina propria
- Inflammatory cells within the urothelium is highly suggestive of a reactive pattern when only mild-moderate atypia exists
- One should exercise extreme caution in rendering a diagnosis of dysplasia or CIS in the setting of inflammation

Characteristic cytologic features of reactive changes may also be helpful in confirming reactive changes. Reactive urothelial cells are only slightly enlarged with vesicular or dispersed chromatin and a central small, but prominent nucleolus, in contrast to the hyperchromatic nuclei of CIS (Figures 2.35 and 2.36). Mitotic figures can be frequent in reactive urothelium, often confined to the basal half of the urothelium. The presence of mitoses does not necessarily connote dysplasia or worse. The routine use of Ki-67 for the assessment of CIS in a specimen with other reactive changes may confuse the issue, as an increased proliferation index is common in reactive specimens.

PEARLS AND PITFALLS: Malakoplakia

- Reactive process in the bladder that can mimic malignancy
- Caused by defective phagocytosis of urinary bacteria, usually *Escherichia coli*
- Classic findings of histiocyte-rich mixed inflammation within the lamina propria (Figures 2.37 and 2.38)
- Michaelis-Gutmann bodies are targetoid inclusions within histiocytes comprised of bacterial products, highlighted by von Kossa calcium or iron stain (Figure 2.39)

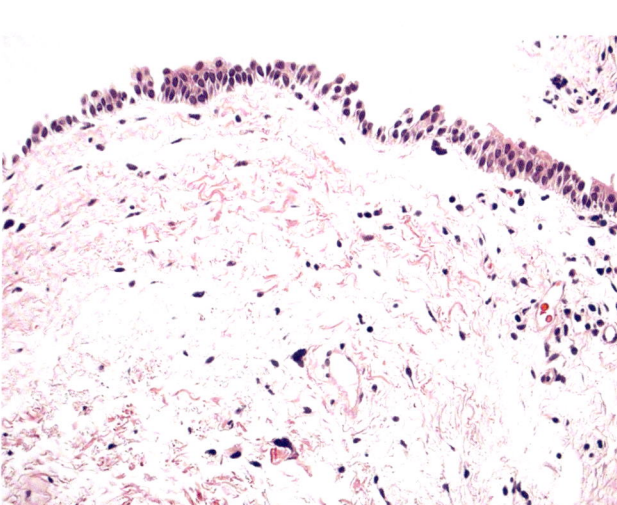

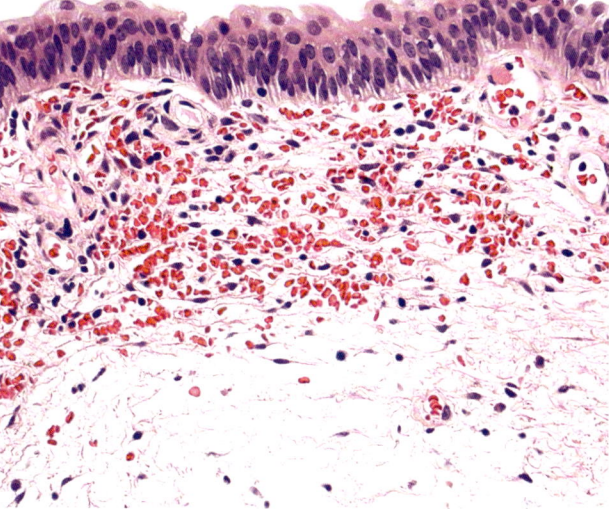

Figure 2.35. Low-power image of reactive urothelium with mild reactive changes. Clues to the reactive nature of the process at low power include maintained polarity and lack of nuclear enlargement. The presence of edema and chronic inflammation within the lamina propria also indicates an inflammatory process.

Figure 2.36. At higher power, the cytologic features of reactive urothelium include single prominent nucleolus within dispersed chromatin background. Hyperchromasia and marked nuclear enlargement are absent, and in this example, mitotic figures are not appreciated.

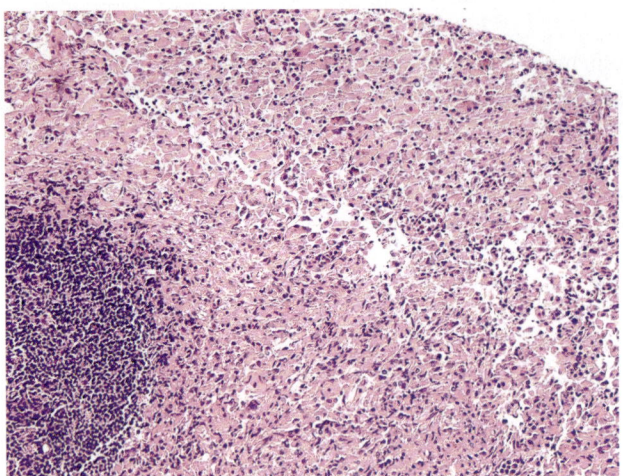

Figure 2.37. Malakoplakia is a reactive inflammatory condition in which histiocytes are unable to fully phagocytose bacteria, especially *Escherichia coli*. The histologic findings include diffuse sheets of histiocytes and mixed inflammation within the lamina propria.

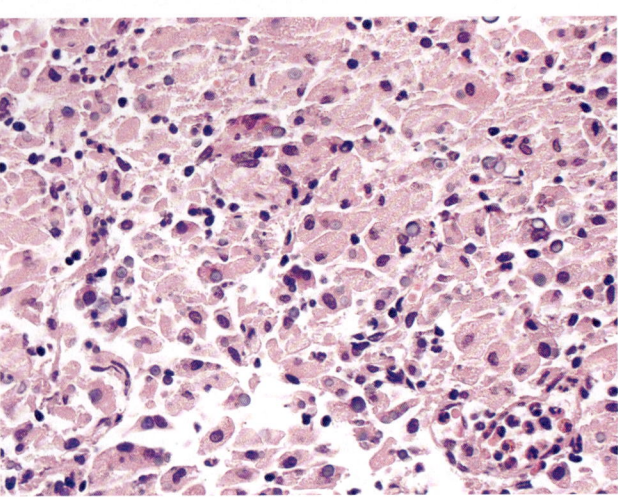

Figure 2.38. At higher power, on hematoxylin and eosin staining targetoid bodies are present within the cytoplasm of the histiocytes. These Michaelis-Gutmann bodies are comprised of undigested bacterial components.

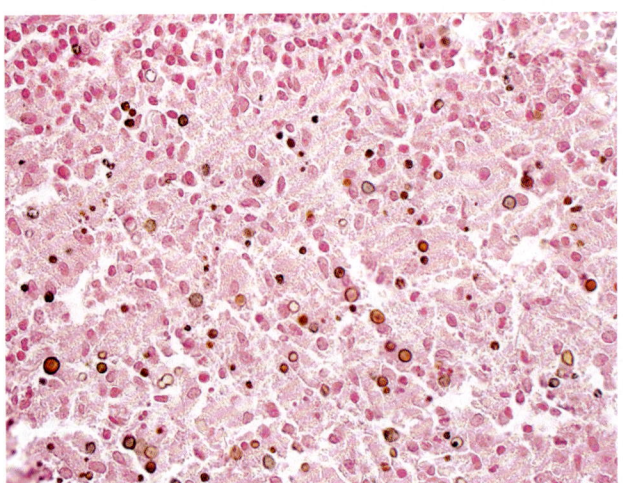

Figure 2.39. von Kossa stain highlights the calcium-rich Michaelis-Gutmann bodies found in malakoplakia.

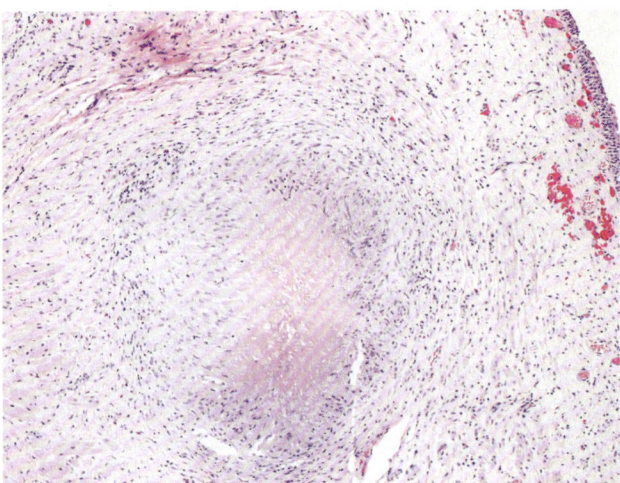

Figure 2.40. Granulomas occurring after TURBT (transurethral resection of bladder tumor) have a distinctive morphologic appearance. Centrally, there is bright eosinophilic material consistent with fibrinoid necrosis. Surrounding the amorphous material are palisading histiocytes.

Iatrogenic and Treatment-Related Cystitis

Iatrogenic causes of cystitis are frequently identified in bladder biopsies, due to the surveillance of many bladder tumors and repeat biopsies. In patients with high-grade urothelial cancer treated with intravesical therapy, BCG, mitomycin C, or gemcitabine may also induce specific changes in the bladder. Granulomatous inflammation is a common response to both prior biopsy and intravesical BCG. Subtle differences in the nature of the granulomas, in addition to good clinical history, can help distinguish between the two causes. Post-TURBT granulomas show central brightly eosinophilic amorphous material, consistent with fibrinoid necrosis, surrounded by palisading histiocytes (Figures 2.40 and 2.41).[10] Foreign body–type giant cells are also a common finding after any surgical procedure (Figure 2.42). A prominent eosinophilic infiltrate is common after TURBT and does not connote allergic response (Figures 2.43 and 2.44). BCG granulomas are more consistent with the small epithelioid granulomas expected in tuberculosis infection, may be caseating or noncaseating, and may extend deep in the bladder wall.[11] If these types of granulomas are observed in a patient without a history of BCG therapy, it is recommended that one perform stains

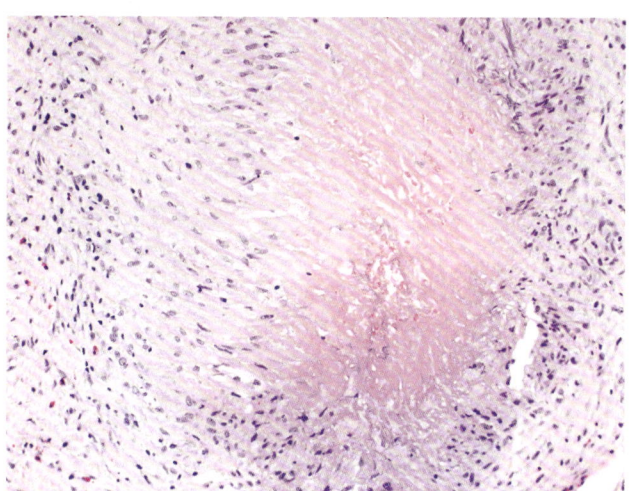

Figure 2.41. At higher power, the palisading nature of the histiocytes in post-TURBT (transurethral resection of bladder tumor) granuloma is evident.

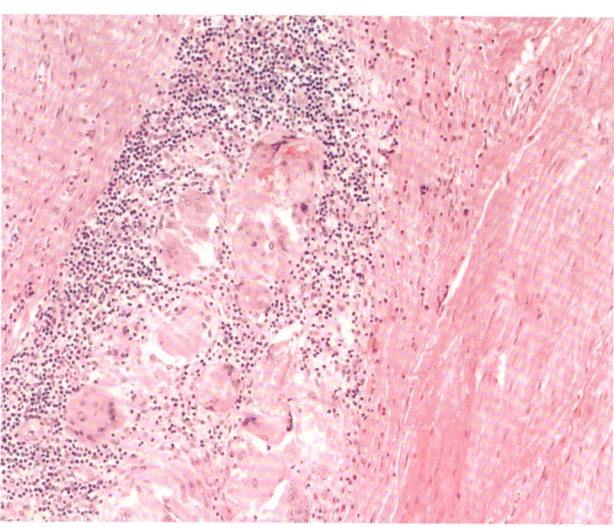

Figure 2.42. Any prior surgical procedure may result in foreign body giant cell reaction, including post-TURBT (transurethral resection of bladder tumor).

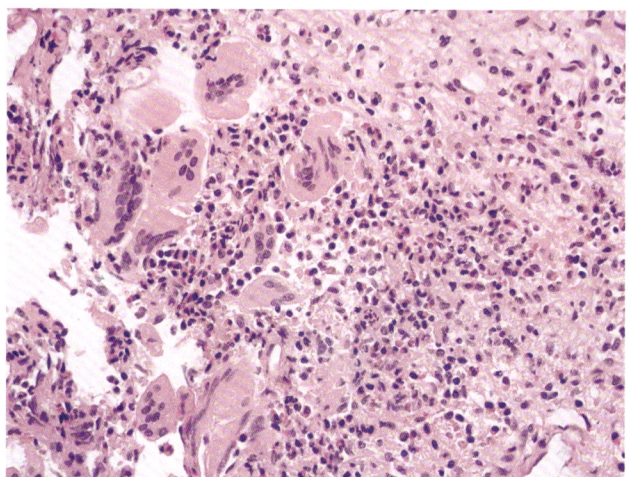

Figure 2.43. In addition to the classic post-TURBT (transurethral resection of bladder tumor) granuloma, giant cells and prominent eosinophilic infiltrate are common findings. Dense eosinophilia in this setting does not connote an allergic response or parasitic process.

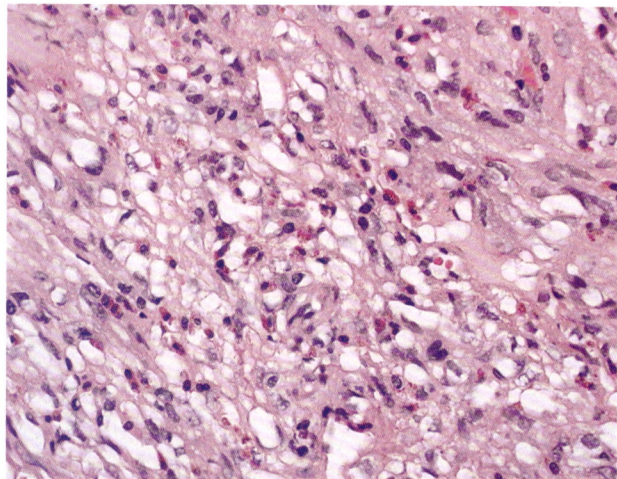

Figure 2.44. Higher power image of numerous eosinophils present in a background of histiocytic inflammation occurring in a post-TURBT (transurethral resection of bladder tumor) granuloma.

for acid-fast and fungal organisms. In a patient with prior BCG treatment, one should not perform acid-fast stains, as they may highlight nonpathogenic acid-fast bacilli and lead to confusion.[12]

Pseudocarcinomatous Urothelial Hyperplasia

A very specific reactive pattern may be observed in urothelium following radiation treatment or other ischemic insult. Pseudocarcinomatous urothelial hyperplasia (PCUH) classically occurs in the setting of pelvic radiation, but can be associated with any vascular insult, and may present clinically with hematuria.[13,14] In addition to the clinical history of radiation, the key to the diagnosis is identifying hemorrhage, fibrin, and fibrin thrombi within the lamina propria and a regenerative appearance to the urothelium (Figures 2.45 and 2.46). PCUH shows atypical urothelial cells which may form small nests and appear to invade the lamina propria (Figures 2.47-2.49). The nests may show retraction artifact, suggestive of invasion.[15] The urothelial nests occupy the superficial lamina propria and show minimal cytologic atypia with absent mitotic activity.

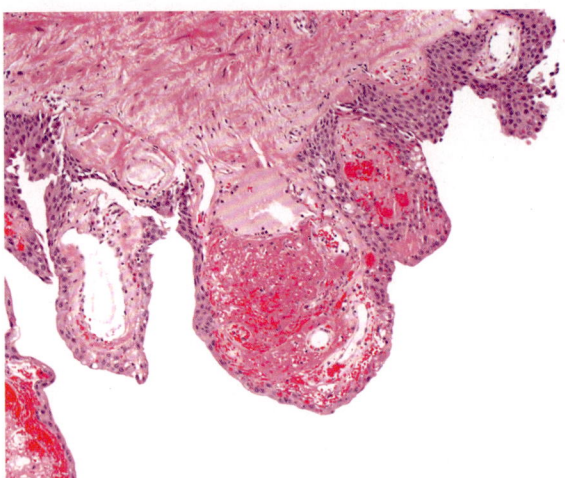

Figure 2.45. Pseudocarcinomatous urothelial hyperplasia (PCUH) occurs in the setting of radiation or ischemic changes in the bladder. At low power, the hallmark feature is hemorrhage and fibrin within the lamina propria.

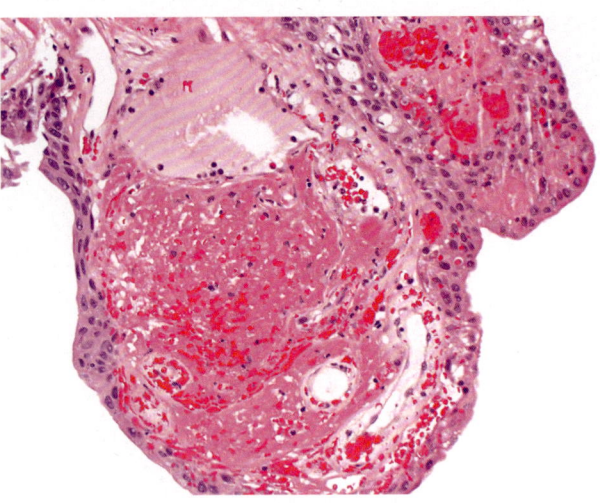

Figure 2.46. At high power, the hemorrhage, extravasated blood cells and organizing fibrin, is evident in the lamina propria, along with scattered hemosiderin deposition.

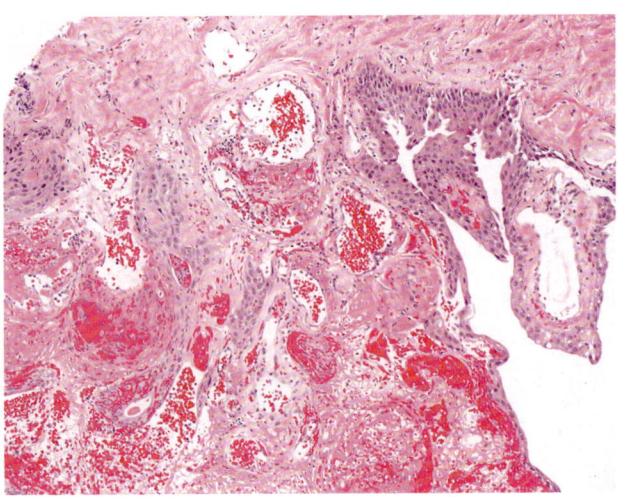

Figure 2.47. In pseudocarcinomatous urothelial hyperplasia (PCUH), the overlying urothelium often has florid regenerative changes conferring some degree of atypia and may show an inverted growth pattern into lamina propria, suspicious for invasive carcinoma. The context of numerous vessels with hemorrhage and fibrin deposition is critical for accurate diagnosis.

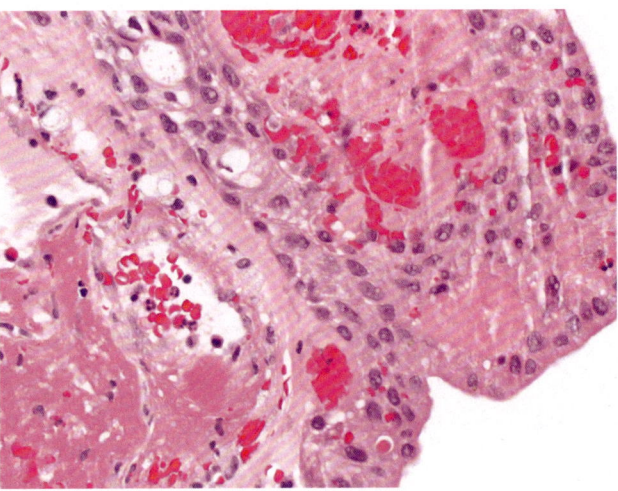

Figure 2.48. Urothelium in pseudocarcinomatous urothelial hyperplasia (PCUH) often shows reactive-type changes, without high-grade atypia. The chromatin pattern is vesicular with a single nucleolus and mitotic figures are scarce. Scattered hemosiderin deposition is also present.

SAMPLE NOTE: Pseudocarcinomatous Urothelial Hyperplasia (See Note)

Note: The specimen demonstrates urothelium with atypia and downward growth into the lamina propria. Numerous vessels and hemorrhage are evident within the lamina propria, many of which show fibrin thrombi. The overall appearance is that of a reactive and regenerative process, consistent with PCUH. This entity is associated with prior radiation, chemotherapy, or other ischemic process.

Reference:
Kryvenko ON, Epstein JI. Pseudocarcinomatous urothelial hyperplasia of the bladder: clinical findings and follow-up of 70 patients. *J Urol.* 2013;189(6):2083-2086.

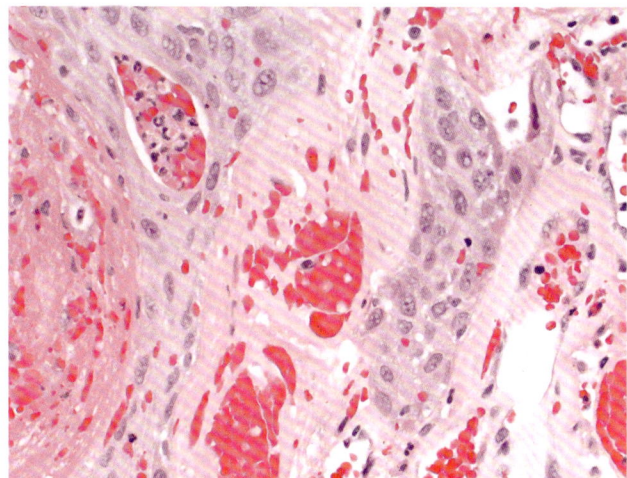

Figure 2.49. Small nests of urothelium present in the lamina propria give the impression of invasive carcinoma, leading to the term "pseudocarcinomatous." The low-power impression of a reactive process and clinical history will help avoid an incorrect diagnosis in this setting.

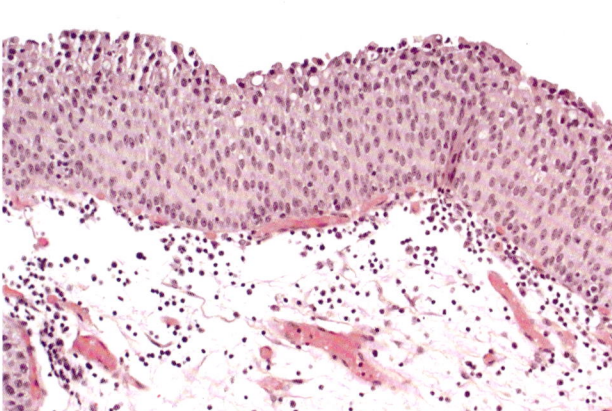

Figure 2.50. Flat urothelial hyperplasia shows thickened urothelium with preserved maturation and relative preservation of polarization. No cytologic atypia or increased mitotic figures are acceptable in this entity.

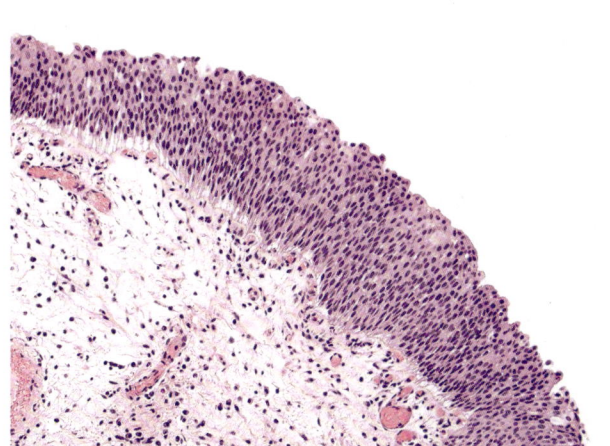

Figure 2.51. Another example of flat urothelial hyperplasia showing well-oriented, but thickened, urothelium without atypia.

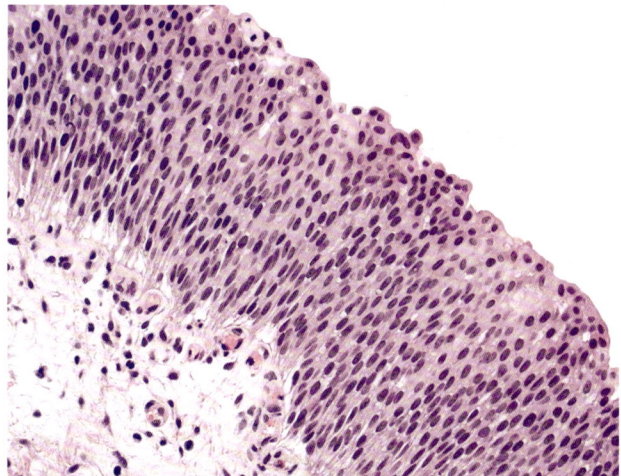

Figure 2.52. At higher power, urothelial hyperplasia shows urothelium of 16 to 20 cell layers thick. Cytologically, the cells have open, dispersed chromatin and small nucleoli without atypia or mitoses.

Flat Urothelial Hyperplasia

Significantly thickened, but flat urothelium with minimal atypia falls into the category of flat urothelial hyperplasia, or urothelial proliferation of uncertain malignant potential (UPUMP) (Figures 2.50 and 2.51). There are no specific symptoms associated with hyperplasia, and it is likely sampled as a subtle irregularity seen on cystoscopy for workup of hematuria or bladder cancer surveillance. In many cases, it is even more likely that it represents an artifact of tangential sectioning of normal urothelium. Flat urothelial hyperplasia may be associated or adjacent to low-grade papillary urothelial carcinoma and is a possible precursor lesion.[16] Cells can show some mild loss of polarity, but maturation is preserved, and there should not be any cytologic atypia or mitotic figures identified (Figure 2.52).[17] This diagnosis should be used sparingly, with more definitive diagnostic categories considered where possible.

Flat Urothelial Lesions With Significant Atypia or Dysplasia

Flat urothelium with atypia raises several diagnostic possibilities, largely dependent on the severity of atypia. If the atypia is significant, i.e., beyond that expected with reactive

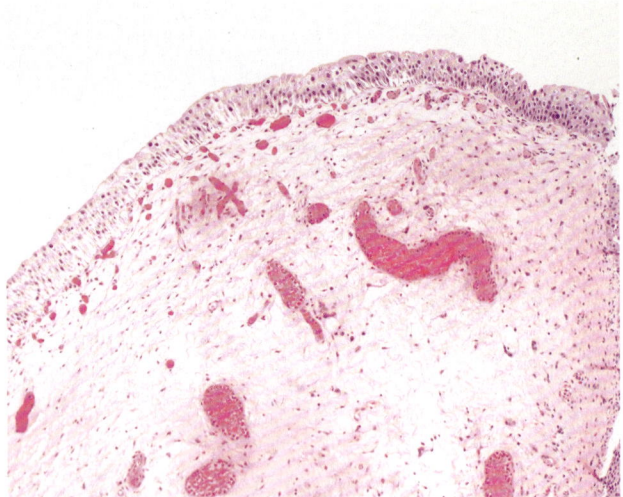

Figure 2.53. Atypia of uncertain significance (AUS) is a highly subjective category representing atypia beyond that expected from reactive changes, but falls short of a diagnosis of dysplasia. This diagnosis should be used sparingly and a more definitive, clinically actionable category assigned when possible.

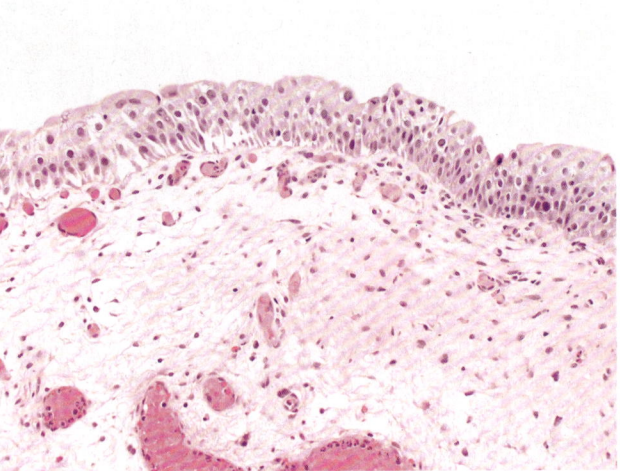

Figure 2.54. In atypia of uncertain significance, scattered larger and darker nuclei are seen in the urothelium, without obvious inflammation or clinical history to explain the changes.

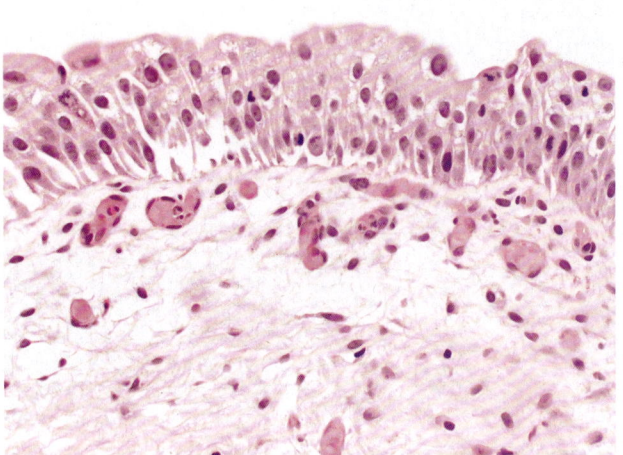

Figure 2.55. At high power, atypia of uncertain significance (AUS) shows scattered hyperchromatic cells and nuclear enlargement. Many of the cells in the background show relatively bland cytology, however.

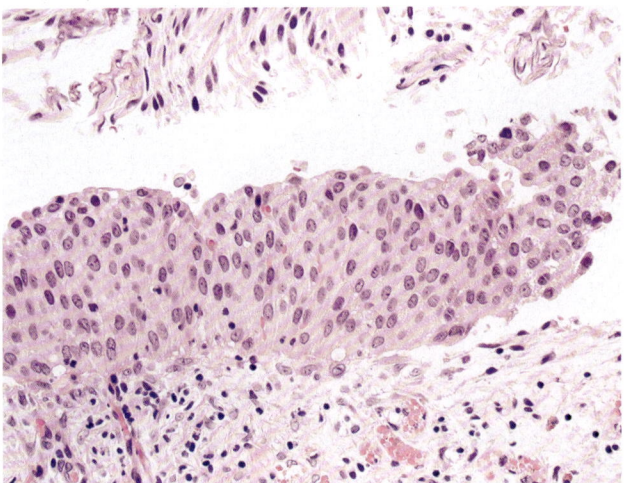

Figure 2.56. Another example of atypia of uncertain significance (AUS) showing mild atypia with the majority of cells demonstrating bland cytologic features, with scattered hyperchromatic cells present along with some loss of polarity.

changes, the spectrum of dysplasia includes atypia of unknown significance, urothelial dysplasia, and urothelial carcinoma in situ.

Atypia of Unknown Significance

When urothelial atypia beyond that expected from reactive changes is present, or no explanation for reactive-type atypia can be readily identified, the lowest level of atypia one can diagnose is atypia of unknown significance. This category was introduced into the ISUP/WHO consensus guidelines in 1998.[18,19] The atypical cells may be slightly enlarged with some hyperchromasia and nuclear pleomorphism (Figures 2.53-2.58). This finding falls short of the diagnosis of dysplasia, but the atypia is concerning or unexplained by other causes (inflammation, instrumentation, stones, radiation, intravesical therapy, etc.). A diagnosis of atypia of unknown significance carries no established risk of adverse outcomes and in general is thought to be equivalent to a diagnosis of reactive atypia.[20] Because of the lack of clinical significance for this diagnosis, every attempt should be made

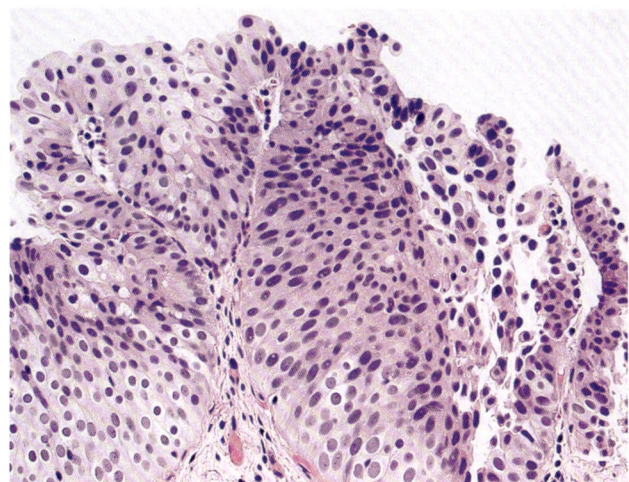

Figure 2.57. Atypia of uncertain significance (AUS) exists on a spectrum with dysplasia, and this image shows a greater degree of atypia than the prior cases. There is significant nuclear enlargement in many of the cells as well as scattered hyperchromasia. These findings are nearing the dysplastic end of the spectrum and different pathologists may disagree on exact classification.

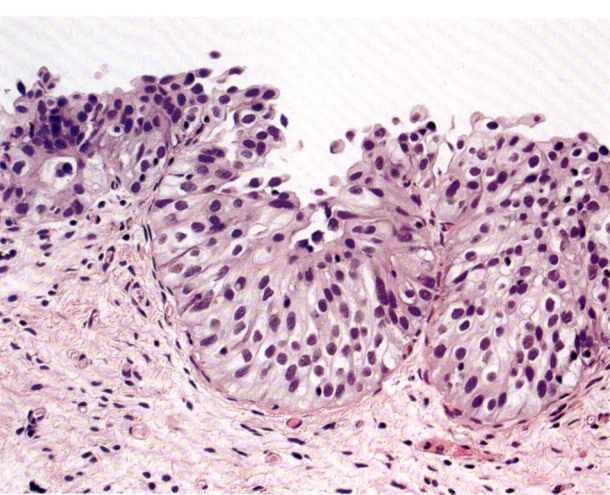

Figure 2.58. Higher power image of Figure 2.57 showing scattered atypical cells in a background of cells with open chromatin and rare nuclear grooves.

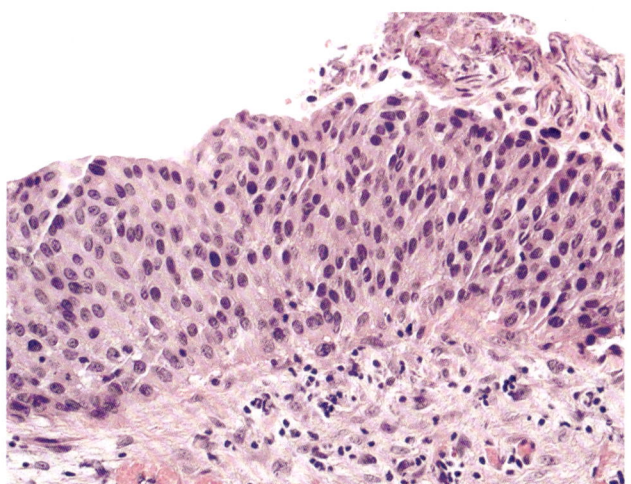

Figure 2.59. Urothelial dysplasia showing a greater degree of atypia, hyperchromasia, and loss of polarity than seen in atypia of uncertain significance. There are no specific diagnostic criteria for this category, but the finding should be reported and warrants clinical follow-up as there is an increased risk for carcinoma in situ (CIS).

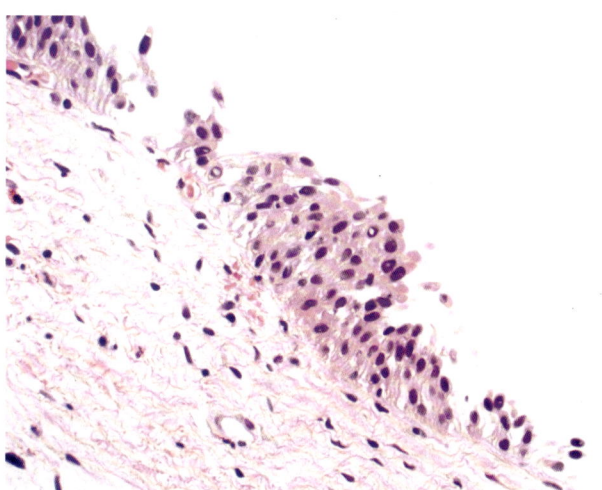

Figure 2.60. Dysplastic urothelium showing hyperchromasia and disorganization, but lacking the nuclear enlargement and increased mitotic figures expected in carcinoma in situ (CIS). On the spectrum of urothelial atypia, dysplasia falls between atypia of uncertain significance and CIS.

to find a more concrete category for these minimal changes when possible. However, in rare cases, such terminology may be necessary to convey a lack of certainty regarding the pathologic findings. Numerous images are included as this diagnosis exists on a spectrum between reactive atypia and dysplasia, and significant subjectivity exists in the diagnosis (Figures 2.57 and 2.58).

Urothelial Dysplasia

Urothelial dysplasia is a histologic term describing flat urothelium with atypia that is beyond reactive changes, but which does not have significant cytologic or architectural disarray to reach a diagnosis of CIS (Figures 2.59 and 2.60).[17] Unfortunately, because it lacks specific diagnostic criteria, this entity suffers from poor interobserver reliability and lacks good data on outcomes. Regardless, it is felt to represent a preneoplastic lesion, with some risk of developing CIS and warrants clinical follow-up.[21]

Urothelial Carcinoma In Situ

At the far end of the spectrum of atypia in flat urothelium, urothelial carcinoma in situ (CIS) shows high-grade cytology with enlarged hyperchromatic cells with obvious disorganization and frequent mitoses (Figures 2.61-2.63). The marked atypia and hyperchromasia in these cases is apparent at scanning power (10×), though more subtle findings may exist in the form of small cell CIS or CIS that is partially or predominantly denuded (Figure 2.64). The loss of orientation of the urothelium to the surface is also evident at low power, with a jumbled appearance and lack of even distribution of cells throughout the urothelium (Figures 2.65 and 2.66). CIS cells are dyscohesive and prone to denudation; identification and close evaluation of denuded urothelium may actually alert the astute pathologist to the possibility of CIS. Various morphologic appearances exist in CIS, including large cell with nuclear pleomorphism, large cell without nuclear pleomorphism, small cell, and clinging and pagetoid spreading type (Figures 2.67-2.69).[22] It is important to note that an intact umbrella cell layer does not exclude the possibility of CIS, especially when present in the pagetoid form.

PEARLS AND PITFALLS: Urothelial Carcinoma In Situ

- CIS is usually evident at 10× scanning magnification. If you are going to high power to convince yourself of atypia, it is probably not CIS!
- Nuclear enlargement of 4 to 5× the size of a resting lymphocyte is a helpful diagnostic criterion for CIS; however, small cell CIS does exist
- Always raise your suspicion for CIS in denuded specimens; hunt around the edges for focally intact urothelium and level into the block if any concerning features are identified (Figure 2.70)
- In denuded specimens, recommending urine cytology may capture dyscohesive CIS cells shed from the bladder wall

Immunohistochemistry for Urothelial Dysplasia/Carcinoma In Situ

In general, immunohistochemistry is not entirely robust for resolving the differential diagnosis between urothelial reactive changes and CIS; however, a number of potential markers have been studied for this purpose. The most commonly used antibodies include cytokeratin 20 (CK20), p53, and sometimes CD44.[22-24] Other markers that have been studied or proposed include cytokeratin 5/6, p16, alpha-methylacyl-CoA racemase (AMACR), HER2, ProEx C, Ki67, among others.[24-29]

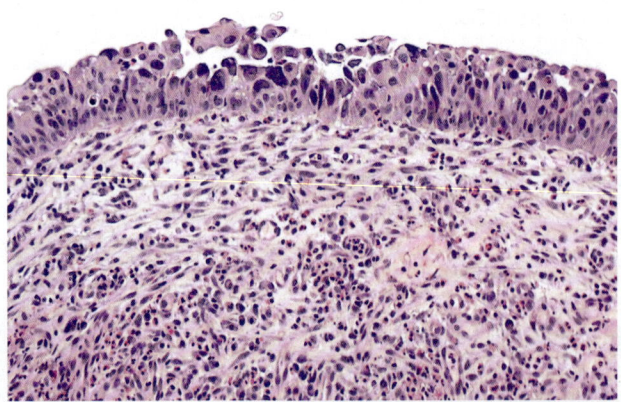

Figure 2.61. Urothelial carcinoma in situ (CIS) showing high-grade atypia, evident at scanning magnification. Hyperchromatic, enlarged nuclei with irregular nuclear membranes are present and the cells are focally dyscohesive.

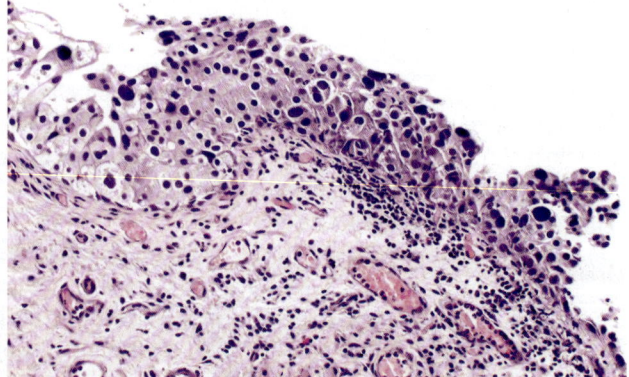

Figure 2.62. Carcinoma in situ (CIS) at higher power illustrating the true hyperchromatic nature of the malignant cells. The chromatin is inky black, to the extent no specific chromatin pattern can be seen and nucleoli are obscured.

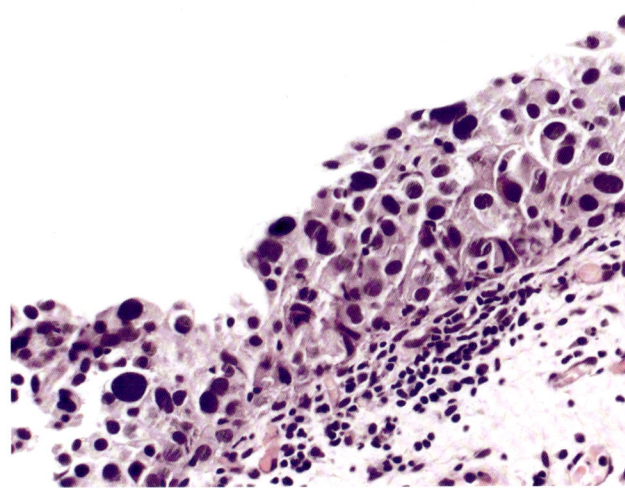

Figure 2.63. Nuclear enlargement is a diagnostic feature of carcinoma in situ (CIS). The largest malignant cell in this image is more than 5× the size of a resting lymphocyte present in the lamina propria.

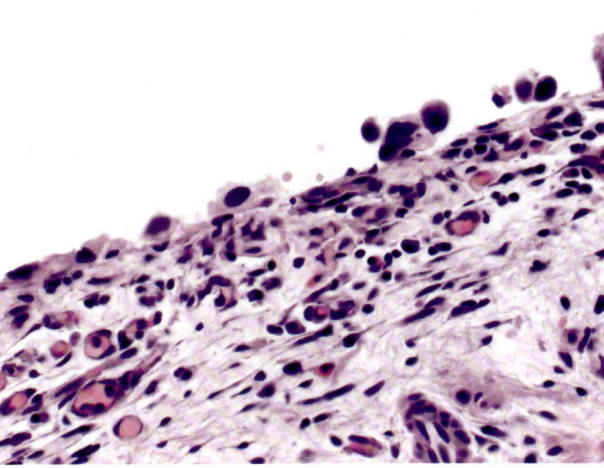

Figure 2.64. Carcinoma in situ (CIS) is often dyscohesive, and only a few malignant cells may remain attached to the surface. Despite the paucity of cells, when they meet the other criteria for CIS (hyperchromasia, nuclear enlargement), it is still possible to call CIS in a scanty specimen.

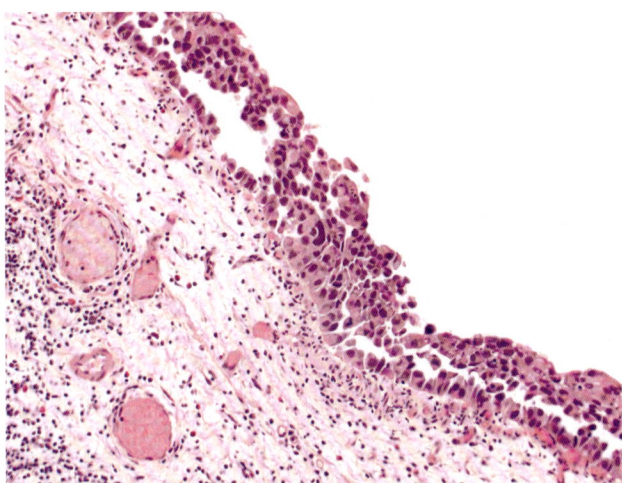

Figure 2.65. Another low-power clue for carcinoma in situ (CIS) is an obvious lack of maturation and disorganization of the urothelium. At scanning magnification, there is no orderly arrangement of cells from the basal to the luminal surface.

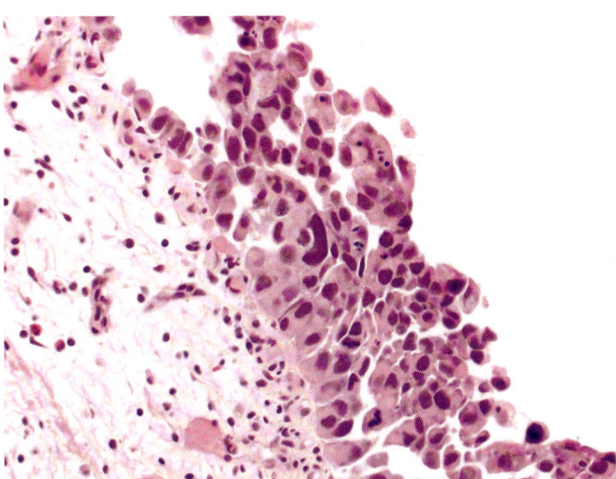

Figure 2.66. Higher power of Figure 2.65 showing marked atypia, nuclear enlargement, and frequent mitotic figures in a disorganized, jumbled urothelium. The cellular dyscohesion is evident, as well as loss of the umbrella cell layer.

With regard to the most common markers, CK20 generally shows negative staining or weak, subset staining of the superficial cells only in benign or reactive epithelium, whereas full-thickness staining favors a neoplastic lesion. For CD44, a reactive pattern is full-thickness staining of the reactive epithelium, whereas reduced staining in the neoplastic cells is found with CIS. For p53, a heterogeneous pattern of variable weak to moderate staining (a wild-type pattern) would be consistent with normal or reactive epithelium, whereas diffuse strong staining (and possibly completely negative/"null" staining) would favor CIS (Figure 2.71, Table 2.1).[30]

However, these stains can be fraught with technical and interpretative challenges, such that in a given patient, the pattern may not be definitive. For example, a moderate degree of p53 staining can be difficult to discern from strong diffuse staining, depending on laboratory technical staining conditions. In one study of diagnostically difficult cases where immunohistochemistry was used, very few patients without a history of prior urothelial

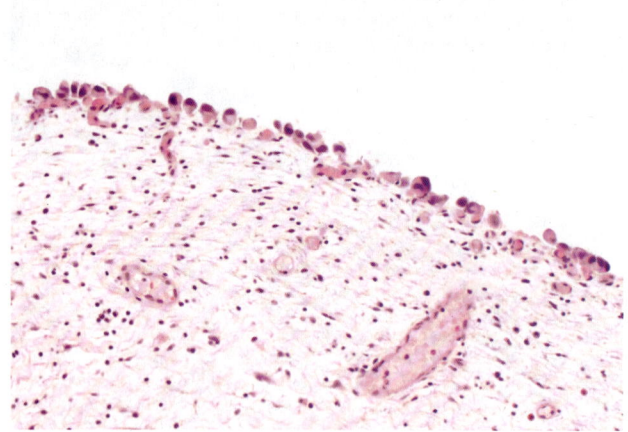

Figure 2.67. Carcinoma in situ (CIS) can have varying morphologic appearances. This image demonstrates a small cell CIS with clinging pattern. Small, hyperchromatic, and dyscohesive cells "cling" to the lamina propria surface.

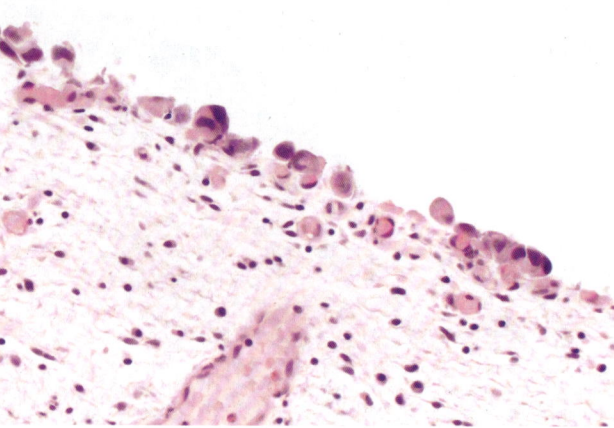

Figure 2.68. Higher power image of clinging nature of carcinoma in situ (CIS), where cells are detaching from the surface and focally denuded.

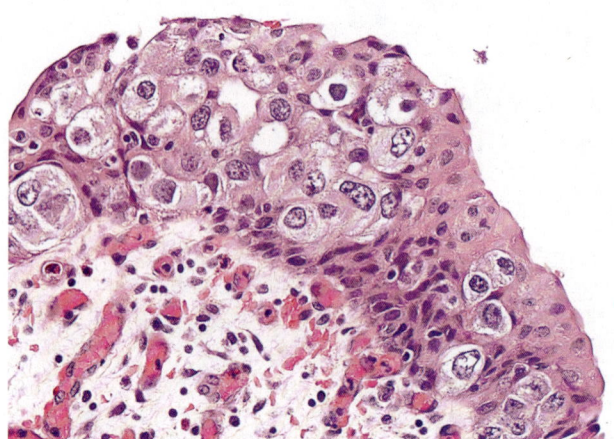

Figure 2.69. Carcinoma in situ (CIS) may spread in a pagetoid fashion, where individual or nests of malignant cells percolate through the benign urothelium.

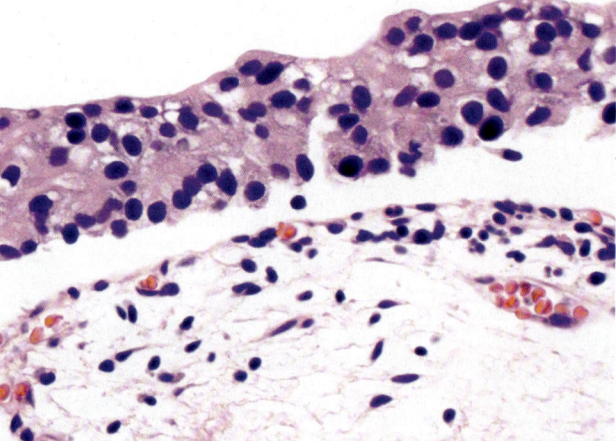

Figure 2.70. This image of carcinoma in situ (CIS) shows the vast degree to which denudation can occur, illustrating the complete detachment of the urothelium from the underlying lamina propria. If the detachment had been more advanced, or a smaller biopsy was taken, it is possible the CIS cells would not have been sampled. Urine cytology can be extremely useful in the setting of denuded urothelium where there is a suspicion of CIS.

TABLE 2.1: Most Common Immunohistochemical Patterns for Distinction of CIS From Reactive Epithelium

	CIS	Reactive
CK20	Full thickness	Superficial ("umbrella") cells only or negative
p53	Strong throughout all atypical cells	Variable weak to moderate (depends on laboratory techniques)
CD44	Decreased in atypical cells	Full thickness

CIS, carcinoma in situ.

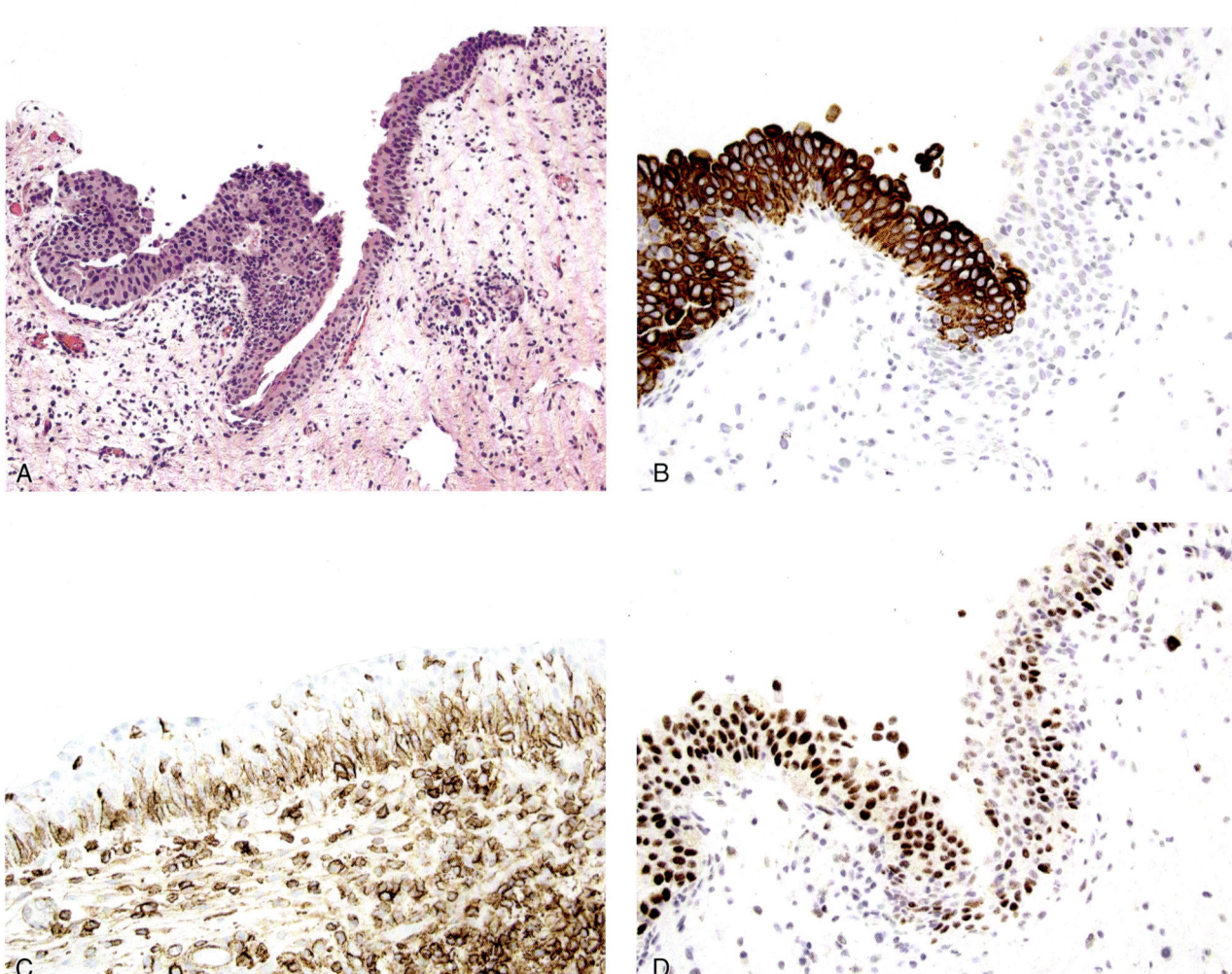

Figure 2.71. In some cases, immunohistochemistry can help in cases with morphology that is equivocal for the diagnosis of CIS. A, shows an atypical urothelial proliferation with some evidence of maturation, but many hyperchromatic atypical cells (primarily on the left side of the image). B, CK20 staining is full thickness in the atypical urothelium, supporting a diagnosis of carcinoma in situ (CIS). Note that the normal urothelium on the right side of the image shows largely negative staining with faint staining in the umbrella cell layer. C, CD44 shows loss of full-thickness staining in the atypical proliferation, supporting a diagnosis of CIS. No normal urothelium is present in this image; however, the expected pattern of CD44 in normal urothelium is staining the full thickness of the urothelium (the opposite pattern of CK20). D, shows strong, diffuse nuclear staining for p53 in all atypical urothelial cells, again supporting a diagnosis of CIS. It is critical to remember that these stains can be fraught with technical and interpretative challenges, such that in a given patient, the pattern may not be definitive. hematoxylin and eosin morphology is key to accurate diagnosis of CIS.

neoplasm went on to develop urothelial carcinoma, suggesting that careful attention to morphology and clinical history is more important than an immunohistochemical staining pattern.[23]

In the absence of thermal injury from electrocautery, it is important to recognize that entirely denuded urothelium should not be diagnosed as benign, and a comment raising the possibility of a denuded CIS with the suggestion of obtaining urine cytology should be included (Figures 2.72-2.74).[31,32]

SAMPLE NOTE: Denuded Urothelial Mucosa (See Note)

Note: Denudation of the urothelium may occur when dyscohesive CIS cells detach from the lamina propria and exfoliate into the urine. Urine cytology or additional sampling may be useful in this setting.

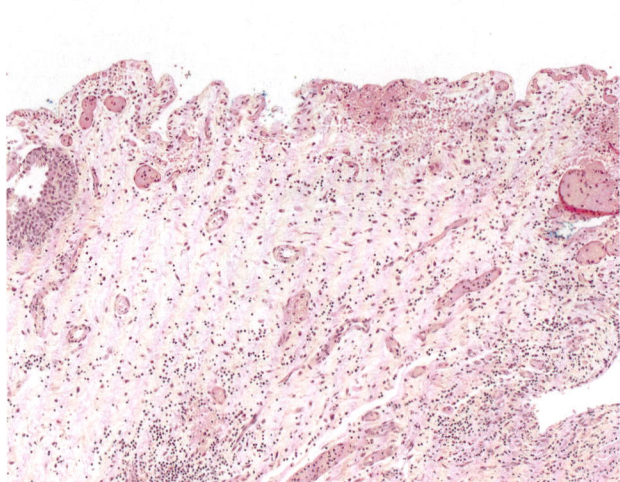

Figure 2.72. Another example of entirely denuded urothelium, raising suspicion for carcinoma in situ (CIS). Close inspection of the surface for rare atypical cells is warranted in these cases, along with suggestion to collect urine cytology.

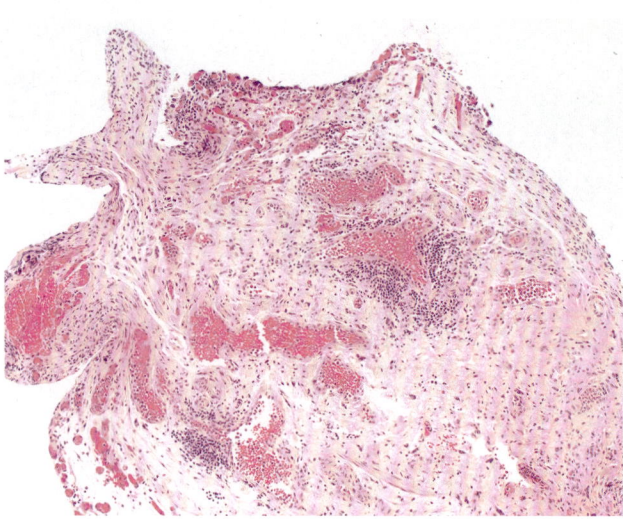

Figure 2.73. Focally denuded urothelium with rare intact atypical urothelial cells.

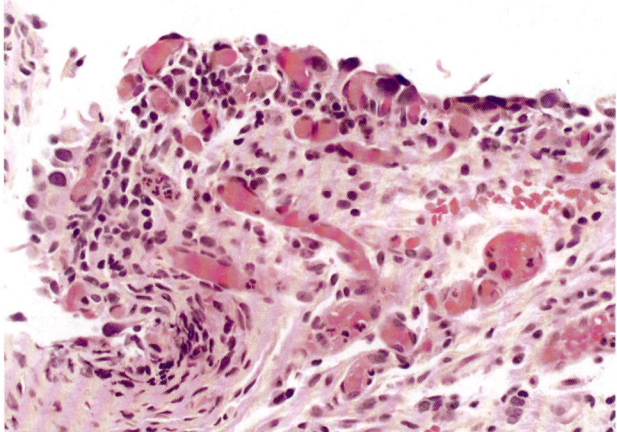

Figure 2.74. At high power, the intact urothelial cells from Figure 2.73 show high-grade atypia with increased nuclear size and hyperchromasia, sufficient for a diagnosis of carcinoma in situ (CIS).

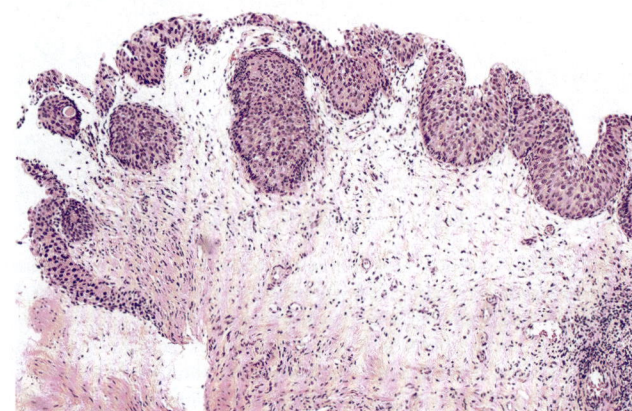

Figure 2.75. Carcinoma in situ (CIS) commonly involves von Brunn nests (VBN) and can be confused for invasive carcinoma. Because VBN represent downward growth of the surface urothelium, this represents extension of malignant cells in continuity with the surface, not invasive growth.

PEARLS AND PITFALLS: CIS Involving von Brunn Nests

- CIS commonly involves VBN, as they represent a downward growth into the lamina propria which is in continuity with the surface (Figures 2.75 and 2.76)
- VBN involved by CIS usually appears as moderate to large nests with rounded contours and lack of specific features of invasion (no retraction artifact, small or irregular nests, or infiltrating single cells)

PAPILLARY LESIONS OF THE BLADDER—UROTHELIAL

Papillary lesions of the bladder are evident by exophytic papillary fronds, projecting into the lumen of the bladder and readily identified on cystoscopic evaluation. The cystoscopy procedure note is of paramount importance when diagnosing papillary lesions, especially if the histologic appearance is equivocal for true papillary architecture. A helpful urologist

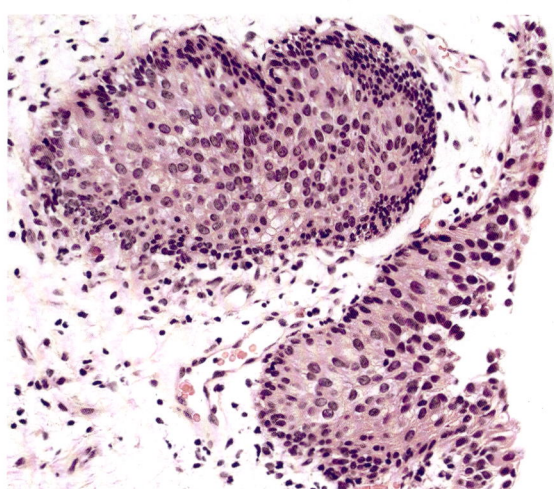

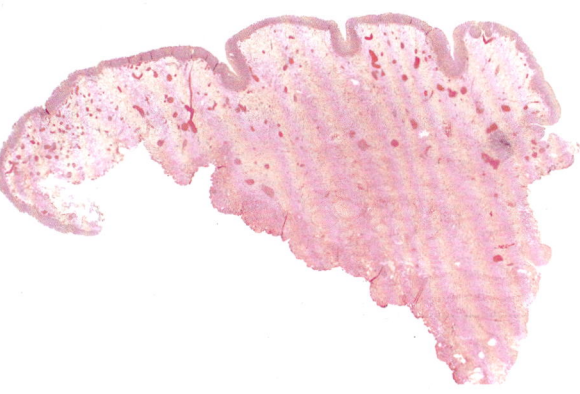

Figure 2.76. Higher power image of carcinoma in situ (CIS) involving von Brunn nests (VBN) with rounded nests of tumor without retraction artifact or irregular contours. The CIS cells show greater atypia than expected in a normal VBN, with nuclear enlargement and hyperchromasia.

Figure 2.77. Whole slide image of a TURBT (transurethral resection of bladder tumor) fragment demonstrating the broad mucosal folds of polypoid cystitis.

will comment on the exact nature of the lesion, often using descriptors such as papillary, polypoid, sessile, low-grade appearing, etc. Their description can help confirm a histologic impression or prompt deeper levels on a specimen to identify a possible small papillary lesion when none is identified on initial sections.

Papillary/Polypoid Cystitis

Before discussion of true urothelial neoplasms, it is important to be aware of the benign mimickers of papillary neoplasms. A true papillary neoplasm is defined by the presence of true fibrovascular cores. Without well-formed papillae, all caution is warranted to avoid overdiagnosis of a neoplasm. Papillary/polypoid cystitis is one potential pitfall in this differential diagnosis.[33] The classic appearance of polypoid cystitis is the presence of broad, edematous folds of urothelial mucosa and lamina propria (Figure 2.77). Unlike a true papillary neoplasm, there are no long, thin papillary projects with fibrovascular cores. The lamina propria is markedly edematous, often appearing as a cleared out space with the urothelium floating above (Figures 2.78 and 2.79). Inflammation is usually evident in both the lamina propria and within the urothelium (Figure 2.80). Given the inflammatory and reactive nature of these lesions, a clinical history of recent catheter use, indwelling catheter, or stones may be solicited from the medical record.

PEARLS AND PITFALLS: Polypoid Cystitis

- Low-power clues include broad folds with pale, edematous lamina propria and inflammatory cells
- Overlying urothelium may be thickened and show reactive epithelial changes; however, no more than minimal atypia should be present in these cases
- Over time, polypoid cystitis may become more papillary in nature as inflammation resolves and fibrosis contracts the broad folds into smaller papillary fronds (Figures 2.81-2.83)
- In papillary/polypoid cystitis, fronds lack the true fibrovascular cores found in papillary neoplasms
- Identifying the overall inflammatory context is important for accurate diagnosis of these lesions

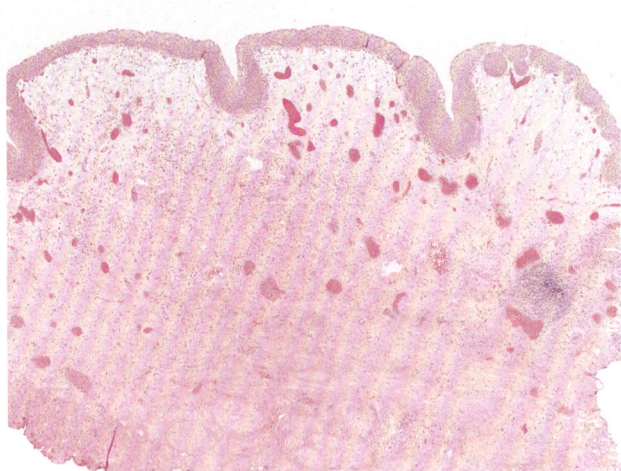

Figure 2.78. At low power, the broad folds and underlying edematous lamina propria are a distinct appearance from a true papillary neoplasm.

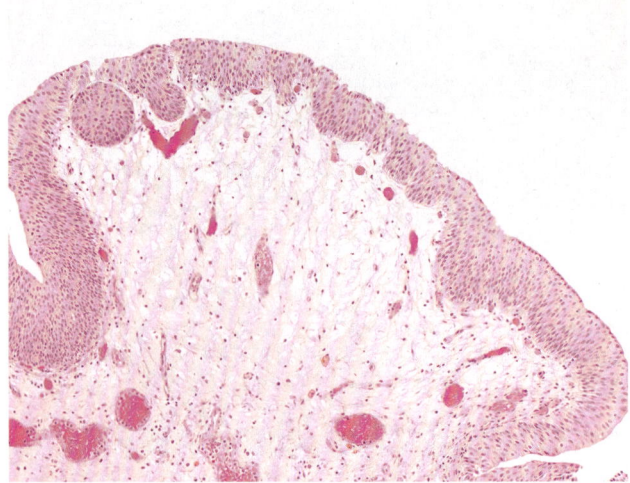

Figure 2.79. At higher power, polypoid cystitis shows only minimal reactive changes in the urothelium. The lamina propria is edematous and pale, bulging into the lumen of the bladder.

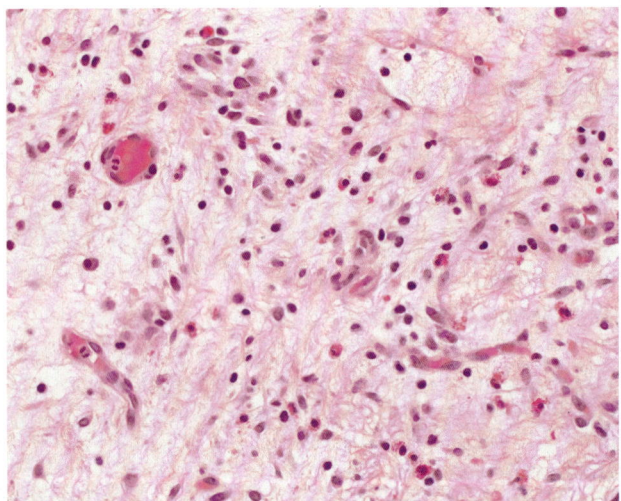

Figure 2.80. Within the lamina propria, a chronic inflammatory infiltrate is readily identifiable in most cases of polypoid cystitis.

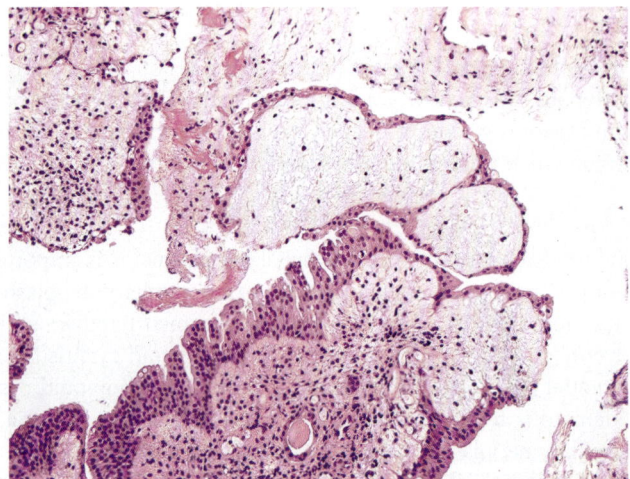

Figure 2.81. In cases of long-standing polypoid cystitis, the broad mucosal folds can undergo fibrosis and become more papillary (smaller, less broad based) fronds. These changes should not be confused for a true papillary lesion. Note that the lamina propria edema and chronic inflammation are still prominent in this case.

Papillary Hyperplasia

Another quasi-papillary lesion to consider in this spectrum of lesions is papillary urothelial hyperplasia, also referred to as urothelial proliferation of uncertain malignant potential by the WHO. While this lesion lacks true fibrovascular cores, it may raise the possibility of a true neoplasm in small biopsy specimens. The diagnosis of papillary urothelial hyperplasia should be used only when limited folds or "tenting" of the urothelium are present. Papillary urothelial hyperplasia will show a wave-like periodicity to the mucosal folds, leading to a corrugated appearance of the urothelium (Figure 2.84). True fibrovascular cores are absent, though small capillary-sized vessels may be present at the tips of the folds. Papillary urothelial hyperplasia may represent a precursor lesion to low-grade papillary urothelial carcinoma and has been noted associated with established low-grade papillary carcinomas as a "shoulder" lesion (Figure 2.85).[34,35] In biopsy settings, the diagnosis of papillary hyperplasia should be reserved for lesions not directly associated with low-grade papillary urothelial carcinoma.

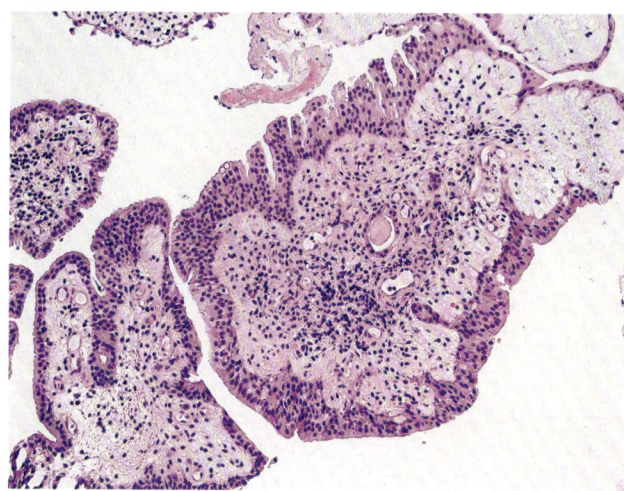

Figure 2.82. At higher power, this polypoid/papillary cystitis frond lacks fibrovascular cores; instead, it shows contracted and fibrotic fronds with lamina propria edema and inflammation.

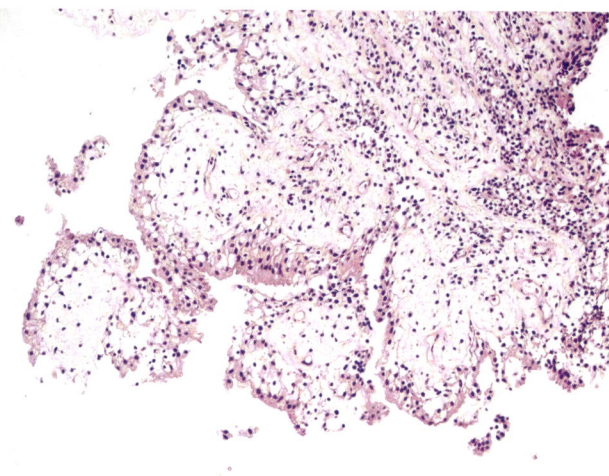

Figure 2.83. Another example of polypoid/papillary cystitis with lamina propria edema and chronic inflammation. While the papillary fronds are somewhat complex in this case, the overall impression is that of a reactive/inflammatory process.

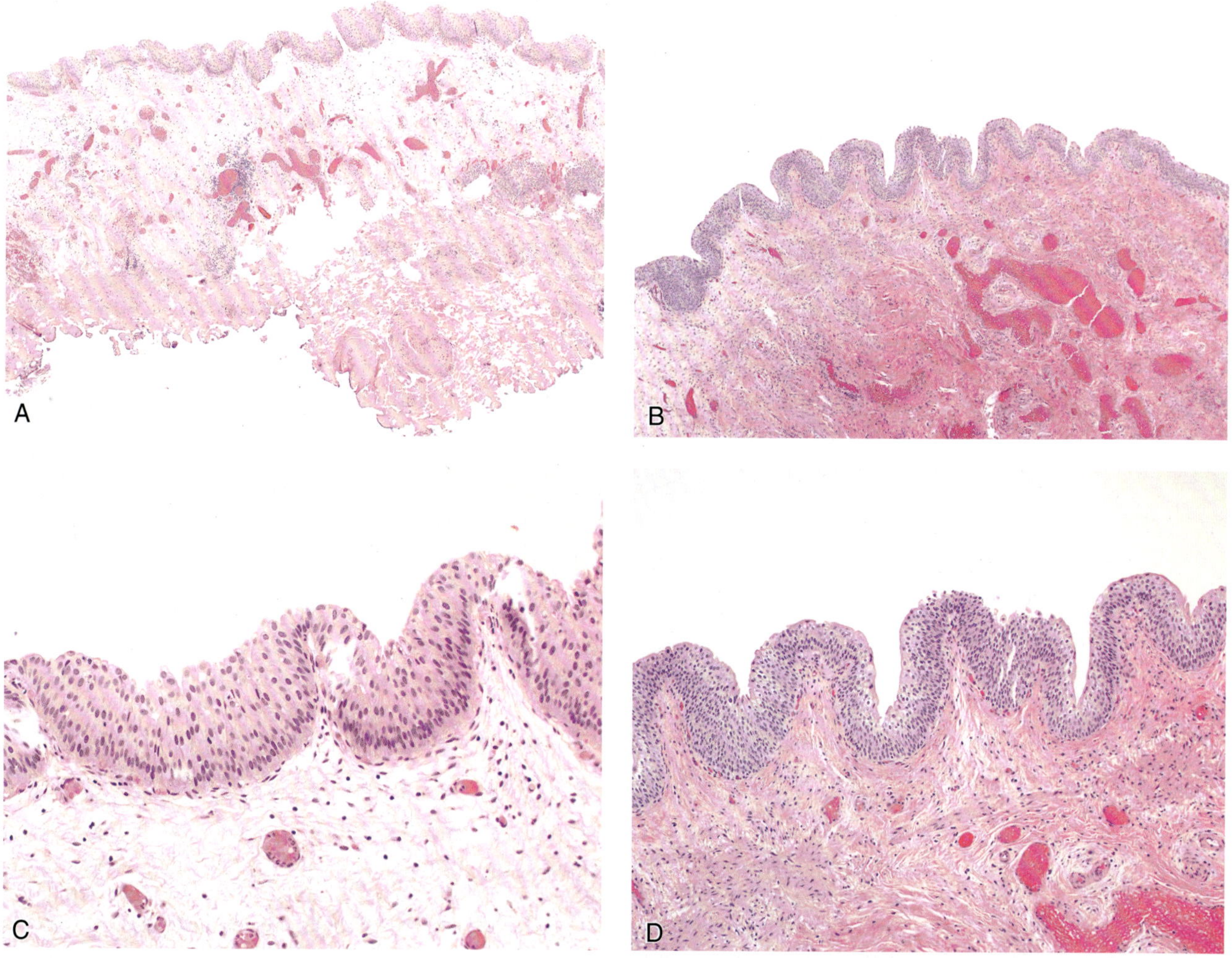

A

B

C

D

Figure 2.84. A and B, show a scanning magnification of papillary hyperplasia with the wave-like periodicity or "corrugation" of the urothelial surface. No discrete papillary fronds have formed, although rarely a small vessel will begin to orient itself toward the tented urothelium. C and D, are higher power images of the lesions, highlighting the lack of fibrovascular cores. The overlying urothelium is of slightly increased thickness and displays only minimal atypia. Papillary hyperplasia may represent a precursor lesion to low-grade papillary urothelial carcinoma and has been noted associated with established low-grade papillary carcinomas as a "shoulder" lesion.

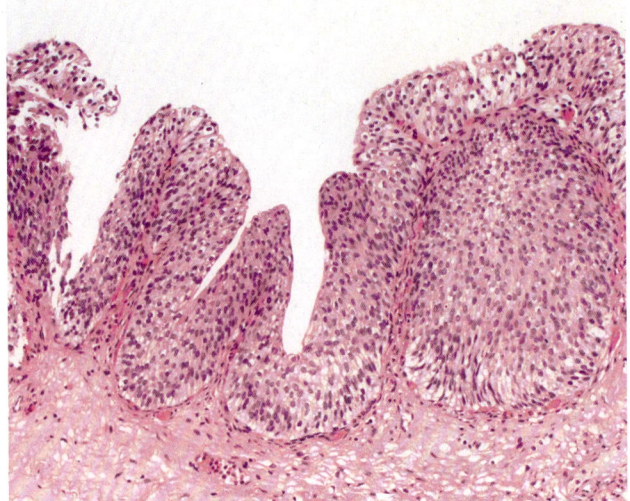

Figure 2.85. The urothelium of papillary hyperplasia shown at high power showing increased thickness and minimal atypia. Papillary hyperplasia may occur adjacent to low-grade papillary urothelial carcinoma ("shoulder" lesion) or unrelated to a papillary lesion. In small biopsy settings, the diagnosis should be reserved for lesions not directly associated with low-grade papillary urothelial carcinoma.

Benign Urothelial Papilloma

Now that we have discussed mimickers of papillary neoplasms, we can begin to address true papillary urothelial neoplasms. These lesions are exophytic lesions with true fibrovascular cores lined by urothelium (Figure 2.86). Referring again to the checklist, diagnosing papillary lesions of the bladder also begins with an assessment of the urothelial thickness. Once the papillary architecture has been identified, the thickness of the urothelium will help to focus the diagnostic possibilities. Papillary lesions with normal thickness urothelium that lacks atypia are considered benign urothelial papillomas. In addition to well-formed papillary cores, papillomas should have a urothelial lining that closely approximates that of normal flat benign urothelium, 5 to 7 cells thick and lacking atypia. At low power, urothelial papillomas often appear as pale eosinophilic to clear lesions, due to the small nuclei and ample cytoplasm that often has clearing (Figures 2.87 and 2.88). If stretched out flat, the urothelial lining of a papilloma looks the same as benign urothelium lining the bladder (Figure 2.89). The papillary fronds are usually very slender and long, a feature that may be remarked on in the cystoscopy note and lead the urologist to suggest a papilloma or "low-grade appearance." Patients with benign papillomas are often younger than those diagnosed with papillary carcinoma, and rarely progress to higher grade disease.[36,37]

Papillary Urothelial Neoplasm of Low Malignant Potential

Papillary lesions with thickened urothelium have a broader differential diagnosis. Relying on the checklist, once you have determined that the urothelium is too thick to qualify as a benign urothelial papilloma, the next step is assessing the presence of atypia. A thickened papillary lesion with minimal atypia and minimal architectural disorganization is best classified as a papillary urothelial neoplasm of low malignant potential (PUNLMP) (Figure 2.90). At low power, these lesions often show a slightly more eosinophilic appearance, with less cytoplasmic clearing than seen in papilloma. Given the thickened urothelium, the papillary fronds also become less slender and elongated overall, giving it a slightly more stumpy appearance (Figure 2.91). At higher power, minimal cellular atypia may be identified in the form of mildly enlarged nuclei, loss of nuclear grooves, and some hyperchromasia. Mitoses should be infrequent and basally oriented (Figure 2.92). The low-power impression of PUNLMP is that of an eosinophilic, "stubby" papillary neoplasm, with less delicate papillary fronds than a benign urothelial papilloma (Figures 2.93-2.95). PUNLMPs recur in approximately 20% of patients and may recur as PUNLMP, low-grade papillary urothelial cancer, or extremely rarely as high-grade papillary urothelial cancer.[38]

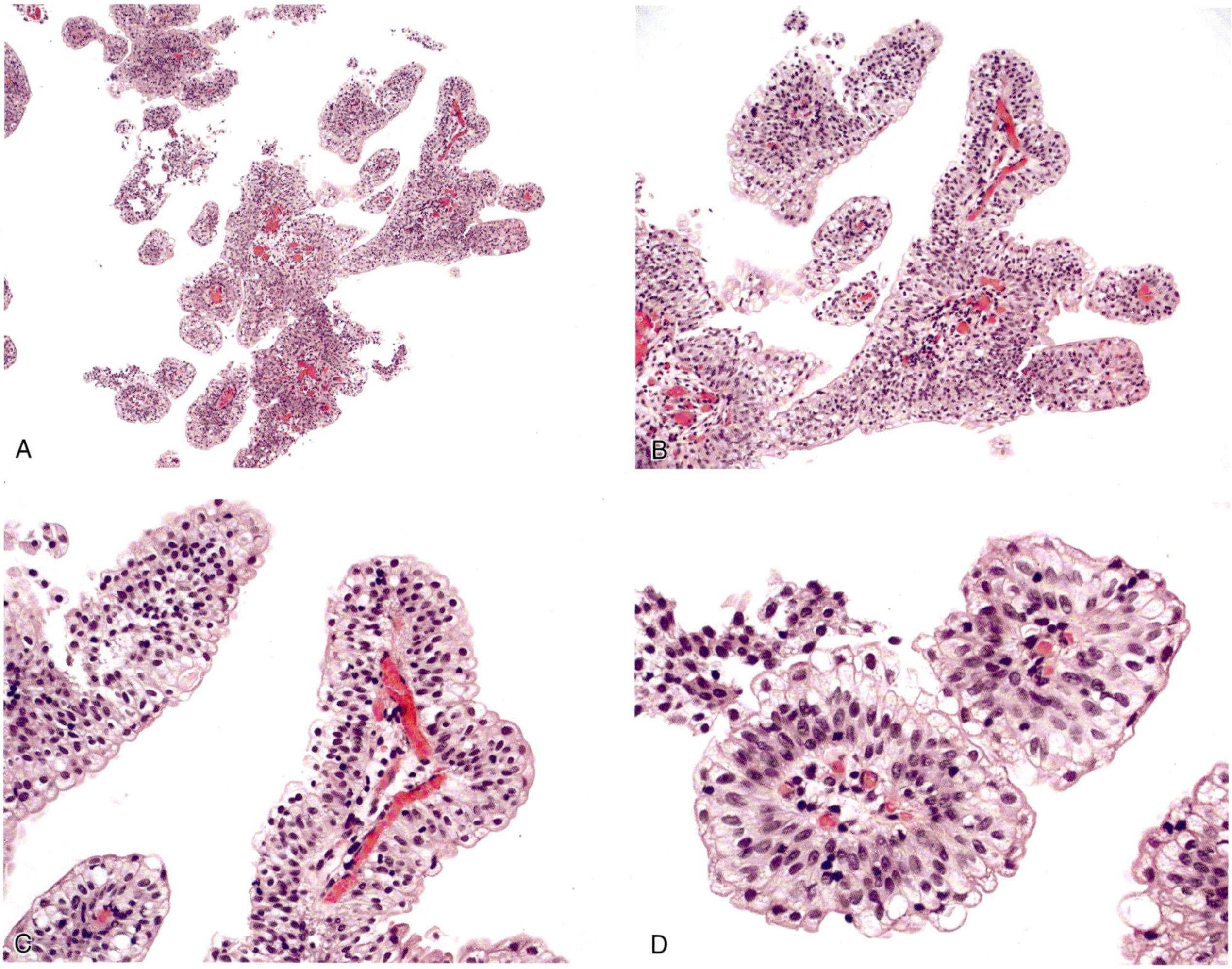

Figure 2.86. A benign urothelial papilloma shows true fibrovascular cores lined by benign urothelium (A). The fronds are usually long and thin and show a relatively simple branching pattern (B). The urothelium is of usual thickness (5-7 cell layers) and lacks atypia (C). High-power examination shown in (D) demonstrates relatively well-oriented cells with occasional nuclear grooves and dispersed chromatin.

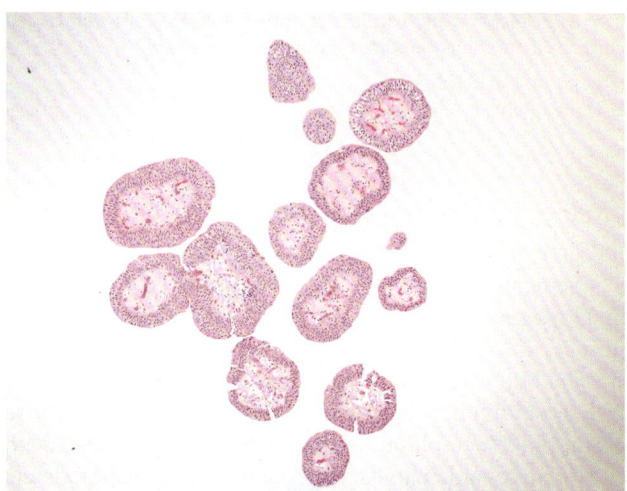

Figure 2.87. Another example of benign urothelial papilloma with simple fibrovascular cores cut perpendicular to the long axis. The overall impression is of a lightly eosinophilic, pale papillary neoplasm.

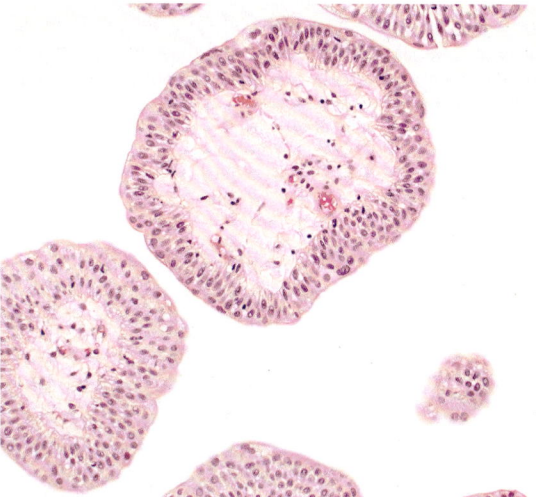

Figure 2.88. Higher power of Figure 2.87 shows the bland, well-oriented urothelial lining without atypia, consistent with benign urothelial papilloma.

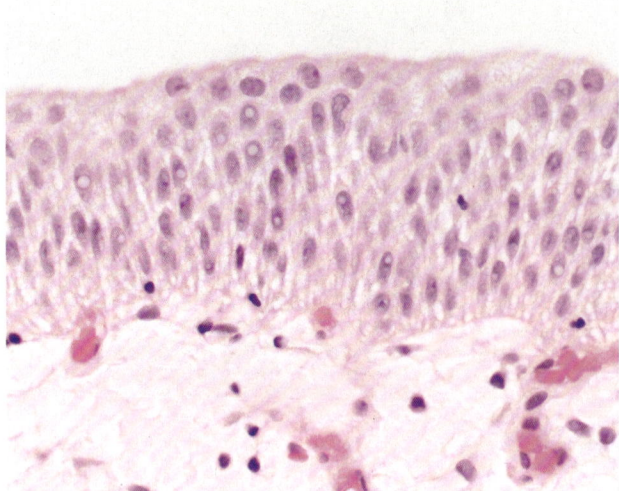

Figure 2.89. A high-power image of one area of the papilloma from Figure 2.87, demonstrating that if the urothelium were stretched out flat, it would look exactly like the normal lining of the bladder.

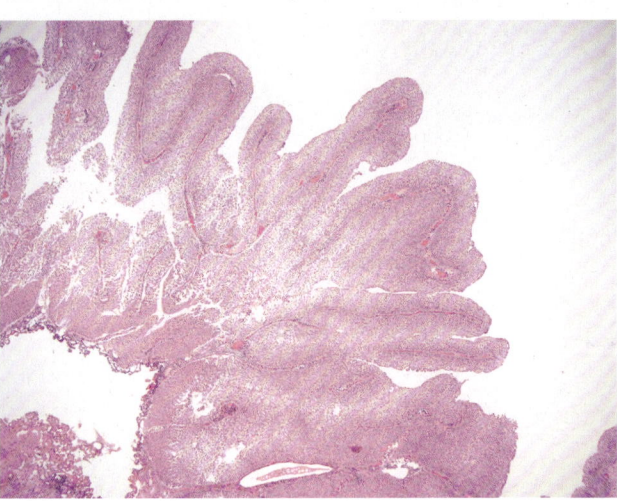

Figure 2.90. A low-power image of papillary urothelial neoplasm of low malignant potential (PUNLMP). Note that even at low power, the urothelial surface is thickened and the papillary fronds appear less delicate and fine than those seen in a papilloma.

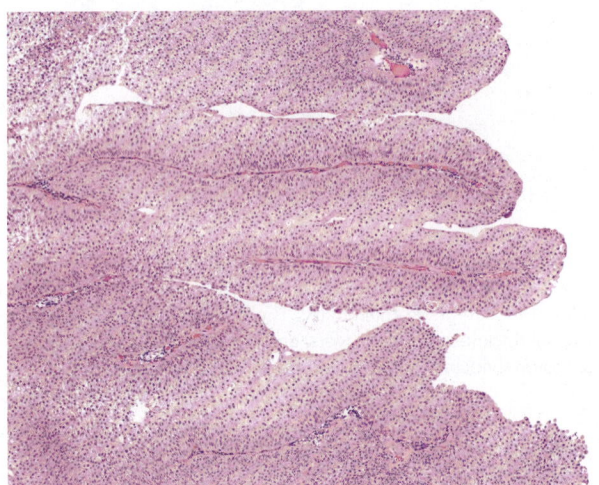

Figure 2.91. Well-formed fibrovascular cores lined by thickened urothelium are present in PUNLMP. Discrimination from a benign urothelial papilloma is based on the thickened urothelium. Discrimination from a low-grade papillary urothelial carcinoma is based on the degree of atypia.

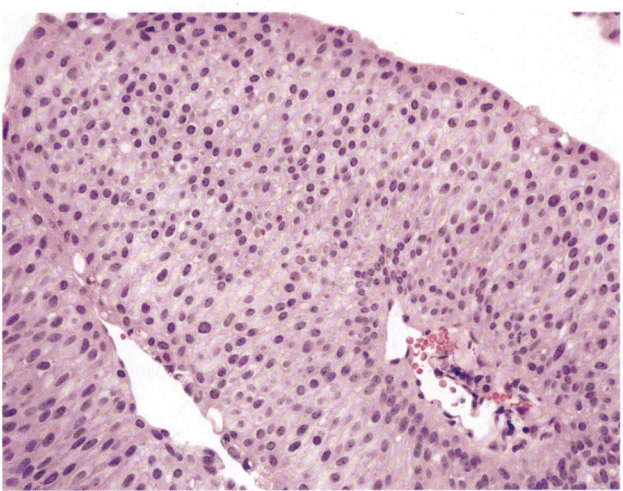

Figure 2.92. At high power, in addition to thickening, the urothelium of PUNLMP demonstrates scattered atypical cells with hyperchromasia and enlargement. Mitotic figures are rare.

Low-Grade Papillary Urothelial Carcinoma

Moving up the scale in terms of degree of cellular atypia, a papillary lesion with thickened urothelium, obvious nuclear enlargement, and scattered hyperchromatic cells with occasional mitoses is consistent with a low-grade papillary urothelial carcinoma (Figure 2.96). With thickened urothelium and more robust papillary fronds, the low-power impression may overlap considerably with a PUNLMP, but does not resemble a papilloma (Figure 2.97). These lesions are usually relatively eosinophilic, consistent with the preserved nuclear to cytoplasmic ratio and ample eosinophilic cytoplasm. At low power, this contrasts with the usual basophilic appearance of a high-grade papillary urothelial carcinoma. Moderate architectural disarray also starts to appear in low-grade papillary urothelial carcinoma. Whereas PUNLMPs tend to maintain a relative perpendicular orientation of the long axis of the nucleus to the basal layer, in a low-grade tumor, you can begin to see the nuclei "turning," where the long axis begins to tilt away from the basal layer to a more angled or

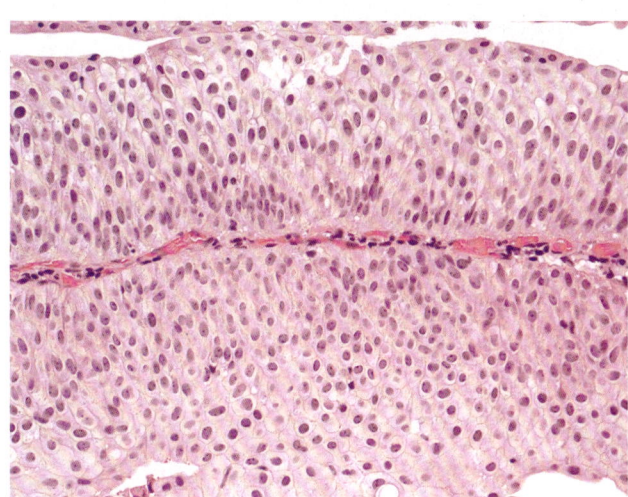

Figure 2.93. A horizontally oriented image of PUNLMP showing both urothelial thickening and scattered atypia. Compare to the horizontally oriented papilloma urothelial lining in Figure 2.89. The PUNLMP does not resemble normal urothelium in the way that papilloma does.

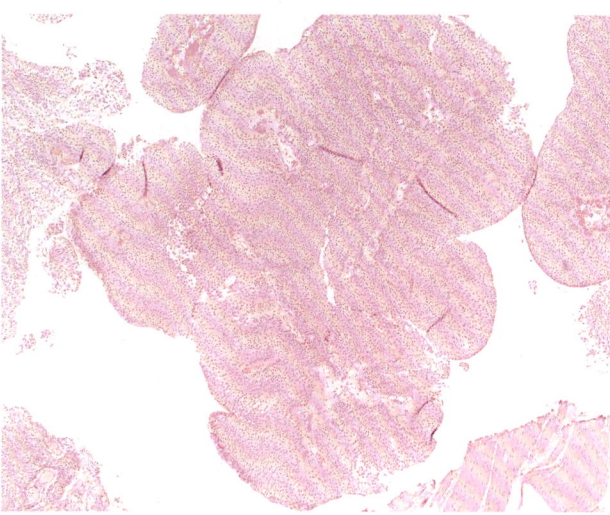

Figure 2.94. Another example of PUNLMP which demonstrates a relatively "pink" low-power impression with thickened, stubby papillary fronds. Compared with a benign urothelial papilloma, the lesion appears less delicate.

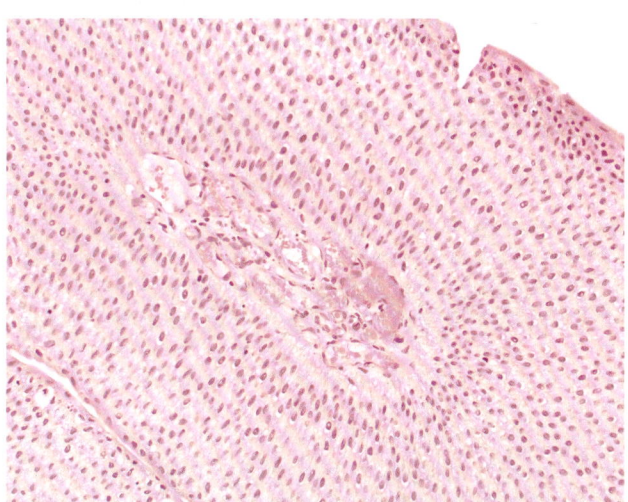

Figure 2.95. High-power image of Figure 2.94 demonstrating markedly thickened urothelium (20-24 cells thick). Cytologically, the cells show less atypia than the PUNLMP in Figures 2.90-2.92, but the urothelial thickening precludes a diagnosis of benign urothelial papilloma.

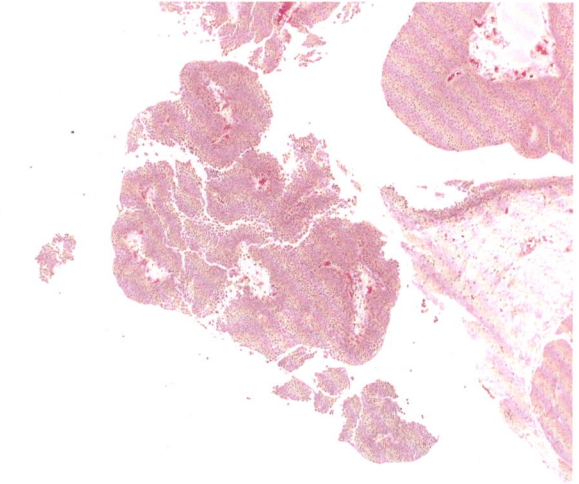

Figure 2.96. Low-grade papillary urothelial carcinoma at low power shows thickened urothelium and a slightly denser eosinophilic appearance than expected in PUNLMP.

even parallel orientation (Figures 2.98-2.100). In a low-grade tumor, it should be easy to identify cells with obvious nuclear enlargement, loss of nuclear grooves, hyperchromasia, and increased mitotic figures, which are less frequent or not identified in PUNLMP (Figures 2.101 and 2.102). Low-grade papillary urothelial carcinomas have a relatively consistent cystoscopic appearance, and cystoscopy notes may comment on a "low grade–appearing" papillary neoplasm. In the setting of a papillary neoplasm identified on cystoscopy, even scant biopsies may be diagnosed as low-grade papillary urothelial carcinoma based on the presence of true fibrovascular cores lined by atypical urothelium (Figures 2.103 and 2.104).

High-Grade Papillary Urothelial Carcinoma

Continuing in the spectrum of atypical papillary neoplasms, high-grade papillary urothelial carcinoma demonstrates severe atypia and marked architectural disarray. Scanning the specimen at low power, the tumor appears more basophilic, often with both elongated and blunted papillary fronds with complex branching patterns, and cytologic atypia is evident

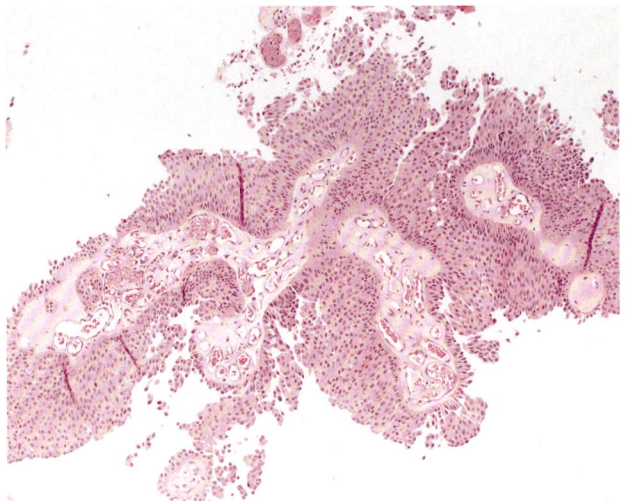

Figure 2.97. Well-formed fibrovascular cores are present in this low-grade papillary urothelial carcinoma, and with thickened urothelium and more complex branching, they may appear short and stubby at low power when compared with the long thin fronds of papilloma.

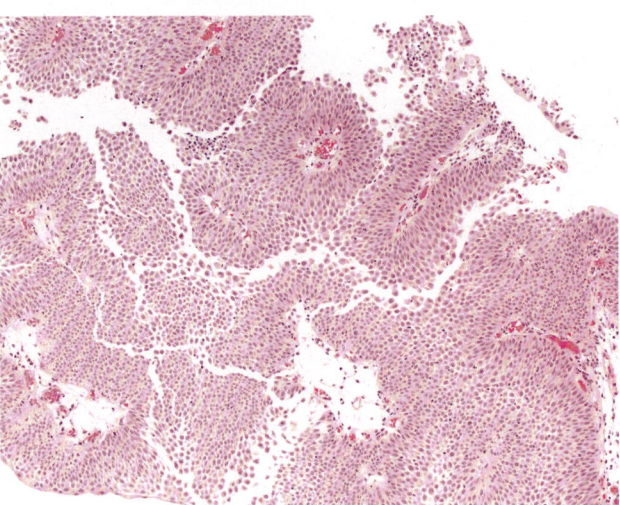

Figure 2.98. Low-grade papillary urothelial carcinoma at medium power showing moderate distortion of cellular polarity in the urothelial lining with scattered atypia. Assessment of polarity should be done in well-oriented cores, such as the one located at 12 o'clock. The tangential sectioning present in the lower right-hand corner creates artifactual disorganization of the urothelium.

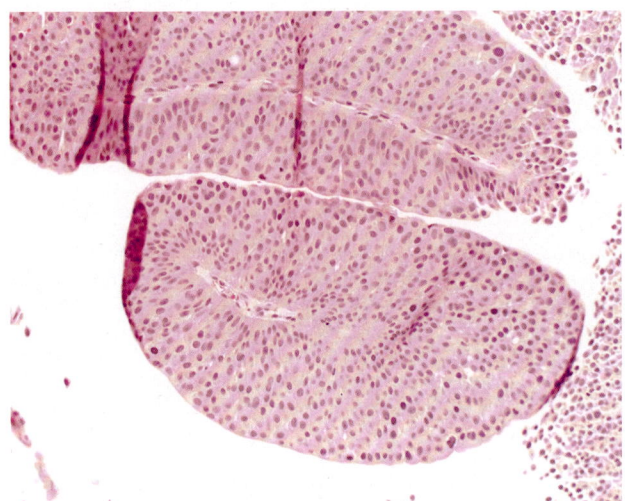

Figure 2.99. At higher power, a well-oriented core shows scattered nuclei with loss of polarity. Rather than pointing in one direction, the nuclei begin to turn off a common axis and orient in different directions. This finding is useful in the diagnosis of low grade papillary urothelial carcinoma.

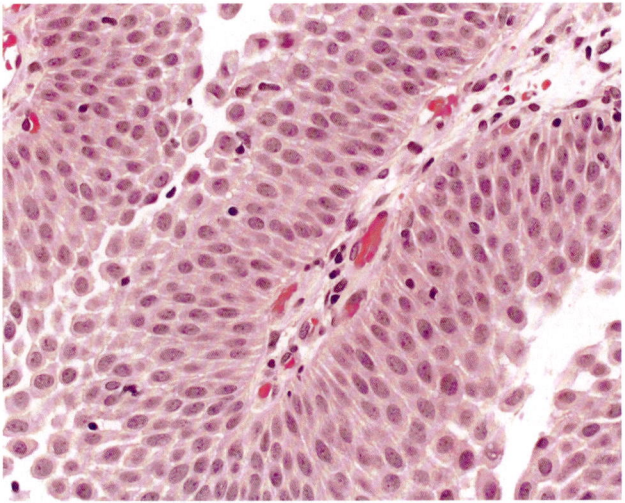

Figure 2.100. Higher power image showing the subtle loss of polarity in low-grade papillary urothelial carcinoma. The majority of the cells show a long axis oriented perpendicular to the surface, but numerous scattered cells deviate from that alignment.

without going to higher power (Figures 2.105 and 2.106). Cells show increased nuclear to cytoplasmic ratio, hyperchromatic nuclei with clumped chromatin, and irregular nuclear membranes (Figures 2.107 and 2.108). Mitotic figures are easily identifiable and present at all layers of the urothelium (Figure 2.109). The same degree of atypia necessary to call CIS should be used for high-grade papillary urothelial carcinoma; one could imagine flattening out a high-grade papillary frond and it would look like CIS.

Similar to CIS, high-grade papillary urothelial carcinoma also has a tendency for denudation and dyscohesion. As such, denuded papillary cores may be seen—either in the presence of obvious high-grade papillary urothelial carcinoma or in isolation (Figure 2.110). Similar to CIS, close inspection of denuded fibrovascular cores is critical for the identification of focal areas of high grade (Figure 2.111).

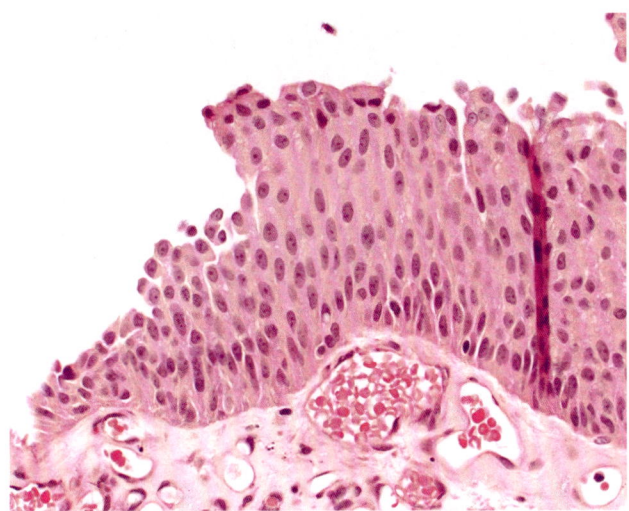

Figure 2.101. Cytologically, the urothelial cells in low-grade papillary urothelial carcinoma lose nuclear grooves, acquire more clumped chromatin with some prominent nucleoli, and nuclear enlargement is easily identified. Mitotic figures are scarce, but more common than expected in PUNLMP.

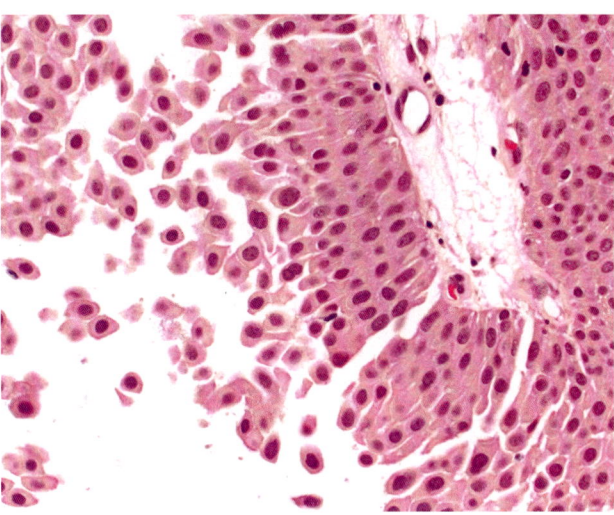

Figure 2.102. Another example of low-grade atypia with numerous cells with enlarged, hyperchromatic nuclei with nuclear membrane irregularities that still retain some eosinophilic cytoplasm, most consistent with low-grade papillary urothelial carcinoma.

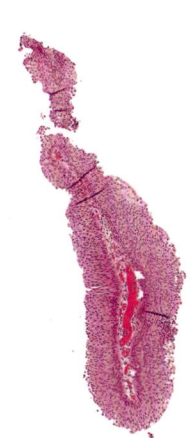

Figure 2.103. Although this biopsy shows only one papillary frond, true fibrovascular cores are evident, and therefore, a papillary neoplasm can be diagnosed in the setting of cystoscopic evidence of papillary neoplasm.

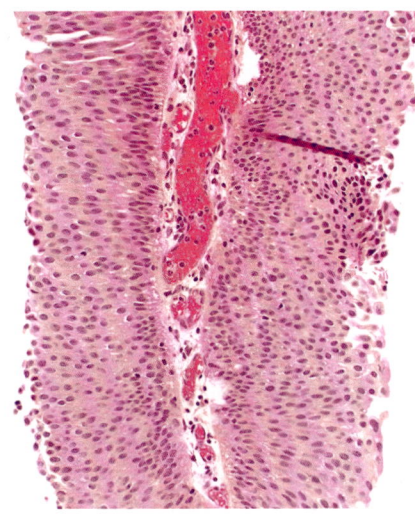

Figure 2.104. At higher power, the papillary neoplasm in Figure 2.103 shows thickened urothelium and scattered atypia, most consistent with a low-grade papillary urothelial carcinoma.

PEARLS AND PITFALLS: Inverted Growth Pattern

- A prominent inverted growth pattern can occur in any papillary lesion, including inverted papilloma and papillary urothelial carcinoma of any grade
- The identification of any exophytic component will exclude the diagnosis of inverted papilloma
- Inverted growth pattern is distinguished from invasion by the bulging and large nature of the nests of urothelium and lack of stromal reaction or retraction artifact

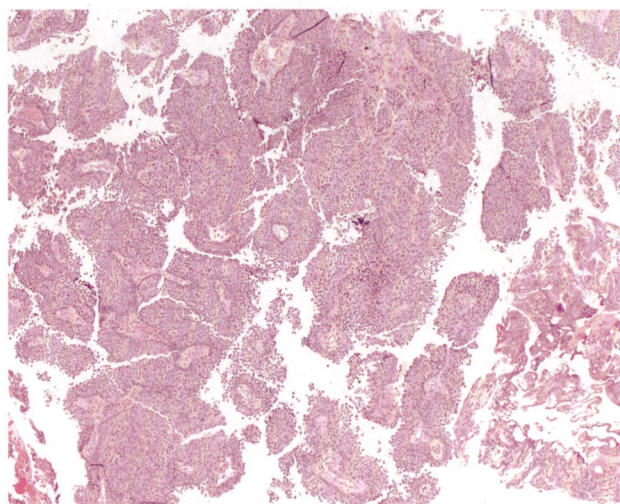

Figure 2.105. High-grade papillary urothelial carcinoma shows basophilia ("blue") at low power due to the increased nuclear to cytoplasmic ratio in the high-grade cells. Atypia is evident even at scanning power, with large dark cells standing out in the background.

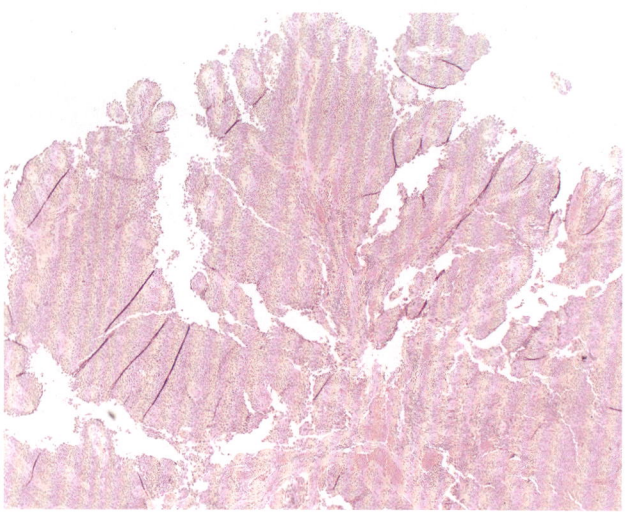

Figure 2.106. Papillary fronds with true fibrovascular cores are thickened and blunt and show complex branching in high-grade papillary urothelial carcinoma.

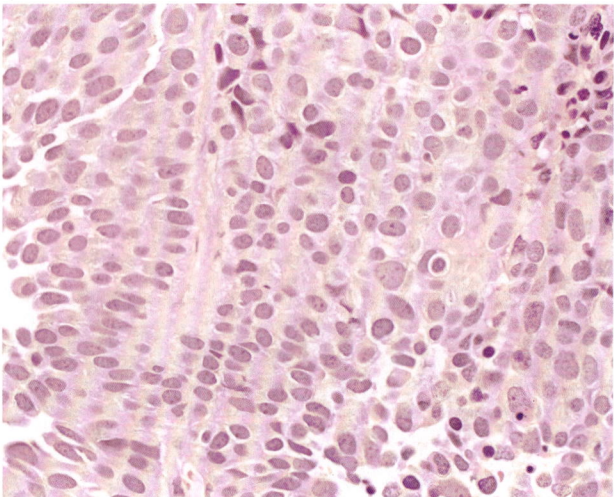

Figure 2.107. At high power, high-grade atypia is evident by marked nuclear pleomorphism and nuclear enlargement. The increased nuclear to cytoplasmic ratio lends a basophilic quality to the tumors. The chromatin is clumped and irregular, rather than evenly dispersed.

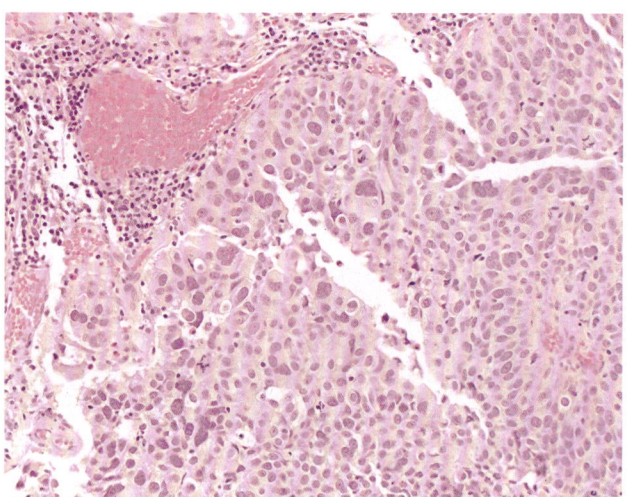

Figure 2.108. Severe nuclear atypia is a hallmark for high-grade papillary urothelial carcinoma and can often be seen at scanning magnification. Large, bizarre nuclei are present in the middle of the field, in a background of less impressively atypical high-grade cells.

When a tumor exhibits a florid inverted growth pattern, it can be easily confused for invasion.[39,40] This pitfall is particularly difficult to avoid in high-grade papillary tumors, where the a priori risk of invasion is much higher. Several findings can help one dodge this pitfall. Firstly, true exophytic papillary fronds must be identified to exclude an inverted papilloma (Figure 2.112) and diagnose a papillary neoplasm. Inverted growth pattern (noninvasive) shows broad-based, rounded invaginations of similar appearance to the surface lesion (Figure 2.113). While there is no true basement membrane in urothelium, a pinkish outline of the lamina propria surrounding these rounded nests may be evident and confer a smooth appearance to the nests. There tends to be a maintained architectural organization to the infolding, giving a vaguely polarized appearance. The surrounding stroma lacks desmoplastic response. Criteria for invasion are similar to those discussed earlier: irregular small nests with jagged, infiltrative borders with potential desmoplasia.[39]

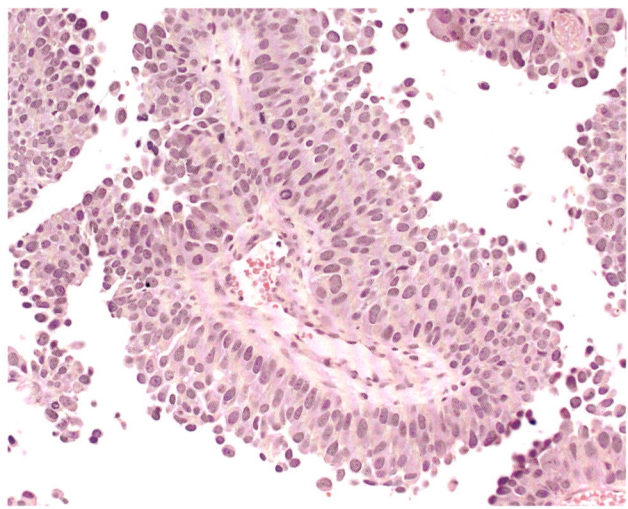

Figure 2.109. In high-grade papillary urothelial carcinoma, mitotic figures are easily identified and occur at all levels of urothelium. Atypical mitotic figures (circular, tripolar) are also common.

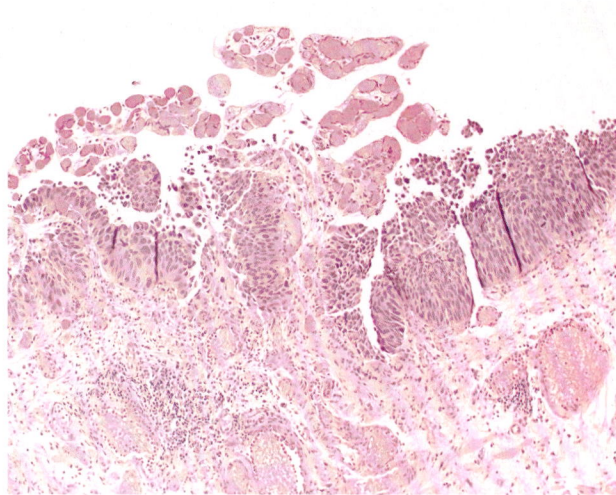

Figure 2.110. Denuded fibrovascular cores are evident at the top of the image. In this case, there is abundant surrounding high-grade urothelial carcinoma that the diagnosis is unequivocal.

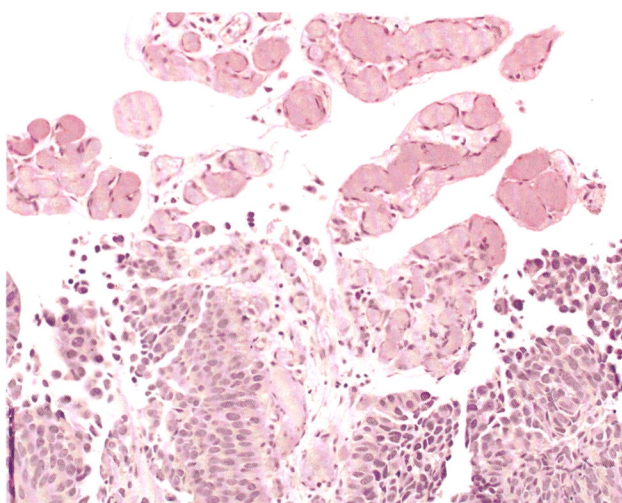

Figure 2.111. Higher power image of denuded fibrovascular cores. If you imagine a biopsy that only samples the top half of the image, you could easily miss the diagnosis of high-grade papillary urothelial carcinoma. Remember to scan closely for detached high-grade cells when denuded cores are seen.

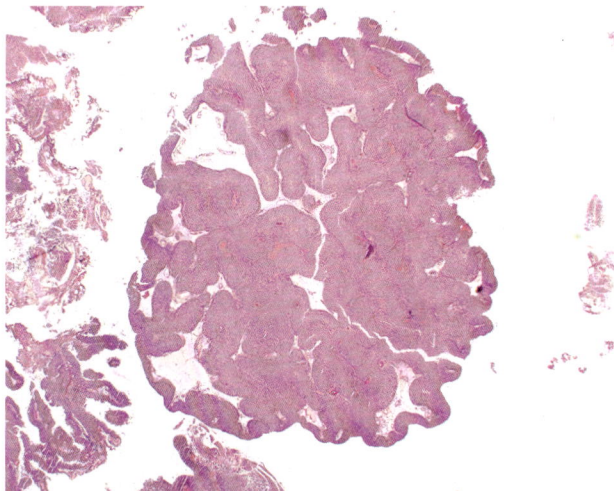

Figure 2.112. Low-grade papillary urothelial carcinoma with inverted growth pattern. Notice in the bottom left of the image, there are well-formed exophytic papillary cores, precluding a diagnosis of benign inverted urothelial papilloma.

CHECKLIST: Systematic Approach to the Evaluation of Inverted Urothelial Lesions

☐ Does the lesion demonstrate a true exophytic papillary component?
   o If yes → true papillary lesion (papilloma, PUNLMP, papillary carcinoma)
   o If no → consider florid VBN, inverted papilloma, or inverted pattern of urothelial carcinoma
☐ Does the lesion have cytologic atypia in the inverted component?
   o If yes → papillary carcinoma
   o If no → VBN, inverted papilloma
☐ Does the lesion involve the muscularis propria?
   o If yes → papillary carcinoma

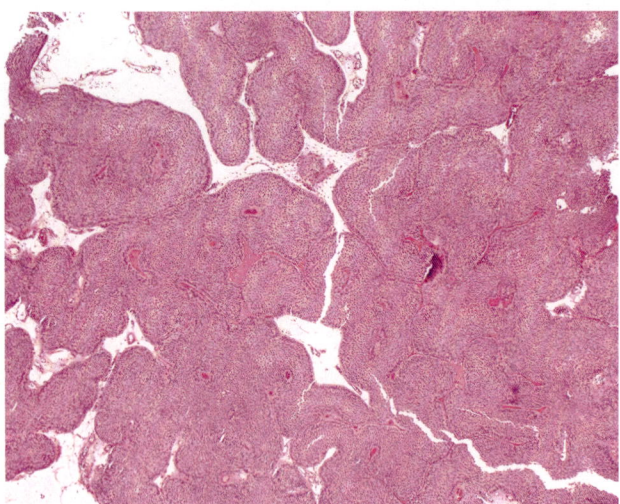

Figure 2.113. At higher power, the inverted component of this noninvasive low-grade papillary urothelial carcinoma shows rounded nests which bulge into the lamina propria. There is no stromal reaction or retraction artifact present.

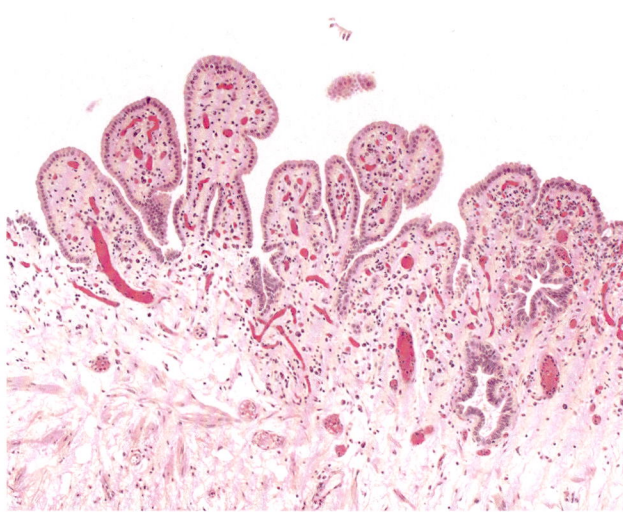

Figure 2.114. Nephrogenic adenomas may present as small papillary lesions on cystoscopy, prompting a biopsy. This image shows a classic papillary nephrogenic adenoma. Clues to the correct diagnosis include the single layer of small, bland low cuboidal cells, rather than multilayered urothelium. The lamina propria often shows some inflammation and edema, suggestive of prior urothelial damage in the area.

PAPILLARY LESIONS OF THE BLADDER—NONUROTHELIAL

Nephrogenic Adenoma

The nonurothelial papillary lesions of the bladder span a wide range of morphologic appearances, some of which overlap with their urothelial counterparts. Nephrogenic adenoma is a reactive lesion that occurs when exfoliated renal tubular epithelial cells are embedded or entrapped in areas of damaged urothelium.[41] A careful examination of damaged or inflamed urothelium, particularly in the setting of past TURBT, catheter use, or stone disease, is essential for identifying and correctly diagnosing these lesions. Before making a diagnosis of a small papillary urothelial carcinoma in an inflamed and denuded surface, always consider nephrogenic adenoma.

A nephrogenic adenoma may be primarily tubular in morphology, recapitulating renal tubules, but there may also be a prominent papillary component. This papillary appearance can be a mimicker for papillary urothelial carcinoma, and the tubular component can even raise the possibility of an invasive glandular urothelial carcinoma.

KEY FEATURES: Nephrogenic Adenoma

- At low-power magnification, a papillary nephrogenic adenoma will often show shorter, poorly formed papillae that may have an overall sessile appearance. In a small sampling, a few papillary fronds can mask the more diffuse nature of the lesion (Figure 2.114)

- Nephrogenic adenoma that are predominantly papillary can be tricky, and identifying any tubular elements will support the diagnosis of nephrogenic adenoma

- Within the tubular lumina, eosinophilic material is often present (Figures 2.115 and 2.116)

- The lamina propria often shows evidence of prior urothelial damage in the form of chronic inflammation, edema, or fibrosis (Figure 2.117). These damaged areas allow the implantation of shed renal tubular epithelial cells

- The cytology of the lining cells is usually small, hyperchromatic cells, which may have a hobnail appearance

- A single layer of cuboidal cells favors nephrogenic adenoma over urothelial carcinoma, which is usually multilayered

- Mitotic figures should not be readily identifiable. If frequently identified, consider the alternative diagnosis of clear cell adenocarcinoma

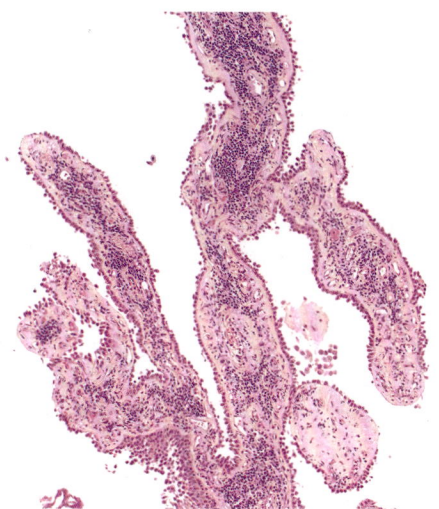

Figure 2.115. Another papillary nephrogenic adenoma showing single layer of cuboidal cells with hobnail appearance. In this case, a tubular component is also present within the lamina propria, along with marked chronic inflammation.

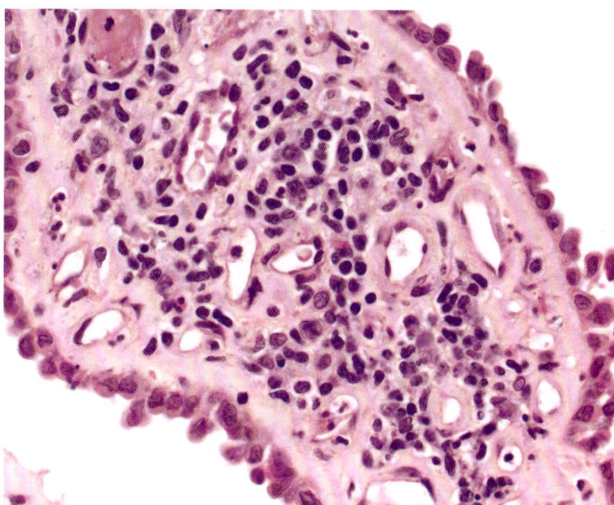

Figure 2.116. At higher power, the tubular components of this papillary nephrogenic adenoma are shown.

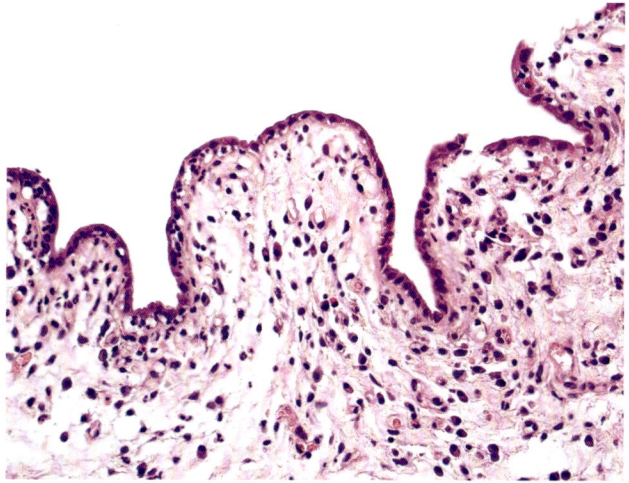

Figure 2.117. Another example of a more sessile papillary adenoma with broad fronds. As a result of urothelial disruption, the lamina propria often shows chronic inflammation, edema, or fibrosis.

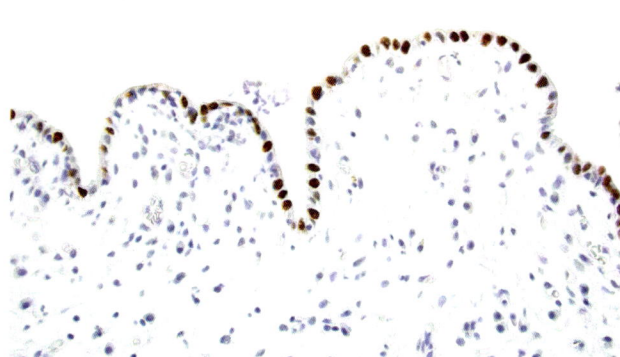

Figure 2.118. PAX-8 is strongly expressed in the nuclei of nephrogenic adenoma, consistent with their renal origin.

- Because these lesions are derived from renal tubular epithelium, they are strongly immunoreactive for PAX8 (Figure 2.118)
- Nephrogenic adenomas are often AMACR positive. Focal prostate specific antigen (PSA) and prostate specific acid phosphatase (PSAP) expression and negative staining for basal cell markers can bring prostatic adenocarcinoma into the differential diagnosis[42,43]

Prostatic Urethral Polyp

The next nonurothelial papillary lesion in this category is the prostatic urethral polyp. These are most commonly identified in the trigone and urethra. Obviously, the location of the lesion is important for making an accurate diagnosis. However, the clinician may not provide this information or the lesion may occur at the bladder neck without definite urethral involvement and, as such, be labeled as bladder. Rarely, true ectopic prostate tissue may be identified in the bladder lending a similar appearance.[44] Regardless, the morphology of the lesion should be sufficiently unusual for a urothelial neoplasm that an alternative diagnosis is considered.

For prostatic urethral polyps, the low-power appearance shows a complex papillary lesion with numerous infoldings and even glandular elements within the stroma at the base of the lesion (Figure 2.119). Cytologically, the cells show ample clear to lightly

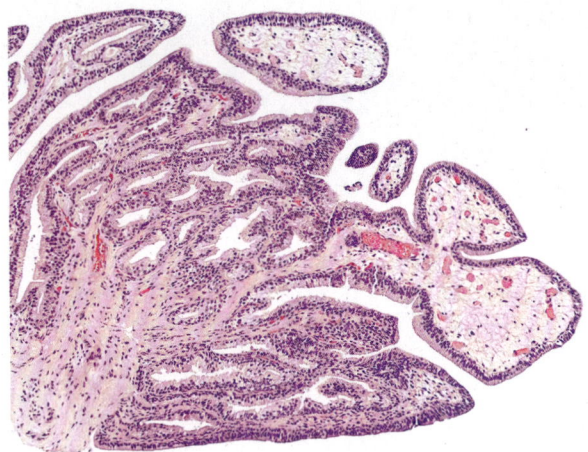

Figure 2.119. A prostatic urethral polyp is a papillary lesion lined by prostatic secretory cells, often with underlying prostatic glands. It represents ectopic prostate tissue. This entity is most commonly identified at the trigone or bladder neck, in addition to the urethra.

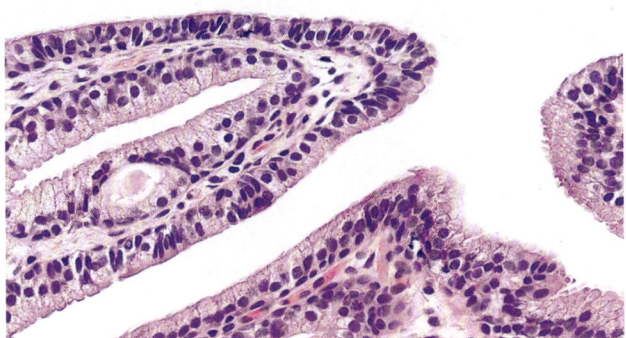

Figure 2.120. The cytologic features of a prostatic urethral polyp include columnar cells with lightly eosinophilic granular cytoplasm containing small round nuclei, with basal cells present.

eosinophilic cytoplasm and small round nuclei (Figure 2.120). Atypia is absent or minimal, and the overall appearance is that of a very bland process. The glands are morphologically identical to prostate glands, with their complex infolding and voluminous cytoplasm; however, there can be a mixture of urothelial elements as well. If the sampling is not sufficient to make the diagnosis on hematoxylin and eosin (H&E) alone, these lesions will stain for classic prostate markers, including PSA, PSAP, and NKX3.1.[45] Basal cells are present and would stain for HMWCK and p63.

PEARLS AND PITFALLS: Prostatic Urethral Polyp

- Morphology is still critical to the correct diagnosis of prostatic urethral polyp; should look like benign prostatic glands
- A polypoid/papillary lesion in the area of the verumontanum with marked atypia and columnar "tubular adenoma–like" cytology may represent a prostatic ductal adenocarcinoma
- The immunoprofile would be similar in prostatic urethral polyp and ductal adenocarcinoma and represents a possible pitfall (especially problematic because ductal adenocarcinoma may retain basal cell staining)

PEARLS AND PITFALLS: Urethral Caruncle

- Urethral caruncle is a common finding in the posterior urethra of middle-aged women
- Commonly identified on workup for urogynecologic examination and may be fulgurated at time of procedure rather than submitted for pathology
- Microscopic appearance is that of granulation tissue with prominent vessels and inflammation (Figure 2.121)

Villous Adenoma

The last nonurothelial papillary lesion in this category is villous adenoma. Villous adenomas may arise anywhere in the urothelial tract, but are most common in the bladder. These lesions will look quite familiar to the general surgical pathologist, as they are morphologically identical to their colonic counterpart (Figure 2.122). The low-power appearance is of a villous papillary lesion with mucinous epithelium and cytologic atypia

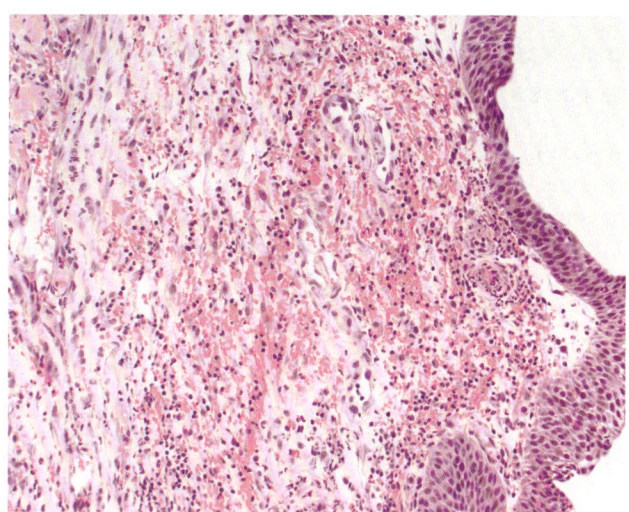

Figure 2.121. Urethral caruncles are most commonly found in the posterior urethra. Histologically, it is comprised of granulation tissue with prominent vessels and inflammation.

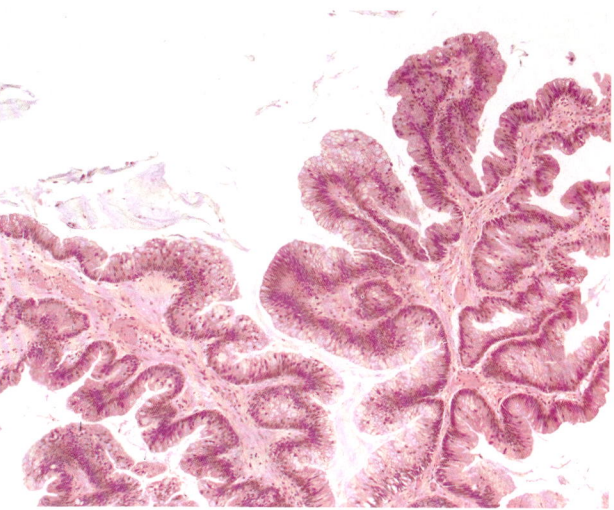

Figure 2.122. Villous adenomas of the bladder are morphologically identical to their counterpart in the colon. At low power, villous adenomas are papillary with mucinous epithelium and low-grade cytologic atypia.

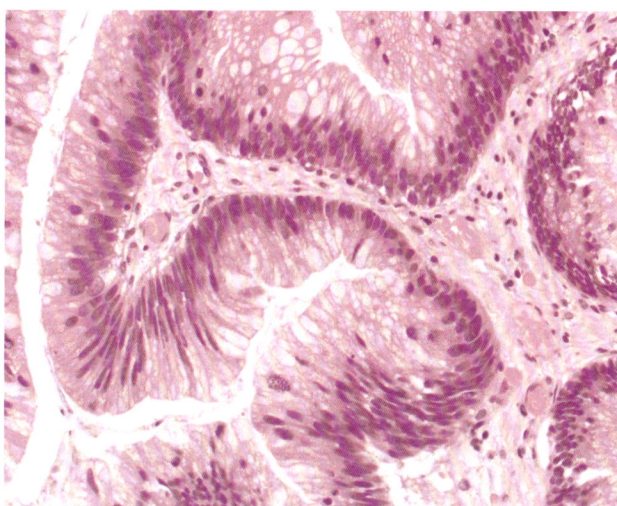

Figure 2.123. At high power, the cytologic features include nuclear pseudostratification, some loss of apical mucin, and occasional mitotic figures. These features are consistent with adenomatous change. High-grade dysplasia is not an acceptable finding in villous adenoma and, when present, should raise the possibility of an unsampled adenocarcinoma.

consistent with the adenomatous changes in a colonic polyp. These changes include nuclear pseudostratification, some loss of apical mucin, and occasional mitotic figures (Figure 2.123).

Adenomatous change is expected as part of the diagnosis, and one should not comment on the finding of low-grade dysplasia in these lesions. Pure villous adenomas that are completely excised have an overall favorable prognosis. However, if true high-grade dysplasia is identified, a risk of invasive disease or recurrence exists.[46] In these cases, a comment should be made stating that high-grade dysplasia is present and the lesion should be completely excised to rule out invasion. When possible, the entire lesion should be removed to minimize the risk of progression to adenocarcinoma.

SAMPLE NOTE: Villous Adenomatous Lesion With High-Grade Dysplasia (See Note)

Note: If metastasis or direct invasion by colon tumor is clinically excluded, this lesion is favored to represent a villous adenoma of the bladder with high-grade dysplasia. No definitive invasion is identified in the sampled tissue; however, recommend complete excision of the tumor to exclude invasion. These lesions may recur or progress to invasive adenocarcinoma, and close clinical follow-up is warranted.

DEEP LESIONS OF THE BLADDER

The first section of this chapter focused on recognizing patterns of superficial lesions of the urothelial tract. In this section, the focus will shift to the deeper components of the bladder—the lamina propria and muscularis propria—and the lesions that can involve these layers. The checklist approach still applies; once we have assessed the surface urothelium, we then turn to the lamina propria. Some tumors discussed above (high-grade papillary urothelial carcinoma, nephrogenic adenoma) may also involve deeper levels, such that each step of the checklist contributes to a differential diagnosis within the deeper components as well. A number of nonneoplastic lesions can also be found in deeper layers of the bladder, and it is critical to recognize these as potential mimickers of invasive carcinoma. Following a stepwise progression when evaluating bladder lesions provides a comprehensive and efficient approach to diagnosing these entities.

INVASIVE UROTHELIAL CARCINOMA

Invasive urothelial carcinoma may arise in the setting of flat CIS or a papillary urothelial carcinoma. While the features of invasion are similar in each setting, the complexity of a papillary lesion makes the identification of invasion much more difficult and time-consuming. Learning to recognize subtle differences in the size of urothelial nests, the cytoplasmic quality of cells, and normal contours of the urothelial surface will assist in the diagnosis of invasion.

However, a low-power scan of TURBT specimens is always an efficient first step. At low power, a determination of architecture (papillary versus flat), grade (high grade versus low grade), and, if you are fortunate, obvious lamina propria or muscularis propria invasion can often be made. In instances where high-grade muscle invasive disease is readily identified, you can verify your low-power impression at high power and scan the remainder of the specimen at intermediate power, looking for variant histology and lymphovascular invasion (Figure 2.124).

More commonly, the evaluation of muscularis propria invasion involves close inspection of the large, rounded muscle bundles for the presence of any infiltrating nests of tumor (Figures 2.125-2.127). Occasionally tumor will splay apart muscle bundles, making it difficult to discern if the muscle represents muscularis mucosae of the lamina propria or muscularis propria. The identification of rounded muscle bundles with multiple fascicles is a helpful feature for muscularis propria (Figure 2.128).

KEY FEATURES: Diagnostic Criteria for Early Invasive Urothelial Carcinoma

- Paradoxical maturation—"pinking up" of invasive nests of tumor relative to surface lesion (Figures 2.129 and 2.130)
- Retraction artifact—clear space surrounding invasive nest, may resemble lymphovascular invasion (Figures 2.131-2.133)
- Small and irregularly shaped nests—unlike the rounded contours of the surface papillary lesion, small and irregularly shaped nests are found in invasive tumor (Figure 2.134)
- Single infiltrating cells (Figure 2.135)
- Desmoplasia

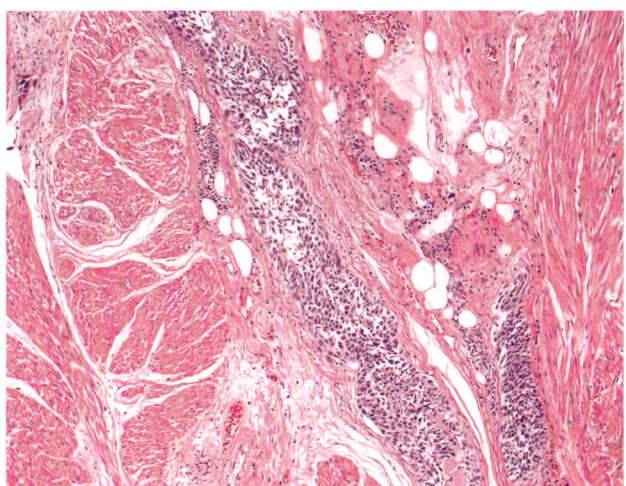

Figure 2.124. The presence of easily identifiable muscularis propria invasion in a TURBT (transurethral resection of bladder tumor) specimen is a low-power finding that can make the task of scanning numerous tissue fragments less onerous.

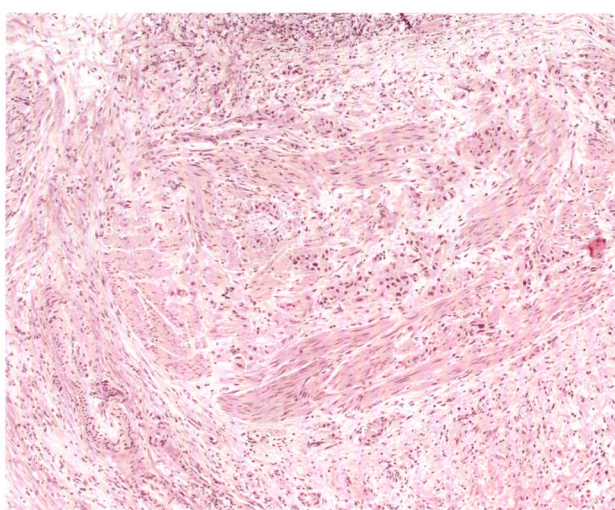

Figure 2.125. More frequently, one will have to closely examine each individual tissue fragment for more subtle muscularis propria invasion, as seen here. A few nests of high-grade urothelial carcinoma are present within the large muscle bundle in the center of the image.

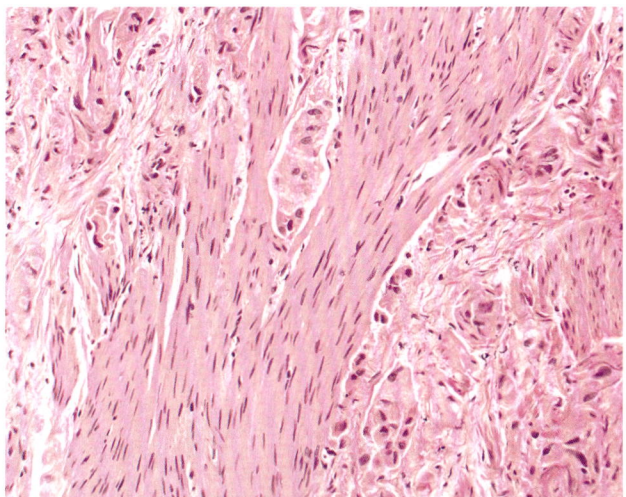

Figure 2.126. At high power, the atypical urothelial nests splay apart a thick bundle of muscularis propria.

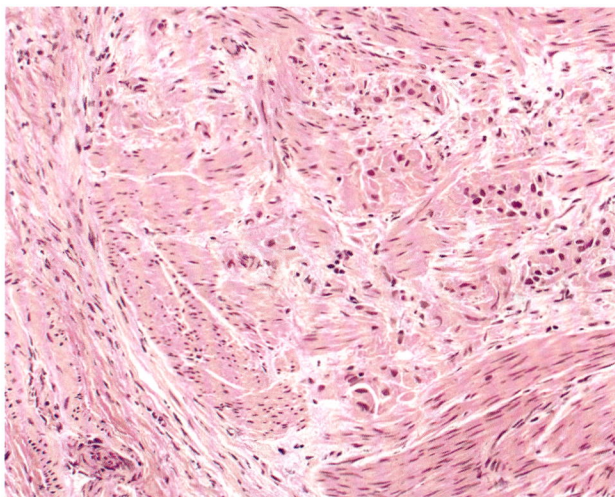

Figure 2.127. Additional image of infiltrating urothelial cells present within the large rounded muscle bundles of the muscularis propria.

Given the morphologic overlap with retraction artifact and its clinical importance, the possibility of lymphovascular invasion in urothelial carcinoma is common. Readily identifiable LVI is demonstrated by large caliber vessels with intact endothelial cells containing red blood cells. Frequently, the tumor within the vessel conforms to the shape of the vessel or may be adherent to the endothelial surface (Figures 2.136 and 2.137). When the finding of LVI is equivocal, vascular markers such as D2-40 or CD31 can be used to highlight the endothelial lining.

When invasion is not readily identified at low power, a much more thorough evaluation of the lesion is necessary. At this point, one must methodically scan just below the urothelial surface looking for alterations in the smooth contour of the urothelial-lamina propria junction. In a papillary lesion, early invasion is most frequently identified in the fibrovascular cores, which means close attention must be taken to scan each frond (Figure 2.138). You can mentally subtract out the surface urothelium, concentrating on the stroma just below the urothelium. The goal is to identify small nests or single cells that infiltrate the lamina propria (Figure 2.139).

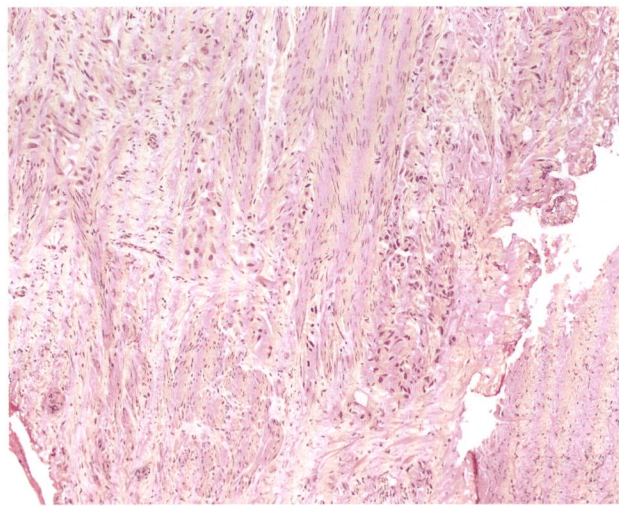

Figure 2.128. Invasive tumor may cause the muscle bundles to splay open and appear thinned out. The differential diagnosis in these cases includes muscularis mucosae of the lamina propria. The identification of a round bundle with multiple fascicles is a helpful feature for muscularis propria.

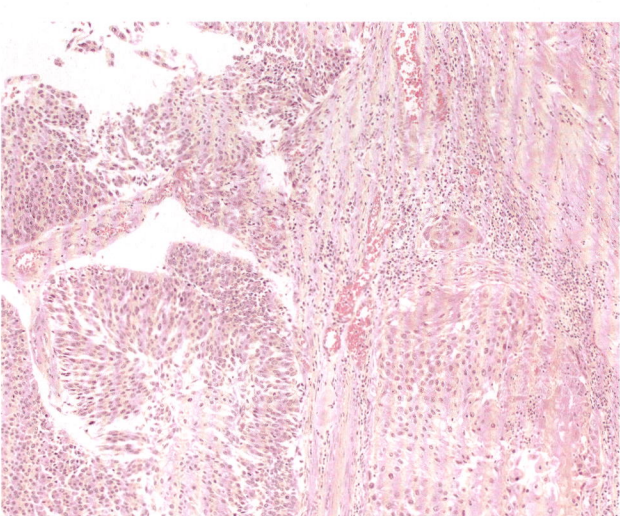

Figure 2.129. This example of invasive tumor also shows paradoxical maturation, with the invasive nests having more voluminous eosinophilic cytoplasm.

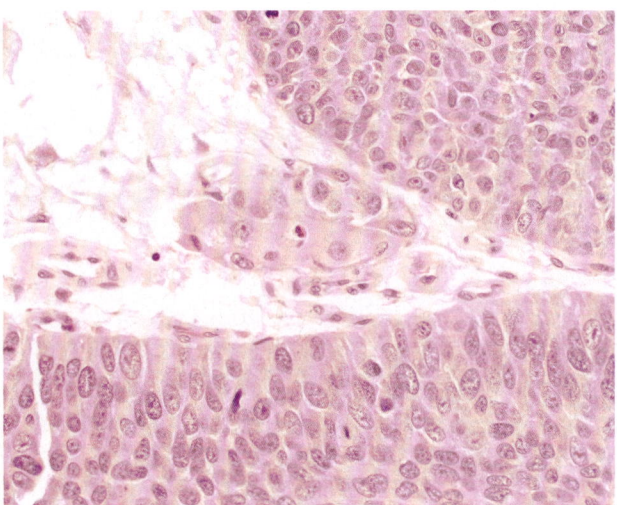

Figure 2.130. Paradoxical maturation in this tumor at high power demonstrating the increased amount of cytoplasm with dense pink cytoplasm. Compare to the surface lesion with darker cells and less cytoplasm.

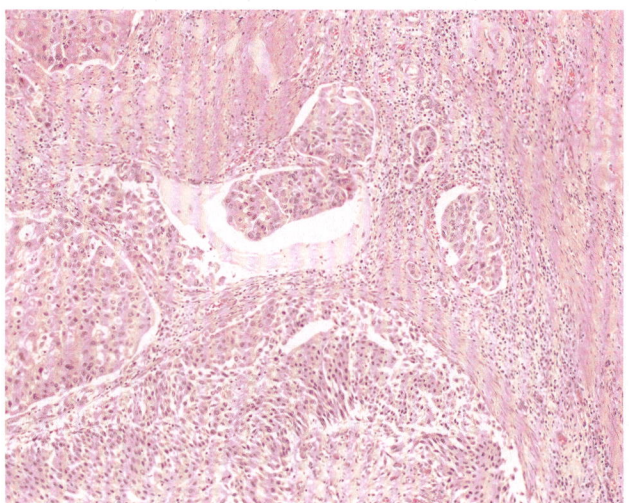

Figure 2.131. Retraction artifact surrounding invasive nests of tumor.

Tangential sectioning of a papillary neoplasm can mimic invasive disease. Clues to the artifactual nature of this finding include lack of invasive features (see Key Features above) and a rounded, bulging contour that lacks sharp borders between the stroma and urothelium (Figures 2.140-2.142). The cytoplasm of these nests often appears to blur into the lamina propria, indicating that the sectioning is going through the cells, rather than intact cells invading into the lamina propria. As previously discussed, one of the most helpful clues for invasive urothelial carcinoma is retraction artifact, where a small nest or single cells will appear floating within a clear space (Figures 2.143 and 2.144). When unsure about the nature of a urothelial nest within the lamina propria, recut levels may show the connection to the surface urothelium and prove tangential sectioning is the explanation for the finding (Figures 2.145 and 2.146).

When lamina propria invasion is identified, your diagnostic line should include whether the invasion is focal or nonfocal. Focal invasion is diagnosed when there is a single, small focus of invasive carcinoma, whereas nonfocal invasion requires a large single focus or multiple foci of invasion. The extent of invasion in early non–muscle-invasive urothelial carcinoma has prognostic significance and should be reported in biopsy and TURBT

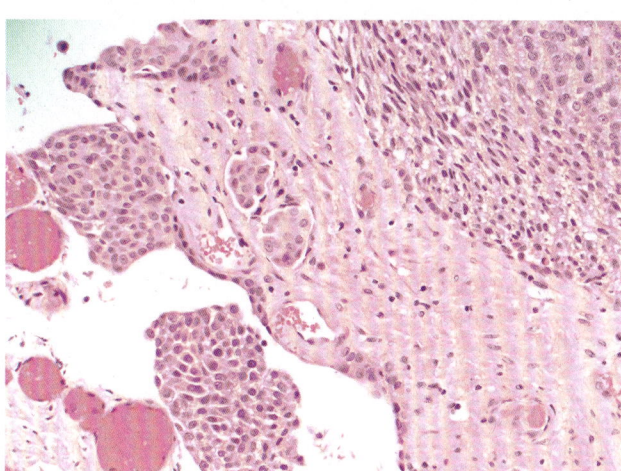

Figure 2.132. Higher power demonstrating the clear area surrounding infiltrating tumor nests. Vascular markers such as D2-40 and CD31 may be useful in distinguishing retraction artifact from lymphovascular invasion.

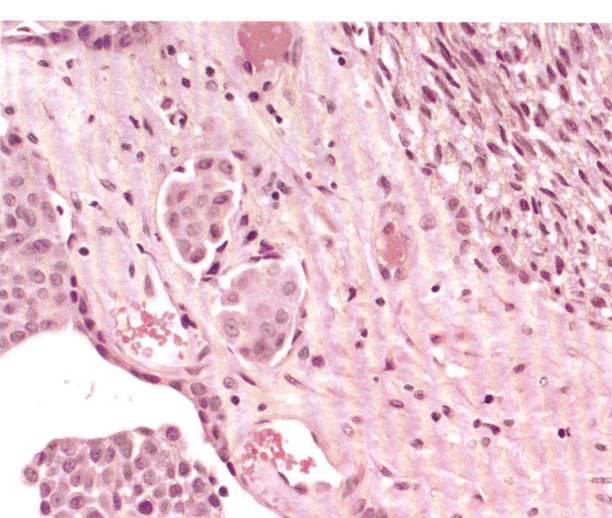

Figure 2.133. High-power image of two nests of tumor with retraction artifact. No endothelial cells are readily identifiable.

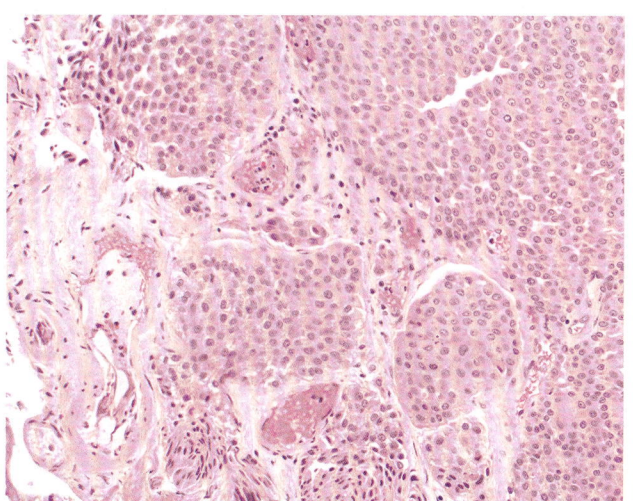

Figure 2.134. Small, irregularly shaped nests within the lamina propria occur in early invasive disease. These nests should be contrasted with the inverted pattern and tangential sectioning often seen in papillary tumors, which result in rounded, large nests.

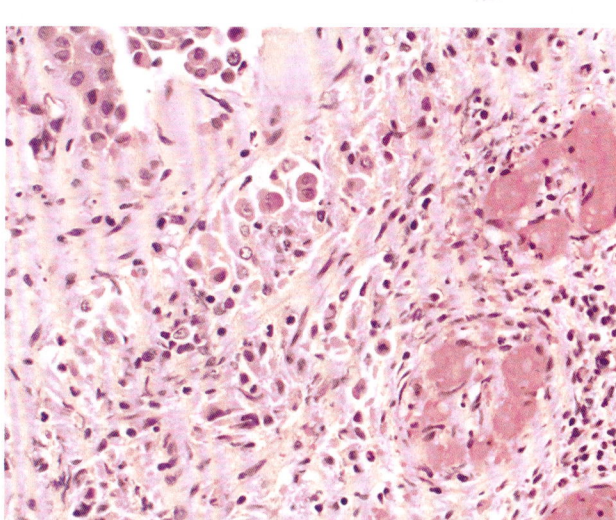

Figure 2.135. Single infiltrating tumor cells are another finding in early invasive urothelial carcinoma. The individual cells are atypical with hyperchromasia and dense cytoplasm and also show retraction.

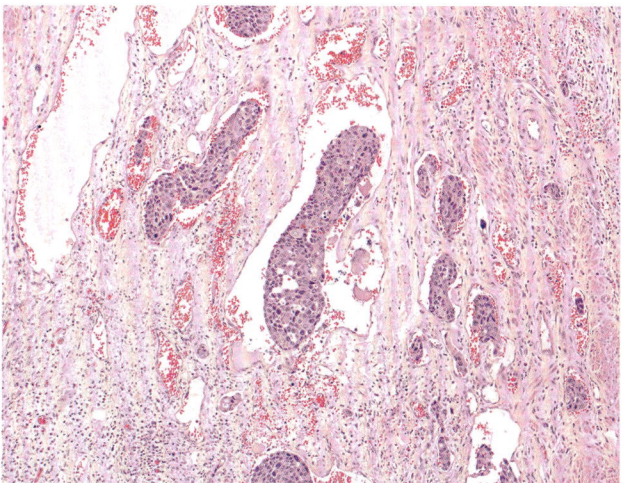

Figure 2.136. Lymphovascular invasion by urothelial carcinoma involving multiple large, thin-walled vessels.

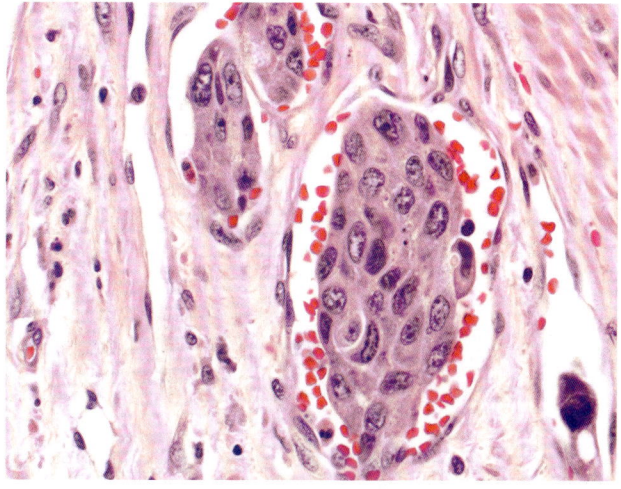

Figure 2.137. At high power, endothelial cells are readily identifiable in the vessel wall. The tumor has conformed to the shape of the vessel.

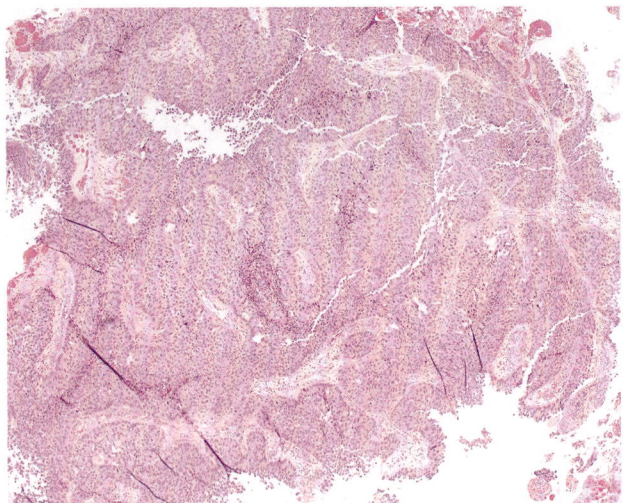

Figure 2.138. Low-power image of high-grade papillary urothelial carcinoma demonstrating the complexity of the fibrovascular cores. In these architecturally complex areas, mental subtraction of the surface urothelium—which is visually dark and busy—to concentrate on the relatively homogenous pink lamina propria will allow for detection of small nests of invasive disease.

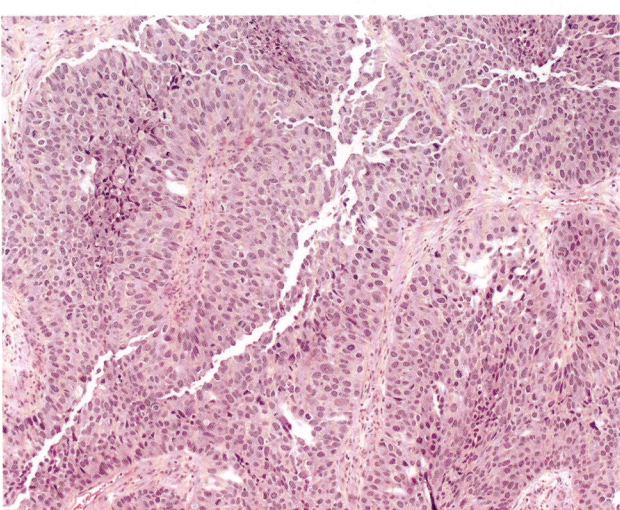

Figure 2.139. Higher power image of fibrovascular cores which lack invasive tumor. Training the eyes to recognize the normal contours of the papillary fronds can help speed up the detection of abnormal cells within the lamina propria.

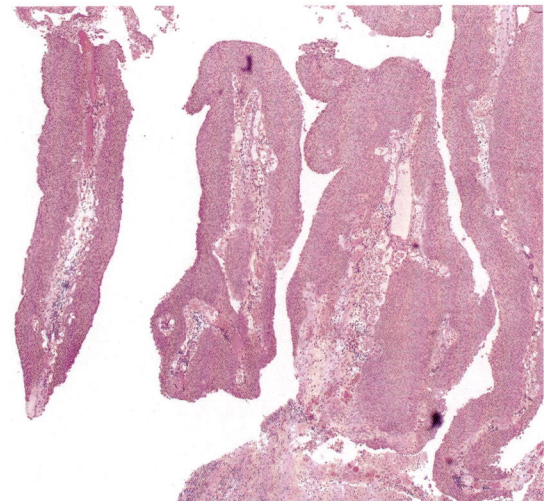

Figure 2.140. At scanning magnification, there is a disruption in the normal contour of the lamina propria and a nest of urothelial cells is present within the stroma. Identifying this difference at low power will prompt evaluation at higher magnification.

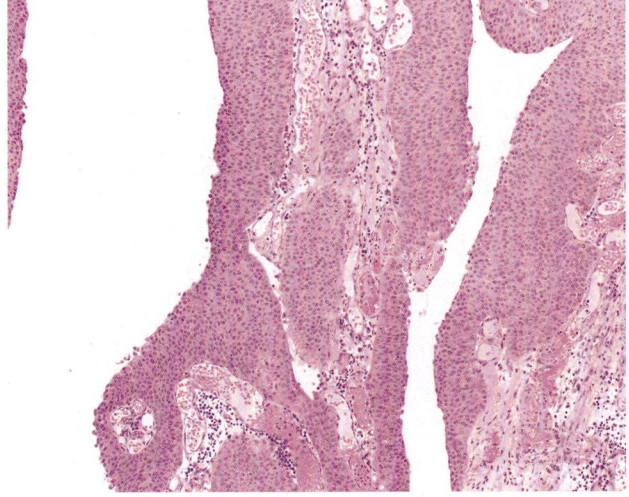

Figure 2.141. At medium power, the nests of urothelium show smooth rounded contours and lack definitive features of invasion. This appearance is most consistent with tangential sectioning of a papillary lesion mimicking invasion.

specimens.[47-49] Extent of lamina propria invasion should be included in the report, and various methods have been proposed.

SAMPLE NOTE: Extent of Lamina Propria Invasion

Invasive high-grade papillary urothelial carcinoma.
Focal lamina propria invasion is identified. Note: There is a single, less than or equal to 40× high-power field focus of invasive tumor. (van Rhijn BW, van der Kwast TH, Alkhateeb SS, et al. A new and highly prognostic system to discern T1 bladder cancer substage. *Eur Urol.* 2012;61(2):378-384.)

OR

Nonfocal lamina propria invasion identified. There is either a single, greater than 40× high-power field focus or multiple foci of invasive tumor. (van Rhijn BW, van der Kwast TH, Alkhateeb SS, et al. A new and highly prognostic system to discern T1 bladder cancer substage. *Eur Urol.* 2012;61(2):378-384.)

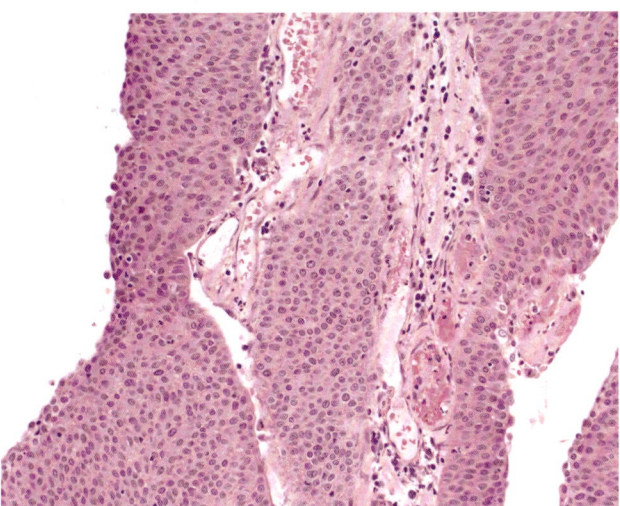

Figure 2.142. High-power examination highlights lack of retraction artifact or single cells, and the edges of the nest show cytoplasm that blur into the surrounding lamina propria. Over multiple levels, actual connection to the urothelial surface may be identified.

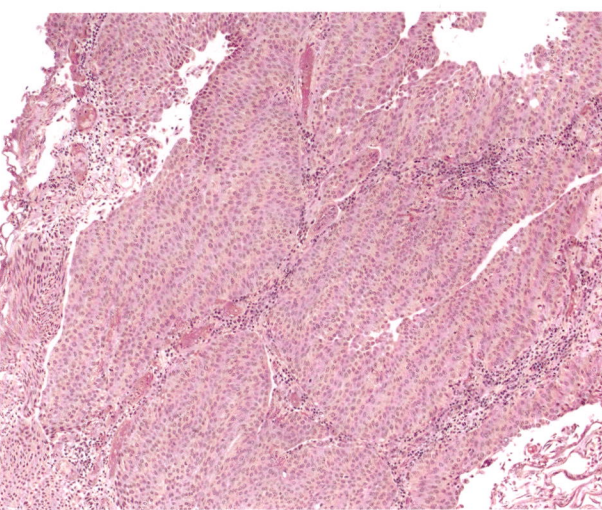

Figure 2.143. In contrast to tangential sectioning, these nests are evident at scanning power with retraction artifact present. Training your eye to identify the differences between inverted growth or tangential sectioning and invasion with the fibrovascular cores is essential to recognizing early invasive disease.

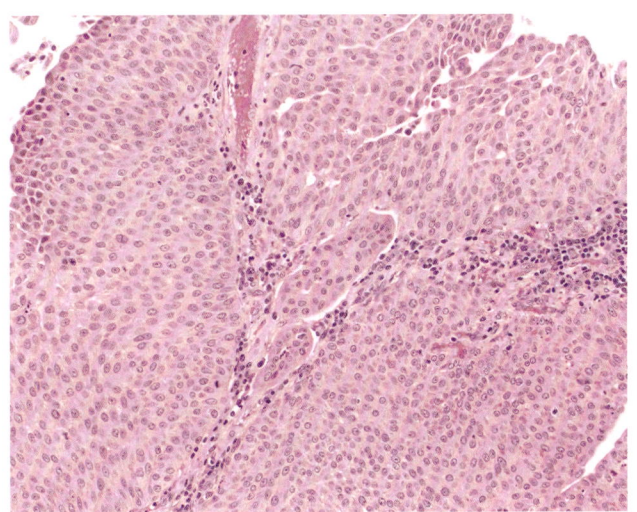

Figure 2.144. Higher power image showing retraction artifact around invasive nests within fibrovascular cores.

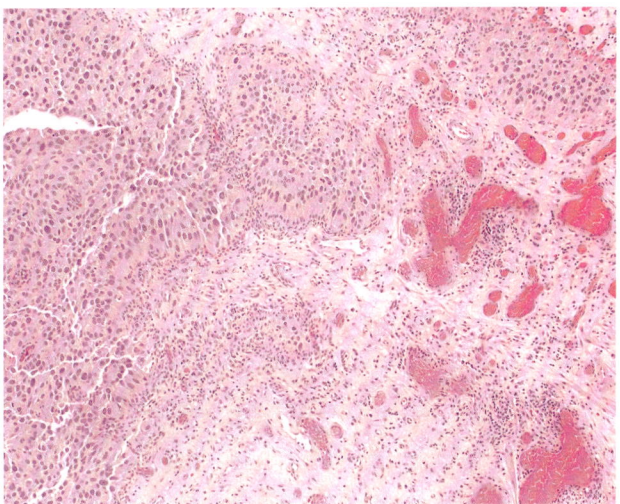

Figure 2.145. Another example of tangential sectioning where the urothelial nest within the lamina propria shows indistinct borders and lacks definitive features of invasion.

Muscularis Propria Invasion

Regardless of the presence or absence of lamina propria invasion, the assessment of muscularis propria invasion is most critical to the clinician's decision-making. Muscle-invasive urothelial cancer connotes aggressive behavior, and the patient becomes a candidate for cystectomy and possible neoadjuvant chemotherapy. Given the significance of muscle invasion, the finding should be unequivocal.

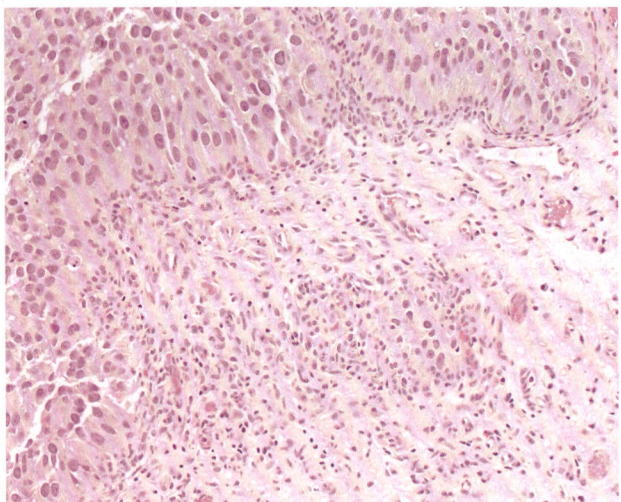

Figure 2.146. Higher power image showing tangential sectioning of atypical urothelium, mimicking invasion. When in doubt, recut levels may help show the connection of the questionable nest to the urothelial surface.

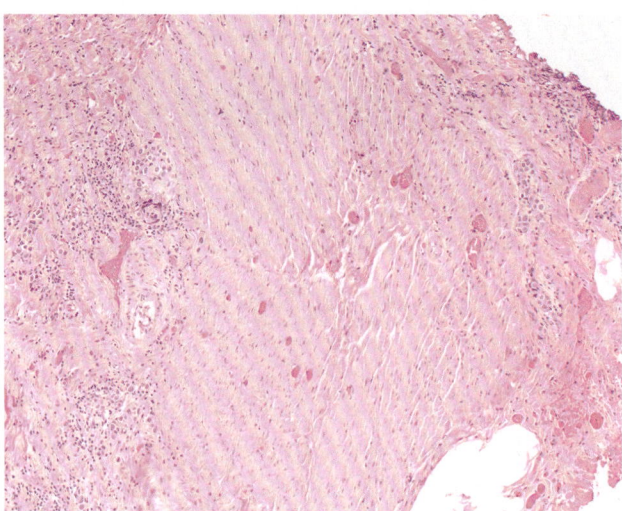

Figure 2.147. Subtle muscularis propria invasion is present in this case with small nests of tumor surrounding a large muscle bundle.

PEARLS AND PITFALLS: Muscularis Propria Invasion

- The presence of muscularis mucosae in the lamina propria complicates the diagnosis, as involvement of these thin, wispy muscle bundles can resemble involvement of muscularis propria (Figures 2.147-2.149)
- When these thin muscle bundles are encountered, scan the surrounding area for clues that you may still be in the lamina propria—large caliber vessels and loose edematous stroma (Figures 2.150-152)
- There is a subtle qualitative difference between muscularis mucosae and muscularis propria in that muscularis propria is present as robust, rounded fascicles. This finding is especially notable when cut in perpendicular cross section, as the muscle bundles appear almost perfectly round. In contrast, muscularis mucosae often appears as short, parallel bundles with tapered ends
- It should also be noted that some regions of the bladder lack muscularis mucosae in the lamina propria, including the bladder neck and trigone. If biopsies are indicated as taken from these regions, any involvement of muscle bundles is consistent with muscularis propria invasion

If uncertain whether the involved muscle is muscularis mucosae or muscularis propria, a note stating that the finding is equivocal for deep muscle involvement is warranted. In certain cases, performing a desmin immunohistochemical stain may help highlight muscle bundles to ascertain overall thickness of the muscle involved. When tumor dissects through numerous bundles which are highlighted by desmin and appear oriented in the same general direction, this can support a diagnosis of muscularis propria invasion.

SAMPLE NOTE: Invasive High-Grade Papillary Urothelial Carcinoma

Nonfocal lamina propria invasion (see note).

Note: The invasive tumor involves small muscle bundles, which may represent muscularis mucosae within the lamina propria or splaying of large muscle bundles of muscularis mucosae. Recommend additional sampling.

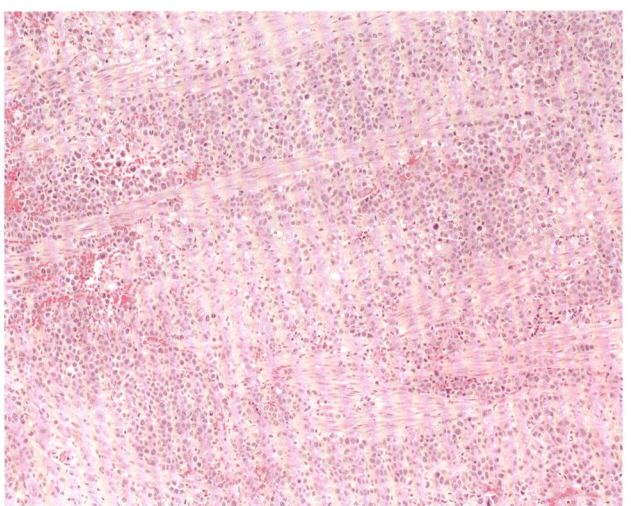

Figure 2.148. In TURBT (transurethral resection of bladder tumor) specimens, a large volume of tumor may massively disrupt the underlying bladder wall. In this image, tumor is involving thin, wispy bundles of muscle. When no definitive large round muscle bundles are present, it is not possible to discriminate between the muscularis mucosae of the lamina propria and muscularis propria that has been partially obliterated by tumor.

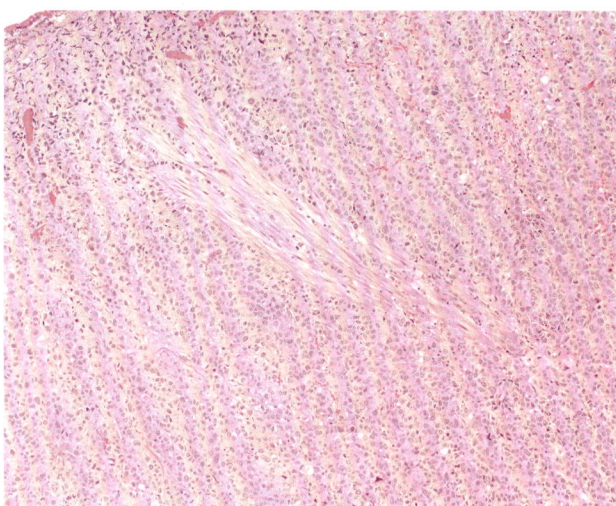

Figure 2.149. Another example of extensive tumor present around a single thin muscle fiber. No definitive features of muscularis propria (rounded muscle bundles with multiple fascicles) are identified in this field.

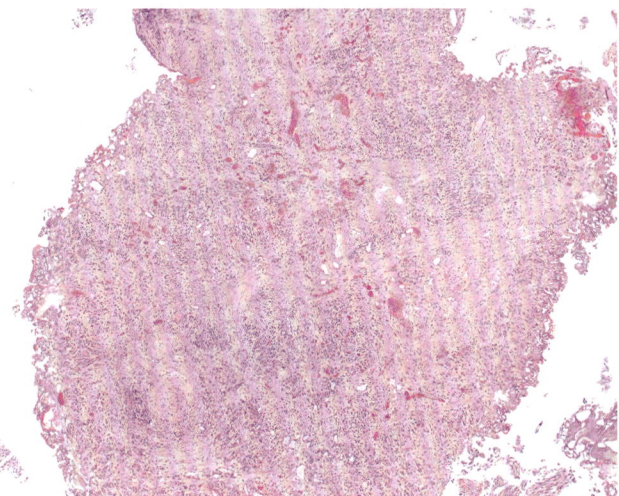

Figure 2.150. A low-power image of invasive tumor involving thin muscle bundles. Subtle clues to the location of these muscle bundles are the numerous large caliber vessels in the background. This finding is not diagnostic of muscularis propria invasion.

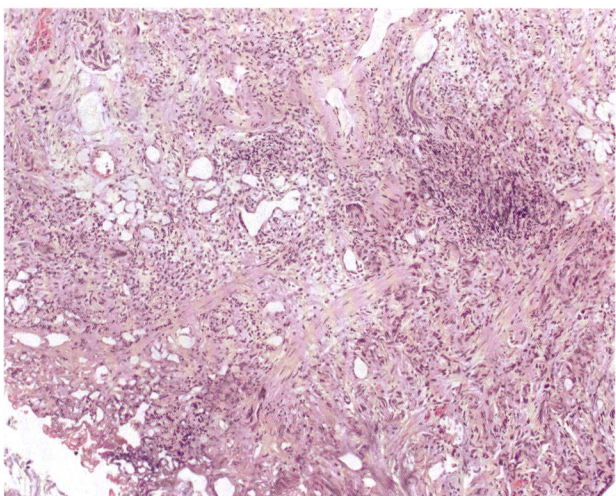

Figure 2.151. Another subtle clue to the possibility that muscle fibers represent muscularis mucosae is the background stroma showing edematous stroma, in addition to larger vessels. These muscle bundles also should not be considered muscularis propria, and a note indicating this possibility is warranted.

The second pitfall for muscularis propria invasion is prominent desmoplastic response to tumor, with the spindled fibroblastic response mimicking muscle that splayed apart by tumor. Identifying the pale to clear cytoplasm of fibroblasts with reactive-appearing nuclear features may aid correct diagnosis. In some instances, immunohistochemistry for muscle markers (desmin) may be of assistance, though it often confuses the issue given admixture of muscle throughout the specimen. Because of the treatment implications of muscle-invasive disease, the diagnosis of muscularis propria invasion should be reserved for definite involvement of large, rounded muscle bundles.

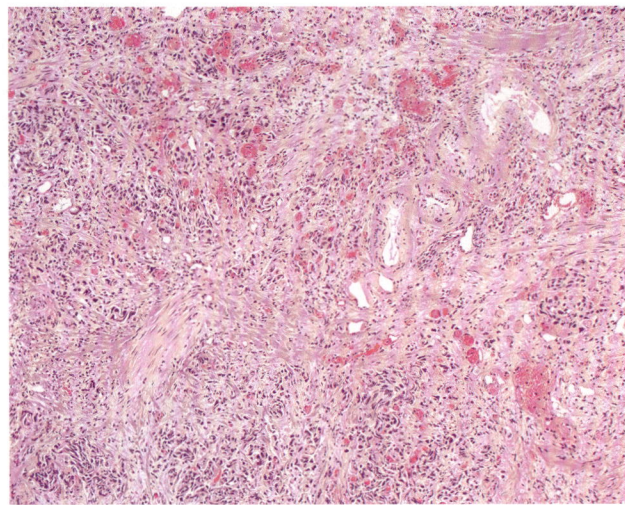

Figure 2.152. The finding of tumor involving thin muscles bundles, especially when large caliber vessels and edematous stroma are present is nondiagnostic of muscularis propria invasion and should not be diagnosed as muscularis propria invasion. The recommendation of additional sampling is reasonable in this situation.

PEARLS AND PITFALLS: Staging Urothelial Carcinoma Involving Prostatic Urethra

- Urothelial carcinoma may involve the prostatic urethra and prostatic ducts by various routes, and different staging systems apply
- Gross examination of the prostatic urethra is critical to accurate staging, and sections of the prostatic urethra should be taken for each case
- Urothelial carcinoma arising in the bladder and directly invading the prostatic stroma is staged as a bladder primary, pT4a
- When involving the prostate via prostatic urethra, complete both the bladder staging and the prostatic urethra staging summaries
- Urothelial carcinoma in situ involving the prostatic urethra and involving the prostatic ducts without stromal invasion is staged as prostatic urethral CIS, pTis (Figure 2.153)
- Urothelial carcinoma in situ that invades through the urothelial surface or prostatic ducts and into the subepithelial connective tissue is staged as prostatic urethral carcinoma, pT1
- Urothelial carcinoma in situ that invades through the urothelial surface or prostatic ducts and into the stroma is staged as prostatic urethral carcinoma, pT2 (Figure 2.154)

FAQ: Metastatic Urothelial Carcinoma and PD-L1

- Tumors with high expression of PD-L1 on their tumor cells are less likely to respond to traditional chemotherapy regimens
- Immune checkpoint therapy with anti-PD-L1 inhibitors has increased efficacy in tumors with high PD-L1 expression
- Immune checkpoint therapy is approved in metastatic or locally advanced urothelial carcinoma

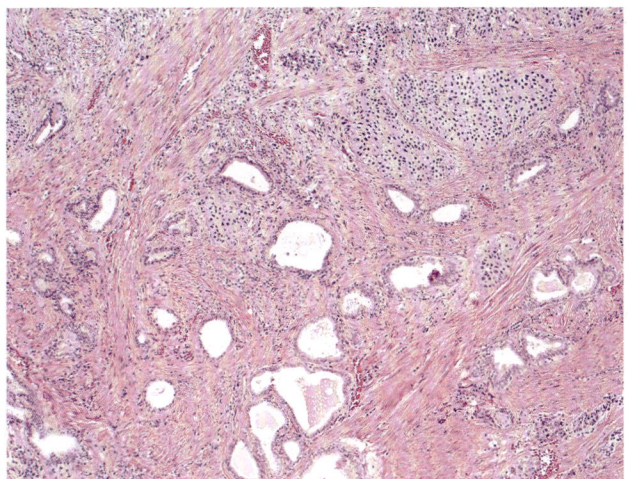

Figure 2.153. Urothelial carcinoma can involve the prostate by carcinoma in situ (CIS) spreading through the ducts and acini via the prostatic urethra as shown here. When there is no stromal involvement identified, this is staged as a prostatic urethral CIS, pTis.

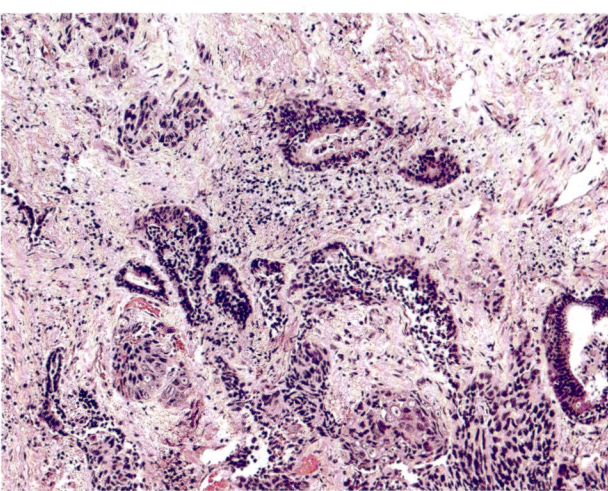

Figure 2.154. When there is stromal involvement of the prostate which appears to originate from the prostatic duct involvement, this is staged as prostatic urethral invasive carcinoma, pT2. Clues to stromal involvement are irregular infiltrating nests and a desmoplastic response.

Histologic Variants of Urothelial Carcinoma

Once a determination of architecture and invasion is made for a specimen, one must also identify any variant histology in the specimen. A histologic variant shows a distinct morphology from usual urothelial carcinoma and frequently is identified in combination with usual urothelial carcinoma. Approximately 25% to 30% of urothelial tumors show some variant histology, and the WHO currently recognizes 10 histologic variants[50] (Table 2.2). These histologic variants are in addition to the broader categories of primary bladder tumors, including squamous cell, glandular, urachal, Mullerian, neuroendocrine, melanocytic, and mesenchymal.

Recognizing and reporting histologic variants is important for a number of reasons. A number of the histologic variants recognized by the WHO have direct prognostic implications, which may drive specific decisions about surgery or chemotherapy. Additionally, unusual variants of urothelial carcinoma may masquerade as other tumor types, especially in metastatic sites. Knowledge of these divergent histologic appearances is critical to accurate diagnosis.[51]

Histologic Variants of Urothelial Carcinoma: Micropapillary

Micropapillary variant of urothelial carcinoma is recognized by the presence of multiple small nests of tumor within cleared out lacunar spaces. Other features include ring-like formations, peripherally oriented nuclei ("reverse polarization"), and extensive stromal reaction. One of the most specific findings for the diagnosis is the presence of multiple small nests within one lacunar space (Figure 2.174).[52] These tumors often present with high-stage disease and lymphovascular invasion and may be widely metastatic. Micropapillary urothelial carcinoma, composing any amount of the tumor, should be included in the top-line diagnosis. Patients with micropapillary carcinoma do not respond well to intravesical therapy, and the recommendation of some clinicians is to proceed directly to cystectomy.

Histologic Variants of Urothelial Carcinoma: Plasmacytoid

Plasmacytoid variant of urothelial carcinoma may also be referred to as signet ring-like or diffuse pattern, given its appearance of single cells that infiltrate in a dyscohesive manner. These infiltrative single cells often have eccentric nuclei (plasmacytoid) and may have intracytoplasmic vacuoles displacing the nucleus (signet ring–like) (Figure 2.175). Regardless of the exact cytologic appearance, the key feature is that these cells infiltrate in a single cell pattern, much like lobular breast carcinoma, and often have a loose myxoid stroma. Plasmacytoid variant also shows aggressive behavior with advanced stage at presentation, frequent local recurrence, and a pattern of spread that may cross fascial planes and lead

TABLE 2.2: Histologic Variants of Infiltrating Urothelial Carcinoma and Their Key Diagnostic and Clinical Features

WHO-Recognized Variant Histology	Key Diagnostic Features	Clinical Features	Reference Image
Nested, including large nested (Figures 2.155-2.160)	Small or large nests of relatively bland, "low-grade" urothelial cells with irregular infiltrating pattern, often involving muscularis propria; TERT promoter mutation may help in diagnosis	Often present at higher stage, though similar stage for stage prognosis as usual urothelial carcinoma	
Microcystic (Figure 2.161)	Round microcysts with thin urothelial lining, irregular infiltrating pattern; also "low-grade" appearance and may be related to nested pattern		
Micropapillary (Figures 2.162 and 2.163)	Minute nests of tumor lacking fibrovascular cores, multiple within single lacunar space; reverse polarity of nuclei	Aggressive disease often presents with high stage and LVI; may warrant immediate cystectomy	
Lymphoepithelioma-like (Figures 2.164 and 2.165)	Undifferentiated epithelial cells growing in syncytial pattern within dense lymphoid infiltrate	EBV negative; may have better response to chemotherapy	
Plasmacytoid/signet ring cell/diffuse (Figures 2.166 and 2.167)	Single cell pattern of infiltration within myxoid background; may be CD138 positive, use pan-keratin	Aggressive disease that may spread across fascial planes with peritoneal involvement. Differential diagnosis includes metastasis from GI or breast	

TABLE 2.2: Histologic Variants of Infiltrating Urothelial Carcinoma and Their Key Diagnostic and Clinical Features   (Continued)

WHO-Recognized Variant Histology	Key Diagnostic Features	Clinical Features	Reference Image
Sarcomatoid (Figure 2.168)	Malignant spindle cell component or other sarcomatous differentiation (may be heterologous); may retain focal cytokeratin positivity in sarcomatous component	Associated with radiation therapy and cyclophosphamide treatment. Aggressive, often presents with metastatic disease	
Giant cell (Figure 2.169)	Numerous pleomorphic giant cells often admixed with poorly differentiated urothelial carcinoma	More common in renal pelvis; highly aggressive	
Poorly differentiated (Figure 2.170)	Poorly differentiated carcinoma without specific morphologic features. May have osteoclast-type giant cells (CD68 positive)	Rare tumors associated with poor outcomes	
Lipid-rich (Figures 2.171-2.172)	"Lipoblast"-like cells with numerous cytoplasmic vacuoles containing lipid	Presents at higher stage with high mortality	
Clear cell (Figure 2.173)	Voluminous clear glycogenated cytoplasm; differential diagnosis includes clear cell adenocarcinoma	Rare variant, prognosis uncertain	

EBV, Epstein-Barr virus; GI, gastrointestinal.

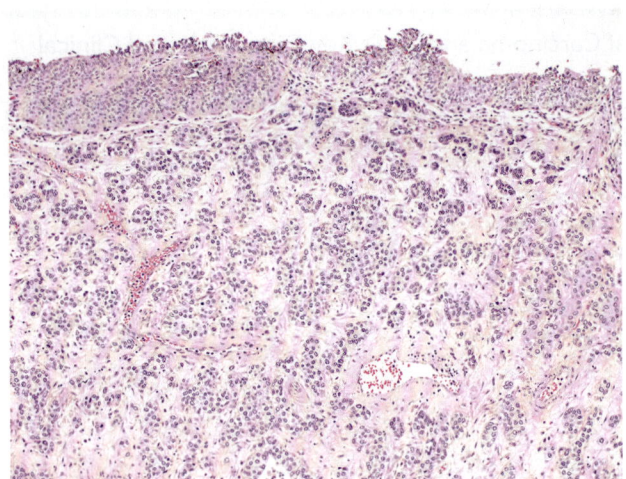

Figure 2.155. Nested variant of urothelial carcinoma demonstrating small nests of tumor infiltrating in an irregular manner deep into the lamina propria. The differential diagnosis includes von Brunn nests, and superficial biopsies may not capture the irregular growth pattern.

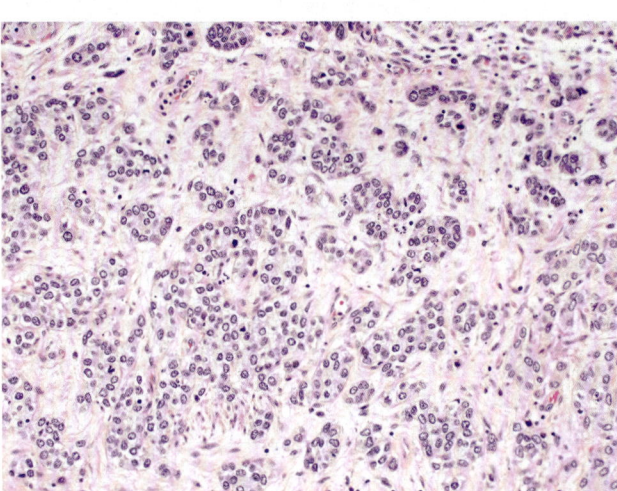

Figure 2.156. At high power, the bland cytologic features of nested variant can be appreciated. Despite the low-grade appearance, scattered atypia is present with rare mitotic figures identified.

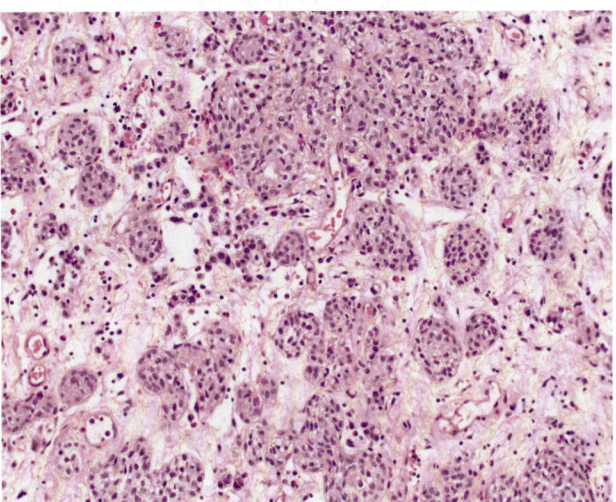

Figure 2.157. Another example of nested variant showing irregular nests of tumor with bland cytology.

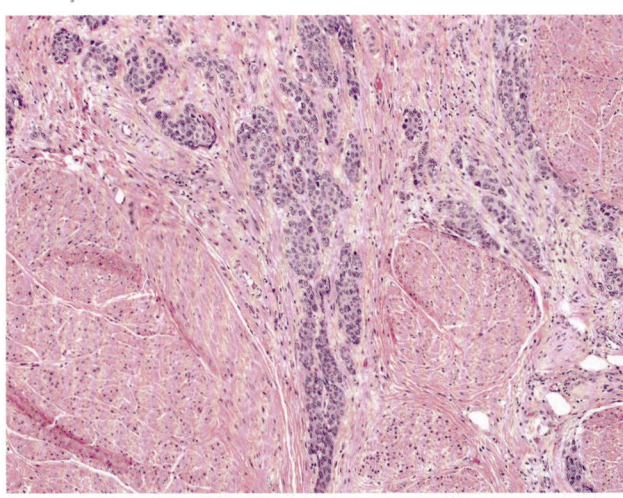

Figure 2.158. Although not always present on biopsy or TURBT (transurethral resection of bladder tumor), the finding of muscle invasion in nested variant eliminates any possibility of a benign mimicker such as von Brunn nests.

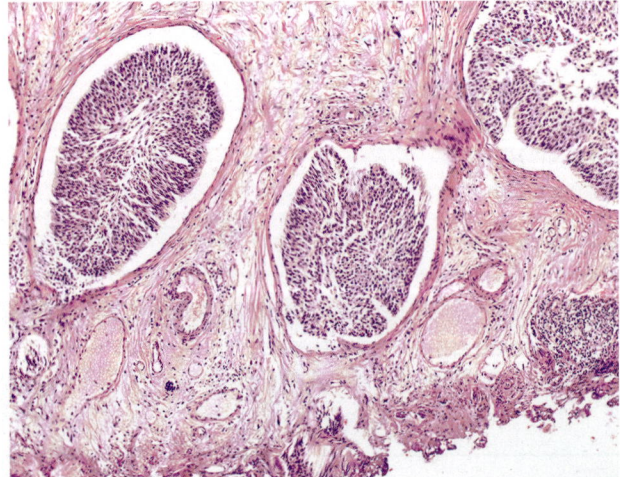

Figure 2.159. Large nested variant of urothelial carcinoma has similarly bland cytologic features, but shows large rounded nests infiltrating the lamina propria.

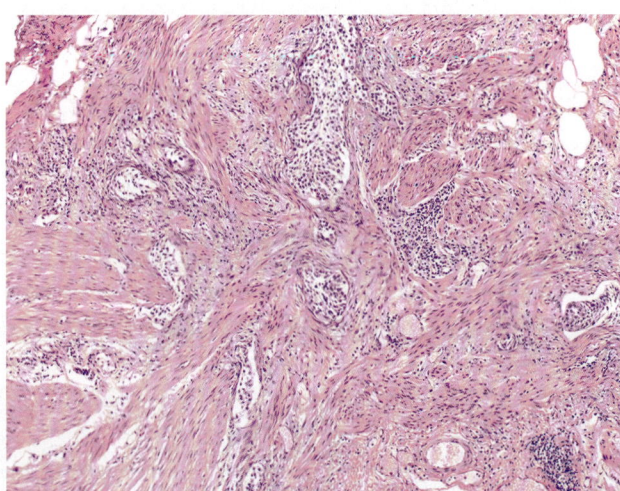

Figure 2.160. Muscularis propria involvement is common in both small and large nested variant of urothelial carcinoma.

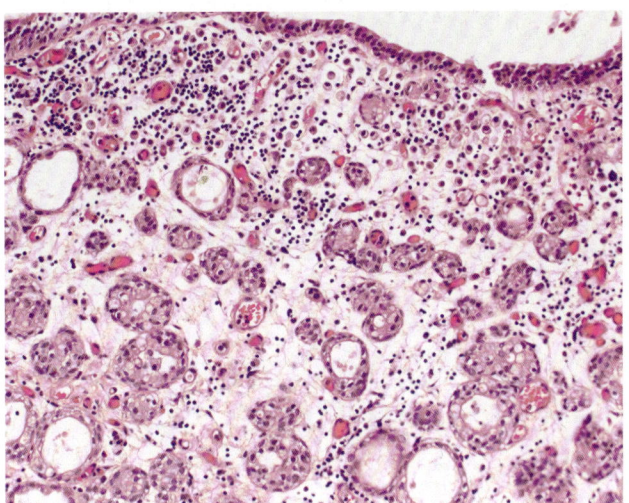

Figure 2.161. Microcystic variant of urothelial carcinoma demonstrating the small round microcysts from which it takes its name. This variant has morphologic overlap with nested variant, with low-grade cytologic features.

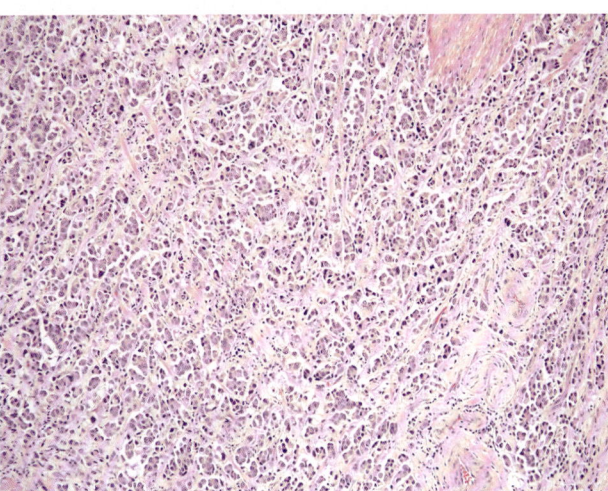

Figure 2.162. Diagnostic features of micropapillary carcinoma include minute nests of urothelial cells without fibrovascular cores, often within lacunar spaces.

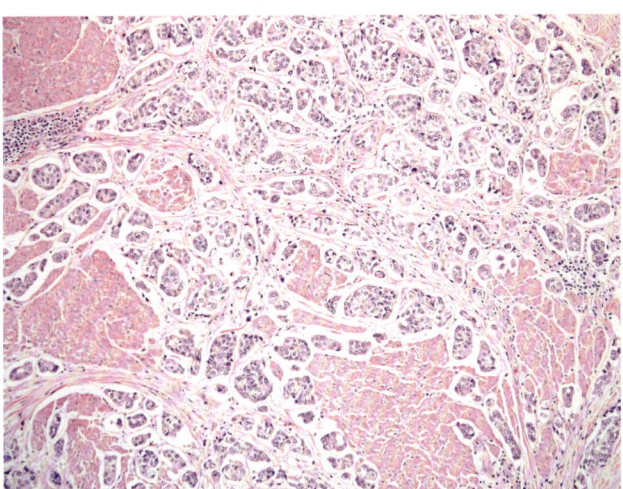

Figure 2.163. Micropapillary variant of urothelial carcinoma is an aggressive tumor with propensity for high stage at diagnosis and lymphovascular invasion. Here it is shown invading muscularis propria.

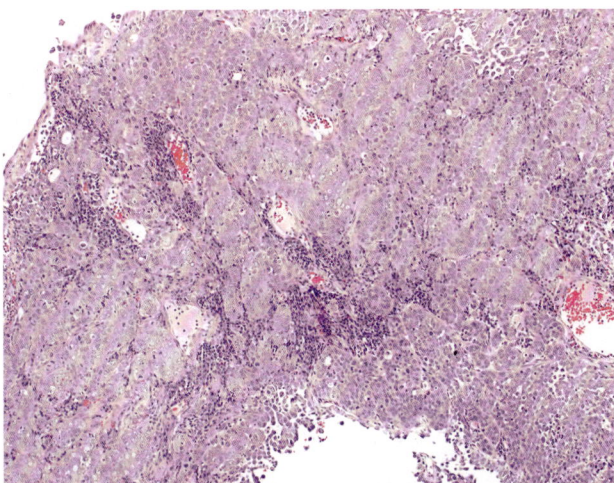

Figure 2.164. Lymphoepithelioma-like carcinoma of the bladder is a variant showing a dense mixed inflammatory infiltrate surrounding syncytial nests of undifferentiated epithelial cells. Given the relative lack of differentiating morphologic features, this tumor may be confused for a lymphoma.

to widespread peritoneal involvement. Interestingly, similar to lobular breast carcinomas, plasmacytoid urothelial carcinomas display mutations in *CDH1*, the gene which encodes e-cadherin.[53] This mutation explains their dyscohesive pattern and is demonstrable with loss of immunohistochemical expression of e-cadherin. In contrast to hereditary gastric cancers, it appears that these mutations are predominantly somatic (not germline).[53]

Because of their dyscohesive single cell pattern, sampling of a relatively pure plasmacytoid component presents a broad differential diagnosis. First, one must recognize the single cells as malignant and, if unsure, perform a pan-keratin immunohistochemical stain to confirm that the cells are in fact carcinoma. The morphology also raises the possibility of a plasmacytoma, melanoma, or sarcoma, which can be assessed by a broader immunohistochemical panel. Even with a positive keratin, the differential includes primary bladder carcinomas (bladder adenocarcinoma and urachal adenocarcinoma) and metastatic carcinomas (lobular breast carcinoma, signet ring–/diffuse-type gastrointestinal carcinoma.)

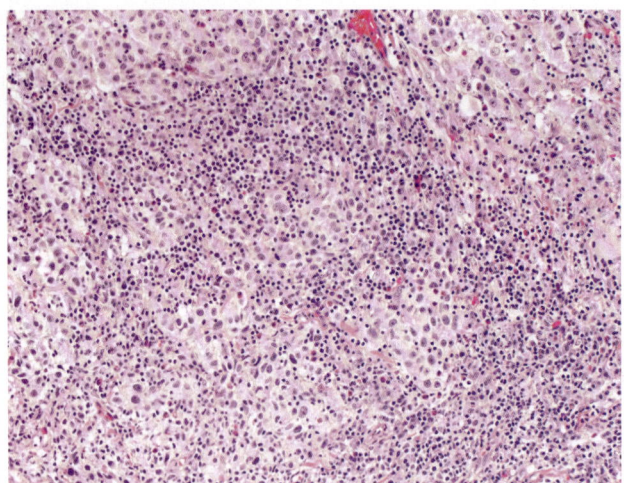

Figure 2.165. Higher power image of lymphoepithelioma-like carcinoma showing nests of epithelial cells with abundant cytoplasm, large pleomorphic nuclei with vesicular chromatin and prominent nucleoli. The background inflammatory infiltrate is comprised of a mixture of B and T lymphocytes, plasma cells, and eosinophils.

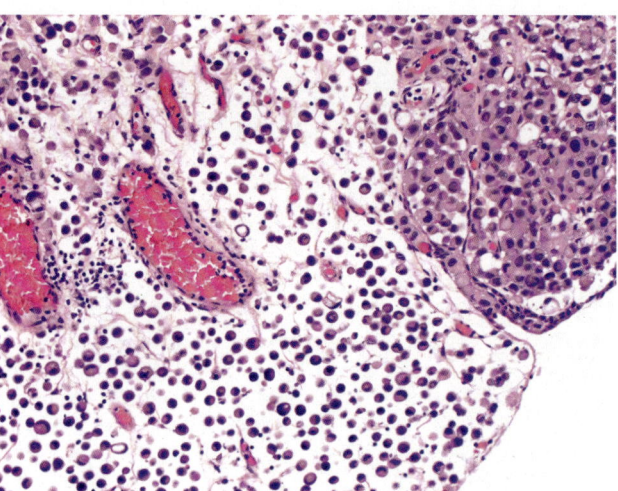

Figure 2.166. Plasmacytoid variant of urothelial carcinoma is recognized by its dyscohesive, single cell infiltration. Tumor cells often show a plasmacytoid morphology with eccentric nucleus and pink cytoplasm, but signet ring cells may also be present.

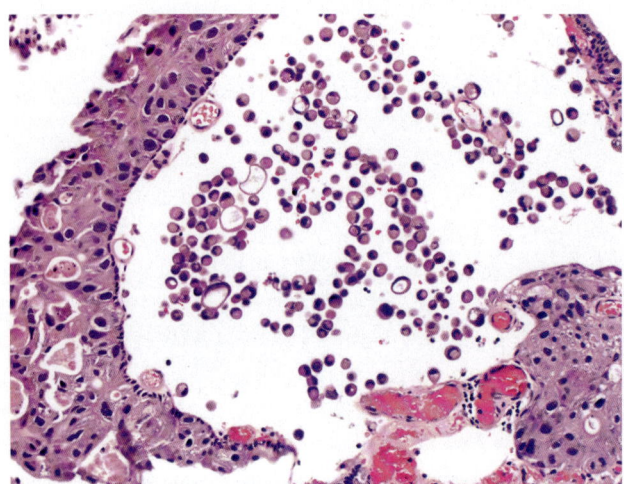

Figure 2.167. Plasmacytoid urothelial cells are commonly identified floating in an edematous or myxoid background. Because their morphology overlaps with other entities, including plasmacytoma and melanoma, immunohistochemistry may be useful in the diagnosis. Beware the finding of CD138 in these urothelial cells and also order a pan-keratin and GATA3. In this case, overlying carcinoma in situ (CIS) helps support a diagnosis of primary urothelial carcinoma.

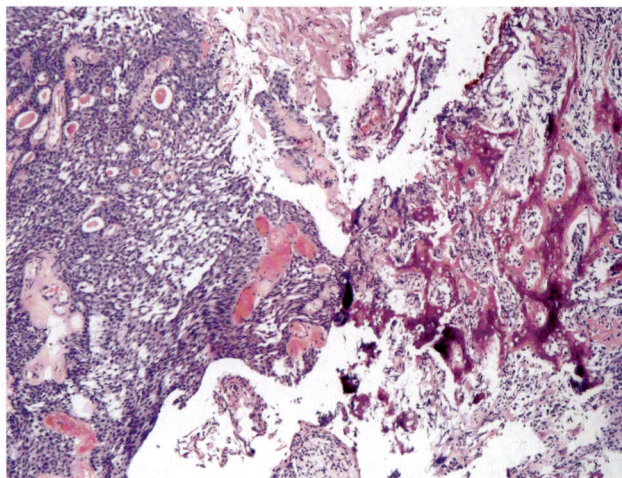

Figure 2.168. Sarcomatoid variant of urothelial carcinoma can have a multitude of morphologic appearances. Most common is a malignant spindle cell pattern, not otherwise specified, but in this case, the tumor shows obvious heterologous differentiation to osteosarcoma. This diagnosis requires identification of both an epithelial and sarcomatous component to distinguish it from a primary sarcoma.

CHECKLIST: Reporting Variant Histology in Bladder Specimens

☐ Before signing out a bladder biopsy, TURBT, or cystectomy, be sure to comment on the presence or absence of a surface lesion (CIS or papillary neoplasm)

☐ Report all variant histology patterns identified in the specimen

☐ Recommend providing rough percentages of each histologic subtype present in the specimen

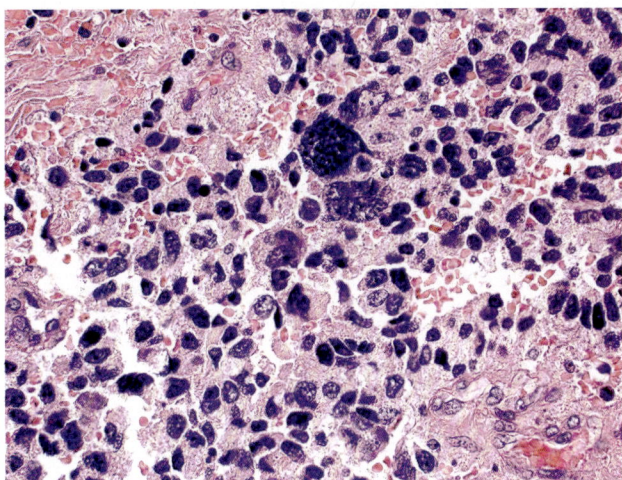

Figure 2.169. Similar to other organ systems, giant cell variant of urothelial carcinoma demonstrates numerous pleomorphic giant cells in a background of undifferentiated urothelial carcinoma.

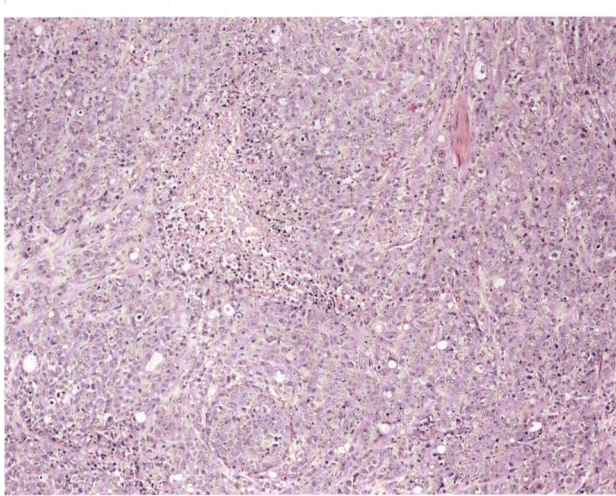

Figure 2.170. Poorly differentiated urothelial carcinoma shows no histologic features suggestive of cell type or other variant histology. While relatively rare, it is associated with poor outcomes.

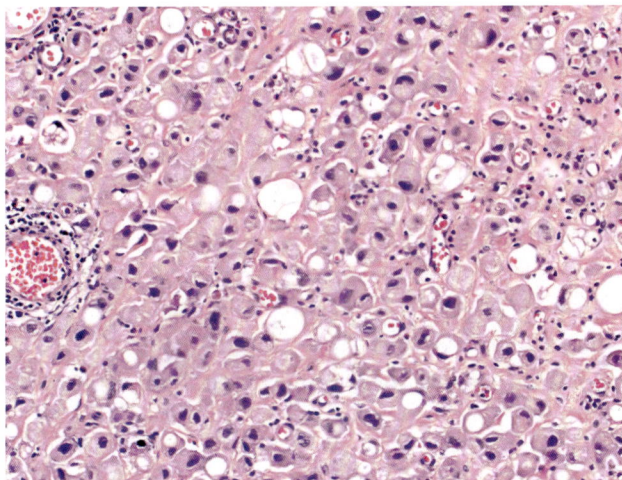

Figure 2.171. Lipid-rich variant of urothelial carcinoma shows numerous clear vacuoles and lipoblast-like cells.

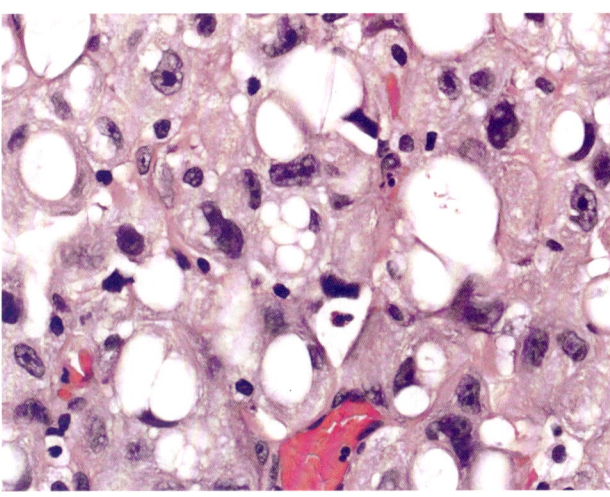

Figure 2.172. High-power image of lipid-rich urothelial carcinoma with several lipoblast-like cells.

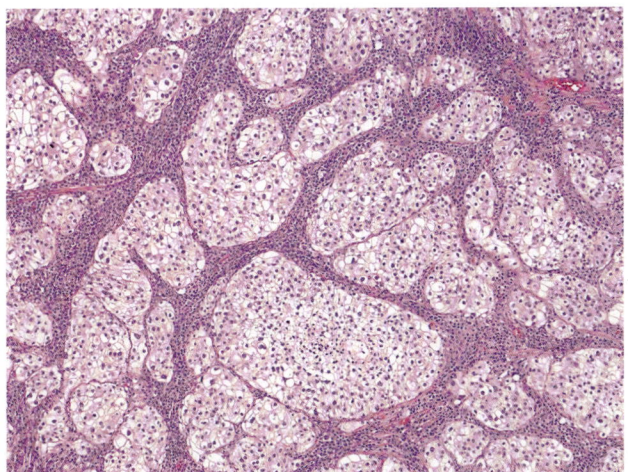

Figure 2.173. Clear cell features in urothelial carcinoma showing voluminous clear cytoplasm. The differential diagnosis of these tumors includes clear cell adenocarcinoma. Immunohistochemistry for GATA-3 and PAX-8 can be helpful in this distinction (along with the finding of usual urothelial carcinoma or a surface urothelial lesion).

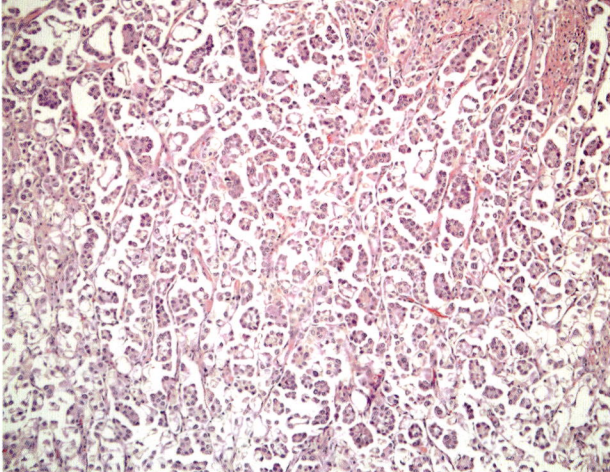

Figure 2.174. Micropapillary urothelial carcinoma is one of the most critical variants to report, as many urologists will proceed directly to cystectomy in patients with this histology. Morphologically, it shows numerous small nests of tumor without fibrovascular cores, often occupying the same lacunar space.

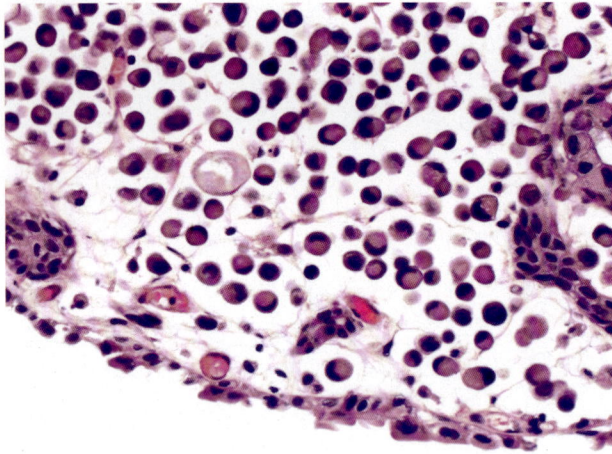

Figure 2.175. Plasmacytoid variant may present a diagnostic challenge—the morphology can overlap with metastatic adenocarcinoma, plasmacytoma, sarcoma, and melanoma. It also presents a unique pattern spread across fascial planes with peritoneal involvement.

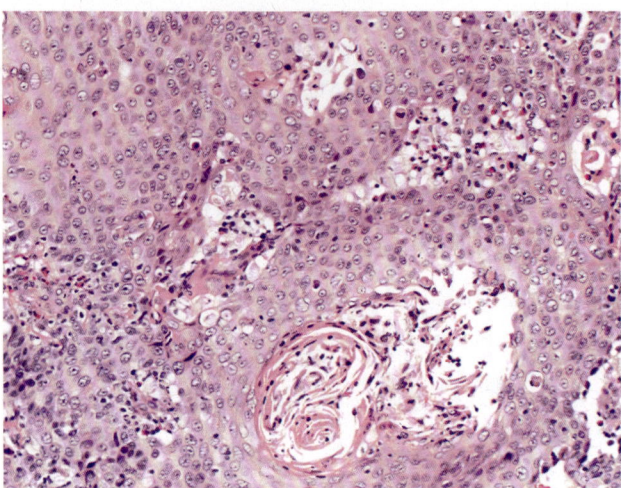

Figure 2.176. Divergent differentiation is seen in urothelial carcinoma with squamous features. Convincing keratinization is necessary for the diagnosis of squamous features, given the morphologic overlap of usual urothelial carcinoma and squamous carcinoma.

FAQ: Lynch Syndrome and Upper Tract Urothelial Carcinoma

- Lynch syndrome (LS) is a germline defect in mismatch repair machinery leading to an increased risk of multiple malignancies
- Upper tract urothelial carcinomas are the third most common type of malignancy to occur in LS after colorectal and endometrial carcinoma
- Bladder urothelial carcinomas also occur with increased frequency in LS
- Upper tract urothelial carcinomas in LS often show an inverted pattern of growth with infiltrating lymphocytes[54]

Divergent Differentiation in Urothelial Carcinoma

Urothelial carcinoma frequently shows divergent differentiation into other tumor morphologies including squamous, glandular, and neuroendocrine types. These divergent morphologies may be admixed with usual urothelial carcinoma or pure subtypes. The identification of unusual histology, especially in pure form, should raise the possibility of secondary involvement by other primary tumors. Primary squamous cell carcinoma of the bladder is most frequently associated with chronic irritation of the bladder from recurrent UTI, indwelling catheter or schistosomiasis. When that history is lacking, other considerations include the possibility of involvement by a primary gynecologic squamous cell carcinoma in a female patient. Unfortunately, human papilloma virus (HPV) in situ hybridization and p16 immunohistochemistry are not entirely reliable in this differential, as rare primary urothelial squamous cell carcinomas have shown HPV and p16 positivity.[55] Clinical and radiographic correlation is essential to establishing the correct diagnosis.

A mixture of usual urothelial carcinoma and squamous differentiation is more common than pure squamous cell carcinoma. True keratinization should be present in order to call squamous features, as usual urothelial carcinoma can have similar cytologic features to squamous carcinoma (Figures 2.176-2.179). The report should include the percent of tumor with squamous differentiation, similar to reporting variant histology.

PEARLS AND PITFALLS: Sarcomatoid Carcinoma With Squamous Features

- Squamous features may also comprise the epithelial component of a sarcomatoid carcinoma (Figure 2.180)
- Report as "Sarcomatoid carcinoma, epithelioid component comprised of squamous cell carcinoma and mesenchymal component comprised of spindle cells, not otherwise specified"

Glandular differentiation of urothelial carcinoma is also relatively common and can lead to diagnostic uncertainty (Figure 2.181). This finding may manifest as the formation of glands with no special epithelial type, presence of mucin and/or intestinal-type epithelium. When presented with a glandular lesion in the bladder, especially in a biopsy or TURBT specimen, the primary differential diagnosis in a male patient is prostate cancer. In a female patient, gynecologic primaries should be considered. Performing GATA3, NKX3.1, and PAX-8 immunohistochemistry depending on the patient is a straightforward, and essential,

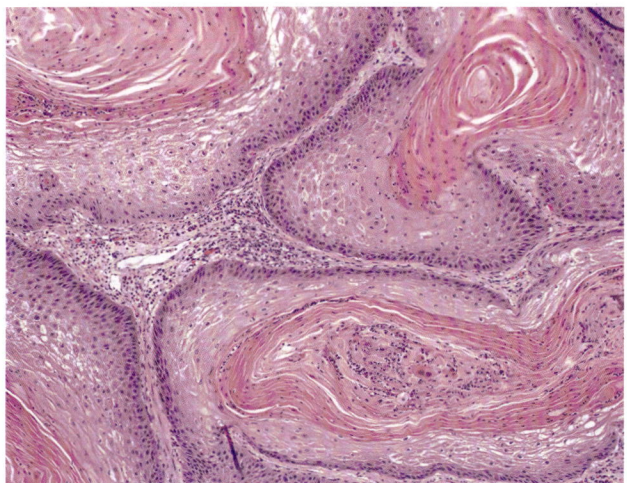

Figure 2.177. This well-differentiated squamous component shows abundant keratin formation. Occasionally, squamous cell features may be suspected by the clinician if the bladder contains keratinous debris at the time of cystoscopy.

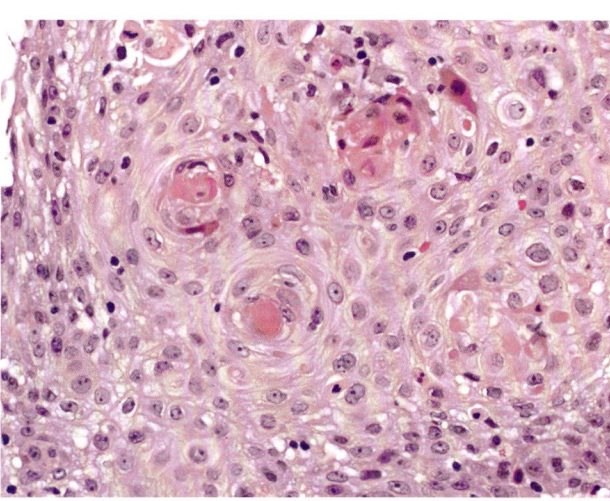

Figure 2.178. Well-formed keratin pearls are present in this urothelial carcinoma with squamous features.

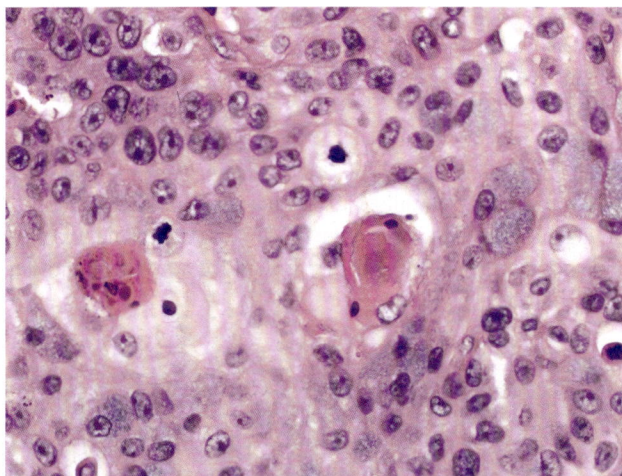

Figure 2.179. High-power image of keratinization in squamous component of urothelial carcinoma.

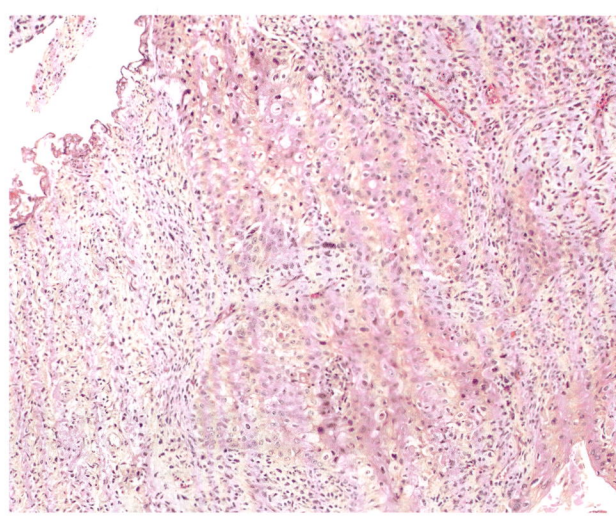

Figure 2.180. Sarcomatoid carcinomas are comprised of both epithelial and mesenchymal components. In this case, the epithelial component is squamous cell carcinoma.

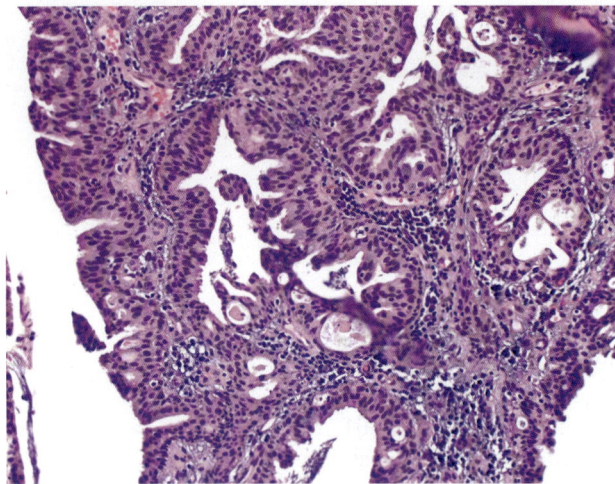

Figure 2.181. Glandular differentiation is another form of divergent differentiation seen in urothelial carcinoma, demonstrated by glands with open lumens, some of which contain mucinous secretions.

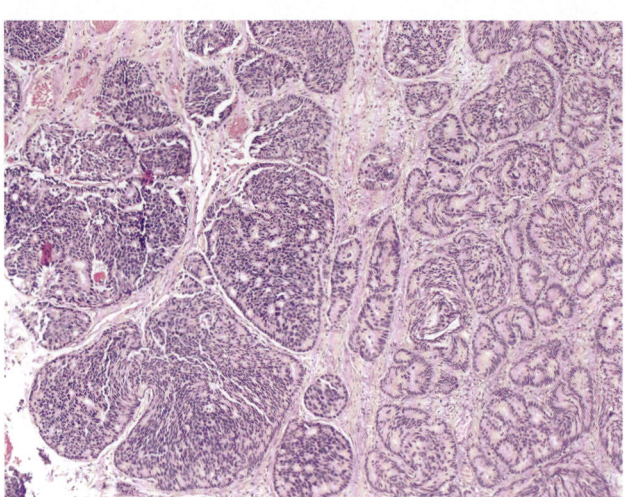

Figure 2.182. Urothelial carcinomas can have extensive glandular differentiation, presenting a diagnostic challenge. Identification of a surface lesion—carcinoma in situ (CIS) or papillary lesion—can assist in the diagnosis. In small biopsies, there may only be the glandular component and immunohistochemistry may be necessary for accurate diagnosis. In this case, the tumor shows a prominent cribriform pattern, raising the possibility of a prostate adenocarcinoma.

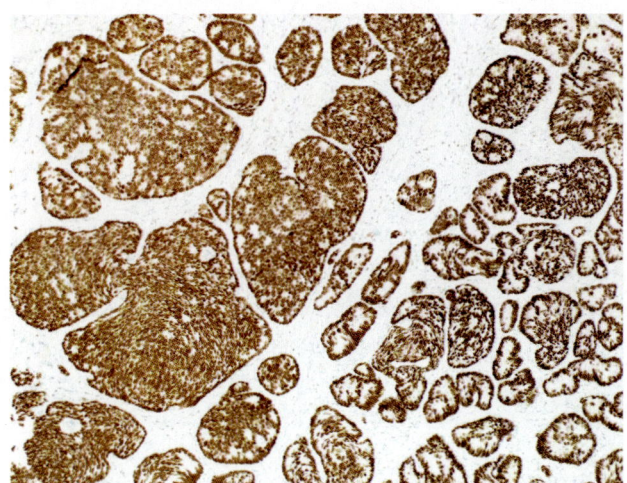

Figure 2.183. GATA3 was performed on the case in Figure 2.181, showing diffuse nuclear positivity and confirming urothelial origin.

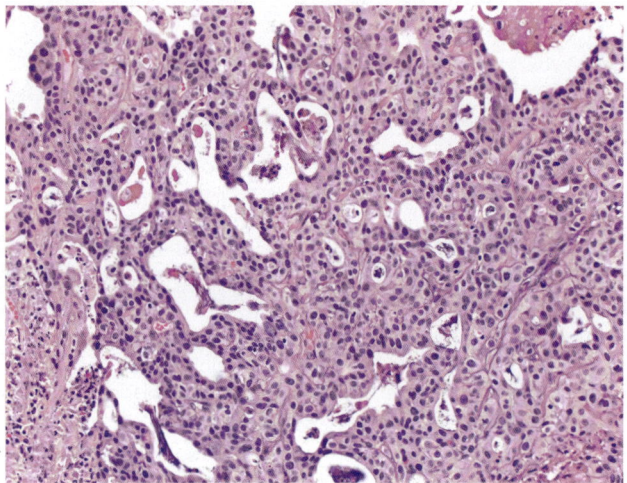

Figure 2.184. Pseudoglandular spaces in an otherwise usual urothelial carcinoma are formed by the drop out of necrotic cells, leading to empty spaces that mimic glands.

means of sorting out the diagnosis (Figures 2.182 and 2.183). When glandular features occur admixed with usual urothelial carcinoma (papillary urothelial carcinoma or urothelial CIS), the diagnosis can be made without the addition of stains. The treatment for a prostate cancer involving the bladder wall is very different from the treatment for a primary bladder cancer, so this diagnosis should not be missed.

PEARLS AND PITFALLS: Pseudoglandular Spaces

- Urothelial carcinoma can show cellular drop out and create pseudoglandular spaces, which should not be confused with glandular differentiation (Figure 2.184)

NEOPLASTIC DEEP LESIONS OF THE BLADDER—GLANDULAR PATTERN

The differential diagnosis of infiltrative glandular lesions of the bladder includes primary bladder adenocarcinoma, urachal carcinoma, and secondary or metastatic involvement of adenocarcinoma from another primary site.[56] Clinical history, cystoscopic appearance, and imaging are especially important in this differential diagnosis.

Primary Bladder Adenocarcinoma

Primary adenocarcinoma arising in the bladder accounts for 2% of all bladder cancers.[57] This diagnosis applies only to pure adenocarcinomas without any usual urothelial carcinoma component. The clinical presentation is similar to conventional urothelial carcinoma, although some unique symptoms may be encountered such as mucosuria. Histologically, the tumors have a glandular growth pattern with intestinal-type, morphologically similar to colorectal adenocarcinomas (Figures 2.185 and 2.186). Extracellular and intracellular mucin (in the form of signet ring cells) is often present (Figures 2.187 and 2.188). Cellular

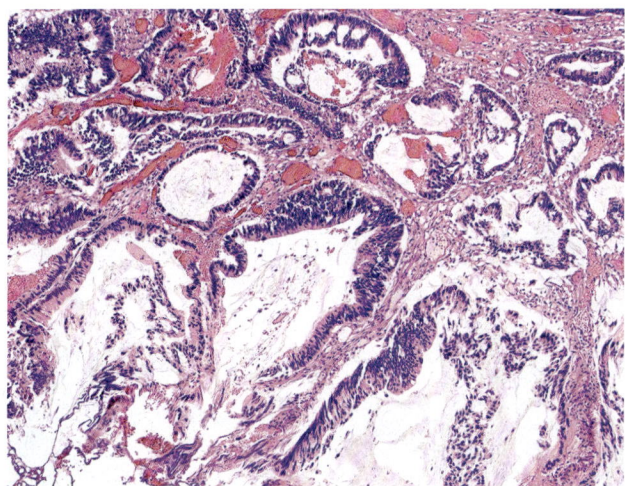

Figure 2.185. Primary bladder adenocarcinoma is morphologically similar to colorectal carcinoma with columnar cells with elongated, hyperchromatic nuclei, and intra- and extracellular mucin.

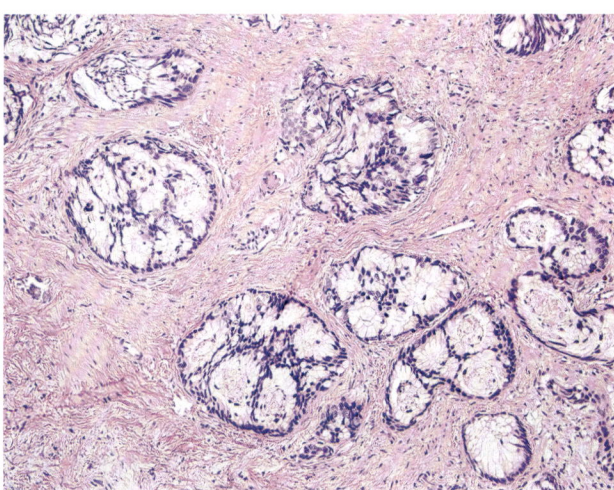

Figure 2.186. Abundant intracellular mucin and cribriform pattern is present in this bladder adenocarcinoma.

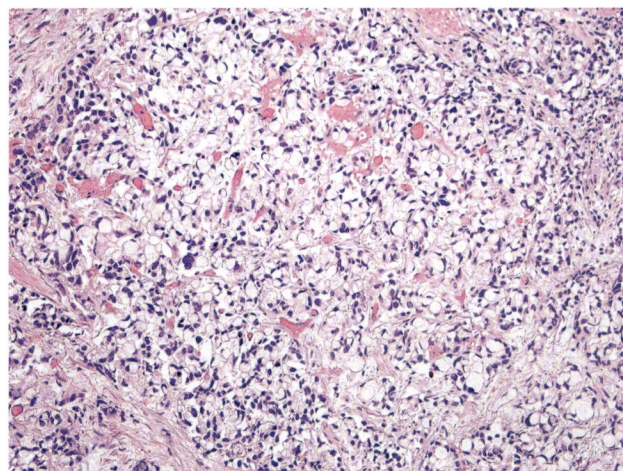

Figure 2.187. Signet ring cell morphology, similar to diffuse-type gastric adenocarcinoma, may predominate in primary bladder adenocarcinoma. All of the morphologic patterns of an intestinal adenocarcinoma may be seen in primary bladder adenocarcinoma, leading to the difficulty in distinguishing these tumors from direct extension or metastasis from another site of origin.

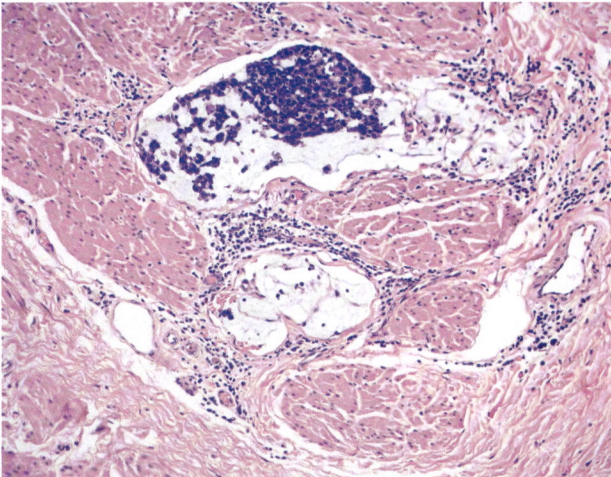

Figure 2.188. Muscle invasion is evident in this primary bladder adenocarcinoma, with extracellular mucin and hyperchromatic tumor cells.

atypia is prominent, with hyperchromasia, nuclear pseudostratification, and numerous mitotic figures. A surface component of glandular CIS may be identified and assist in the diagnosis of a bladder primary; however, in rare circumstances, adenocarcinoma of other sites may involve surface urothelium in a pagetoid manner (Figures 2.189 and 2.190). Similarly, primary bladder adenocarcinoma may arise in the setting of florid intestinal metaplasia. No specific immunoprofile exists for these tumors, which overlaps with intestinal adenocarcinoma of other sites showing variable expression of CK7, CK20, and CDX-2 and often are negative for GATA3 (Figures 2.191-2.194). Thorough review of clinical history, cancer history, and imaging are essential to the accurate diagnosis of primary bladder adenocarcinoma.

Secondary and Metastatic Adenocarcinoma Involving Bladder

Adenocarcinomas may involve the bladder via direct extension (e.g., colorectal carcinoma) or as a site of metastatic disease. Before diagnosing a primary bladder adenocarcinoma, attempt to rule out alternative sites of origin through a search of the medical record for prior

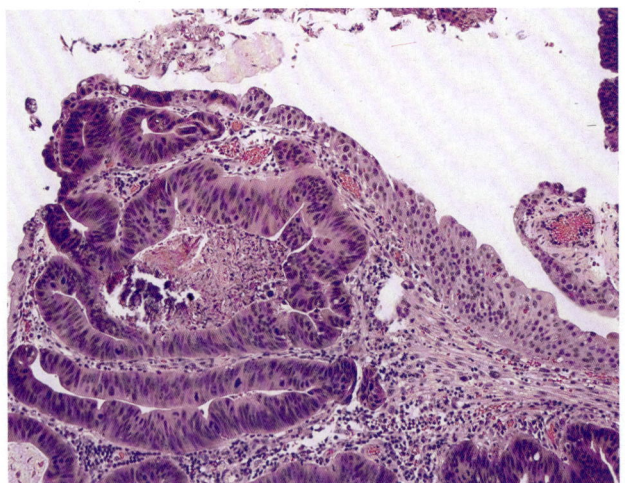

Figure 2.189. Surface involvement in the form of glandular carcinoma in situ may help support a diagnosis of primary bladder adenocarcinoma; however, metastatic or secondary involvement of other tumors can colonize the surface in a pagetoid manner. Other clues to the tumor growing from "outside in" or "inside out" may be useful in these situations.

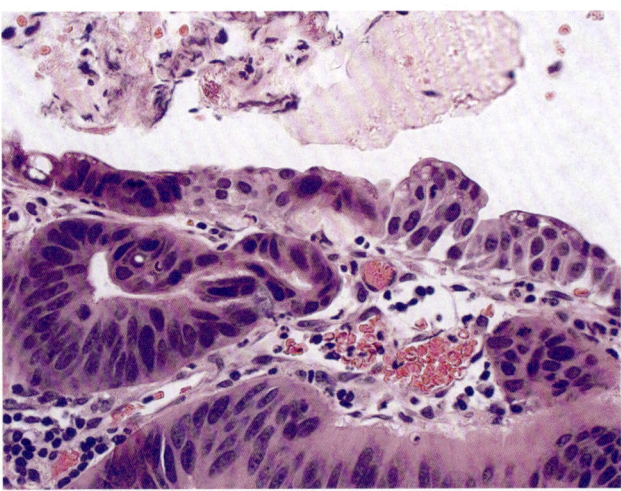

Figure 2.190. Higher power image of adenocarcinoma from Figure 2.189 showing colonization of urothelial surface with malignant glandular cells.

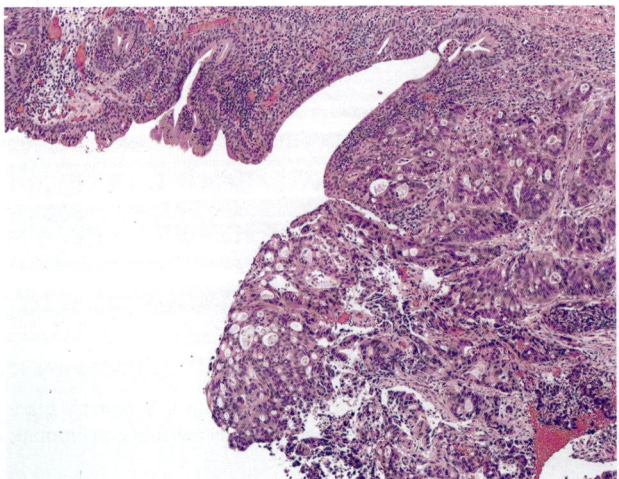

Figure 2.191. Metastatic colonic adenocarcinoma involving lamina propria and extending onto urothelial surface.

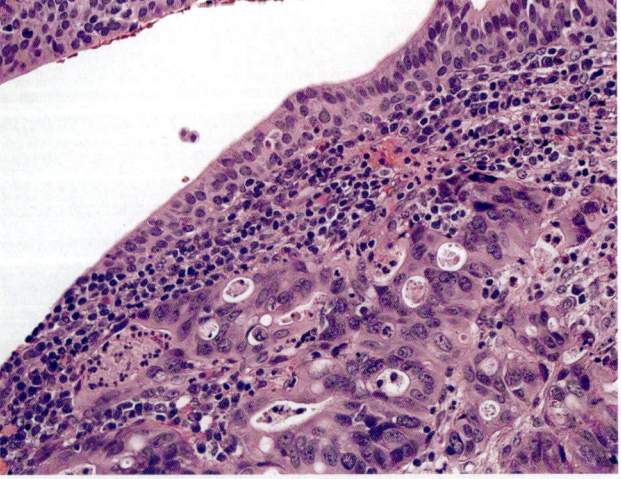

Figure 2.192. Higher power image of metastatic colonic adenocarcinoma with dirty necrosis and intraluminal mucin.

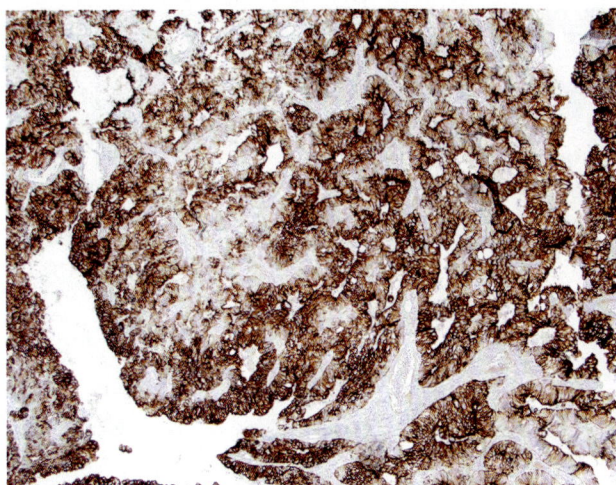

Figure 2.193. CK20 is usually positive in primary bladder adenocarcinoma and is not a differential marker in distinguishing primary bladder adenocarcinoma from other sites.

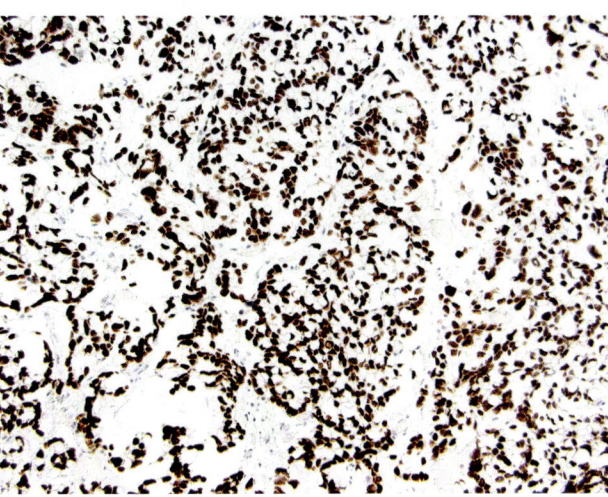

Figure 2.194. Similarly, most primary bladder adenocarcinomas are also positive for CDX-2, similar to colonic adenocarcinoma.

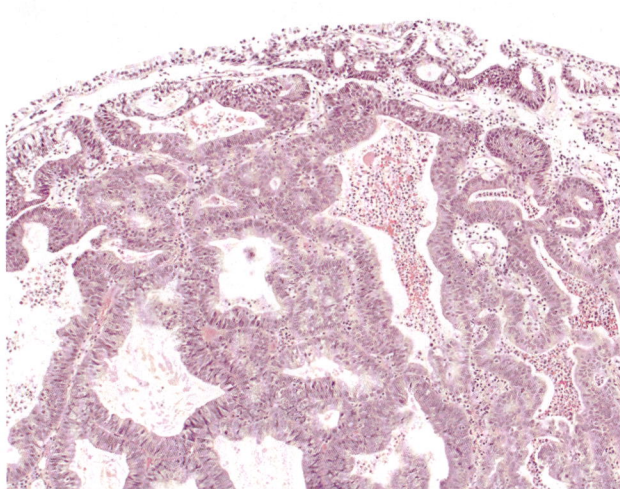

Figure 2.195. Metastatic endometrial carcinoma involving the bladder can be deceptively bland. Clinical correlation is necessary for accurate diagnosis, although estrogen receptor/progesterone receptor (ER/PR) immunohistochemistry is helpful in this differential diagnosis.

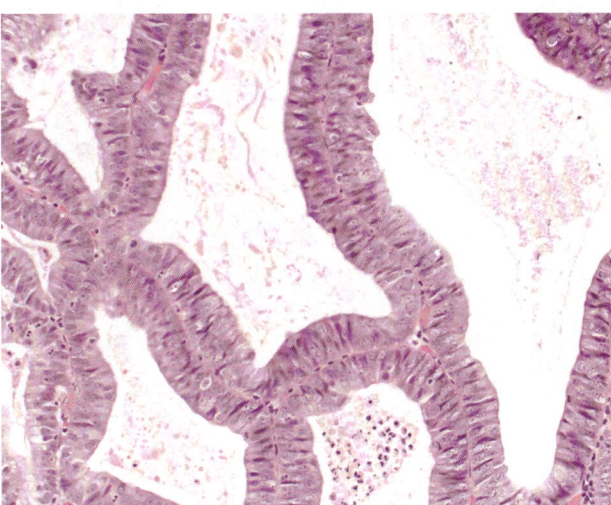

Figure 2.196. Higher power image of endometrial carcinoma with atypical columnar nuclei with stratification and frequent mitotic figures.

cancer history and a review of any available imaging studies. Most intestinal-type adenocarcinomas are morphologically indistinguishable, so incorporating history and imaging may be the only way to make an accurate diagnosis. The finding of relatively bland, nondescript glands that are deeply infiltrating in the muscularis propria should raise the possibility of metastatic or secondary invasion by adenocarcinoma of another origin. Specifically, pancreatic and gynecologic tumors can be deceptively low grade despite aggressive metastatic disease (Figures 2.195 and 2.196).

To complicate the situation, primary bladder adenocarcinoma has an immunoprofile that overlaps with primary gastrointestinal adenocarcinomas, often displaying CK20 and CDX-2 positivity. Beta-catenin positivity has been proposed as a differential marker in distinguishing primary bladder adenocarcinoma from colorectal adenocarcinoma, with colon cancer more frequently showing strong nuclear and cytoplasmic staining (Figures 2.197-2.200).[58,59]

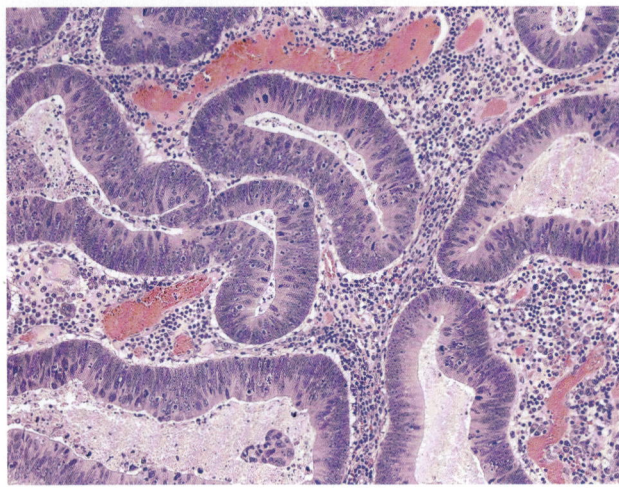

Figure 2.197. A moderately differentiated adenocarcinoma involving the bladder has no specific morphologic features to indicate site of origin, as seen in this case.

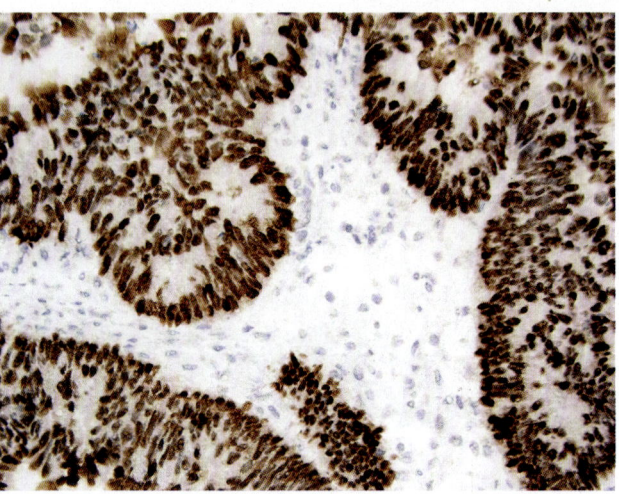

Figure 2.198. Immunohistochemistry for CDX-2 showing diffuse nuclear positivity, which indicates intestinal-type differentiation and is nonspecific for site of origin.

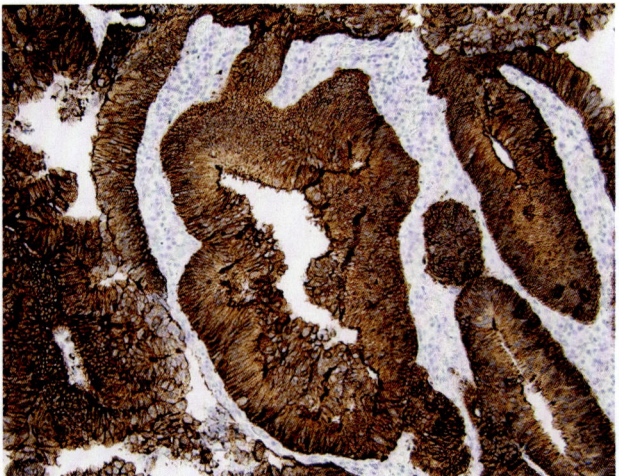

Figure 2.199. Immunohistochemistry for CK20 showing strong, diffuse positivity, which is also nonspecific for site of origin and expected to be positive in both primary bladder adenocarcinoma and gastrointestinal (GI) origin.

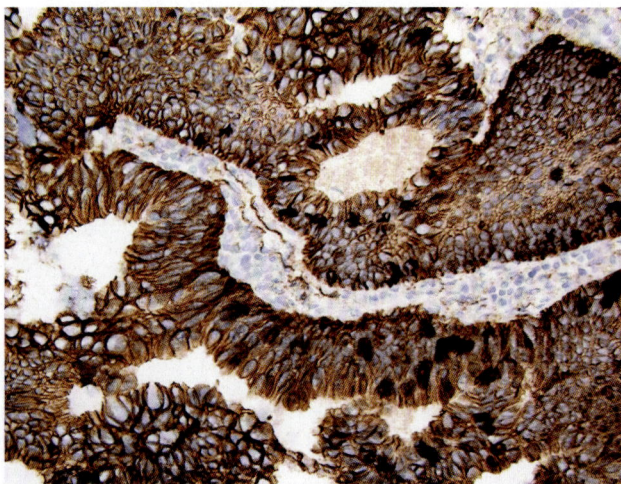

Figure 2.200. Nuclear and cytoplasmic expression of beta-catenin has been proposed as a differential marker for metastatic colorectal carcinoma involving the bladder. Strong expression favors secondary/metastatic involvement by colorectal carcinoma over a primary bladder adenocarcinoma.

SAMPLE NOTE: Mucinous Adenocarcinoma Involving Bladder

Bladder, TURBT: Invasive mucinous adenocarcinoma (see note)
- Note: There is no specific immunohistochemical profile for primary adenocarcinoma of the bladder, and secondary involvement from a gastrointestinal, gynecologic, or other primary must be excluded clinically and radiographically. In the absence of evidence of another primary source, the findings would be consistent with a primary bladder adenocarcinoma.

Urachal Carcinoma

Urachal carcinoma is an exceedingly rare type of bladder cancer with several specific diagnostic criteria. Most importantly, these tumors must arise in the muscular wall in the dome or anterior wall, as this is the anatomic location of the embryogenic remnant of the urachus, the median umbilical ligament. Histologically, they are similar to other intestinal-type adenocarcinomas and may show enteric, mucinous/colloid, signet ring cell or mixture of these appearances (Figures 2.201 and 2.202). Calcifications are common in these tumors, and finding calcifications on imaging studies may suggest urachal carcinoma (Figure 2.203). An accurate diagnosis of urachal carcinoma is important because the surgical treatment of these tumors differs from primary bladder adenocarcinomas. For complete resection of urachal carcinoma, a partial cystectomy and excision of the median umbilical ligament (site of former urachus and allantois) and umbilicus is necessary.

KEY FEATURES: Diagnostic Criteria for Urachal Carcinoma

- Located in anterior wall or dome of bladder
- Involves muscularis propria or deeper tissues that undermines, rather than directly involves, the surface urothelium
- No in situ component present in the surface urothelium
- No other source of primary adenocarcinoma known

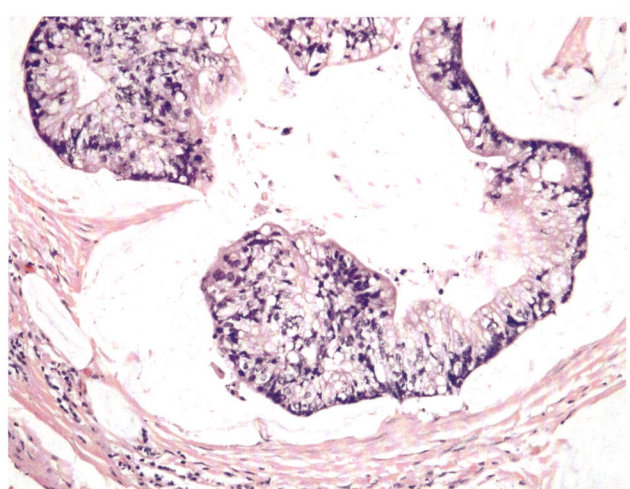

Figure 2.201. Urachal adenocarcinoma is a rare type of bladder adenocarcinoma with specific diagnostic criteria. Histologically, it is an adenocarcinoma which may have intestinal/mucinous differentiation as seen here.

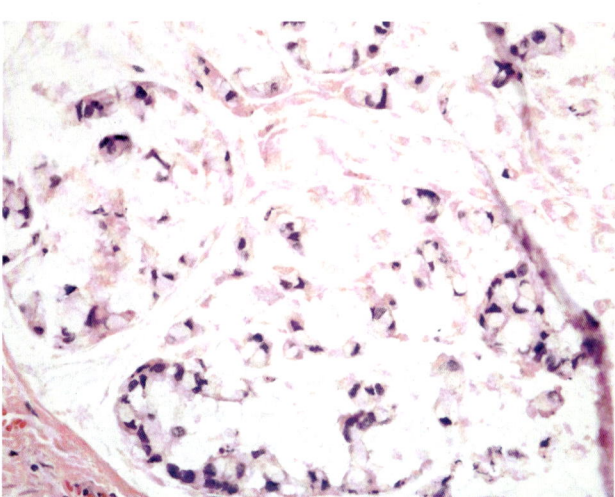

Figure 2.202. Signet ring cells may also be identified in urachal adenocarcinoma.

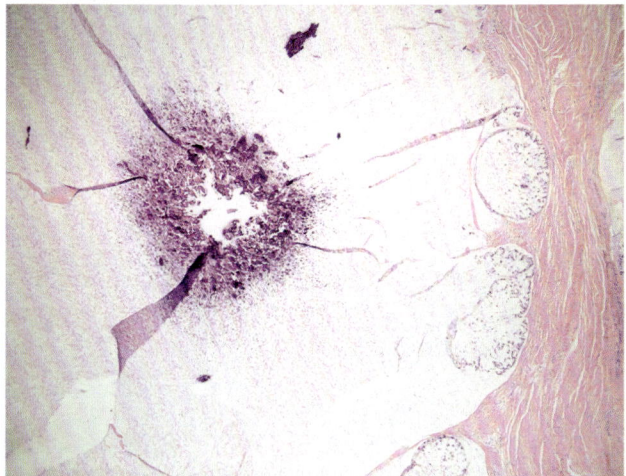

Figure 2.203. Calcifications are commonly present in urachal adenocarcinoma and may be identified in radiologic studies, hinting at the diagnosis.

Prostatic Ductal Adenocarcinoma

A rare type of primary prostatic adenocarcinoma can mimic a bladder primary cancer when it presents as a papillary lesion in the urethra. Prostatic ductal adenocarcinoma may develop in the periurethral ducts near the verumontanum and be seen on cystoscopy as a papillary mass. When biopsied in this location, the site will be often listed as "urethra" and it is easy to overlook the possibility of a nonurothelial origin. These tumors are often villoglandular or cribriform, with slit-like spaces, rather than the rounded lumina seen in usual acinar prostate cancer (Figure 2.204). By definition, the nuclei of ductal adenocarcinoma are columnar and pseudostratified and show prominent nucleoli (Figure 2.205). When encountering a papillary lesion in the urethra of a male, a limited immunohistochemical panel of NKX3.1, PSA, and GATA3 will help distinguish between a prostatic origin and urothelial origin. Basal cell markers may be absent in ductal adenocarcinoma, but be aware that these tumors may also grow intraductally and retain basal cells in a patchy distribution. Regardless of basal cell presence, they still represent invasive tumors.

CHECKLIST: Differential Diagnosis of Glandular Lesions of Deep Bladder

☐ Primary bladder adenocarcinoma
☐ Urachal carcinoma
☐ Metastatic adenocarcinoma involving bladder
☐ Prostatic adenocarcinoma involving bladder
☐ Cystitis cystica et glandularis (with florid intestinal metaplasia)
☐ Nephrogenic adenoma
☐ Mullerianosis
☐ Urachal remnants

OTHER PATTERNS OF NEOPLASTIC DEEP LESIONS OF THE BLADDER

Invasive urothelial carcinoma is not the only process that can involve the deep (lamina propria or muscularis propria) layers of the bladder. Several entities should be included in the differential diagnosis of invasive urothelial cancer, including the neoplastic lesions inverted papilloma, paraganglioma, inflammatory myofibroblastic tumor, leiomyoma,

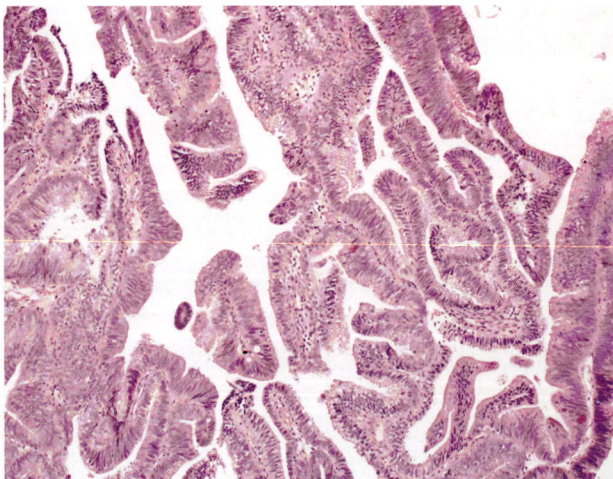

Figure 2.204. Prostatic ductal adenocarcinoma can present as a papillary lesion in the prostatic urethra and mimic papillary urothelial carcinoma. The tumors have a villoglandular appearance and the cribriform spaces are more slit-like than rounded.

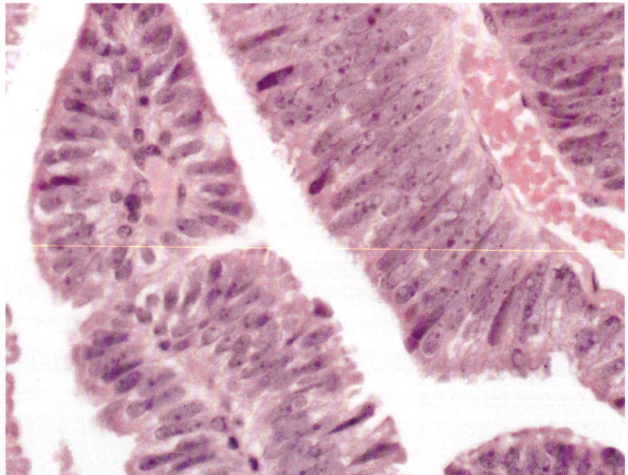

Figure 2.205. Higher power image detailing the cytologic features of prostatic ductal adenocarcinoma. The nuclei are columnar, similar to endometrioid carcinoma. Pseudostratification and prominent nucleoli are evident.

leiomyosarcoma, and sarcomatoid carcinoma. Each of these processes has an overall architectural pattern that drives the differential diagnosis. Nonneoplastic processes can also appear to infiltrate into the bladder wall, particularly cystitis glandularis, urachal remnants, nephrogenic adenoma, and Mullerianosis. Because all of these entities represent potential pitfalls for overdiagnosis of invasive carcinoma, they should be considered every time a deep bladder lesion is encountered.

Inverted Papilloma—Inverted Pattern

Inverted papilloma is a benign entity with a somewhat ominous histologic appearance. At low power, these tumors are often very blue and show a highly complex infiltrative pattern that expands the lamina propria. Knowing the key features of these tumors will prevent the overdiagnosis of invasive urothelial carcinoma. The identification of any true exophytic papillary component is not consistent with an inverted papilloma, and a true papillary lesion should be diagnosed in these cases. In a limited sampling, the distinction between a low-grade papillary urothelial carcinoma with prominent inverted growth pattern and an inverted papilloma may be extremely difficult. Often, an inverted papillary urothelial carcinoma will show large broad-based nests, compared with the thinner anastomosing cords in an inverted papilloma.

KEY FEATURES: Histologic Features of Inverted Urothelial Papilloma

- No established exophytic component; rare papillary frond acceptable (Figure 2.206)
- Interlocking or anastomosing cords of tumor (Figures 2.207 and 2.208)
- Peripheral palisading and swirling of urothelial cells with bland cytologic features resembling normal urothelium, including nuclear grooves (Figure 2.209)
- Microcystic lumina containing eosinophilic material, "colloid cyst" (Figure 2.210)
- No or exceedingly rare mitotic figures
- Papillary urothelial carcinoma can have a prominent inverted pattern—scan thoroughly for the presence of any established papillary component (Figure 2.211)

Paraganglioma—Nested Pattern

A neoplastic proliferation of paraganglion cells can occur in the bladder and is commonly identified in the muscularis propria, consistent with the anatomic location of the paraganglia (Figure 2.212). Paraganglioma should form a true mass, so as not to overdiagnose normal paraganglia as a tumor. Patients may present with hematuria alone, or the classic

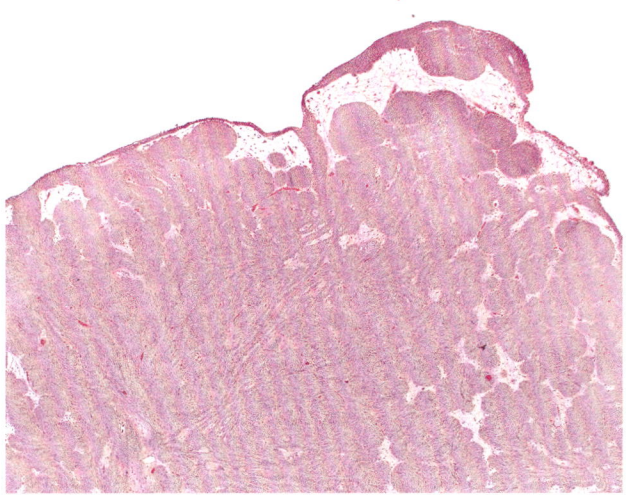

Figure 2.206. At low power, a benign inverted urothelial papilloma has no established exophytic papillary component. A rare papillary frond is acceptable.

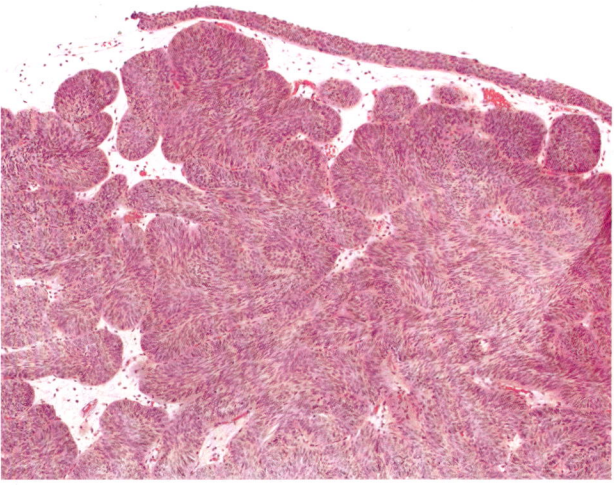

Figure 2.207. The growth pattern of inverted papilloma is cords and trabeculae of urothelial cells that interlock or anastomose, reminiscent of a jigsaw puzzle.

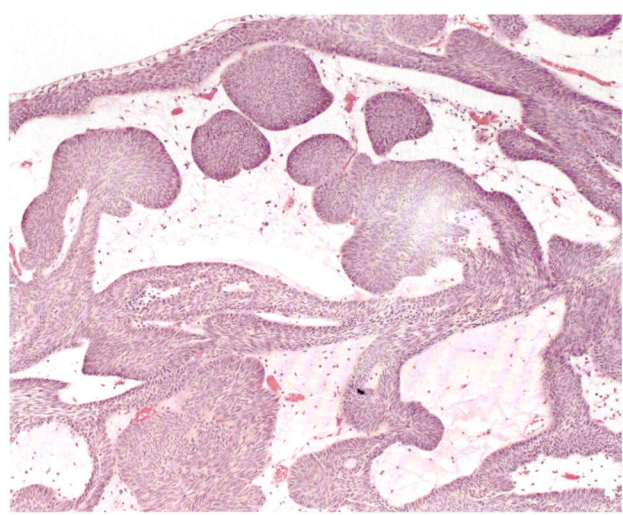

Figure 2.208. At higher power, the interlocking nature is evident as cords of tumor separate and rejoin to other nests of papilloma.

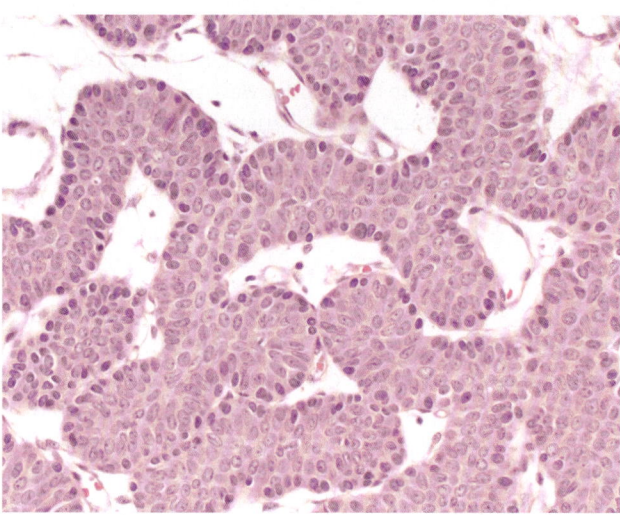

Figure 2.209. At high power, the bland cytology of inverted papilloma is demonstrated with rare nuclear grooves identified. There is palisading or condensation of cells at the periphery of the cords.

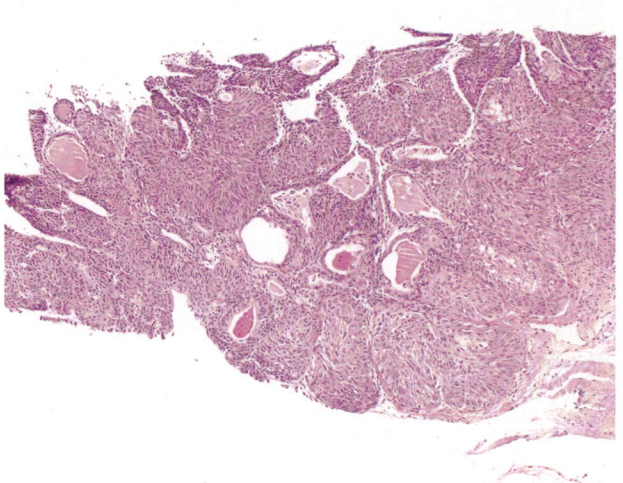

Figure 2.210. Eosinophilic material is commonly present within microcystic lumina in inverted papilloma.

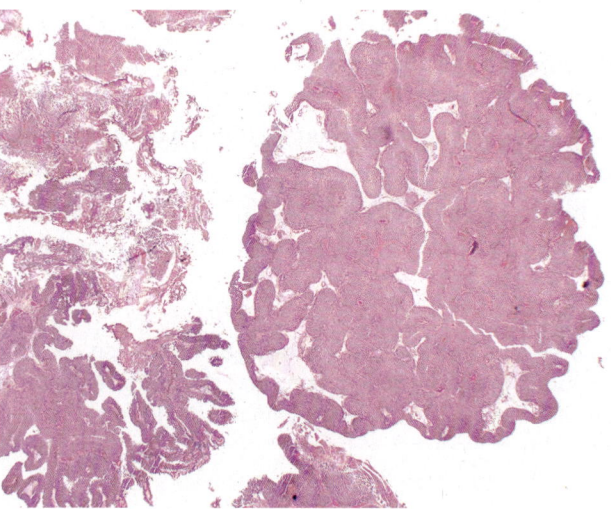

Figure 2.211. Low-grade papillary urothelial carcinoma mimicking inverted papilloma with a prominent inverted growth pattern in the fragment in the middle-right portion of the image. In the lower left, there are well-established papillary fronds, leading to the diagnosis of low-grade papillary urothelial carcinoma.

finding of "micturition attack." A micturition attack is an episodic headache, anxiety, and increase in blood pressure with potential for syncope when a patient urinates. Clinical laboratory values may demonstrate elevated vanillylmandelic acid in the urine of affected patients.

Histologically, these tumors are similar to their adrenal counterparts, pheochromocytomas. They display a nested architecture with intervening fine capillary vessels, the same "zellballen" pattern seen in pheochromocytomas (Figure 2.213). Cells are generally round to polygonal with abundant amphophilic cytoplasm, imparting a somewhat purple granular appearance to the tumors (Figures 2.214 and 2.215). Neuroendocrine-type chromatin pattern is identified in paraganglioma, with finely stippled or "salt and pepper" appearance. Occasionally, the cytoplasm can demonstrate clearing and lack of granular appearance. The nuclei can be relatively monotonous, although endocrine atypia is common, with nuclear inclusions and degenerative changes.

PEARLS AND PITFALLS: Paraganglioma

- Paragangliomas can easily be confused with invasive urothelial carcinoma due to their location in the muscularis propria (Figure 2.216)
- Recognition of zellballen pattern, granular cytoplasm, and vascular network can prevent a misdiagnosis (Figure 2.217)
- Urothelial carcinomas also can have a very nested appearance and abundant eosinophilic cytoplasm, which can mimic paraganglioma (Figure 2.218)
- Paragangliomas are GATA3 positive, and performing only a single immunohistochemical stain may lead to incorrect diagnosis; should use a panel of immunohistochemistry for the diagnosis including pan-keratin, p40 (both negative in paraganglioma), synaptophysin, chromogranin, and S100 (positive in paraganglioma) (Figures 2.219-2.222)

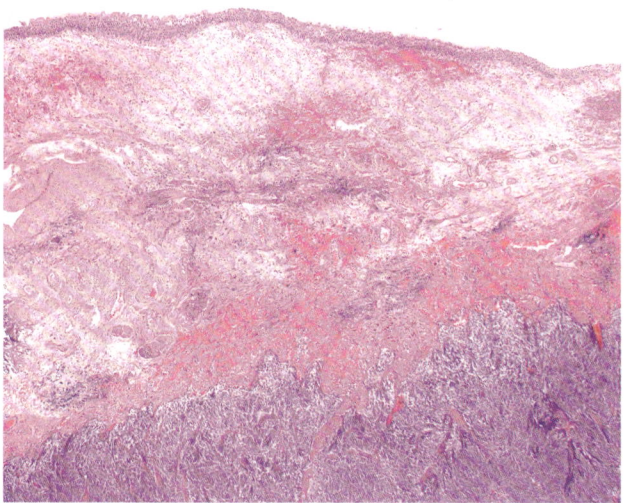

Figure 2.212. Paragangliomas are usually centered in the muscularis propria, the anatomic location of the nerves and paraganglia from which they arise.

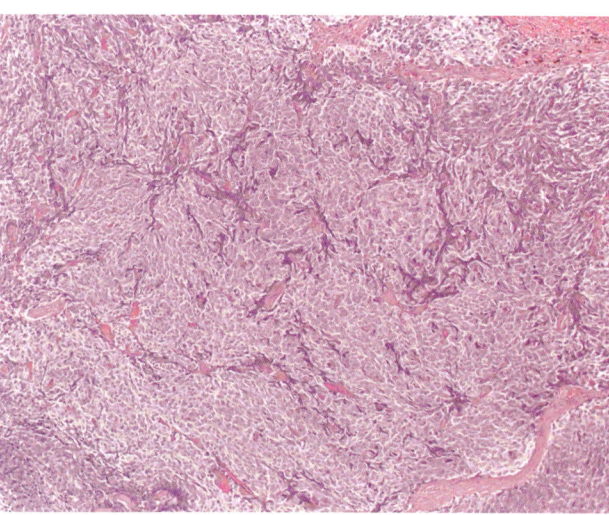

Figure 2.213. The characteristic nested or "zellballen" architecture of pheochromocytomas is also present in paragangliomas of the bladder. Small capillary vessels are seen between the nests of tumor cells.

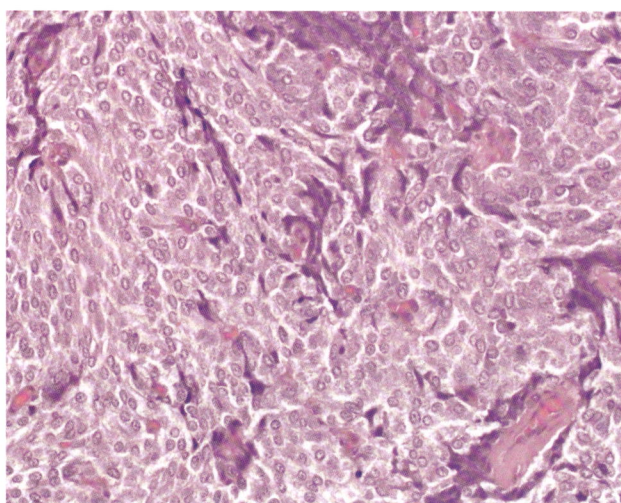

Figure 2.214. The classic amphophilic, granular cytoplasm of paraganglioma is demonstrated in this image. It imparts a purple appearance to these tumors.

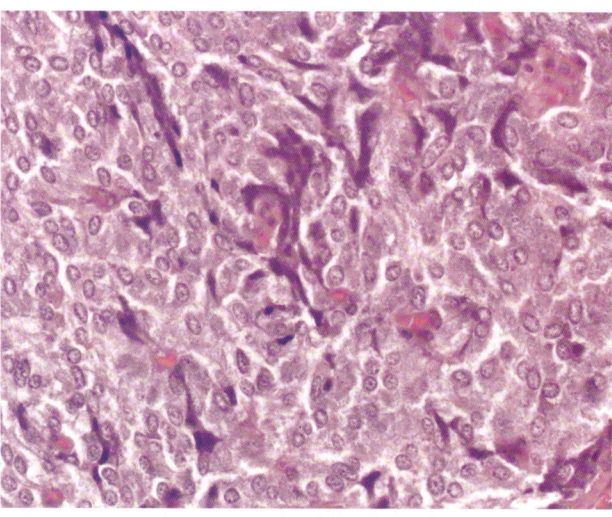

Figure 2.215. The neuroendocrine chromatin pattern of paraganglioma showing finely speckled "salt and pepper" appearance.

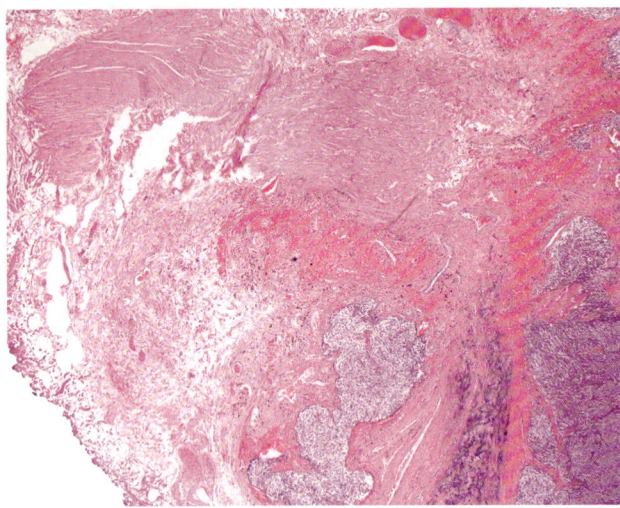

Figure 2.216. The classic location of paraganglioma located in the deep muscle wall can lead to a reflexive diagnosis of invasive carcinoma. Recognition of the zellballen pattern, granular cytoplasm, and immunohistochemistry can help avoid a misdiagnosis.

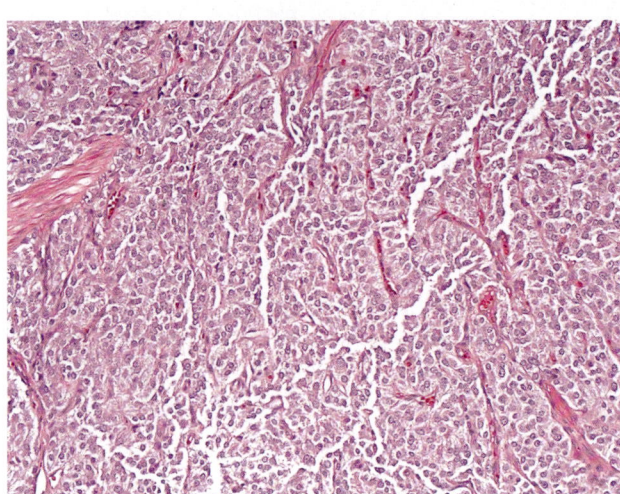

Figure 2.217. The classic amphophilic granular cytoplasm of paraganglioma is an important feature to recognize in the diagnosis.

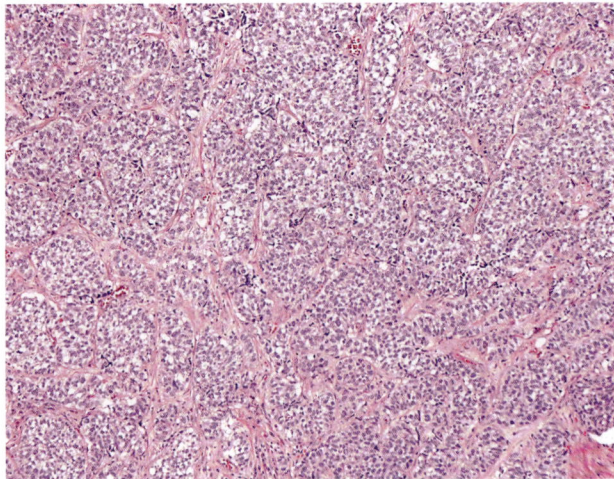

Figure 2.218. Urothelial carcinoma mimicking paraganglioma by virtue of its nested architecture and finely granular and clear cytoplasm. If no surface lesion is present to indicate a primary urothelial process, immunohistochemistry is warranted.

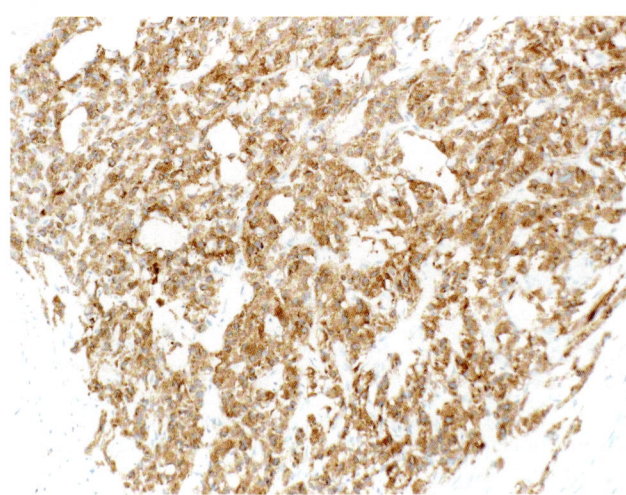

Figure 2.219. As neuroendocrine tumors, paragangliomas show diffuse expression of synaptophysin.

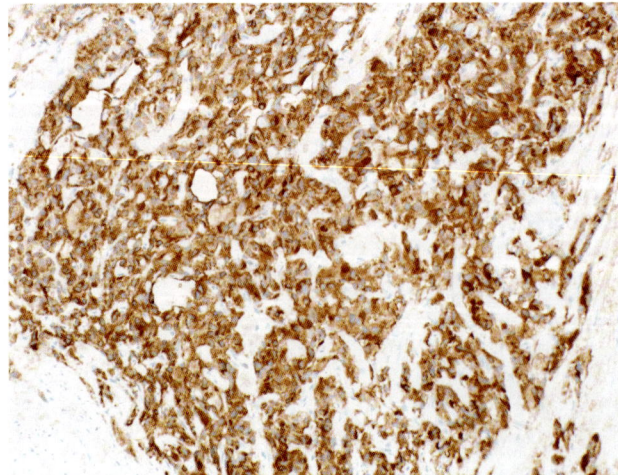

Figure 2.220. The neuroendocrine marker chromogranin is also diffusely positive in paragangliomas.

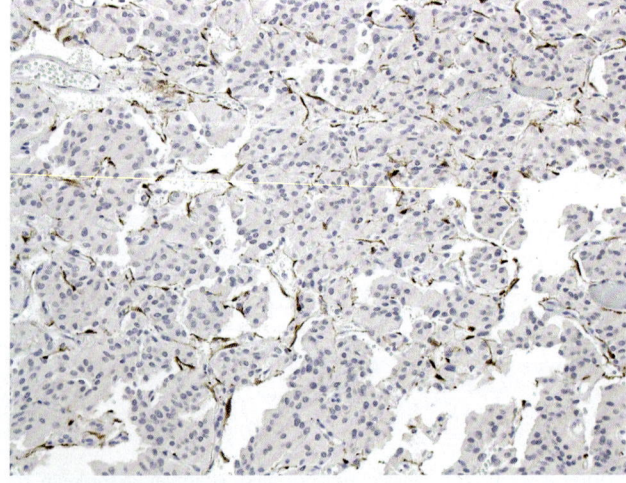

Figure 2.221. S100 highlights sustentacular cells between the nests of paraganglioma.

NEOPLASTIC DEEP LESIONS OF THE BLADDER—SPINDLE PATTERN

Inflammatory Myofibroblastic Tumor

Inflammatory myofibroblastic tumors (IMTs) are neoplastic spindle cell lesions that can infiltrate the bladder wall, involving the muscularis propria (Figure 2.223). These tumors may occur because of prior trauma and can be associated with prior biopsy or resection. Histologically, these tumors are comprised of a spindled, patternless fibroblastic proliferation set within a loose myxoid stroma (Figure 2.224). IMTs are richly vascular, and extravasated red blood cells are easily identified (Figure 2.225). Within the myxoid stroma, inflammatory cells are easily identified (Figure 2.226). Cytologically, the spindled cells demonstrate reactive nuclear features with open chromatin and prominent nucleoli (Figure 2.227). IMTs are proliferative lesions and mitotic figures may be prominent; however, atypical mitotic figures are not compatible with the diagnosis.

Up to two-thirds of IMTs are positive for anaplastic lymphoma kinase (ALK), and this is considered a confirmatory stain when positive (Figure 2.228). Overlapping and potentially related entities include postoperative spindle cell nodule (when the myofibroblastic

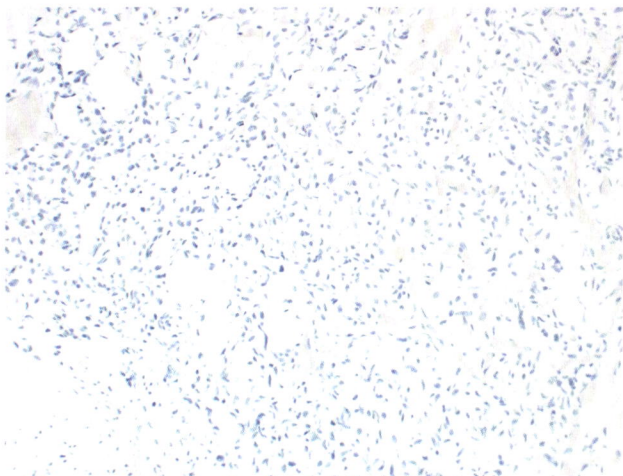

Figure 2.222. Pan-keratin is negative in paraganglioma, distinguishing it from urothelial carcinoma. GATA3 is not a useful marker in this differential diagnosis, as GATA3 is also expressed in paragangliomas.

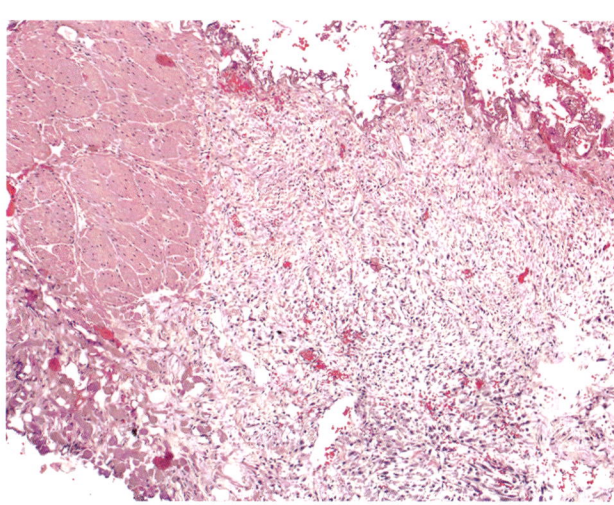

Figure 2.223. Inflammatory myofibroblastic tumor (IMT) seen here involving muscularis propria.

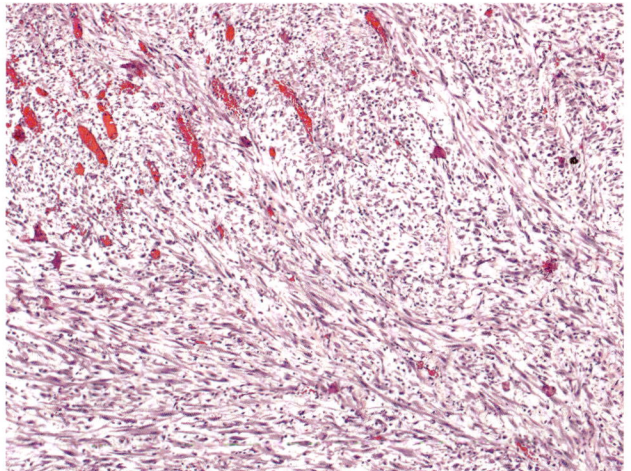

Figure 2.224. At medium power, the spindle cells of this inflammatory myofibroblastic tumor (IMT) show intersecting fascicles without distinctive pattern.

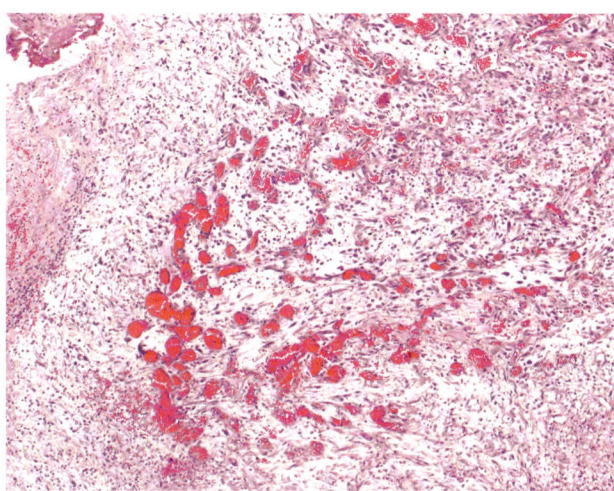

Figure 2.225. Inflammatory myofibroblastic tumors (IMTs) are highly vascular tumors, with multiple intact vessels and extravasated red blood cells present within the myxoid background.

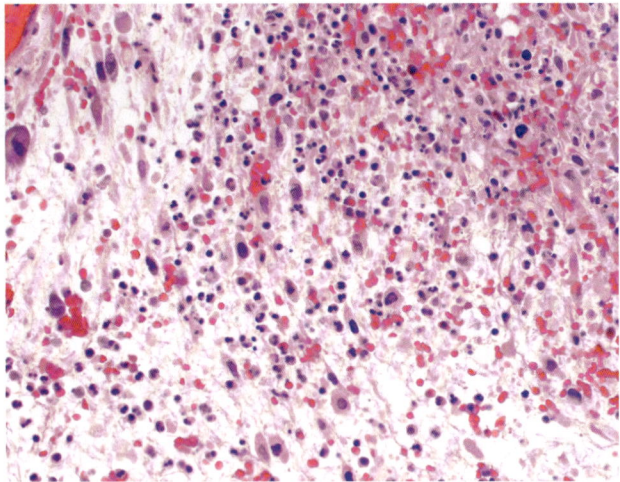

Figure 2.226. Mixed inflammatory cells are one of the diagnostic features of inflammatory myofibroblastic tumor (IMT) and are easily identified within the myxoid stroma, along with extravasated red blood cells.

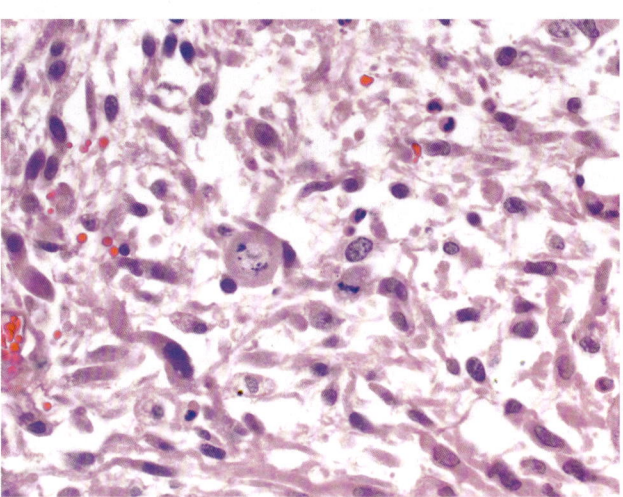

Figure 2.227. At high power, inflammatory myofibroblastic tumor (IMT) cytology can be concerning with mitotic figures frequently identified in these proliferative lesions. The spindled cells show open chromatin and prominent nucleoli, consistent with a reactive pattern.

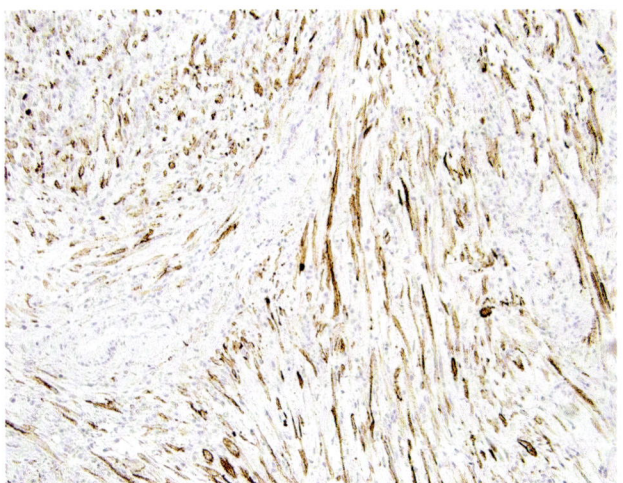

Figure 2.228. ALK immunohistochemistry showing diffuse expression within the spindle cells. Up to two-thirds of inflammatory myofibroblastic tumor (IMT) are positive for ALK, and it is a useful adjunct to the diagnosis.

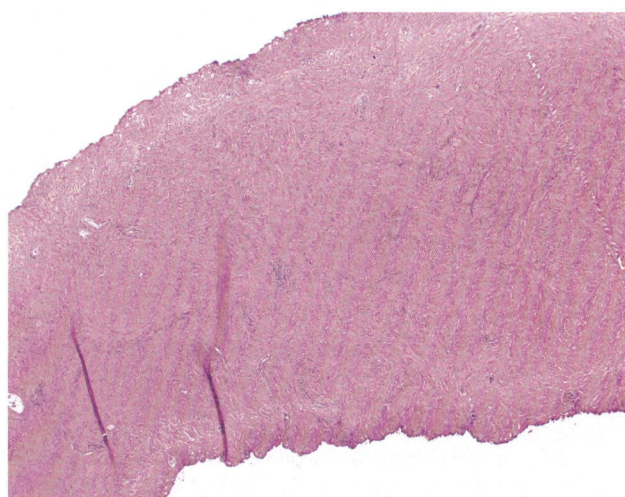

Figure 2.229. Leiomyoma of the bladder is a difficult diagnosis to make, given that the normal bladder is made up of bundles of smooth muscle. This image demonstrates diffuse sheets of smooth muscle without the usual distinct muscle bundles of muscularis propria. When a clinical correlate of a well-circumscribed mass is identified, the diagnosis of leiomyoma of the bladder is possible.

proliferation occurs after a known procedure) and pseudosarcomatous myofibroblastic proliferation.[60] Terminology in this situation can be controversial, with some authors preferring to designate all such lesions as IMTs, whereas others would consider those that are ALK negative to be different. Although the ALK-negative tumors have a number of similarities to nodular fasciitis, they have been recently found to be negative for the *USP6* gene rearrangement that is characteristic of nodular fasciitis.[61]

Leiomyoma

Leiomyoma is a benign proliferation of the smooth muscle bundles of the bladder. It is exceedingly difficult to make this diagnosis, given that the muscularis propria of the bladder demonstrates a fascicular arrangement of smooth muscle bundles (Figures 2.229 and 2.230). The diagnostic criteria for distinguishing leiomyoma from leiomyosarcoma are similar to those in other sites: no nuclear atypia, no increased mitotic activity, and no tumor necrosis (Figure 2.231). Correlation with clinical information is generally helpful,

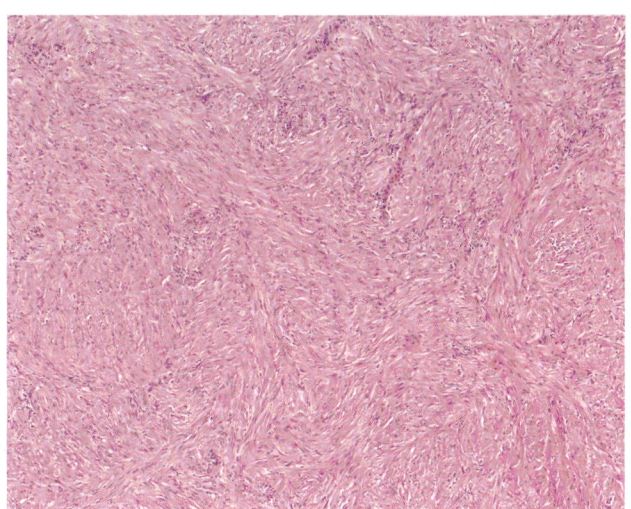

Figure 2.230. Intersecting fascicles of smooth muscle without organization into discrete bundles, consistent with leiomyoma.

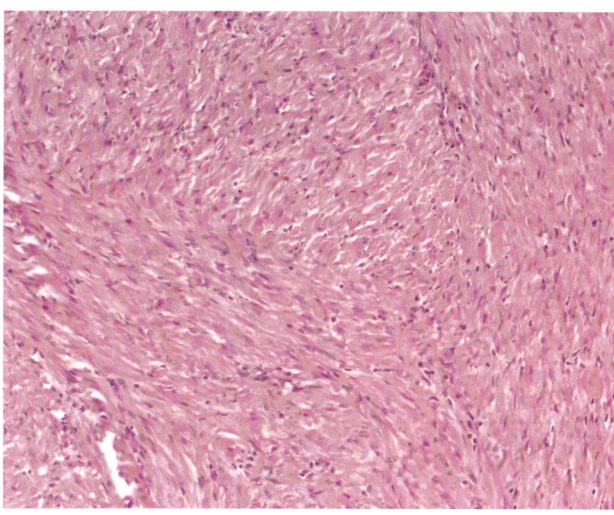

Figure 2.231. The diagnostic features of leiomyoma are similar to those in other sites: eosinophilic cytoplasm, blunt cigar–shaped nuclei, occasional perinuclear vacuoles, no nuclear atypia, no appreciable mitotic activity, and no necrosis.

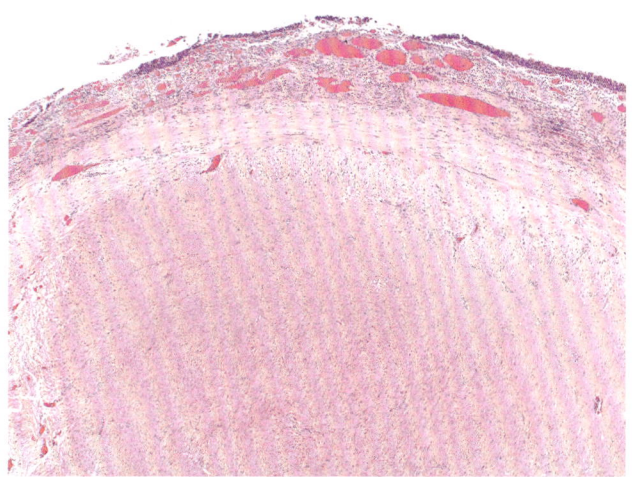

Figure 2.232. Leiomyosarcoma of the bladder at low power, showing a domed lesion bulging the overlying urothelial surface.

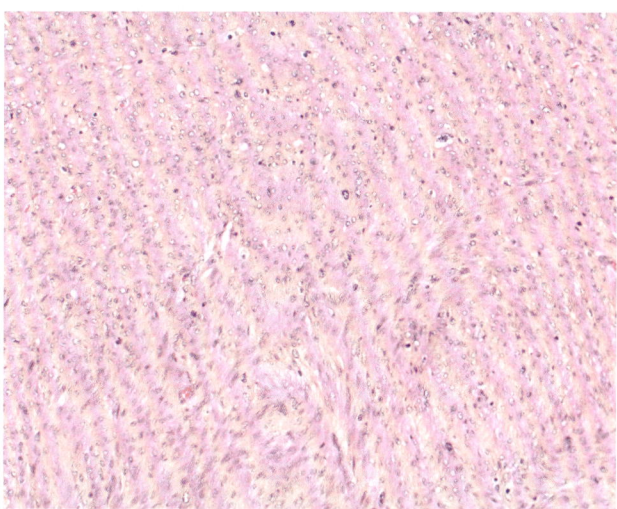

Figure 2.233. At medium power, leiomyosarcoma maintains a fascicular pattern of growth and eosinophilic, spindled cells. However, nuclear atypia is evident with hyperchromasia and pleomorphism.

to ensure that a mural nodule or mass was noted, to avoid overdiagnosing normal muscularis propria as a lesion. When a circumscribed, rounded nodule of muscle is present that clearly deviates from the configuration of adjacent normal muscularis propria, this can be a helpful clue.[62]

Leiomyosarcoma

Leiomyosarcoma is the most common primary sarcoma to arise in the bladder. Similar to its benign counterpart, leiomyosarcoma is a malignant proliferation of smooth muscle demonstrating a fascicular pattern of intersecting bundles of spindle cells (Figure 2.232). However, the cytology is markedly atypical, with hyperchromasia, increased mitotic activity, and occasional necrosis identified (Figure 2.233-2.236). The criteria for diagnosing leiomyosarcoma in the bladder are the same as in other soft tissue regions.

Sarcomatoid Urothelial Carcinoma

A major pitfall in the diagnosis of spindle cell neoplasms of the bladder is sarcomatoid variant of urothelial carcinoma. In a biopsy or TURBT specimen, a limited sampling of a malignant spindle cell proliferation should prompt a broad differential diagnosis, with

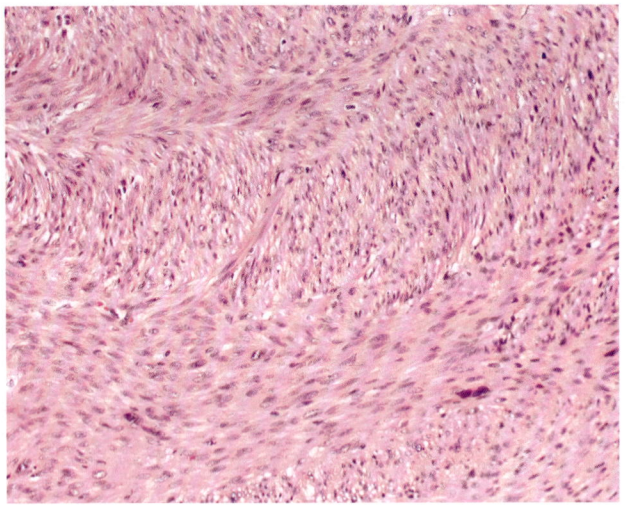

Figure 2.234. Large, dark nuclei are evident in this leiomyosarcoma, deviating from the cigar-shaped bland nuclei of a leiomyoma.

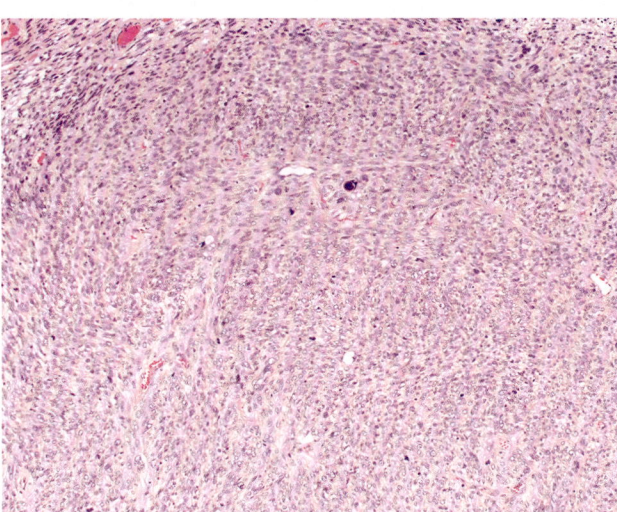

Figure 2.235. At scanning magnification, numerous large atypical cells and frequent mitotic figures are present in this leiomyosarcoma.

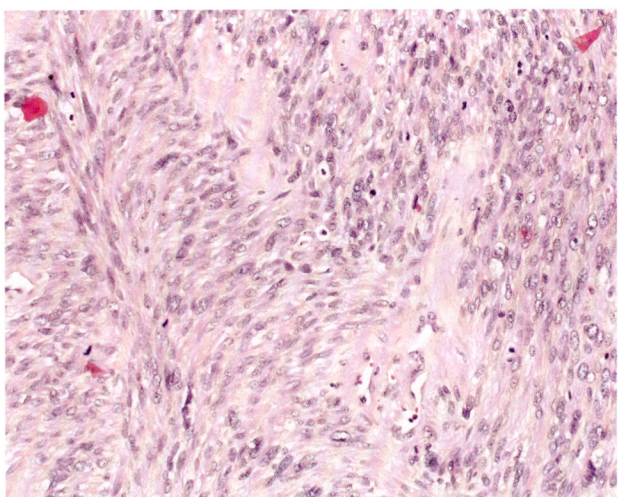

Figure 2.236. Numerous mitotic figures are scattered throughout this high-power field, which far exceed the acceptable number in a leiomyoma.

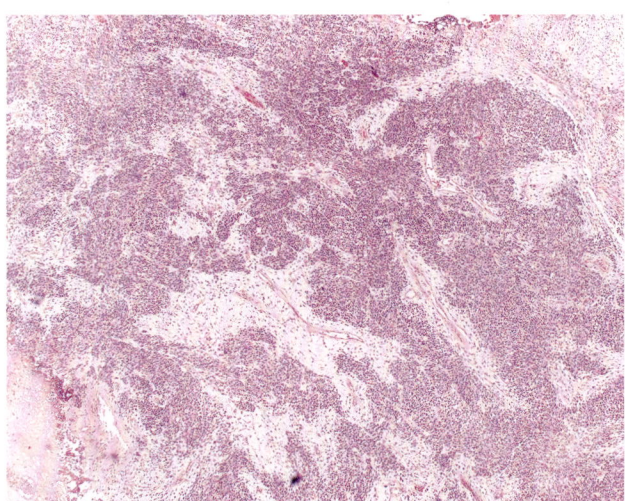

Figure 2.237. Low-power image of sarcomatoid carcinoma showing obvious epithelial and mesenchymal components. Sarcomatoid carcinoma occurs much more frequently than primary sarcoma of the bladder, so should always be the primary consideration when a spindle cell neoplasm is identified.

sarcomatoid carcinoma topping the list, as primary sarcomas of the bladder are far less common. A urothelial carcinoma with sarcomatoid features may have both components evident in the same specimen; however, a limited sampling of the sarcomatoid morphology is not uncommon (Figures 2.237 and 2.238). Often, the sarcomatoid component will retain pan-keratin or high-molecular-weight cytokeratin (34betaE12) staining, and this should be the first immunostain performed on the specimen.[63] Any surface component such as urothelial CIS or papillary urothelial carcinoma in the specimen would also favor a sarcomatoid carcinoma.

NONNEOPLASTIC DEEP LESIONS OF THE BLADDER— GLANDULAR PATTERN

Cystitis Cystica et Glandularis

Cystitis cystica et glandularis (CCG) is a very common finding in normal bladders, though it may also be associated with recurrent infection, bladder exstrophy, or trauma. Effectively anything that causes irritation to the urothelium and its underlying VBN can develop into CCG. CCG is most frequently identified in the trigone, but is also very common in the

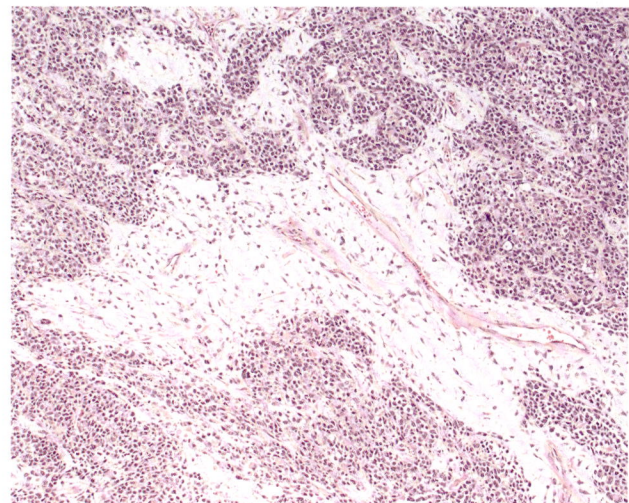

Figure 2.238. Higher power image of the spindle cell component of a sarcomatoid carcinoma. When the majority or sole component of a biopsy shows a spindle cell neoplasm, sarcomatoid carcinoma may be confused for a primary sarcoma.

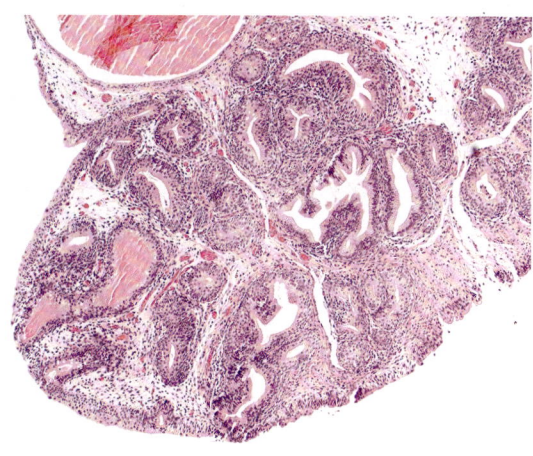

Figure 2.239. Cystitis cystica et glandularis (CCG) comprised of small nests of urothelial cells with open lumina. The benign lesions are confined to the lamina propria, in the same distribution as von Brunn nests.

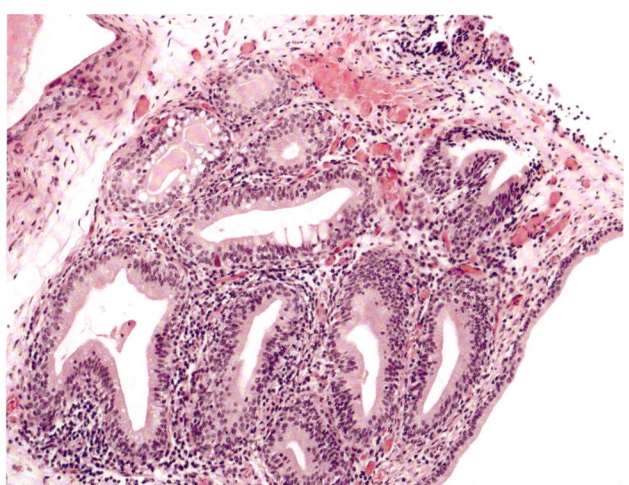

Figure 2.240. At high power, rare goblet cells with intracytoplasmic mucin are present in this glandular component of cystitis cystica et glandularis (CCG).

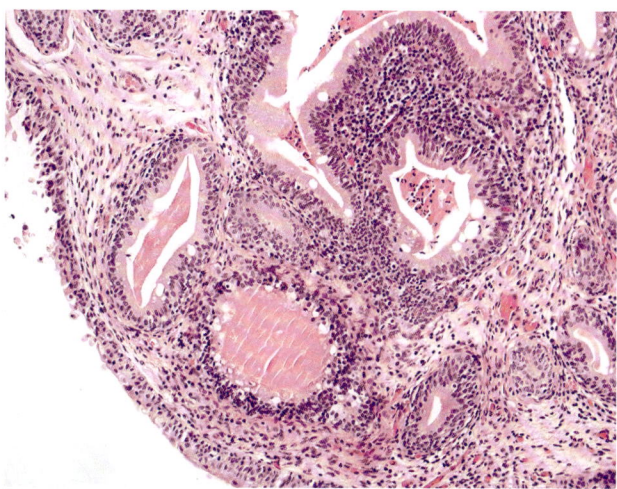

Figure 2.241. Prominent eosinophilic secretions are present in the lumina of this section of cystitis cystica et glandularis (CCG).

ureter. Histologically, CCG shows small nests of urothelium within the lamina propria that show open lumens (cystica) often containing eosinophilic material and occasional areas with columnar or mucinous lining (glandularis) (Figures 2.239-2.241). CCG is generally confined to the lamina propria and often clusters as small nests beneath the urothelium, the expected pattern as it arises from the VBN. It should not involve the deep muscularis propria.

VBN, and as a result CCG, are frequently identified in the ureters. In small ureteral biopsies, these nests and microcysts with open lumina should not be confused for an invasive process. Bland cytology, confinement to the lamina propria, and lack of stromal response are expected in ureteritis cystica et glandularis (Figures 2.242 and 2.243).

Occasionally, this mucinous metaplasia can become very extensive and form a mass. When this occurs, the term florid intestinal metaplasia (IM) is used and the differential diagnosis includes adenocarcinoma. Florid intestinal metaplasia is a benign process that can have a worrisome appearance with prominent mucin extravasation, giving

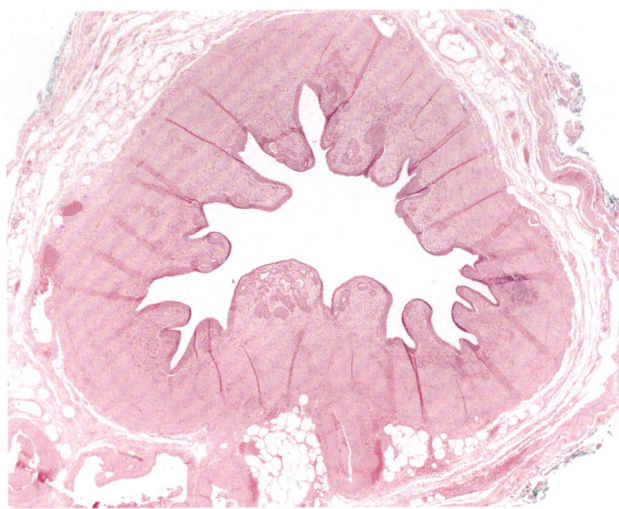

Figure 2.242. Low-power image of ureter with ureteritis cystica et glandularis (UCG). The ureters are frequently involved with UCG, arising from the von Brunn nests present in this location.

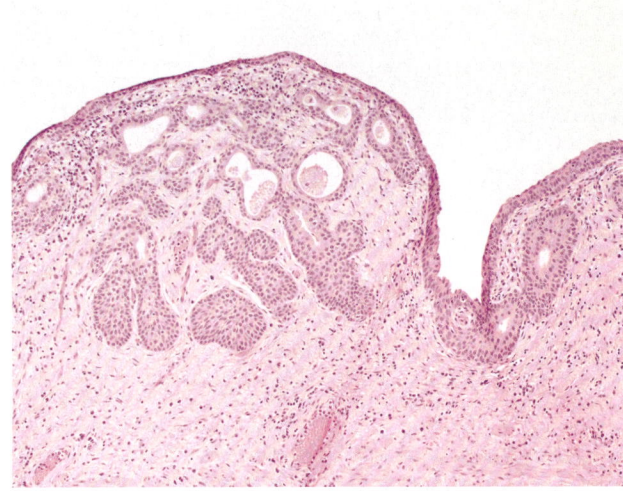

Figure 2.243. At higher power, ureteritis cystica et glandularis (UCG) has the same appearance as cystitis cystica et glandularis (CCG). In small biopsies, it should not be confused for an invasive process.

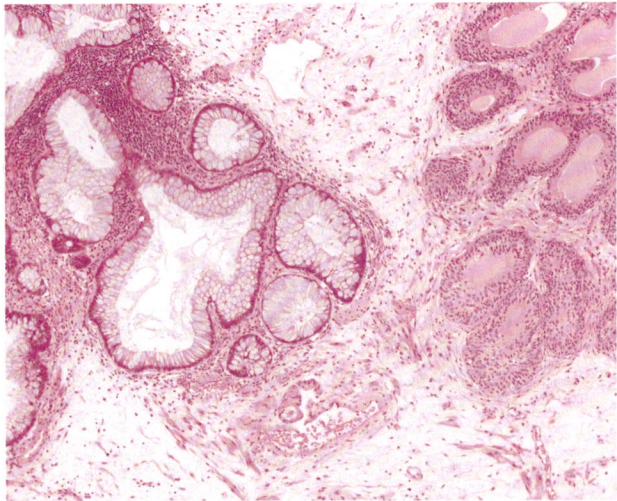

Figure 2.244. Intestinal metaplasia may arise from cystitis cystica et glandularis (CCG) and become so florid that it forms a mass lesion. This image demonstrates intestinal metaplasia on the left and CCG on the right. The intestinal metaplasia appears well organized and lacks nuclear atypia, without increased mitotic figures or architectural disarray.

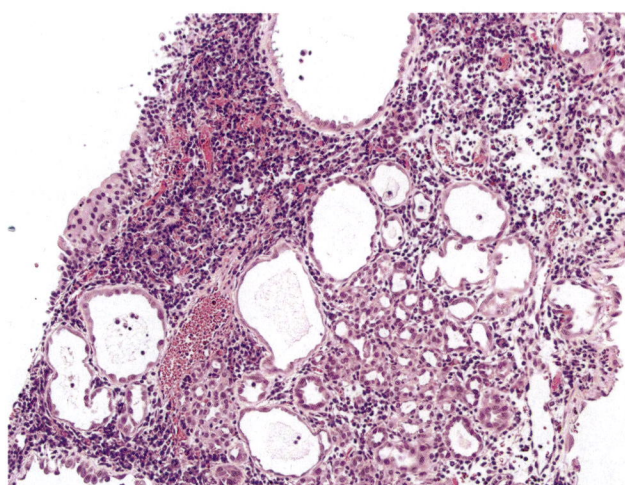

Figure 2.245. Nephrogenic adenoma may present with a predominantly tubular pattern that can mimic an invasive glandular neoplasm.

the appearance of glands floating within the mucin (Figure 2.244). IM lacks marked nuclear atypia, glandular disarray, or necrosis; conversely, these features are expected in adenocarcinoma.

Nephrogenic Adenoma

In addition to its papillary form, nephrogenic adenoma can present as a tubular proliferation in the lamina propria and occasionally involving the muscularis propria (Figure 2.245). As discussed in the section on papillary lesions, nephrogenic adenoma is derived from renal tubular epithelium and the glandular form recapitulates those renal tubules. The key features for identifying nephrogenic adenoma are the hobnail-shaped cells projecting into the tubular lumina and the thickened eosinophilic basement membrane that surrounds the tubules (Figures 2.246-2.248). The lumina may contain brightly eosinophilic material. If the H&E appearance is equivocal and the differential includes a glandular urothelial carcinoma, a limited

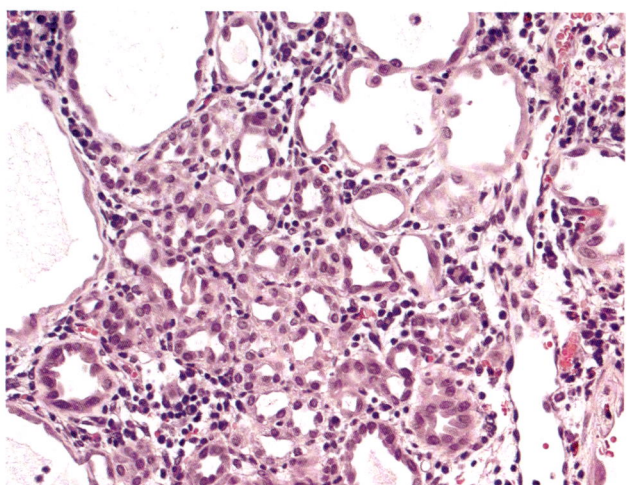

Figure 2.246. Compact nests of small tubules in nephrogenic adenoma, some of which show a basement membrane–like material at the periphery. The background inflammation is also a soft feature for nephrogenic adenoma, as these tend to occur in areas of mucosal damage.

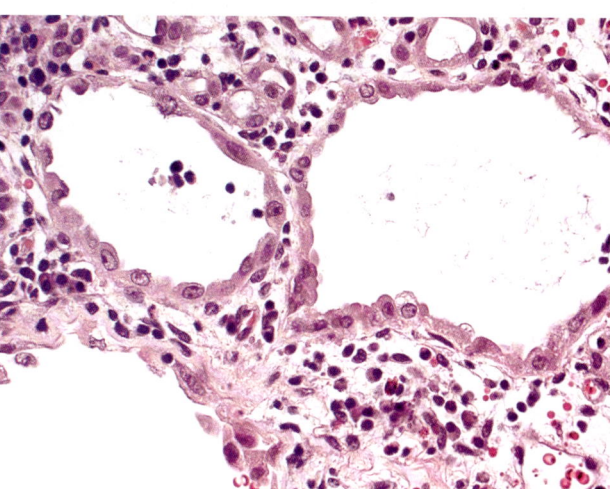

Figure 2.247. Hobnail cytology is classic for nephrogenic adenoma. While some mild nuclear atypia is acceptable, mitotic figures should not be present. If increased mitotic figures are identified, clear cell adenocarcinoma should be considered in the differential.

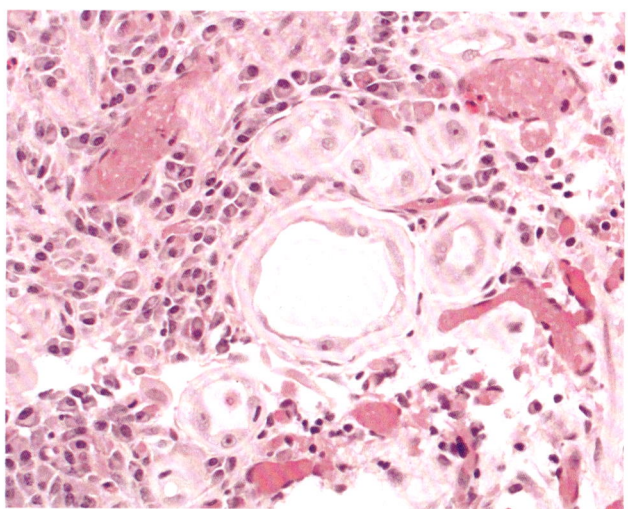

Figure 2.248. Distinct eosinophilic basement membrane–like material surrounds these tubules of nephrogenic adenoma, a helpful feature in distinguishing between glandular lesions and nephrogenic adenoma.

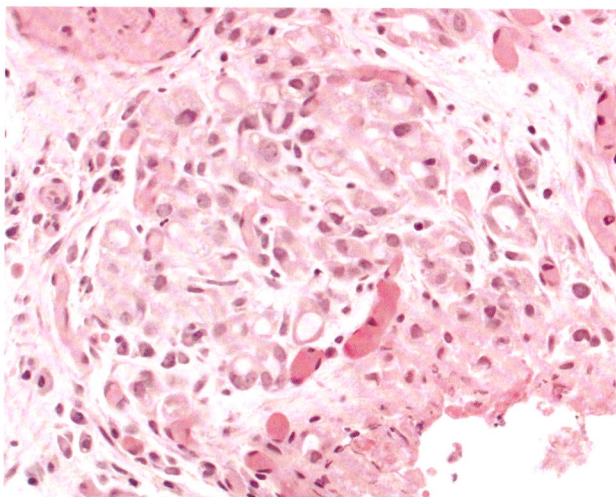

Figure 2.249. This focus of small tubules and nests displays some cells with an almost signet ring–like pattern. This focus had fewer well-formed tubules than expected in nephrogenic adenoma and warranted immunohistochemistry workup.

immunohistochemical panel may be useful. Nephrogenic adenoma will express CK7 and PAX-8, and urothelial carcinoma will express GATA3 (Figures 2.249 and 2.250). Occasionally, the tubules and inflammation may raise the possibility of granulation tissue. In these instances, the CK7 positivity in the tubular component will confirm nephrogenic adenoma.

Mullerianosis

Mullerianosis is a broad term used when glands with features of Mullerian remnants are identified in the bladder wall. Specific entities in this category are endometriosis, endocervicosis, and endosalpingiosis. The glands in these processes may involve any level of the bladder, including the muscularis propria. The finding of glandular elements in the muscularis may raise suspicion for a malignant process; however, there will be no atypia, stromal reaction, or necrosis. The usual diagnostic features of endometriosis apply in this setting. Specimens should show at least two of the following: endometrial-type glands, endometrial stroma, and hemosiderin (Figures 2.251-2.254). Endosalpingiosis contains ciliated tubal type epithelium (Figures 2.255-2.257). PAX-8 immunohistochemistry is useful to support

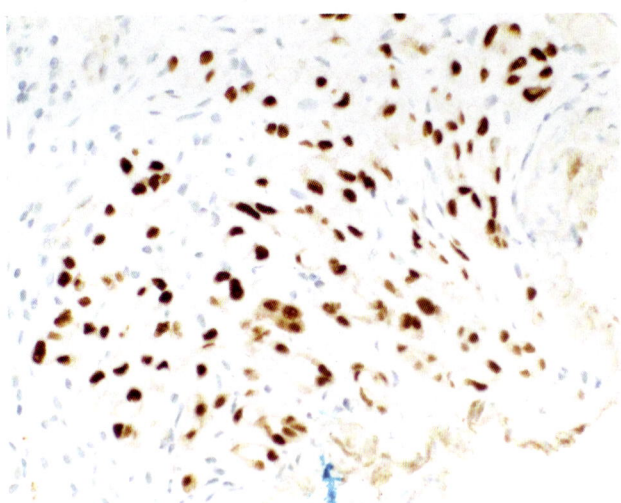

Figure 2.250. PAX-8 is strongly expressed in the nuclei of this nephrogenic adenoma, helping to exclude a glandular urothelial carcinoma or other neoplasm.

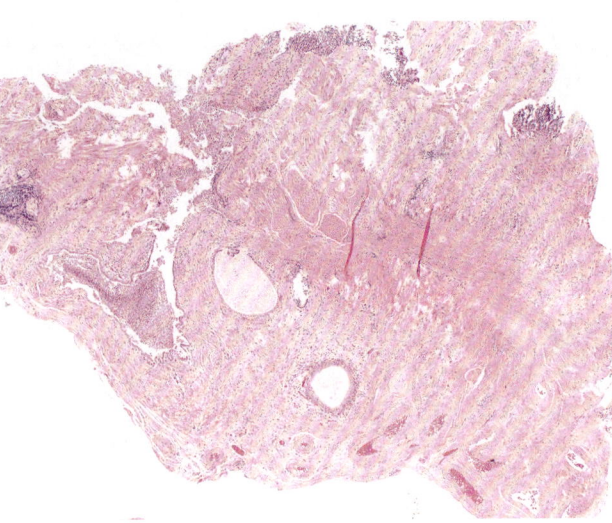

Figure 2.251. Low-power image of glandular process involving deep bladder wall. Secretions are present in many of the glands. Mullerianosis should be considered in bland glandular lesions, even if they involve the deep bladder.

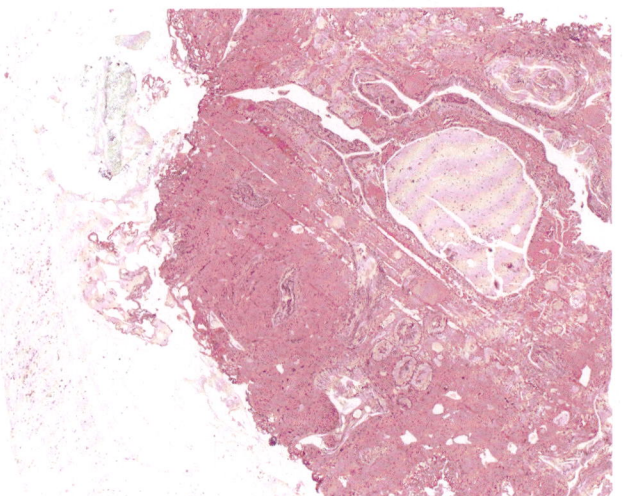

Figure 2.252. Additional image of mucinous glands with secretions growing in an infiltrative pattern in this example of Mullerianosis.

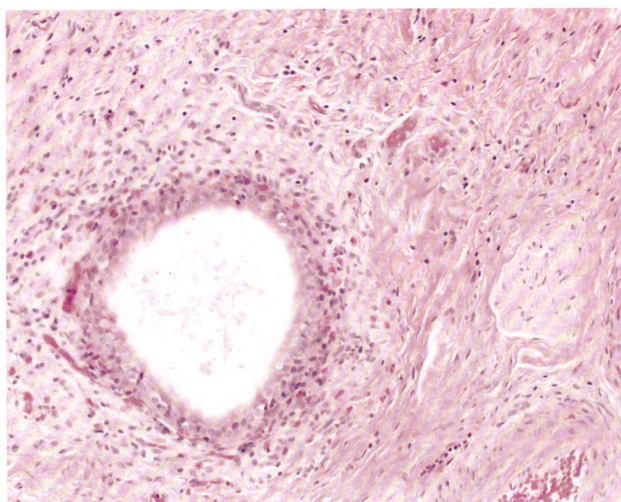

Figure 2.253. At high power, hemosiderin-laden macrophages are present surrounding the endometrial gland, which lacks any cytologic atypia. This finding is consistent with endometriosis.

a Mullerian origin (Figure 2.258 and 2.259). If marked nuclear atypia is appreciated in a glandular lesion, the differential diagnosis includes primary bladder adenocarcinoma, secondary/metastatic adenocarcinoma, or clear cell adenocarcinoma, which may arise in the setting of Mullerianosis. While PAX-8 will help prove Mullerian origin, remember that other benign (nephrogenic adenoma) and malignant (clear cell adenocarcinoma) are also PAX-8 positive.

Urachal Remnants

The urachus is the embryologic remnant of the allantois, located at the dome of the bladder. Because the allantois combined both urothelial and intestinal-type epithelium when functional, urachal remnants often show a combination of urothelial and intestinal epithelial lining. A distinct muscular layer is often present around the epithelial elements (Figures 2.260 and 2.261). The anatomic and cystoscopic location of the biopsy will help with a correct diagnosis, as these lesions are invariably found at the dome and may show some cystic changes prompting biopsy (Figure 2.262).

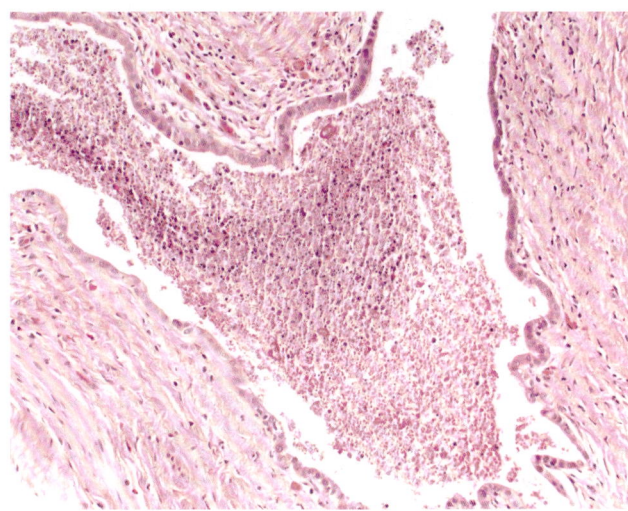

Figure 2.254. Endometriosis showing glandular secretions, indicative of response to hormonal cycling.

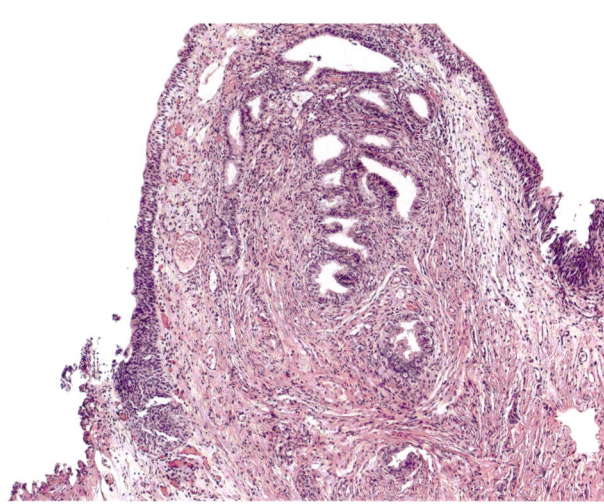

Figure 2.255. Another form of Mullerianosis is endosalpingiosis. At low power, infiltrating glands are seen within the lamina propria.

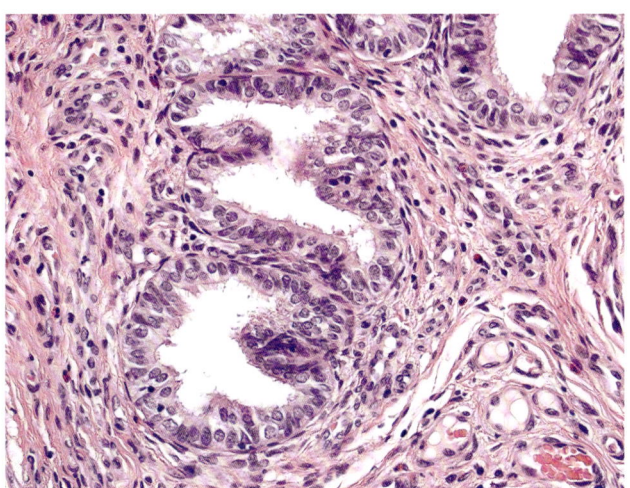

Figure 2.256. Endosalpingiosis lacks cytologic atypia. Any significant atypia should raise suspicion for a malignant process.

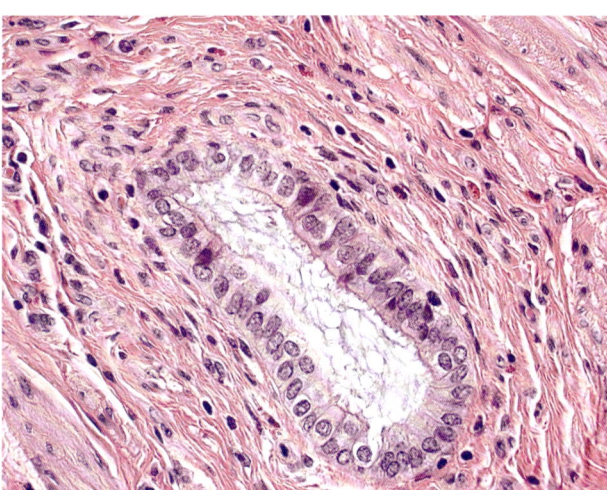

Figure 2.257. Distinct ciliated cells are evident in this high-power image of endosalpingiosis.

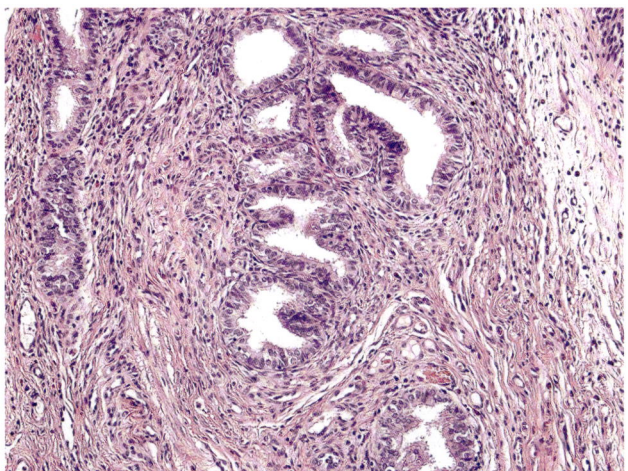

Figure 2.258. In this image of endosalpingiosis, the ciliated tubular epithelium is bland and rare peg cells are present in the lower middle gland.

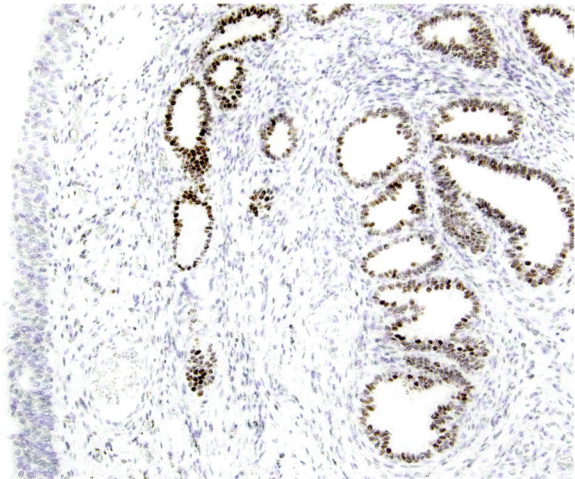

Figure 2.259. PAX-8 immunohistochemistry shows diffuse nuclear positivity, consistent with Mullerian origin. Note that the overlying urothelium is negative for PAX-8.

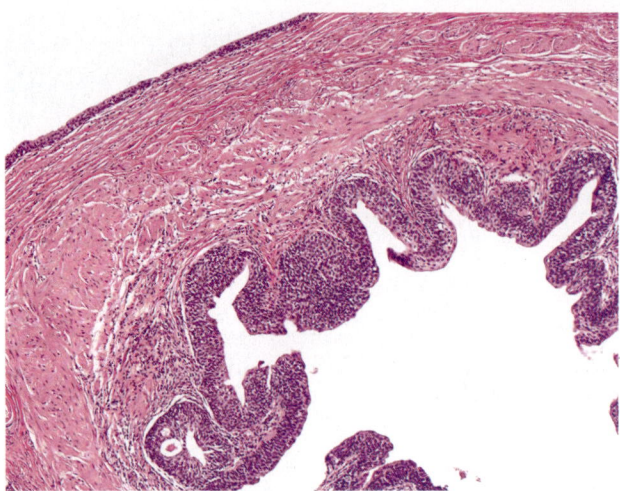

Figure 2.260. Urachal remnants are found in the bladder dome and are comprised of urothelial and intestinal type epithelium, often with their own distinct muscular layer. The urothelial surface of the bladder is present at the top left of the image.

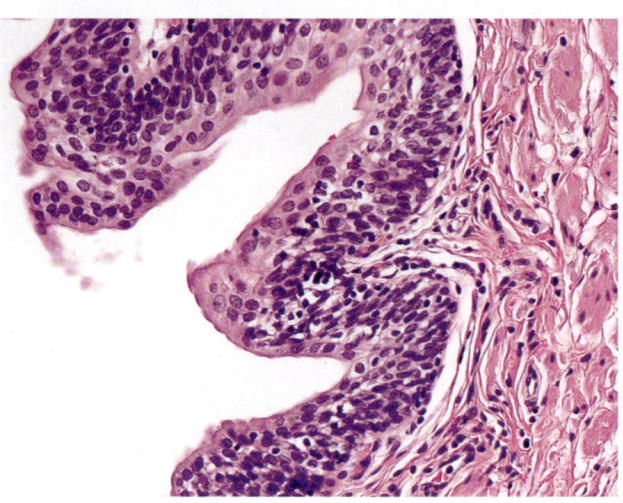

Figure 2.261. High-power image of completely benign urothelial lining of the urachal remnant.

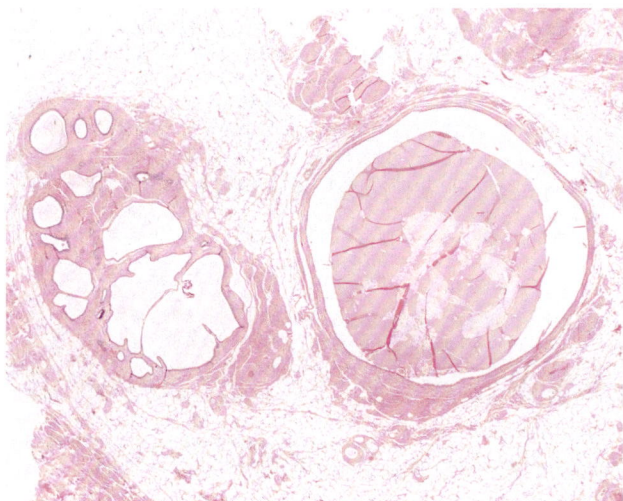

Figure 2.262. A mixture of urothelial and intestinal lining is present in this urachal remnant. Dilated glands may contribute to a tumor-like appearance.

NONNEOPLASTIC DEEP LESIONS OF THE BLADDER—SPINDLE PATTERN

Stromal Predominant Benign Prostatic Hyperplasia

Another spindle-shaped cell lesion that may be sampled in a TURBT is actually not primary to the bladder at all. The median lobe of the prostate is often involved by benign prostatic hyperplasia (BPH), and when it becomes very enlarged, it is sometimes mistaken as a mass originating from the bladder and biopsied. In these instances, the specimen will come labeled as "bladder" and confuse the diagnosis even more. Histologically, stromal predominant BPH is a bland proliferation of spindle-shaped cells with a relatively patternless pattern, small vessels with hyalinization, and scattered lymphocytes (Figures 2.263 and 2.264). See additional discussion in the Prostate Chapter 1, Page 8.

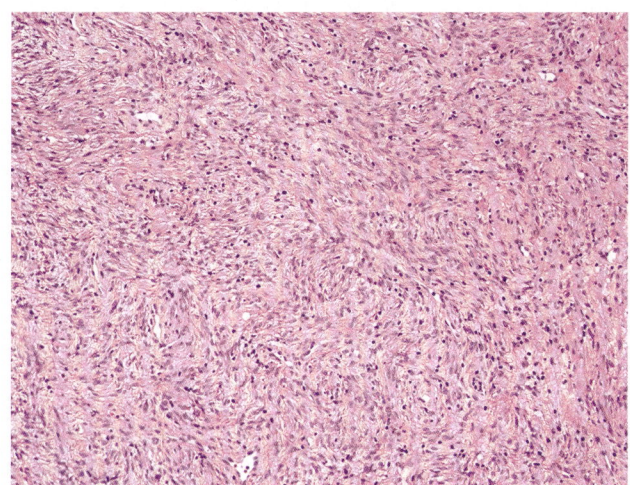

Figure 2.263. Stromal predominant benign prostatic hyperplasia is a mimicker of a primary spindle cell lesion in the bladder. These lesions are sampled when the medial lobe protrudes into the bladder, and the requisition states "bladder tumor."

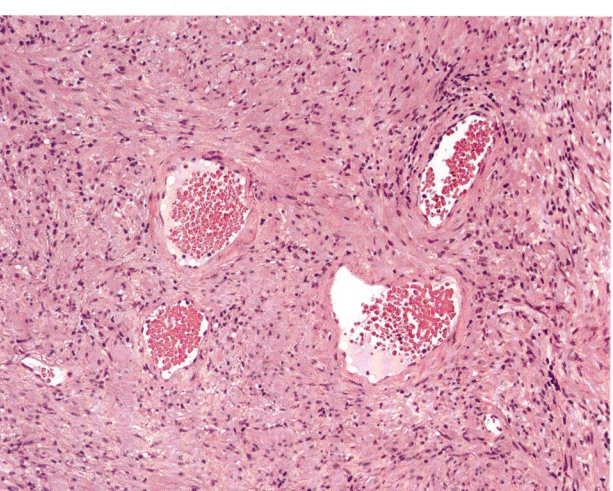

Figure 2.264. Small capillary vessels and scattered lymphocytes (in addition to clinical and cystoscopic information) support the diagnosis of stromal predominant benign prostatic hyperplasia (BPH).

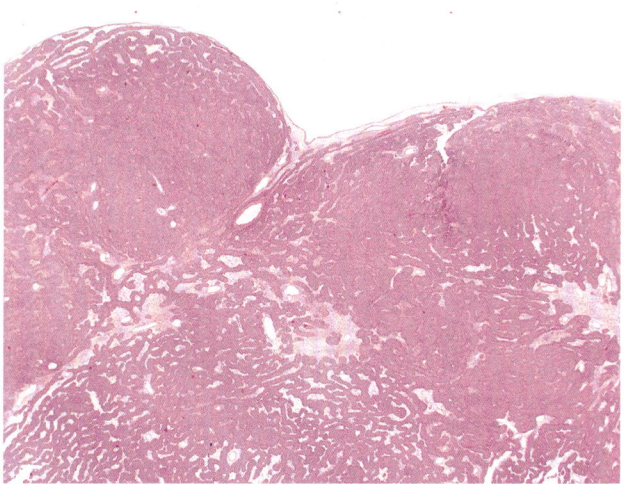

Figure 2.265. Inverted papillomas lack true exophytic papillary fronds. They exhibit a downward growth of nests and cords of urothelial cells, which interlock in a jigsaw pattern.

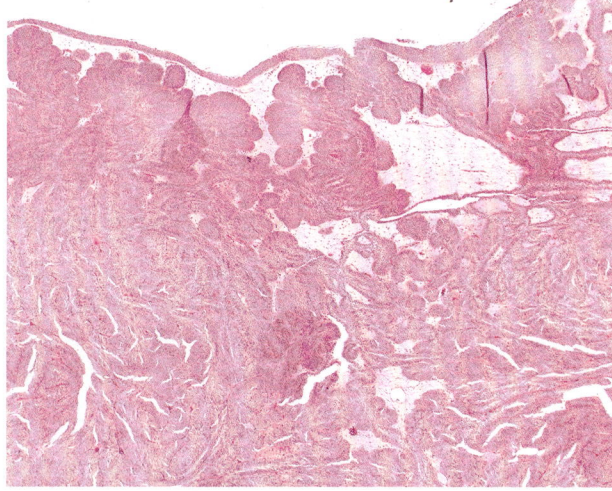

Figure 2.266. The cords of urothelium are invested in a loose myxoid stroma. The classic features of invasion are absent.

NEAR MISSES

INVERTED PAPILLOMA

This lesion was identified in the bladder on cystoscopy, and a TURBT was performed. The morphology shows a highly cellular proliferation of urothelium, which is very basophilic and striking at low power. The growth pattern demonstrates downward growth of anastomosing cords of tumor expanding the lamina propria of the bladder. At first glance, an inverted growth pattern of urothelial carcinoma or invasive urothelial carcinoma could be considered due to the expansile nature of the lesion. These tumors occur most frequently in the bladder neck and trigone.

These images represent an example of inverted papilloma. The low-power appearance shows a jigsaw puzzle–like arrangement of nests and cords of urothelium, which interdigitate within the lamina propria that is often loose and myxoid (Figures 2.265 and 2.266). While the neoplasm is cellular and basophilic, at higher power the cytology is bland and monotonous without frequent mitotic figures, nuclear atypia, or stromal response. The edges of the nests show peripheral palisading of the nuclei, and the cells appear to swirl or make eddies in the more central areas (Figure 2.267 and 2.268). To exclude a papillary carcinoma with invasion, it is important to note the lack of a true exophytic component or any small, irregular

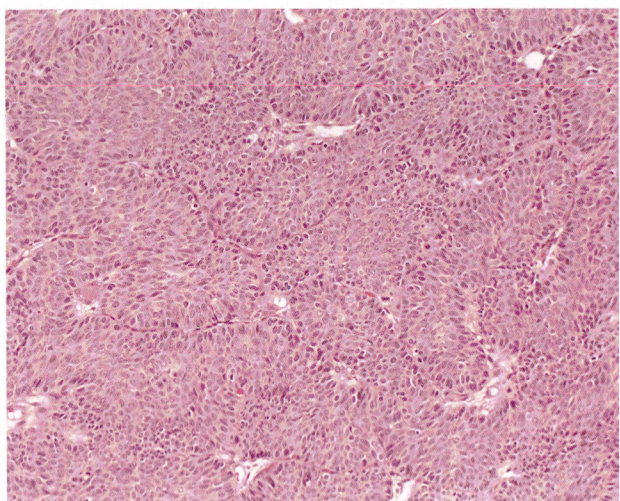

Figure 2.267. Cytologically, inverted papillomas demonstrate bland urothelial cells that often retain nuclear grooves. Peripheral palisading is a helpful feature.

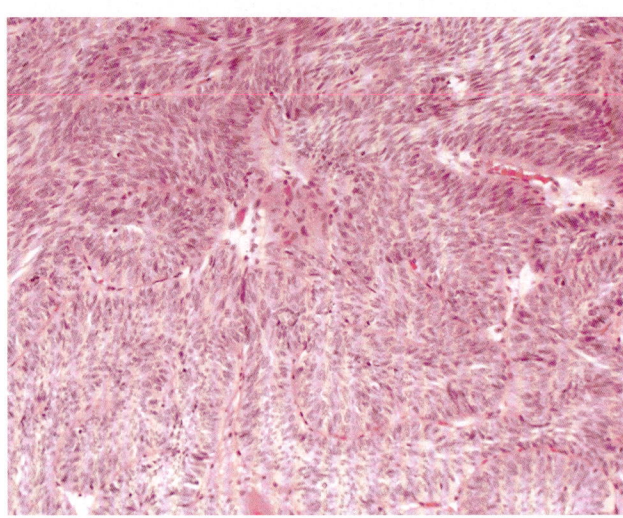

Figure 2.268. Pronounced peripheral palisading is present in this high-power image of inverted papilloma.

nests with retraction artifact. While nested variant of urothelial carcinoma may have a similar appearance, there is usually some cytologic atypia in this entity, possible muscularis propria invasion, and a lack of the palisading and unique thin anastomosing cords.

The key to making this diagnosis is to keep in mind that not all expansile lesions in the lamina propria are invasive carcinomas, and use the key diagnostic features of anastomosing cords, peripheral palisading, and lack of atypia to make the diagnosis of inverted papilloma.

METASTATIC COLORECTAL ADENOCARCINOMA

This mass was identified on cystoscopy as an ulcerated, bulging mass. Microscopically, the lesion is frankly malignant with a glandular architecture. Without clinical history, the differential diagnosis includes primary bladder adenocarcinoma, urachal adenocarcinoma, or a secondary/metastatic adenocarcinoma from another primary site. A urachal adenocarcinoma would be favored if the mass is centered on the dome of the bladder. In this case, the patient has a known history of colorectal adenocarcinoma and this mass represents metastatic involvement.

There are no definitive morphologic findings distinguishing a bladder adenocarcinoma from an adenocarcinoma of another site. However, bladder adenocarcinomas are often high grade/poorly differentiated, whereas some metastatic adenocarcinomas are deceptively low grade (such as pancreatic adenocarcinoma and gynecologic malignancies) (Figure 2.269). In this case, the tumor is moderately to poorly differentiated with a glandular/cribriform appearance and dirty necrosis. In most epithelial organs, a primary site of origin is suggested by the finding of a superficial component (CIS); however, this finding is not entirely reliable, as a metastatic tumor may grow to involve the surface as it does in this case.

As with most mucinous adenocarcinomas, immunohistochemistry is not particularly helpful in the differential diagnosis of primary bladder adenocarcinoma and colorectal adenocarcinoma. The immunoprofile overlaps significantly, with both tumors exhibiting CK20 and CDX2 positivity, with CK7 negative (Figures 2.270 and 2.271). The finding of diffuse beta-catenin positivity supports a colorectal primary.[64] Clinical, radiographic, and endoscopic correlation is necessary to ascertain site of origin in adenocarcinomas involving the bladder. Given the relative rarity of primary bladder adenocarcinomas, consider secondary/metastatic disease first when working up these tumors.

MULLERIANOSIS

The patient presented with a ureteral stone and was found to have an incidental bladder dome mass. Cystoscopy showed a large protuberant bladder mass on anterior dome, which was clinically worrisome for adenocarcinoma, possibly urachal origin due to the location. A TURBT was performed. The specimen showed a proliferation of glands with bland cytology and mucinous secretions. The glands were present deep in the muscularis propria; however, no cytologic atypia was appreciated in the glands.

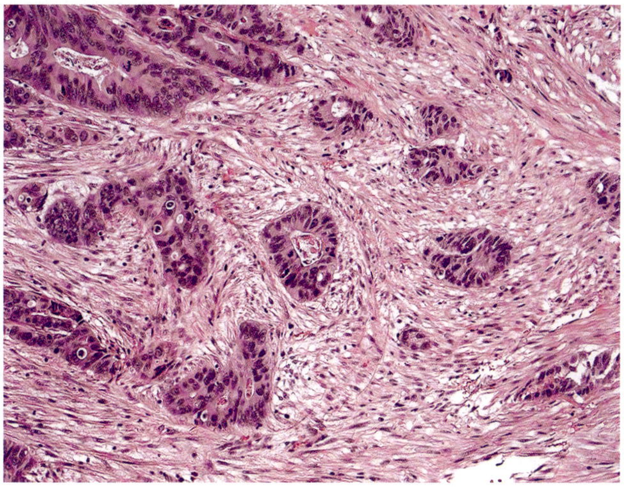

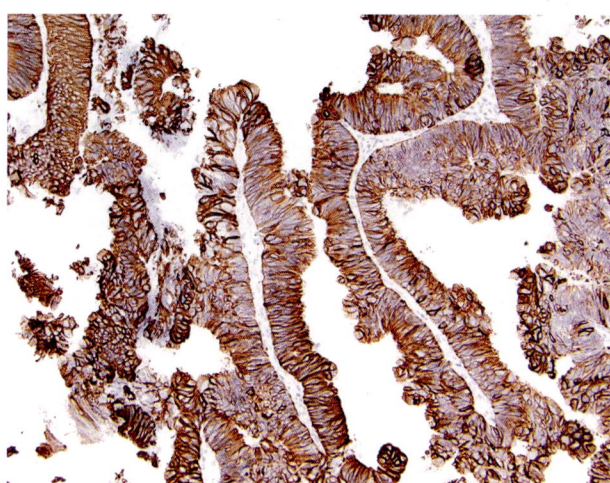

Figure 2.269. An invasive mucinous adenocarcinoma involving the bladder raises a broad differential. No specific morphologic features exist to predict site of origin; however, metastatic adenocarcinomas are often deceptively low grade. In general, primary bladder adeno-carcinomas are high-grade lesions.

Figure 2.270. Immunohistochemistry for CK20 shows diffuse positivity, a nonspecific finding in intestinal-type adenocarcinomas.

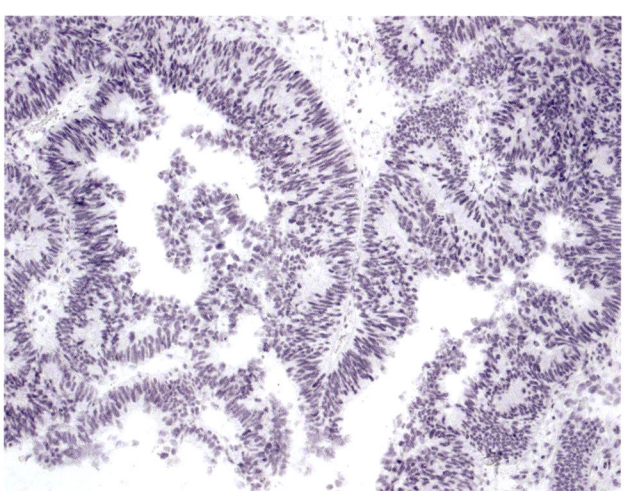

Figure 2.271. CK7 is negative, which would be consistent with a lower gastrointestinal (GI) origin combined with the CK20 positivity. Given this patient's known history of colorectal carcinoma, secondary involvement by that tumor is favored. Clinical, radiographic, and endoscopic correlation is necessary to ascertain site of origin in bladder adenocarcinomas.

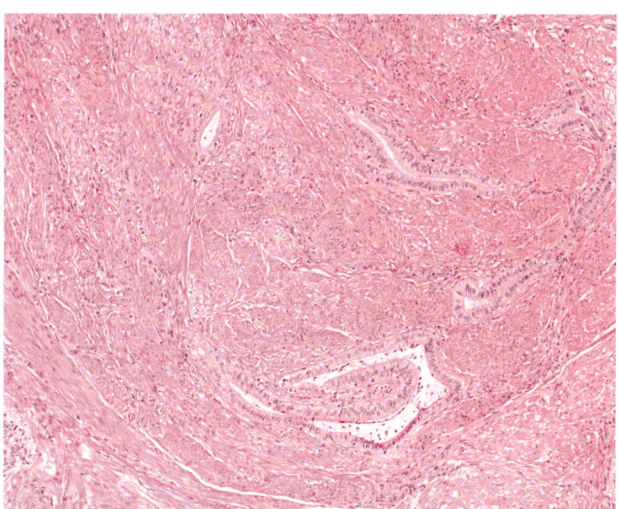

Figure 2.272. Mullerianosis is one of the glandular lesions that can involve muscularis propria, mimicking an invasive neoplasm.

Despite involvement of muscularis propria, a benign lesion was favored in this patient. The possibility of Mullerianosis was considered, and a panel of immunostains was performed on the TURBT specimen. The glands showed strong positivity for CK7, ER, and PR and were negative for GATA3, p63, CK20, and CDX2 (Figures 2.272-2.276). Overall, the morphology and immunoprofile supported a diagnosis of Mullerianosis, as markers of urothelial and glandular differentiation were negative and did not support the possibility of urachal remnants.

Specifically, this case predominantly represents endocervicosis with bland mucinous endocervical-type glands and mucinous secretions reminiscent of tunnel clusters in the cervix. Rare glands show ciliated epithelium, also consistent with a Mullerian origin. Endocervicosis occurs most commonly in women of reproductive age, located in the anterior wall or dome of the bladder.

The key to making the correct diagnosis in this case is to recognize that benign glandular processes can involve muscularis propria and not overcall an adenocarcinoma. Cystitis cystica, Mullerianosis, and nephrogenic adenoma are glandular lesions that all involve muscularis propria. These entities all have bland cytologic features and do

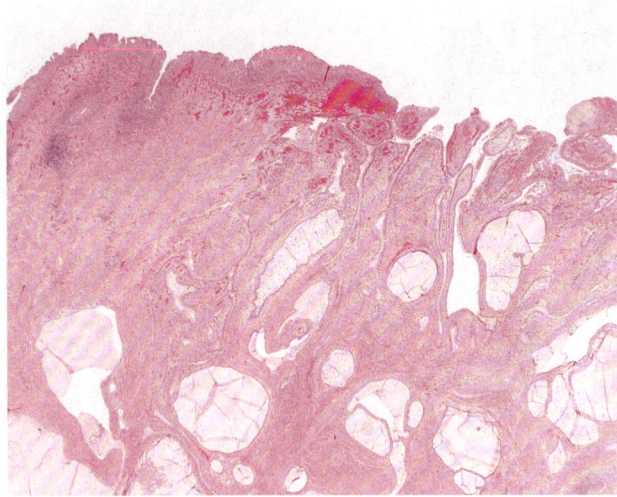

Figure 2.273. In this image, Mullerian mucinous endocervical-type glands extend from the ulcerated surface down into the muscularis propria. The presence of surface involvement can also increase the likelihood of calling this a malignant process.

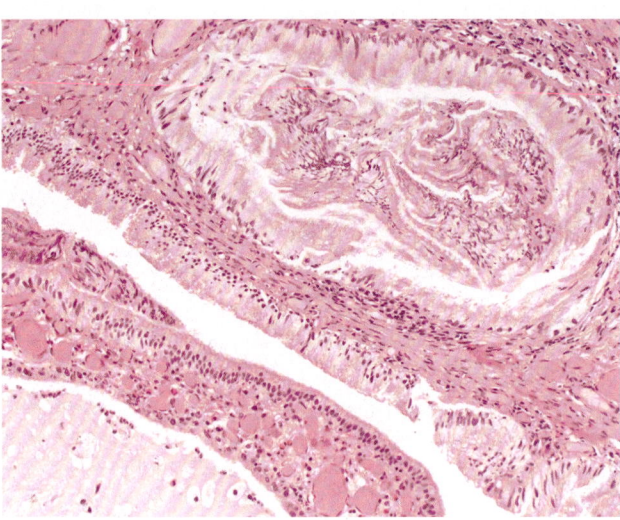

Figure 2.274. Close examination of the glands reveals no significant atypia, with small monotonous nuclei that are basally oriented. Cilia are also present, which are rarely identified in malignant glands.

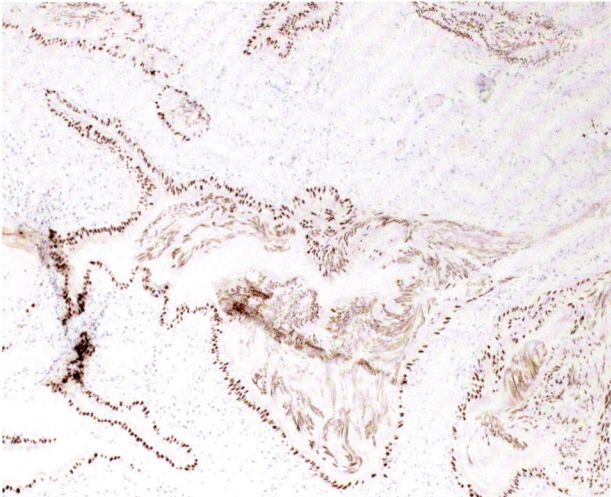

Figure 2.275. Estrogen receptor (ER) immunohistochemistry confirms that the glands are of Mullerian origin.

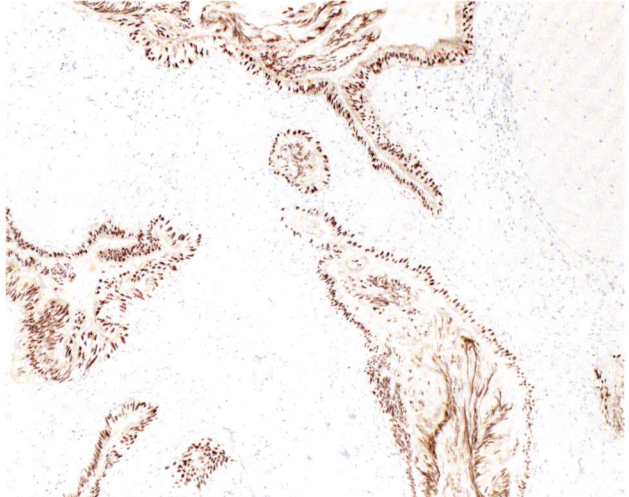

Figure 2.276. Progesterone receptor (PR) immunohistochemistry also shows strong diffuse nuclear positivity.

not elicit a stromal response. The identification of high-grade atypia, increased mitotic figures, apoptotic debris, or necrosis should exclude the possibility of Mullerianosis (Figures 2.277 and 2.278).

MELANOMA

The patient presented with hematuria and underwent a cystoscopy, which demonstrated mildly atypical urothelium with bulging surface. The mass was biopsied, and microscopic sections showed a solid growth pattern of malignant cells. Scattered atypical cells were present in the surface urothelium. On higher power, coarsely granular brown pigment was identified in some of the malignant cells (Figures 2.279-2.281).

Without clinical history, the differential diagnosis is broad in this case. A sheet-like proliferation of malignant cells without obvious surface component could represent urothelial carcinoma, lymphoid malignancy, sarcoma, or, rarely, melanoma. A broad immunohistochemical panel was performed which showed that the malignant cells were pan-keratin, CD45, and vimentin negative and strongly and diffusely S100 positive (Figure 2.282).

The patient had no known history of skin lesions or melanoma excision. In this case, a primary bladder melanoma was favored. Although it is more common for the bladder to be involved as a metastatic site, primary melanoma can occur in the bladder. In women, it is also possible for direct spread from a gynecologic/vaginal mucosal melanoma to involve the bladder.

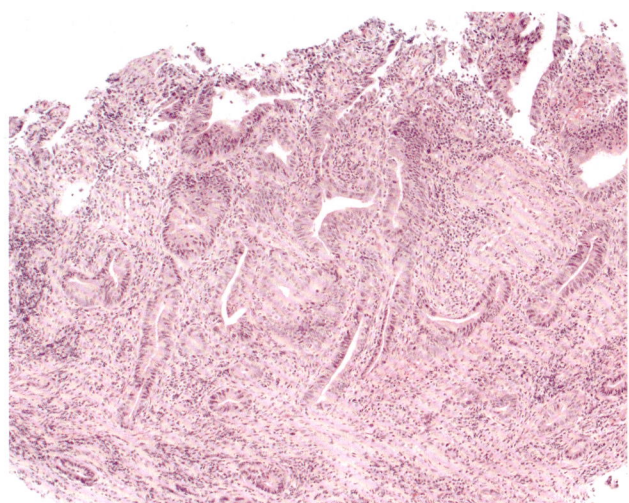

Figure 2.277. Bladder TURBT (transurethral resection of bladder tumor) showing invasive adenocarcinoma. At low power, the glands are irregular, with focal cribriform pattern. Nuclear atypia is evident at scanning magnification with hyperchromasia and pseudostratification.

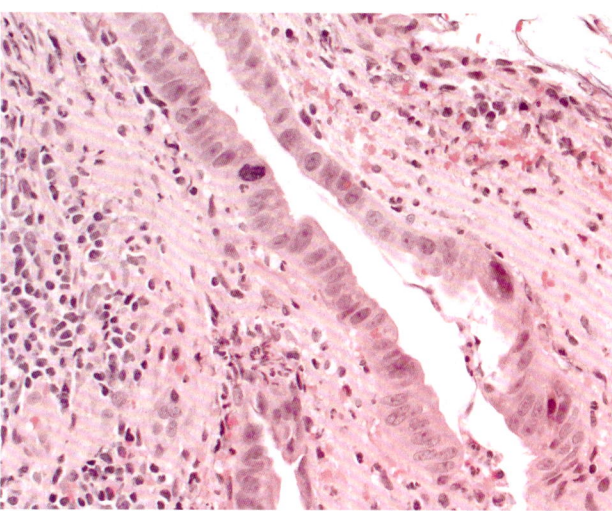

Figure 2.278. Marked nuclear pleomorphism and increased mitotic figures are not compatible with a diagnosis of Mullerianosis. This case is an invasive adenocarcinoma, and clinical and radiographic correlation is necessary to determine the site of origin.

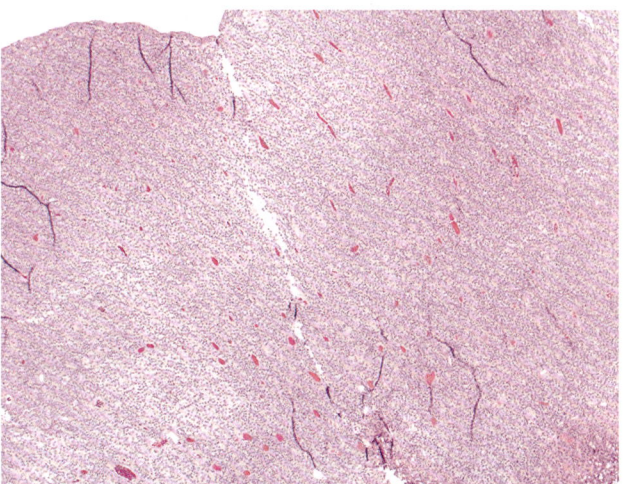

Figure 2.279. At low power, the lamina propria of this bladder shows a highly cellular infiltrate without obvious architectural pattern.

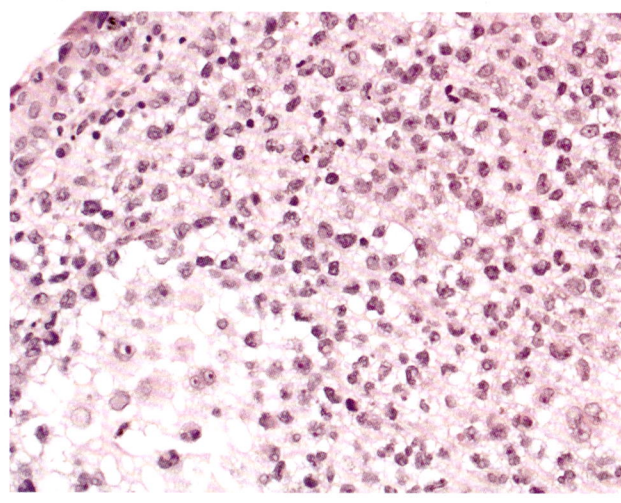

Figure 2.280. The medium-power impression raises the possibility of lymphoma, poorly differentiated carcinoma, small round blue cell tumor, or melanoma.

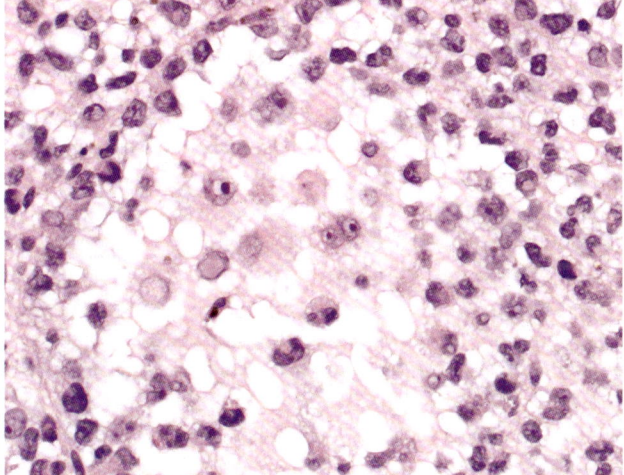

Figure 2.281. Scattered cells show large nucleoli and occasional binucleation (so called "bug-eyed demons"). Brown pigment is present in the background, strongly suggesting that this tumor is a melanoma.

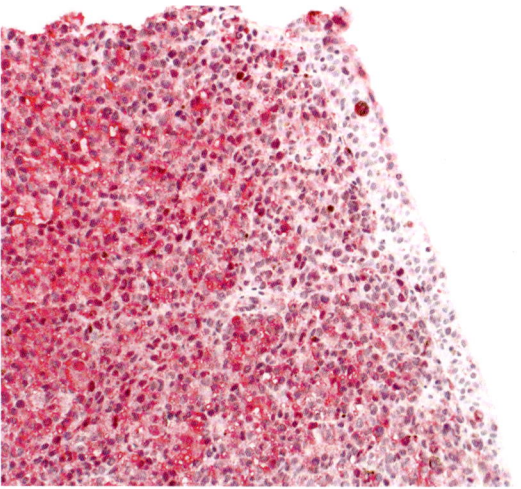

Figure 2.282. S100 is strongly and diffusely positive in the tumor cells and even highlights a few cells transmigrating through the urothelium.

The key to making the correct diagnosis is recognizing the pigment as unusual and working up a relatively undifferentiated, sheet-like malignant proliferation with a broad immunohistochemical panel.

References

1. Reuter VE, Al-ahmadie H, Tickoo SK. In: Mills SE, ed. *Histology for Pathologists*. 4th ed.Philadelphia: Lippincott Williams and Wilkins; 2012.

2. Volmar KE, Chan TY, De Marzo AM, Epstein JI. Florid von Brunn nests mimicking urothelial carcinoma: a morphologic and immunohistochemical comparison to the nested variant of urothelial carcinoma. *Am J Surg Pathol*. 2003;27(9):1243-1252.

3. Daneshmand S, Patel S, Lotan Y, et al. Efficacy and safety of blue light flexible cystoscopy with hexaminolevulinate in the surveillance of bladder cancer: aphase III, comparative, multicenter study. *J Urol*. 2018;199(5):1158-1165. doi:10.1016/j.juro.2017.11.096.

4. Fradet Y, Grossman HB, Gomella L, et al. A comparison of hexaminolevulinate fluorescence cystoscopy and white light cystoscopy for the detection of carcinoma in situ in patients with bladder cancer: aphase III, multicenter study. *J Urol*. 2007;178(1):68-73. doi:10.1016/j.juro.2007.03.028.

5. NCCN. *Bladder Cancer Guidelines Version 3.2019*. 2019. Available at https://www.nccn.org/professionals/physician_gls/pdf/bladder.pdf. Accessed June 26, 2019.

6. Chan AWH, Tong JHM, Pan Y, et al. Lymphoepithelioma-like hepatocellular carcinoma.*Am J Surg Pathol*. 2015;39(3):304-312. doi:10.1097/PAS.0000000000000376.

7. Denson MA, Griebling TL, Cohen MB, Kreder KJ. Comparison of cystoscopic and histological findings in patients with suspected interstitial cystitis. *J Urol*. 2000;164(6):1908-1911.

8. Thilagarajah R, Vale JA, Witherow RO, Walker MM. A clinicopathological approach to cystitis–recommendations for simplified pathology reporting. *Br J Urol*. 1997;79(4):567-571.

9. Sanfrancesco J, Jones JS, Hansel DE. Diagnostically challenging cases: what are atypia and dysplasia?*Urol Clin North Am*.2013;40(2):281-293. doi:10.1016/j.ucl.2013.01.006.

10. Eble JN, Banks ER. Post-surgical necrobiotic granulomas of urinary bladder. *Urology*. 1990;35(5):454-457.

11. Betz SA, See WA, Cohen MB. Granulomatous inflammation in bladder wash specimens after intravesical bacillus Calmette-Guerin therapy for transitional cell carcinoma of the bladder. *Am J Clin Pathol*. 1993;99(3):244-248.

12. LaFontaine PD, Middleman BR, Graham SD, Sanders WH. Incidence of granulomatous prostatitis and acid-fast bacilli after intravesical BCG therapy. *Urology*. 1997;49(3):363-366.

13. Kryvenko ON, Epstein JI. Pseudocarcinomatous urothelial hyperplasia of the bladder: clinical findings and followup of 70 patients. *J Urol*. 2013;189(6):2083-2086. doi:10.1016/j.juro.2012.12.005.

14. Lane Z, Epstein JI. Pseudocarcinomatous epithelial hyperplasia in the bladder unassociated with prior irradiation or chemotherapy. *Am J Surg Pathol*. 2008;32(1):92-97. doi:10.1097/PAS.0b013e3180eaa1dc.

15. Chan TY, Epstein JI. Radiation or chemotherapy cystitis with "pseudocarcinomatous" features. *Am J Surg Pathol*. 2004;28(7):909-913.

16. Khani F, Robinson BD. Precursor lesions of urologic malignancies. *Arch Pathol Lab Med*. 2017;141(12):1615-1632. doi:10.5858/arpa.2016-0515-RA.

17. Hodges KB, Lopez-Beltran A, Davidson DD, Montironi R, Cheng L. Urothelial dysplasia and other flat lesions of the urinary bladder: clinicopathologic and molecular features. *Hum Pathol*. 2010;41(2):155-162. doi:10.1016/j.humpath.2009.07.002.

18. Amin MB, McKenney JK. An approach to the diagnosis of flat intraepithelial lesions of the urinary bladder using the World Health Organization/ International Society of Urological Pathology consensus classification system. *Adv Anat Pathol*. 2002;9(4):222-232.

19. Epstein JI, Amin MB, Reuter VR, Mostofi FK. The World Health Organization/International Society of Urological Pathology consensus classification of urothelial (transitional cell) neoplasms of the urinary bladder. Bladder Consensus Conference Committee. *Am J Surg Pathol*. 1998;22(12):1435-1448.

20. Cheng L, Cheville JC, Neumann RM, Bostwick DG. Flat intraepithelial lesions of the urinary bladder. *Cancer*. 2000;88(3):625-631.

21. Cheng L, Cheville JC, Neumann RM, Bostwick DG. Natural history of urothelial dysplasia of the bladder. *Am J Surg Pathol*. 1999;23(4):443-447.

22. McKenney JK, Gomez JA, Desai S, Lee MW, Amin MB. Morphologic expressions of urothelial carcinoma in situ: a detailed evaluation of its histologic patterns with emphasis on carcinoma in situ with microinvasion. *Am J Surg Pathol*. 2001;25(3):356-362.

23. Arias-Stella JA, Shah AB, Gupta NS, Williamson SR. CK20 and p53 immunohistochemical staining patterns in urinary bladder specimens with equivocal atypia. *Arch Pathol Lab Med*. 2018;142(1):64-69. doi:10.5858/arpa.2016-0411-OA.

24. Aron M, Luthringer DJ, McKenney JK, et al. Utility of a triple antibody cocktail intraurothelial neoplasm-3 (IUN-3-CK20/CD44s/p53) and α-methylacyl-CoA racemase (AMACR) in the distinction of urothelial carcinoma in situ (CIS) and reactive urothelial atypia. *Am J Surg Pathol*. 2013;37(12):1815-1823. doi:10.1097/PAS.0000000000000114.

25. Edgecombe A, Nguyen BN, Djordjevic B, Belanger EC, Mai KT. Utility of cytokeratin 5/6, cytokeratin 20, and p16 in the diagnosis of reactive urothelial atypia and noninvasive component of urothelial neoplasia. *Appl Immunohistochem Mol Morphol*. 2012;20(3):264-271. doi:10.1097/PAI.0b013e3182351ed3.

26. Gunia S, Koch S, Hakenberg OW, May M, Kakies C, Erbersdobler A. Different HER2 protein expression profiles aid in the histologic differential diagnosis between urothelial carcinoma in situ (CIS) and non-CIS conditions (dysplasia and reactive atypia) of the urinary bladder mucosa. *Am J Clin Pathol*. 2011;136(6):881-888. doi:10.1309/AJCPKUZ69LXZGFEA.

27. Moatamed NA, Vergara-Lluri ME, Lu D, Apple SK, Kerkoutian S, Rao J-Y. Utility of ProEx C in the histologic evaluation of the neoplastic and nonneoplastic urothelial lesions. *Hum Pathol*. 2013;44(11):2509-2517. doi:10.1016/j.humpath.2013.06.011.

28. Sun W, Zhang PL, Herrera GA. p53 protein and Ki-67 overexpression in urothelial dysplasia of bladder. *Appl Immunohistochem Mol Morphol AIMM*. 2002;10(4):327-331.

29. Yin M, Bastacky S, Parwani AV, McHale T, Dhir R. p16ink4 immunoreactivity is a reliable marker for urothelial carcinoma in situ. *Hum Pathol*. 2008;39(4):527-535. doi:10.1016/j.humpath.2007.08.005.

30. Hodgson A, Xu B, Downes MR. p53 immunohistochemistry in high-grade urothelial carcinoma of the bladder is prognostically significant. *Histopathology*. 2017;71(2):296-304. doi:10.1111/his.13225.

31. Levi AW, Potter SR, Schoenberg MP, Epstein JI. Clinical significance of denuded urothelium in bladder biopsy. *J Urol*. 2001;166(2):457-460.

32. Parwani AV, Levi AW, Epstein JI, Ali SZ. Urinary bladder biopsy with denuded mucosa: Denuding cystitis?Cytopathologic correlates. *Diagn Cytopathol*. 2004;30(5):297-300. doi:10.1002/dc.10406.

33. Lane Z, Epstein JI. Polypoid/papillary cystitis: a series of 41 cases misdiagnosed as papillary urothelial neoplasia. *Am J Surg Pathol*. 2008;32(5):758-764. doi:10.1097/PAS.0b013e31816092b5.

34. Readal N, Epstein JI. Papillary urothelial hyperplasia: relationship to urothelial neoplasms. *Pathology*. 2010;42(4):360-363. doi:10.3109/00313021003767322.

35. Taylor DC, Bhagavan BS, Larsen MP, Cox JA, Epstein JI. Papillary urothelial hyperplasia. A precursor to papillary neoplasms. *Am J Surg Pathol*. 1996;20(12):1481-1488.

36. Magi-Galluzzi C, Epstein JI. Urothelial papilloma of the bladder: a review of 34 de novo cases. *Am J Surg Pathol*. 2004;28(12):1615-1620.

37. McKenney JK, Amin MB, Young RH. Urothelial (transitional cell) papilloma of the urinary bladder: a clinicopathologic study of 26 cases. *Mod Pathol*. 2003;16(7):623-629. doi:10.1097/01.MP.0000073973.74228.1E.

38. Maxwell JP, Wang C, Wiebe N, Yilmaz A, Trpkov K. Long-term outcome of primary Papillary Urothelial Neoplasm of Low Malignant Potential (PUNLMP) including PUNLMP with inverted growth. *Diagn Pathol*. 2015;10(1):3. doi:10.1186/s13000-015-0234-z.

39. Hodges KB, Lopez-Beltran A, Maclennan GT, Montironi R, Cheng L. Urothelial lesions with inverted growth patterns: histogenesis, molecular genetic findings, differential diagnosis and clinical management. *BJU Int*. 2011;107(4):532-537. doi:10.1111/j.1464-410X.2010.09853.x.

40. Jones TD, Zhang S, Lopez-Beltran A, et al. Urothelial carcinoma with an inverted growth pattern can be distinguished from inverted papilloma by fluorescence in situ hybridization, immunohistochemistry, and morphologic analysis. *Am J Surg Pathol*. 2007;31(12):1861-1867. doi:10.1097/PAS.0b013e318060cb9d.

41. Mazal PR, Schaufler R, Altenhuber-Müller R, et al. Derivation of nephrogenic adenomas from renal tubular cells in kidney-transplant recipients. *N Engl J Med*. 2002;347(9):653-659. doi:10.1056/NEJMoa013413.

42. Kunju LP. Nephrogenic adenoma: report of a case and review of morphologic mimics. *Arch Pathol Lab Med*. 2010;134(10):1455-1459. doi:10.1043/2010-0226-CR.1.

43. Allan CH, Epstein JI. Nephrogenic adenoma of the prostatic urethra: a mimicker of prostate adenocarcinoma. *Am J Surg Pathol*. 2001;25(6):802-808.

44. Remick DG, Kumar NB. Benign polyps with prostatic-type epithelium of the urethra and the urinary bladder. A suggestion of histogenesis based on histologic and immunohistochemical studies. *Am J Surg Pathol*. 1984;8(11):833-839.

45. Walker AN, Mills SE, Fechner RE, Perry JM. Epithelial polyps of the prostatic urethra. A light-microscopic and immunohistochemical study. *Am J Surg Pathol*. 1983;7(4):351-356.

46. Seibel JL, Prasad S, Weiss RE, Bancila E, Epstein JI. Villous adenoma of the urinary tract: a lesion frequently associated with malignancy. *Hum Pathol*. 2002;33(2):236-241.

47. van Rhijn BWG, van der Kwast TH, Alkhateeb SS, et al. A new and highly prognostic system to discern T1 bladder cancer substage. *Eur Urol*. 2012;61(2):378-384. doi:10.1016/j.eururo.2011.10.026.

48. Brimo F, Wu C, Zeizafoun N, et al. Prognostic factors in T1 bladder urothelial carcinoma: the value of recording millimetric depth of invasion, diameter of invasive carcinoma, and muscularis mucosa invasion. *Hum Pathol*. 2013;44(1):95-102. doi:10.1016/j.humpath.2012.04.020.

49. Orsola A, Werner L, de Torres I, et al. Reexamining treatment of high-grade T1 bladder cancer according to depth of lamina propria invasion: a prospective trial of 200 patients. *Br J Cancer*. 2015;112(3):468-474. doi:10.1038/bjc.2014.633.

50. Humphrey PA, Moch H, Cubilla AL, Ulbright TM, Reuter VE. The 2016 WHO classification of tumours of the urinary system and male genital organs-part b: prostate and bladder tumours. *Eur Urol*. 2016;70(1):106-119. doi:10.1016/j.eururo.2016.02.028.

51. Amin MB. Histological variants of urothelial carcinoma: diagnostic, therapeutic and prognostic implications. *Mod Pathol*. 2009;22 suppl 2(S2):S96-S118. doi:10.1038/modpathol.2009.26.

52. Sangoi AR, Beck AH, Amin MB, et al. Interobserver reproducibility in the diagnosis of invasive micropapillary carcinoma of the urinary tract among urologic pathologists. *Am J Surg Pathol*. 2010;34(9):1367-1376. doi:10.1097/PAS.0b013e3181ec86b3.

53. Al-Ahmadie HA, Iyer G, Lee BH, et al. Frequent somatic CDH1 loss-of-function mutations in plasmacytoid variant bladder cancer. *Nat Genet*. 2016;48(4):356-358. doi:10.1038/ng.3503.

54. Harper HL, McKenney JK, Heald B, et al. Upper tract urothelial carcinomas: frequency of association with mismatch repair protein loss and lynch syndrome. *Mod Pathol*. 2017;30(1):146-156. doi:10.1038/modpathol.2016.171.

55. Blochin EB, Park KJ, Tickoo SK, Reuter VE, Al-Ahmadie H. Urothelial carcinoma with prominent squamous differentiation in the setting of neurogenic bladder: role of human papillomavirus infection. *Mod Pathol*. 2012;25(11):1534-1542. doi:10.1038/modpathol.2012.112.

56. Zhong M, Gersbach E, Rohan SM, Yang XJ. Primary Adenocarcinoma of the Urinary Bladder Differential Diagnosis and Clinical Relevance. 2013;137(3):371-381. doi:10.5858/arpa.2012-0076-RA.

57. Grignon DJ, Ro JY, Ayala AG, Johnson DE, Ordóñez NG. Primary adenocarcinoma of the urinary bladder. A clinicopathologic analysis of 72 cases. *Cancer*. 1991;67(8):2165-2172.

58. Wang HL, Lu DW, Yerian LM, et al. Immunohistochemical distinction between primary adenocarcinoma of the bladder and secondary colorectal adenocarcinoma. *Am J Surg Pathol*. 2001;25(11):1380-1387.

59. Roy S, Smith MA, Cieply KM, Acquafondata MB, Parwani AV. Primary bladder adenocarcinoma versus metastatic colorectal adenocarcinoma: a persisting diagnostic challenge. *Diagn Pathol*. 2012;7(1):151. doi:10.1186/1746-1596-7-151.

60. Harik LR, Merino C, Coindre J-M, Amin MB, Pedeutour F, Weiss SW. Pseudosarcomatous myofibroblastic proliferations of the bladder. *Am J Surg Pathol*. 2006;30(7):787-794. doi:10.1097/01.pas.0000208903.46354.6f.

61. Jebastin JAS, Smith SC, Perry KD, et al. Pseudosarcomatous myofibroblastic proliferations of the genitourinary tract are genetically different from nodular fasciitis and lack *USP6, ROS1* and *ETV6* gene rearrangements. *Histopathology*. 2018;73(2):321-326. doi:10.1111/his.13526.

62. Lee TK, Miyamoto H, Osunkoya AO, Guo CC, Weiss SW, Epstein JI. Smooth muscle neoplasms of the urinary bladder: a clinicopathologic study of 51 cases. *Am J Surg Pathol*. 2010;34(4):502-509. doi:10.1097/PAS.0b013e3181cf326d.

63. Jones EC, Young RH. Myxoid and sclerosing sarcomatoid transitional cell carcinoma of the urinary bladder: a clinicopathologic and immunohistochemical study of 25 cases. *Mod Pathol*. 1997;10(9):908-916.

64. Roy S, Parwani AV. Adenocarcinoma of the urinary bladder. *Arch Pathol Lab Med*. 2011;135(12):1601-1605. doi:10.5858/arpa.2009-0713-RS.

KIDNEY

3

CHAPTER OUTLINE

THE UNREMARKABLE AND NONNEOPLASTIC KIDNEY

Entire volumes are written on the subject of nonneoplastic renal disease,[1] so this chapter will not attempt to cover medical renal disease in its entirety. However, a few aspects of normal renal anatomy and histology are very relevant to renal cancer staging. Likewise, a few of the more common medical renal diseases may be relevant to the surgical or genitourinary pathologist when evaluating kidney specimens for surgical or oncologic disease.

ANATOMY AND HISTOLOGY

The Glomerulus

The glomerulus is composed of a complex network of capillaries that plays a key role in the kidney's filtration of blood. The normal adult glomerulus is composed of numerous capillary loops with thin walls and open lumens (Figures 3.1 and 3.2). The mesangium or mesangial matrix shows pale eosinophilic staining in hematoxylin and eosin sections and in the normal state should be inconspicuous with usually only one to two mesangial cell nuclei (not more than three, Figure 3.3). Blood enters and leaves the glomerulus through the afferent and efferent arterioles, although only one or neither may be visualized in a given tissue section due to the plane of cutting (Figure 3.4).[2] For the surgical pathologist examining tissue adjacent to a tumor, usually it is reasonable to briefly assess the glomeruli in tissue away from the tumor. (Tissue immediately adjacent to the tumor can have unusual changes that may be difficult to assess as indicative of systemic disease or not.) If the glomeruli appear largely normal, in most cases more extensive evaluation (with special stains or full medical renal evaluation) is probably unnecessary. When the amount of mesangial matrix is increased, the most common etiology is diabetic nephropathy, discussed later.[3-6] Global glomerular sclerosis or obsolescence results in a consolidated nodule with complete loss of the glomerular architecture (Figure 3.5). It is relatively common to have some degree of global glomerular sclerosis that increases with age; however, evaluating areas immediately adjacent to the renal mass likely would be an overestimate due to compressive mass effect. At the same time, we have encountered end-stage or atrophic kidneys that histologically have large areas of tissue appearing near-normal, so detailed quantification of glomerular sclerosis is probably unnecessary for routine cases.

KEY FEATURES: The Normal Glomerulus

- Capillary loops with thin walls
- Mesangial matrix material not conspicuous
- Maximum of two to three nuclei in mesangial areas
- Inflammatory cells rare in capillary lumens, if any
- No fibrin thrombi in arteriolar or capillary lumens (Figure 3.6)

Renal Tubules

The proximal tubules have taller and more eosinophilic epithelial cells than those of the distal nephron (Figure 3.7). Over the years, most subtypes of renal neoplasm have been assigned a putative "cell of origin" from one of the renal tubular compartments, in which most renal cell carcinomas (RCCs) are regarded as of proximal tubular origin or phenotype.[7] Oncocytoma and chromophobe RCC are hypothesized to be of intercalated cell origin or phenotype, whereas a few aggressive carcinomas are thought to have the phenotype of the principal cells of the distal nephron, including collecting duct carcinoma and renal medullary carcinoma.[7] For routine surgical pathology practice, there is not usually great significance to recognizing proximal versus distal tubules; however, the proximal tubules may serve as a helpful internal control for immunohistochemistry, usually showing very strong staining for alpha-methylacyl-CoA racemase (AMACR, Figure 3.8), which corresponds to what is expected in papillary RCC.

Renal Arteries and Veins

Renal blood vessels have major significance for staging of renal cancer, especially involvement of veins. Therefore, it is worthwhile for the surgical pathologist handling renal specimens to be familiar with their normal structure and appearance.[8] Although there is classically a main artery and vein which are taken as margin sections in staging of a renal cancer, numerous anatomic variations can occur, with additional arteries or vein branches present at the specimen margin. The larger veins and tributaries will have a recognizable smooth muscle media histologically (Figure 3.9); however, smaller vein tributaries will not necessarily have smooth muscle in their walls (Figures 3.10 and 3.11), which has led to the removal of the requirement from the American Joint Committee on Cancer (AJCC) staging system[9] that vein invasion be into "muscle-containing" branches. Staging is discussed more in a section on renal cancer staging.

PEARLS AND PITFALLS: Identifying Veins in Renal Histology Sections

- Typically adjacent to a paired artery (Figures 3.9-3.11)
- Elastic layer present in paired artery (Figure 3.12)
- Larger vein tributaries will have smooth muscle, but smaller ones will not (Figures 3.10 and 3.11)

The Renal Sinus

The renal sinus is the central compartment of adipose tissue that contains the renal vasculature around the hilum of the kidney (Figures 3.13-3.15). Since the renal sinus does not have a discrete capsule separating the kidney from the fat and since this contains the renal vein and tributaries, this is one of the most common pathways for extrarenal spread of renal cancer.[10,11] As discussed in the section on renal cancer staging, multiple sections should be submitted from the renal sinus, especially for larger renal tumors. In radical nephrectomy specimens, often there are few or no lymph nodes in the hilar area unless specifically dissected by the surgeon, often as separate specimens. Therefore, attempt should be made to identify any readily appreciable lymph nodes; however, it is not a failure if none are identified in a radical nephrectomy specimen without a specified lymph node dissection.

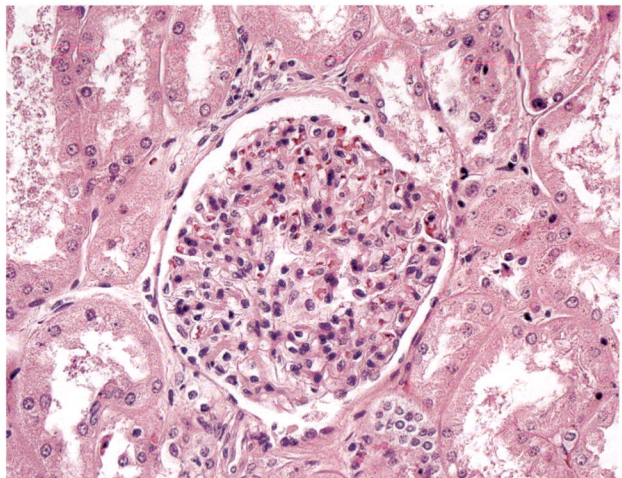

Figure 3.1. The normal glomerulus is composed of multiple capillary loops with thin walls. The Bowman capsule separating the glomerulus from the renal tubules and interstitium is also thin and inconspicuous.

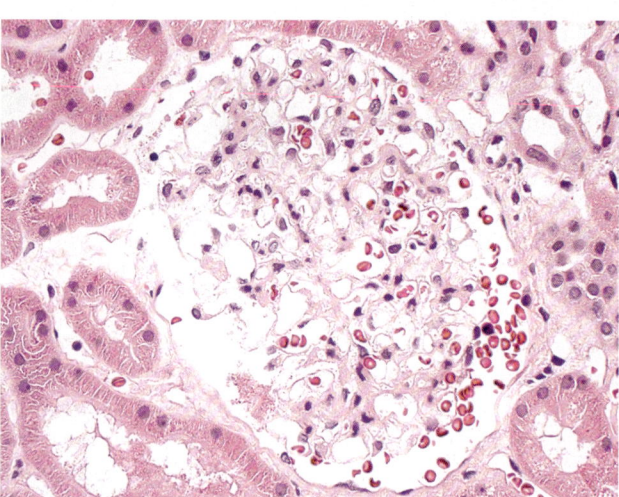

Figure 3.2. In this high magnification H&E stain of a glomerulus, the mesangial matrix is light pink with a normal number of nuclei (1-2 cells).

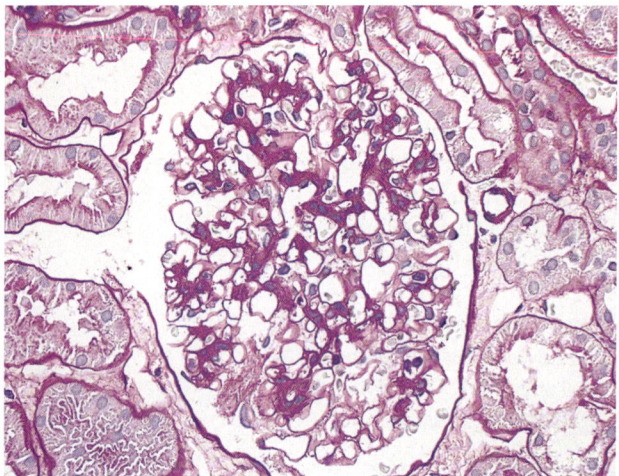

Figure 3.3. The mesangial matrix stains red-purple in this periodic acid Schiff–stained section. It should be relatively inconspicuous in normal kidneys, whereas it is increased with diabetes. There are only two to three nuclei at most in the mesangial areas. Four or more cells are generally considered abnormal.

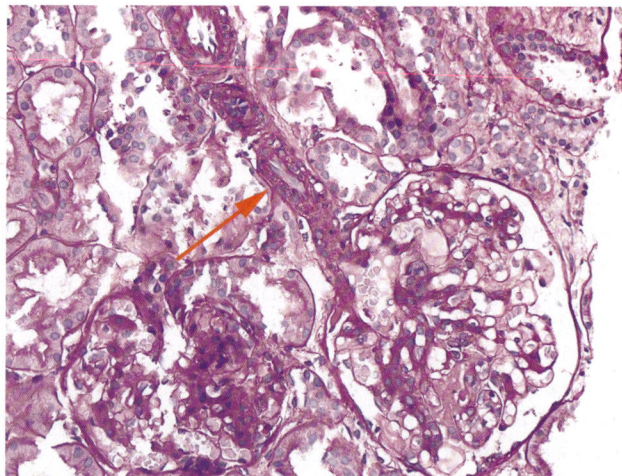

Figure 3.4. In this periodic acid Schiff–stained section, the arteriole (arrow) is well visualized, although only one (afferent or efferent) is visible due to the plane of section.

NONNEOPLASTIC RENAL DISEASE

Several studies have investigated the incidence of nonneoplastic renal disease in tumor nephrectomy specimens, finding mostly that diabetic nephropathy and vascular disease (hypertensive changes, etc.) are the most common incidental abnormalities.[3-6,12] However, a variety of other diseases have been reported, including amyloidosis (Figures 3.16 and 3.17), focal segmental glomerular sclerosis (FSGS, Figure 3.18), atheroembolism, and thrombotic microangiopathy, among others.[3-6,12] Ideally, if a suspicion of medical renal disease is known at the time of surgery for a renal mass, coordination between the pathologist and surgeon can facilitate collection of samples for full medical renal evaluation (including direct immunofluorescence and electron microscopy). However, in the vast majority of cases, medical renal disease is not particularly suspected and no such samples are taken. If the surgical pathologist is familiar with some general principles, then the appropriate cases for medical renal consultation can be selected. It is worthwhile to submit at least one to two sections of normal appearing renal parenchyma away from the neoplasm in specimens with sufficient tissue, to aid in screening for clinically relevant medical renal disease. If more

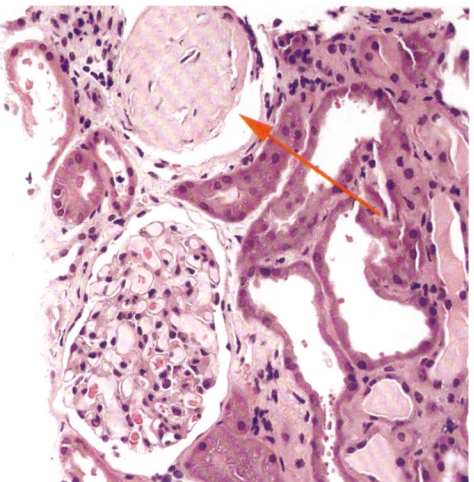

Figure 3.5. Global glomerular sclerosis is a generally nonspecific pattern of injury. This glomerulus (arrow) is consolidated into a nonspecific fibrous nodule in a patient with hypertension as the presumed etiology of renal disease. The below glomerulus is largely normal.

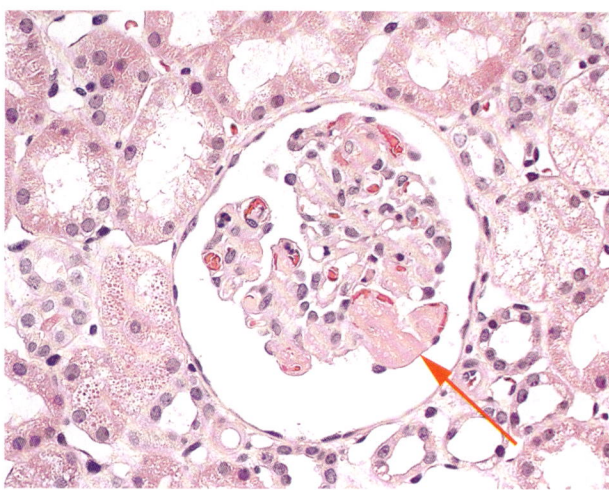

Figure 3.6. Fibrin thrombi can sometimes be encountered in glomerular capillary loops or arterioles. This generally is considered a thrombotic microangiopathy pattern. In the setting of kidneys collected for organ donation, it is thought that this often results from donor head trauma and does not necessarily contraindicate use of the kidney for transplantation. The fibrin (arrow) is a light pink color, in contrast to erythrocytes, which are darker red.

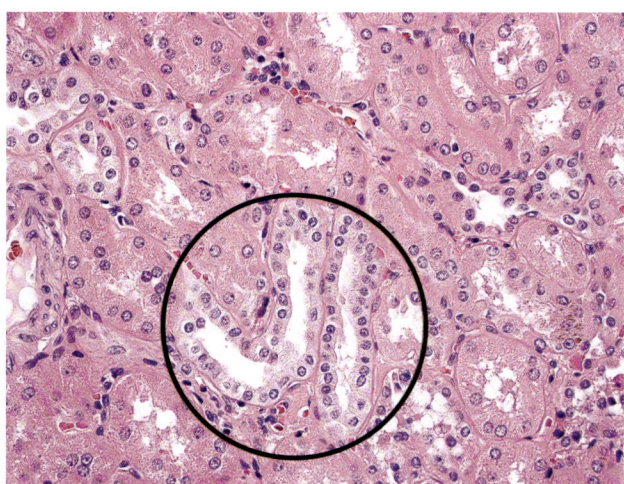

Figure 3.7. Proximal tubules, occupying most of this field, typically have voluminous eosinophilic cytoplasm. Distal tubules (circled) have slightly less cytoplasm and more cuboidal cells.

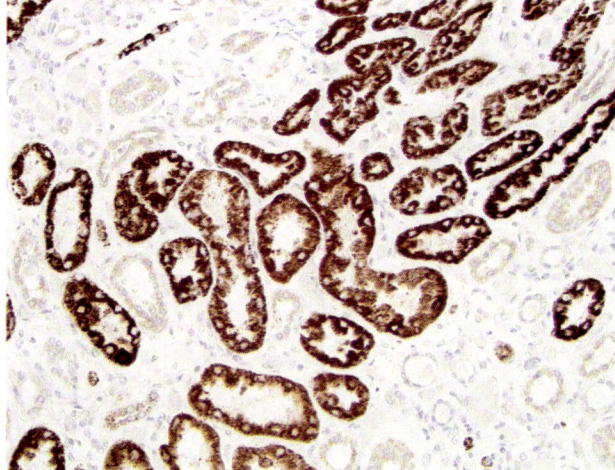

Figure 3.8. Using immunohistochemistry, this stain for AMACR shows extremely bright staining in the proximal tubules, which would mirror that seen in papillary renal cell carcinomas.

thorough medical renal evaluation is needed, some laboratories can perform immunofluorescence from formalin-fixed, paraffin-embedded tissues, and tissue for electron microscopy can be either extracted from the paraffin block (with some artifact) or processed from the gross specimen.

Hypertensive Changes/Arterial Thickening

Some degree of arterial thickening is quite common in nephrectomy specimens (Figure 3.19) and generally considered to reflect hypertensive changes. The elastic layer may be irregular or duplicated. In addition to intimal thickening of large arteries, arterioles may show hyalinosis, which is associated most often with hypertension or diabetes (Figure 3.20). These findings may be documented either in the main diagnoses or in the nonneoplastic disease section of cancer checklists,[13] since hypertension is relatively common in patients with typical demographics for renal cancer (i.e., age 50+). Hypertension, obesity, smoking, etc. are also considered risk factors for renal cancer.[14]

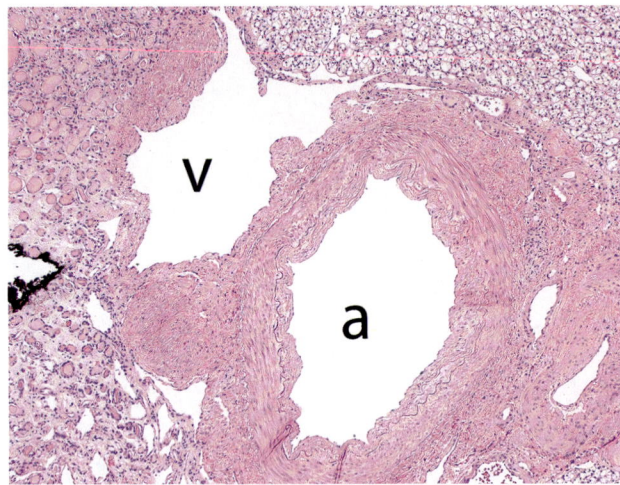

Figure 3.9. This field shows a paired renal artery (a) and vein (v). Both have smooth muscle in their walls, although the smooth muscle of the vein is variable in thickness and focally absent.

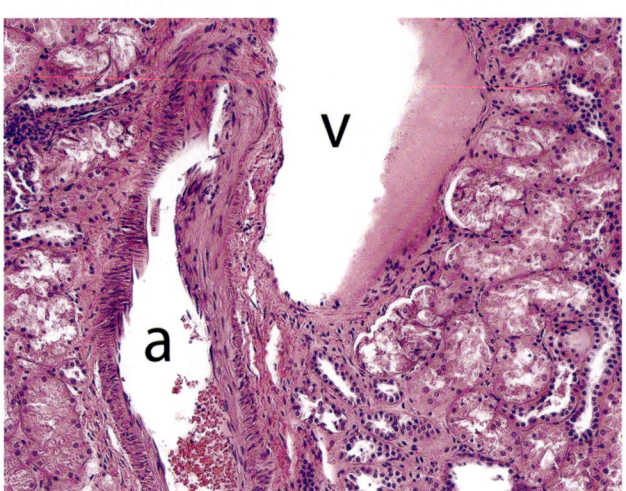

Figure 3.10. This smaller paired artery (a) and vein (v) shows no significant smooth muscle in the vein wall. The requirement that veins contain muscle to diagnose pT3a vein branch invasion has been removed in the 8th edition AJCC staging, as even grossly visible renal vein branches may have inconspicuous muscle.

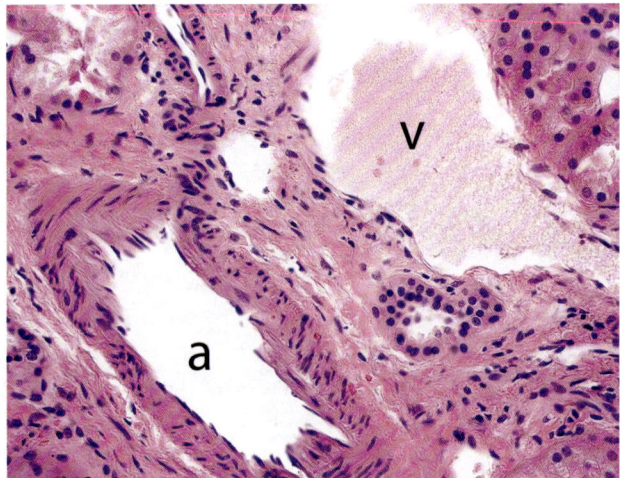

Figure 3.11. At high magnification, this artery (a) and vein (v) pair shows no muscle in the small vein.

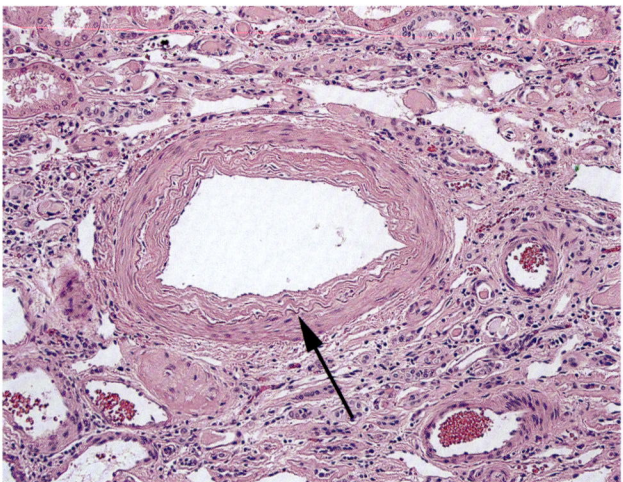

Figure 3.12. An elastic layer (arrow) can be helpful in recognizing arteries. This example shows some multilayering, suggesting hypertension.

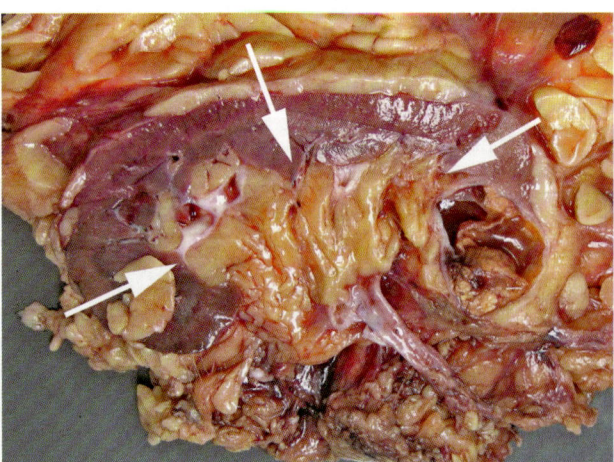

Figure 3.13. The renal sinus is the fatty compartment that surrounds the renal hilar vasculature and renal pelvis (arrows). This area should be carefully examined for staging renal cancer.

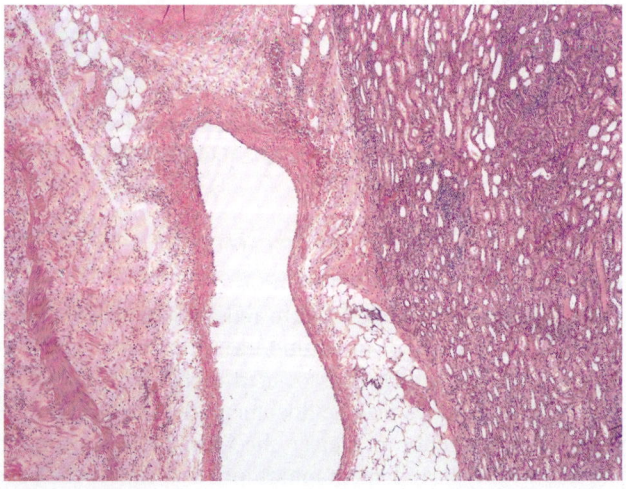

Figure 3.14. Microscopically, the renal sinus is composed of loose fibrous tissue, fat, and vascular structures. This large vein branch has a thin wall.

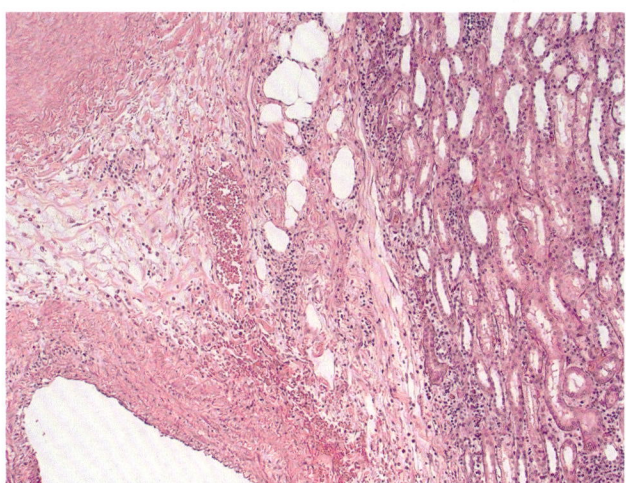

Figure 3.15. Higher magnification of the interface of the kidney and renal sinus shows loose fibrous tissue, fat, and a vein wall.

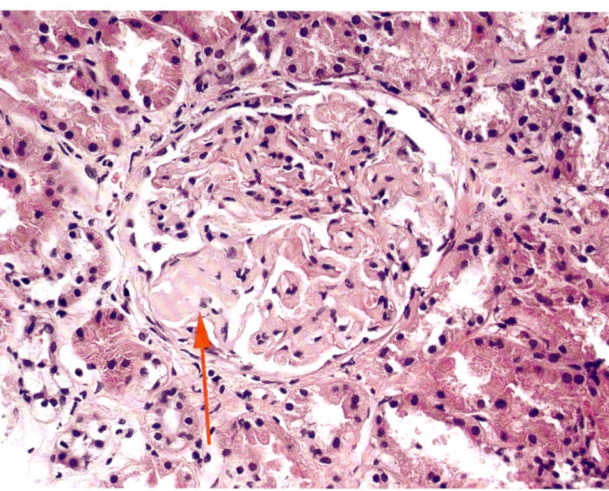

Figure 3.16. This case of amyloidosis shows focal eosinophilic nodularity (arrow) within the glomerulus.

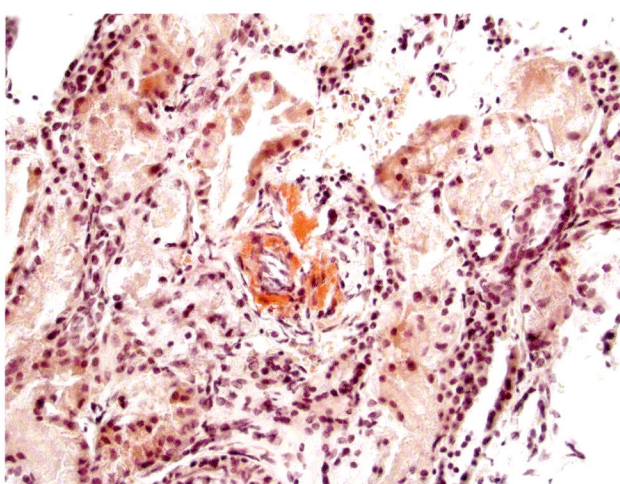

Figure 3.17. Congo red staining in the same case from Figure 3.16 shows positive staining of an arteriole, supporting amyloidosis. This case was AL (light chain type).

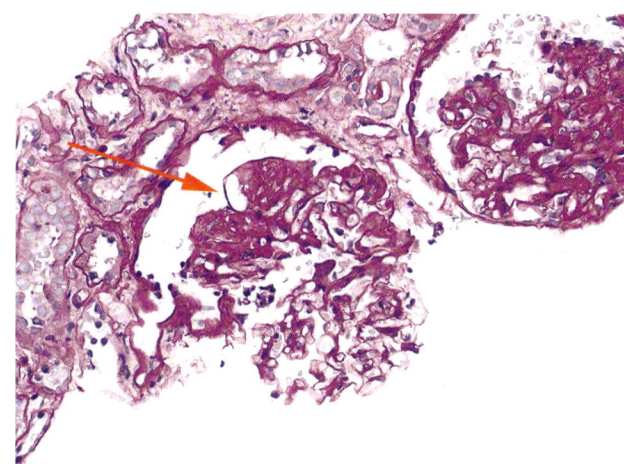

Figure 3.18. Focal segmental glomerular sclerosis is characterized by partial sclerosis of the glomerulus (arrow). In this example, the opposite side of the same glomerulus is essentially normal.

Diabetic Nephropathy

Diabetic nephropathy is one of the most common incidental abnormalities in tissue from tumor nephrectomy specimens.[3-6,12] Typical features include expansion of the mesangial matrix. If severe, mesangial matrix is expanded to the point of forming nodules (Kimmelstiel-Wilson nodules, Figure 3.21). There may also be capillary microaneurysms in which the capillaries form wide, flat loops, in contrast to the normal thin individual loops, presumably from loss of connection to the mesangium, in which multiple loops become confluent (Figure 3.22). Other classic features of diabetic nephropathy include "capsular drop" with nodules of hyalinosis on the Bowman capsule and "hyaline cap" with hyalinosis in the glomerulus (Figure 3.23).

KEY FEATURES: Diabetic Nephropathy

- Mesangial matrix expanded or nodular (Kimmelstiel-Wilson nodules)
- Hyalinosis in both afferent and efferent arterioles (if both are visualized, Figure 3.24)
- Glomerular or Bowman capsule hyalinosis

- Mesangial matrix positive (black) on silver stain (Figure 3.25), in contrast to amyloid (pink)
- Congo red negative in nodules, in contrast to amyloid (positive)

Changes Adjacent to Tumor

Several morphologic changes can be found in the renal parenchyma adjacent to a neoplasm, and therefore we would hesitate to make overarching diagnoses for findings that are only present immediately around the mass. For example, there can be more prominent tubulointerstitial inflammation in the areas around the mass. We have also encountered glomerular abnormalities resembling those of FSGS, which we would again hesitate to diagnose as the disease FSGS if not present in tissue away from the mass (Figure 3.26), and especially so if there is not clinically appreciable proteinuria.

Focal Segmental Glomerular Sclerosis

FSGS is a pattern of glomerular injury caused by diverse potential etiologies,[15] ranging from glomerulonephritis to FSGS as a primary disease. This injury pattern is characterized histologically by segmental scarring of the glomerular tuft, such that part of the glomerulus appears relatively normal and another part is sclerotic (Figure 3.27). FSGS as a disease is classically associated with significant proteinuria. As noted in the previous paragraph, we have encountered some lesions that resemble glomerular segmental sclerosis in the tissue immediately adjacent to a mass. If the patient has no definite chronic renal disease or proteinuria and these are found only adjacent to the mass, then it is probably reasonable to disregard them. If there is clinical evidence of renal disease or these lesions are found away from the mass (Figure 3.26), it is likely worthwhile to comment on them or request a more detailed medical renal evaluation of the specimen, either internally or externally.

Inflammation

It is not unusual to find some inflammation in the tissue adjacent to a renal mass, which again may be related to compressive or obstructive mass effect (Figure 3.28). We generally avoid use of the term tubulointerstitial nephritis or similar to avoid potentially implying acute tubulointerstitial nephritis, which is presumptively an allergic-type reaction. Instead, terminology such as chronic interstitial inflammation can be used descriptively to indicate the lack of a definite etiology. Several inflammatory pseudotumors and other distinct entities are discussed later in the inflammatory pattern section.

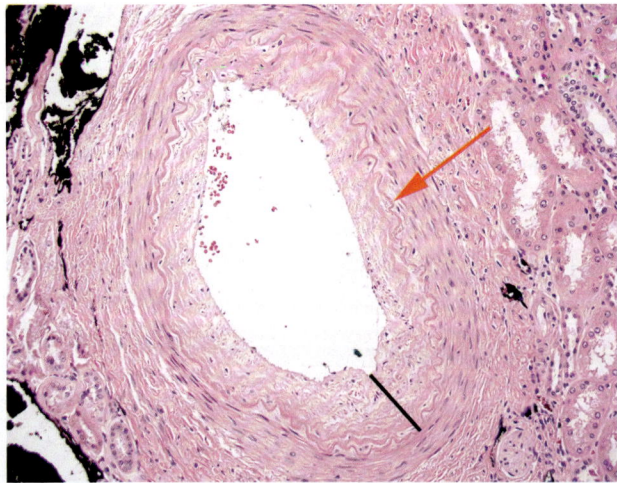

Figure 3.19. This artery with hypertensive changes shows multilayering of the elastic layer (red arrow). Normally, the intima should be inconspicuous, with endothelial cells just above the elastic layer; however, this case shows substantial intimal thickening (black bar).

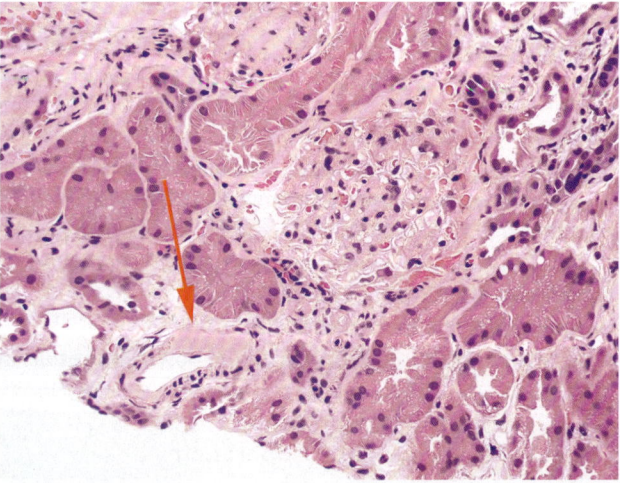

Figure 3.20. Hyaline arteriolosclerosis (arrow) is associated with diabetes and hypertension. This arteriole shows asymmetrical thickening with eosinophilic material. There are small "bubbles" which differ from the usual pattern of amyloid.

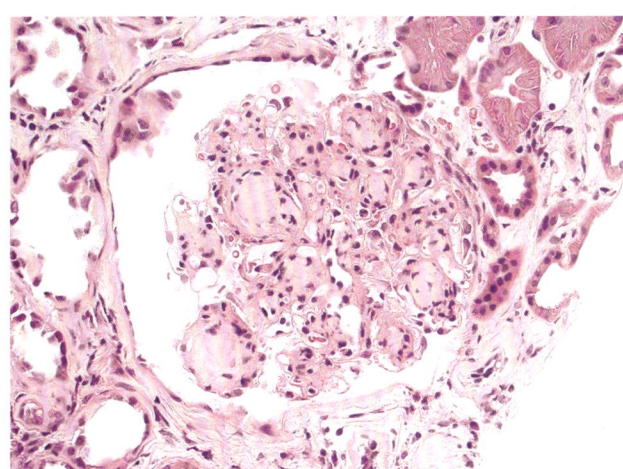

Figure 3.21. In diabetic nephropathy, the mesangial matrix is expanded, forming Kimmelstiel-Wilson nodules.

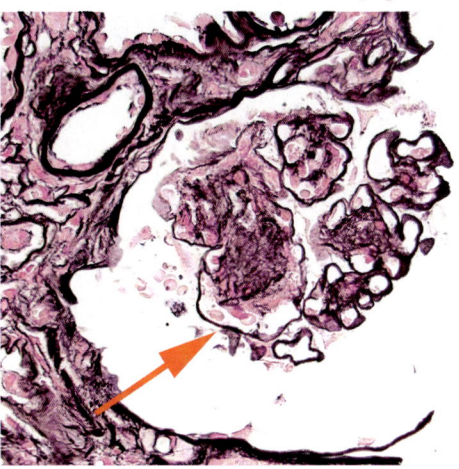

Figure 3.22. Microaneurysms are a feature of diabetic nephropathy, in which it appears that multiple capillary loops have merged to form one large loop (arrow), shown in this Jones silver stain.

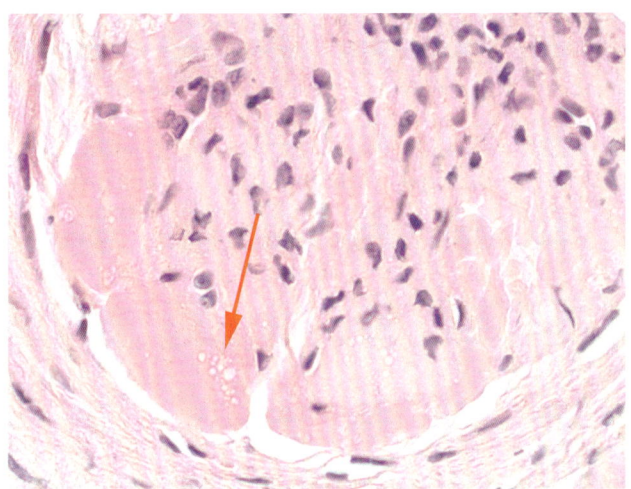

Figure 3.23. Hyalinosis can also be present in glomeruli with diabetic nephropathy. This example shows eosinophilic material with "bubbles," (arrow) differing from the waxy/cracked appearance of amyloid.

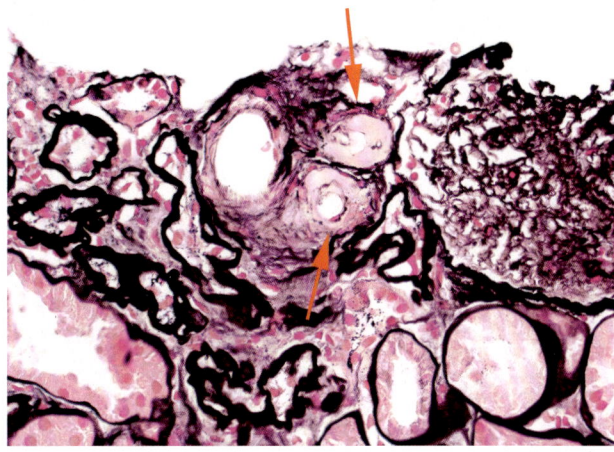

Figure 3.24. Classically, diabetic nephropathy will show hyaline arteriolosclerosis of both the afferent and efferent arterioles (arrows), although both cannot always be visualized due to the plane of sectioning.

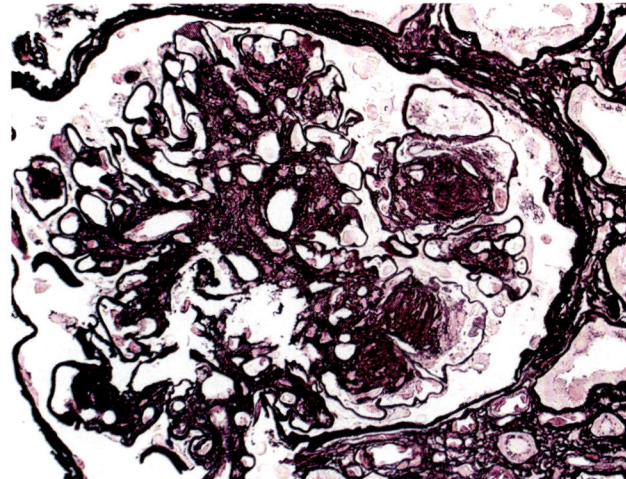

Figure 3.25. The expanded mesangial matrix in diabetic nephropathy is black in Jones silver stain, compared with pink in amyloidosis.

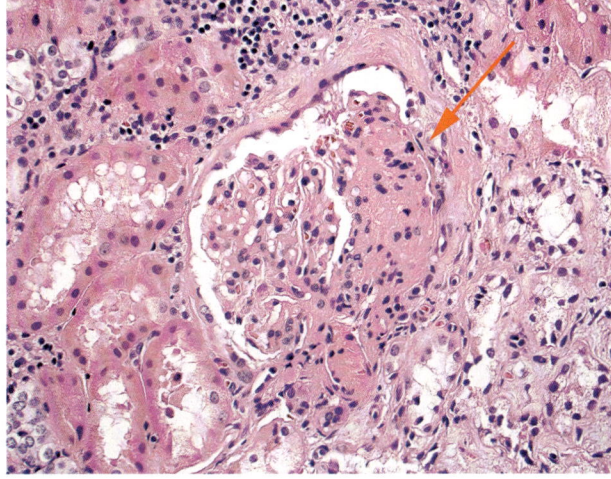

Figure 3.26. With focal segmental glomerular sclerosis, part of the glomerulus is sclerotic (arrow), whereas the remainder appears relatively normal. This biopsy came from a 16-year-old with proteinuria.

TUMORS

RENAL CANCER GENERAL

FAQ: What are the Most Important Aspects of Renal Cancer Classification for Clinical Treatment?

Although the classification of renal cancer has expanded greatly with numerous recognized subtypes and variants, in general there are only a few major diagnostic branch points that have significant implications for treatment at present. Unless specified here, most other subtypes of RCC are currently categorized with "non–clear cell" for treatment purposes.

- Clear cell versus non–clear cell: Clinical guidelines do distinguish clear cell from non–clear cell RCC for treatment pathways in the metastatic setting.[16] So, pathologists should make the best attempt possible to discern clear cell from non–clear cell RCC. In some cases, this may not be possible, however, especially for small biopsies of a metastatic lesion with atypical morphology (Figures 3.29 and 3.30). One of the most helpful immunohistochemical markers for this purpose is carbonic anhydrase IX (showing diffuse membrane labeling in clear cell RCC); however, this should be interpreted with caution in the setting of unknown primary cancer or absence of a renal mass, as its specificity is lower in these scenarios.

- RCC versus urothelial carcinoma: RCC will typically be treated markedly differently than urothelial carcinoma (such as with tyrosine kinase inhibitors, vascular endothelial growth factor (VEGF) or mammalian target of rapamycin (MTOR) pathway agents, in contrast to conventional chemotherapy, i.e., gemcitabine/cisplatin for urothelial carcinoma). In most cases, the clinical impression of a renal pelvis mass versus spherical renal mass will correctly predict urothelial carcinoma versus RCC, but occasionally patterns of growth can be deceptive. Helpful immunohistochemical markers are

  - PAX8—in general favors RCC; however, caution is necessary, as upper tract urothelial carcinoma can also be positive[17]

  - GATA3—favors urothelial carcinoma[18]

  - P63—strongly favors urothelial carcinoma[19]

- Fumarate hydratase–deficient/hereditary leiomyomatosis and renal cell carcinoma syndrome (HLRCC)–associated renal cancer: This aggressive form of renal cancer, discussed later, is beginning to be recognized as potentially necessitating specific therapy.[16] In brief, findings that suggest this diagnosis include an eosinophilic ("type 2") papillary RCC with extremely prominent nucleoli or heterogeneous architectural patterns, such as tubulocystic, papillary, and infiltrative growth.[20-22]

- Renal medullary carcinoma: Cytotoxic chemotherapy, such as platinum-based regimens, is generally recommended for this aggressive and rare form of renal cancer.[16]

- Sarcomatoid RCC: A specific treatment is not explicitly recommended for sarcomatoid RCC at present; however, some studies have investigated a conventional chemotherapy approach (such as gemcitabine, sometimes in combination with RCC-directed therapies, such as sunitinib or bevacizumab).[16] Distinguishing sarcomatoid RCC from mimics is discussed further under the spindle cell tumors pattern.

- Hereditary syndromes: Renal cancers of hereditary syndromes are generally treated similarly to their sporadic counterparts. However, multiple masses, such as in von Hippel-Lindau (VHL) disease or other syndromes, may be treated with more conservative renal sparing surgery, such as enucleation. Conversely, HLRCC-associated tumors require aggressive treatment, even if solitary, and may require specific chemotherapeutic considerations.[16] Finally, pathologist recognition of hereditary renal cancer syndromes is important to trigger follow-up for metachronous tumors and tumors of other organs in the patient and family members. A summary of the best established syndromes associated with renal tumors is listed in Table 3.1.[14,23]

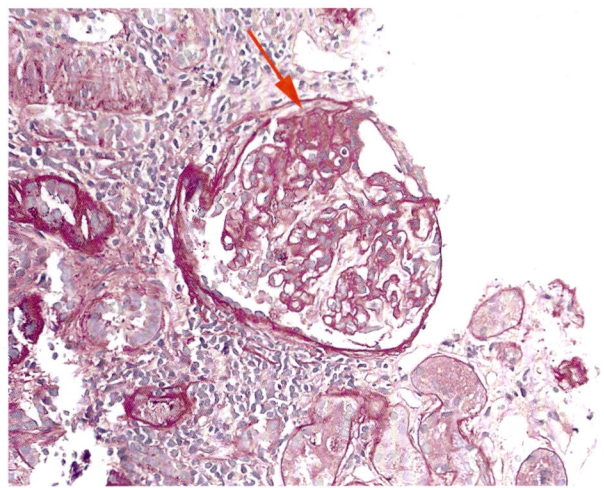

Figure 3.27. In this case of focal segmental glomerular sclerosis, the periodic acid Schiff stain highlights the area of segmental sclerosis (arrow).

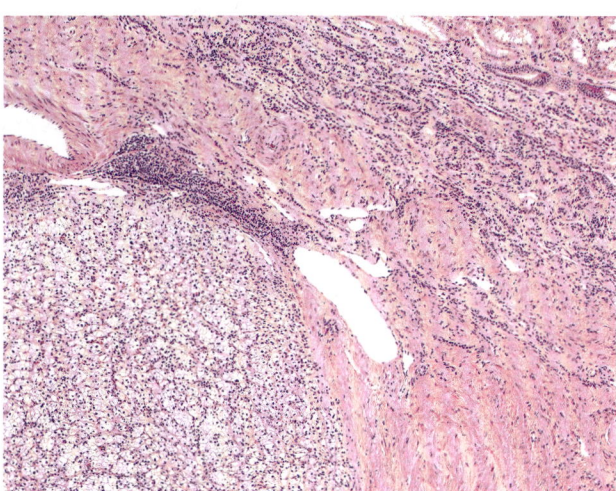

Figure 3.28. Interstitial inflammation is relatively common in the areas immediately around a renal mass, and we generally do not use the terminology "interstitial nephritis" to avoid confusion with allergic-type reactions to drugs.

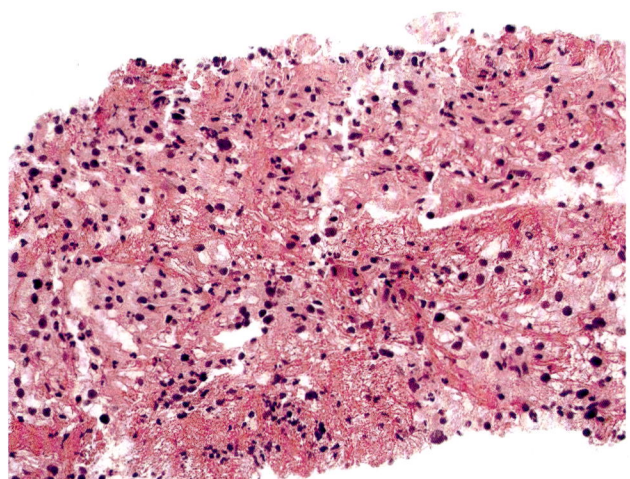

Figure 3.29. This renal mass biopsy shows a renal cell carcinoma tumor that was positive for PAX8 and negative for AMACR and cytokeratin 7.

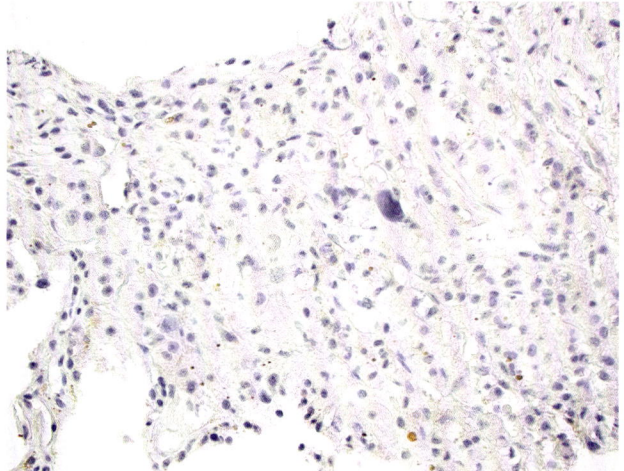

Figure 3.30. Immunohistochemistry of the same biopsy from Figure 3.29 shows negative staining for carbonic anhydrase IX. Although this does not lend support to diagnosis of clear cell renal cell carcinoma (RCC), a comment was given for this specimen indicating that clear cell RCC was favored based on the morphology and difficult to entirely exclude due to the small amount of tissue.

CLEAR/PALE CELL PATTERN

Clear Cell Renal Cell Carcinoma

Clear cell RCC is overwhelmingly the most common subtype of renal cancer, typically accounting for at least 60% to 70% of adult renal tumors.[24] However, with increasing understanding of the molecular features of renal cancer and immunohistochemistry, it is now known that there are several other "clear cell" tumors that must be distinguished from clear cell RCC.[25] Clear cell RCC characteristically has a golden-yellow or orange cut surface grossly (Figure 3.31), although this can be variable, depending on features such as hemorrhage or sarcomatoid dedifferentiation, which may influence the gross appearance to more red-brown (Figure 3.32) or white-tan (Figure 3.33). Microscopically, clear cell RCC can have many patterns, some of which can be diagnostically deceptive.

TABLE 3.1: Hereditary Renal Cancer Syndromes

	Gene/Chromosome	Renal Tumors	Other Manifestations
Von Hippel-Lindau disease	VHL/3p25	Clear cell renal cell carcinoma (RCC), multiple, and renal cysts	Hemangioblastoma (nervous system and retina), pheochromocytoma, pancreatic neuroendocrine tumors, pancreatic cysts, cystadenomas of epididymis/broad ligament, endolymphatic sac tumor of inner ear
Hereditary leiomyomatosis and renal cell carcinoma syndrome	FH/1q42	Aggressive RCC with prominent nucleoli, multiple patterns (papillary, infiltrative, tubulocystic)	Cutaneous leiomyomas, uterine leiomyomas (at a young age)
Hereditary papillary RCC	MET/7p31	Papillary RCC, type 1, numerous	
Birt-Hogg-Dubé syndrome	FLCN/17p11	Oncocytic neoplasms, multiple	Lung cysts, skin fibrofolliculomas
Tuberous sclerosis	TSC1/9q34 TSC2/16p13	Angiomyolipomas, renal cysts, and RCCs (eosinophilic solid and cystic RCC, smooth muscle stroma, and oncocytic)	Cardiac rhabdomyoma, intestinal polyps, pulmonary cysts, brain tubers and subependymal giant cell astrocytoma
Hereditary pheochromocytoma/paraganglioma syndromes	Succinate dehydrogenase subunits (most common SDHB)	SDH-deficient RCC (oncocytic with cytoplasmic vacuoles)	Paraganglioma/pheochromocytoma, gastrointestinal stromal tumor
Constitutional chromosome 3 translocations	3p	Clear cell RCC	
Cowden syndrome	PTEN/10q23	Clear cell, papillary, chromophobe RCC	Cancers of breast, thyroid, endometrium, and prostate; colon polyps, facial trichilemmomas, macrocephaly
Hyperparathyroid jaw tumor syndrome	CDC73/1q31.2	Papillary RCC, mixed epithelial and stromal tumor	Parathyroid tumors, jaw fibromas
BAP1 cancer syndrome	BAP1/3p21	Clear cell RCC	Melanoma and mesothelioma
MITF cancer syndrome	MITF/3p14	Unknown	Melanoma, pancreatic cancer, pheochromocytoma

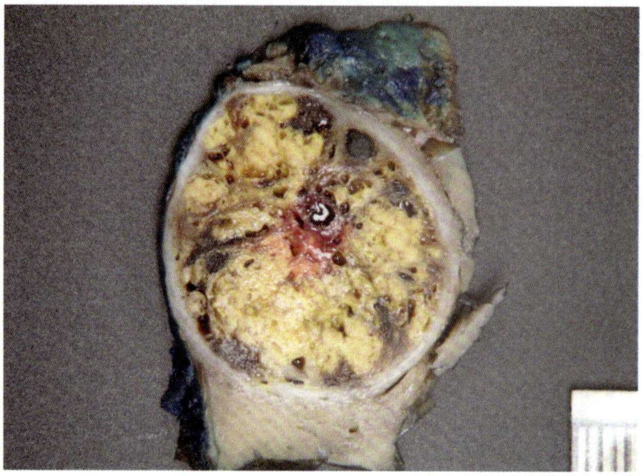

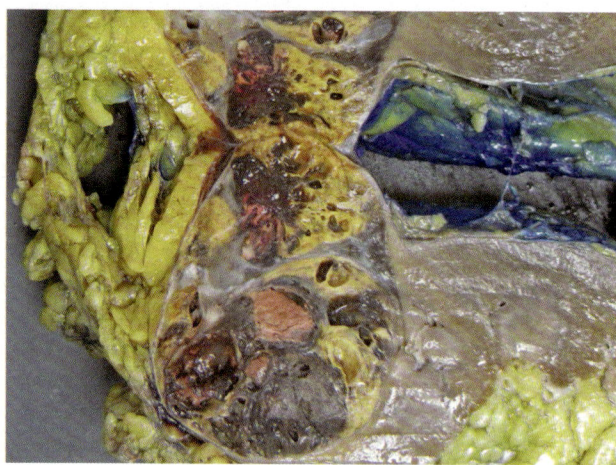

Figure 3.31. The classic gross appearance of clear cell renal cell carcinoma is golden-yellow or orange. This tumor also has some small hemorrhagic areas. It is circular and very well circumscribed.

Figure 3.32. This clear cell renal cell carcinoma shows a mixture of yellow and red-brown gross appearances, likely resulting from hemorrhage.

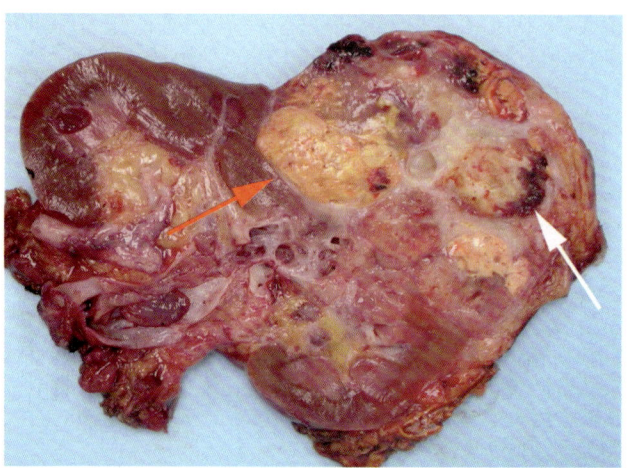

Figure 3.33. This large clear cell renal cell carcinoma includes yellow areas (red arrow) but also white-tan areas (white arrow). The latter should always be sampled histologically, as this can represent higher-grade areas or sarcomatoid change.

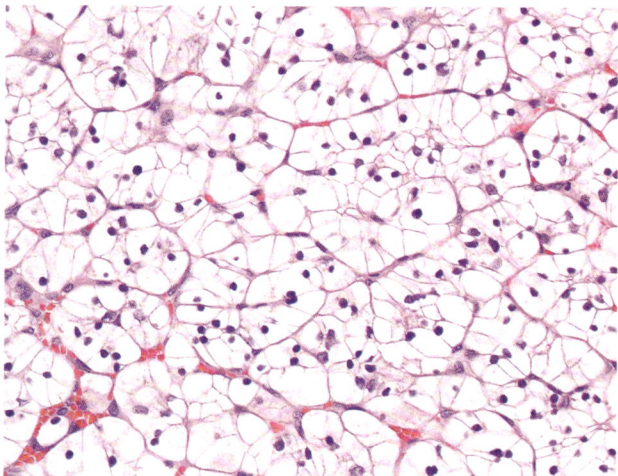

Figure 3.34. The classic appearance of clear cell renal cell carcinoma histologically is nested growth of cells with optically clear cytoplasm and an extremely intricate capillary fibrovascular network.

KEY FEATURES: Clear Cell Renal Cell Carcinoma

- Nested or alveolar architecture, composed of cells with clear cytoplasm (Figures 3.34 and 3.35)

- May have eosinophilic cytoplasm (Figures 3.36 and 3.37) or bizarre features[26,27] (Figures 3.38-3.42) with higher-grade tumors

- Scarring, infarct-type necrosis, or fibrosis is common,[28] which may contain inconspicuous tumor cells and may be deceptive if captured in a biopsy (Figures 3.43 and 3.44)

- Cystic changes may be variably present (Figures 3.45 and 3.46)

- Immunohistochemistry is consistently positive for carbonic anhydrase IX with membranous pattern (Figure 3.47), but may be decreased or negative in high-grade areas (Figure 3.48)[26]

- Cytokeratin 7 staining usually negative, minimal, or focal (Figure 3.49), but rarely can be more diffuse in true clear cell RCC (Figure 3.50)[29]

- Often positive for vimentin, especially higher-grade tumors (Figure 3.51)

- Negative for KIT (contrasting to oncocytoma/chromophobe RCC)[30]

- Minimal or negative staining for high molecular weight cytokeratin (contrasting to clear cell papillary RCC)

- PAX8 consistently positive, supporting renal cell origin[31-33]

- *VHL* gene mutation or promoter hypermethylation via molecular testing[24,34]
- Chromosome 3p loss detected via fluorescence in situ hybridization (FISH) or copy number assessment techniques is very common and often used as a surrogate (Figure 3.52)[35] but may not be 100% specific for clear cell RCC[36-38]
- Has a tendency to grow into veins and renal sinus tissue,[8,10,11,39-42] discussed more with renal cancer staging

The behavior of clear cell RCC is known to be deceptive. Although small tumors of stage pT1a often have favorable outcomes, it is also known that recurrences can occur many years after the original diagnosis, including metastases to unusual sites, such as the skin, pancreas (Figure 3.53), or gallbladder.[24,43,44] Interestingly, although it might intuitively suggest advanced disseminated disease, there is evidence that surgical resection of isolated pancreatic metastases of RCC is clinically warranted and may be associated with long-term survival.[44] In general, clear cell RCC is considered to be a less favorable histologic subtype when compared to chromophobe or papillary subtypes.[45,46]

PEARLS AND PITFALLS: Pathology of Metastatic Clear Cell RCC for Guiding Clinical Treatment

- Much of the molecular knowledge of renal cancer comes from clear cell RCC, particularly the role of the *VHL* gene and chromosome 3p25 where it is located, which is often deleted as a "second hit"[47]
- Multiple treatment approaches have been established based on key molecular pathways in clear cell RCC, especially those targeting VEGF, tyrosine kinases in general, and the MTOR pathway[16]
- It is therefore relatively important for the pathologist to attempt to subtype metastatic renal cancer, as the treatment algorithms are different for clear cell and non–clear cell tumors[16]
- PAX8 is currently the most helpful marker to support a metastasis being of renal origin (Figure 3.54),[48] although this should be interpreted cautiously if there is not clinical evidence of a renal mass or a known history of a high-stage (or large) renal mass, as it is rare for RCC to present with metastases and a subtle or unidentified primary tumor
- Carbonic anhydrase IX diffuse membrane immunohistochemical staining is supportive of clear cell subtype of RCC[49-52]
  - However, staining can be found in nonrenal cancers,[53] so this should again be interpreted cautiously if there is no renal mass
  - Staining can also be decreased or negative in the poorly differentiated component of clear cell RCC tumors. Therefore, a negative result does not entirely exclude clear cell RCC

SAMPLE NOTE: Metastatic Renal Cell Carcinoma With Minimal or Negative Carbonic Anhydrase IX Staining

- Metastatic renal cell carcinoma—see Comment

Comment: The findings are in keeping with metastatic renal cell carcinoma. Carbonic anhydrase IX, a marker of the *VHL* and hypoxia pathway, shows minimal staining, which does not lend support to clear cell subtype; however, staining can be decreased or absent in poorly differentiated or metastatic tumors.[a]

[a]If a nephrectomy has been previously performed elsewhere, recommendation can be made to obtain the original pathology slides. If the primary tumor has never been sampled histologically, molecular analysis, such as *VHL* sequencing, could be considered if necessary for treatment selection.

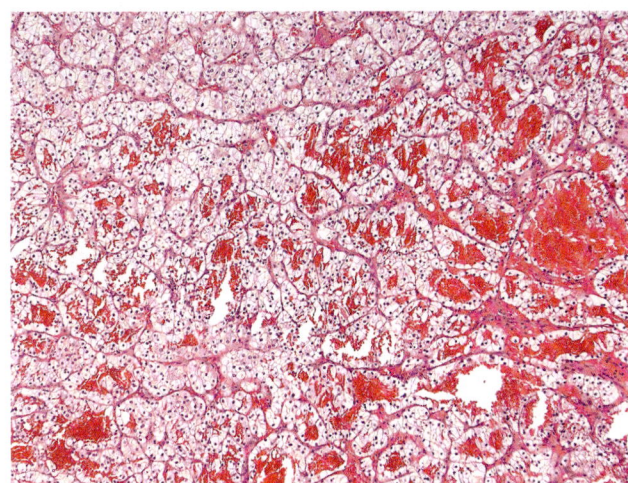

Figure 3.35. Other patterns in clear cell renal cell carcinoma can also include an alveolar hemorrhagic growth pattern.

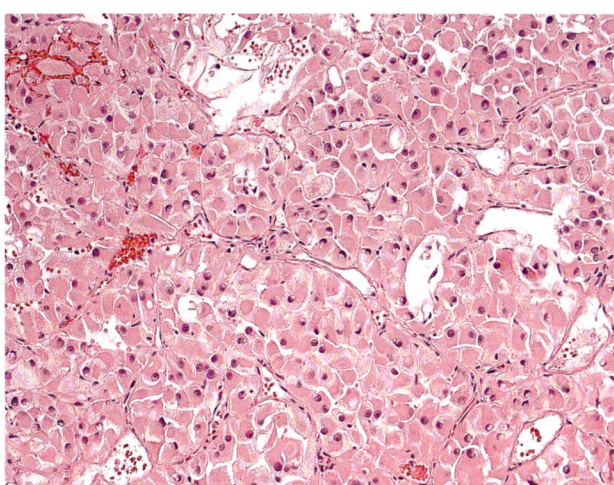

Figure 3.36. Rarely clear cell renal cell carcinoma (RCC) can have large areas of eosinophilic cell pattern, mimicking an oncocytic neoplasm. This tumor also had classic areas of clear cell RCC elsewhere in the tumor.

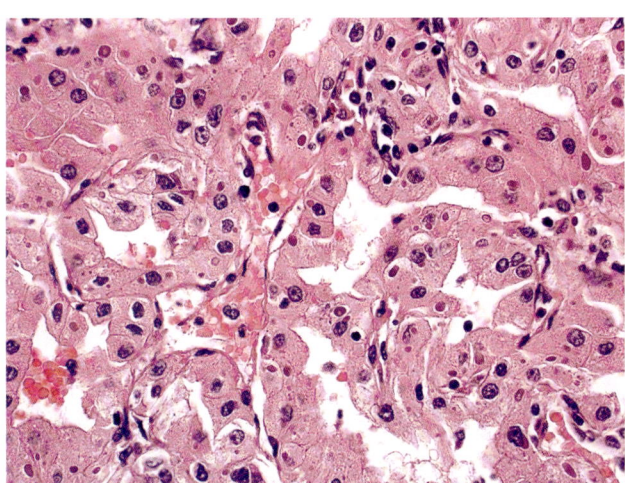

Figure 3.37. Eosinophilic areas of clear cell renal cell carcinoma can contain hyaline globules of various sizes and shapes. This case includes dense globules of variable size.

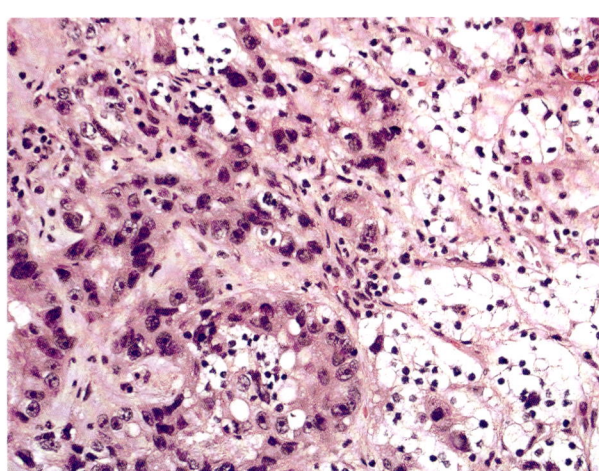

Figure 3.38. Rare examples of clear cell renal cell carcinoma can transition to a poorly differentiated component that may mimic a nonrenal adenocarcinoma. Differential diagnosis for this pattern could include urothelial carcinoma or metastatic adenocarcinoma of another origin, if viewed in isolation.

Papillary Renal Cell Carcinoma With Clear Cell Change

Papillary RCC is the second most common subtype of adult renal cancer, after clear cell RCC. Its prototypical features are discussed in more detail under the section on the papillary pattern. However, in some cases, possibly as much as 39%, papillary RCC can contain cells with clear cytoplasm, mimicking clear cell RCC (Figures 3.56-3.60).[37,54] Fortunately, awareness of a few clues can help distinguish these two entities.

PEARLS AND PITFALLS: Papillary Renal Cell Carcinoma With Clear Cell Change (Figures 3.55-3.61)

- Cells often have vacuolated rather than empty cytoplasm (Figure 3.56)
- Foamy macrophages often present, with similar consistency of cytoplasm compared to the tumor cells (Figure 3.57)[54]
- Psammoma bodies may be present (Figure 3.56) (very rare in clear cell RCC)
- Very strong immunohistochemical staining for AMACR (Figure 3.59), similar intensity to proximal tubules, supports papillary RCC
- Cytokeratin 7 often diffusely positive, contrasting to true clear cell RCC (Figure 3.60)[37]
- Carbonic anhydrase IX usually negative or minimal (labeling only areas of necrosis or hypoxia) (Figures 3.61 and 3.62)
- Trisomy of chromosome 7 or 17 by FISH or copy number assessment would favor papillary RCC, but likely not necessary in most cases[54]
- Loss of chromosome 3p, although generally favoring clear cell RCC, may not be entirely specific, with some losses reported in papillary RCC with clear cell change[37,54]
- Markers of MITF family translocation RCC negative (TFE3 or TFEB proteins, cathepsin K, melanocytic markers)[55]

Chromophobe Renal Cell Carcinoma, Classic Type

Chromophobe RCC is usually considered the third most common subtype of renal cancer, at approximately 5% or less of adult renal cancers.[56] Grossly, it typically forms a tan-colored mass, which may have a central scar (Figures 3.63 and 3.64), or for eosinophilic variant, the color may be red-brown, more similar to that of oncocytoma (Figure 3.65).

KEY FEATURES: Chromophobe Renal Cell Carcinoma

- Often unencapsulated or incompletely encapsulated (Figure 3.66)[57]
- Cells with pale staining or flocculent eosinophilic cytoplasm, often with admixture of both cell types (Figure 3.67)
- Often prominent cell borders, resembling plant cells (Figure 3.66)

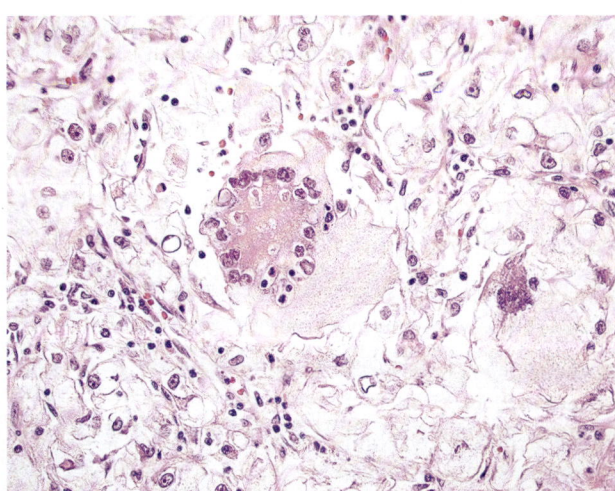

Figure 3.39. Occasional high-grade clear cell renal cell carcinoma tumors can contain syncytial-type giant cells with numerous nuclei.

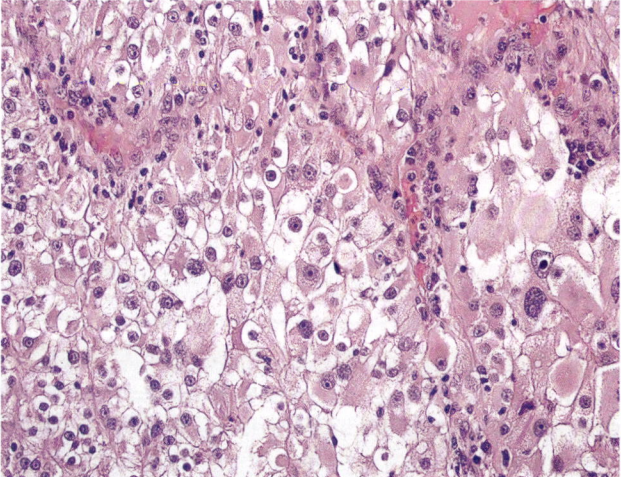

Figure 3.40. Rhabdoid features in clear cell renal cell carcinoma manifest as central eosinophilic globules within the cytoplasm that mimic rhabdomyoblastic cells (although without immunohistochemical evidence of skeletal muscle differentiation).

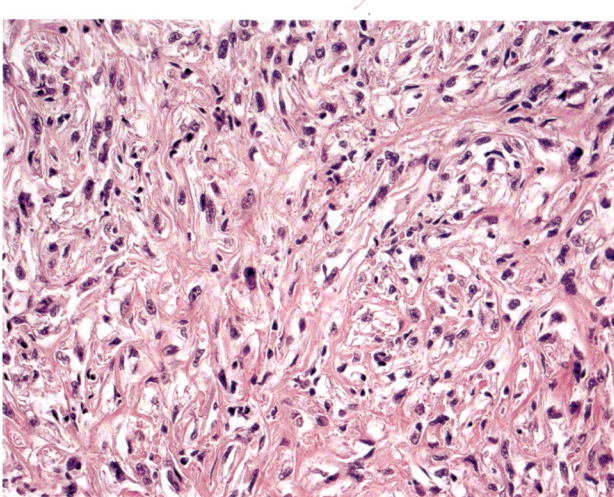

Figure 3.41. Higher magnification in this case of rhabdoid clear cell renal cell carcinoma shows clear cytoplasm with central eosinophilic material, mimicking rhabdomyoblasts.

Figure 3.42. Sarcomatoid changes in renal cell carcinoma may also be deceptive. This case shows a hint of clear cytoplasm but otherwise resembles a spindle cell sarcoma.

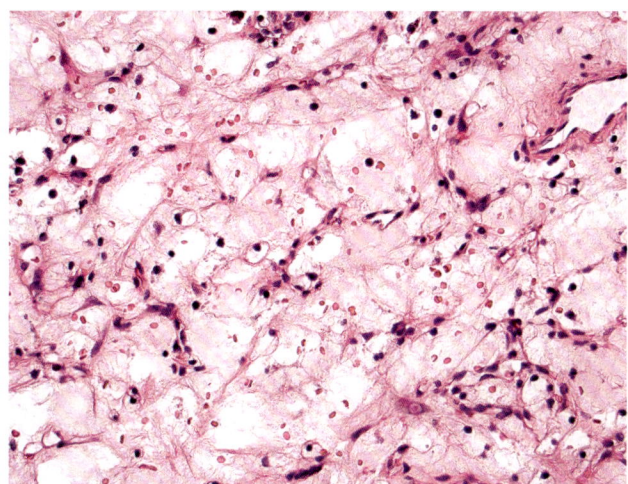

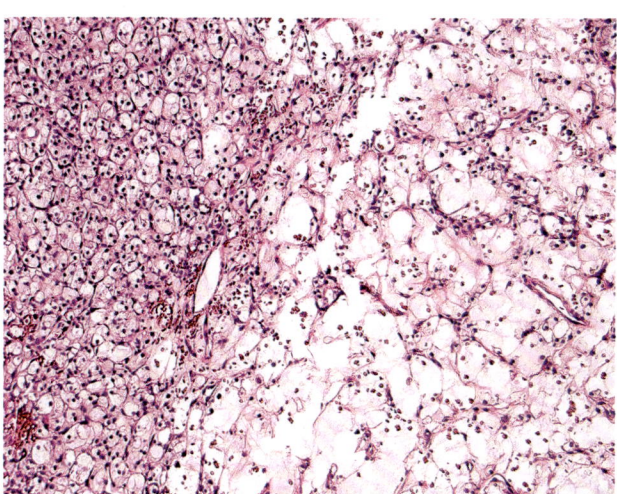

Figure 3.43. Degenerative changes or scar in clear cell renal cell carcinoma (RCC) can be deceptive if encountered in a biopsy sample. This field comes from the center of a clear cell RCC tumor and contains vasculature with inconspicuous tumor cells, mimicking lymphocytes or capillaries.

Figure 3.44. Other areas of the same tumor from Figure 3.43 show transition to typical clear cell renal cell carcinoma.

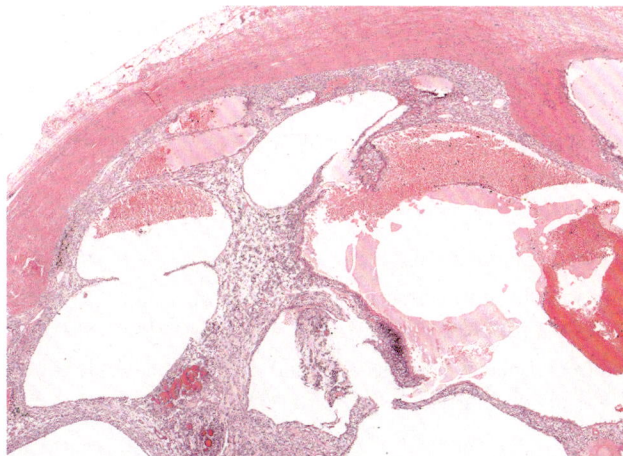

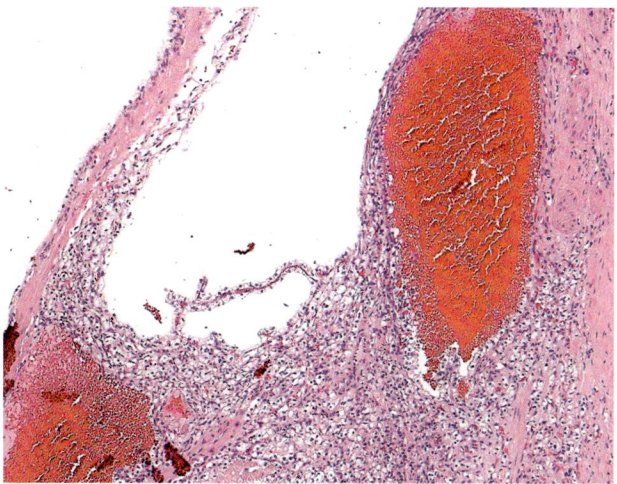

Figure 3.45. Cystic changes can be variably present in clear cell renal cell carcinoma (RCC), which some authors have associated with favorable behavior. This tumor is predominantly cystic but contains solid areas within the walls, consistent with cystic clear cell RCC.

Figure 3.46. Higher magnification of cystic clear cell renal cell carcinoma shows solid areas adjacent to cysts lined by similar cells.

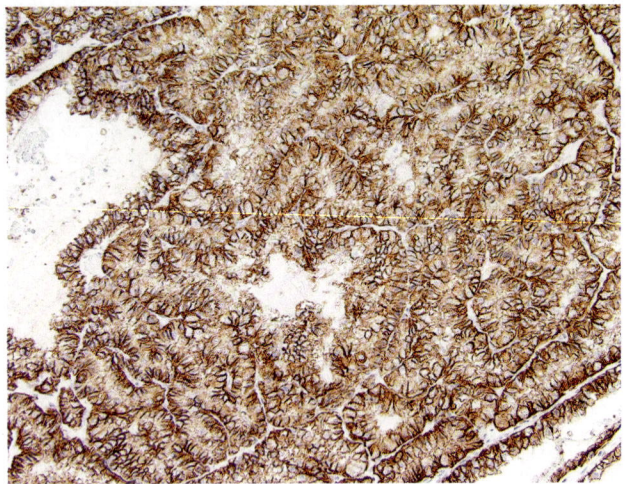

Figure 3.47. Carbonic anhydrase IX typically shows diffuse membranous staining in clear cell renal cell carcinoma.

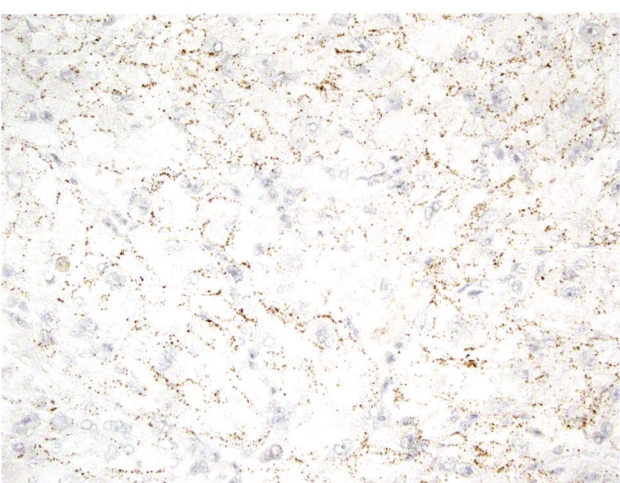

Figure 3.48. Carbonic anhydrase IX staining can be decreased in high-grade, poorly differentiated, or sarcomatoid clear cell renal cell carcinoma (RCC) tumors. This example included spindle cell and rhabdoid components with markedly decreased carbonic anhydrase IX staining in those areas, compared to diffuse staining in typical clear cell RCC areas.

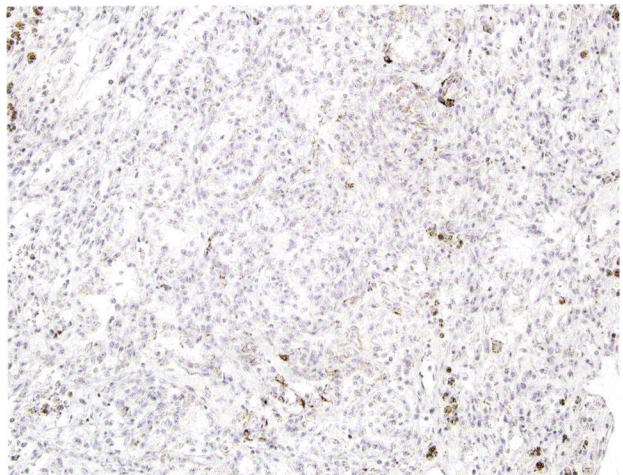

Figure 3.49. Cytokeratin 7 staining is usually minimal in clear cell renal cell carcinoma, if any.

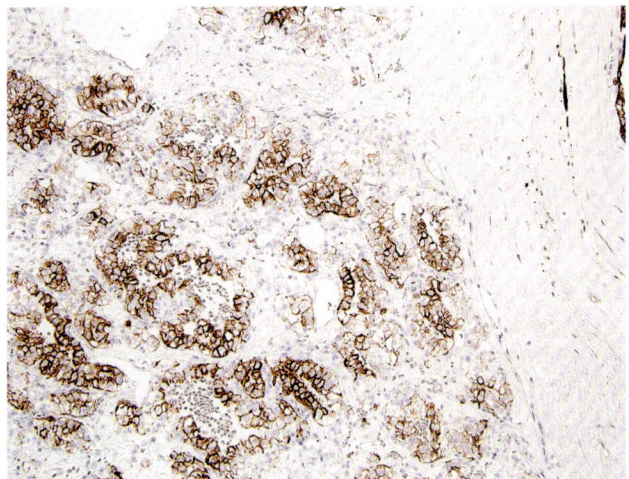

Figure 3.50. Rarely, clear cell renal cell carcinoma can have greater amounts of cytokeratin 7 staining.

- Nuclear size variation, from small to large (Figure 3.68)
- Large, wrinkled nuclei with dark, smudged nuclear chromatin ("raisinoid") (Figure 3.66)
- May have intranuclear cytoplasmic invaginations (Figure 3.69)
- Perinuclear clearing ("halo") (Figure 3.70)
- Solid or trabecular growth pattern (Figure 3.71)
- "Missing nuclei:" cytoplasm is so voluminous that some cells appear to have no nuclei (plane of section entirely misses the nucleus, Figure 3.72)
- Colloidal iron stain—positive in cytoplasm (Figures 3.73 and 3.74) but variable results depending on laboratory technical conditions
- Immunohistochemistry[58]
  - Negative for vimentin, in contrast to clear cell or papillary RCC (Figure 3.75)
  - Often substantial staining for cytokeratin 7 (but decreased in eosinophilic variant) (Figure 3.76)

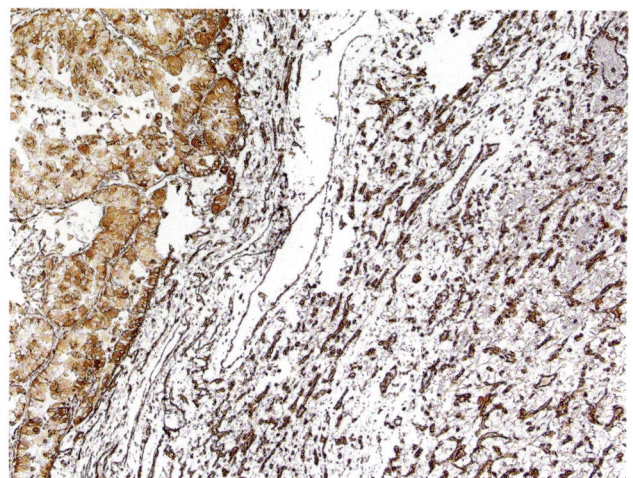

Figure 3.51. Vimentin is often positive in clear cell renal cell carcinoma, especially higher-grade areas. In this case, low-grade areas (right) are negative, whereas high-grade areas (left) are positive.

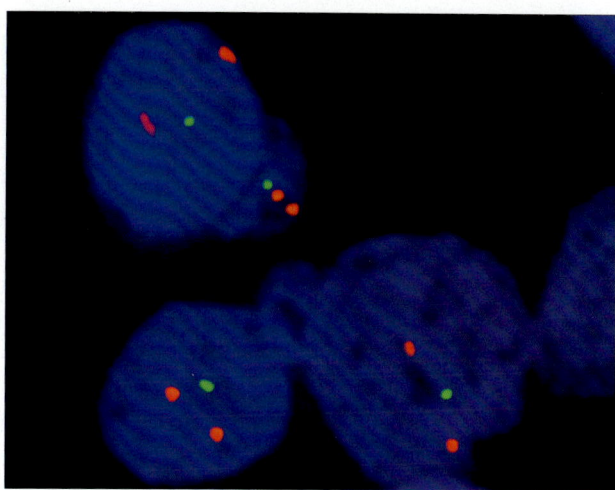

Figure 3.52. Copy number analyses or fluorescence in situ hybridization (FISH) can be used to support a diagnosis of clear cell renal cell carcinoma in difficult cases. This example shows 3p25 deletion via FISH with two copies of the centromere (red) but only one copy of the 3p25 region (green).

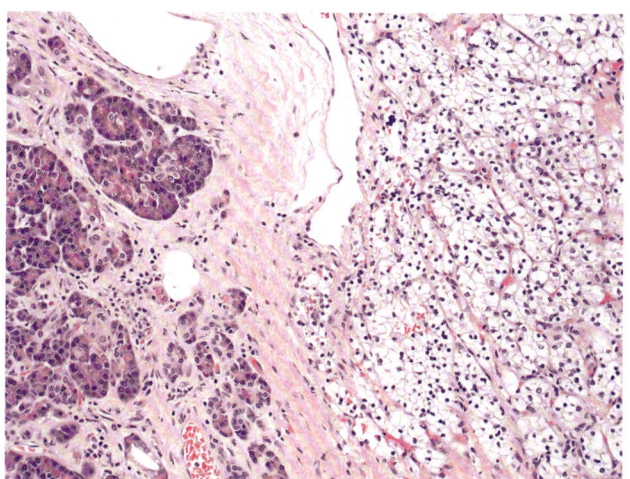

Figure 3.53. Clear cell renal cell carcinoma has an unusual predilection to metastasize to the pancreas (left).

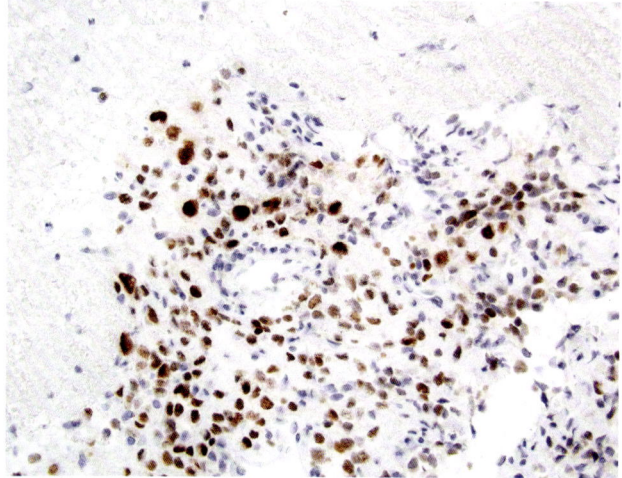

Figure 3.54. Nuclear staining for PAX8 is generally supportive of metastatic renal cell carcinoma in the appropriate context. This patient had metastatic disease involving bone with a suspicious renal lesion.

- Positive for KIT (CD117, Figure 3.77)
- Carbonic anhydrase IX negative or minimal, in contrast to clear cell RCC (Figure 3.78)

The behavior of chromophobe RCC is generally favorable[45,46]; however, aggressive behavior is possible, especially with sarcomatoid change (Figure 3.79), necrosis (Figure 3.80), or vascular invasion (Figure 3.81).[59,60] Some prior studies have suggested that the rate of sarcomatoid change is higher in chromophobe RCC than other RCC types (despite the much lower prevalence of the tumor type overall)[59,61]; however, this has been challenged by other large series finding low rates of sarcomatoid change.[60] Since the nuclei are inherently atypical in chromophobe RCC, grading using the typical system does not appear to have value and is not recommended.[62-65] Some novel systems of grading have been proposed, the most well-known being the chromophobe tumor grade described by Paner et al.[66] This system divides tumors with the typical pattern of widely spaced nuclei (grade 1) from tumors with more overlapping and crowding of nuclei (grade 2) and those

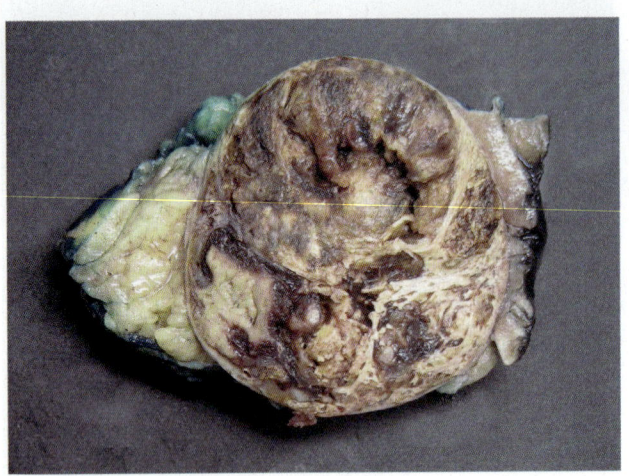

Figure 3.55. This papillary renal cell carcinoma (RCC) has heterogeneous gross cut surfaces with some areas appearing yellow, mimicking clear cell RCC, likely due to foamy cells.

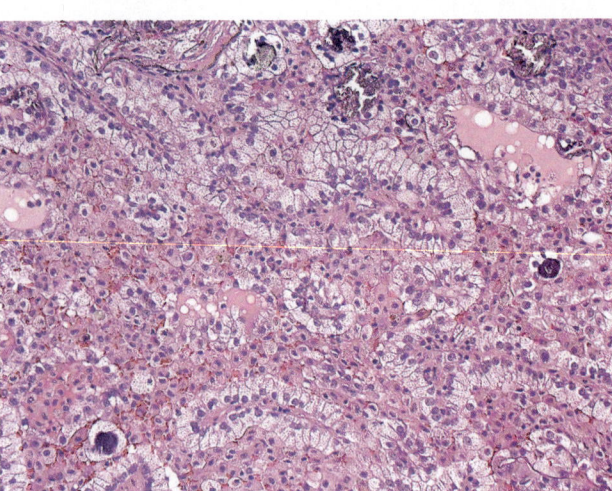

Figure 3.56. In contrast to clear cell renal cell carcinoma (RCC), the cytoplasm of papillary RCC with clear cell change is usually highly vacuolated. This example also has psammoma bodies, which are rare for clear cell RCC.

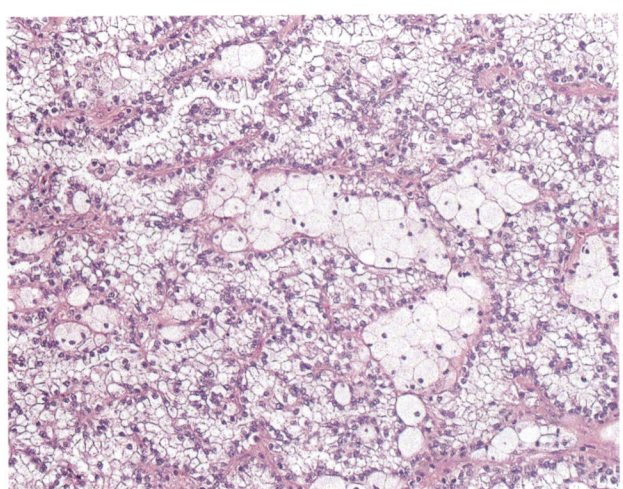

Figure 3.57. In this papillary renal cell carcinoma with clear cell change, the tumor cells have a similar cytoplasmic quality to intermingled foamy macrophages.

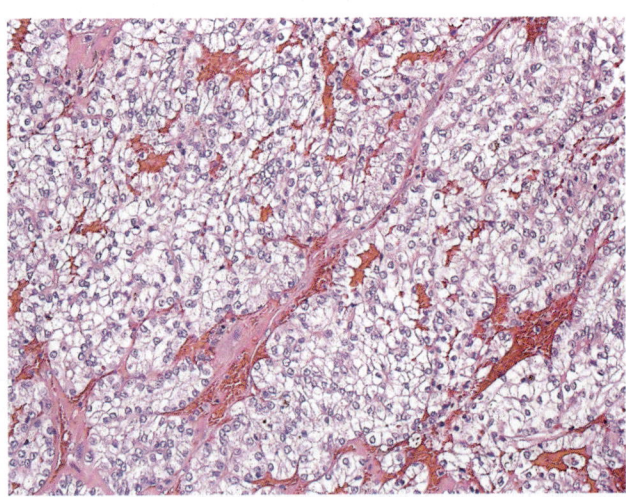

Figure 3.58. This case of papillary renal cell carcinoma (RCC) with clear cell change could be easily mistaken for clear cell RCC if this area were encountered in isolation. Sampling additional areas of the tumor, or for a biopsy sample, immunohistochemistry, may be helpful to recognize the correct classification.

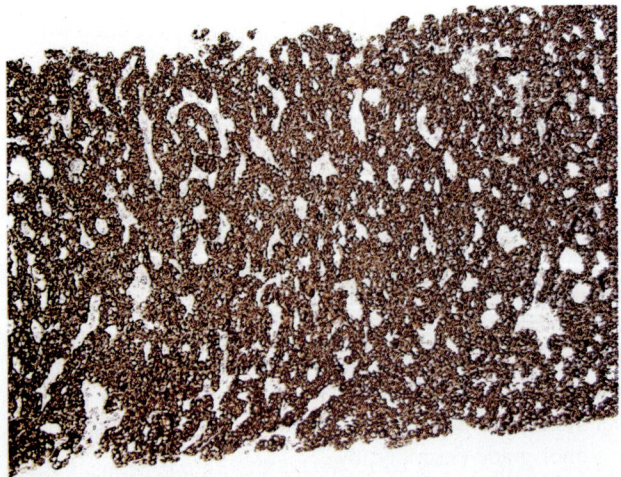

Figure 3.59. AMACR is diffusely positive in this papillary renal cell carcinoma with clear cell change in a core biopsy sample.

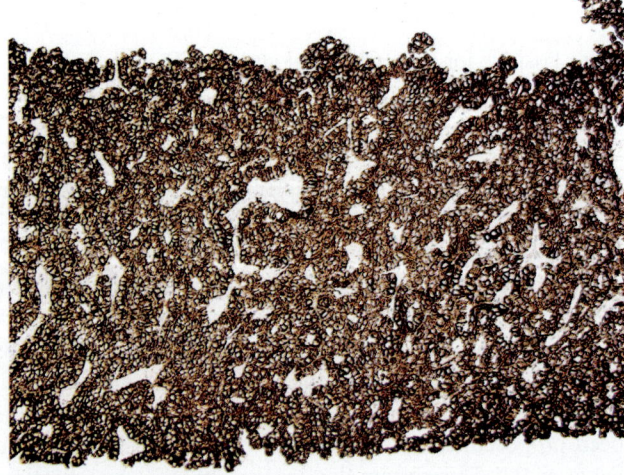

Figure 3.60. Cytokeratin 7 staining is also diffuse in the same case from Figure 3.59.

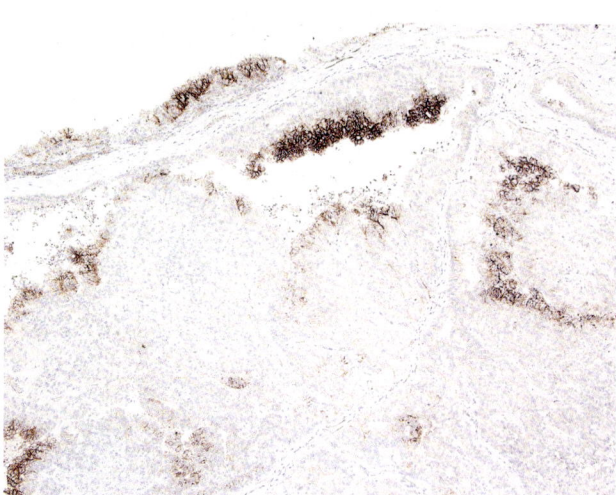

Figure 3.61. Carbonic anhydrase IX staining is negative in the papillary renal cell carcinoma (RCC) with clear cell change from Figures 3.59 and 3.60, contrasting to clear cell RCC.

Figure 3.62. Focal staining for carbonic anhydrase IX can be observed in non–clear cell renal cell carcinomas, usually in areas of ischemia or necrosis. In this case, there is some staining in cystic areas, but large solid areas are negative.

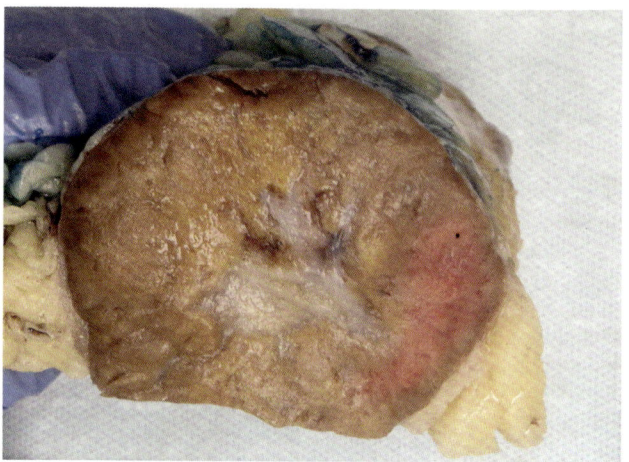

Figure 3.63. This chromophobe renal cell carcinoma has a central scar, which is not specific for oncocytoma.

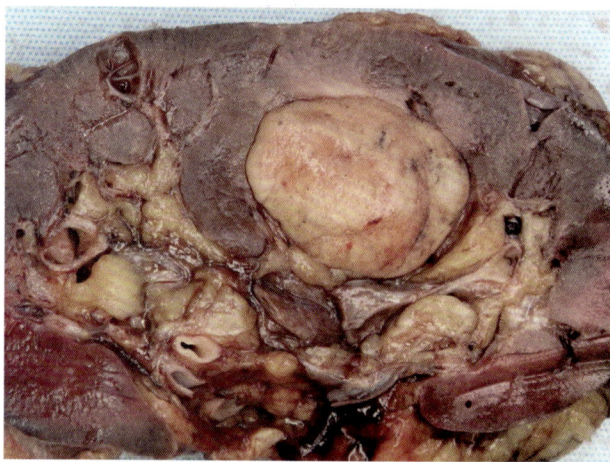

Figure 3.64. Some chromophobe renal cell carcinomas (RCCs) have a pale tan color that differs from the golden-yellow or orange cut surface of clear cell RCC.

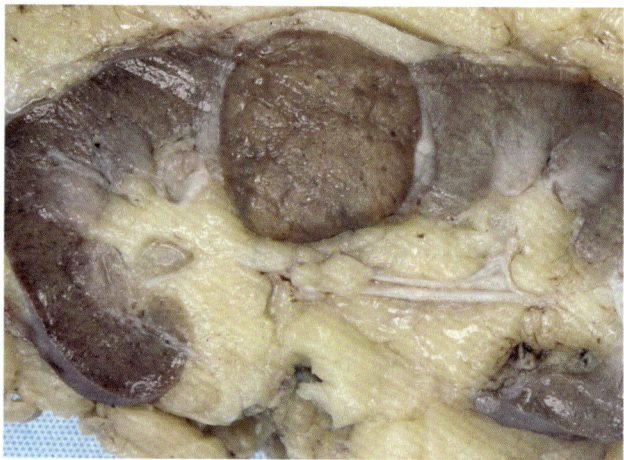

Figure 3.65. This chromophobe renal cell carcinoma has a red-brown color, similar to the normal renal parenchyma, which would raise a differential diagnosis with oncocytoma.

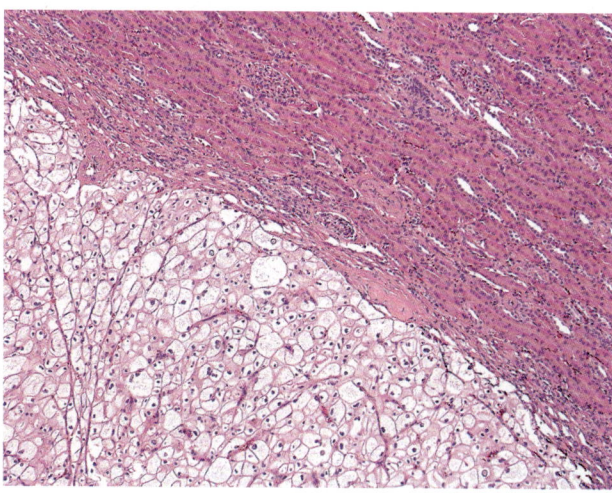

Figure 3.66. Chromophobe tumors are often unencapsulated or incompletely encapsulated, contrasting to clear cell renal cell carcinoma, which usually has a fibrous pseudocapsule.

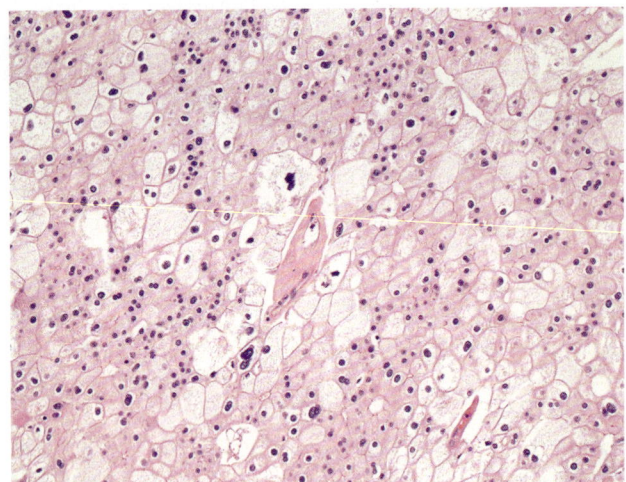

Figure 3.67. Typical cytologic features of chromophobe renal cell carcinoma include cells with prominent borders (resembling plant cells), variable pale to eosinophilic cytoplasm, and scattered wrinkled nuclei ("raisinoid").

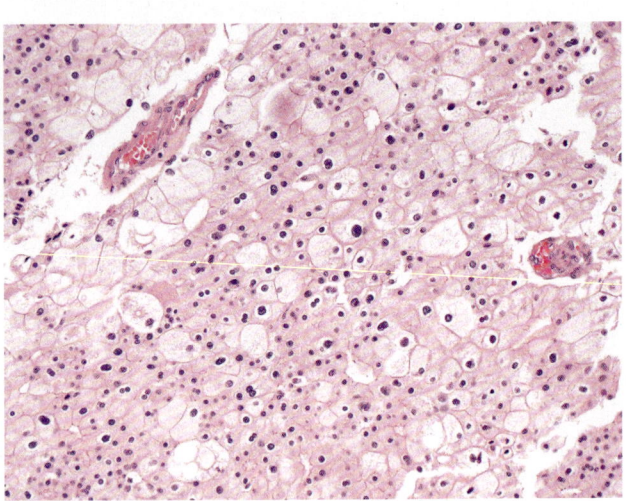

Figure 3.68. Nuclei of chromophobe renal cell carcinoma often vary considerably in size.

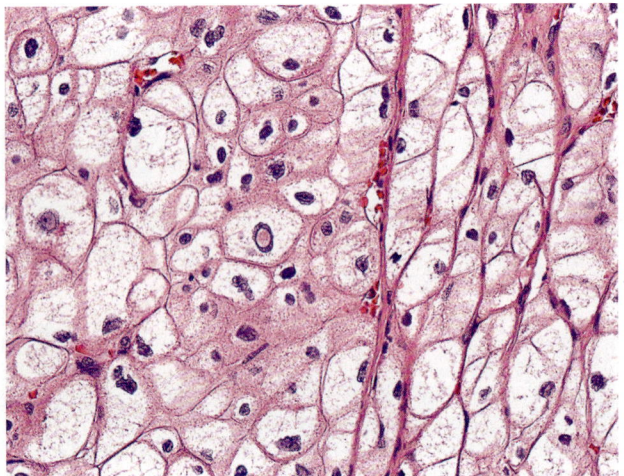

Figure 3.69. Intranuclear cytoplasmic invaginations (pseudoinclusions) are sometimes present in chromophobe renal cell carcinoma.

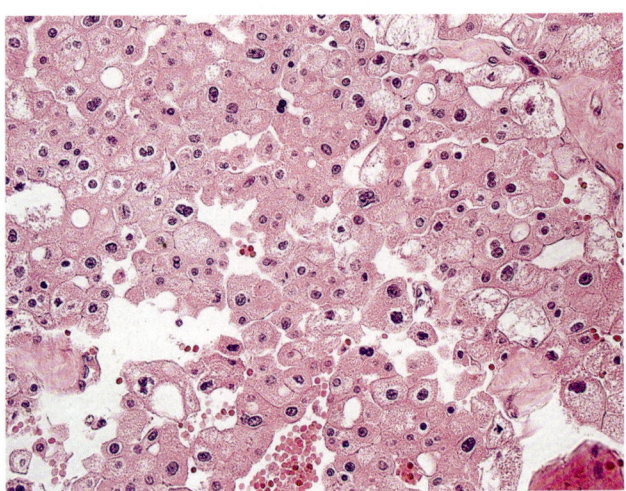

Figure 3.70. Perinuclear cytoplasmic clearing ("halos") are often present in chromophobe cells with eosinophilic cytoplasm.

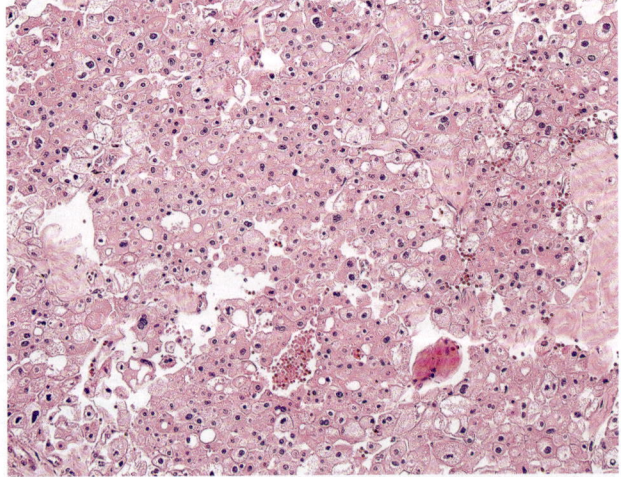

Figure 3.71. The growth of chromophobe renal cell carcinoma (RCC) may be diffuse or trabecular, contrasting to the discrete packets of cells circumscribed by a capillary vascular network in clear cell RCC.

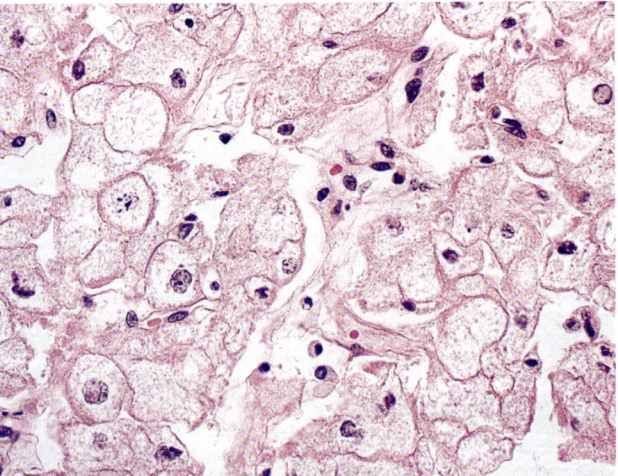

Figure 3.72. In chromophobe tumors, some cells often appear to have no nuclei, likely because the cytoplasm is so voluminous the nucleus was entirely missed in the plane of section.

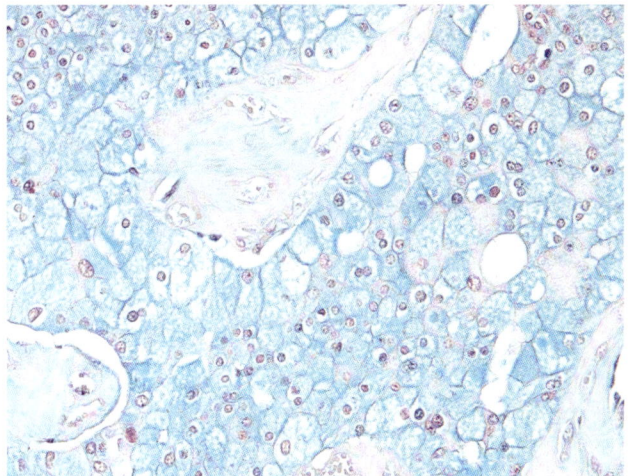

Figure 3.73. Classically, the colloidal iron stain (modified Mowry shown here) will show diffuse cytoplasmic staining of chromophobe renal cell carcinoma, although ideal staining conditions can be technically challenging.

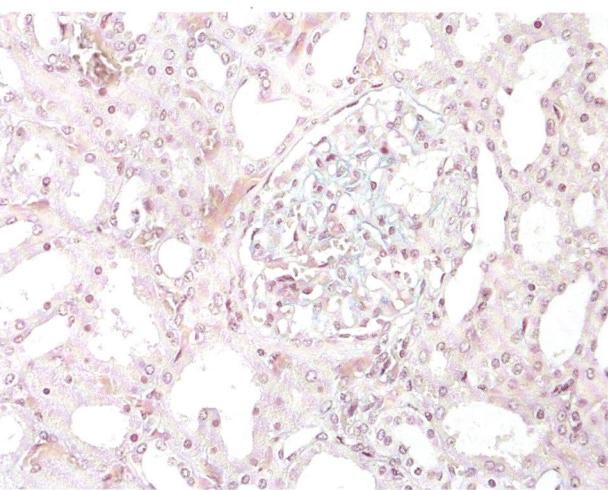

Figure 3.74. To verify a well-stained colloidal iron stain, there should be outlining of glomerular cells with minimal to no staining of proximal tubules.

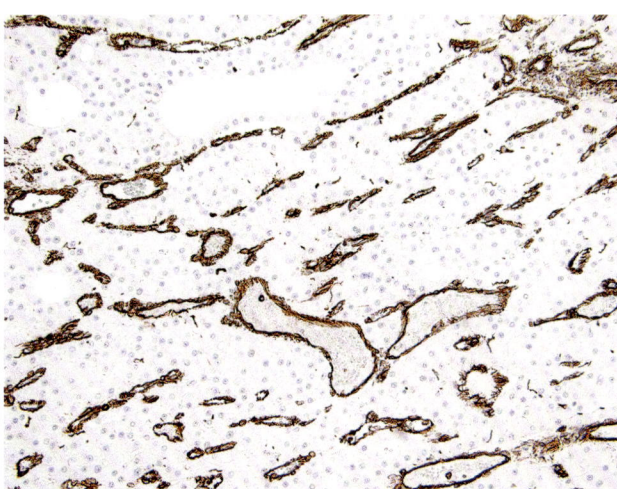

Figure 3.75. Vimentin immunohistochemistry is consistently negative in chromophobe renal cell carcinoma (RCC), contrasting to the expected pattern of many other RCC types.

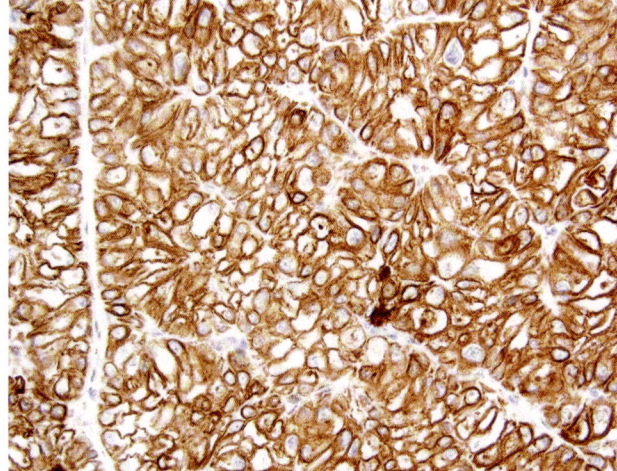

Figure 3.76. In classic chromophobe renal cell carcinoma, cytokeratin 7 often shows diffuse staining with membranous accentuation. However, the extent of staining is often markedly lower in eosinophilic chromophobe tumors.

with anaplastic nuclear features.[66] However, this system has not gained widespread usage at present and is not required in reporting schemes.[13]

Genetically, chromophobe RCC most commonly has rearrangements of the *TERT* promoter, mutations of mitochondrial genes, and mutations of *TP53* or *PTEN*.[58,67] With respect to copy number pattern, chromophobe RCC tends to have copy losses of chromosomes Y, 1, 2, 6, 10, 13, 17, and 21 and lesser rates of loss for chromosomes 3, 5, 8, 9, 11, and 18.[56,58] However, chromosomal gains have also been noted by some authors.[68] For difficult cases, particularly with respect to the eosinophilic variant, some form of copy number assessment may be helpful, such as conventional cytogenetic karyotyping, FISH, or copy number assays; however, this is less necessary for distinction between chromophobe and clear cell RCC, which can usually be resolved with morphology and immunohistochemistry (especially KIT, carbonic anhydrase IX, vimentin, and cytokeratin 7). Distinction of eosinophilic chromophobe from oncocytoma is discussed further under the oncocytic/eosinophilic pattern.

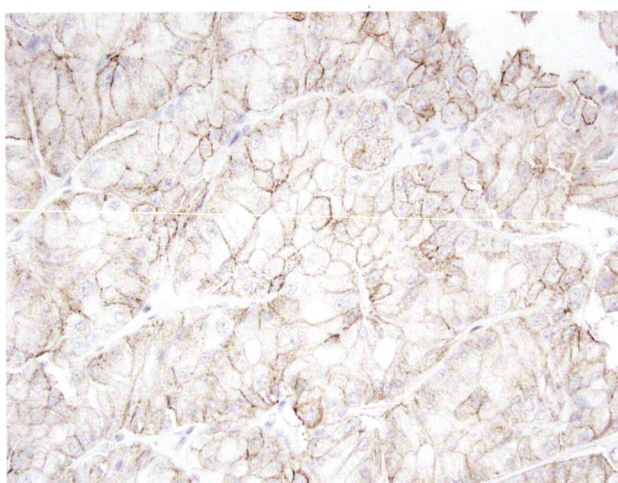

Figure 3.77. KIT (CD117) staining is often positive with a membranous pattern in chromophobe renal cell carcinoma (RCC), contrasting to clear cell RCC.

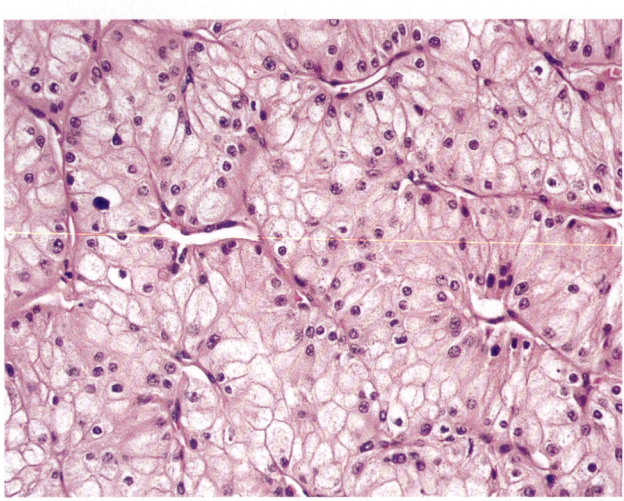

Figure 3.78. This case of chromophobe renal cell carcinoma (RCC) (same case from Figures 3.76 and 3.77) raised a differential diagnosis with clear cell RCC due to the nested arrangement of cells with prominent capillary vascular network and less conspicuous nuclear size variation than usual. However, the immunohistochemistry in this case clarified the diagnosis.

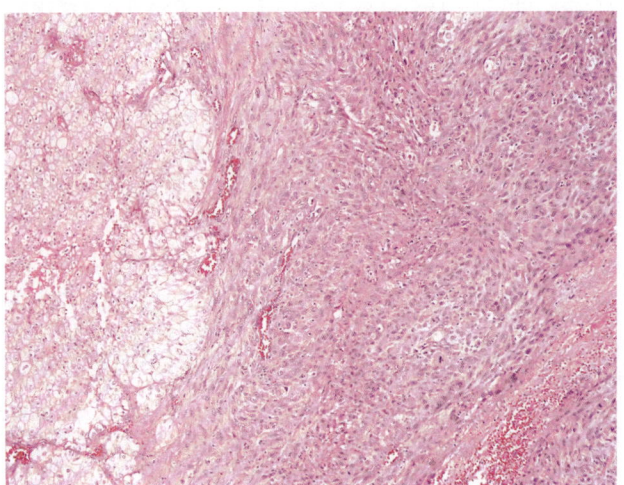

Figure 3.79. Aggressive features in chromophobe renal cell carcinoma include sarcomatoid change, as shown in this case with transition from chromophobe morphology (left) to spindle cell pattern (right).

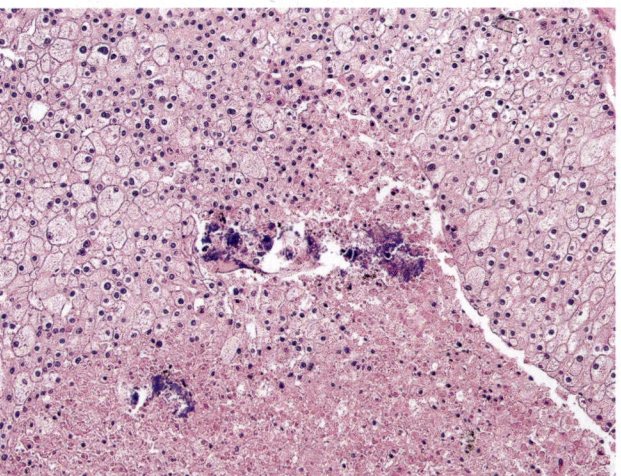

Figure 3.80. Necrosis has also been associated with more aggressive behavior from chromophobe renal cell carcinoma in some studies. This example shows coagulative necrosis with calcification at bottom center.

Clear Cell Papillary Renal Cell Carcinoma

Clear cell papillary RCC is interesting in that it is a distinct entity in renal tumor classification[69,70] that was only recognized as different from clear cell RCC in 2006.[71] Now, with increased recognition, it is thought that this makes up as much as 3% to 4% of adult RCC, making it likely the fourth most common RCC subtype, approaching the incidence of chromophobe RCC.[72,73] These tumors are almost always small (predominantly stage pT1a) and low grade (grade 1-2).[72] Although they microscopically resemble clear cell RCC, they often do not grossly have its golden-yellow or orange color (Figures 3.82-3.84).

KEY FEATURES: Clear Cell Papillary Renal Cell Carcinoma

- Composed of
  - Solid areas nearly identical to clear cell RCC (Figure 3.85)
  - Glandular structures with a branching configuration (Figures 3.86-3.88), in contrast to solid round nests of clear cell RCC

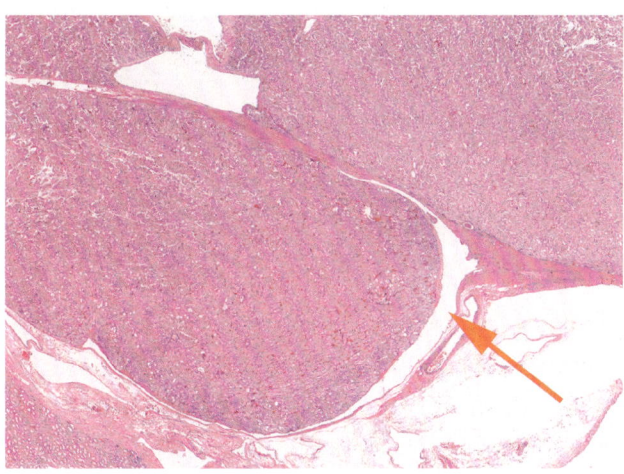

Figure 3.81. Vascular invasion is also a potential adverse feature in chromophobe renal cell carcinoma. This example shows a large polypoid protrusion of tumor into a renal sinus vein (arrow).

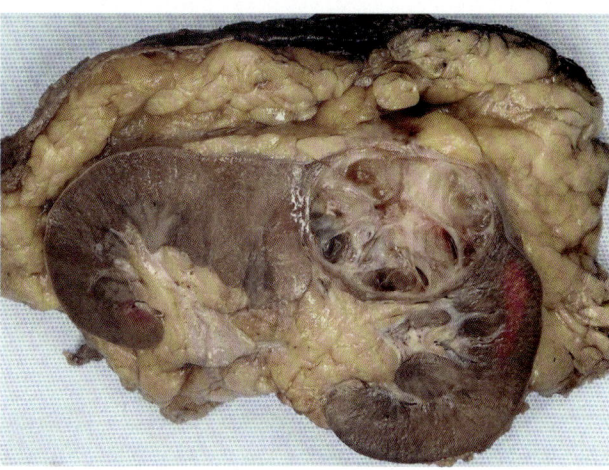

Figure 3.82. Clear cell papillary renal cell carcinoma (RCC) may form solid or cystic tumors that are not necessarily golden-yellow like clear cell RCC. This mass forms a solid and cystic lesion with white areas that slightly bulges beyond the contour of the kidney.

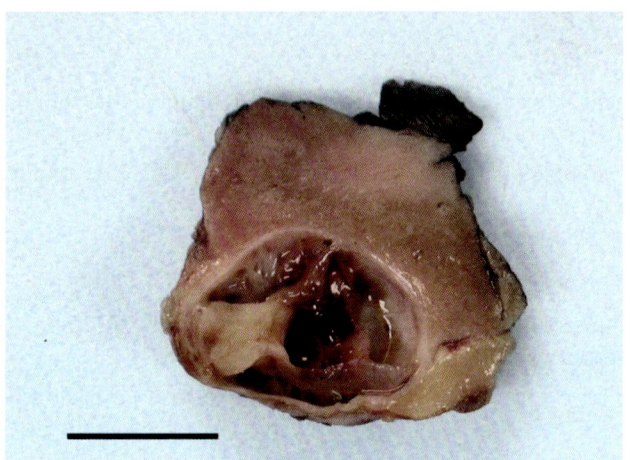

Figure 3.83. This example of clear cell papillary renal cell carcinoma in a partial nephrectomy forms a small extensively cystic mass with almost no grossly appreciable solid component (scale bar 1 cm).

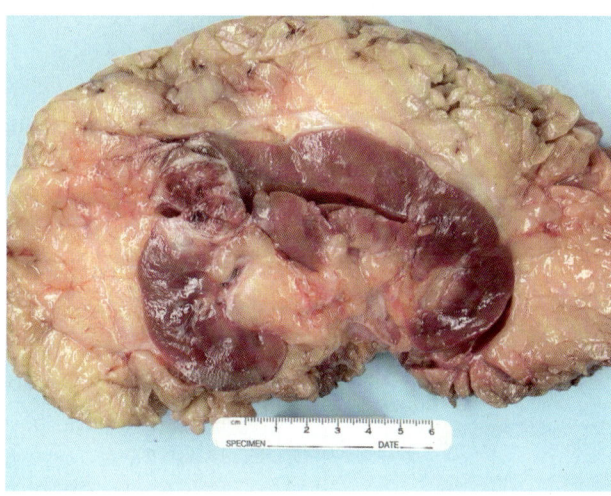

Figure 3.84. This example of clear cell papillary renal cell carcinoma shows a more solid white-tan to red mass.

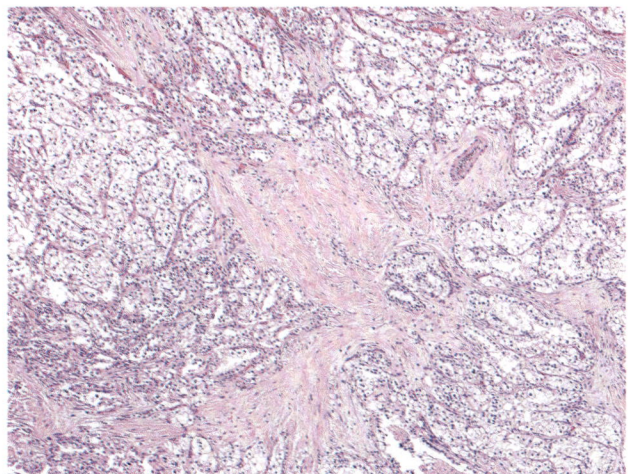

Figure 3.85. Some areas of clear cell papillary (RCC) may be difficult or impossible to distinguish from clear cell RCC based on morphology alone. This example shows solid nests resembling clear cell RCC. The stroma is slightly prominent, which may be a clue, although this alone is not specific.

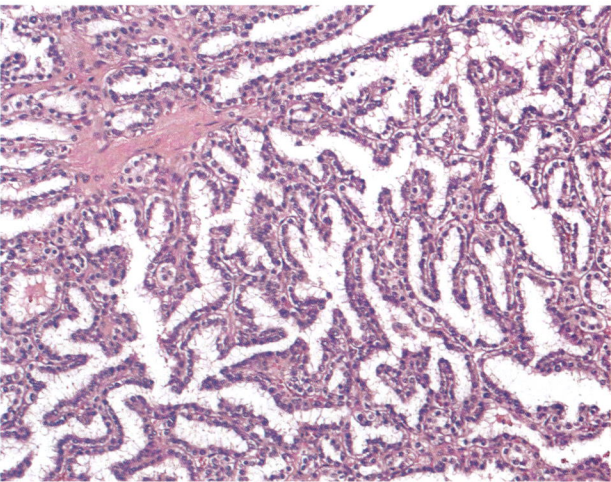

Figure 3.86. Branched glandular structures are a clue to possible recognition of clear cell papillary renal cell carcinoma.

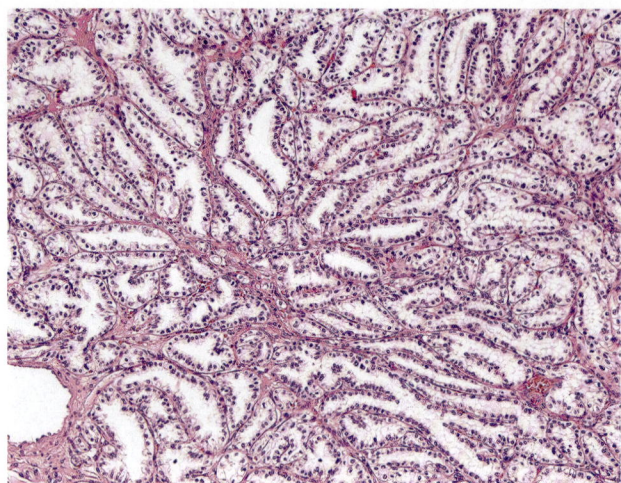

Figure 3.87. This field of a clear cell papillary renal cell carcinoma (RCC) shows tubular or glandular structures with predominantly clear cytoplasm. There is slightly more branching than a usual clear cell RCC, which may be a clue to the diagnosis.

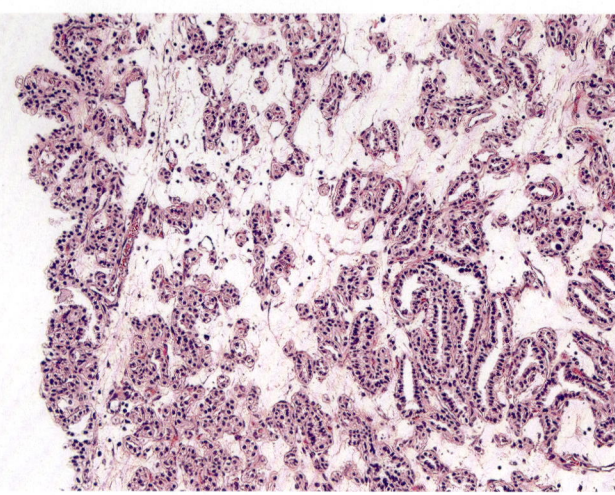

Figure 3.88. This clear cell papillary renal cell carcinoma demonstrates some branching glands, edematous stroma, and focal papillary structures in a cystic space at the left edge.

- Cells with nuclear alignment above the basement membrane, resembling the subnuclear vacuoles of early secretory endometrium or "piano keys" (Figures 3.89-3.91)
- Cysts with small or more complex papillary structures (Figures 3.92-3.95), usually blunt rather than elongated
- Fibrous stroma between glands (Figure 3.85)
- Immunohistochemistry[72,74-79]
  - Carbonic anhydrase IX diffuse membrane staining, similar to clear cell RCC, sometimes with "cup-shaped" pattern (Figure 3.96)
  - Diffuse, uniform positive for cytokeratin 7 (Figure 3.97), unexpected for clear cell RCC
  - Negative for CD10 (Figure 3.98), in contrast to clear cell RCC
  - Negative or minimal weak staining for AMACR (Figure 3.99), contrasting to papillary RCC
  - Often staining for GATA3 (Figure 3.100), suggesting distal nephron phenotype
  - Often staining for high molecular weight cytokeratin (Figure 3.101), suggesting distal nephron phenotype
- Genetics:
  - Despite resemblance to clear cell RCC, almost all clear cell papillary RCCs have been found to lack chromosome 3p25 deletion or *VHL* mutations,[80-85] with rare exceptions of uncertain significance[86]

The importance of clear cell papillary RCC is that it has exceedingly favorable behavior.[87,88] To date, no definite examples with well-characterized pathology from multiple series have been proven to metastasize, and the overwhelming majority have been pT1a. However, a recent case report documented a metastatic lesion with features in keeping with clear cell papillary RCC, including absence of *VHL* mutation/chromosome 3p25 loss. For this case, the corresponding primary tumor was never resected.[89] However, this does raise the question of whether rare metastasis from clear cell papillary RCC is possible, or if primary tumors left untreated can progress to a more aggressive carcinoma. For as yet not understood reasons, clear cell papillary RCC does have a tendency to be multiple and/or bilateral, even in the absence of end-stage renal disease.[72] In general, thinking is that this entity may be a candidate for reclassification as a benign or low malignant potential tumor in future schemes, although additional data are needed.

PEARLS AND PITFALLS: Clear Cell Papillary-Like Tumors With Imperfect Features

- Occasional clear cell RCCs can have overlapping features of clear cell papillary RCC,[29,90,91] such as branched glands, nuclear alignment, and focal papillary structures (Figures 3.102-3.104)
- Typically, the immunohistochemistry in these tumors does not show the expected pattern of clear cell papillary RCC, such as with positive AMACR or CD10 (Figure 3.103)
- This has a high rate of correlation with chromosome 3p deletion using FISH,[29,91] suggesting that these are better classified as clear cell RCCs
- Aggressive behavior, higher tumor stage, and necrosis have also been noted in these tumors with imperfect features,[90] supporting classification as clear cell RCC
- Patients with VHL disease may also have tumors resembling clear cell papillary RCC (Figure 3.105), but similarly the immunohistochemical profile usually shows an imperfect staining pattern, favoring classification as clear cell RCC[91]
- Some translocation RCCs, such as those with *NONO* fusion, may have nuclear alignment mimicking clear cell papillary RCC (Figure 3.106), although usually accompanied by higher-grade nuclear features
  - Psammoma bodies would be atypical for clear cell papillary RCC

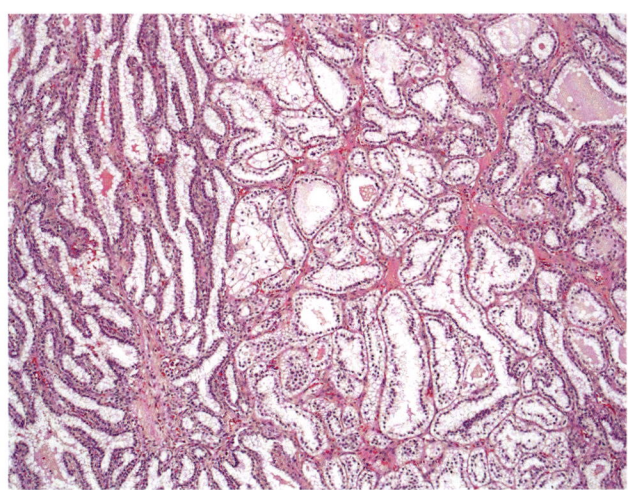

Figure 3.89. This clear cell papillary renal cell carcinoma shows a branched glandular configuration. At left, the cells have less cytoplasm, and at right the cells have more cytoplasm. Especially prominent at right is alignment of the nuclei at the same height in the cytoplasm.

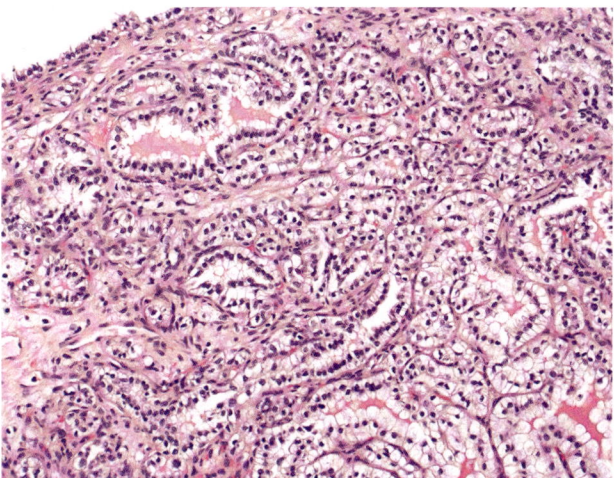

Figure 3.90. Nuclear alignment is a clue to the diagnosis of clear cell papillary renal cell carcinoma. This has been compared to the subnuclear vacuoles of early secretory phase endometrium. The cells resemble piano keys (where the nuclei are the black keys and the cytoplasm makes up the white keys).

SAMPLE NOTE: Clear Cell Papillary RCC

- Kidney, left, partial nephrectomy:
  - Clear cell papillary RCC, 2.5 cm greatest dimension
  - ISUP/WHO grade 2
  - Confined to the kidney (pT1a)
  - Margins negative

Comment: Clear cell papillary RCC is a recently recognized renal tumor that morphologically resembles clear cell RCC but using immunohistochemistry and molecular analysis

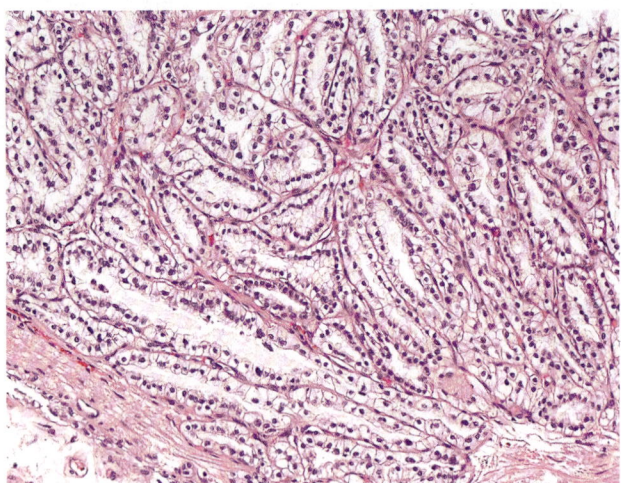

Figure 3.91. This example of clear cell papillary renal cell carcinoma demonstrates prominent nuclear alignment and slight branching of the glands.

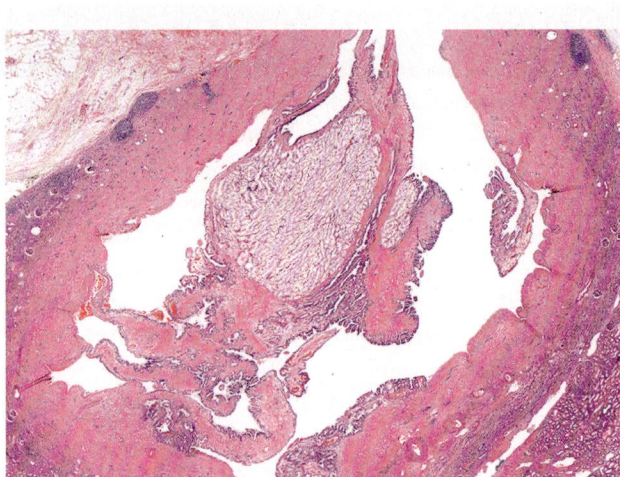

Figure 3.92. Many clear cell papillary renal cell carcinoma tumors are cystic. This example shows predominantly cystic architecture with some small papillae protruding into the cysts. There is a central solid nodule, which would preclude a diagnosis of multilocular cystic neoplasm of low malignant potential.

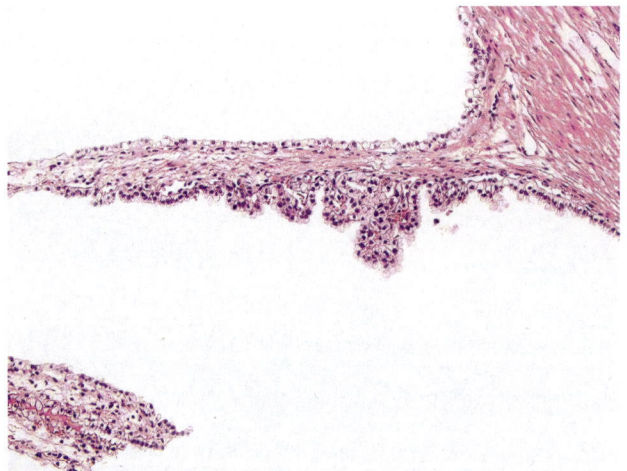

Figure 3.93. In extensively cystic examples of clear cell papillary renal cell carcinoma, there are often small stubby papillae that protrude into the cystic spaces.

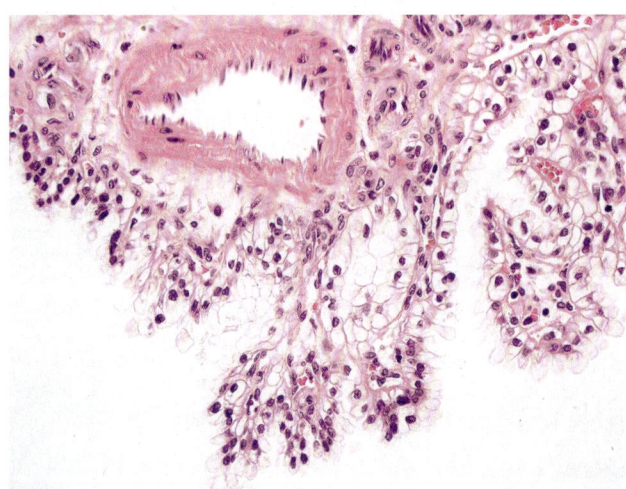

Figure 3.94. Papillary structures in clear cell papillary renal cell carcinoma are often small, with branching resembling fingers from a hand.

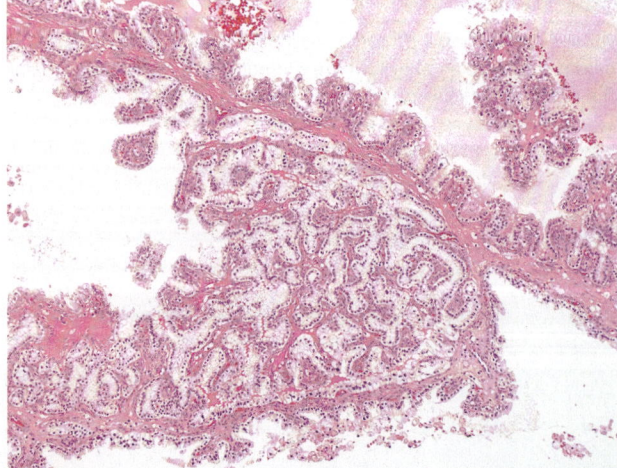

Figure 3.95. Occasional clear cell papillary tumors can have more florid papillary architecture, leading to confusion with papillary renal cell carcinoma.

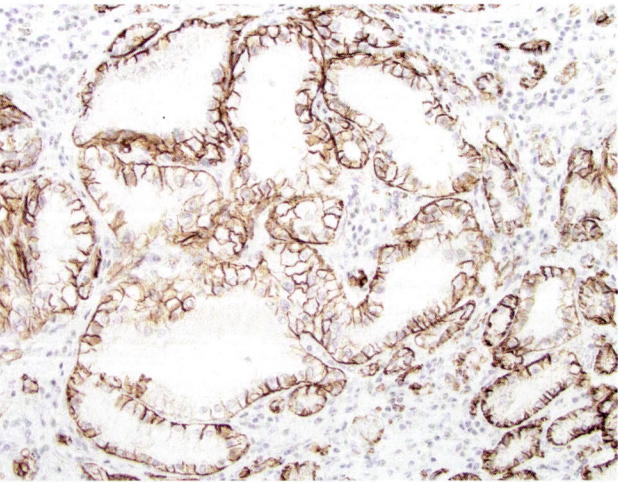

Figure 3.96. Carbonic anhydrase IX is diffusely positive in clear cell papillary renal cell carcinoma and sometimes shows a "cup-shaped" staining pattern, where the basal and lateral cell borders are positive but the apical staining is absent.

CHAPTER 3 KIDNEY **223**

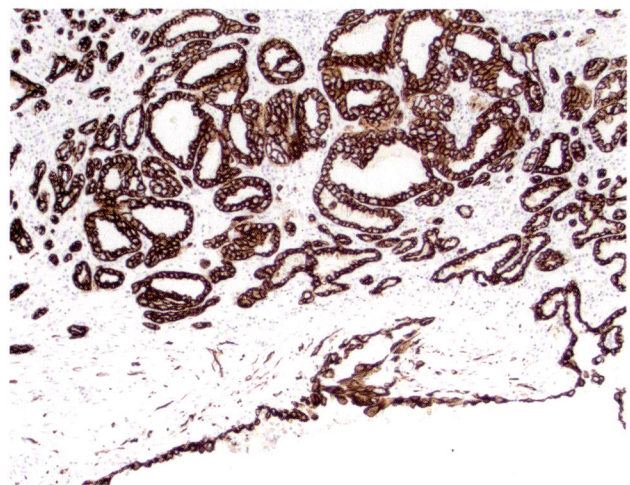

Figure 3.97. Cytokeratin 7 consistently shows diffuse positive staining in clear cell papillary renal cell carcinoma.

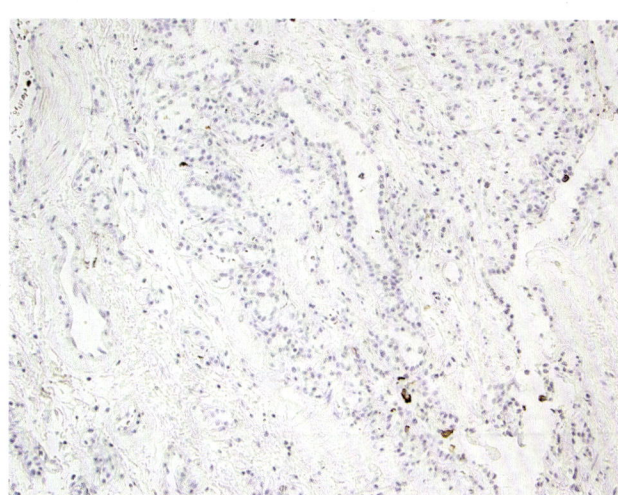

Figure 3.98. CD10 is negative in clear cell papillary renal cell carcinoma, although focal labeling of cystic areas has been reported.

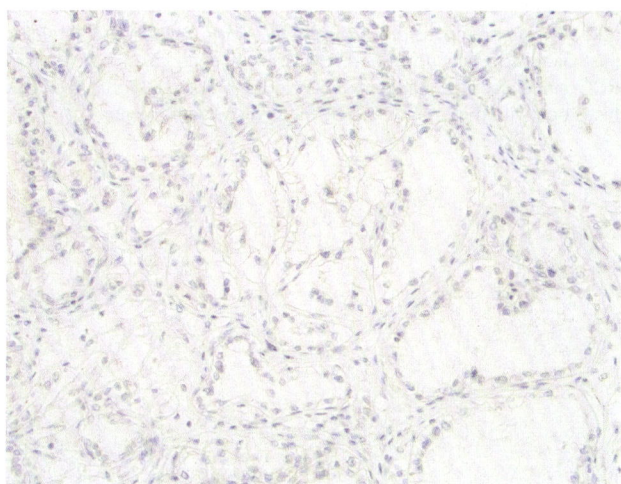

Figure 3.99. AMACR is consistently negative or extremely minimal in clear cell papillary renal cell carcinoma.

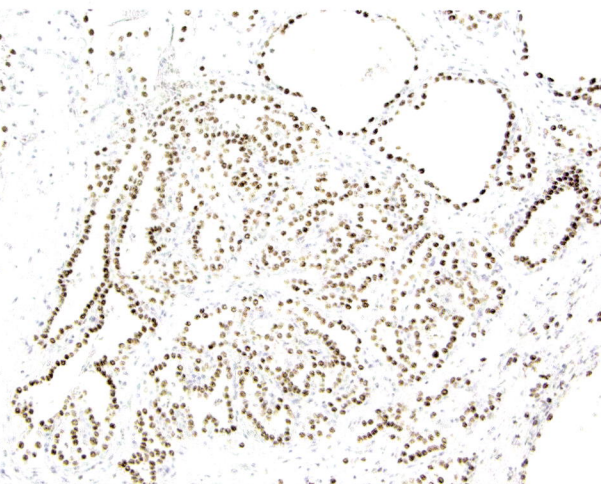

Figure 3.100. GATA3 is often positive in clear cell papillary renal cell carcinoma, suggesting a possible distal nephron phenotype.

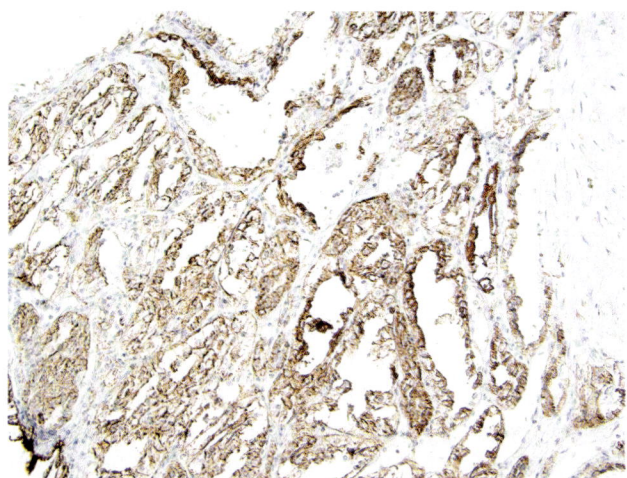

Figure 3.101. Like GATA3, high molecular weight cytokeratin positivity in clear cell papillary is suggestive of a distal nephron phenotype.

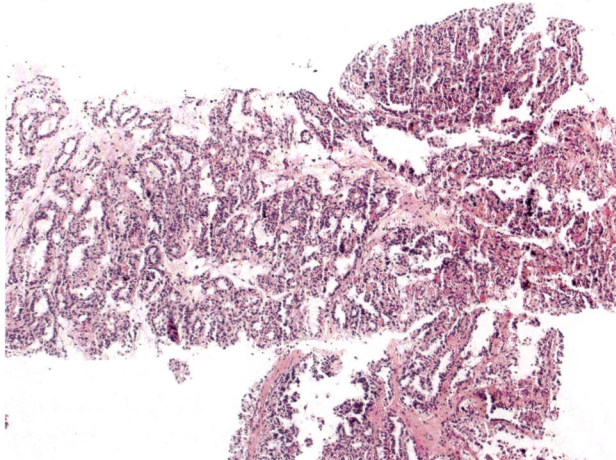

Figure 3.102. This renal mass biopsy case shows a tumor with branched glands and prominent stroma, suggestive of clear cell papillary renal cell carcinoma (RCC). Although substantial cytokeratin 7 staining was present (not pictured), there was strong staining for AMACR (Figure 3.103), arguing against clear cell papillary RCC.

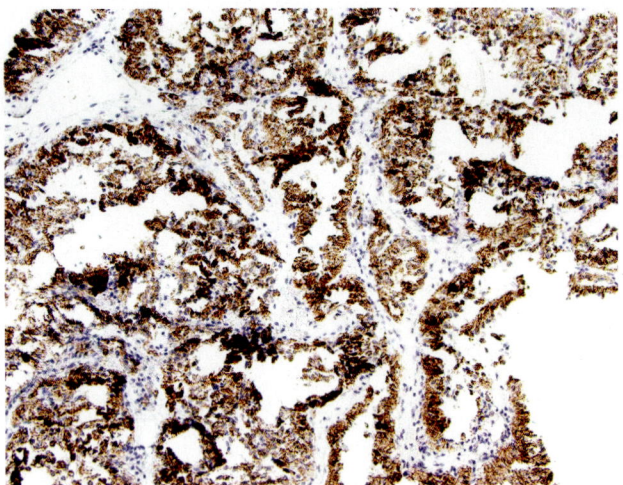

Figure 3.103. The same biopsy from Figure 3.102 shows strong staining for AMACR, arguing against clear cell papillary renal cell carcinoma (RCC). Our approach is to regard tumors with imperfect features as clear cell RCCs due to the greater potential for aggressive behavior. This tumor also showed diffuse membranous staining for carbonic anhydrase IX and negative staining for high molecular weight cytokeratin in the final resection, which had a similar borderline morphology.

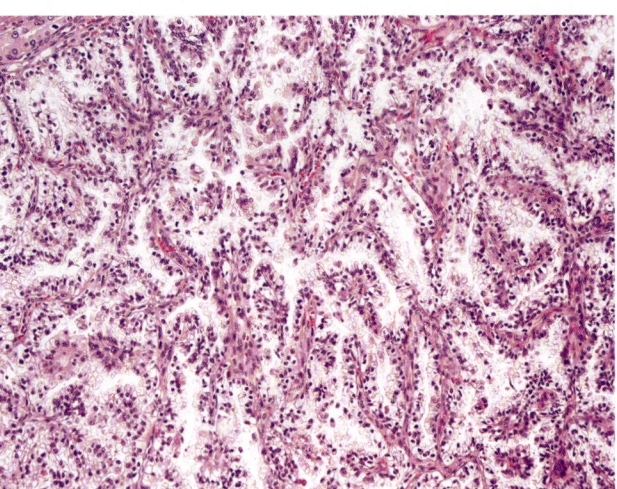

Figure 3.104. This renal neoplasm shows prominent branched glandular configuration morphologically, raising consideration of clear cell papillary renal cell carcinoma (RCC). However, several atypical features were present, including a size of 9 cm with renal sinus and vein branch invasion, and patchy AMACR and CD10 staining (not pictured). Our approach is to classify such cases as clear cell RCC, since clear cell papillary RCC would indicate a highly favorable histology with minimal or no known aggressive behavior.

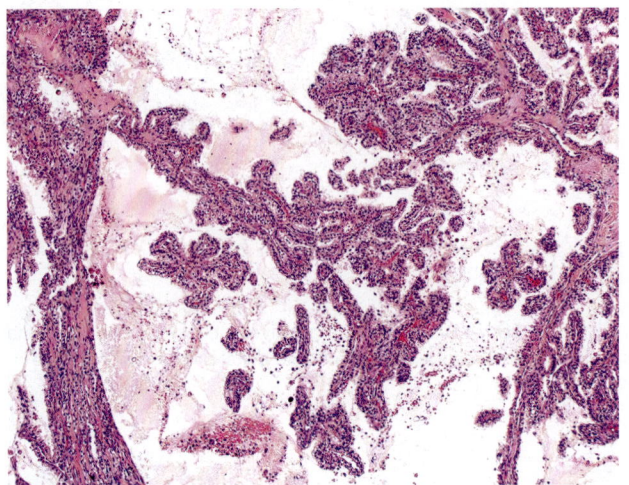

Figure 3.105. This tumor closely resembles clear cell papillary renal cell carcinoma (RCC), occurring in a young man in his 20s. Although immunohistochemistry showed diffuse carbonic anhydrase IX staining and substantial cytokeratin 7 staining, other markers showed imperfect results, including strong AMACR staining, substantial CD10 staining, and negative GATA3 and high molecular weight cytokeratin. This constellation of features, including the young age, is suspicious for VHL disease, in which tumors can mimic clear cell papillary RCC.

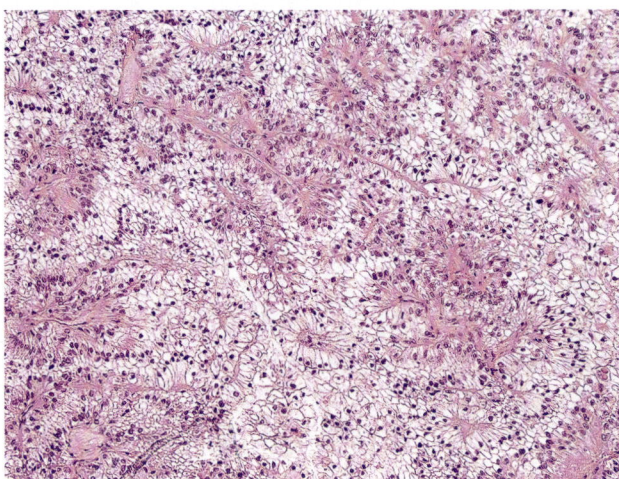

Figure 3.106. Some translocation renal cell carcinomas (RCCs), such as RCC with *NONO-TFE3* fusion in this case, can show nuclear alignment mimicking clear cell papillary RCC. Psammoma bodies or higher nuclear grade (grade 3 or higher) would be unusual for clear cell papillary RCC.

appears distinct from both clear cell RCC and papillary RCC. To date, we are not aware of any tumor with this constellation of features that has metastasized or otherwise demonstrated aggressive behavior, suggesting that the malignant potential of these tumors is low, if any. It is estimated that these tumors make up as much as 4% of adult RCCs. Previously most were likely classified as low-grade, low-stage clear cell RCCs.

References:

Williamson SR, Eble JN, Cheng L, et al. Clear cell papillary renal cell carcinoma: differential diagnosis and extended immunohistochemical profile. *Mod Pathol*. 2013;26:697-708.

Tickoo SK, dePeralta-Venturina MN, Harik LR, et al. Spectrum of epithelial neoplasms in end-stage renal disease: an experience from 66 tumor-bearing kidneys with emphasis on histologic patterns distinct from those in sporadic adult renal neoplasia. *Am J Surg Pathol.* 2006;30:141-153.

Srigley JR, Delahunt B, Eble JN, et al. The International Society of Urological Pathology (ISUP) Vancouver classification of renal neoplasia. *Am J Surg Pathol.* 2013;37:1469-1489.

MITF Family Translocation RCC, Clear Cell Pattern

Translocation-associated RCC is best known for its occurrence in children and young adults, and indeed if a child or young adult develops RCC, the likelihood of an MITF family translocation tumor is higher. However, since RCC is rare in young patients, there are likely more MITF family translocation cancers in the typical age range for renal cancer (50 years and above).[92,93] Most of these tumors have translocations of *TFE3*, located at Xp11.2. Hence, these tumors are sometimes referred to as Xp11 translocation carcinomas or similar names. Less frequently, translocations involve *TFEB*, located at 6p21,[92,93] and very recently, rare translocations of the *MITF* gene itself have been reported.[94,95] It is common for these tumors to have a prominent clear cell component, such that they could be confused with clear cell RCC.

PEARLS AND PITFALLS: MITF Family Translocation RCC

- May have abnormally voluminous clear cytoplasm, greater than expected for clear cell RCC
- Alternating between clear cell and papillary patterns, or clear cell and eosinophilic patterns, raises consideration of MITF family translocation RCC (Figures 3.107 and 3.108)
- Rarely may have multilocular cystic-like morphology (Figure 3.109)
- Other clues to MITF family translocation RCC:
  - Psammoma bodies (Figure 3.110)
  - Pigment deposition
  - Young age (suggestive but not necessary) (Figure 3.111)
  - Stromal hyalinization (Figures 3.112 and 3.113)
- Helpful immunohistochemistry:
  - Carbonic anhydrase IX—negative or minimal, in contrast to clear cell RCC[96]
  - HMB45 or melan-A—positivity may be a clue to the diagnosis (Figure 3.114)
  - TFE3 or TFEB proteins—positive, depending on the fusion (although optimal staining may be technically challenging)[92,93] (Figure 3.115)
  - Cathepsin K—frequently positive, but depends on the fusion[97,98]
  - Keratin, EMA, or vimentin—may be negative or decreased (but not required, may be positive)[96]
- Molecular markers:
  - *TFE3* or *TFEB* break-apart FISH (Figure 3.116)—typically shows an abnormal split signal pattern; however, a few translocations occur by chromosomal inversion and may have a false-negative result, particularly *NONO*, *GRIPAP1*, *RBMX*, and *RBM10* partners of *TFE3*[99-104]
  - Reverse transcriptase polymerase chain reaction or next-generation sequencing—may detect those with false-negative FISH. Depending on the assay, this may require knowledge of both partners

TFE3 RCC is best known; however, tumors with *TFEB* fusions, also known as t(6;11) RCC for the most common fusion between *TFEB* on chromosome 6 and *MALAT1* on chromosome 11, also occur. These have been noted at their original description to have nests

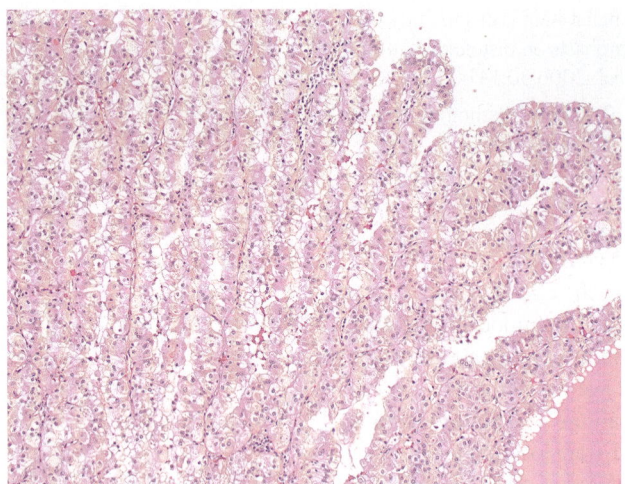

Figure 3.107. This translocation renal cell carcinoma shows papillary architecture with mixed eosinophilic and clear cells.

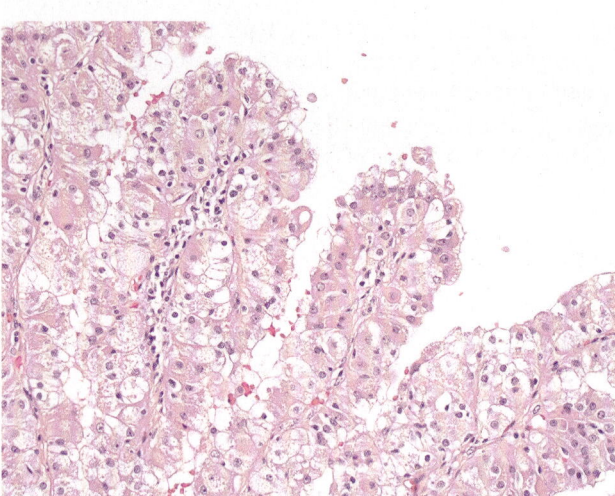

Figure 3.108. Higher magnification of the same case from Figure 3.107 shows papillary architecture and a mixture of clear and eosinophilic cells in translocation renal cell carcinoma.

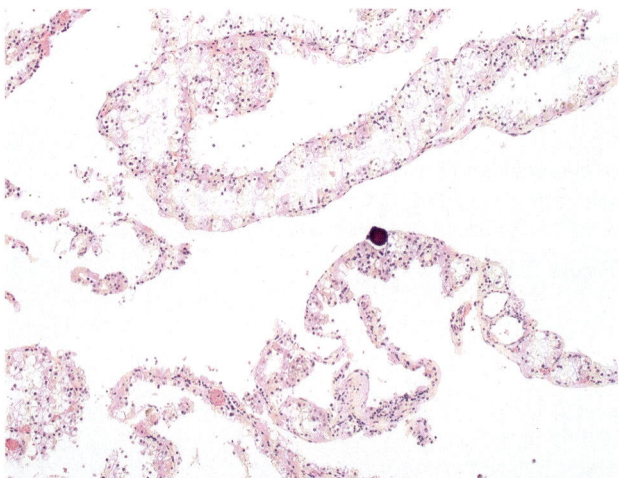

Figure 3.109. Some MITF family translocation renal cell carcinomas may have a multilocular cystic morphology. This case resembled multilocular cystic neoplasm of low malignant potential; however, there is a psammoma body within one of the septa.

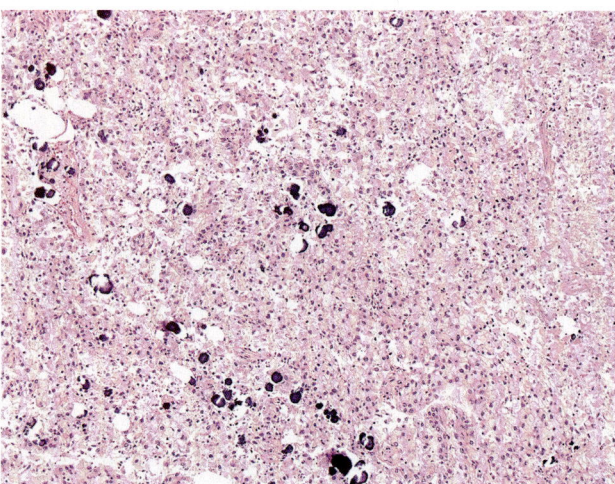

Figure 3.110. This MITF family translocation renal cell carcinoma (RCC) closely resembles clear cell RCC; however, numerous psammoma bodies are a clue to the diagnosis.

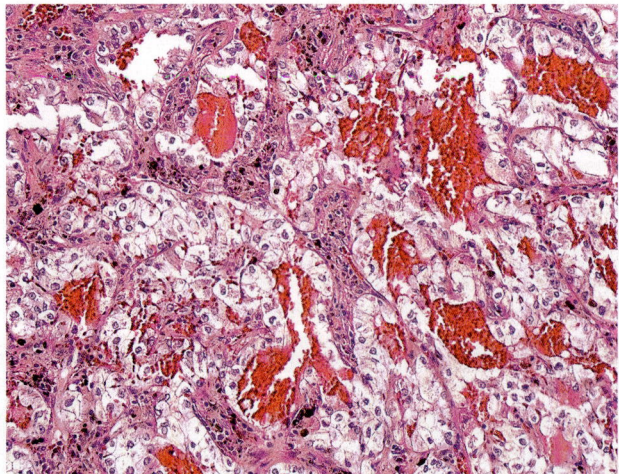

Figure 3.111. This MITF family translocation-associated renal cell carcinoma (RCC) occurred in a child, which is a clue to distinction from clear cell RCC.

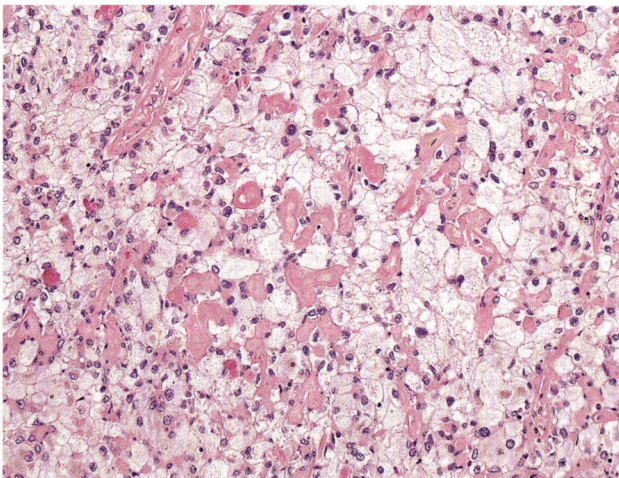

Figure 3.112. Stromal hyalinization can be a clue to the diagnosis of translocation (*TFE3* or *TFEB*) renal cell carcinoma (RCC). This example has subtly increased stromal hyalinization between the cells, which otherwise would resemble clear cell RCC.

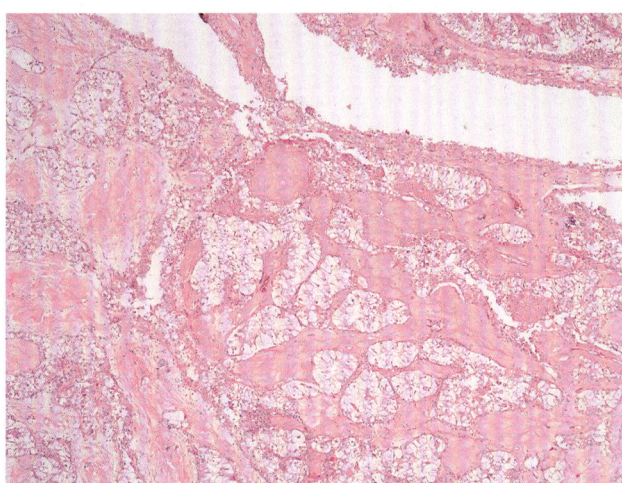

Figure 3.113. This translocation renal cell carcinoma (RCC) from a child has very abundant uniform hyalinization around the nests, which would be an odd pattern in clear cell RCC and should prompt consideration of MITF family translocation RCC.

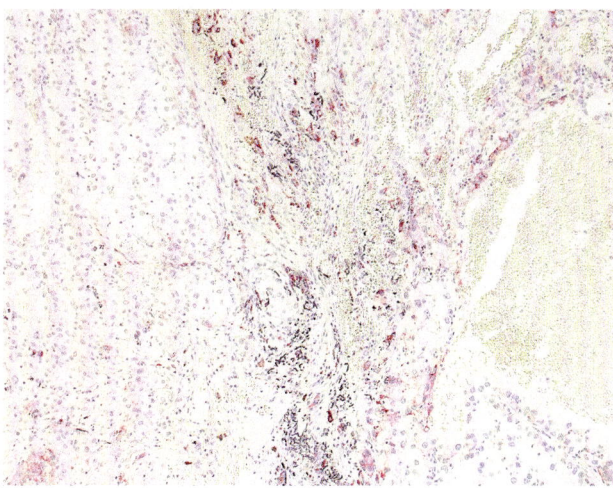

Figure 3.114. Melanocytic marker positivity raises suspicion for MITF family translocation renal cell carcinoma. This example shows focal staining for HMB45 (red chromogen).

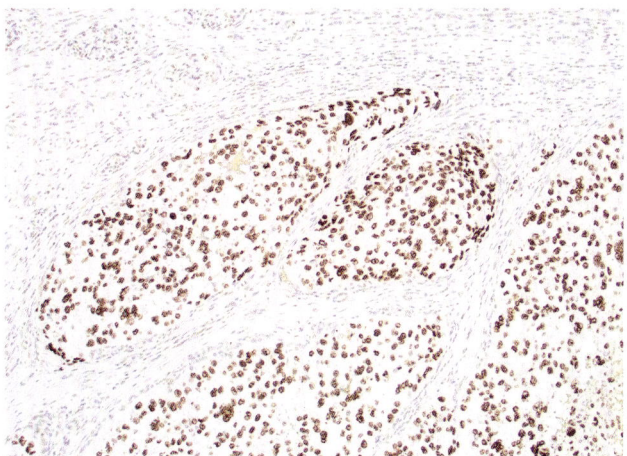

Figure 3.115. Immunohistochemistry for the TFE3 or TFEB proteins can be technically challenging to optimize. However, a strong nuclear staining reaction can be supportive of the diagnosis of MITF family translocation renal cell carcinoma. This example shows strong nuclear TFE3 staining in a tumor with negative/minimal staining in adjacent normal tissue.

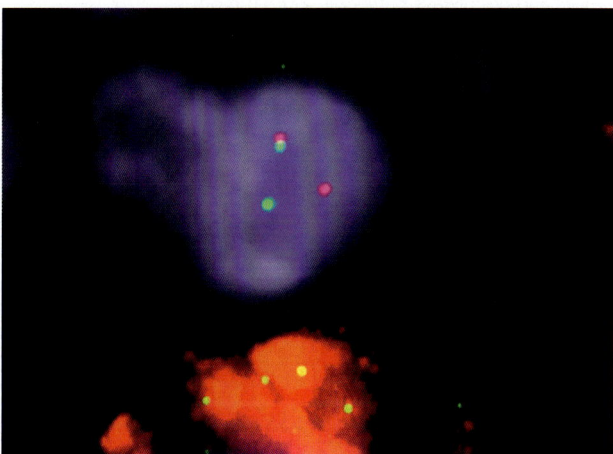

Figure 3.116. Break-apart fluorescence in situ hybridization in this example of *TFEB* rearrangement-associated renal cell carcinoma shows one copy of the *TFEB* gene with closely juxtaposed red and green signals (top). The other copy shows widely separated signals, supporting rearrangement.

of cells with clear cytoplasm surrounding smaller cells with hyaline globules, forming a rosette-like pattern (Figure 3.117).[105] This finding is neither uniformly present, nor is it entirely specific for the diagnosis, as it can sometimes be mimicked in *TFE3* tumors and is not always observed (Figure 3.118).[93] The optimal treatment for translocation RCC is not entirely known at present, due to their rarity.

Adrenal Cortical Lesions Involving the Kidney

A rare consideration for a renal tumor with a clear cell pattern is an adrenal cortical lesion. This can represent either a developmental rest or remnant, in which adrenal tissue is present within the kidney or fused to the renal capsule, or inadvertent sampling of adjacent adrenal tissue, such as in a core biopsy. If the differential diagnosis for a tumor within the adrenal gland itself includes metastatic RCC, the same principles also apply. Most adrenal cortical rests or remnants are small lesions (less than 2 cm) that are incidentally identified,[106] such as upon evaluation of a potential donor kidney (Figures 3.119 and 3.120) or at autopsy. However, rarely larger lesions can be encountered such as adrenal cortical adenoma that is fused with the kidney (Figure 3.121).

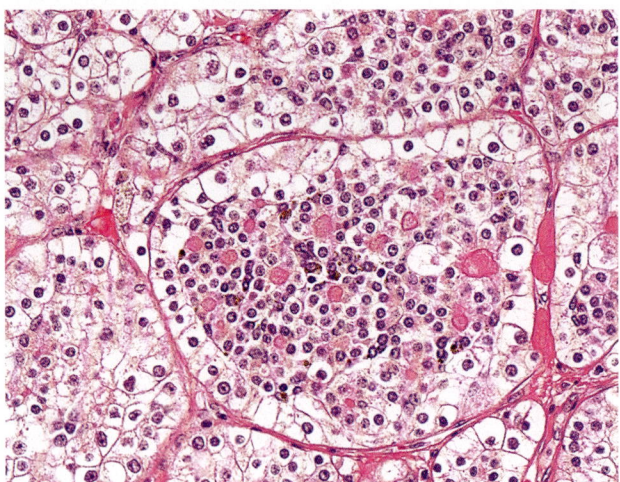

Figure 3.117. The prototypical pattern of *TFEB* rearrangement renal cell carcinoma shows large nests of cells with clear cytoplasm containing a rosette-like formation of smaller cells with hyaline globules, as shown here. However, this pattern is not entirely specific for *TFEB* rearrangement, having been occasionally observed in *TFE3* tumors and not always present in *TFEB* tumors.

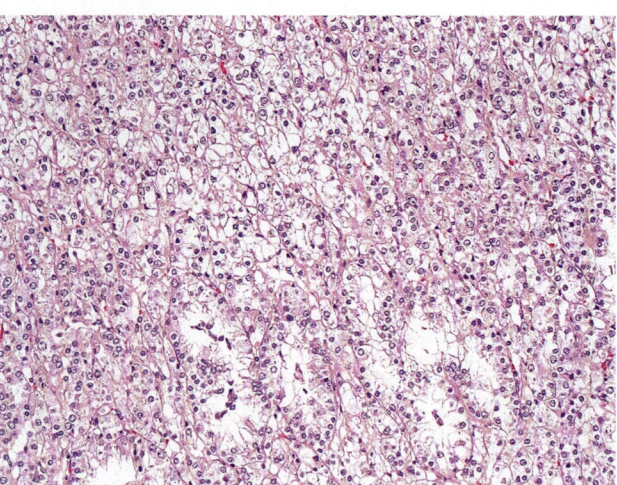

Figure 3.118. This *TFEB* translocation tumor otherwise would be most likely confused with clear cell renal cell carcinoma, as the rosette-like pattern is not conspicuous.

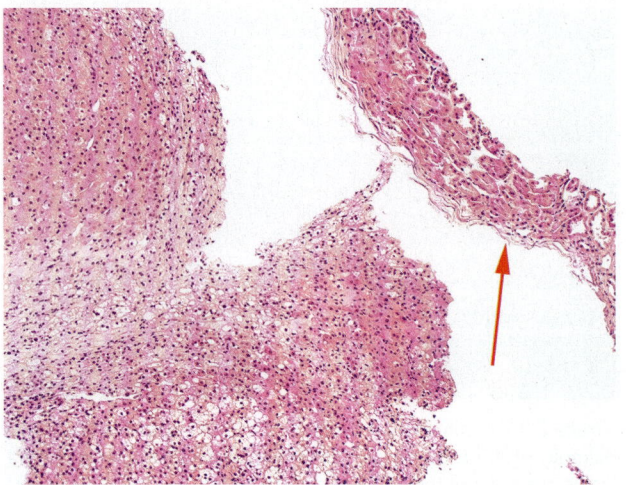

Figure 3.119. Adrenal cortical rests in renal specimens could lead to confusion with renal cell carcinoma (RCC). This biopsy of a possible transplant kidney contains a small amount of renal parenchymal tissue (arrow). The rest of the field is composed of adrenal cortical tissue, which could be misconstrued as RCC.

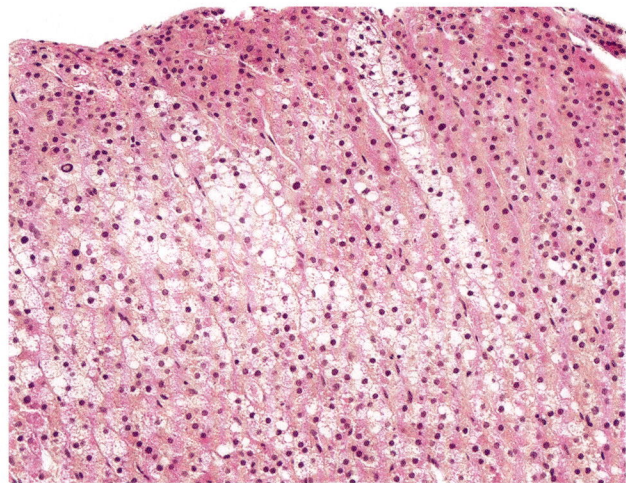

Figure 3.120. At higher magnification, adrenal rests are composed of cells with numerous cytoplasmic vacuoles rather than entirely clear cytoplasm.

KEY FEATURES: Distinguishing Adrenal Cortical Lesions From RCC

- Adrenal cortical cells are typically highly vacuolated (Figures 3.120 and 3.123) rather than entirely optically clear, contrasting to clear cell RCC
- Adrenal cortical tissue is often positive for inhibin, steroidogenic factor 1, calretinin, or melan-A, and negative for PAX8 and epithelial membrane antigen, with the opposite results in clear cell RCC, although rare PAX8 positivity has been reported[106-108]

Hemangioblastoma

Hemangioblastoma is a benign neoplasm of uncertain histogenesis that is overwhelmingly more common in the central nervous system; however, it has been recently recognized that it can occur at other soft tissue sites and rarely the kidney.[109-117] In the kidney, this poses a tremendous diagnostic challenge, as it so closely mimics the morphology of clear cell RCC. In fact, it is well known that metastatic RCC versus hemangioblastoma is a diagnostic

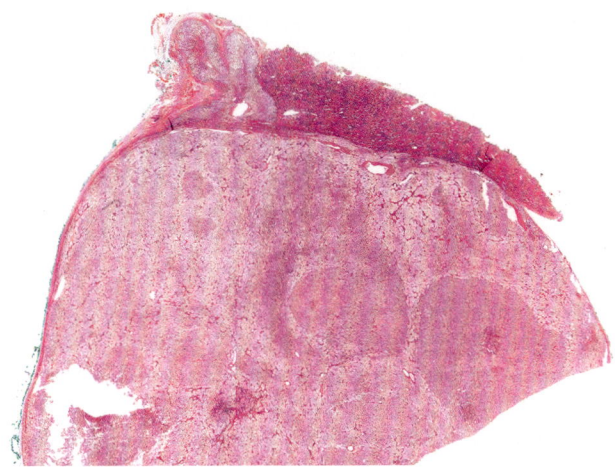

Figure 3.121. This adrenal cortical adenoma is fused with the kidney and presented as a possible renal mass by diagnostic imaging. The surgeon recognized intraoperatively that it likely originated from the adrenal gland and resected the adrenal gland with a small rim of kidney tissue.

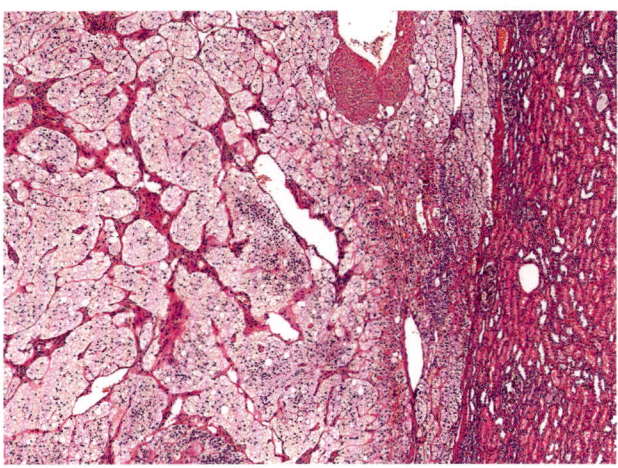

Figure 3.122. Higher magnification of the same case from Figure 3.121 shows the adrenal cortical adenoma abutting benign renal parenchyma without a clear plane of separation.

difficulty in the brain.[118-122] Hemangioblastomas are associated with VHL syndrome, which may raise both clear cell RCC and hemangioblastoma in the differential diagnosis of a renal mass in such a patient.

PEARLS AND PITFALLS: Renal hemangioblastoma Versus RCC[109-117]

- Hemangioblastoma cells may be more flocculent or vacuolated (Figures 3.124-3.126) than the entirely clear pattern of clear cell RCC
- Inhibin is characteristically positive; S100 or neuron-specific enolase is often present in hemangioblastoma
- Lesser staining for keratin or epithelial membrane antigen is often found in hemangioblastoma
- Paradoxically, PAX8 may be positive in renal hemangioblastoma,[109-117] contrasting to the brain, in which this is typically used to support metastatic RCC. Therefore, PAX8 should not be used in isolation to argue against renal hemangioblastoma

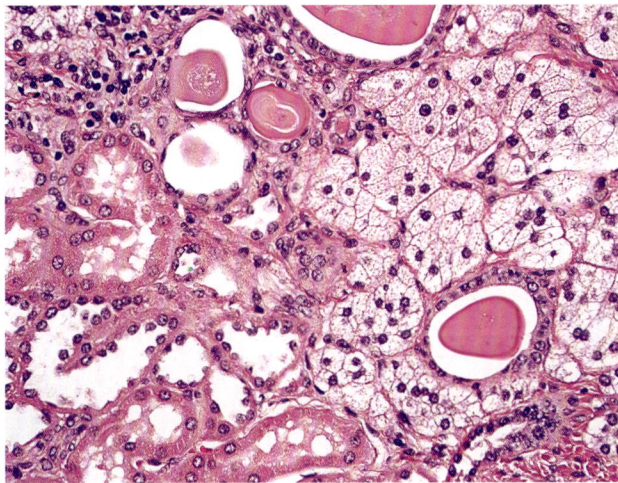

Figure 3.123. In some areas of the same case from Figures 3.121 and 3.122, adrenal cortical tissue intermingles with renal tubules.

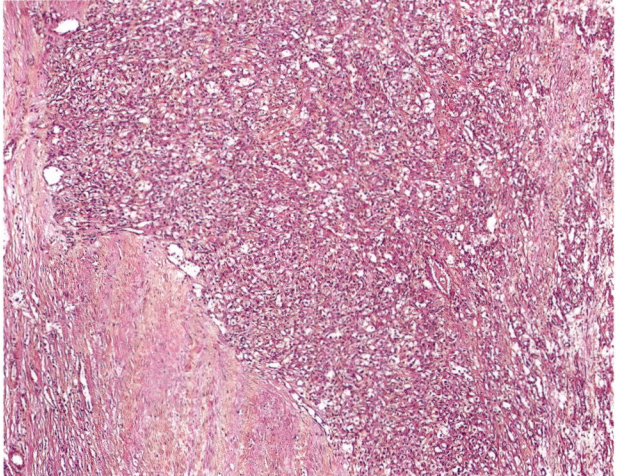

Figure 3.124. Rarely hemangioblastomas may occur in the kidney, which is especially deceptive in distinguishing from renal cell carcinoma. A potential clue in this case is the predominant solid architecture without arrangement into separate nests.

An unusual phenomenon that has been recently recognized is that rare RCCs can have overlapping features of hemangioblastoma, including positivity for inhibin.[123,124] The significance of this is not well understood at present, but likely will be better characterized with the increasing awareness of renal hemangioblastoma and increasing use of immunohistochemistry.

Epithelioid Angiomyolipoma/Perivascular Epithelioid Cell Tumor (PEComa), Clear Cell Pattern

Angiomyolipoma is primarily discussed under the section on spindle cell pattern; however, a rare subset of tumors of the kidney within the angiomyolipoma/PEComa family of tumors are predominantly epithelioid and can closely resemble clear cell RCC (Figures 3.127 and 3.128).[125-131] In contrast to conventional angiomyolipoma, which is well established as a benign neoplasm, epithelioid angiomyolipoma is considered to have malignant potential (Figure 3.129). However, the precise criteria for distinguishing epithelioid angiomyolipoma from conventional angiomyolipoma with focal epithelioid cells are not always well agreed upon.[128] Our approach is to reserve the diagnosis of epithelioid angiomyolipoma (which may have malignant potential) for tumors that are overwhelmingly epithelioid, to the point that they would be easily mistaken for RCC and that conventional angiomyolipoma would barely be a diagnostic consideration (Figures 3.127 and 3.128). Focal epithelioid features are not unusual in conventional angiomyolipoma (Figures 3.130 and 3.131) and need not be mentioned, as this might cause unnecessary concern for aggressive behavior from a benign neoplasm.

Precise criteria for malignancy are somewhat variable between studies. One series proposed that three or more of the following findings would be concerning for malignant behavior: 70% atypical epithelioid cells, two mitotic figures per 10 high-power fields, atypical mitotic figures, or necrosis.[125] Another series noted that associated tuberous sclerosis complex or concurrent angiomyolipoma, tumor size >7 cm, extrarenal extension or renal vein involvement, and carcinoma-like growth pattern were additional concerning features.[131] Interestingly, a recent series found only 20 epithelioid angiomyolipomas (>80% epithelioid morphology) from a series of over 400 tumors from three institutions, with only one developing distant metastasis, suggesting that aggressive behavior may be rare in an unselected patient population.[127]

KEY FEATURES: Recognizing Epithelioid Angiomyolipoma

- May have a sheet-like growth pattern, lacking the discrete nests of clear cell RCC
- Cells may be partly clear and partly eosinophilic (Figure 3.132), sometimes with a central eosinophilic globule

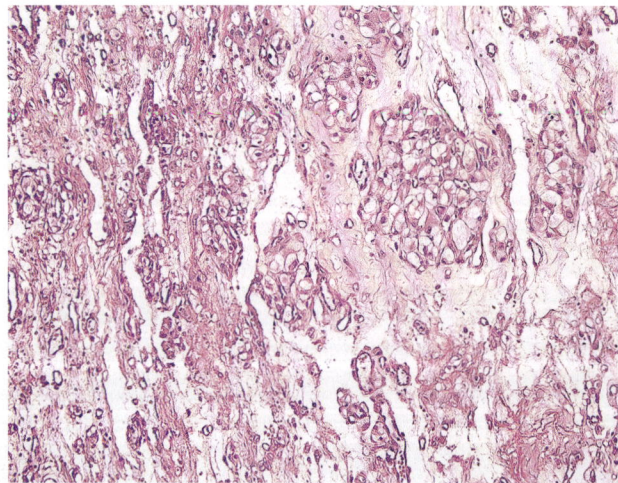

Figure 3.125. Other areas of hemangioblastoma may have edematous or fibrotic stroma, which can also be found in sclerotic areas of renal cell carcinoma.

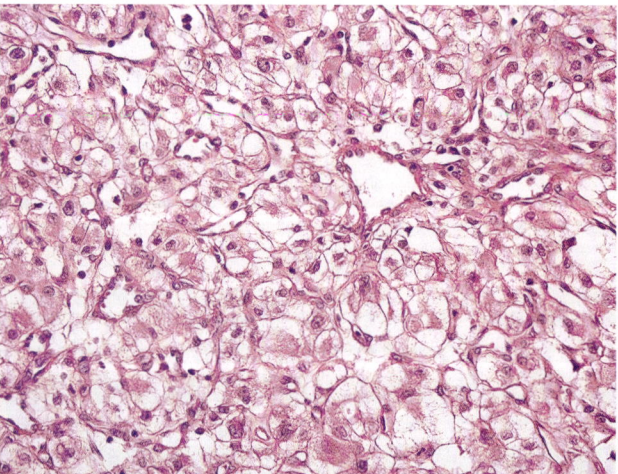

Figure 3.126. At high magnification, this renal hemangioblastoma is composed of cells with clear to flocculent eosinophilic cytoplasm. There is a prominent vascular network, mimicking that of clear cell renal cell carcinoma (RCC). A low threshold to further investigate unusual RCC cases that are lacking obvious epithelial formations may be helpful in recognizing this benign neoplasm.

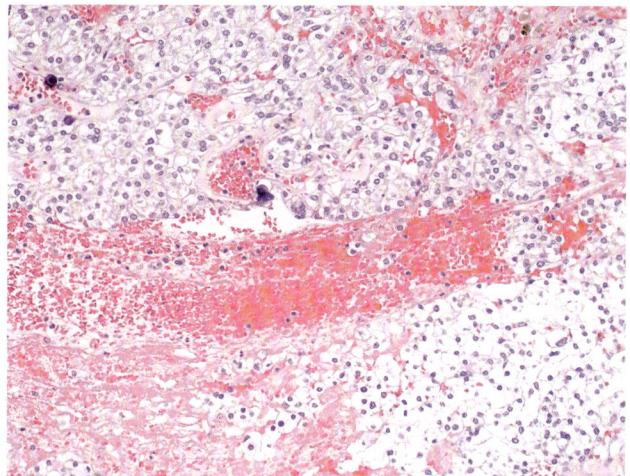

Figure 3.127. Epithelioid angiomyolipoma may closely mimic a clear cell renal cell carcinoma (RCC). This tumor occurred in a very young patient and contains scattered calcifications, which are atypical for clear cell RCC.

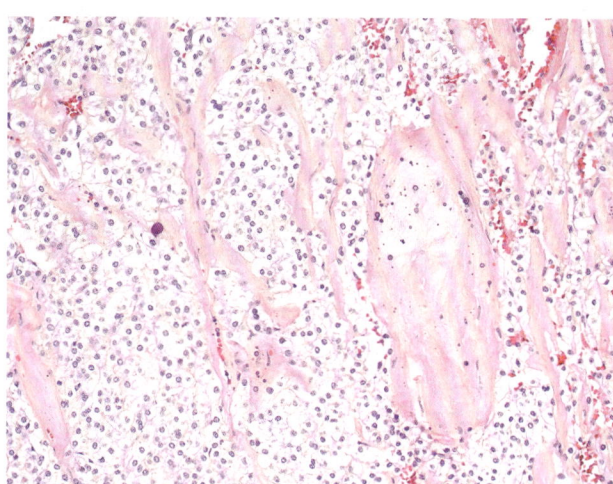

Figure 3.128. Prominent stromal hyalinization in this case of epithelioid angiomyolipoma/PEComa is a clue to the diagnosis, similar to MITF family translocation renal cell carcinoma.

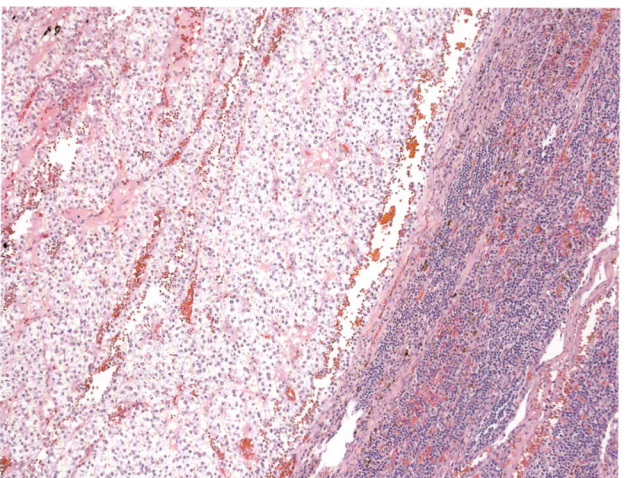

Figure 3.129. In contrast to conventional angiomyolipoma, epithelioid angiomyolipoma/PEComa is considered as having malignant potential. This case metastasized to lymph nodes (lymph node tissue at right).

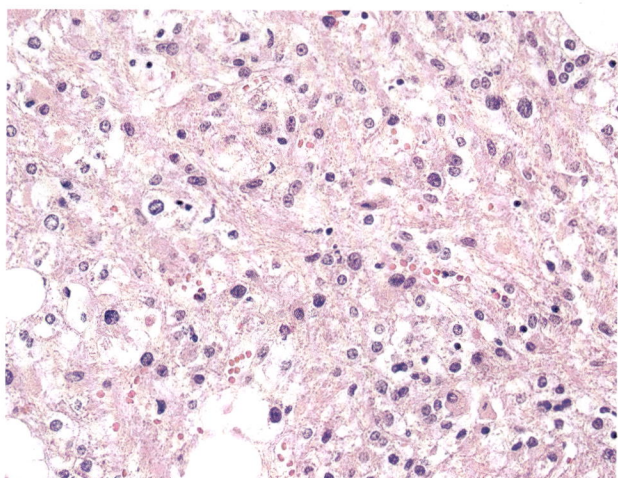

Figure 3.130. Focal epithelioid features in a typical angiomyolipoma generally should not be referred to as epithelioid angiomyolipoma, to avoid implying potential malignant behavior. At high magnification, this example includes clear to eosinophilic epithelioid cells; however, focal fat is appreciable at lower left. The overall pattern of this tumor was readily recognizable as angiomyolipoma, arguing against epithelioid designation.

- May contain multinucleated tumor giant cells (Figure 3.132)
- May have a lesser spindle-shaped cell component, focal thick blood vessels or fat
- Immunohistochemical reactivity:
  - Melanocytic markers positive
  - Cathepsin K positive[132] (Figure 3.133)
  - Often positive for smooth muscle markers, such as smooth muscle actin and less frequently desmin[127]
  - Cytokeratin negative
  - Scant data available, but likely PAX8 and carbonic anhydrase IX negative
- Molecular: subset has *TFE3* rearrangements, like MITF family translocation RCC (distinguished from translocation RCC by lack of epithelial marker staining)[133,134]

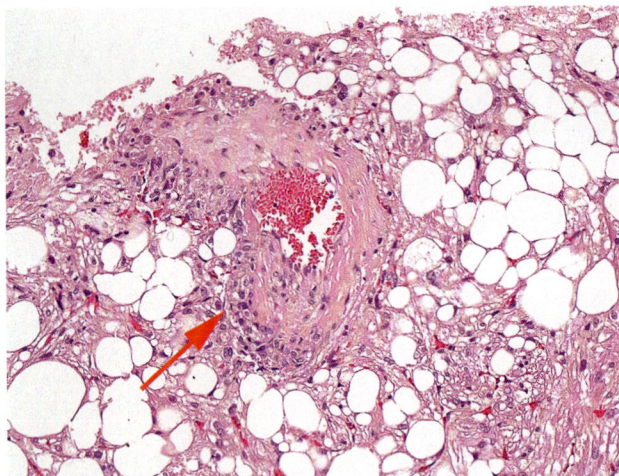

Figure 3.131. In angiomyolipoma, epithelioid cells are most often arranged around blood vessels (arrow), giving rise to the "perivascular epithelioid" name of this tumor family.

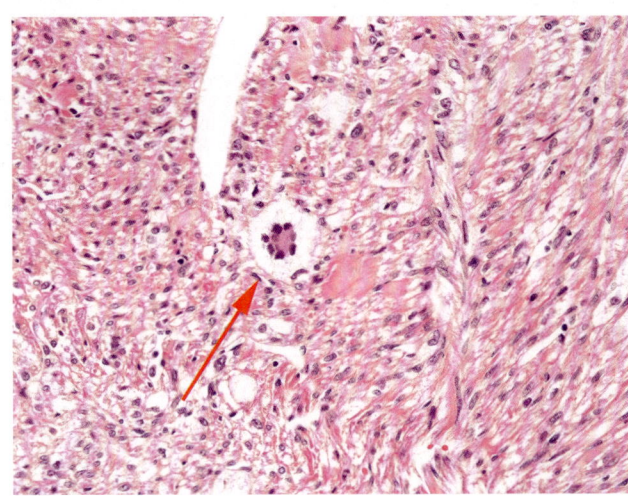

Figure 3.132. Occasional cells in angiomyolipoma can have a Touton cell-like appearance (arrow) with a central globule of hyaline material surrounded by a pale/clear zone.

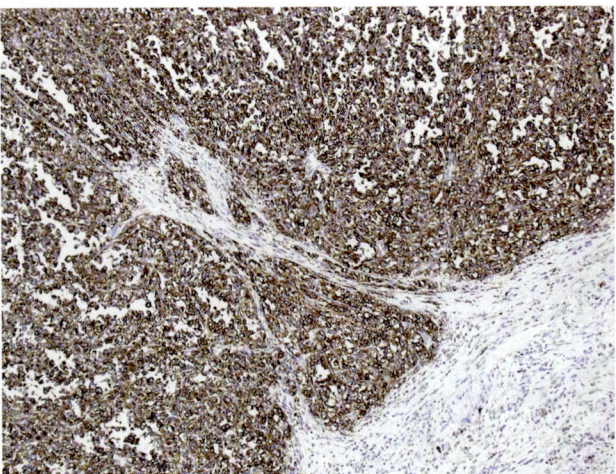

Figure 3.133. Cathepsin K staining in angiomyolipoma and PEComas is typically diffuse and strong (shown here), in contrast to melanocytic marker labeling, which may be focal. This case showed negative staining for cytokeratin AE1/AE3 and EMA and was positive for TFE3 protein, supporting a *TFE3* rearrangement PEComa.

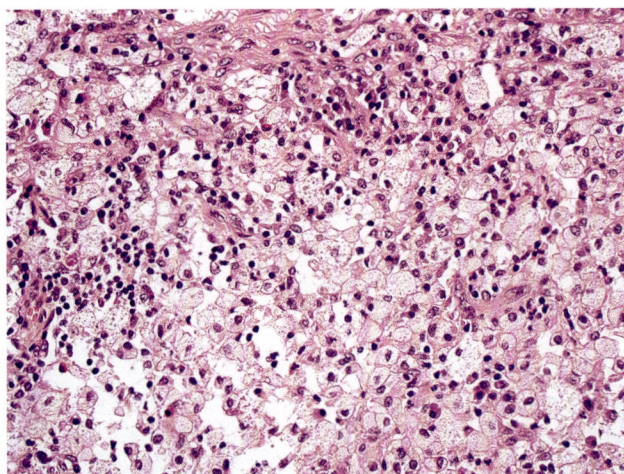

Figure 3.134. Foamy cells in xanthogranulomatous pyelonephritis can lead to confusion with renal cell carcinoma. Admixture of other inflammatory cells may be a clue to the diagnosis.

Although data are scant, discriminating epithelioid angiomyolipoma from RCC may have some potential implications for treatment purposes in the metastatic setting, as MTOR pathway inhibitors may be more likely considered than the typical VEGF pathway drugs or other tyrosine kinase inhibitors used for RCC.

Xanthogranulomatous Pyelonephritis

Xanthogranulomatous pyelonephritis is discussed in more detail under the inflammatory pattern and nonneoplastic pseudotumors. However, it is worth mentioning that this process may be confused for clear cell RCC when the foamy histiocyte component is predominant (Figure 3.134). Likewise, a spindle cell-like pattern may mimic sarcomatoid RCC (Figure 3.135). As long as this possibility is considered, immunohistochemical markers such as histiocytic markers (CD68 or CD163) and epithelial markers (keratin, PAX8) should resolve this distinction easily. Xanthogranulomatous pyelonephritis typically will have a more diffuse growth pattern, lacking the discrete nests of cells observed in clear cell RCC, and other inflammatory cell components are clues to the diagnosis (such as neutrophils, plasma cells, lymphocytes, or histiocytic giant cells).

PAPILLARY PATTERN

Papillary Adenoma

Papillary adenoma is, by definition, a small renal neoplasm with features resembling type 1 papillary RCC.[135] The 2016 World Health Organization (WHO) Classification increased the allowable size for this diagnosis from 5 mm (in the 2004 scheme) to 15 mm. Therefore, a papillary renal cell neoplasm may be classified as an adenoma, as long as it is 15 mm (1.5 cm) or smaller (Figure 3.136). Two limitations were given for this definition, that (1) the lesion must be unencapsulated (Figures 3.137 and 3.138) and (2) the nuclear grade must be 1 or 2 (not 3 or higher).[135] That said, we are not aware of any data indicating that papillary RCCs of this size (<15 mm) with nuclear grade 3 or encapsulation behave aggressively; however, these are reasonable working limits for the definition of papillary adenoma at present.

FAQ: Should I Change My Practice for Diagnosis of Papillary RCC in Renal Mass Biopsy in View of the Larger Allowable Size for Papillary Adenoma?

The larger allowable size for papillary adenoma does increase the potential that an adenoma may be sampled in a core biopsy specimen, in contrast to the historical 5 mm size, which would often be more difficult to visualize by imaging and biopsy. In most cases, masses will be larger than 15 mm based on clinical or imaging findings, so it is likely reasonable to continue to diagnose these as papillary RCC in the biopsy setting. If clinical findings indicate that the mass may be 15 mm or smaller, it would be reasonable to diagnose "papillary renal cell neoplasm" with a comment that distinction of adenoma from RCC would depend on size, grade, and encapsulation.

Papillary Renal Cell Carcinoma

Type 1

Papillary RCC, type 1, is the best characterized form of papillary RCC at present, composed of papillary or compact glandular structures, typically lined by cuboidal or columnar cells with an overall basophilic appearance at low magnification.[136]

KEY FEATURES: Type 1 Papillary Renal Cell Carcinoma

- Gross appearance may be variable: yellow (foamy cells or necrosis), red (hemorrhage), or brown (hemosiderin), usually round and well circumscribed (Figures 3.139-3.142)
- Often basophilic appearance at low magnification microscopically (Figure 3.143)
- Variable encapsulation, sometimes with tumor herniating through the pseudocapsule (Figure 3.144)
- Cells cuboidal or low columnar (Figures 3.145 and 3.146)
- Cytoplasm variable from pale eosinophilic to clear (vacuolated)[37,54] or containing hemosiderin (Figure 3.147)
- Architecture: papillary, glomeruloid structures, solid, or cystic
- Immunohistochemistry[19,48,137]
  - Cytokeratin 7—typically substantial positivity (but may be decreased with eosinophilic cells) (Figures 3.148 and 3.149)
  - AMACR—consistently diffuses strong staining, with intensity similar to that of proximal tubules (Figure 3.150)
  - Carbonic anhydrase IX—negative or minimal staining in areas of necrosis/ischemia (Figure 3.151)
  - Vimentin—often positive
  - High molecular weight cytokeratin—variable positive[137]

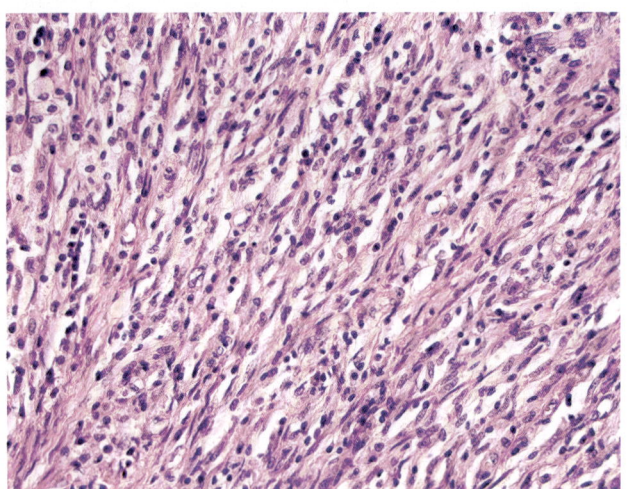

Figure 3.135. Xanthogranulomatous pyelonephritis can also include spindle cell areas, which could lead to confusion with sarcomatoid renal cell carcinoma.

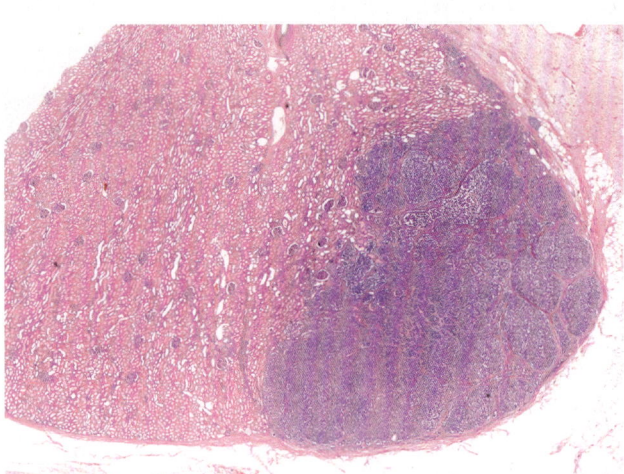

Figure 3.136. The 2016 WHO Classification now allows papillary adenomas to be up to 15 mm. This is a large papillary adenoma diagnosed under these new criteria.

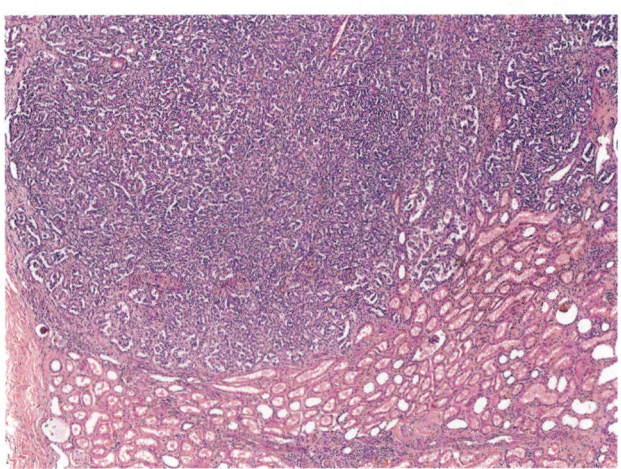

Figure 3.137. Requirements for papillary adenoma include lack of encapsulation and nuclear grade 1 to 2.

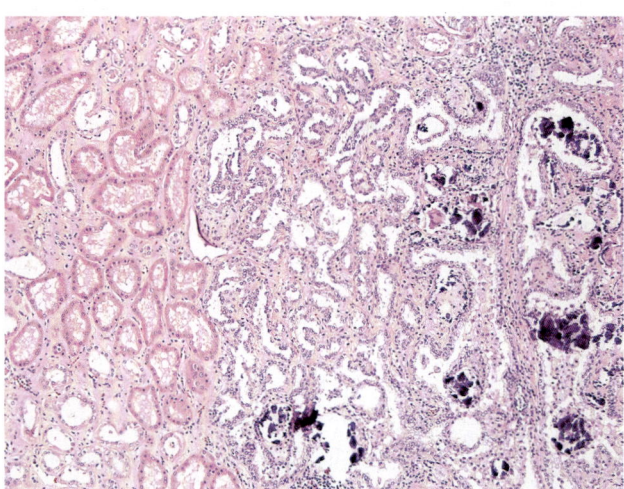

Figure 3.138. This small papillary adenoma includes psammoma bodies, like papillary renal cell carcinoma, and blends with the adjacent benign renal tissue.

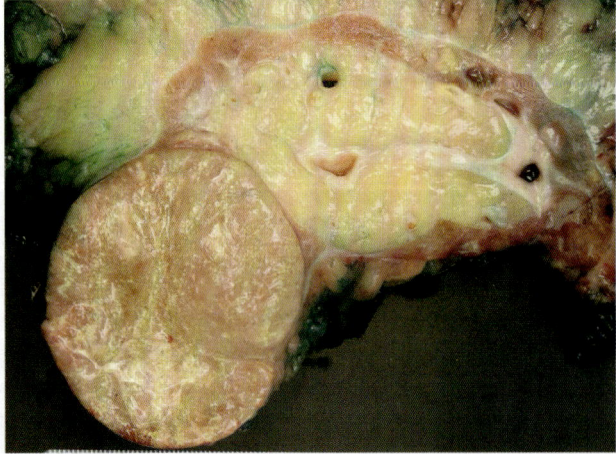

Figure 3.139. Papillary renal cell carcinoma can have variable gross appearances. This example is predominantly pink-tan with some yellow streaks likely corresponding to foamy cells.

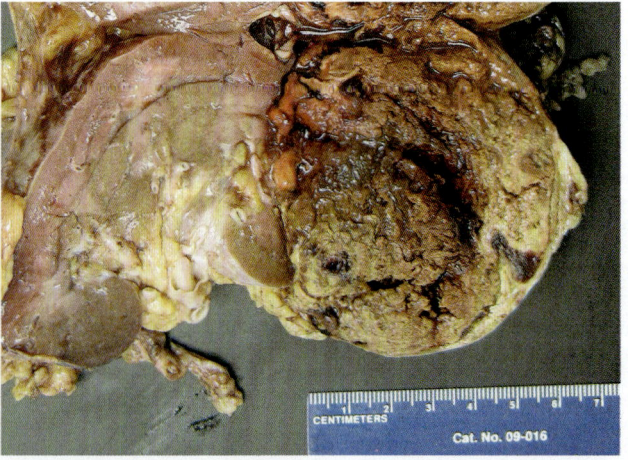

Figure 3.140. This large papillary renal cell carcinoma is grossly friable-appearing and hemorrhagic centrally, corresponding to necrosis.

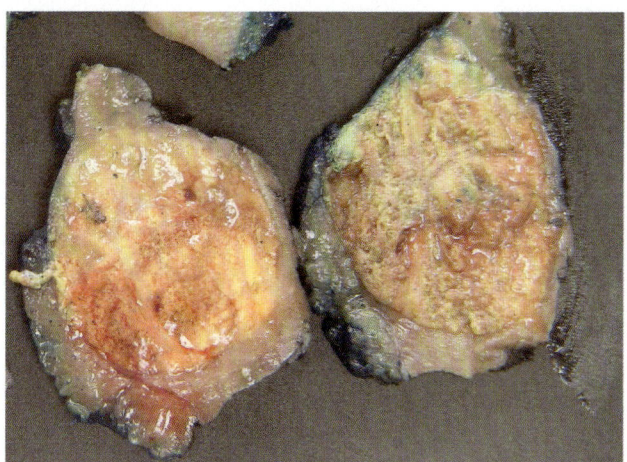

Figure 3.141. This papillary renal cell carcinoma (RCC) appears yellow, mimicking the gross appearance of clear cell RCC.

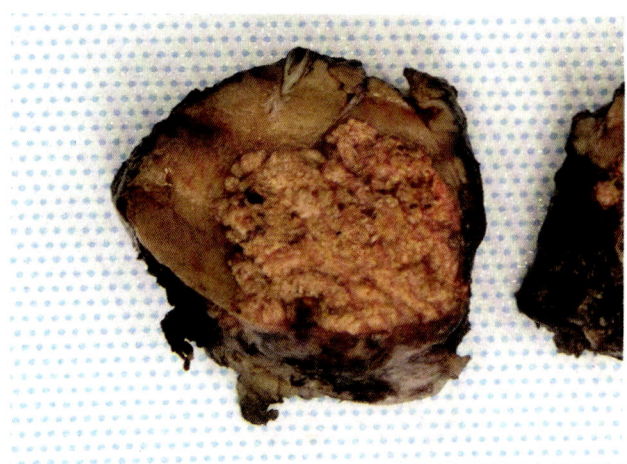

Figure 3.142. Some papillary renal cell carcinomas can be recognized grossly as very granular, a hint to their papillary architecture.

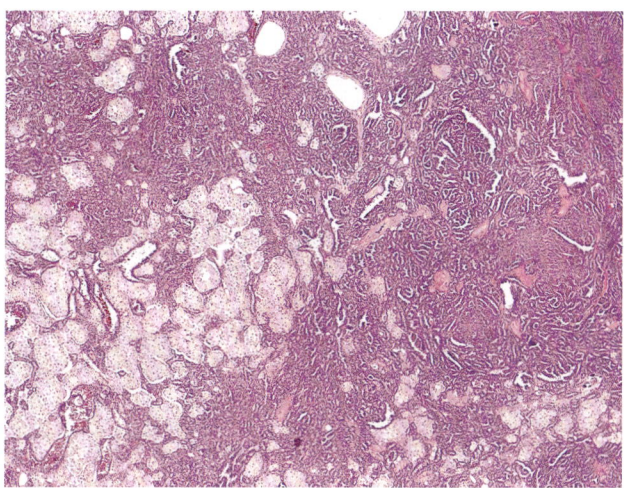

Figure 3.143. At low magnification, type 1 papillary renal cell carcinoma is typically basophilic. This tumor has some foamy macrophages at left.

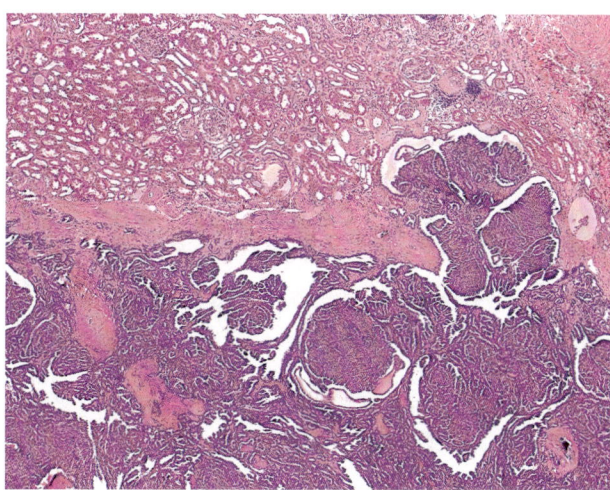

Figure 3.144. Papillary renal cell carcinoma is variably encapsulated and sometimes herniates beyond the tumor capsule.

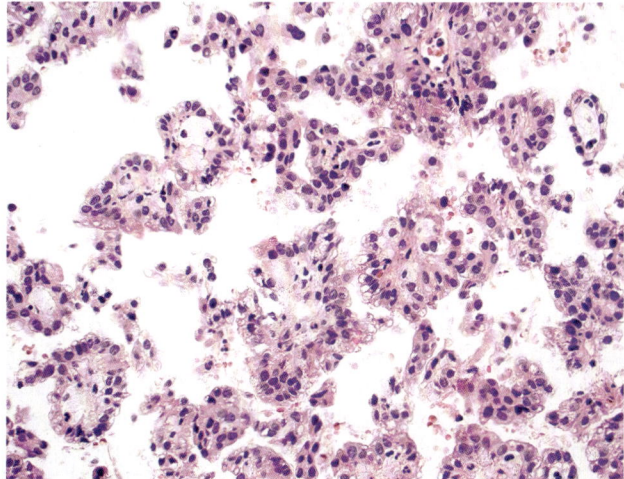

Figure 3.145. Tumor cells in papillary renal cell carcinoma are often cuboidal or low columnar. This example shows classic papillary formations.

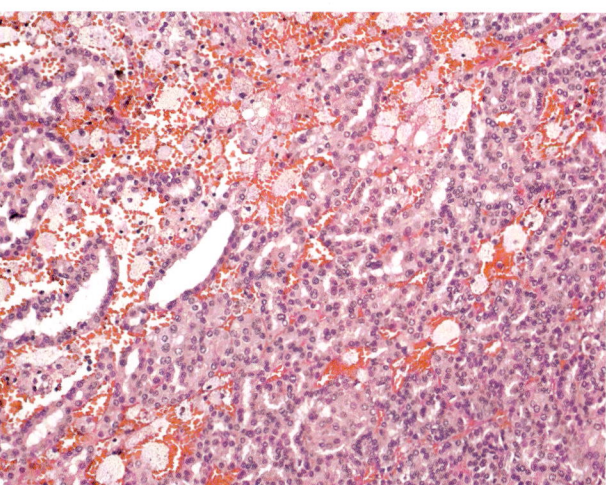

Figure 3.146. This papillary renal cell carcinoma is composed of cuboidal eosinophilic cells with focal foamy macrophages.

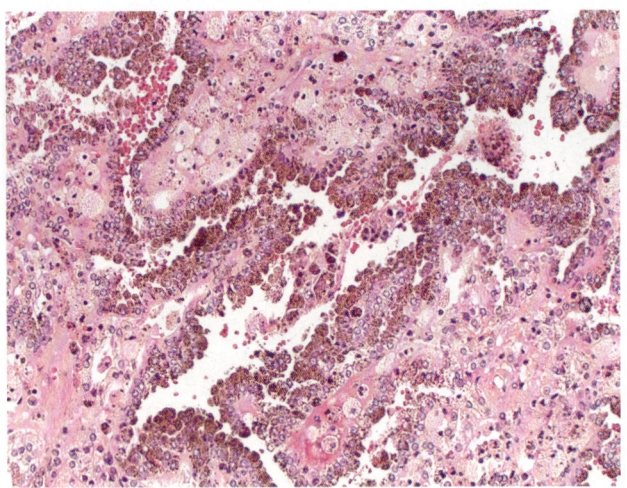

Figure 3.147. Some papillary renal cell carcinoma tumors contain prominent intracytoplasmic hemosiderin.

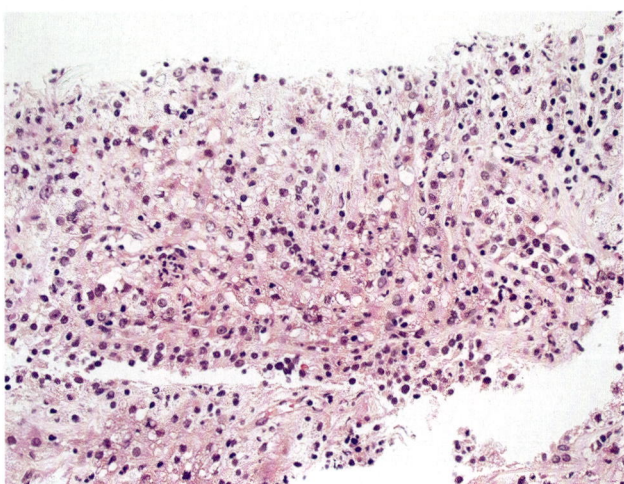

Figure 3.148. This renal mass biopsy shows a papillary renal cell carcinoma with somewhat deceptive morphology, raising a differential diagnosis of clear cell renal cell carcinoma.

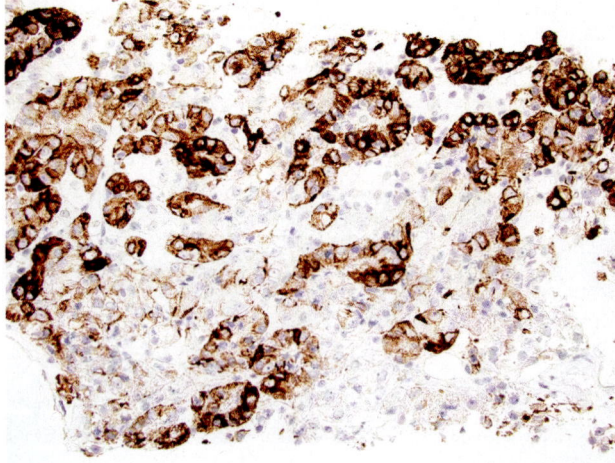

Figure 3.149. Immunohistochemistry shows substantial staining for cytokeratin 7 in the same tumor from Figure 3.148.

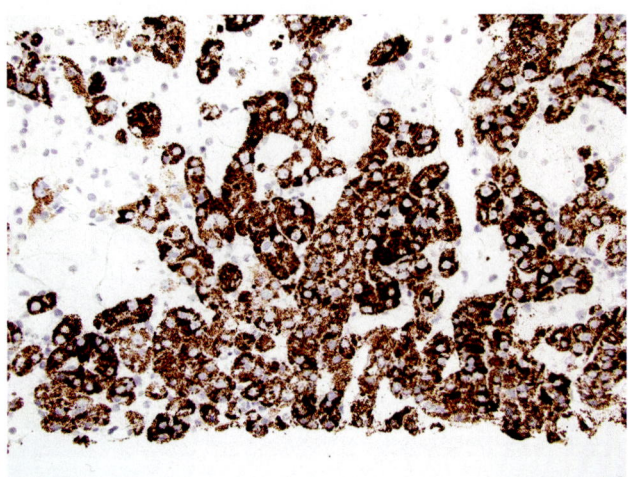

Figure 3.150. AMACR staining is very strong in the tumor from Figures 3.148 and 3.149, supporting papillary renal cell carcinoma.

Several unusual variants of type 1 papillary RCC have been described, ranging from those that resemble Warthin tumor with prominent inflammation[138] to predominantly solid tumors (Figures 3.152 and 3.153).[139] A recently described unusual pattern includes "squamoid" cells (Figure 3.154). Although this was initially proposed as an unusual RCC variant (biphasic alveolosquamoid RCC and similar terminology), recent work has shown that this is essentially an odd morphology of type 1 papillary RCC, with similar immunohistochemical findings. An unusual phenomenon in this variant is that cyclin D1 shows increased staining of the "squamoid" areas, for unknown reasons.[140-142] Other unusual morphologies include mucin in the papillary cores (Figure 3.155).[143]

Genetically, type 1 papillary RCC often shows trisomy of chromosome 7 or 17 and loss of the Y chromosome, which are not entirely specific findings but have been used in some contexts to support the diagnosis, such as by karyotyping or FISH.[35] The hereditary papillary RCC syndrome, in which patients develop numerous multifocal type 1 papillary RCCs, is characterized by germline mutations of *MET*; however, the rate of *MET* mutations appears lower in sporadic papillary RCC than in the hereditary population,[144] contrasting to *VHL*, which is frequently mutated in both sporadic and hereditary clear cell RCC. For practical purposes, molecular testing is rarely necessary in diagnostic practice to distinguish papillary RCC from mimics, as the morphology and immunohistochemistry is usually sufficient to confirm the diagnosis. Most relevant differential diagnoses for type 1 papillary RCC are shown in Table 3.2.

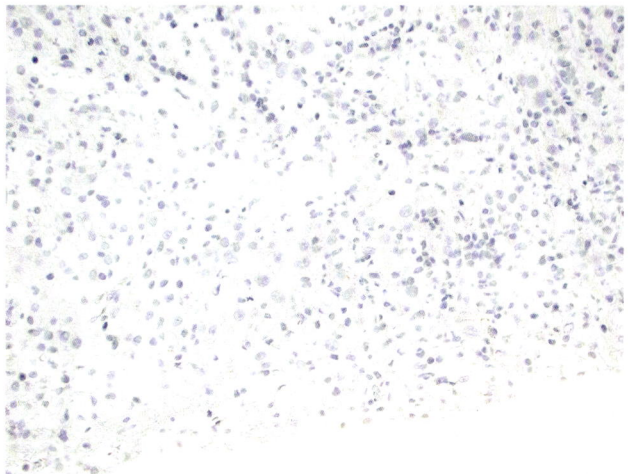

Figure 3.151. Carbonic anhydrase IX staining is negative in the tumor from Figures 3.148-3.150, arguing against clear cell renal cell carcinoma.

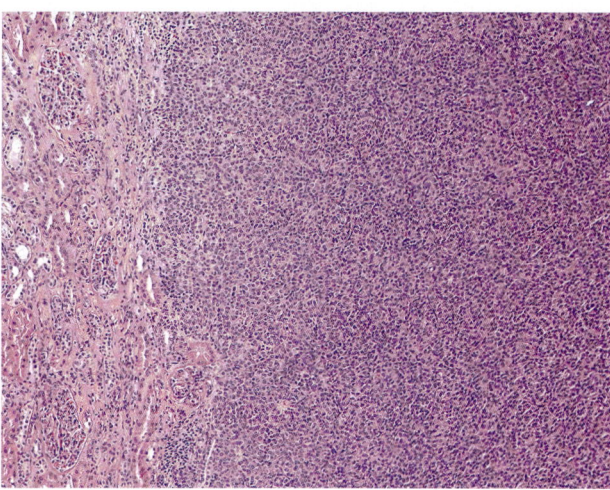

Figure 3.152. Occasional papillary renal cell carcinomas can be predominantly solid, potentially obscuring the diagnosis.

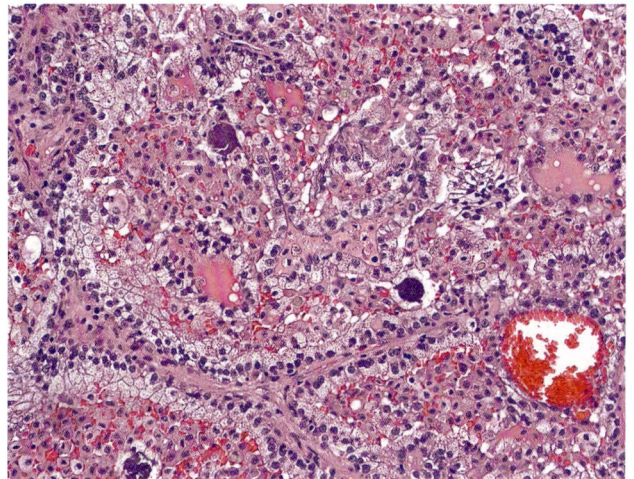

Figure 3.153. The same tumor from Figure 3.152 also contained more classic areas of papillary morphology with foamy cells and psammoma bodies.

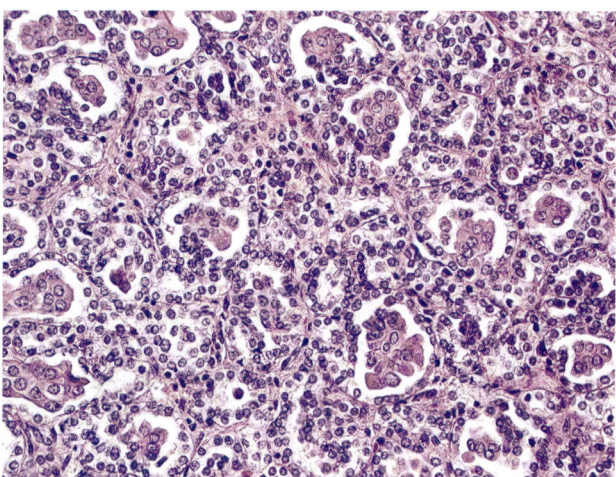

Figure 3.154. A recently recognized variant of papillary renal cell carcinoma (RCC) contains clusters of cells with more eosinophilic cytoplasm within tubular structures that resemble typical type 1 papillary RCC. When extreme, these structures can appear almost squamous, although they are negative for squamous markers. This has been termed "biphasic" papillary RCC.

Type 2 and Related Tumors

Papillary RCC was originally split into type 1 and type 2 based on the distinctive findings of eosinophilic cytoplasm and cells with prominent nucleoli and pseudostratified nuclei in the latter (Figure 3.156)[145]; however, it is now increasingly recognized that type 2 tumors represent a heterogeneous category of neoplasms with differing genetics and potentially significant implications for treatment.[144] Most prominent among these are fumarate hydratase (*FH*)–deficient RCC/HLRCC syndrome–associated tumors, discussed in the next section. As such, we would consider type 2 papillary RCC to be almost a diagnosis of exclusion that should be used only after several considerations are argued against (Table 3.3).

Papillary Renal Cell Neoplasm With Reverse Polarity/Oncocytic Papillary RCC

In the past, oncocytic papillary RCC has been put forward as an additional possible subtype of papillary RCC, although it has not gained traction in classification schemes due to lack of agreement about its features.[146-149] However, recent studies have suggested that there is a distinct subtype of neoplasm, characterized by oncocytic cells and papillary architecture with nuclei aligned toward the apex of the cells (Figures 3.157 and 3.158).[150-152]

TABLE 3.2: Differential Diagnosis of Type 1 Papillary Renal Cell Carcinoma (RCC)

	Key Features	Pitfalls	Immunohistochemistry
Papillary RCC	Papillary architecture, usually at least focally conspicuous nucleoli. May have foamy macrophages, psammoma bodies, vacuolated cells, intracytoplasmic hemosiderin	May have clear cells or solid growth	**Positive:** cytokeratin 7 (decreased if eosinophilic), strong AMACR, often vimentin **Variable:** high molecular weight cytokeratin **Negative:** WT1, CD57, carbonic anhydrase IX (or focal)
Metanephric adenoma	Very uniform bland nuclei	May have papillary component or calcifications	**Positive:** WT1, CD57 **Negative:** AMACR, cytokeratin 7 (or minimal)
Thyroid-like RCC	Colloid-like secretions		**Positive:** variable PAX8 (supporting primary renal cell lineage) **Negative:** TTF1 or thyroglobulin (to exclude metastatic thyroid cancer), AMACR usually negative or much less than that of papillary RCC
Clear cell RCC with papillary or pseudopapillary structures	Usually classic clear cell areas evident with thorough sampling		**Positive:** carbonic anhydrase IX (diffuse membrane) **Variable:** AMACR **Negative:** cytokeratin 7 (or focal)
MITF family translocation RCC	Mixed papillary and clear cell features, voluminous cytoplasm. May have: psammoma bodies, pigment	Varied patterns	**Positive:** often melanocytic markers, TFE3 or TFEB protein, often cathepsin K **Variable:** AMACR, cytokeratin, EMA, vimentin **Negative:** usually cytokeratin 7
Clear cell papillary RCC	Branched glandular structures, clear cytoplasm, nuclei aligned above basement membrane	Can closely mimic clear cell RCC	**Positive:** cytokeratin 7 (diffuse), carbonic anhydrase IX (cup-shaped pattern), high molecular weight cytokeratin, GATA3 **Negative:** AMACR, CD10
Mucinous tubular and spindle cell carcinoma	Mixture of areas resembling type 1 papillary RCC with spindle cell component and mucinous material	Can be mistaken for sarcomatoid change in papillary RCC	Similar to papillary RCC

TABLE 3.3: Differential Diagnosis of Type 2 Papillary Renal Cell Carcinoma (RCC)

	Key Features	Pitfalls	Immunohistochemistry
Type 2 papillary RCC	Papillary architecture, eosinophilic cells, nuclear pseudostratification	Diagnosis of exclusion after the others are argued against	**Positive:** PAX8 (supporting renal origin), AMACR strong **Negative:** p63, GATA3
Fumarate hydratase (FH)–deficient RCC	Mixed architectural patterns: papillary, tubular, infiltrative Very prominent nucleoli with perinucleolar clearing	Morphology can be heterogeneous and not exclusively papillary	**Positive:** 2-succino-cysteine **Negative:** abnormal negative FH, usually negative cytokeratin 7
MITF family translocation RCC	Mixed papillary and clear cell features, voluminous cytoplasm May have psammoma bodies, pigment	Varied patterns	**Positive:** often melanocytic markers, TFE3 or TFEB protein, often cathepsin K **Variable:** AMACR, cytokeratin, EMA, vimentin **Negative:** usually cytokeratin 7
Medullary carcinoma	Infiltrative carcinoma, sometimes prominent inflammation, occurring in patient with sickle trait or other hemoglobinopathy	Rare cases recently described in patients without hemoglobinopathy, referred to as RCC, unclassified with medullary phenotype	**Positive:** OCT3/4 often **Negative:** abnormal negative SMARCB1 (INI1)
Urothelial carcinoma	Infiltrative growth pattern, invading around normal renal structures, usually more pleomorphism than RCC	PAX8 may be positive in upper tract urothelial carcinoma	**Positive:** GATA3, p63, high molecular weight cytokeratin **Variable:** PAX8
Metastatic carcinoma of another origin	Resembles carcinoma of organ of origin, lung cancer most common	Can mimic a primary tumor (solitary, unilateral, circumscribed)	**Positive:** organ-specific markers (TTF1, others)
Collecting duct carcinoma	Infiltrative carcinoma of renal origin not meeting criteria for any of the others		**Positive:** PAX8 **Negative:** p63, GATA3

In one classification scheme, this was referred to as oncocytic low-grade papillary RCC (type 4),[150] and recently another group has proposed the name "papillary renal cell neoplasm with reverse polarity" for this entity.[151,152] These have been found to be negative for vimentin, contrasting to usual papillary RCC, and negative for KIT, contrasting to oncocytoma and chromophobe RCC, with the unusual finding of GATA3 positivity that seems

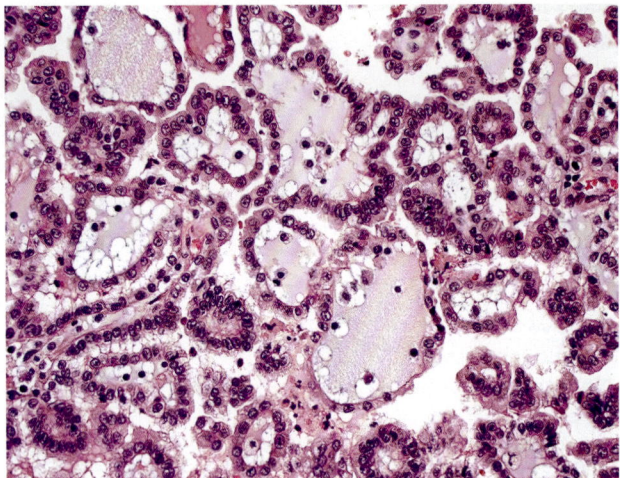

Figure 3.155. Occasional papillary renal cell carcinomas contain mucin, as in this example, within the fibrovascular cores.

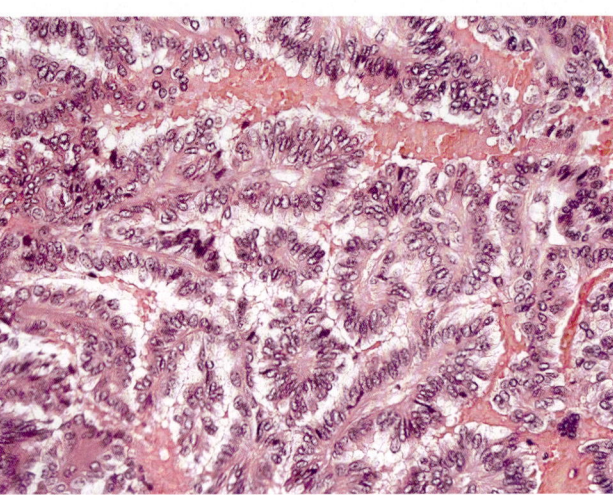

Figure 3.156. Type 2 papillary renal cell carcinoma has become almost a diagnosis of exclusion in current practice. It is composed of columnar eosinophilic cells with pseudostratified nuclei.

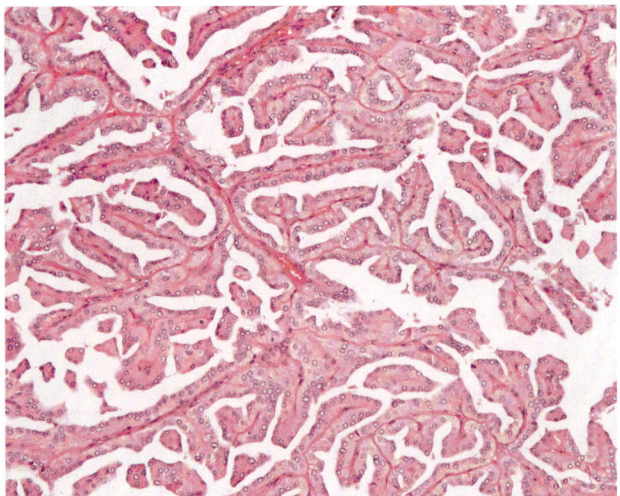

Figure 3.157. Papillary renal neoplasm with reverse polarity has been recently recognized as composed of oncocytic cells lining papillary structures, with nuclei aligned at the cell apex. (Courtesy of Khaleel Al-Obaidy, MD, Indiana University.)

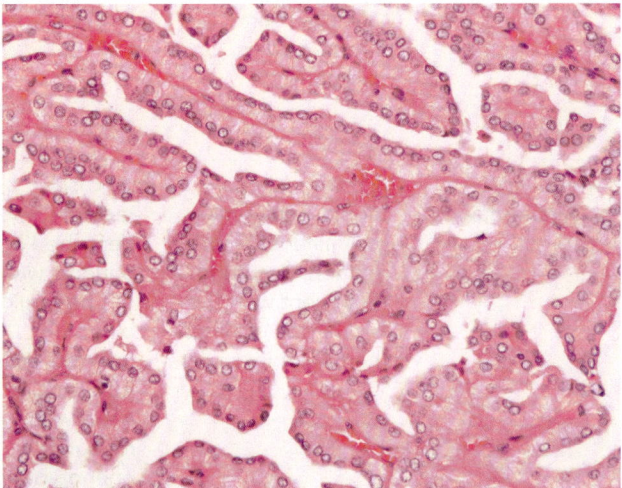

Figure 3.158. Higher magnification of this papillary renal neoplasm with reverse polarity shows the apical nuclear alignment. (Courtesy of Khaleel Al-Obaidy, MD, Indiana University.)

to discriminate them from other papillary RCCs (Figure 3.159). Staining for cytokeratin 7 is frequently present but variable in extent and AMACR does not always show the diffuse strong pattern of typical papillary tumors (Figure 3.160).[150,152] Recent work has found frequent *KRAS* mutations, which contrasts to type 1 and type 2 papillary RCC, supporting the consideration of this as a distinct type of renal neoplasm.[151]

FH-Deficient RCC/Hereditary Leiomyomatosis and RCC Syndrome

There has been an explosion of knowledge recently regarding FH-deficient RCC and the HLRCC syndrome–associated tumors.[22,153-158] The HLRCC syndrome is characterized by germline mutations of the *FH* gene, which leads to the development of renal cancer as well as multiple uterine and cutaneous leiomyomas. More recently, the term FH-deficient RCC has been proposed as a designation for renal cancer that is abnormal for the FH protein but in which definite germline mutation of the gene is not yet established. This avoids labeling patients who have not yet been proven to have a germline mutation as having the syndrome and allows for the possibility that occasional somatic mutations in *FH* in renal cancer might occur. FH-deficient renal cancer is known to be highly aggressive. In contrast to other hereditary renal cancer syndromes, in which the clinical paradigm is usually to preserve

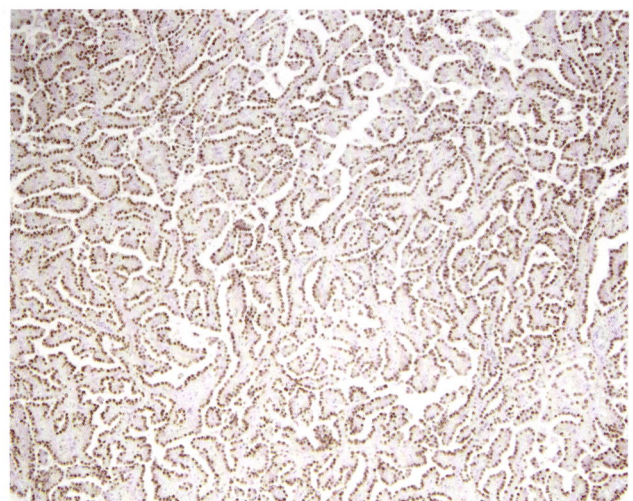

Figure 3.159. Papillary renal neoplasm with reverse polarity shows characteristic positive immunohistochemistry for GATA3, which is absent in most type 1 and type 2 papillary renal cell carcinomas. (Courtesy of Khaleel Al-Obaidy, MD, Indiana University.)

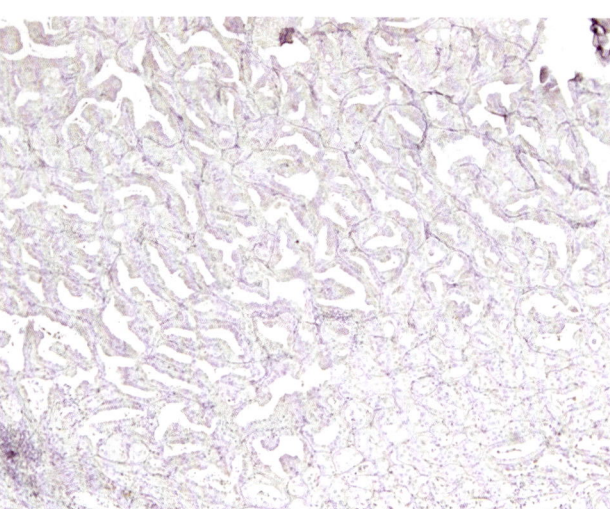

Figure 3.160. In contrast to most type 1 and 2 papillary renal cell carcinomas, AMACR staining may be limited or negative in papillary renal neoplasm with reverse polarity. (Courtesy of Khaleel Al-Obaidy, MD, Indiana University.)

the kidney as much as possible by performing nephron-sparing surgery with a close margin (such as enucleation), radical nephrectomy is typically recommended for even clinically localized or small HLRCC tumors.[159]

It was first recognized that HLRCC tumors resemble type 2 papillary RCCs and typically have extremely prominent nucleoli with perinucleolar clearing, resembling a cytomegalovirus inclusion.[20] However, subsequent studies have found that the morphology can be highly variable and sometimes deceptive.[21,22,160]

KEY FEATURES: FH-Deficient/HLRCC Tumors

- "Type 2" papillary RCC morphology, but variable patterns (Figures 3.161 and 3.162):
  - Tubulocystic-like (Figure 3.163)
  - Infiltrative adenocarcinoma (see Infiltrative Pattern section)
  - Solid
  - Cribriform
  - Cystic
- Cells with eosinophilic cytoplasm
- Nucleoli very prominent with perinucleolar clearing (can resemble viral inclusion)
  - However, not entirely specific alone[22,157] (Figure 3.164)
- Immunohistochemistry:
  - Abnormal negative staining for FH protein (Figure 3.165)
  - Positive staining for 2 succino-cysteine (Figure 3.166)
  - Usually negative for cytokeratin 7
- Deceptive/unusual patterns
  - Tubulocystic RCC with "dedifferentiation" (transition to an extensively infiltrative adenocarcinoma)[21] (Figures 3.167 and 3.168)
  - Rarely, low-grade oncocytic morphology, mimicking succinate dehydrogenase (SDH)–deficient RCC[160]

MITF Family Translocation RCC, Papillary Pattern

MITF family translocation RCC is also discussed under the clear cell pattern; however, a papillary component is also common (Figures 3.169 and 3.170). In general, a diagnosis of translocation-associated RCC should be a consideration for any unusual RCC with multiple

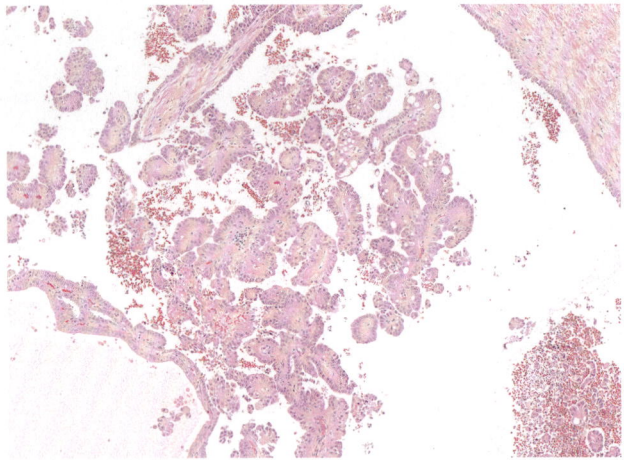

Figure 3.161. Fumarate hydratase–deficient or HLRCC-associated tumors prototypically are thought of as having papillary architecture; however, many patterns can be observed. This example shows intracystic papillary proliferation. (Courtesy of Steven C. Smith, MD, PhD, Virginia Commonwealth University.)

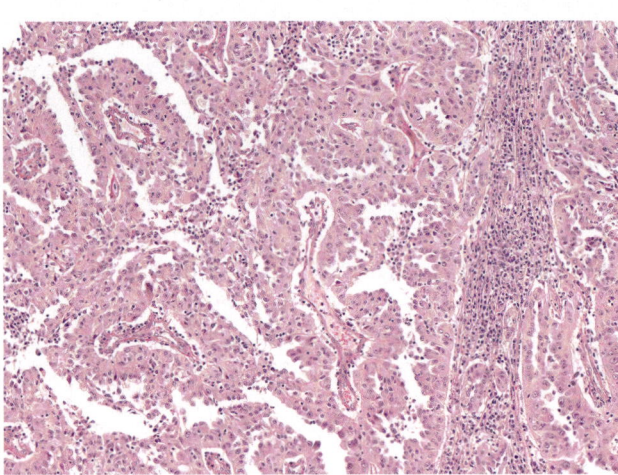

Figure 3.162. Another field of fumarate hydratase–deficient renal cell carcinoma shows complex papillary architecture with eosinophilic cells. (Courtesy of Steven C. Smith, MD, PhD, Virginia Commonwealth University.)

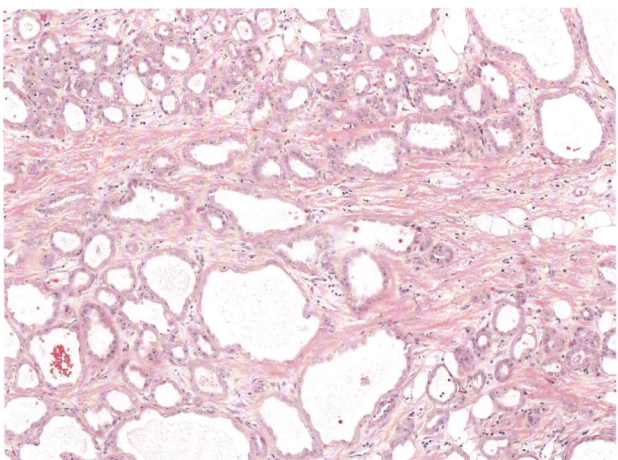

Figure 3.163. A pattern mimicking tubulocystic renal cell carcinoma can also be observed in fumarate hydratase–deficient renal cancer. (Courtesy of Steven C. Smith, MD, PhD, Virginia Commonwealth University.)

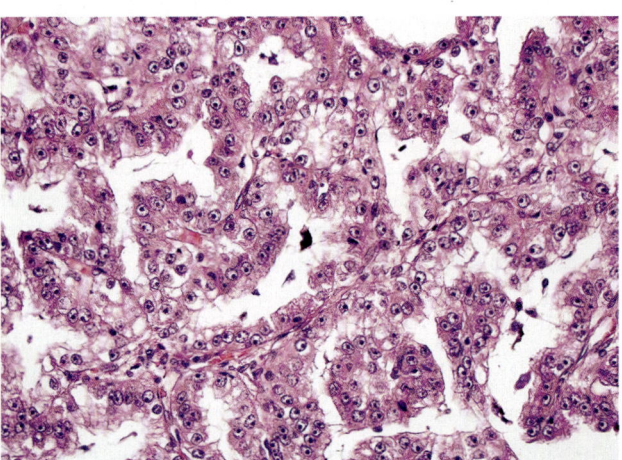

Figure 3.164. Extremely prominent nucleoli are a hallmark of fumarate hydratase (FH)–deficient renal cell carcinoma; however, this finding is not entirely specific. This example shows eosinophilic cells with prominent nucleoli; however, immunohistochemistry showed normal FH staining (not pictured). Normal immunohistochemical staining also does not entirely rule out mutation, as antibody labeling of a dysfunctional protein is also conceivable.

or mixed patterns, especially (but not exclusively) if the patient is young. Features of MITF tumors are discussed more extensively under the clear cell pattern, but in general, clues to a diagnosis of MITF family translocation RCC (*TFE3* or *TFEB* RCC) include mixed clear cell and eosinophilic cell patterns, psammoma bodies, abnormally voluminous cytoplasm, hyalinized stroma, and pigment deposition.[92,93] Helpful immunohistochemistry includes frequent positivity for melanocytic markers (HMB45 or melan-A), positivity for the TFE3 or TFEB proteins (although these stains may be technically challenging), positive cathepsin K, and sometimes unexpectedly negative or minimal reactivity for general epithelial markers (keratin) or vimentin.[96] Break-apart FISH is usually helpful to resolve the diagnosis; however, specific fusions that result from chromosomal inversion (*NONO*, *GRIPAP1*, *RBMX*, and *RBM10* partners of *TFE3*)[99-104] may be misleadingly negative using FISH or show only very slight break of the signals. Sequencing techniques may aid in confirming these deceptive cases.

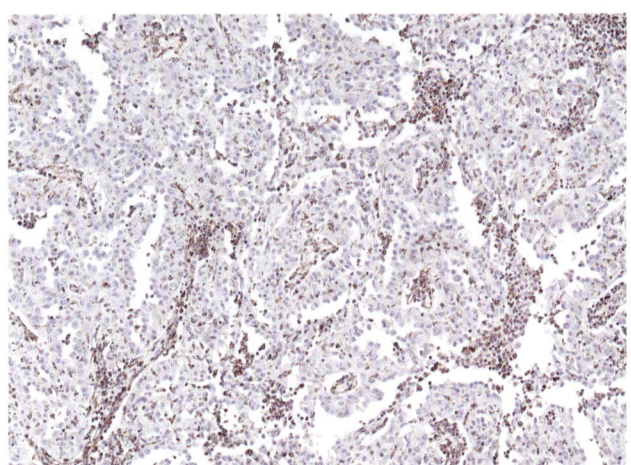

Figure 3.165. This fumarate hydratase (FH)–deficient renal cell carcinoma (RCC) shows abnormal negative staining for FH protein in the tumor cells, with a positive internal control of stromal cells showing normal reactivity. (Courtesy of Steven C. Smith, MD, PhD, Virginia Commonwealth University.)

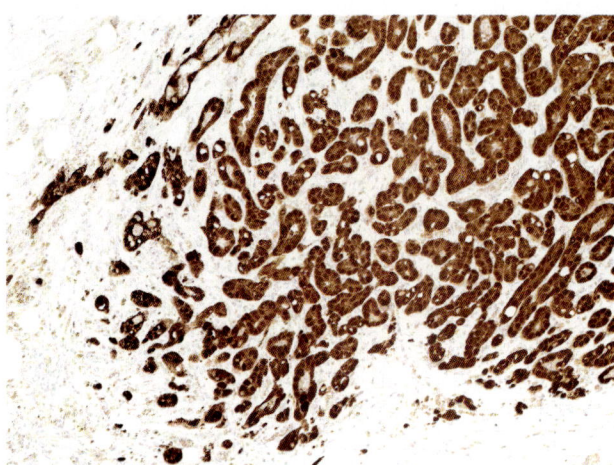

Figure 3.166. 2SC staining shows a positive reaction in fumarate hydratase–deficient renal cancers. (Courtesy of Steven C. Smith, MD, PhD, Virginia Commonwealth University.)

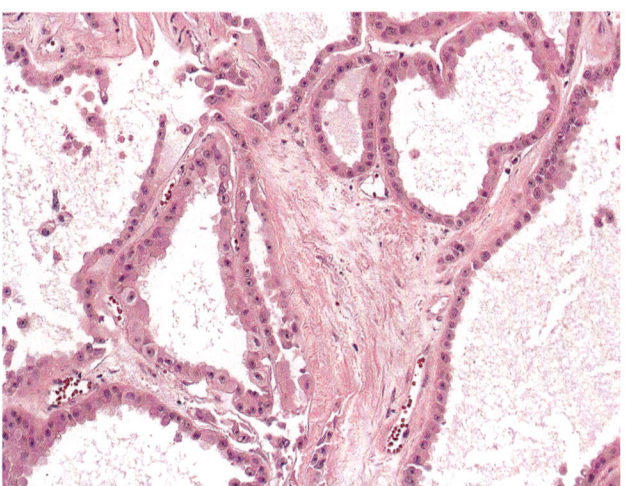

Figure 3.167. It has recently been found that many tumors previously thought to be "dedifferentiated" tubulocystic renal cell carcinoma (RCC) are fumarate hydratase–deficient renal cancers. This example includes areas resembling tubulocystic RCC and aggressive infiltrative adenocarcinoma (Figure 3.168).

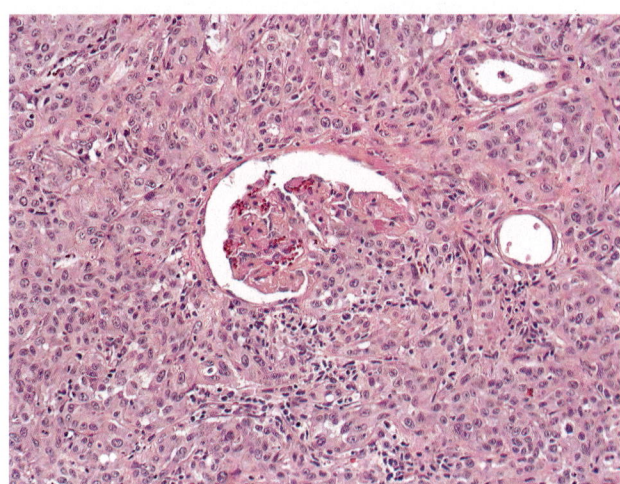

Figure 3.168. The same tumor from Figure 3.167 shows an aggressive adenocarcinoma overgrowing a normal glomerulus.

ONCOCYTIC/EOSINOPHILIC CELL PATTERN

Oncocytoma

Oncocytoma is the prototypical tumor in the category of oncocytic renal neoplasms.[161] Being one of the few benign renal epithelial neoplasms, distinguishing it from mimics, almost all of which are malignant, can be a great consternation for the practicing pathologist.[58,162] Despite being a benign neoplasm, oncocytomas can reach considerable size of greater than 10 cm (Figure 3.171), such that the presumed diagnosis would be unquestionably RCC.[163-165]

KEY FEATURES: Oncocytoma

- Gross appearance: often red-brown, sometimes central scar (although not specific for oncocytoma) (Figures 3.171 and 3.172)
- Architecture: round nests, solid growth, occasional cysts, prominent loose fibrous or edematous stroma (Figures 3.173-3.176)

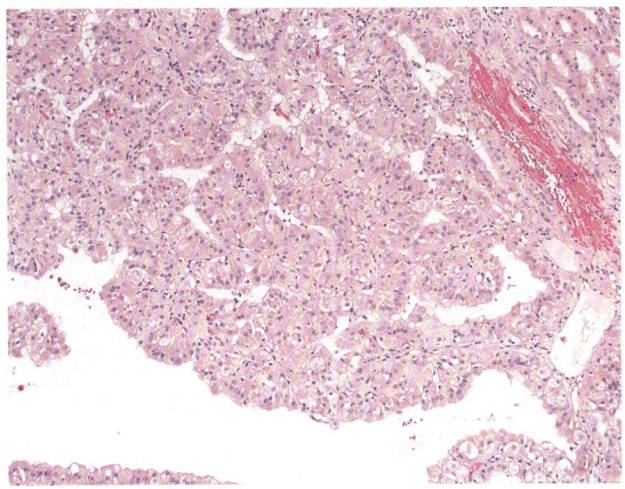

Figure 3.169. MITF family translocation renal cell carcinoma can show a papillary pattern. This tumor shows papillary structures formed by eosinophilic cells.

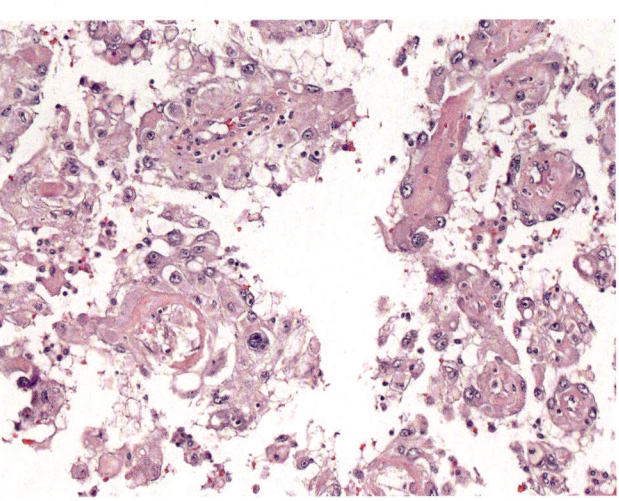

Figure 3.170. This MITF family translocation renal cell carcinoma is a high-grade carcinoma with papillary formation.

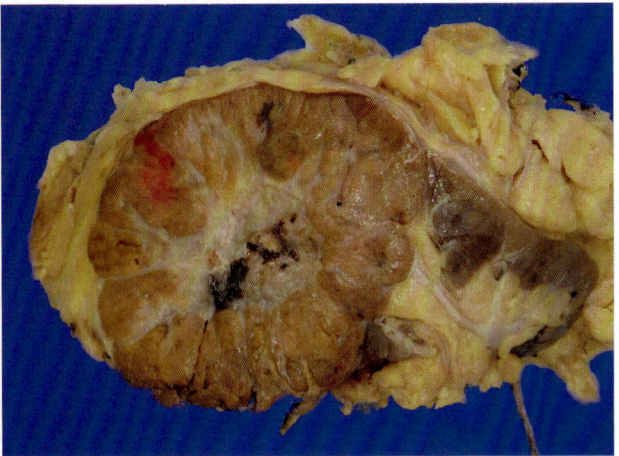

Figure 3.171. Oncocytomas may demonstrate a range of gross appearances. This tumor has the relatively classic brown cut surface, similar to the normal kidney, and central scar.

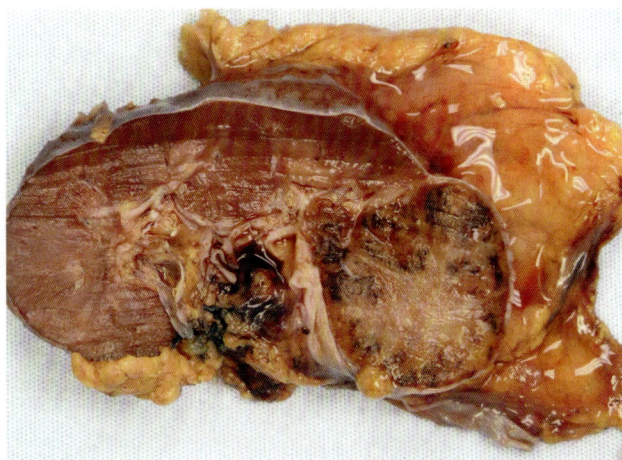

Figure 3.172. This oncocytoma may be more difficult to distinguish from renal cell carcinoma grossly, with dark red-brown hemorrhagic areas.

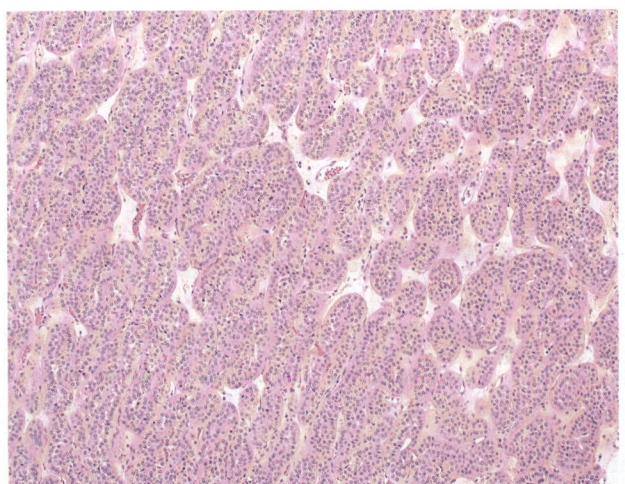

Figure 3.173. The classic architecture of oncocytoma includes discrete round nests of cells.

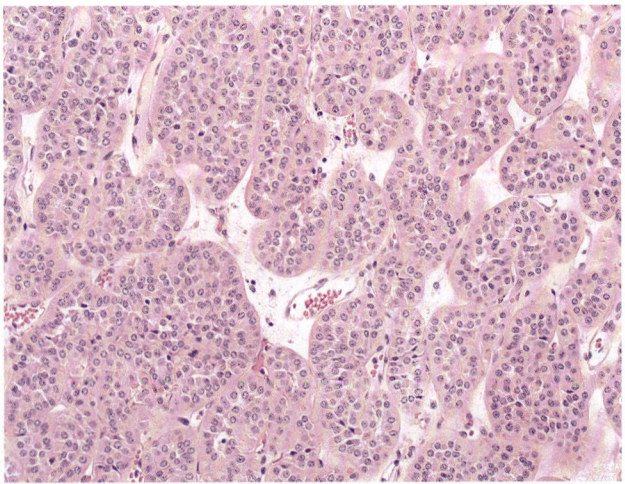

Figure 3.174. At higher magnification, nests of cells in oncocytoma are composed of uniform eosinophilic cells with round, regular nuclei.

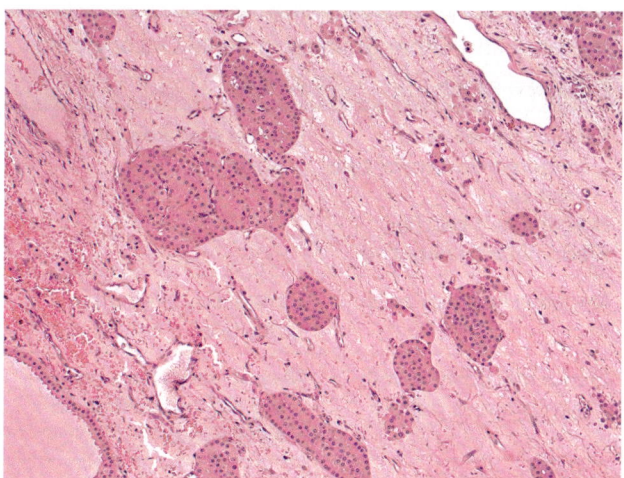

Figure 3.175. Often oncocytomas include areas of edematous or fibrous stroma with islands of cells "floating" in the stroma.

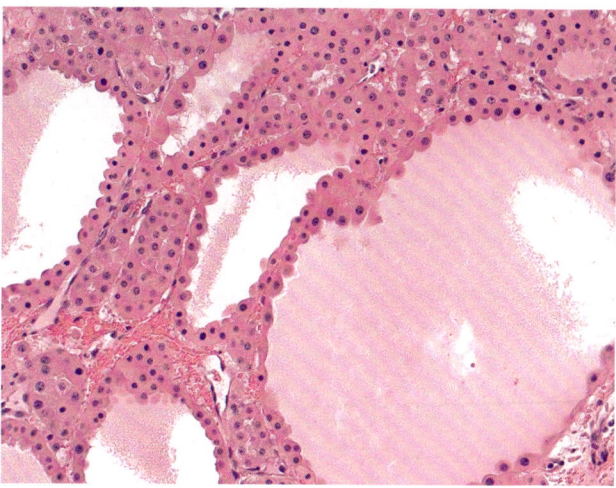

Figure 3.176. Cystic spaces are sometimes present in oncocytoma. Both the cysts and solid areas are lined by similar cells with uniform round nuclei and eosinophilic cytoplasm.

- Cytology: uniform cells with eosinophilic granular cytoplasm and round nuclei (Figures 3.177 and 3.178)
- Mitotic activity extremely rare (more than one on thorough search noted to be highly concerning in an expert survey)[162]
- Histochemical staining: colloidal iron (Hale or modified Mowry stain) is commonly discussed[166] but technically difficult and not used by many laboratories; should show negative staining in oncocytoma (Figure 3.179), contrasting to cytoplasmic staining of chromophobe RCC
- Immunohistochemistry (Table 3.4):
  - Cytokeratin 7—labels rare single cells and clusters of cells (exact percentage not entirely established but likely much less than 5%, typically no confluent patches) (Figure 3.180)[48]
    - Exception: "scar" areas often positive
  - KIT/CD117—often positive with membranous pattern, but may be weak (Figure 3.181)
  - Vimentin—consistently negative (Figure 3.182)
    - Exception: "scar" areas often positive

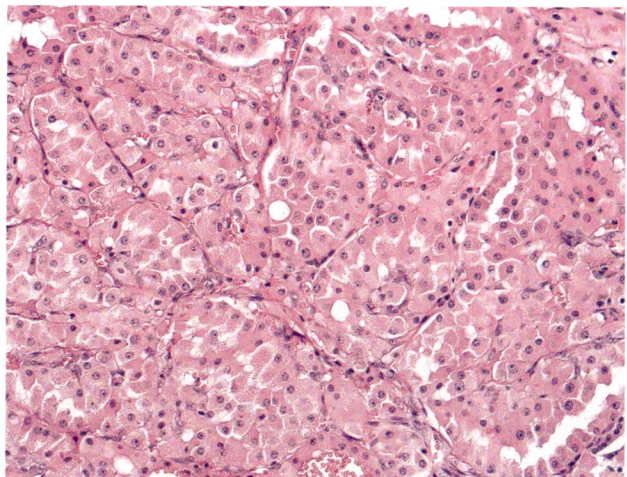

Figure 3.177. In this oncocytoma, cells are arranged in compact nests, imparting a solid appearance. Nuclei are round with uniform nucleoli.

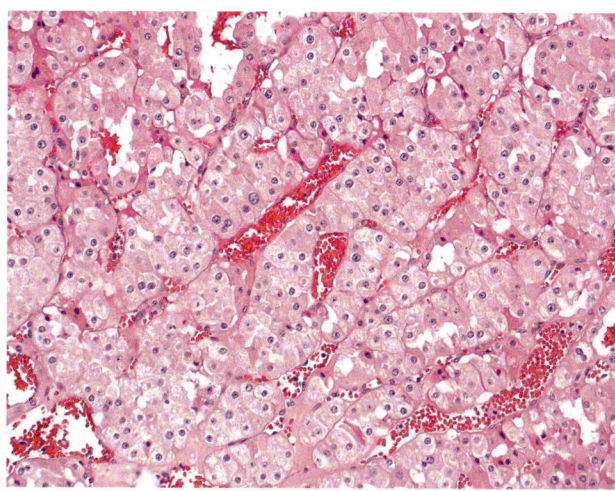

Figure 3.178. This field of oncocytoma shows cells with voluminous cytoplasm and variably prominent nucleoli.

TABLE 3.4: Immunohistochemistry and Other Staining in Renal Oncocytoma

	Expected Result	Pitfalls
Cytokeratin 7	Rare single cells and scattered clusters of cells positive No confluent patches Predominantly negative	Central scar area often positive
Vimentin	Negative in tumor cells	Central scar area often positive
KIT (CD117)	Frequently positive with membranous pattern	May be very weak, requiring high magnification to visualize
Succinate dehydrogenase B	Normal strong granular cytoplasmic staining	
Colloidal iron	Negative cytoplasm of tumor cells	Some authors allow an apical bar pattern of staining as compatible with oncocytoma Technically difficult, not used in all laboratories

- SDHB—normal positive granular cytoplasmic staining (Figure 3.183)
- Carbonic anhydrase IX—negative or minimal
- Various other markers have been explored but few in widespread use[162,167,168]
- Cytogenetics/molecular—generally not necessary in most diagnostic cases but may be a consideration for difficult cases, if FISH or comparative genomic hybridization (CGH) is available
  - May have diploid karyotype, loss of chromosome 1, loss of Y, or rearrangement of 11q13, including t(5;11)(q35;q13)[169]
  - 11q13 rearrangements likely represent *CCND1* gene (cyclin D1) rearrangement[170,171]
  - Multiple chromosomal losses would favor chromophobe RCC, particularly Y, 1, 2, 6, 10, 13, 17, and 21,[56] and lesser rates of 3, 5, 8, 9, 11, and 18[67]
  - Mutations in mitochondrial genes are also noted in both oncocytoma and chromophobe RCC[56,67,171]

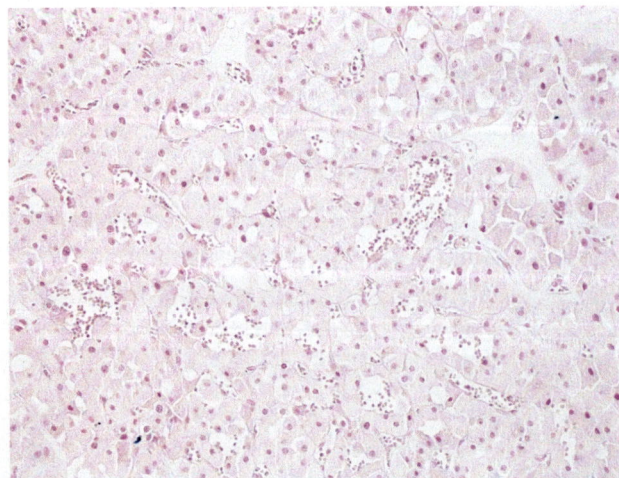

Figure 3.179. Colloidal iron stains are not always easy to calibrate in terms of technical staining conditions. The classic result should be negative staining in oncocytoma.

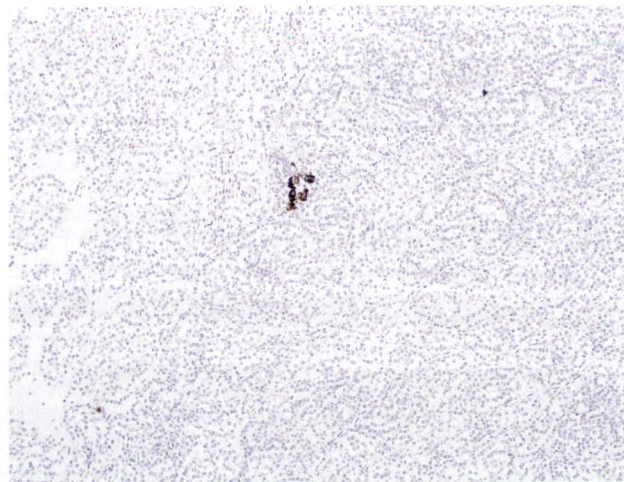

Figure 3.180. Cytokeratin 7 staining typically demonstrates rare scattered cells and clusters of cells positive in oncocytoma, with most areas appearing largely negative.

PEARLS AND PITFALLS: Deceptive Features of Oncocytoma

Oncocytoma can have several features that can cause concern to the pathologist, yet which do not appear to alter its benign behavior:

- Involvement of fat—relatively well characterized that extension into fat is compatible with a diagnosis of oncocytoma (Figures 3.184 and 3.185), despite qualifying for pT3a for renal cancer[58,163,172]

- Involvement of veins—although some pathologists are uncomfortable with this finding in oncocytoma (Figures 3.186 and 3.187),[162] all existing literature suggests that it does not alter the benign behavior[173,174]

- Nuclear atypia—"degenerative" nuclear atypia with large cells showing smudged nuclear chromatin (Figure 3.188) is considered compatible with oncocytoma, as long as it is not associated with increased mitotic activity

- Cytokeratin 7 staining in "central scar"—although the classic staining pattern shows only scattered individual cells positive for cytokeratin 7 in oncocytoma, the central scar area is frequently positive, for unknown reasons (Figures 3.189-3.192)

- Vimentin staining in "central scar"—although vimentin is consistently negative in oncocytoma, the central scar area is frequently positive, for unknown reasons (Figure 3.193)[175]

- Papillary adenoma or RCC entrapped within oncocytoma—rarely papillary tumors can become "entrapped" within an oncocytic tumor (Figure 3.194).[176] If the immunohistochemical features support two distinct processes, these can usually be diagnosed as separate lesions

- Rare oncocytomas can have small papillary tufts in cystic spaces (Figure 3.195). If papillary growth is more extensive, immunohistochemistry may be helpful. Positive staining for vimentin, very strong staining for AMACR, or negative staining for KIT would raise suspicion for papillary RCC with oncocytic cells.

FAQ: Can Oncocytoma Be Diagnosed in a Biopsy Specimen?

It is debated whether the pathologist should report an outright diagnosis of oncocytoma in a biopsy sample, or if instead a general "oncocytic neoplasm" with explanatory comment should be used. Some authors believe that due to the overlap of eosinophilic chromophobe RCC and oncocytoma and so-called "hybrid tumors" that it is impossible to be sure in a biopsy specimen.[162] Others would argue that if the features are entirely consistent with those of oncocytoma, there is no need to issue an equivocal diagnosis. Similarly, it would be unusual to issue an equivocal diagnosis for every colon polyp based on the logic that there may be unsampled adenocarcinoma. Either approach is reasonable, if the findings are accurately communicated to clinicians with appropriate communication as to the clinical needs from the biopsy results. Some data do indicate that surveillance is a viable option for both oncocytoma and eosinophilic chromophobe RCC.[177]

Chromophobe RCC, Eosinophilic Variant

The classic pattern of chromophobe RCC was previously discussed under the clear/pale cell pattern; however, the pattern known to cause a greater amount of diagnostic difficulty is the eosinophilic variant. These tumors inherently closely resemble oncocytoma, and in fact the precise cut-point between the diagnosis of oncocytoma and eosinophilic chromophobe RCC can be subjective.[162] It is a subject of debate whether oncocytoma and chromophobe RCC represent a spectrum of related tumors, or if these are entirely unrelated neoplasms that can mimic each other. On the one hand, there is little similarity between a classic chromophobe RCC and an oncocytoma; however, eosinophilic chromophobe tumors can very closely mimic oncocytoma (Figures 3.196-3.204).

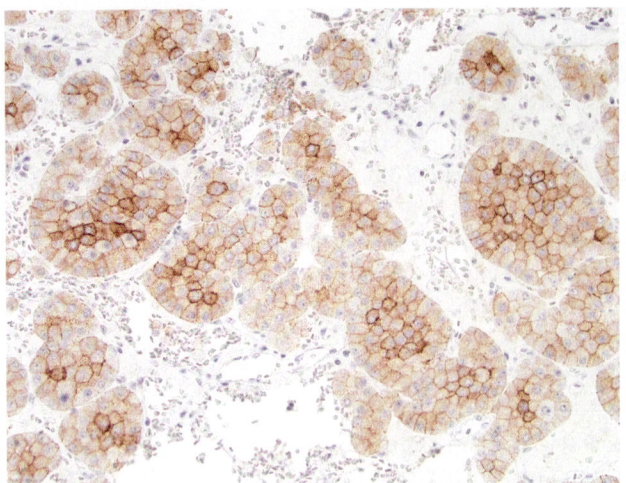

Figure 3.181. KIT (CD117) is often positive in oncocytoma, with a membranous staining pattern. This contrasts to most renal cell carcinoma (RCC) types, which are usually negative (except for chromophobe RCC).

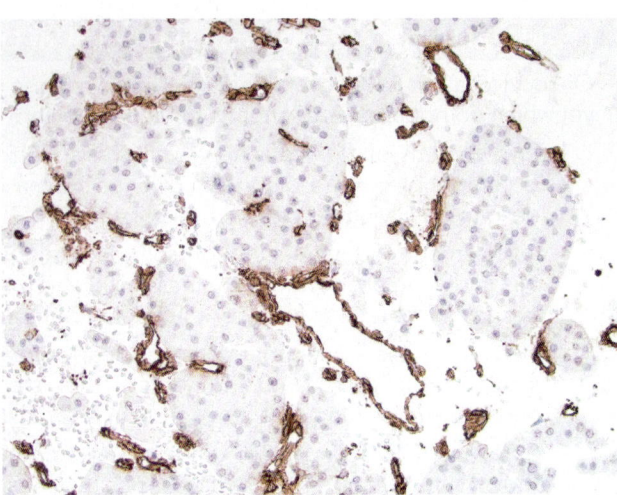

Figure 3.182. Vimentin immunohistochemistry is typically negative in oncocytoma, here highlighting only the blood vessels.

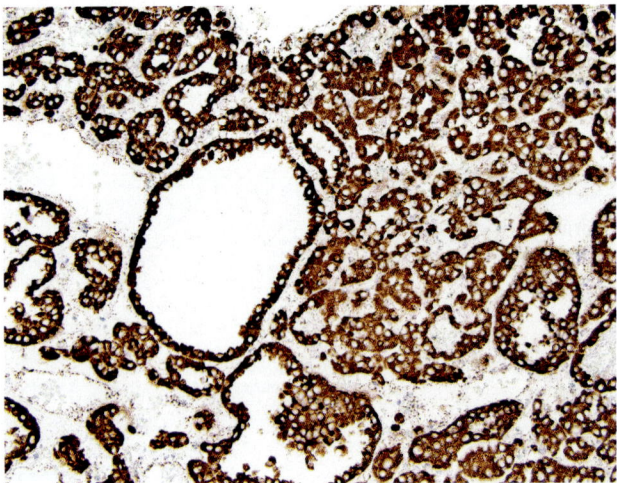

Figure 3.183. SDHB immunohistochemistry is strongly positive (a normal pattern) in this oncocytoma, contrasting to SDH-deficient renal cell carcinoma.

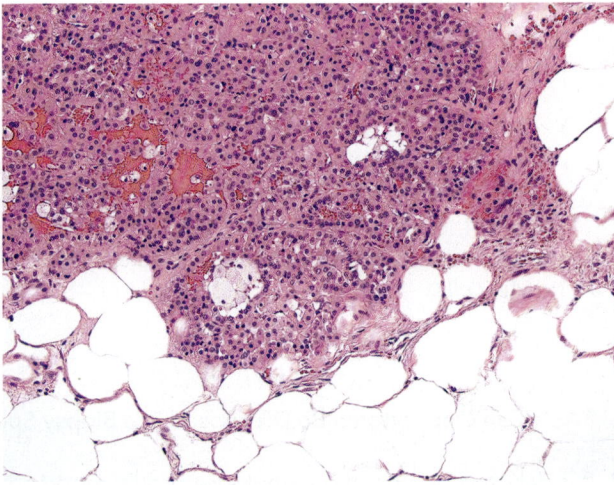

Figure 3.184. Oncocytomas may extend into fat, typically with no fibrosis or stromal reaction, as in this case. This does not appear to alter the benign behavior of oncocytoma, despite that it would be pT3a in renal cancer.

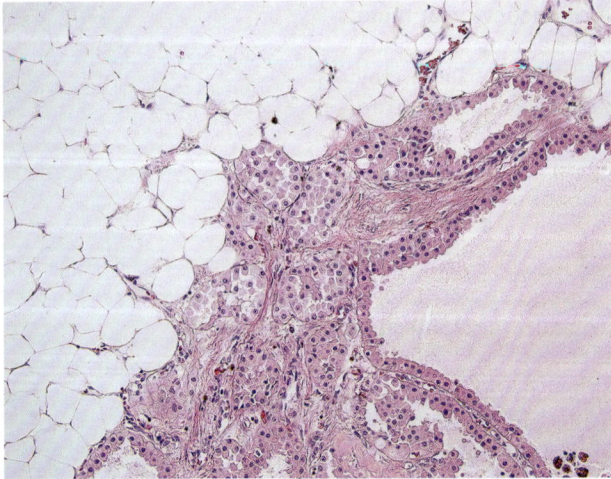

Figure 3.185. In this oncocytoma, cystic structures and small nests of tumor cells abut fat with no stromal reaction.

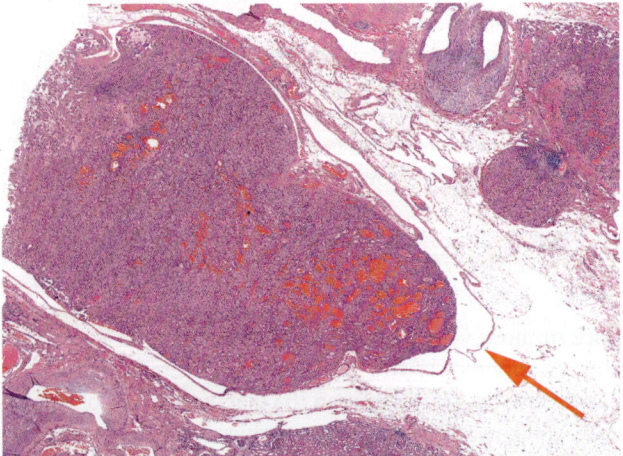

Figure 3.186. Rare oncocytomas have been reported to invade renal vein branches. Here a large polypoid projection fills most of a renal sinus vein (residual lumen at arrow). Despite that this would appear worrisome, all data to date indicate that the behavior of such tumors is still benign.

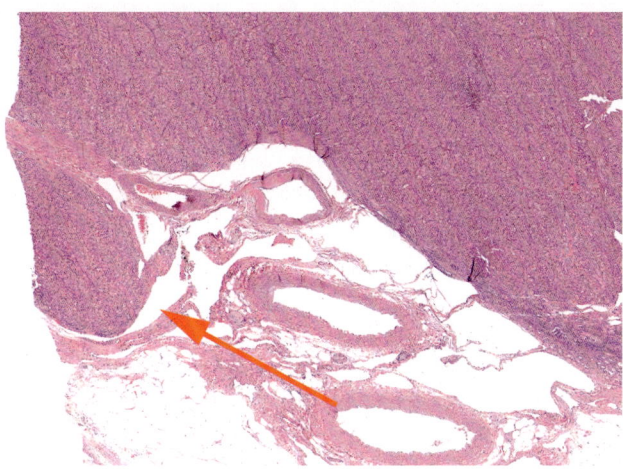

Figure 3.187. This oncocytoma shows a small polypoid protrusion into a renal sinus vein (arrow).

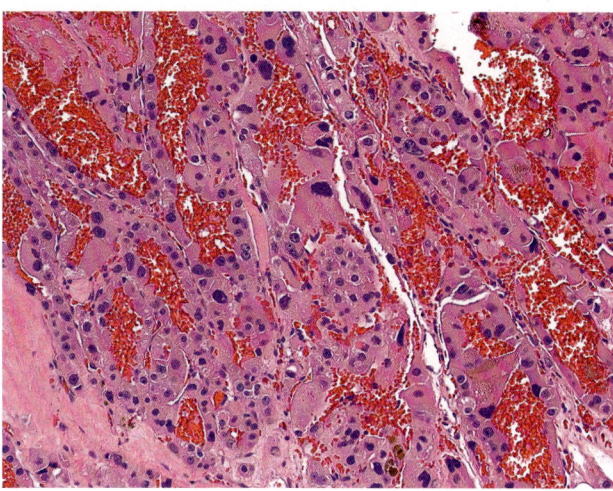

Figure 3.188. Patchy areas of smudgy nuclear atypia can be found in occasional oncocytomas. This is thought to be degenerative in nature and does not appear to alter the benign behavior of oncocytoma.

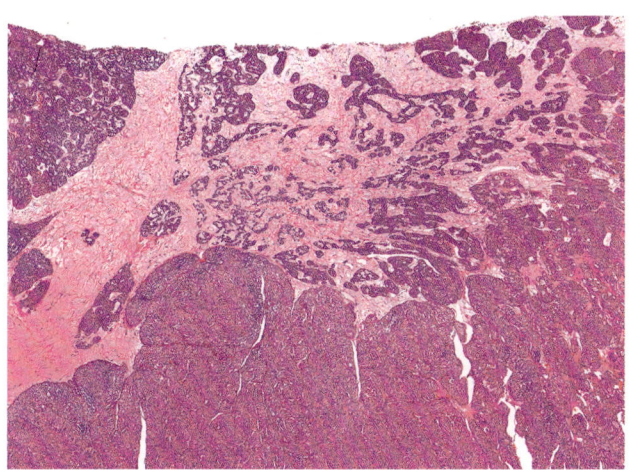

Figure 3.189. Histologically, the central scar of oncocytoma manifests as fibrous tissue, sometimes with the nests of tumor cells having a slightly different appearance.

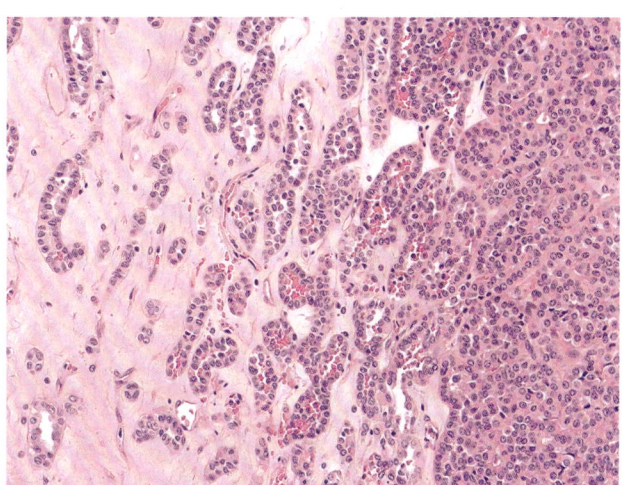

Figure 3.190. At higher magnification, the tubular structures in the central scar of an oncocytoma have a generally similar appearance to the rest of the tumor.

FAQ: How Do I Handle Borderline Cases Between Oncocytoma and Eosinophilic Chromophobe RCC?

In general, our approach to tumors that show borderline features between oncocytoma and chromophobe RCC is to either err toward a diagnosis of chromophobe RCC (if there are atypical features imperfect for that of oncocytoma) or to issue a borderline diagnosis with a comment that it would be reasonable to manage the patient as for a diagnosis of eosinophilic chromophobe RCC. This terminology usually includes oncocytic renal cell neoplasm, and various modifier terms have been proposed such as "low-grade," "borderline features," "unclassified," "low malignant potential," "uncertain malignant potential," or "hybrid tumor."[162] Our preference is to avoid using the terminology "unclassified" whenever possible, as there is sometimes a clinical perception that unclassified RCC is highly aggressive.[178,179] This would likely be a misrepresentation in the case of a tumor that is borderline between a benign neoplasm and a generally nonaggressive carcinoma. This type of diagnosis indicates that the patient can be followed as for a nonaggressive RCC (eosinophilic chromophobe), despite not fitting criteria perfectly for oncocytoma.

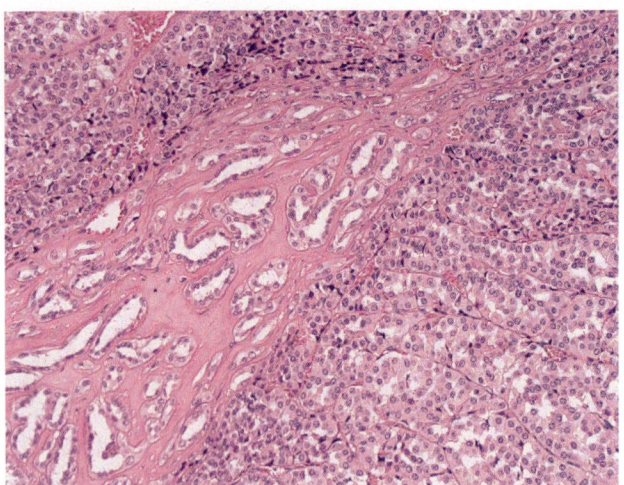

Figure 3.191. Occasionally the oncocytoma tubules entrapped in the central scar will appear more basophilic or have a pale/clear cell appearance, as in this case. The immunohistochemistry may show different results in these areas (Figures 3.192 and 3.193), which remains consistent with an oncocytoma diagnosis.

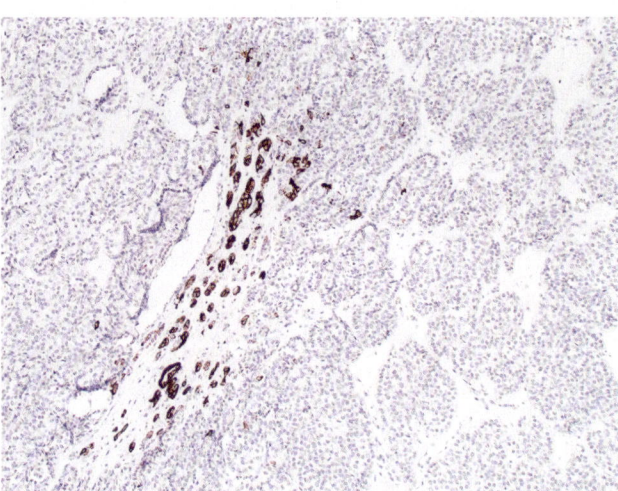

Figure 3.192. In this oncocytoma, cytokeratin 7 staining is increased in the scar areas but shows a normal pattern of only rare positive cells in other areas, which should be expected in oncocytoma.

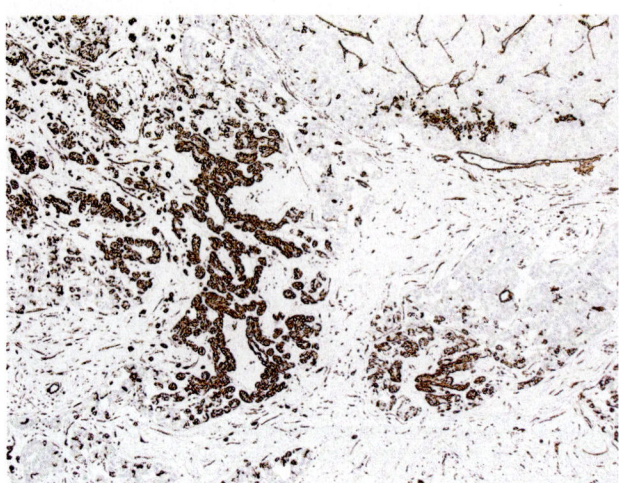

Figure 3.193. Vimentin staining can show the same phenomenon as cytokeratin 7, with increased staining in the scar areas of oncocytoma.

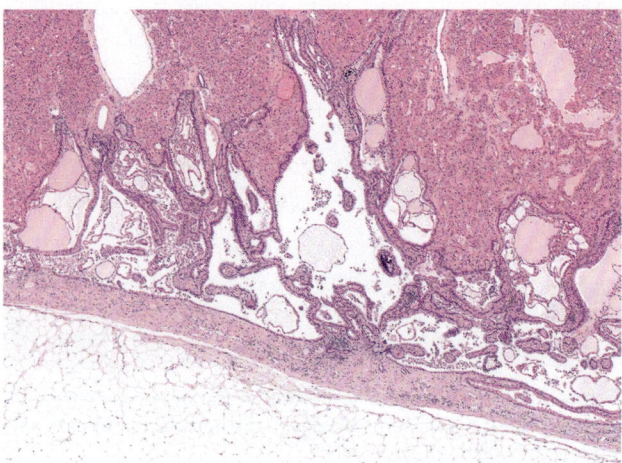

Figure 3.194. An unusual finding in some oncocytomas is entrapment of papillary lesion within the tumor. This may reflect that oncocytomas are often unencapsulated and sometimes entrap benign tubules as well. If the immunohistochemical findings support two distinct processes, this is thought to be compatible with a diagnosis of oncocytoma and concurrent papillary lesion (adenoma or renal cell carcinoma).

Our approach is that patchy contiguous areas of staining for cytokeratin 7 are outside of the spectrum of oncocytoma (Figures 3.205-3.207), which would support a diagnosis of eosinophilic chromophobe. Morphologically, areas of perinuclear clearing, nuclear size variation, and other findings that are typically associated with chromophobe RCC would typically tip the scale toward a diagnosis of chromophobe RCC. In general, chromophobe RCC is considered a favorable histology, and this is especially true for eosinophilic chromophobe.

SAMPLE NOTE: Oncocytic Renal Neoplasm With Borderline Features

Kidney, left, partial nephrectomy:
• Oncocytic renal neoplasm with borderline features—see Comment

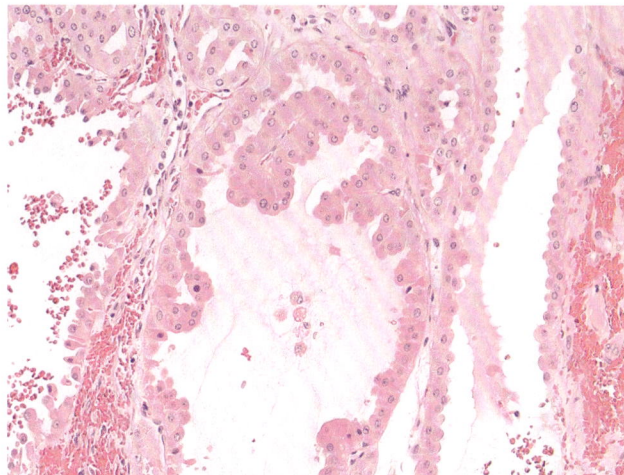

Figure 3.195. Occasionally oncocytomas can have focal small papillary tufts in cystic spaces. Diffuse papillary formation should not be present, and immunohistochemistry can be helpful if features are atypical.

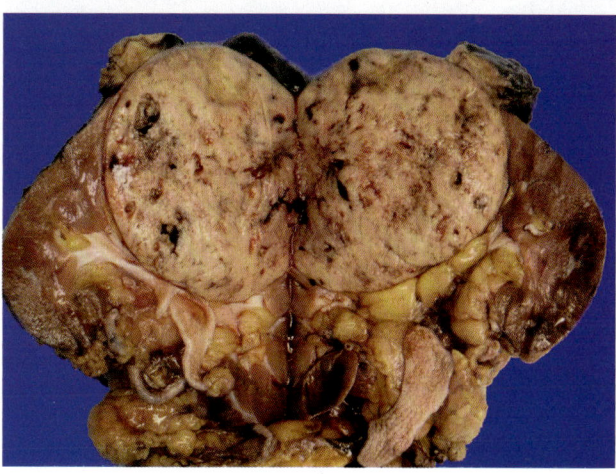

Figure 3.196. This eosinophilic chromophobe renal cell carcinoma (RCC) forms a pale tan mass, similar to conventional chromophobe RCC and less brown than a typical oncocytoma.

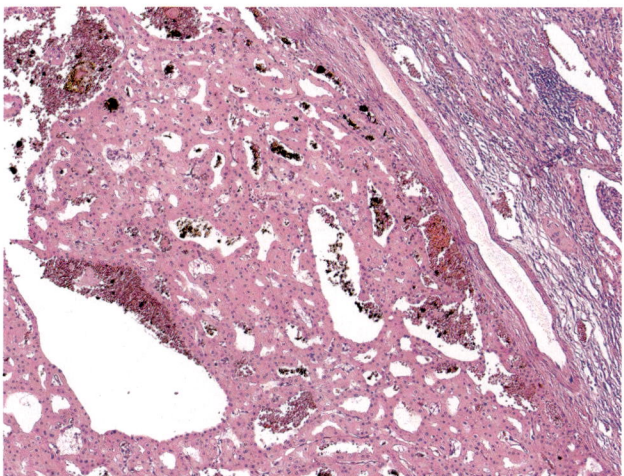

Figure 3.197. Microscopically, distinguishing chromophobe renal cell carcinoma from oncocytoma can be difficult. This example forms multiple confluent tubular structures, which would be atypical for oncocytoma.

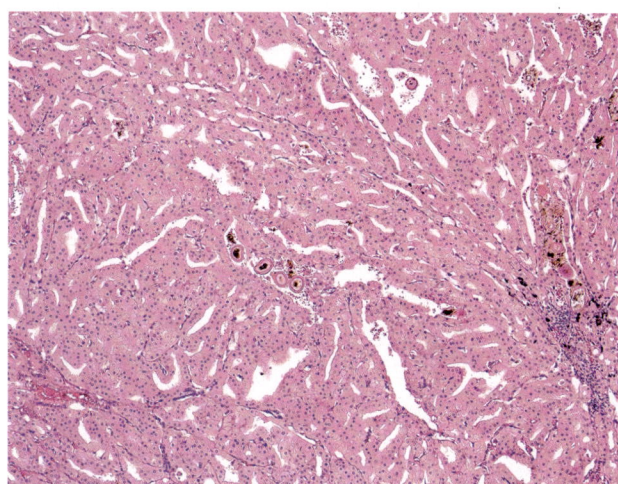

Figure 3.198. This confluent tubular growth would be unusual for oncocytoma and favors eosinophilic chromophobe renal cell carcinoma.

- 3.5 cm greatest dimension, confined to the kidney (pT1a)
- Margins negative

Comment: The features are borderline between oncocytoma and eosinophilic variant chromophobe RCC. Clinical follow-up as for eosinophilic chromophobe RCC would likely be reasonable.

Hybrid Tumors

The terminology of hybrid tumor or hybrid oncocytoma-chromophobe tumor has been used relatively extensively in the literature. However, a problem with this nomenclature is that it lacks a rigorous definition. In a survey of urologic pathologists, it was found that some used this for a mosaic pattern with some areas typical of oncocytoma and others typical of chromophobe RCC; however, others would use this term when there is an apparent syndrome, such as Birt-Hogg-Dubé or renal oncocytosis. Still others would use it for any borderline tumor or not at all, suggesting that there is not a clear definition of this entity. The 2016 WHO Classification discusses it under chromophobe RCC for lack of definitive

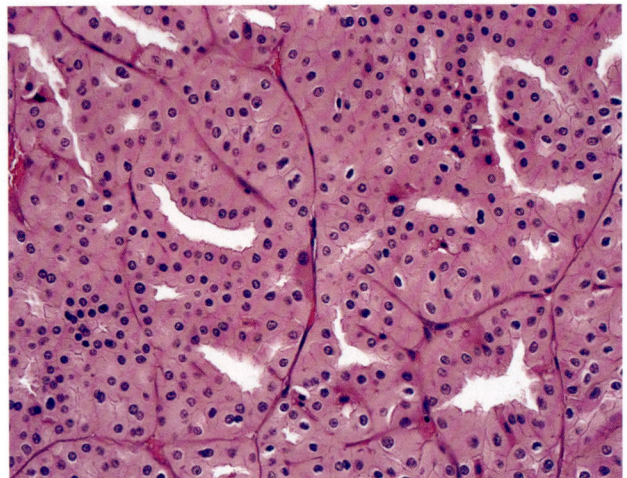

Figure 3.199. At high magnification, this eosinophilic chromophobe renal cell carcinoma forms many tubular structures. There are patchy perinuclear "halos" or areas of clearing, and the nuclei are more ovoid with nuclear grooves, contrasting to the uniform round nuclei of oncocytoma.

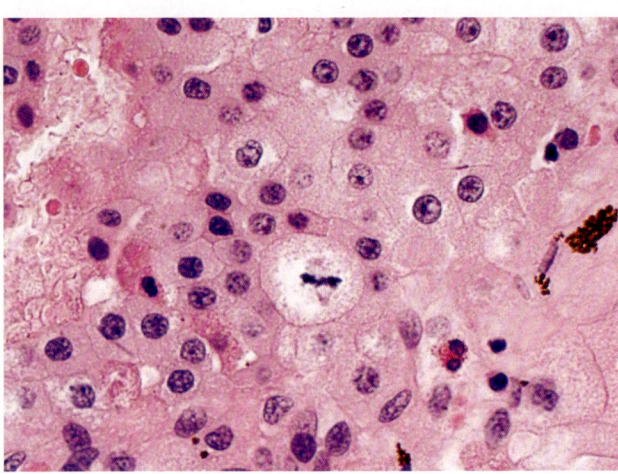

Figure 3.200. This eosinophilic chromophobe renal cell carcinoma contains a mitotic figure. Urologic pathologists generally consider that one mitotic figure on thorough search could potentially be compatible with oncocytoma; however, multiple mitotic figures would be very worrisome or incompatible with this diagnosis.

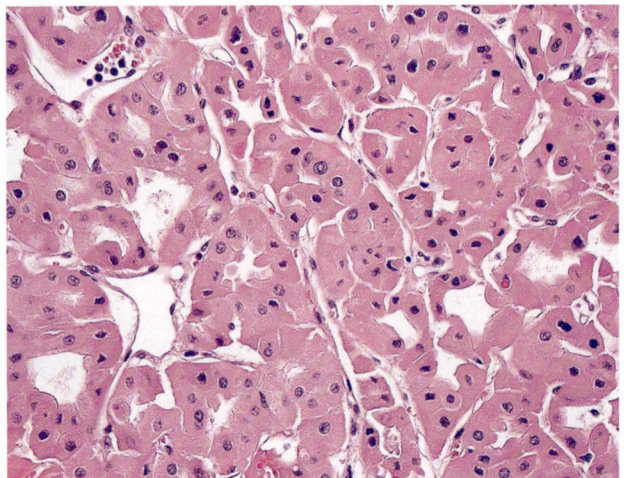

Figure 3.201. At high magnification, this eosinophilic chromophobe renal cell carcinoma demonstrates a predominance of wrinkled nuclei with focal intranuclear cytoplasmic invaginations.

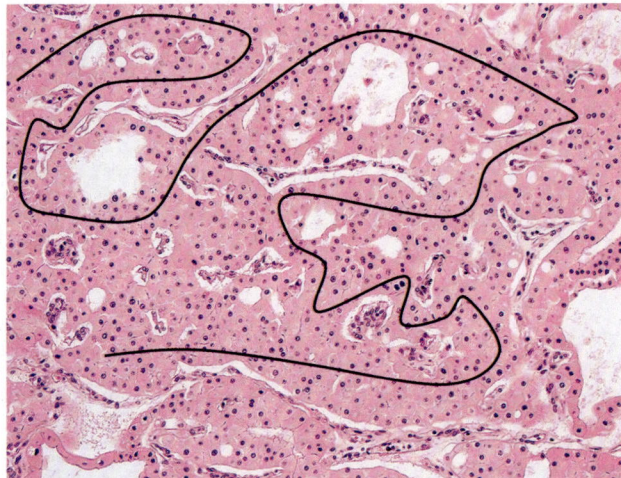

Figure 3.202. A trabecular growth pattern would favor a diagnosis of chromophobe renal cell carcinoma (RCC). In this case, one could draw a line through tumor cells (like solving a maze on paper) without crossing stromal cells or blood vessels. This pattern would be very atypical for oncocytoma or other RCC types, such as clear cell RCC, in which almost every packet of cells appears invested by capillaries.

understanding at present.[56] Our approach is to typically reserve this term for tumors that have clear transition between oncocytoma-like and chromophobe-like components (Figures 3.208-3.211). These patterns have been noted in the settings of syndromes (Birt-Hogg-Dubé or renal oncocytosis), and so a comment regarding the possibility of such a syndrome may be reasonable, particularly when multiple tumors are noted and certainly when there are numerous microscopic oncocytic tumors found incidentally in the grossly normal renal parenchyma.[180-182]

Clear Cell RCC With Eosinophilic Cells

Clear cell RCC may have eosinophilic cells (Figures 3.212-3.215), usually not more than focally mimicking an oncocytic neoplasm. It would be quite unusual for a clear cell RCC to show these changes so diffusely in multiple sections of a resection specimen that the diagnosis is almost entirely obscured. However, in a biopsy specimen with limited visualization, this may be a greater diagnostic problem. In such cases, immunohistochemistry is

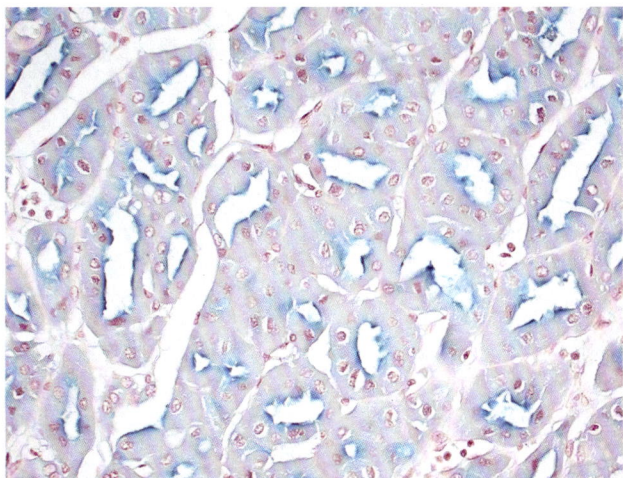

Figure 3.203. The classic colloidal iron staining reaction in chromophobe renal cell carcinoma shows diffuse cytoplasmic staining. This example also has luminal accentuation.

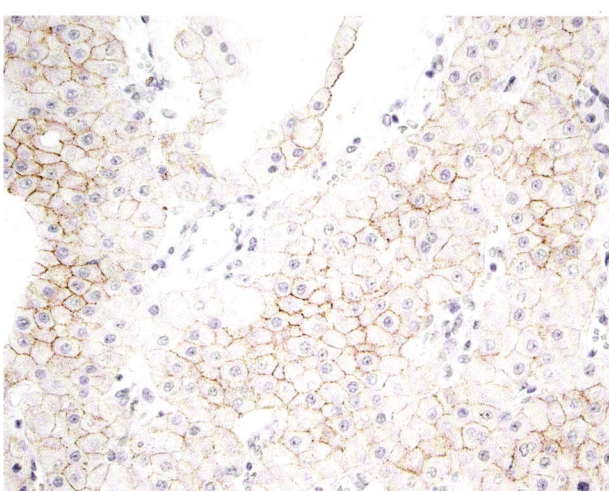

Figure 3.204. Like oncocytoma, KIT staining (CD117) is typically positive in chromophobe renal cell carcinoma. Sometimes the intensity may be weak in both tumors, requiring inspection at high magnification.

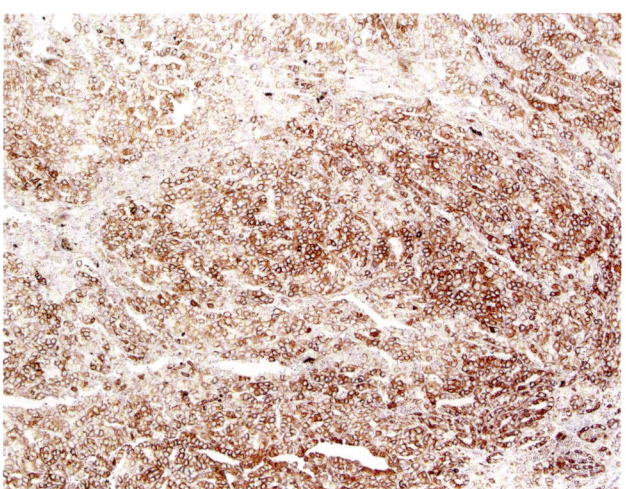

Figure 3.205. Cytokeratin 7 staining can be variable in chromophobe renal cell carcinoma. Diffuse staining would argue against oncocytoma strongly.

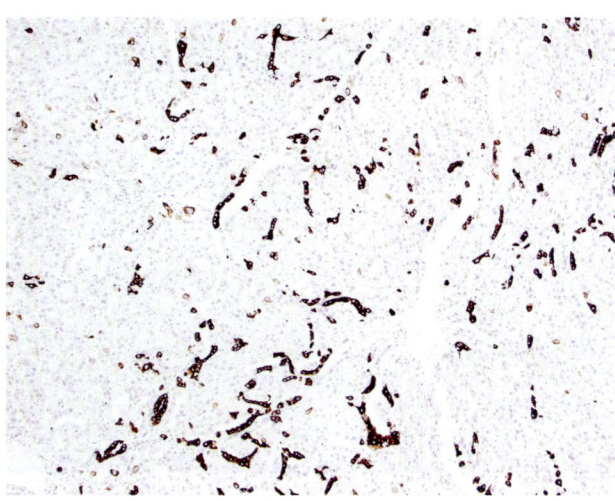

Figure 3.206. This example of chromophobe renal cell carcinoma shows limited cytokeratin 7 staining, although the patches of several cells confluently is more than typically found in oncocytoma.

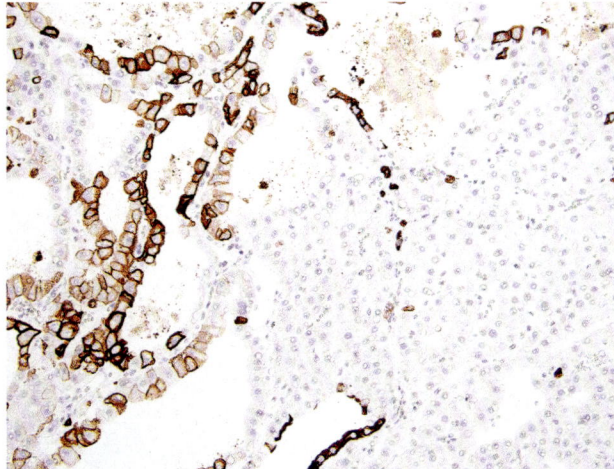

Figure 3.207. This chromophobe renal cell carcinoma shows predominantly negative staining for cytokeratin 7 with an oncocytoma-like pattern (right side). However, confluent patches (left) argue against a diagnosis of oncocytoma.

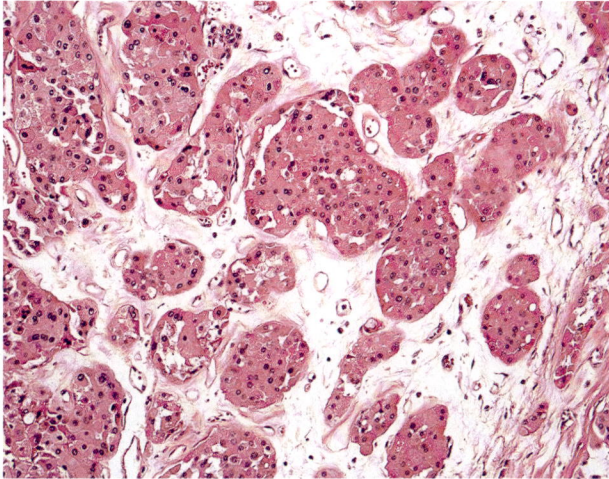

Figure 3.208. "Hybrid" tumors are not very well defined. This example shows a mixture of patterns resembling oncocytoma with nests of eosinophilic cells. Other areas are more chromophobe-like, in Figure 3.209.

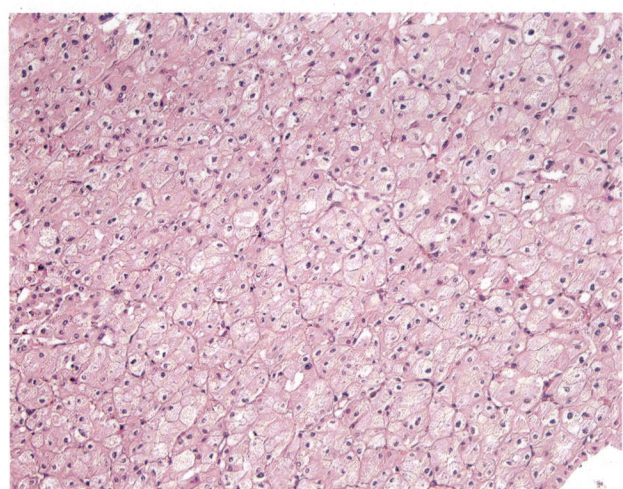

Figure 3.209. Other areas of the same tumor from Figure 3.208 are more chromophobe-like, with ovoid to wrinkled nuclei and variably voluminous cytoplasm, supporting a diagnosis of "hybrid tumor" for this case.

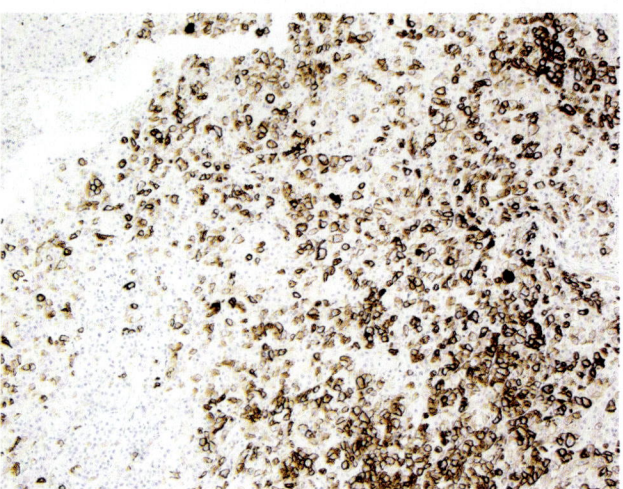

Figure 3.210. The hybrid oncocytoma-chromophobe tumor from Figures 3.208 and 3.209 demonstrates prominent cytokeratin 7 staining in the chromophobe-like areas, whereas other areas showed only scattered cells staining, resembling oncocytoma (not pictured).

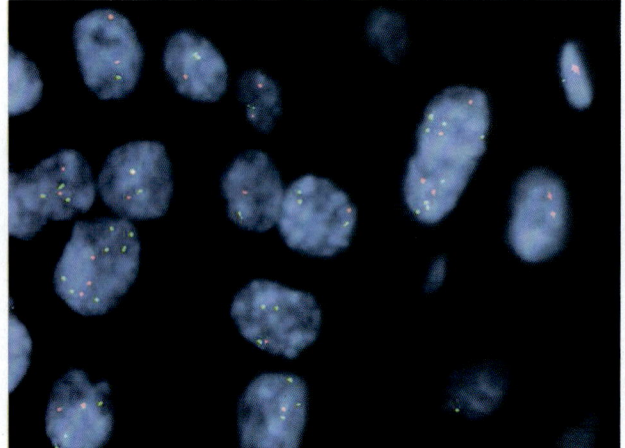

Figure 3.211. In the same tumor from Figures 3.208-3.210, fluorescence in situ hybridization (FISH) was used to assess for the common copy number abnormalities of oncocytoma and chromophobe renal cell carcinoma. In this FISH slide with probes to 1p (orange) and 1q (green), there are multiple copies of both probes, suggesting chromosomal gain, which has been reported in "hybrid" tumors.

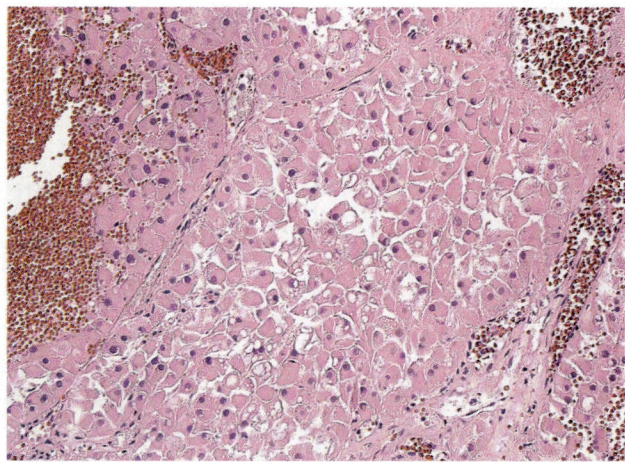

Figure 3.212. This clear cell renal cell carcinoma contains areas of oncocytic cells, which could mimic an oncocytic neoplasm. However, this change is usually focal and not diffuse. The same tumor contained typical clear cell areas, as shown in Figure 3.213.

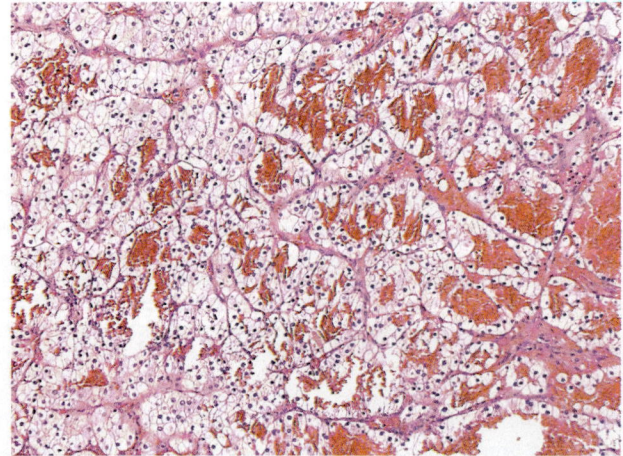

Figure 3.213. The same tumor from Figure 3.212 includes typical clear cell areas, making the diagnosis straightforward.

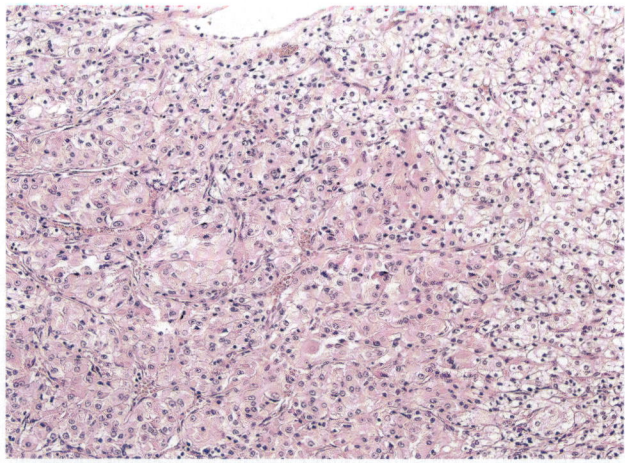

Figure 3.214. In this clear cell renal cell carcinoma, transition between areas of eosinophilic cells (usually higher-grade) and cells with clear cytoplasm is evident.

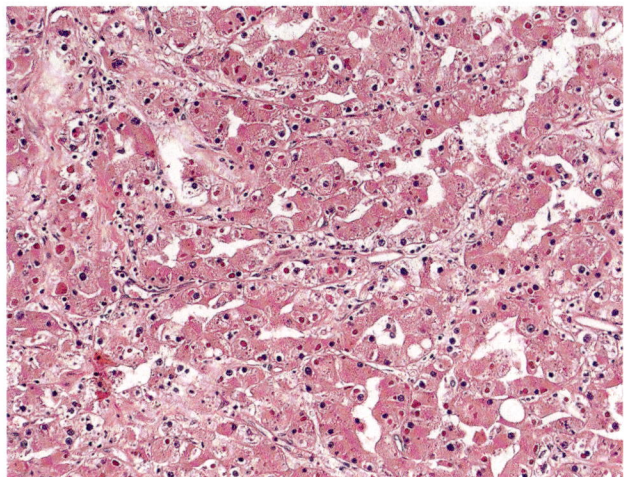

Figure 3.215. This clear cell renal cell carcinoma (RCC) includes eosinophilic cells with globules of hyaline material in the cytoplasm. The same tumor included multiple patterns, including classic clear cell RCC, as well as sarcomatoid and high-grade components (not pictured).

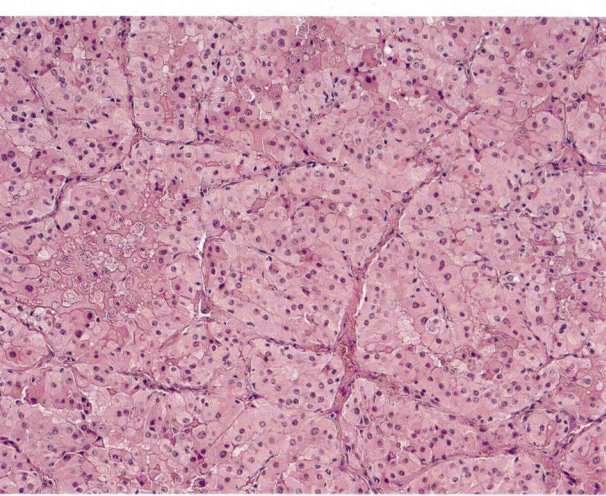

Figure 3.216. This papillary renal cell carcinoma (RCC) with oncocytic cells includes areas that could mimic an oncocytoma or chromophobe RCC.

usually of great help, as carbonic anhydrase IX typically still demonstrates the usual diffuse membranous staining pattern of clear cell RCC. Vimentin is usually positive, especially with nuclear grade 3 or higher (which is almost always the case for eosinophilic tumors),[183] contrasting to oncocytoma and chromophobe RCC. KIT (CD117) is consistently negative in clear cell RCC,[30] the opposite of that expected in oncocytoma and chromophobe RCC. AMACR staining can be variable in high-grade clear cell RCC, so a moderate or strong positive reaction should not be interpreted alone as definitive for papillary RCC. Cytokeratin 7 is usually negative or minimal in clear cell RCC, although in the case of eosinophilic renal cell neoplasms, there is usually minimal staining regardless of the histologic type, and therefore this may not be helpful alone.

Papillary RCC With Eosinophilic Cells

A subset of papillary RCCs are composed of cells with abundant eosinophilic cytoplasm. As noted previously, papillary renal cell neoplasm with reverse polarity/oncocytic papillary RCC appears to be an emerging category of neoplasm with recurring histologic, immunohistochemical, and genetic features; however, this only accounts for a subset of papillary RCCs with eosinophilic cells. Other papillary RCCs, typically with nuclear grade 3, can have abundant eosinophilic cytoplasm (Figures 3.216 and 3.217). In general, the immunohistochemical staining characteristics of these tumors are similar to other papillary RCCs (strong AMACR staining, frequently vimentin positivity, and negative KIT, Figures 3.218-3.220); however, an exception is that with increasing amounts of eosinophilic cells, the amount of cytokeratin 7 staining typically decreases. If the tumor does not have the nuclear pseudostratification described in "type 2" papillary RCC, our approach is to diagnose these as papillary RCC with eosinophilic cells. As noted previously, the category of "type 2" papillary tumors is now thought to be clinically and molecularly heterogeneous. If such a neoplasm demonstrates exceptionally prominent nucleoli or mixed morphologic patterns, FH-deficient RCC/HLRCC should be considered, as previously discussed under the papillary pattern.

Succinate Dehydrogenase–Deficient RCC

SDH-deficient RCC has now been recognized as a distinct renal tumor type in the WHO Classification,[184] following several large series describing its recurring pathologic features.[185,186] These tumors often resemble more common oncocytic neoplasms at the gross level, forming red-brown or tan masses. Microscopically, the prototypical and most common pattern demonstrates solid growth of cells with eosinophilic cytoplasm (Figures 3.221-3.224), characteristically containing cytoplasmic vacuoles or globules,[185,186] which likely represent giant abnormal mitochondria.[187] In contrast to oncocytoma, the growth pattern is

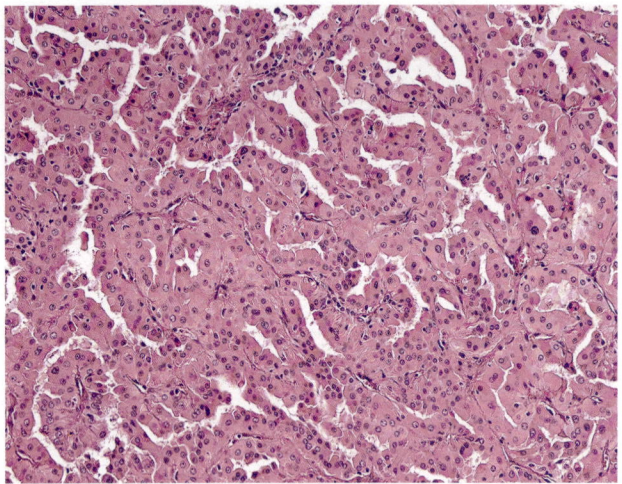

Figure 3.217. The same papillary renal cell carcinoma tumor from Figure 3.216 includes other areas of confluent papillary growth.

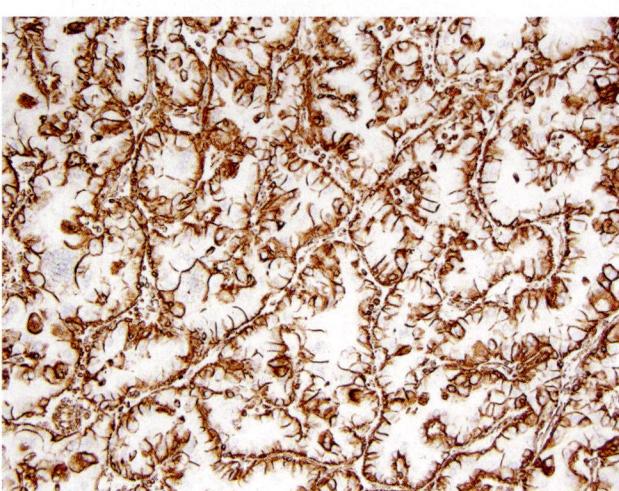

Figure 3.218. Vimentin immunohistochemistry is positive in the tumor from Figures 3.216 and 3.217, arguing against oncocytoma or chromophobe renal cell carcinoma.

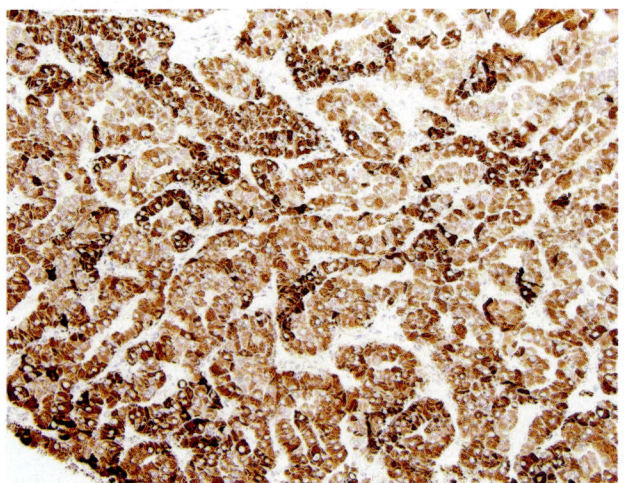

Figure 3.219. AMACR staining is very strong in the same tumor from Figures 3.216-3.218, which is not entirely specific but compatible with papillary renal cell carcinoma.

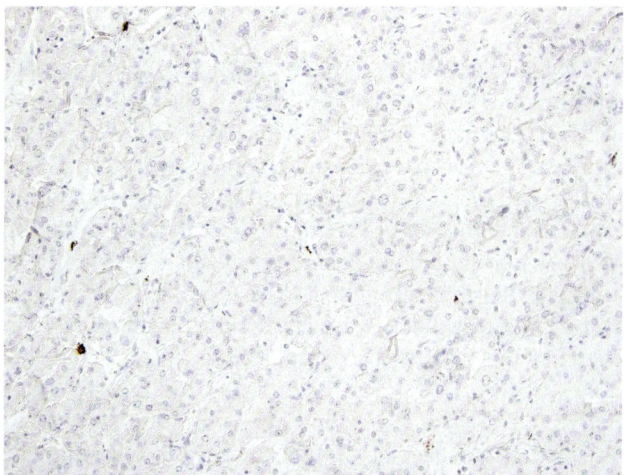

Figure 3.220. KIT (CD117) staining is negative in the papillary renal cell carcinoma (RCC) with eosinophilic cells from Figures 3.216-3.219, arguing against oncocytoma or chromophobe RCC. A few rare mast cells are highlighted.

usually very solid or sheet-like with sometimes a paucity of tubular or glandular structures, and the pattern of solid nests dispersed in loose fibrous or edematous stroma is typically lacking in SDH RCC.

KEY FEATURES: Recognizing SDH-Deficient RCC

- Eosinophilic cells, usually in a diffuse arrangement
- Cytoplasmic vacuoles or globules, likely representing giant mitochondria
- Immunohistochemistry:
  - Cytokeratin 7—usually entirely negative, contrasting to the rare positive cells of oncocytoma (and may highlight entrapped benign tubules)
  - KIT—usually negative, contrasting to oncocytoma and chromophobe RCC (but often highlights many mast cells)
  - Vimentin—usually negative (may highlight mast cells)
  - PAX8—positive, supporting renal tubular origin
  - Keratin or EMA—variable, may be minimal

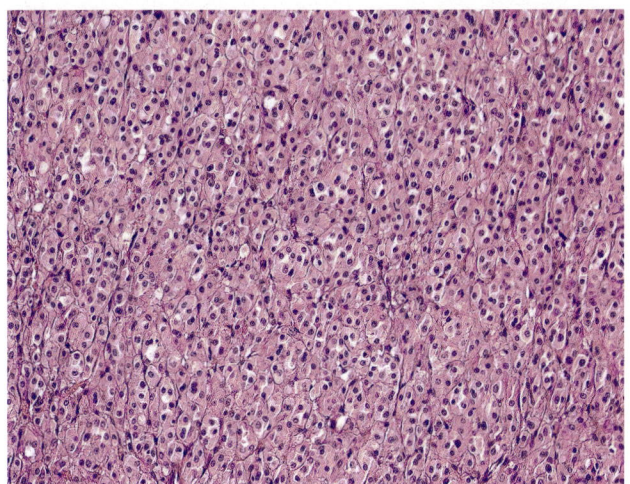

Figure 3.221. SDH-deficient renal cell carcinoma is typically composed of solid growth of eosinophilic cells, usually without the nested arrangement of oncocytoma.

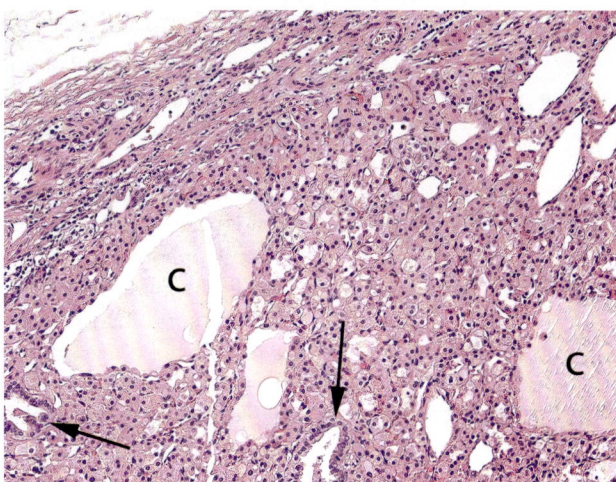

Figure 3.222. Occasional cysts (c) or tubular structures are present, and entrapped nonneoplastic tubular (arrows) are common in SDH-deficient renal cell carcinoma.

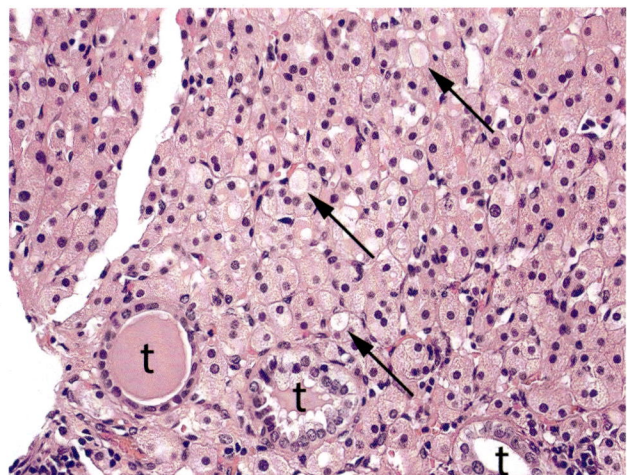

Figure 3.223. The characteristic cytology of SDH-deficient renal cell carcinoma includes cytoplasmic vacuoles (arrows) that likely represent enlarged abnormal mitochondria. Entrapped renal tubules are also present (t).

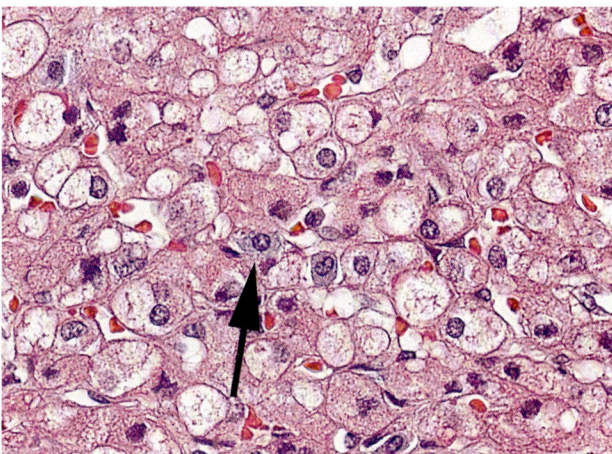

Figure 3.224. This high magnification field of SDH-deficient renal cell carcinoma shows numerous cytoplasmic vacuoles. Mast cells (arrow) are often prominent.

- SDHB—abnormal negative staining (requires verification of normal positive internal control, such as adjacent tissue or tumor endothelial cells, vascular walls, Figure 3.225)

Immunohistochemistry for SDHB protein is a helpful tool in diagnosing these neoplasms.[188-192] Although rare tumors may be mutated for another subunit of the SDH complex, such as *SDHA*, mutations of any of the subunits appear to destabilize the enzyme complex, resulting in the abnormal negative immunohistochemical pattern for SDHB. In contrast, SDHA immunohistochemistry is only negative when the tumor is mutated for *SDHA*. Therefore, SDHB staining is a helpful screening tool, largely independent of which subunit bears a mutation. The behavior of these tumors is somewhat unpredictable. Despite their usual bland histologic appearance, distant metastases and death from disease have been reported.[186] Although the classic morphology of SDH-deficient RCC is recognizable, rare variant morphologies that would be difficult to recognize have also been reported.[185] The patients with germline mutations of the SDH genes are typically regarded as having the pheochromocytoma and paraganglioma syndromes, which also include development of pheochromocytoma, paraganglioma, and gastrointestinal stromal tumor. Awareness of this combination of tumors may also be helpful in identifying patients with germline SDH subunit gene mutations.

Emerging Entities With Oncocytic Pattern

Very recently, several studies have described novel types of renal tumors with oncocytic patterns that appear distinct from previously established entities, although not yet officially included in current classification schemes. The best established of these so far is eosinophilic solid and cystic RCC (Figures 3.226 and 3.227). This tumor pattern was first recognized in the setting of tuberous sclerosis complex.[193] However, it has been subsequently realized that it occurs sporadically as well and preferentially in women.[169] Unique characteristics of these neoplasms include cysts and solid areas both formed by cells with voluminous eosinophilic cytoplasm, often having granular cytoplasmic stippling (Figure 3.228). Interestingly, these tumors often show some degree of positivity for cytokeratin 20 (Figure 3.229), which is usually not a marker associated with renal cell tumors.[194] Initial studies suggested that these neoplasms are likely nonaggressive; however, recent reports of metastases have been published, supporting their consideration as carcinomas.[195-197] It has now been found that even the sporadic tumors typically harbor mutations of the tuberous sclerosis genes (*TSC1* or *TSC2*),[198-200] which suggests that like clear cell RCC, there is a hereditary and sporadic counterpart of this tumor, both of which have mutations in the same genes.

Two other patterns of oncocytic neoplasms that have been recently described have been referred to as low-grade oncocytic tumor (LOT) and high-grade oncocytic tumor (HOT). LOT was recognized for its uniform oncocytic morphology (Figures 3.230 and 3.231), combined with diffuse reactivity for cytokeratin 7 and negative staining for KIT (Figure 3.232).[201] Although these most likely would have been historically classified as chromophobe RCC, the negative reaction for KIT is unusual, and staining for cytokeratin 7 is typically patchy in most eosinophilic renal cell neoplasms including eosinophilic chromophobe RCC. More data will be necessary to verify the status of this neoplasm as a distinct tumor type; however, it currently appears a candidate for consideration as a distinct entity. Finally, two groups simultaneously described neoplasms with oncocytic vacuolated cell morphology.[202-204] One study used the nomenclature of high-grade oncocytic tumor for this pattern, whereas the other study used descriptive terminology of RCC with "eosinophilic and vacuolated cytoplasm" harboring *TSC2* and *MTOR* mutations; however, in our view these both represent the same diagnostic entity (Figure 3.233). The clinical significance of these entities remains to be fully characterized due to their only recent recognition. Key features of these tumors are shown in Table 3.5.

Other Differential Diagnoses for Oncocytic Pattern

Other considerations that may be relevant to the oncocytic pattern are discussed in more detail in other sections. Tubulocystic RCC and acquired cystic kidney disease–associated RCC may come into consideration for differential diagnosis of oncocytic neoplasms. These are covered in the next section, under the tubular/solid patterns, although they are often oncocytic as well.

TUBULAR/SOLID PATTERNS
Tubulocystic Renal Cell Carcinoma

Tubulocystic RCC is a rare RCC variant composed of tubular and cystic structures lined by cells with eosinophilic cytoplasm (Figures 3.234 and 3.235). The lining cells have consistent prominent nucleoli and a hobnail-shaped configuration. Grossly, the classic description of tubulocystic RCC is that it resembles bubble wrap, with a uniform solid cut surface punctuated by numerous cysts.[205] Since several features overlap with papillary RCC,[206] including strong staining for AMACR,[69,207] and tumors with overlapping patterns have been described, it has been speculated that these may be part of a spectrum with each other. For practical purposes, however, tubulocystic RCC is recognized as a distinct entity in current classification schemes.[69] Although positivity for cytokeratin 7 may be minimal, this is again not unusual when considering that most renal neoplasms with oncocytic features have minimal staining for cytokeratin 7, almost regardless of type.[145] As discussed previously under the papillary pattern and FH-deficient RCC, a tumor with an abrupt transition from tubulocystic morphology to high-grade infiltrative carcinoma, or mixed with multiple heterogeneous patterns, is very suspicious for FH-deficient renal cancer.[21,208] The behavior of tubulocystic RCC is most commonly nonaggressive; however, extrarenal extension and

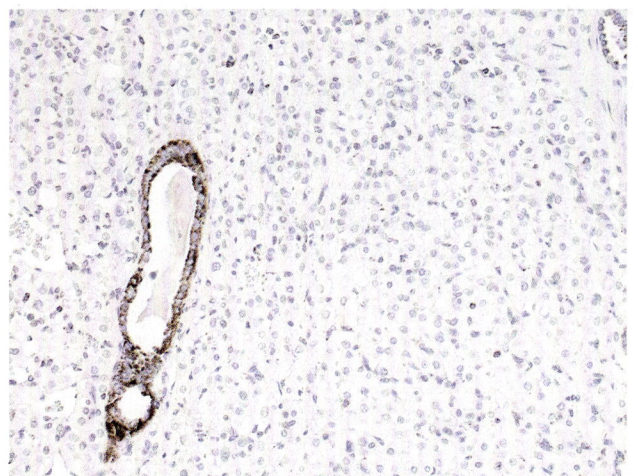

Figure 3.225. Immunohistochemistry for SDHB protein will show an abnormal negative result in the tumor cells of SDH-deficient neoplasms, although it is necessary to verify a positive internal control, such as the entrapped normal tubule that is positive in this field.

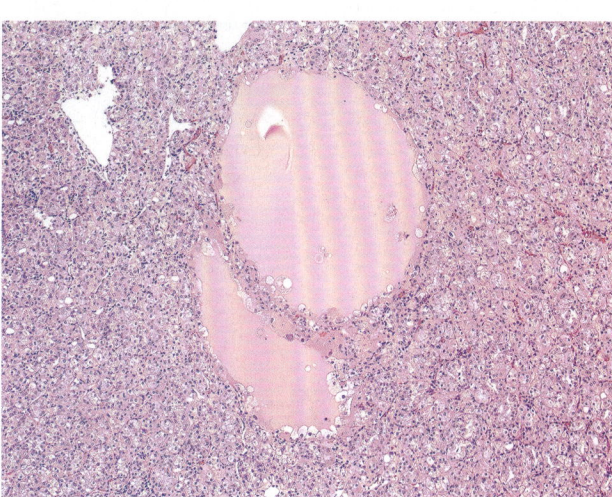

Figure 3.226. Eosinophilic solid and cystic renal cell carcinoma (RCC) has been recently recognized as an emerging RCC type. It typically is composed of solid growth of eosinophilic cells with scattered cysts.

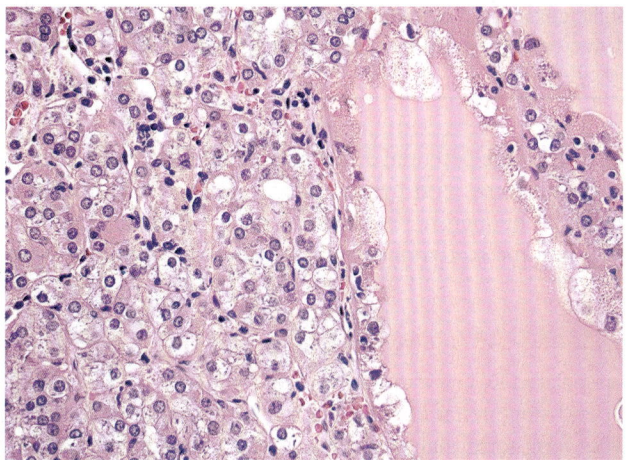

Figure 3.227. At higher magnification, the solid areas and cysts of eosinophilic solid and cystic renal cell carcinoma are lined by similar cells with voluminous eosinophilic to pale cytoplasm.

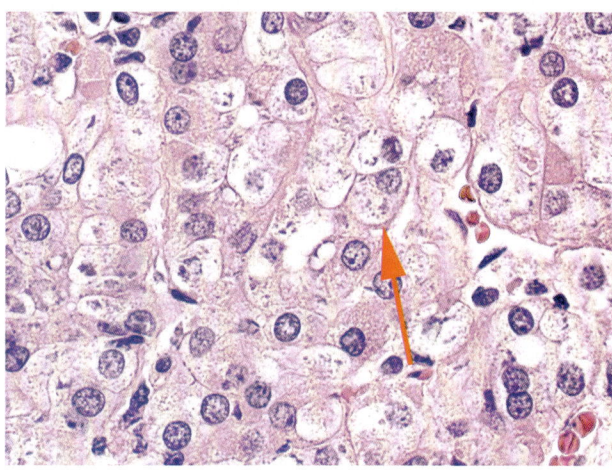

Figure 3.228. Eosinophilic solid and cystic renal cell carcinoma typically has cytoplasmic stippling (arrow), which can be a clue to recognition of this entity.

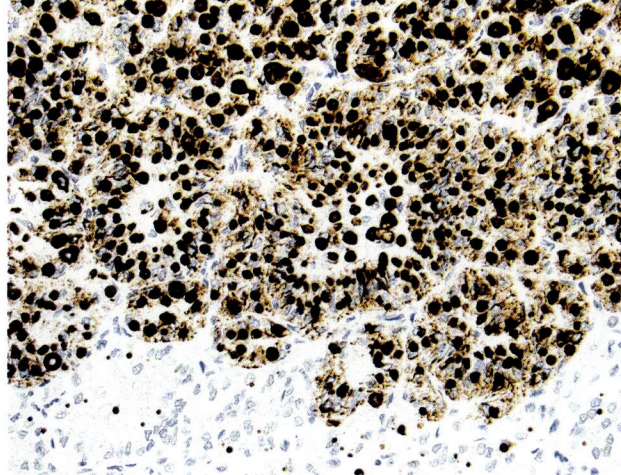

Figure 3.229. Eosinophilic solid and cystic renal cell carcinoma often demonstrates some degree of positivity for cytokeratin 20. The same example from Figures 3.226-3.228 shows an interesting large globular pattern of cytokeratin 20 staining.

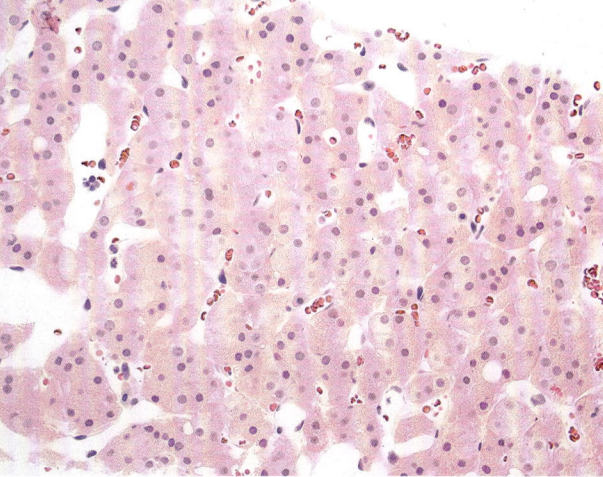

Figure 3.230. The entity recently proposed as "low-grade oncocytic tumor" is composed of uniform eosinophilic cells with bland cytologic features.

TABLE 3.5: Emerging Neoplasms With Oncocytic Pattern

	Histology	Immunohistochemistry	Genetics
Eosinophilic solid and cystic renal cell carcinoma (RCC)	Solid and cystic areas with eosinophilic cells with voluminous cytoplasm Frequent cytoplasmic stippling with basophilic material	Frequently positive for cytokeratin 20 (focal or diffuse) Variable positivity for other RCC markers (AMACR, CD10, vimentin, minimal cytokeratin 7)	*TSC1* or *TSC2* mutations in sporadic tumors Subset associated with tuberous sclerosis complex
Low-grade oncocytic tumor	Uniform oncocytic solid morphology Edematous areas with cells "stretched" and loosely connected	Diffuse labeling for cytokeratin 7 Negative for KIT (CD117)	Chromosomal deletions 19p13.3, 1p36.33, and 19q13.11
High-grade oncocytic tumor (*TSC2/MTOR* mutated)	Solid and nested architecture with eosinophilic cells Prominent nucleoli Vacuolated cytoplasm	Nonspecific with positive PAX8 and minimal cytokeratin 7 or 20 staining, variable KIT	*TSC2* or *MTOR* mutations

metastatic disease have been reported.[69] One potential differential diagnostic consideration for tubulocystic RCC would be oncocytoma with cystic changes.[209] To resolve this distinction, tubulocystic tumors are more frequently positive for vimentin, CD10, AMACR, and cytokeratin 7 (showing more than the scattered cells expected of oncocytoma), with typically negative KIT staining.[209]

Acquired Cystic Kidney Disease–Associated Renal Cell Carcinoma

Acquired cystic kidney disease–associated RCC is a unique type of renal tumor that appears to be restricted to the setting of end-stage renal disease with acquired cystic kidney disease, typically occurring following long-term dialysis, although dialysis is not a requirement (Figure 3.236). The characteristic features of these tumors include cribriform growth composed of eosinophilic cells with intratumoral calcium oxalate crystals (Figures 3.237-3.241).[69,210] Like tubulocystic RCC, there is some overlap between this entity and papillary RCC, such that it could be debated whether they are parts of a spectrum. Tumors with

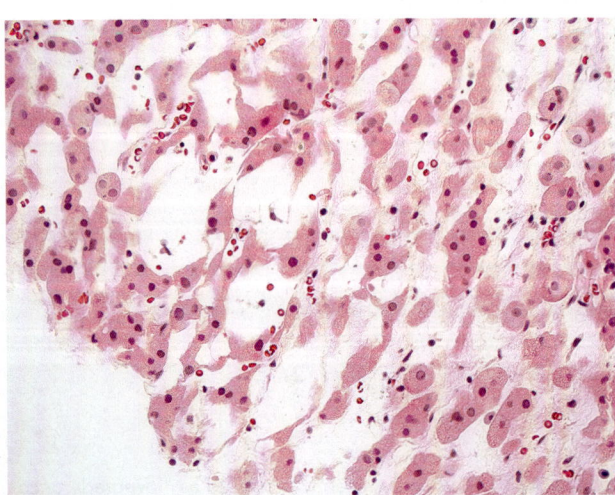

Figure 3.231. In some areas of low-grade oncocytic tumor, the tumor cells appear stretched apart in an edematous background.

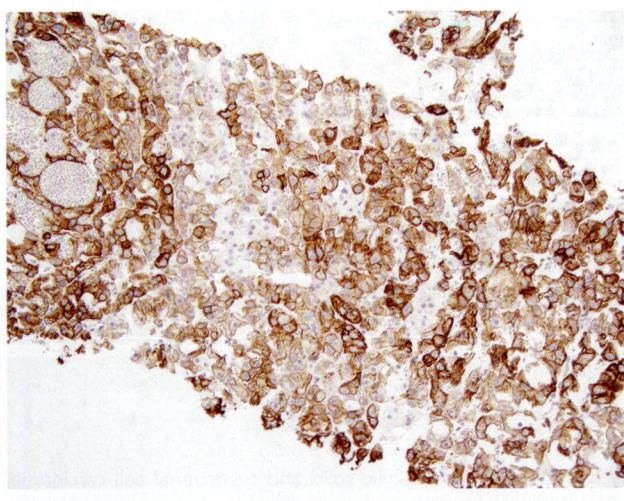

Figure 3.232. Low-grade oncocytic tumor is diffusely positive for cytokeratin 7 but negative for KIT (not pictured).

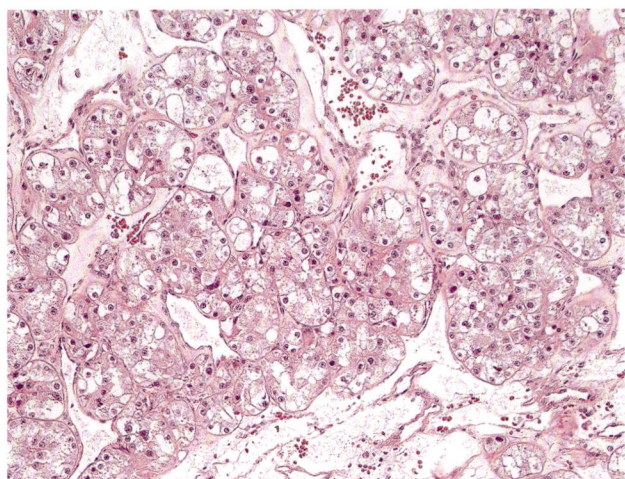

Figure 3.233. A potential emerging entity has been recognized by two different groups. One group proposed the nomenclature "high-grade oncocytic tumor" for this entity and another used descriptive designation of renal cell carcinomas with eosinophilic and vacuolated cytoplasm. These were found to harbor *TSC2* or *MTOR* mutations. These tumors have eosinophilic to pale cells with cytoplasmic vacuoles and prominent nucleoli. Their immunohistochemical profile is not entirely specific.

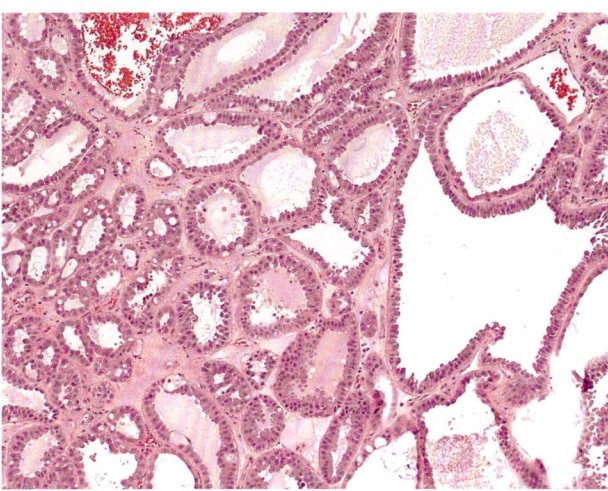

Figure 3.234. Tubulocystic renal cell carcinoma is composed of tubular and cystic structures lined by eosinophilic cells.

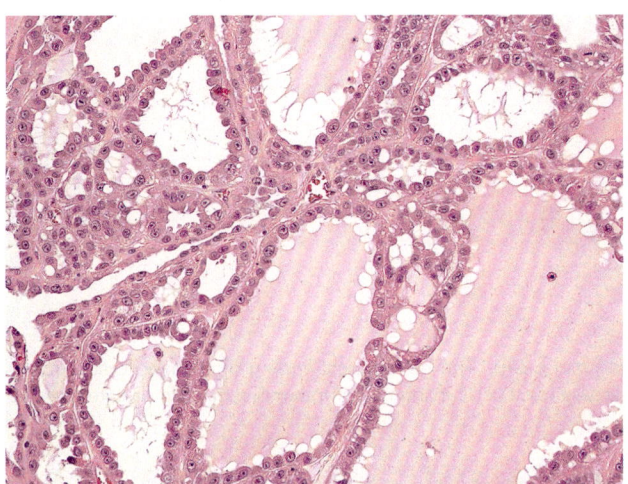

Figure 3.235. At higher magnification, tubulocystic renal cell carcinomas (RCCs) are composed of hobnail-shaped cells lining cystic and tubular spaces with prominent nucleoli. The designation of tubulocystic RCC is best reserved for tumors with this uniform constellation of features, excluding those that have papillary areas or transition to a poorly-differentiated carcinoma. The latter may represent fumarate hydratase–deficient RCC.

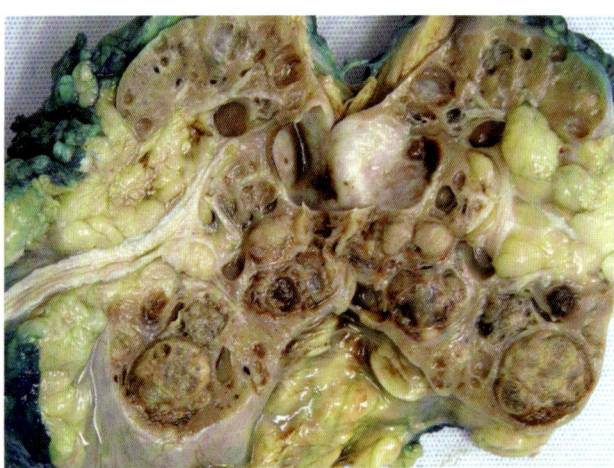

Figure 3.236. This kidney with acquired cystic kidney disease is relatively normal in size with numerous cysts and multiple solid neoplasms.

mixed patterns of papillary RCC and acquired cystic kidney disease–associated tumors have been encountered (Figure 3.242). Occasionally, cysts with proliferative epithelium yet not forming a definitive mass can occur in the setting of acquired cystic kidney disease (Figure 3.243).[69,211] Although specific terminology has not been definitively established for these lesions in major classification schemes, the terminology "atypical cyst" has been proposed, which indicates that these are likely a precursor lesion but not yet fulfilling criteria for carcinoma.[212] Like tubulocystic RCC, behavior of these neoplasms has been mostly nonaggressive, as many are identified incidentally during surveillance of patients with renal disease; however, tumors with sarcomatoid or rhabdoid features have been reported, and metastatic disease has been described.[69]

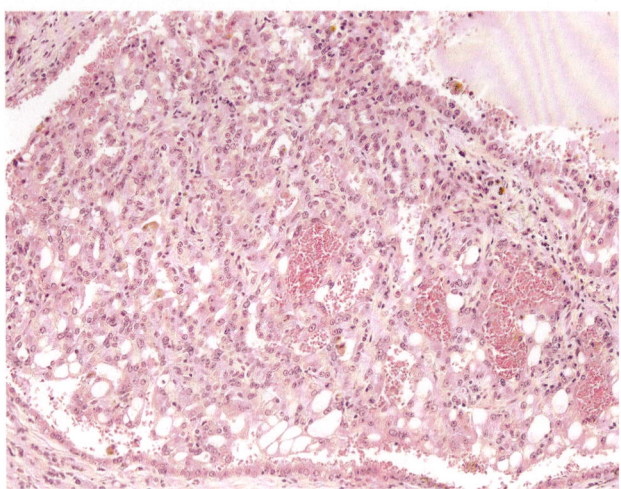

Figure 3.237. The classic morphology of acquired cystic kidney disease–associated renal cell carcinoma is cribriform, with multiple punched-out lumens.

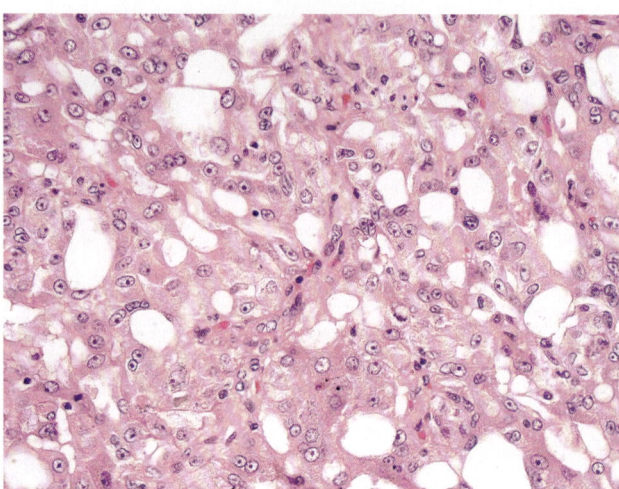

Figure 3.238. At higher magnification, this acquired cystic kidney disease–associated renal cell carcinoma is composed of eosinophilic with variable nucleoli and multiple cribriform lumens.

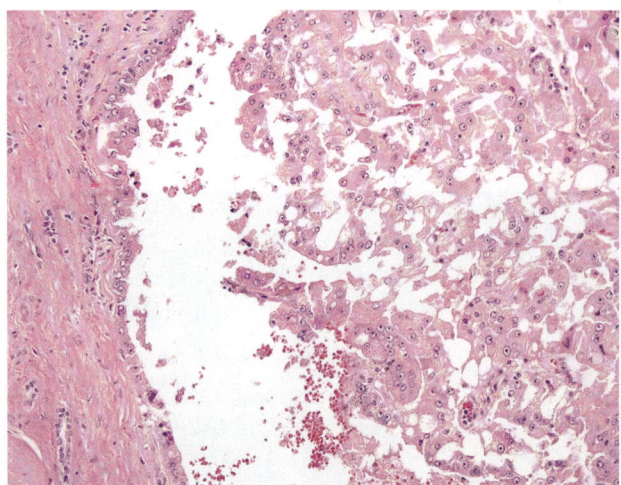

Figure 3.239. This example of acquired cystic kidney disease renal cell carcinoma is a solid cribriform nodule growing within a cyst.

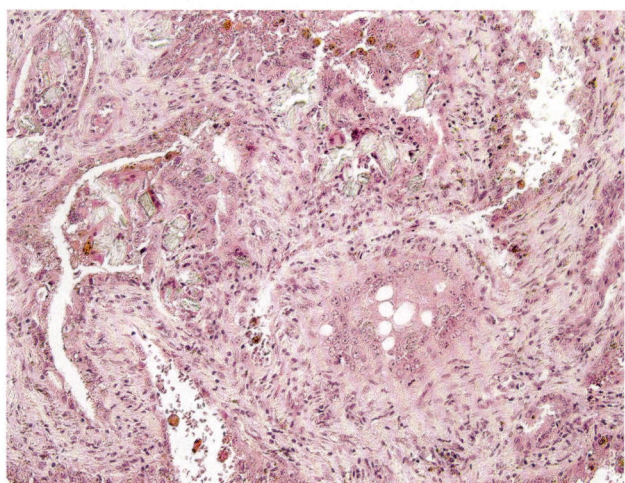

Figure 3.240. The prototypical finding of acquired cystic kidney disease renal cell carcinoma is intratumoral calcium oxalate crystals.

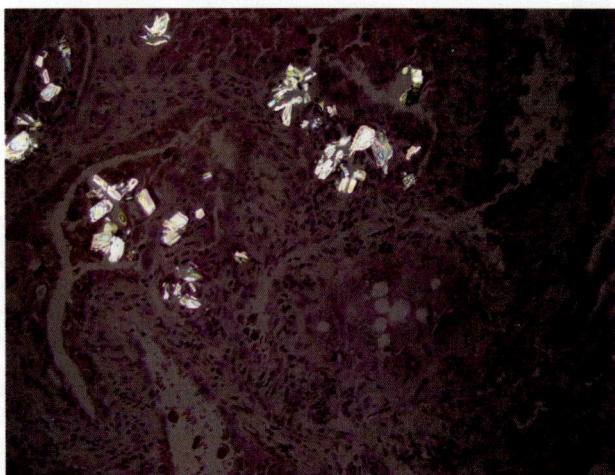

Figure 3.241. The same field as Figure 3.240 under polarization highlights the calcium oxalate crystals.

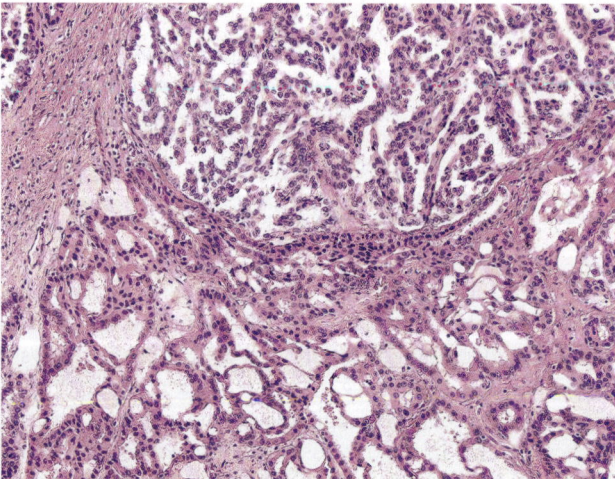

Figure 3.242. It is debatable whether there is a relationship between acquired cystic kidney disease renal cell carcinoma (RCC) and papillary RCC. This example has typical eosinophilic cribriform morphology at bottom but morphology resembling type 1 papillary RCC at top.

Thyroid-Like Renal Cell Carcinoma

Thyroid-like or thyroid follicular–like RCC is a rare variant of renal carcinoma that may mimic a thyroid follicular neoplasm (Figures 3.244 and 3.245). It is possible for thyroid cancer to metastasize to the kidney, although this is also rare (Figure 3.246), so it would typically be prudent to argue against thyroid origin with immunohistochemistry (TTF1, thyroglobulin) before making this diagnosis (Figure 3.247). Although studies have found variable results for PAX2 and PAX8 staining in thyroid-like RCC,[213,214] a substantial number have been shown to be PAX8 positive.[214,215] Therefore, PAX8 would be helpful in supporting a renal cell neoplasm in general but not for distinguishing from metastatic thyroid cancer. Otherwise, the immunohistochemical features of these tumors are relatively nonspecific. Although there is not much published regarding immunohistochemistry for AMACR in these tumors, our experience with a few cases is that they may be negative for AMACR (Figure 3.248),[216] which would contrast markedly to that expected of papillary RCC. Like tubulocystic RCC, acquired cystic kidney disease RCC, and other subtypes, it is possible to encounter follicular areas in a tumor that otherwise resemble papillary RCC (Figures 3.249 and 3.250). Therefore, it seems best at present to reserve this diagnosis for tumors with pure thyroid-like morphology.[214]

PEARLS AND PITFALLS: Thyroid-Like Renal Cell Carcinoma

- Mimics a thyroid neoplasm (follicular adenoma or carcinoma)
- Rarely thyroid cancer can metastasize to the kidney, so immunohistochemistry (TTF1, thyroglobulin) should be used to exclude this possibility
- Colloid-like material in follicular spaces
- Relatively nonspecific immunohistochemistry with variable PAX8, cytokeratin 7
- AMACR may be decreased compared to papillary RCC but limited data
- Tumors with mixed features of papillary RCC and thyroid-like RCC likely better diagnosed as papillary RCC

Recent reports have described a rare renal tumor morphology as atrophic kidney-like.[217] Although on the surface it would be tempting to assume that this is also a variant of thyroid-like RCC, due to the frequent description of atrophic kidney as resembling thyroid follicles, a recent larger series proposed that this may be unrelated to thyroid-like RCC and may be more in keeping with an organizing form of tubular atrophy with glomerulocystic change (Figures 3.251 and 3.252).[218]

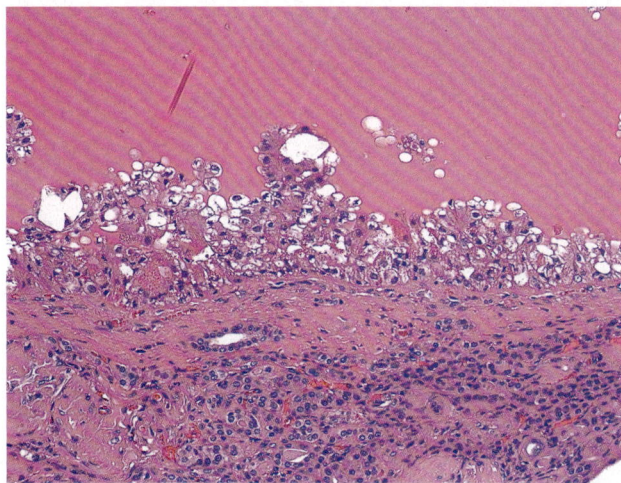

Figure 3.243. The cysts without discrete masses in acquired cystic kidney disease can show thickening and tufting of the epithelium, which is thought to represent a precursor to the neoplasms. This has been termed "atypical cyst" by some authors.

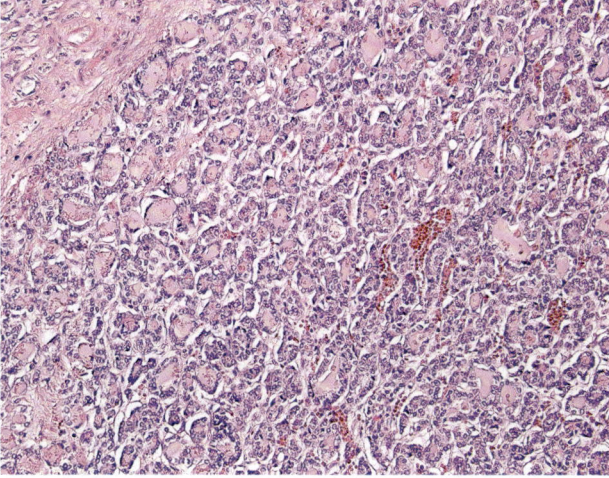

Figure 3.244. Thyroid-like renal cell carcinoma is composed of tubular or follicular structures with colloid-like material, resembling a thyroid neoplasm.

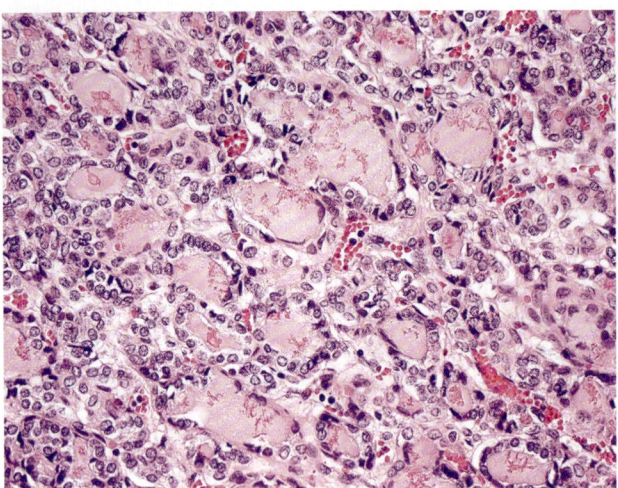

Figure 3.245. At higher magnification, this thyroid-like renal cell carcinoma contains pale eosinophilic material resembling colloid.

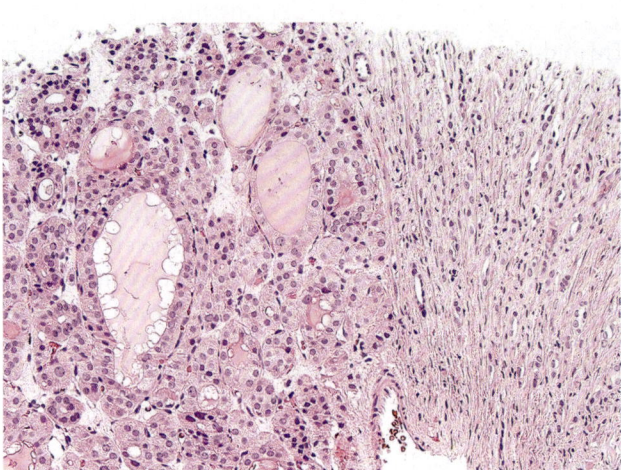

Figure 3.246. Rarely, thyroid cancer can metastasize to the kidney. This core biopsy was taken from a patient with known thyroid cancer and a renal mass.

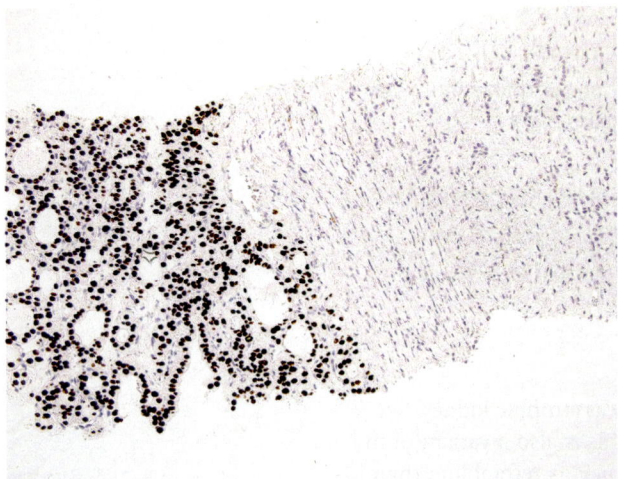

Figure 3.247. The same biopsy from Figure 3.246 shows immunohistochemical positivity for TTF1, supporting metastatic thyroid cancer rather than thyroid-like renal cell carcinoma.

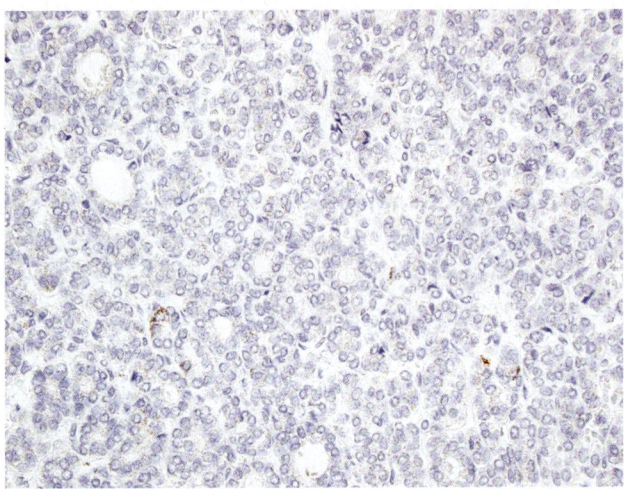

Figure 3.248. This thyroid-like renal cell carcinoma (RCC) shows minimal to no staining for AMACR, which would contrast markedly to type 1 papillary RCC.

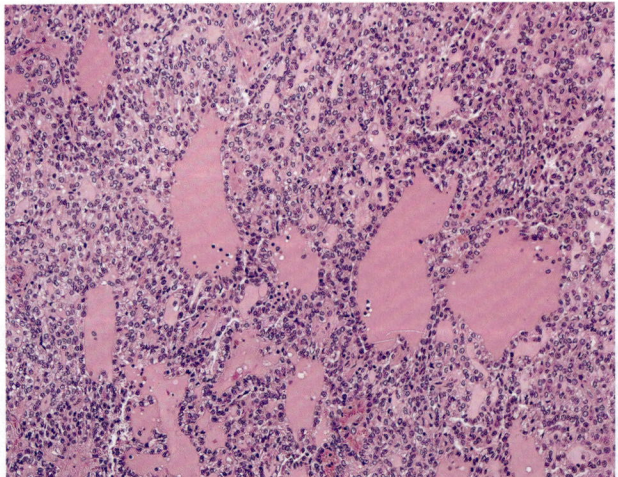

Figure 3.249. Some papillary renal cell carcinomas (RCCs) can have focal thyroid-like features, which are likely best classified as papillary rather than thyroid-like RCC. This example shows colloid-like material; however, other areas were more in keeping with papillary RCC (Figure 3.250).

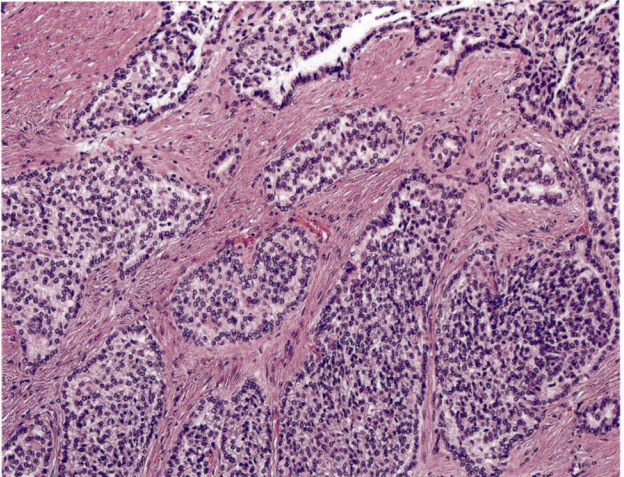

Figure 3.250. The same tumor from Figure 3.249 also contains areas more in keeping with type 1 papillary renal cell carcinoma (RCC). This tumor was strongly positive for AMACR and cytokeratin 7, and there were adjacent papillary adenomas, all favoring type 1 papillary RCC (not pictured).

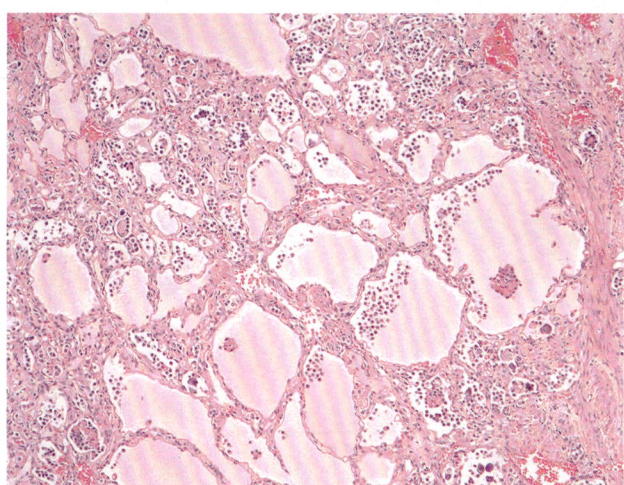

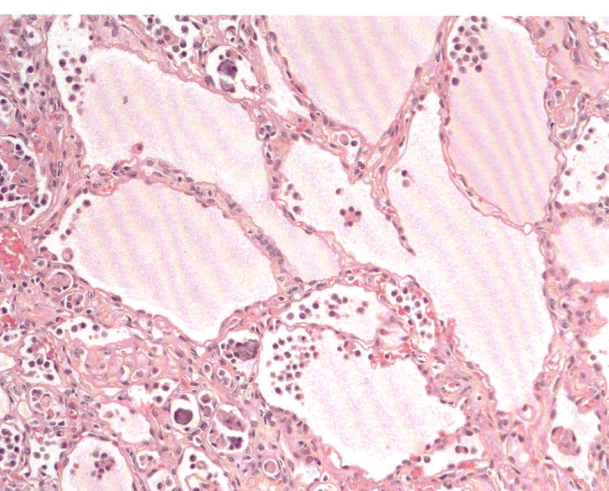

Figure 3.251. Atrophic kidney-like lesions have been recently described. Although it was initially considered that this may be part of the spectrum of thyroid-like renal cell carcinoma, a recent series proposed that this may represent an organizing form of tubular atrophy with glomerulocystic change. (Courtesy of Jesse K. McKenney, MD, Cleveland Clinic.)

Figure 3.252. At higher magnification, atrophy kidney-like tumors are composed of cystic structures with calcification, which has been hypothesized to be related to glomerulocystic change. (Courtesy of Jesse K. McKenney, MD, Cleveland Clinic.)

Other Unusual Patterns of Renal Cell Carcinoma

Several other patterns of RCC have been increasingly recognized recently, yet not currently accepted in major classification schemes, mostly due to recent recognition and uncertainty regarding potential heterogeneity of morphology and genetics. Several discussed here include RCC with 6p21/*TFEB/VEGFA* amplification,[38,219-223] RCC with *ALK* rearrangement,[224-232] and RCC with smooth muscle stroma (see also the section on biphasic/triphasic neoplasms).[142,233] These all show promise for consideration as distinct tumor types, although some limitations have prevented them from being definitively established so far. RCC with 6p21/*TFEB/VEGFA* amplification appears based on present data to be aggressive, which may be important for treatment purposes, and treatment with VEGF targeting agents has been proposed, although not definitively proven to be effective.[221] Likewise, ALK inhibition therapy has been proposed for treatment of *ALK* rearranged RCC, with some success.[234] Features of these neoplasms are summarized in Table 3.6 (Figures 3.253-3.256).

Renal Cell Carcinoma Unclassified

RCC unclassified is not a specific subtype of RCC but rather a category for tumors that are consistent with renal cell origin, yet which do not fit well into a specific subtype based on available data. Different institutions may have different thresholds for using this diagnosis; however, it should be kept in mind that clinicians may perceive unclassified RCC as indicating an aggressive tumor.[178,179] Therefore, our approach is to attempt to avoid using this diagnosis for tumors that closely approximate a specific subtype with minor atypical features. For example, as discussed in the oncocytic tumor section, it may be misleading if a tumor that is borderline between oncocytoma and chromophobe RCC is diagnosed as unclassified RCC due to its imperfect features of the two.[162] However, there do remain many unusual patterns of primary renal cell tumors that are difficult to classify, necessitating this diagnosis (Figures 3.257-3.261). At present, it is recommended that an extensively sarcomatoid tumor for which the originating subtype cannot be discerned be placed in this category.

Epithelioid Angiomyolipoma/Perivascular Epithelioid Cell Tumor (PEComa), Solid Pattern

In addition to epithelioid angiomyolipoma/PEComa resembling clear cell RCC, other unusual patterns of epithelioid angiomyolipoma have been reported, which may show a more solid or eosinophilic pattern (Figures 3.262-3.265). Like other forms of PEComa, these show the phenotype of dual positivity for smooth muscle and melanocytic markers, such as a combination of smooth muscle actin, desmin, melan-A, or HMB45 staining.[130,235,236] Rare examples mimicking oncocytoma have been reported.[237] Epithelioid angiomyolipoma/PEComa is covered in greater detail under the clear/pale cell pattern.

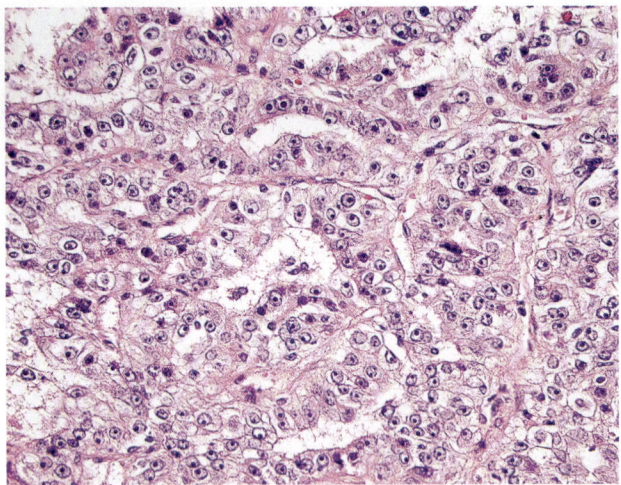

Figure 3.253. Renal cell carcinoma (RCC) with amplification of 6p21 including *TFEB* and *VEGFA* manifests variable patterns. This example has pale to eosinophilic cells with nuclei containing very prominent nucleoli, resembling those of HLRCC tumors.

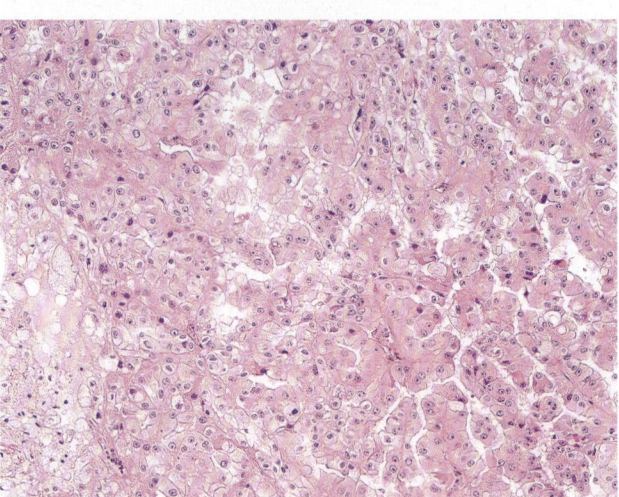

Figure 3.254. Other patterns of renal cell carcinoma with amplification of 6p21 can include more eosinophilic papillary growth.

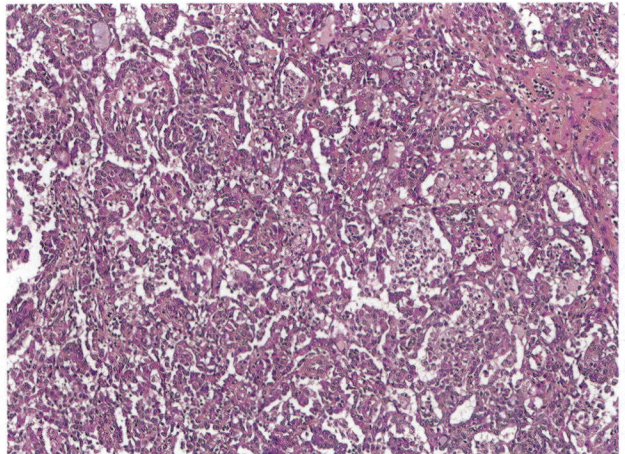

Figure 3.255. Renal cell carcinoma (RCC) with *ALK* rearrangement can have variable patterns. This example shows eosinophilic complex papillary morphology. Other patterns that have been described include cribriform growth, intracytoplasmic lumens, and mucin production (not pictured). (Courtesy of Ondrej Hes, MD, PhD, Charles University, Plzen, Czech Republic.)

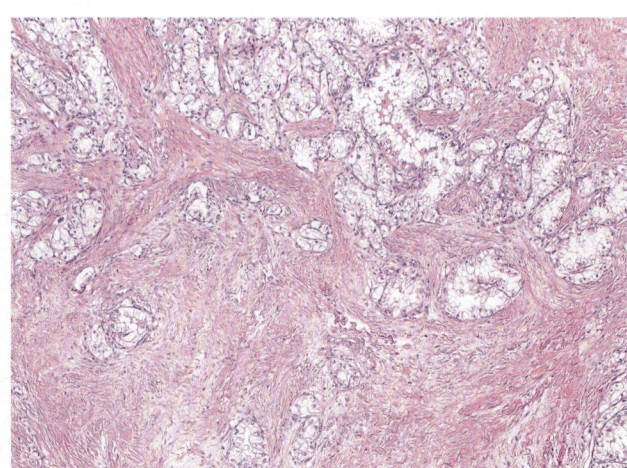

Figure 3.256. Renal cell carcinoma (RCC) with smooth muscle stroma typically forms clear cell RCC-like glandular structures that appear to be "floating" in smooth muscle stroma.

Juxtaglomerular Cell Tumor and Pericytic Tumors

Juxtaglomerular cell tumor is a very rare renal neoplasm that is thought to recapitulate the phenotype of the smooth muscle of the juxtaglomerular apparatus.[238] As such, it is thought that the tumors produce renin, resulting in uncontrollable hypertension. Classically, the hypertension resolves with resection of the tumor.[238-240] Histologically, these tumors are composed of polygonal or spindle-shaped cells containing central round nuclei with variable eosinophilic cytoplasm (Figures 3.266 and 3.267).[238] Deceptive patterns can include papillary formation and entrapment of normal tubules (Figure 3.268). Immunohistochemistry shows positivity for renin, coupled with other less specific markers such as smooth muscle actin, CD34, and KIT.[238] Using electron microscopy, these tumors characteristically contain rhomboid-shaped renin protogranules (Figure 3.269). These are generally considered benign neoplasms; however, a rare example with metastasis has been reported.[241]

Recently it has been better recognized that pericytic tumors can also occur in the kidney, particularly glomus tumor (Figures 3.270-3.272), and less commonly myopericytoma or angioleiomyoma (Figures 3.273 and 3.274).[242-246] Whereas myopericytoma or

TABLE 3.6: Features of Emerging Unusual Renal Cell Carcinoma (RCC) Types

	Morphology	Immunohistochemistry	Behavior	Genetics	Putative Treatment
RCC with 6p21/*TFEB*/*VEGFA* amplification	Clear cell to eosinophilic, variable tubular and papillary, occasionally chromophobe-like (Figures 3.253 and 3.254)	**Positive:** often melanocytic markers (especially melan A), often cathepsin K **Negative:** carbonic anhydrase IX	Highly aggressive	Multiple copies (>10) of 6p21, including *TFEB* and *VEGFA* genes, usually without *TFEB* rearrangement. Can be detected with *TFEB* break-apart fluorescence in situ hybridization	VEGF inhibition, but unproven
ALK rearranged RCC	Variable, papillary, cribriform, intracytoplasmic lumina, mucin production, or myxoid changes (Figure 3.255)	Often positive for ALK immunohistochemistry, may also be positive for TFE3 immunohistochemistry despite lack of rearrangement, other RCC markers generally nonspecific (focal cytokeratin 7, positive vimentin)	May have metastatic disease	Rearrangement of *ALK* gene, various partners described	*ALK* inhibition (alectinib)
RCC with smooth muscle stroma	Clear cell nests and glands dispersed in abundant smooth muscle stroma (Figure 3.256) Smooth muscle may extent away from the epithelium to involve perinephric fat or normal kidney	**Positive:** cytokeratin 7, high molecular weight cytokeratin, CD10, carbonic anhydrase IX **Negative:** AMACR	Generally not aggressive but few cases with lymph node involvement reported Subset of patients have tuberous sclerosis complex	Mutations of *TSC1*, *TSC2*, *MTOR*, or *ELOC* (formerly *TCEB1*)	Unknown

angioleiomyoma would be more obvious as a spindle cell mesenchymal tumor, glomus tumor, due to its epithelioid cells, may be more difficult to discern from a renal cell neoplasm or juxtaglomerular cell tumor. Immunohistochemistry shows most commonly positivity for smooth muscle actin, collagen IV, calponin, CD34, and less frequently desmin.[242] Interestingly, focal staining for renin was noted in a large recent series, although not in a diffuse distribution compared to juxtaglomerular cell tumor.[242] Despite that large size would be considered atypical in subcutaneous glomus tumors, it appears that those of deep abdominal organs are often large and most show benign behavior; however, metastatic examples have been reported.[247] Therefore, it is uncertain if the criteria for malignancy used in soft tissue sites can be extrapolated to those of the kidney.

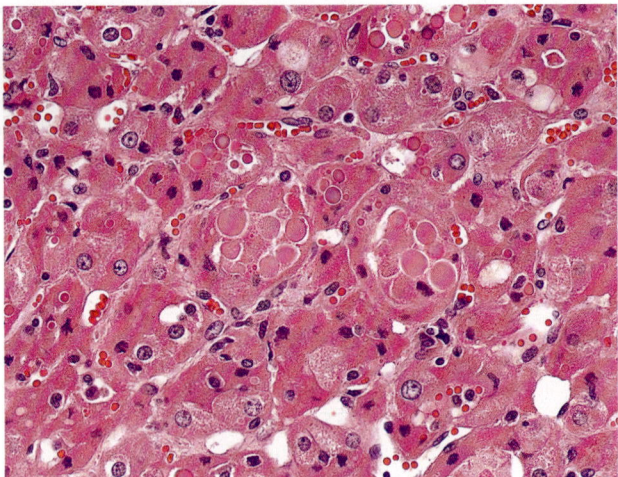

Figure 3.257. This renal cell carcinoma was diagnosed as unclassified due to the unusual oncocytic pattern with large hyaline globules. The immunohistochemical staining pattern (not pictured) was unusual with diffuse cytokeratin 7 staining and negative KIT and vimentin. This occurred in the background of acquired cystic kidney disease. This diagnosis predated the description of low-grade oncocytic tumor, discussed previously, which may be a consideration; however, the morphology is somewhat atypical with prominent nucleoli and hyaline globules.

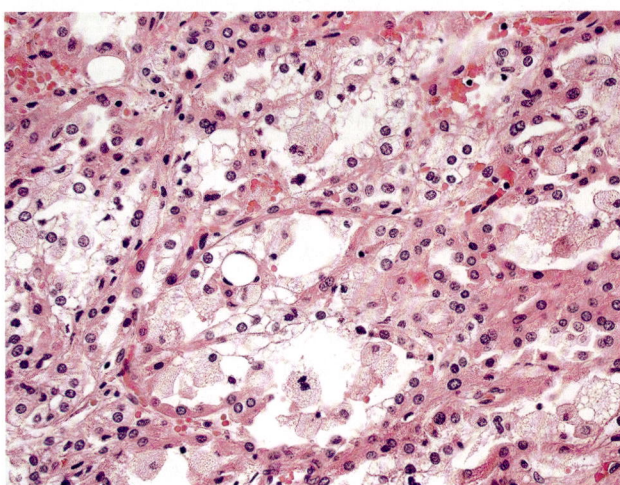

Figure 3.258. This 2.5-cm tumor was diagnosed as renal cell carcinoma (RCC) unclassified. Although the cells have clear cytoplasm, suggesting clear cell RCC, carbonic anhydrase IX staining (Figure 3.259) was entirely negative. There are also cells with foamy cytoplasm, which could raise consideration of papillary RCC; however, the staining for AMACR (not pictured) was variable with some areas being negative or weak, unusual for papillary RCC.

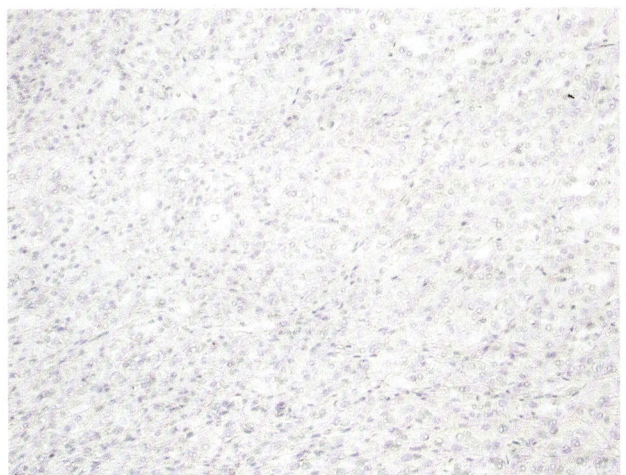

Figure 3.259. Carbonic anhydrase IX staining in the same tumor from Figure 3.258 is entirely negative, which would be unusual for a small, well-differentiated clear cell renal cell carcinoma tumor.

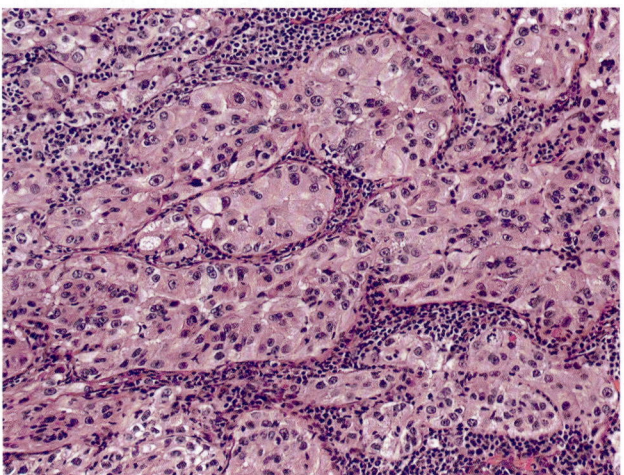

Figure 3.260. This renal cell carcinoma unclassified is involving a lymph node. The cells are eosinophilic with prominent nucleoli. It could not be confidently classified via the morphology and immunohistochemistry.

Neuroendocrine Tumors

Neuroendocrine tumors can occur in the kidney (Figure 3.275), similar to other much more common sites, like the lung and gastrointestinal tract.[248-255] In this context, probably the most important step for the pathologist is to remember that neuroendocrine tumors can occur at that site and to consider the diagnosis, in contrast to the overwhelmingly more common renal cell neoplasms. Neuroendocrine tumors of the kidney can span the spectrum from well-differentiated neuroendocrine tumors (formerly carcinoid tumor) to small and large cell neuroendocrine carcinomas. Small and large cell carcinomas are much more likely to be of urothelial/renal pelvic origin than renal parenchymal origin. Patterns formed by renal well-differentiated neuroendocrine tumors can include compact trabecular structures or ribbons, sheet-like growth, or solid or cribriform architecture, sometimes mimicking the tubular or glandular architecture of RCC. Like other neuroendocrine

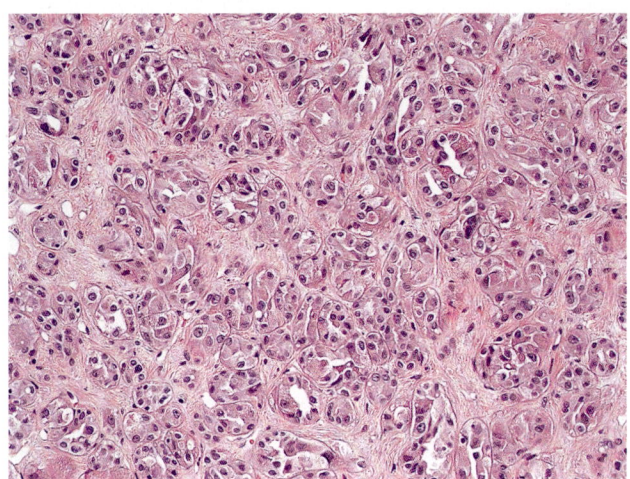

Figure 3.261. This tumor formed an incidental small nodule in a nephrectomy specimen. However, it could not be confidently classified based on this unusual pattern of tubular proliferation in fibrotic stroma and was regarded as unclassified renal cell carcinoma.

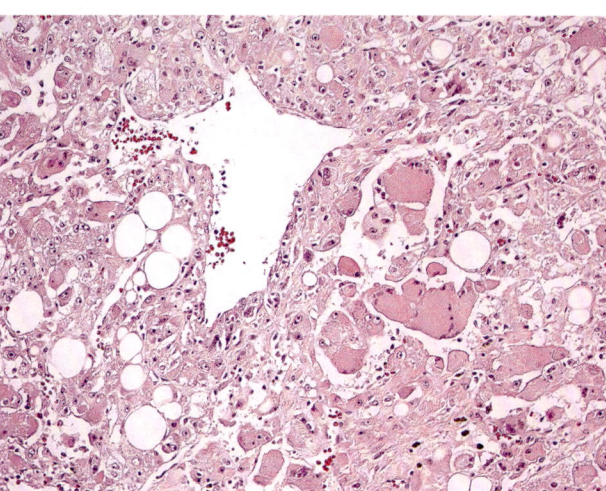

Figure 3.262. This epithelioid angiomyolipoma is composed of pleomorphic giant cells with eosinophilic cytoplasm. A clue to the diagnosis is the presence of focal lipid droplets.

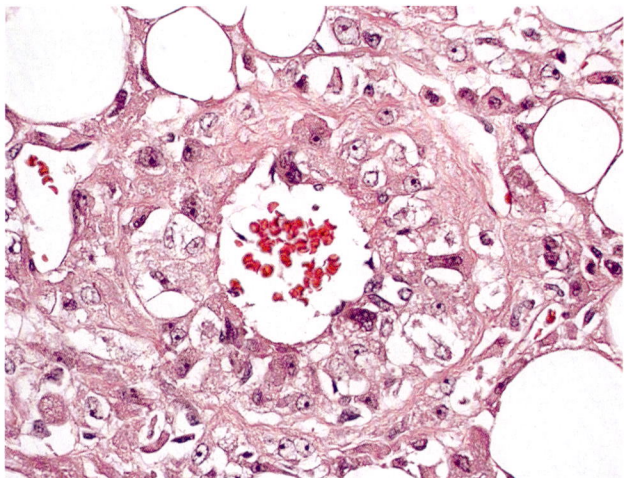

Figure 3.263. In the same tumor from Figure 3.262, epithelioid cells arranged in the wall of a blood vessel are also a clue to the diagnosis of epithelioid angiomyolipoma/PEComa.

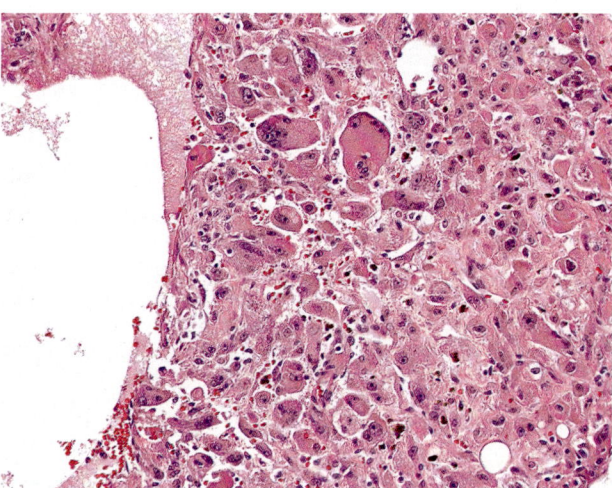

Figure 3.264. This epithelioid angiomyolipoma is composed of a sheet-like arrangement of pleomorphic giant cells. The main differential diagnosis would be high-grade renal cell carcinoma.

tumors, they are typically positive with immunohistochemistry for synaptophysin (Figure 3.276), less frequently chromogranin, and often cytokeratin or vimentin. TTF1 is typically negative in well-differentiated neuroendocrine tumors, contrasting to small cell carcinoma, which may be positive in small cell carcinoma of any origin (lung or otherwise).[248] PAX8 negativity would likely be helpful to distinguish from renal cell tumors,[255] although this may be dependent on antibody, as positivity has been reported in neuroendocrine tumors, particularly with polyclonal antibodies.[256] Due to the rarity of renal well-differentiated neuroendocrine tumors, it is less clear if prognostic parameters similar to neuroendocrine tumors of other organs are applicable. Of course, the best predictor of survival is stage, and for neuroendocrine tumors it is noted that a substantial subset of patients has regional lymph node involvement at nephrectomy. Other studies have correlated mitotic activity and cytologic atypia with behavior.[257]

Metanephric Adenoma

Metanephric adenoma is a rare benign renal neoplasm that typically forms small tubules and papillary structures, lined by exceptionally bland, monotonous epithelial cells with an embryonic-like appearance (yet without substantial mitotic activity) and small round or oval nuclei (Figures 3.277-3.280). Although most examples are relatively small (3-6 cm),

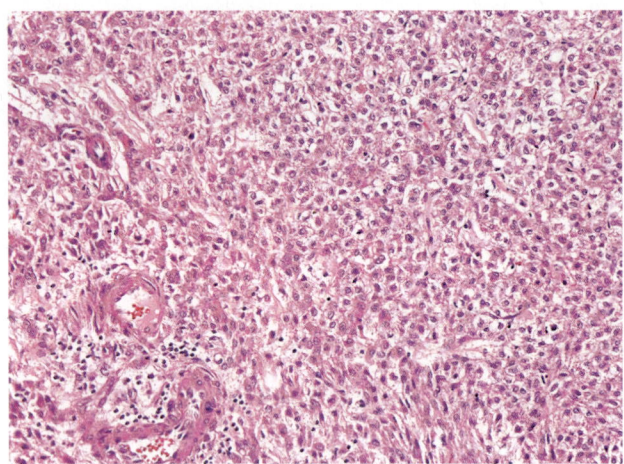

Figure 3.265. This angiomyolipoma is composed of a monomorphic population of bland epithelioid cells. It is **debatable whether** this should be considered epithelioid or conventional angiomyolipoma, as it lacks the features of malignancy discussed previously in the chapter.

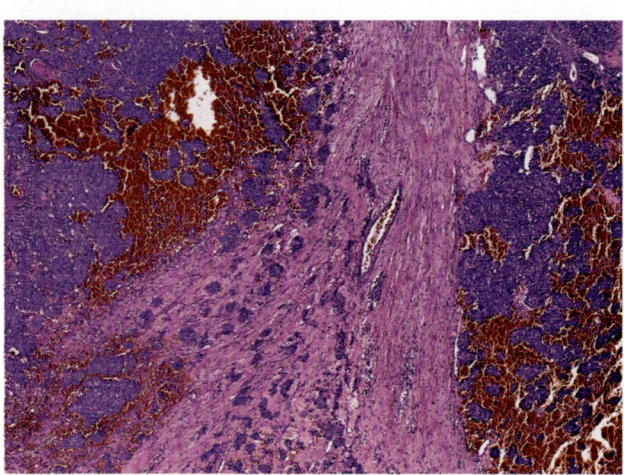

Figure 3.266. Juxtaglomerular cell tumor is composed of epithelioid to spindle-shaped cells with variable fibrous stroma.

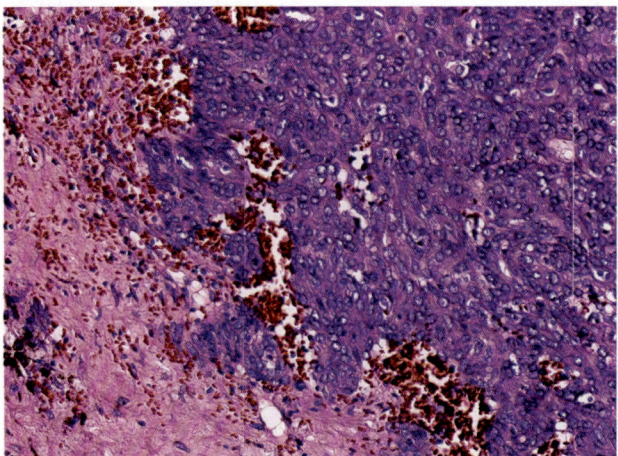

Figure 3.267. This juxtaglomerular cell tumor **shows cells with** small amounts of eosinophilic cytoplasm and bland, **monotonous** nuclei.

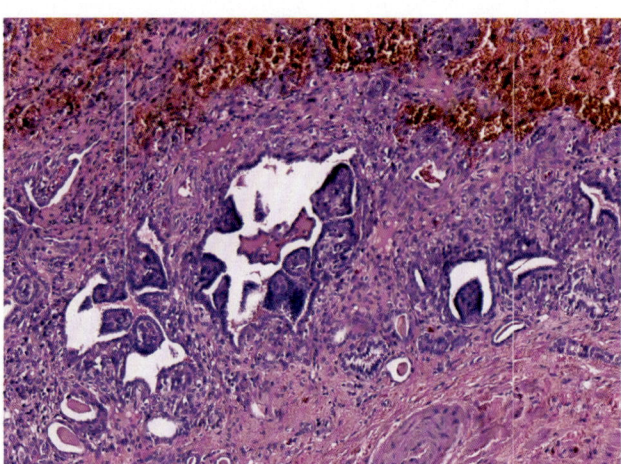

Figure 3.268. Focal papillary formations can be found in juxtaglomerular cell tumor.

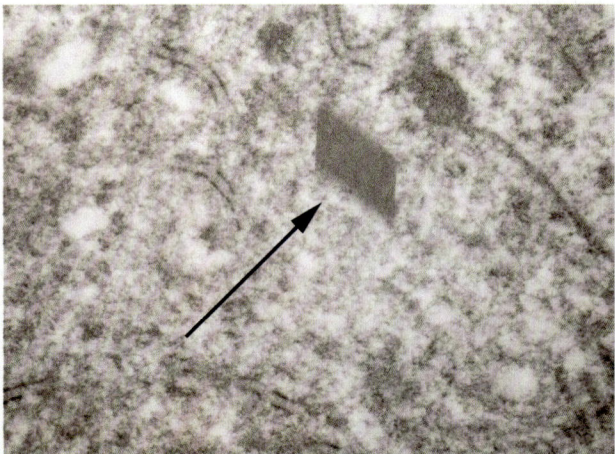

Figure 3.269. The characteristic finding using **electron microscopy** in juxtaglomerular cell tumor is the **rhomboid-shaped renin** protogranule (arrow).

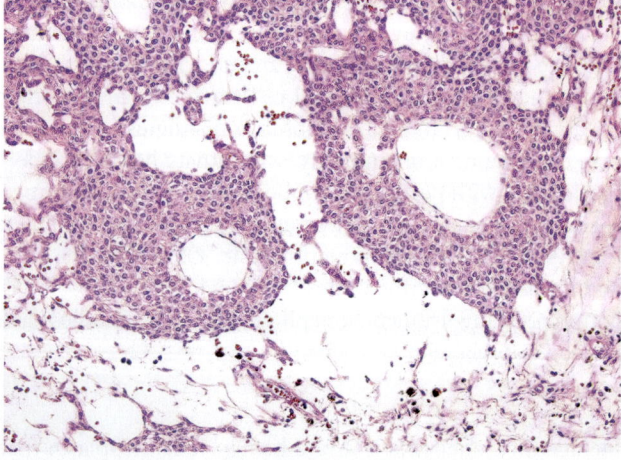

Figure 3.270. It has been recently recognized that renal glomus tumors can occur. This example shows edematous stroma with pericytic cellularity, similar to glomus tumor of soft tissue.

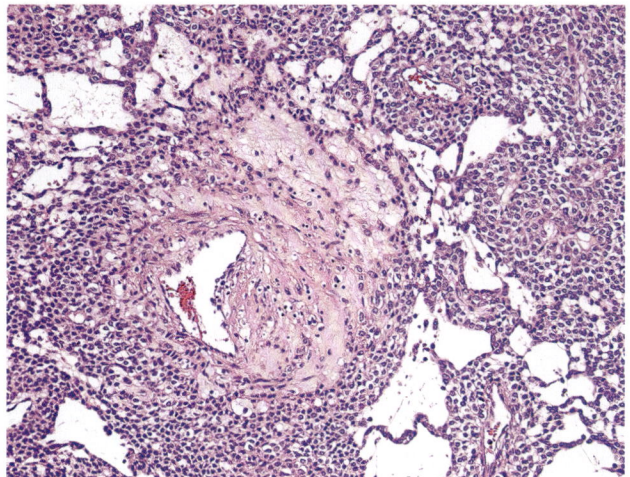

Figure 3.271. This renal glomus tumor shows monotonous epithelioid cells arranged around blood vessels with interconnecting strands of tumor cells separated by edema. Renal glomus tumors are often much larger than those of the superficial skin and soft tissue.

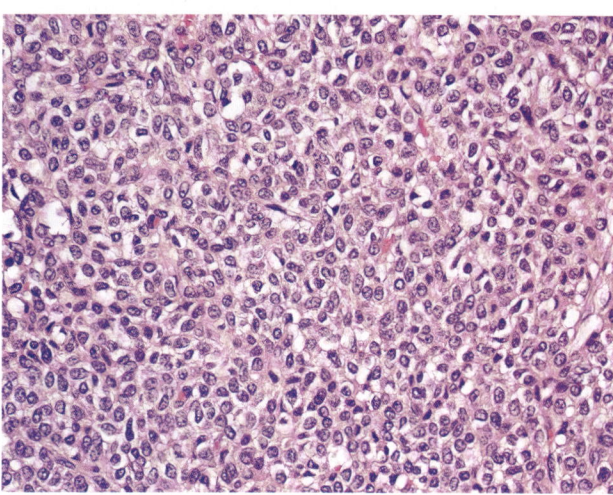

Figure 3.272. At high magnification, this renal glomus tumor shows bland ovoid nuclei with inconspicuous cytoplasm arranged in a sheet-like growth pattern.

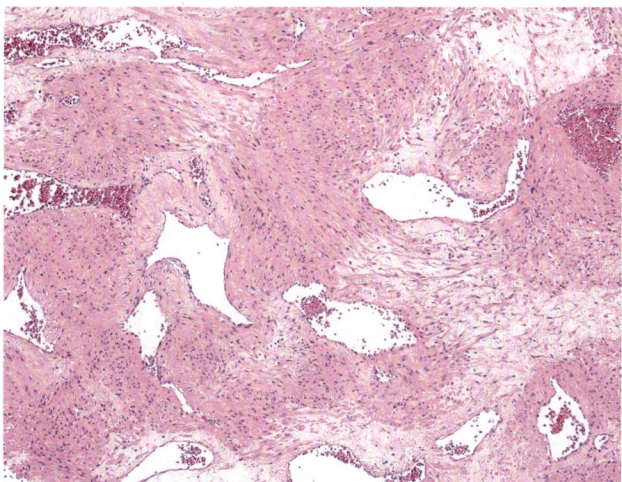

Figure 3.273. Although not epithelioid, it has been recently found that other pericytic tumors can rarely occur in the kidney, such as angioleiomyoma (shown here) or myopericytoma (not pictured).

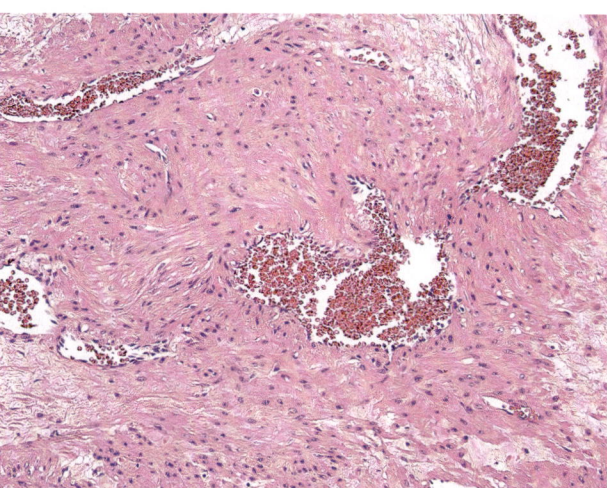

Figure 3.274. At higher magnification, this angioleiomyoma is composed of smooth muscle cells arranged around blood vessels.

those as large as 15 cm have been reported.[258] Due to the rarity of this tumor, a major differential diagnostic consideration would be the much more common papillary RCC (type 1), which can also have tubular and solid components (Figures 3.281 and 3.282).

KEY FEATURES: Metanephric Adenoma

- Variable in size, usually small but rarely can be >10 cm
- Small acini and papillary structures
- Nuclei small, only slightly larger than lymphocytes, with inconspicuous nucleoli
- Psamomma bodies may be present
- Often no pseudocapsule
- Immunohistochemistry[259]
  - WT1 positive (Figure 3.283)
  - CD57 positive

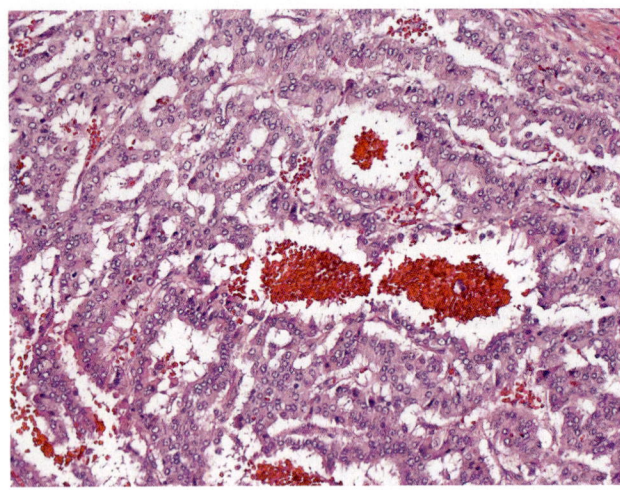

Figure 3.275. Well-differentiated neuroendocrine tumors (carcinoid tumors) can occur in the kidney. This example shows a trabecular or ribbon-like architecture. Confusion with renal cell carcinoma would be very possible due to the rarity of neuroendocrine tumors in the kidney.

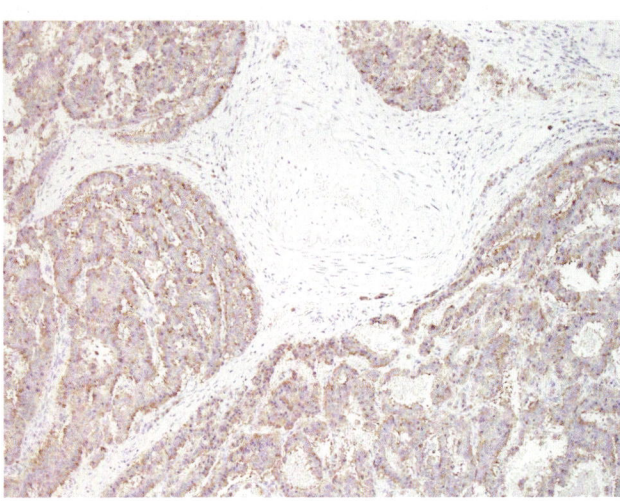

Figure 3.276. The same well-differentiated neuroendocrine tumor from Figure 3.275 shows diffuse synaptophysin immunohistochemical staining.

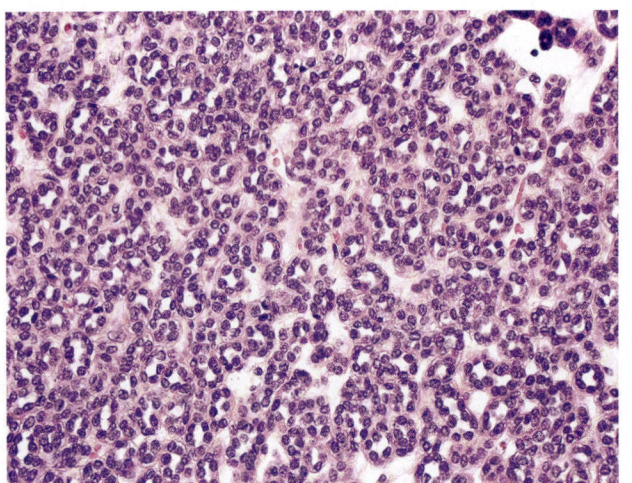

Figure 3.277. Metanephric adenoma is composed of uniform small tubular structures lined by bland cells.

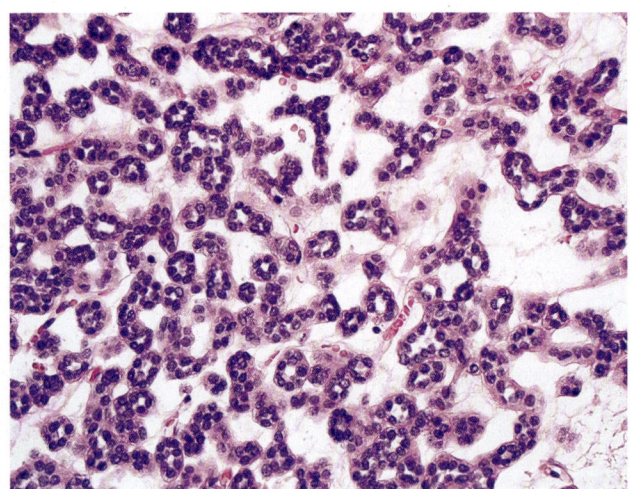

Figure 3.278. At high magnification, the cells of metanephric adenoma have very small nuclei, like those of lymphocytes.

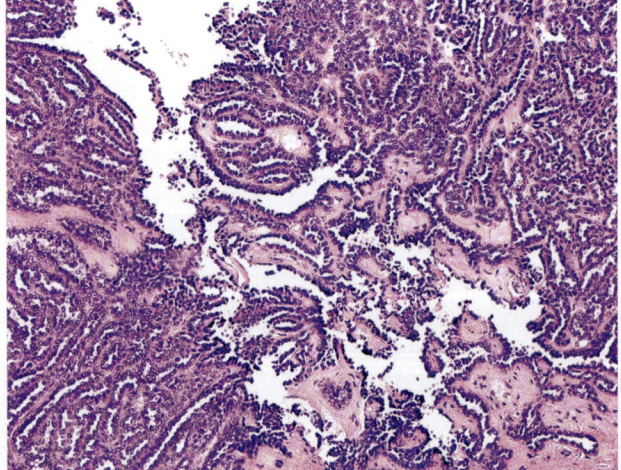

Figure 3.279. Papillary architecture in metanephric adenoma can lead to confusion with papillary renal cell carcinoma.

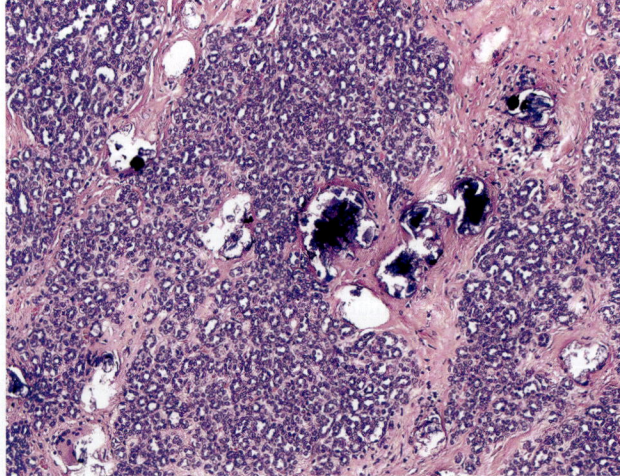

Figure 3.280. Psammoma bodies can be present, sometimes numerous in metanephric adenoma, which also overlaps with papillary renal cell carcinoma.

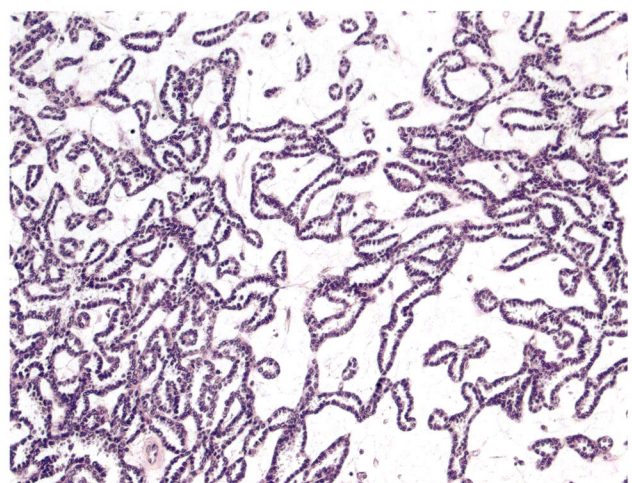

Figure 3.281. This papillary renal cell carcinoma (RCC) contains areas that could be confused for metanephric adenoma with interconnecting tubules lined by small cells. However, typical papillary RCC areas were also present (Figure 3.282).

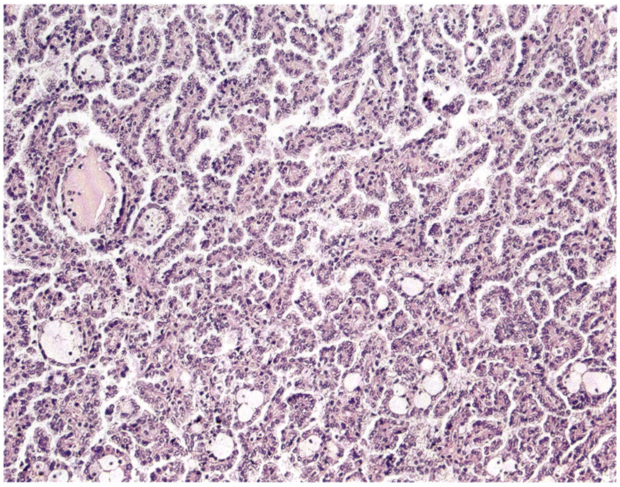

Figure 3.282. The same tumor from Figure 3.281 includes areas of typical papillary renal cell carcinoma.

- AMACR negative or minimal (contrasting to papillary RCC, Figure 3.284)
- Cytokeratin 7 negative or minimal (contrasting to papillary RCC, Figure 3.285)

CHECKLIST: Metanephric Adenoma Versus Other "Blue Cell Tumors"

☐ Small uniform nucleoli

☐ Tubular or papillary architecture (psammoma bodies possible)

☐ Mitotic activity/atypia not conspicuous (if present, consider papillary RCC or nephroblastoma)

☐ No solid/blastemal component (if present, consider nephroblastoma)

☐ AMACR negative or minimal (if strong, consider papillary RCC)

☐ Cytokeratin 7 negative or minimal (if strong, consider papillary RCC)

☐ WT1 positive

☐ CD57 positive

CYSTIC LESIONS

Multilocular Cystic Neoplasm of Low Malignant Potential

The entity formerly known as multilocular cystic RCC has been renamed in the 2016 WHO Classification as a low malignant potential neoplasm, based on long-standing evidence that tumors with this predominant cystic pattern have highly favorable behavior without evidence of metastatic disease. The WHO criteria for this diagnosis dictate an entirely cystic neoplasm with only individual cells scattered in the cyst walls (Figures 3.286-3.288) but lacking any solid areas that would be evident as a gross mass.[260] Despite this strict definition, there is some evidence that extensively cystic clear cell RCC not meeting these criteria is still favorable.[28,261,262] As such, it may be reasonable to give a diagnostic comment for tumors that are cystic but not meeting these criteria to highlight their favorable behavior.

SAMPLE NOTE: Extensively Cystic Clear Cell RCC

- Kidney, left, partial nephrectomy:
  - Clear cell RCC, with extensive cystic changes—see Comment
  - 3.5 cm greatest dimension

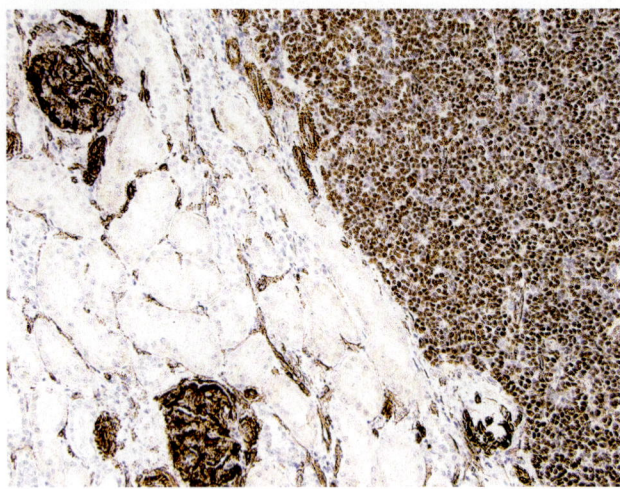

Figure 3.283. WT1 immunohistochemical staining is typically diffusely positive in the tumor cell nuclei of metanephric adenoma (right). Glomerular cells are also labeled (left).

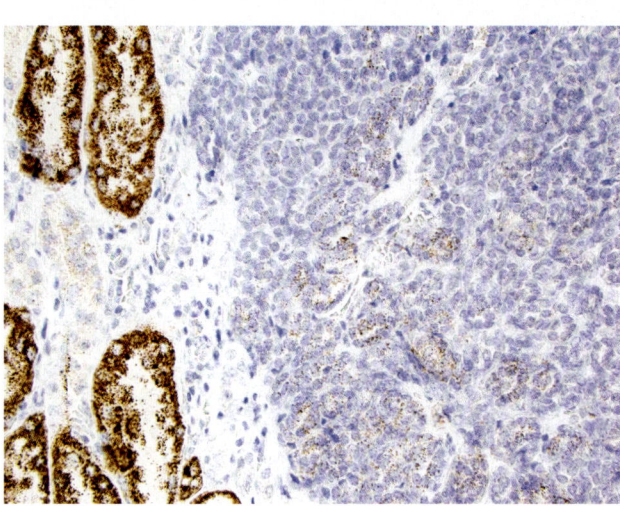

Figure 3.284. AMACR staining is typically minimal in metanephric adenoma (right), contrasting to papillary renal cell carcinoma or the staining pattern of proximal tubules (left).

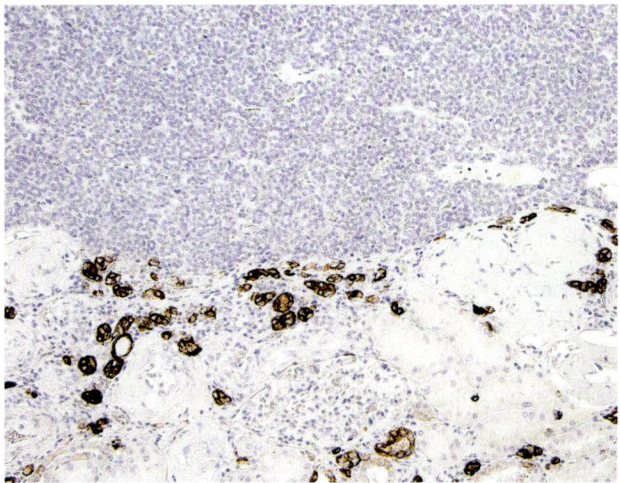

Figure 3.285. Cytokeratin 7 staining is typically minimal in metanephric adenoma, contrasting to type 1 papillary renal cell carcinoma. Normal renal tubules at bottom show patchy staining as well.

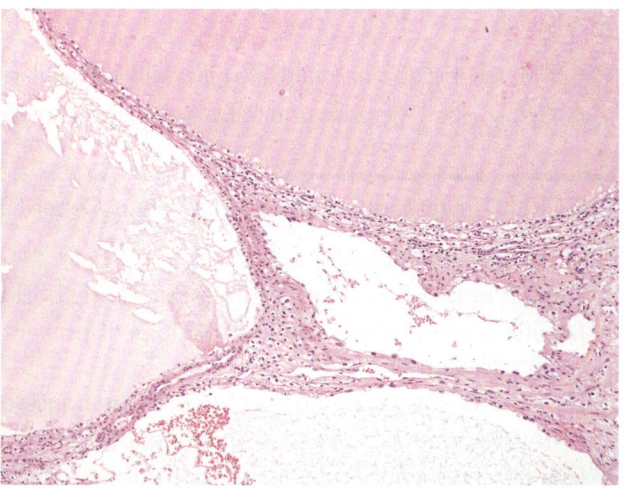

Figure 3.286. Multilocular cystic renal neoplasm of low malignant potential is composed of multiple cysts lined by cells with clear cytoplasm. No solid mass-forming areas should present that could be appreciable grossly.

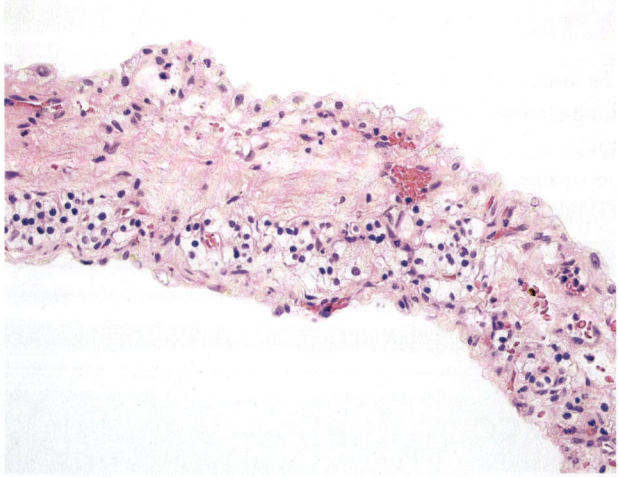

Figure 3.287. At high magnification, the cyst walls of multilocular cystic renal neoplasm of low malignant potential are lined by cells with clear cytoplasm and there are small aggregates of epithelial cells within the wall.

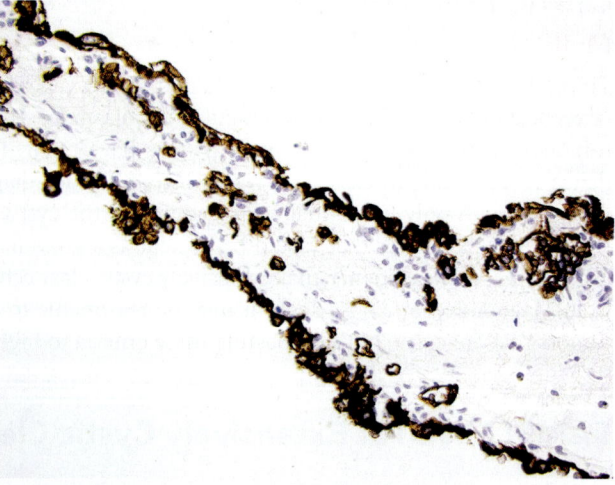

Figure 3.288. Immunohistochemistry for cytokeratin CAM 5.2 shows some epithelial cells within the cyst wall in a multilocular cystic renal neoplasm of low malignant potential.

- ISUP/WHO grade 2
- Confined to the kidney (pT1a)
- Margins negative

Comment: Although the tumor does not meet criteria for multilocular cystic renal neoplasm of low malignant potential, there is some evidence that extensively cystic clear cell RCC has a favorable prognosis.

Immunohistochemistry in general is not necessary for diagnosis of multilocular cystic renal neoplasm of low malignant potential; however, it may be worthwhile to note that there may be increased staining for cytokeratin 7 (Figure 3.289), which overlaps with the phenotype of clear cell papillary RCC.[263] In fact, some authors have suggested that there is substantial overlap between these two diagnostic entities.[264] Distinguishing between these two is likely not of critical importance, as they both have highly favorable behavior, with multilocular cystic neoplasms being longer established and officially regarded as a low malignant potential tumor, in contrast to clear cell papillary RCC, which remains currently considered a nonaggressive carcinoma.

Clear Cell Papillary RCC, Cystic

Some examples of clear cell papillary RCC can be extensively cystic (Figures 3.290 and 3.291), to the point that distinction from multilocular cystic neoplasm of low malignant potential is almost arbitrary. A comparison of the features of these two entities is shown in Table 3.7.[263,265,266] In general, we would favor a diagnosis of clear cell papillary RCC if there are clusters of tubules in the septa with branched glandular configuration or nuclear alignment, as the typical pattern of multilocular cystic neoplasms is usually individual cells and clusters of cells. Likewise, small papillary formations would also favor a clear cell papillary diagnosis. Fortunately, this distinction is not critical, as both neoplasms have highly favorable behavior. In fact, clear cell papillary RCC may eventually be reclassified also as a low malignant potential tumor.[87,88]

Atypical Renal Cyst and Benign Cysts

Atypical cyst has been proposed as a term to encompass some cystic lesions that have no solid mass component to warrant a carcinoma diagnosis, yet which have atypical features raising concern for a precursor lesion.[212] The main forms described in the study of Matoso et al. included cysts lined by (1) clear cells, sometimes with focally papillary tufting, (2)

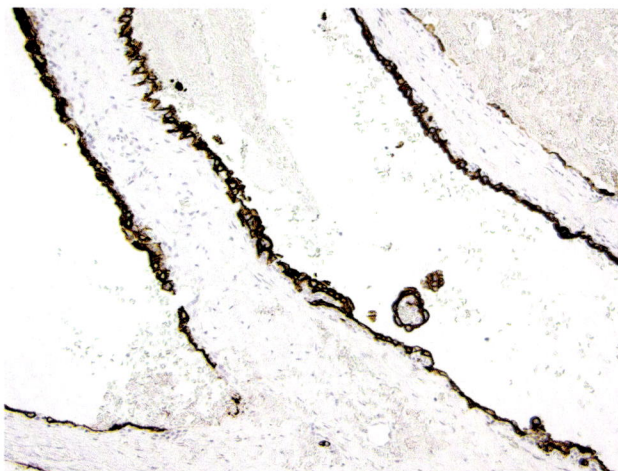

Figure 3.289. Immunohistochemistry for cytokeratin 7 may be substantially positive in multilocular cystic renal neoplasm of low malignant potential, which is therefore not very helpful in differentiating from clear cell papillary renal cell carcinoma.

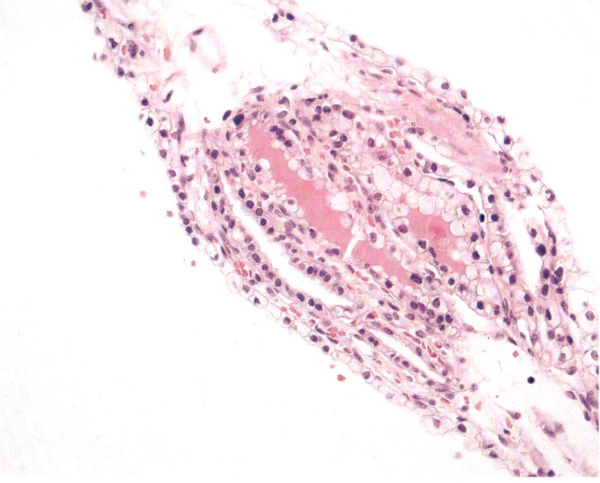

Figure 3.290. Clear cell papillary renal cell carcinoma (RCC) can be extensively cystic, to the point that distinction from multilocular cystic neoplasm of low malignant potential is almost arbitrary. This example of clear cell papillary RCC has small glandular formations within the cyst wall, with a hint of nuclear alignment, contrasting to the individual cells of multilocular cystic neoplasms.

TABLE 3.7: Features Distinguishing Cystic Clear Cell Papillary Renal Cell Carcinoma From Multilocular Cystic Neoplasm of Low Malignant Potential

Clear Cell Papillary	Multilocular Cystic
Solid areas with branched tubules	No solid areas
Papillary tufts into cysts	No papillary tufts
Individual cells in septa not typical	**Cells and clusters of cells in septa**
No 3p deletion or *VHL* abnormality	**3p deletion and *VHL* gene abnormalities**
CK7 positive	CK7 often positive
No known malignant behavior to date	Reclassified as low malignant potential tumor

eosinophilic stratified cells, or (3) eosinophilic cells with papillary proliferation.[212] The clear cell pattern appears to bear resemblance to clear cell papillary RCC, with frequent labeling for both cytokeratin 7 and carbonic anhydrase IX, and indeed some patients with clear cell papillary tumors have multiple tumors, including small incipient tumors or cysts (Figures 3.292 and 3.293). The pattern of papillary proliferation within cysts described by Matoso et al. was noted in several patients with autosomal dominant (adult) polycystic kidney disease,[212] which we have also noted in this setting and typically refer to as papillary hyperplasia of the cyst lining (see next section). In the setting of acquired cystic kidney disease, as noted previously, cysts can also occur with small punched-out lumens within thickened eosinophilic lining (see section on acquired cystic kidney disease), which is thought to be a precursor lesion to the associated tumors.[211] In our experience it is rare to see a kidney resected that contains only such cysts without a tumor, probably because development of a tumor is one of the most common indications for the nephrectomy in this setting; however, in such cases, it would be reasonable to use a designation such as atypical cyst or cyst with epithelial proliferation, with a comment that these may be a precursor lesion to renal neoplasms.

When encountering a cystic lesion that consists of one or multiple cysts without the above features (not lined by clear cells, pseudostratified cells, or papillary proliferation) and lined by flat or cuboidal cells, similar to those of benign tubules, a diagnosis of a

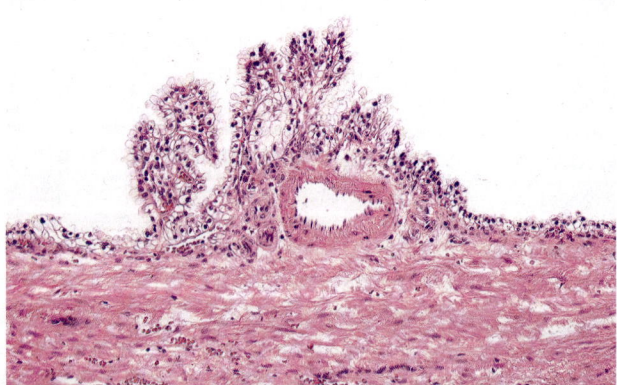

Figure 3.291. The same clear cell papillary tumor from Figure 3.290 also demonstrates small foci of branching papillae, favoring clear cell papillary renal cell carcinoma over multilocular cystic neoplasm. Distinction between these two entities can be difficult in some cases; however, this is likely of minimal clinical significance, as both are nonaggressive.

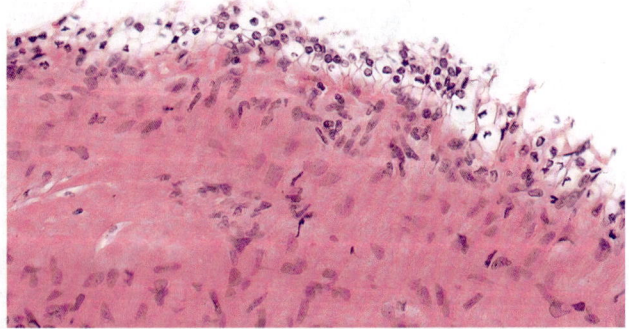

Figure 3.292. This cyst in a patient with multiple clear cell papillary renal cell carcinomas is lined by cells with clear cytoplasm but includes no definite mass-forming component itself. It would be reasonable to consider such lesions as "atypical cyst," which may be a precursor to neoplasms.

benign cortical cyst or aggregate of multiple cysts is reasonable. Often such aggregates of benign cysts will have normal tubules or sometimes glomeruli in the tissue between the cysts (Figure 3.294), contrasting to the neoplastic individual cells or glands in multilocular cystic neoplasms or clear cell papillary RCCs. If there is a question of clear cell lining, immunohistochemistry for carbonic anhydrase IX may be helpful, as substantial membranous labeling would favor a neoplastic or preneoplastic lesion, such as the atypical cysts described previously.

Autosomal Dominant (Adult) Polycystic Kidney Disease

Like medical renal disease, the study of cystic kidney disease is complex on its own; however, since polycystic kidneys are relatively commonly encountered by the urologic or general surgical pathologist, brief discussion of highest yield points is included here. Kidneys with autosomal dominant polycystic kidney disease (Figure 3.295), also known as adult polycystic kidneys, are classically massively enlarged in the range of 1 to 2 kg or more and extensively replaced by cysts.[267] Patients most commonly have *PKD1* gene mutation or less commonly *PKD2* mutation. In addition to the kidney disease, patients also may have heart valve abnormalities, central nervous system vascular aneurysms, and liver or pancreatic cysts. Papillary proliferation of the cyst lining in this form of cystic kidney disease is common, which we usually report as papillary hyperplasia of cysts (Figures 3.296 and 3.297).

SAMPLE NOTE: Autosomal Dominant Polycystic Kidney Disease

Kidney, left, nephrectomy:
- Massively enlarged (# grams), polycystic kidney, consistent with autosomal dominant (adult) polycystic kidney disease
- Papillary hyperplasia of cyst lining epithelium

Acquired Cystic Kidney Disease

In contrast to autosomal dominant polycystic kidney disease, acquired cystic kidney disease is more often small and only partially replaced by cysts (Figure 3.298).[267] This cyst formation occurs with chronic renal disease, usually after prolonged dialysis, although this is not a requirement. Various unusual morphologies in the cyst lining can be encountered, including multilayering or small lumens suggesting early cribriform formation (Figures 3.299 and 3.300). This is the presumptive precursor lesion to acquired cystic kidney disease–associated RCC.[211] However, the precise point at which a cyst with this epithelial proliferation becomes a neoplasm is difficult to pinpoint. We would generally reserve diagnosis of a neoplasm for when this becomes solid, with either a cribriform mass-forming lesion or confluent tubular proliferation. In contrast to autosomal dominant polycystic kidneys, which may be resected due to their large size or when causing pain, acquired cystic disease kidneys are less frequently resected unless they develop a lesion concerning for a mass. Therefore, it is infrequent to encounter only these "atypical" cysts with no mass in our experience.

INFILTRATIVE PATTERN
Urothelial Carcinoma

When encountering a carcinoma with infiltration through the kidney, such that normal glomeruli or tubules are overrun by tumor cells, urothelial carcinoma should be a major consideration, as it usually has markedly different treatment implications than renal cell neoplasms. If there is a papillary urothelial carcinoma component or urothelial carcinoma in situ in the renal pelvis, then the diagnosis is typically straightforward (Figure 3.301); however, this may be lacking in some cases, making the diagnosis more difficult (Figures 3.302 and 3.303). Areas of squamous differentiation (Figure 3.304) would also favor urothelial carcinoma. Of note, however, it is possible for renal cell neoplasms to erode into

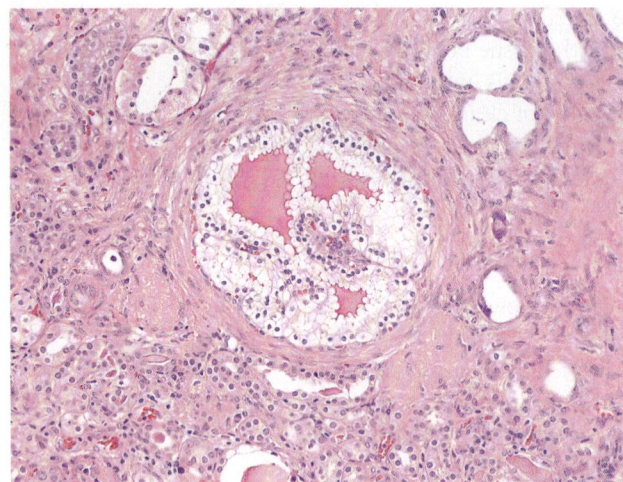

Figure 3.293. This cluster of tubules with clear cytoplasm in a patient with multiple clear cell papillary renal cell carcinomas likely represents a precursor lesion or incipient tumor.

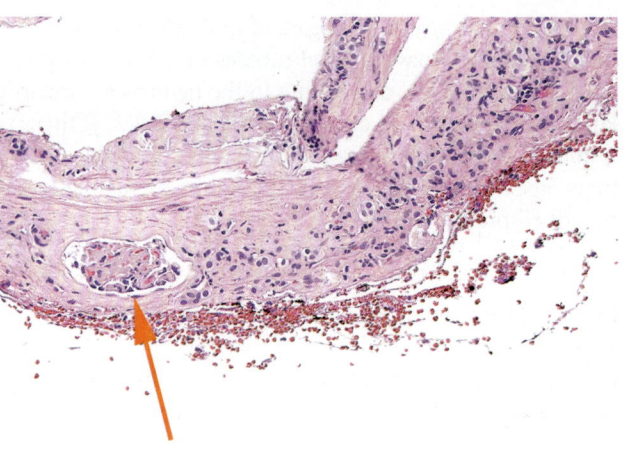

Figure 3.294. In this section of two juxtaposed benign cortical cysts, the cyst lining is not conspicuous. A glomerulus (arrow) and atrophic tubules within the cyst wall contrast to the neoplastic cells of clear cell papillary renal cell carcinoma or multilocular cystic neoplasm of low malignant potential.

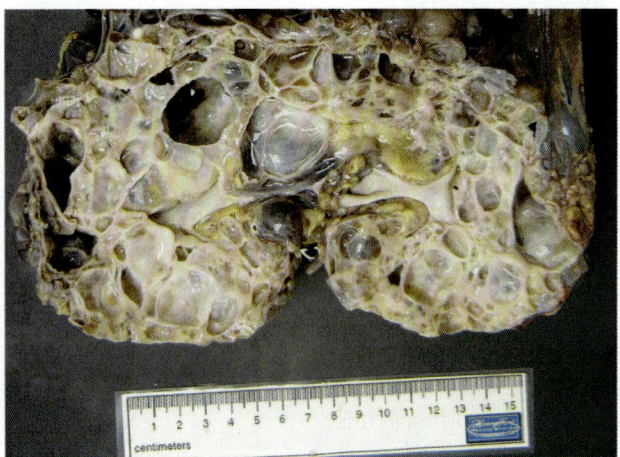

Figure 3.295. Kidneys with autosomal dominant (adult) polycystic kidney disease are often massively enlarged (1-2 kg) and extensively replaced by cysts.

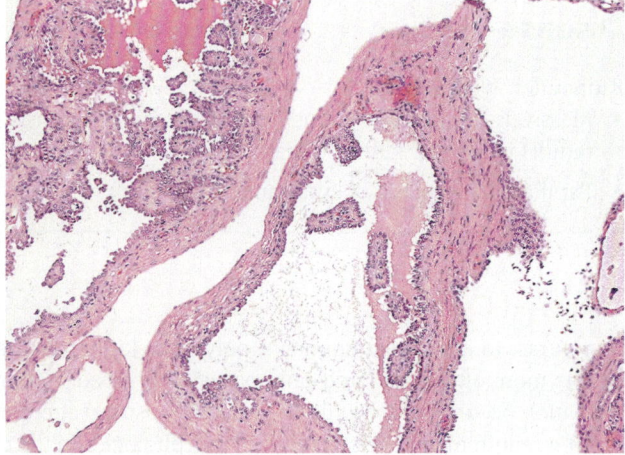

Figure 3.296. Cysts in autosomal dominant polycystic kidney disease are usually lined by bland cuboidal epithelial cells; however, papillary hyperplasia is a relatively frequent finding.

the renal pelvis and to be biopsied via an ureteroscopic approach, and we have encountered RCC, including papillary RCC, presenting this way (Figures 3.305 and 3.306), so a diagnosis of RCC should not be automatically excluded due to pelvic involvement. Urothelial carcinomas of the renal pelvis can spread in a retrograde fashion into medullary tubules at the tip of the renal papilla, and there can be substantial erosion of the medulla, which is not necessarily evidence of invasion in isolation (see staging section). Immunohistochemistry is usually quite helpful for distinguishing RCC from urothelial carcinoma. Urothelial carcinoma is typically positive for p63 or p40, GATA3, and high molecular weight cytokeratin (Figures 3.307 and 3.308). Other emerging markers, such as uroplakin II, may be helpful in especially difficult cases.[268,269] In general, PAX8 positivity would favor RCC; however, some overlap in the phenotype of upper urinary tract urothelial carcinoma and RCC has been reported, especially for PAX8 (i.e., PAX8 positivity has been described in upper tract urothelial carcinoma, Figure 3.309).[17] Therefore, immunohistochemistry should typically be used as a panel of several markers in this scenario, not relying on a single marker in isolation. To a lesser extent, GATA3 can be positive in some renal cell neoplasms, although this has been found mostly to date in well-differentiated patterns, such as chromophobe RCC, clear cell papillary RCC, and a subset of papillary neoplasms.[76,270] Some authors have

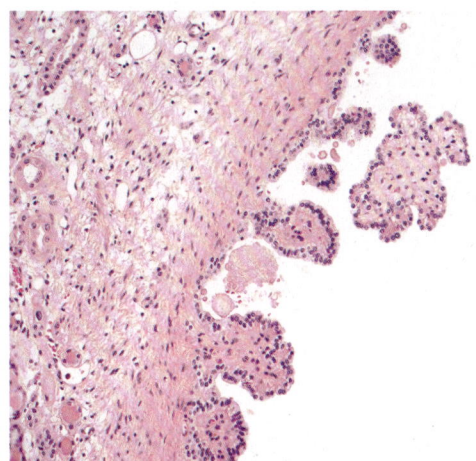

Figure 3.297. At higher magnification, papillary hyperplasia of the cyst lining in autosomal dominant polycystic kidney disease is somewhat reminiscent of papillary nephrogenic adenoma.

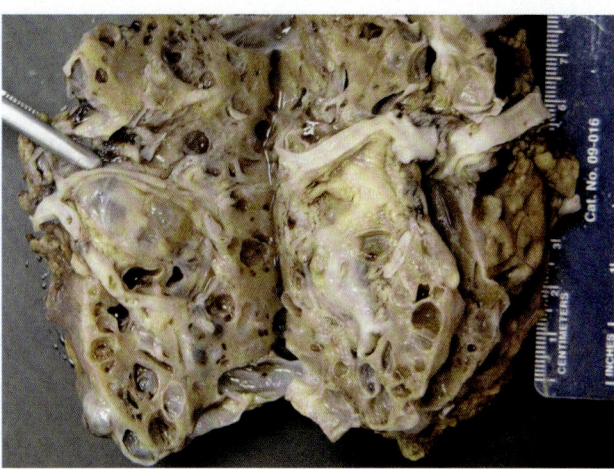

Figure 3.298. In contrast to autosomal dominant polycystic kidney disease (Figure 3.295), kidneys with acquired cystic kidney disease are often small to normal-sized and only partly replaced by cysts.

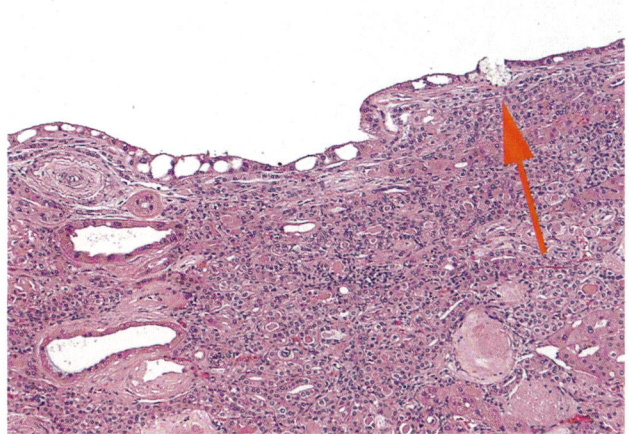

Figure 3.299. This cyst in acquired cystic kidney disease has small, early cribriform lumens and a calcium oxalate crystal (arrow). This is thought to be a precursor to acquired cystic kidney disease renal cell carcinoma.

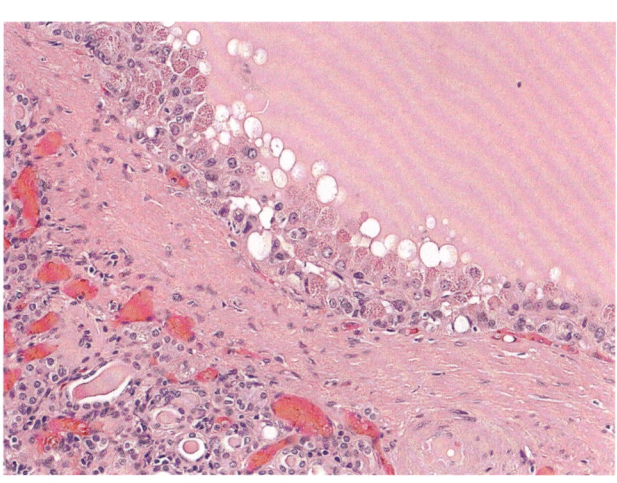

Figure 3.300. This cyst in acquired cystic kidney disease has pseudostratified epithelium with plump cells of different cytoplasmic colors. It would be reasonable to regard this as an "atypical cyst" in the setting of acquired cystic kidney disease.

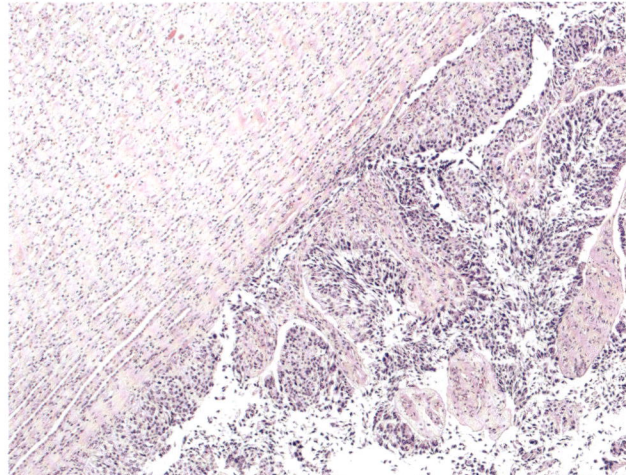

Figure 3.301. Diagnosis of urothelial carcinoma involving the kidney is usually straightforward when there is renal pelvis or ureter involvement by papillary urothelial carcinoma.

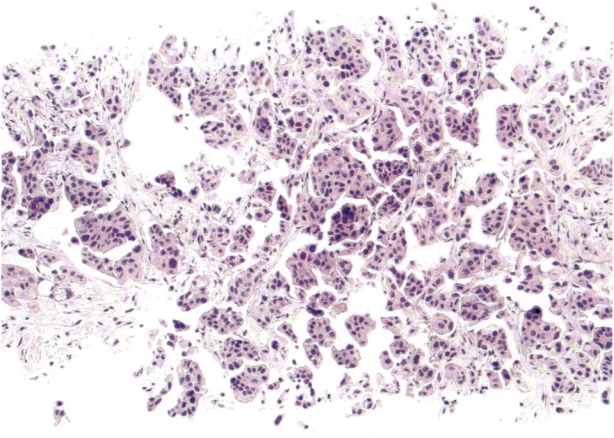

Figure 3.302. This renal mass biopsy shows carcinoma with micropapillary features. This case showed positive staining for GATA3 and p63 (not pictured), supporting renal invasion by urothelial carcinoma.

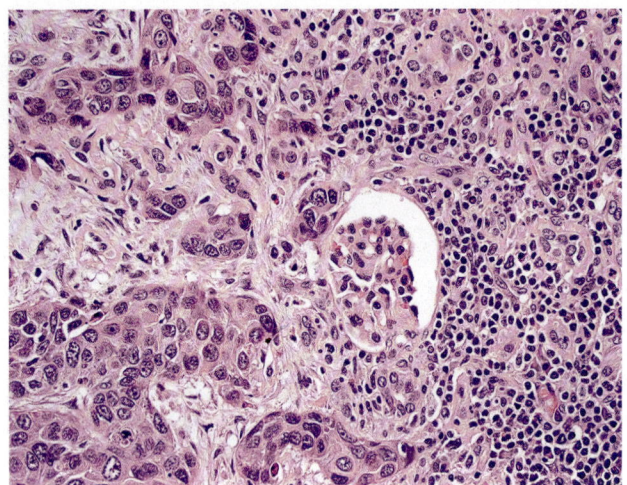

Figure 3.303. Urothelial carcinoma can mimic collecting duct carcinoma by growing as an infiltrative mass that invades around renal structures, such as glomeruli.

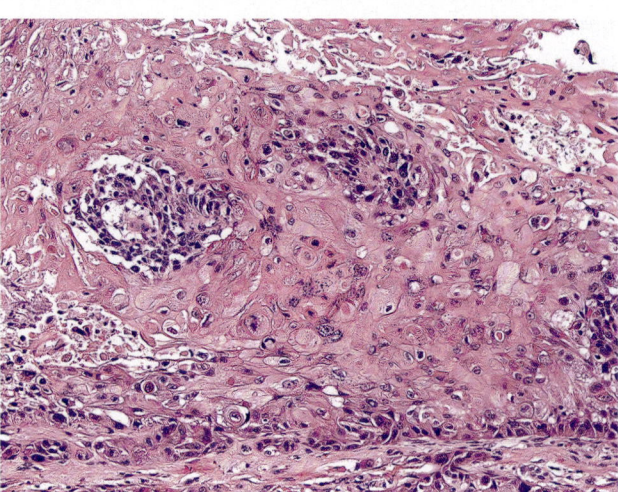

Figure 3.304. Squamous differentiation in a renal mass would favor urothelial carcinoma with squamous differentiation rather than a renal cell tumor.

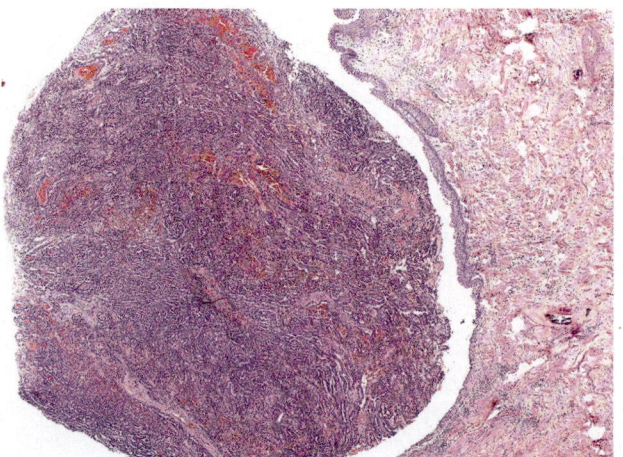

Figure 3.305. Although pelvic involvement generally supports urothelial carcinoma, this papillary renal cell carcinoma grew as a polypoid nodule into the renal pelvis.

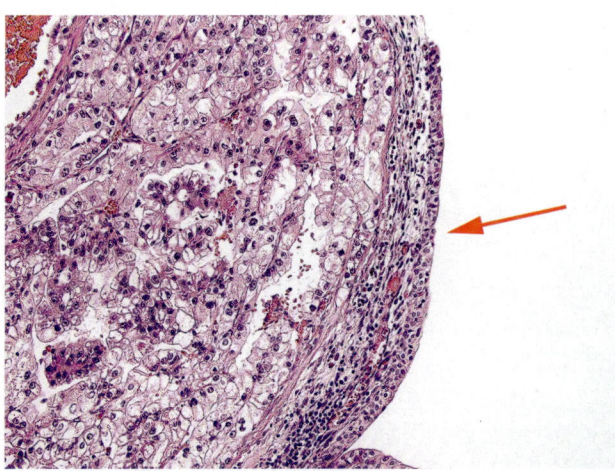

Figure 3.306. This renal cell carcinoma is growing just beneath the urothelial lining of the renal pelvis (arrow).

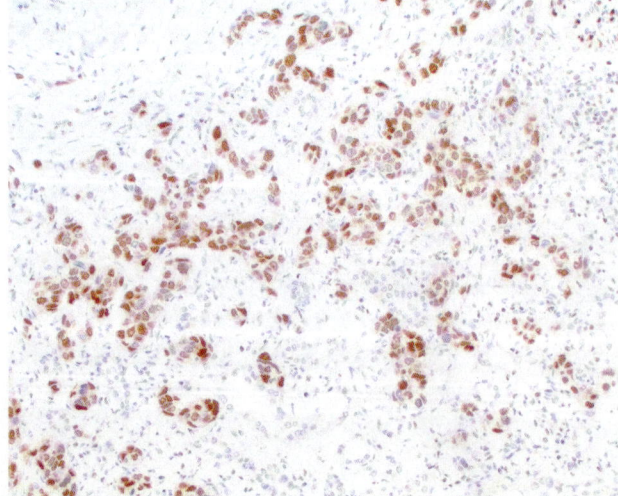

Figure 3.307. Positive immunohistochemistry for GATA3 supports urothelial carcinoma in an infiltrative renal parenchymal mass, mimicking collecting duct carcinoma.

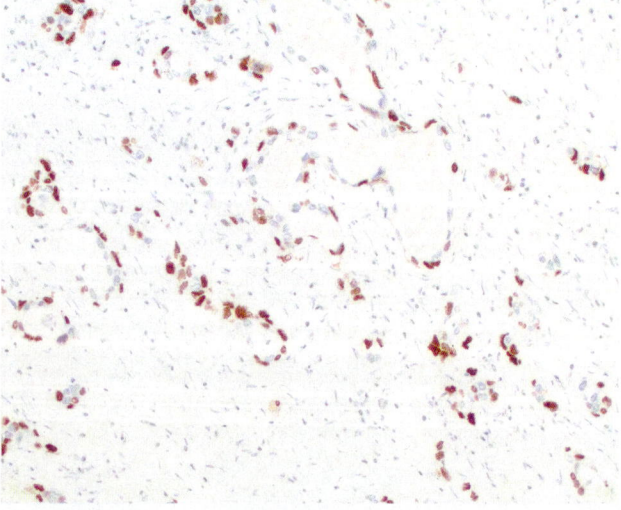

Figure 3.308. This urothelial carcinoma invading the kidney is positive for p63, supporting the diagnosis.

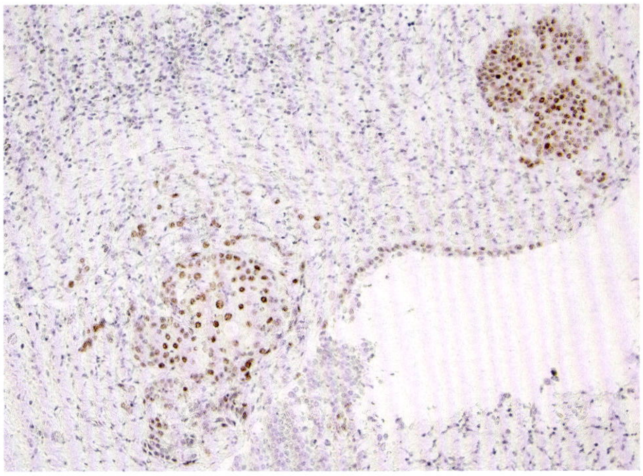

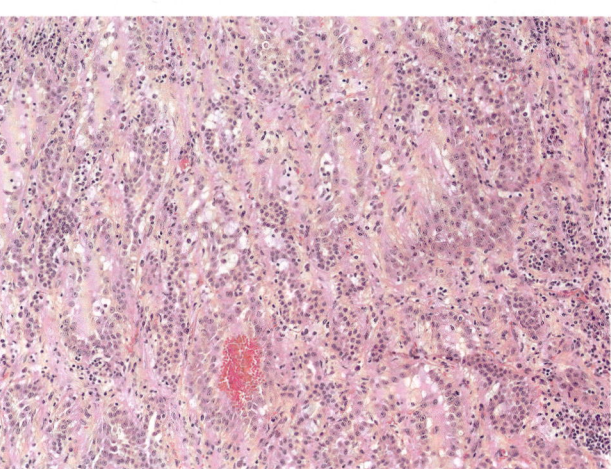

Figure 3.309. This urothelial carcinoma of the renal pelvis shows patchy staining for PAX8, which, although a renal tubular marker, has been described in upper tract urothelial carcinoma.

Figure 3.310. This fumarate hydratase–deficient renal cell carcinoma grows in an infiltrative configuration, resembling collecting duct carcinoma. (Courtesy of Steven C. Smith, MD, PhD, Virginia Commonwealth University.)

allowed p63 positivity in tumors regarded as collecting duct carcinoma.[271,272] We would approach this cautiously, usually considering p63 positivity to strongly favor urothelial carcinoma; however, rare p63 positivity has been reported in renal cell neoplasms, again supporting that several markers should be used in combination rather than putting all emphasis on a single one.[153]

PEARLS AND PITFALLS: Urothelial Carcinoma Involving the Kidney

- Should be a major consideration for infiltrative carcinoma involving the kidney
- Treated differently than most RCCs
  - Nephroureterectomy versus radical nephrectomy
  - Cytotoxic chemotherapy versus tyrosine kinase/VEGF/MTOR inhibitors
- Search for renal pelvis surface (papillary or carcinoma in situ) component may be helpful, including additional gross sampling, if necessary
- Immunohistochemistry is helpful, but some pitfalls are possible:
  - p63 positive usually strongly favors urothelial carcinoma but possible rare positivity in RCC described
  - PAX8 generally favors RCC but can be positive in upper tract urothelial carcinoma
  - GATA3 and high molecular weight cytokeratin usually favor urothelial carcinoma but can be positive in select RCCs
  - Emerging markers such as uroplakin II may be helpful in especially difficult cases

---

FH-Deficient/Hereditary Leiomyomatosis and RCC Syndrome

FH-deficient RCC is primarily discussed under the papillary pattern; however, with the increasing recognition of its morphologic heterogeneity, it is important to remember that it can also manifest as an infiltrative carcinoma that overruns normal structures, resembling collecting duct or medullary carcinoma (Figures 3.310 and 3.311).[21,158] At present, it appears that the best tool for the pathologist to identify potential FH-deficient RCC is immunohistochemistry for the FH protein, which usually shows an abnormal negative staining result (Figure 3.312).

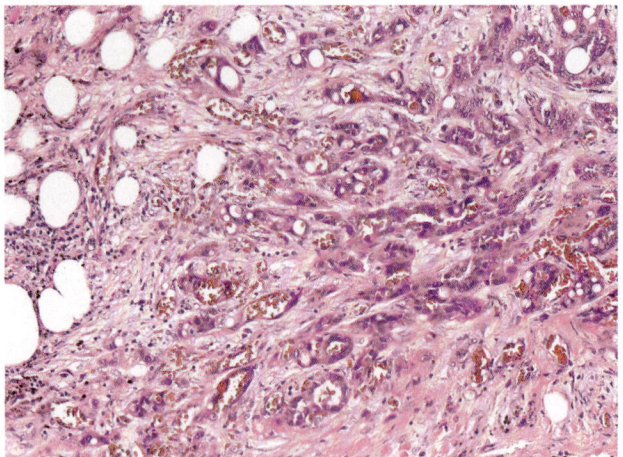

Figure 3.311. This fumarate hydratase–deficient renal cell carcinoma shows infiltration into adjacent fat. (Courtesy of Steven C. Smith, MD, PhD, Virginia Commonwealth University.)

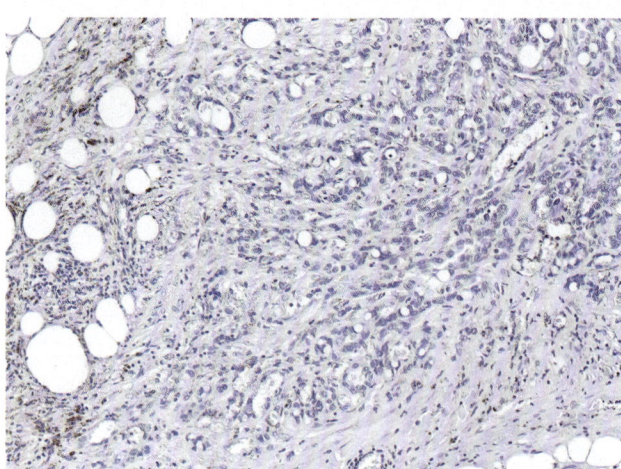

Figure 3.312. The same field from Figure 3.311 shows abnormal negative staining for the fumarate hydratase protein. (Courtesy of Steven C. Smith, MD, PhD, Virginia Commonwealth University.)

Renal Medullary Carcinoma

Medullary carcinoma is another form of aggressive renal cancer that is characteristically found in the setting of sickle cell trait, or less commonly other hemoglobinopathy, often at a younger age than RCC in general. These tumors form infiltrative tubular, papillary, solid, or cribriform structures that overgrow normal renal structures,[158,273,274] sometimes associated with substantial inflammation (Figures 3.313 and 3.314). Sickle trait or other hemoglobinopathy is almost required for diagnosis. Recently it has been noted that disruption of the *SMARCB1* gene (formerly INI1) is a key mechanism in pathogenesis of these tumors, and therefore, abnormal negative immunohistochemistry for SMARCB1 protein can serve as a tool for the pathologist to diagnose these tumors.[158,273-280] Positive OCT3/4 staining, which is more commonly used for diagnosis of testicular seminoma and embryonal carcinoma, has also been noted in medullary carcinoma and may be a diagnostic tool.[280]

FAQ: Is It Possible to Have Medullary Carcinoma in a Patient Without Sickle Trait?

It has recently been noted that rare tumors with *SMARCB1* loss can occur in patients without sickle trait or hemoglobinopathy (Figure 3.315). It has been proposed for this scenario that the term "RCC unclassified with medullary phenotype" be used.[158,281,282] Although data on this phenomenon are scant at present, all evidence suggests that these tumors are highly aggressive, like medullary carcinoma.

Collecting Duct Carcinoma

Collecting duct carcinoma has been historically spoken of among the five or so most common forms of renal cancer; however, now with increasing understanding of RCC subtypes and improved subclassification with immunohistochemistry, this is essentially a diagnosis of exclusion after several relevant differential diagnoses are excluded (see Checklist). As such, our experience is that collecting duct carcinoma is now extremely rare in current practice, much in the way that fibrosarcoma has gone from being one of the most common sarcomas to being almost nonexistent in soft tissue pathology.[283] However, rare cases meeting these criteria do likely occur (Figure 3.316).[284] Classically, the tumor epicenter would be located in the medulla for both collecting duct carcinoma and medullary carcinoma.[284] A recent study evaluating the molecular features of collecting duct carcinoma found genomic alterations in *NF2*, *SETD2*, and *CDKN2A*, as well as alterations of *SMARCB1* or *FH* homozygous loss.[285] Those with the latter findings likely represent either medullary carcinoma or FH-deficient renal cancer, respectively.

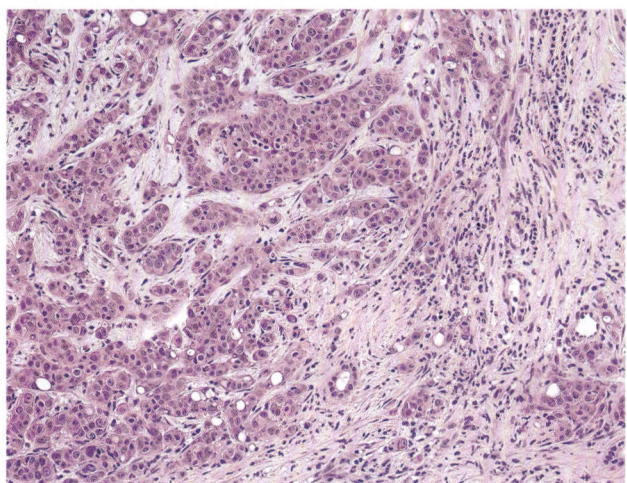

Figure 3.313. This renal medullary carcinoma from a young man with sickle trait demonstrates infiltrative growth within fibrotic stroma, resembling collecting duct carcinoma or urothelial carcinoma.

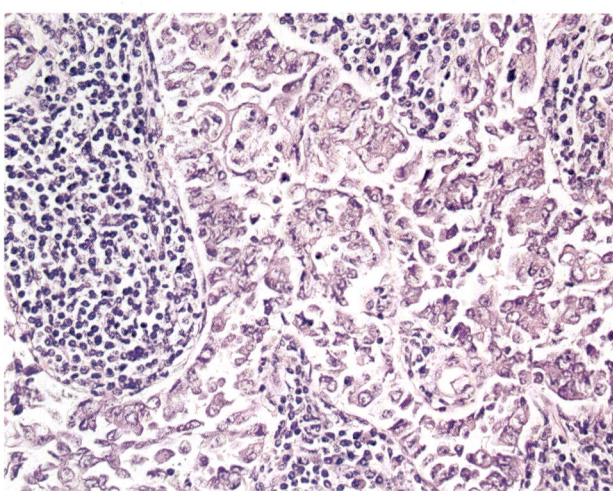

Figure 3.314. This medullary carcinoma shows prominent peritumoral chronic inflammation.

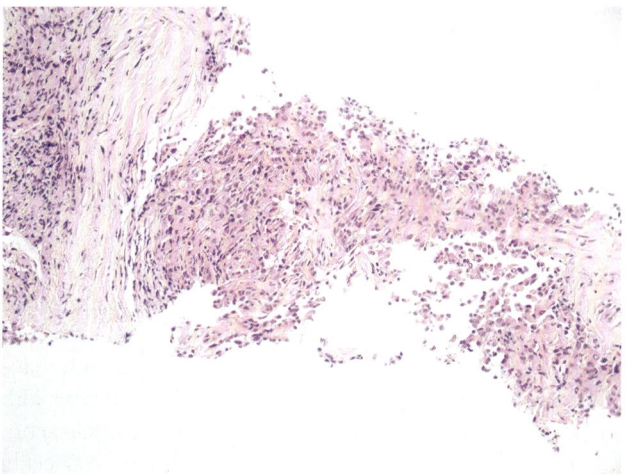

Figure 3.315. This renal mass biopsy shows a high-grade renal cell carcinoma. Immunohistochemistry revealed positivity for PAX8, supporting a primary renal cell neoplasm (not pictured). Comprehensive genomic profiling was performed in search of actionable targets for therapy, which found *SMARCB1* (INI1) mutation. The patient had no known hemoglobinopathy but unfortunately the cancer progressed and he died rapidly after diagnosis.

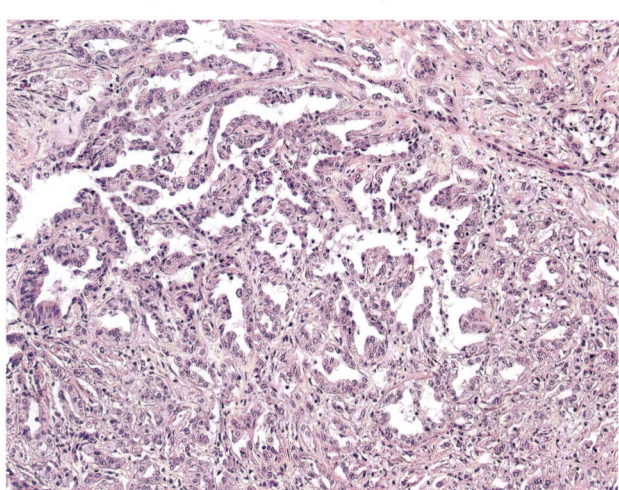

Figure 3.316. This renal mass was diagnosed as collecting duct carcinoma after extensive evaluation was performed to argue against other considerations. AMACR immunohistochemistry showed minimal patchy staining, arguing against papillary renal cell carcinoma, and fumarate hydratase immunohistochemistry showed a normal (intact) pattern. Other considerations that should be argued against would include urothelial carcinoma or metastasis of another cancer to the kidney.

CHECKLIST: Diagnosis of Collecting Duct Carcinoma

- ☐ Infiltrative tubular/papillary/solid carcinoma overrunning the kidney
- ☐ Evidence of renal cell origin (usually PAX8 positive)
- ☐ Patient without sickle trait or hemoglobinopathy (otherwise, likely medullary carcinoma)
- ☐ Normal SMARCB1 (INI1) immunohistochemistry (otherwise, likely medullary carcinoma or RCC unclassified with medullary phenotype)
- ☐ Normal FH immunohistochemistry and/or negative genetic studies for *FH* (otherwise, consistent with FH-deficient RCC/HLRCC)
- ☐ No urothelial carcinoma component (usually negative results for urothelial markers p63/GATA3, but some overlap has been reported)
- ☐ Metastatic carcinoma from another organ argued against with clinical and immunohistochemical data

Metastases to the Kidney

Although the vast majority of renal neoplasms are primary renal cell or urothelial neoplasms, occasionally other cancers do metastasize to the kidney. Interestingly, these can be deceptive and mimic a primary renal mass by being solitary and unilateral, occurring many years after the primary cancer diagnosis, or growing into the renal pelvis, mimicking an in situ component, or involving renal veins, mimicking the behavior of RCC.[286-288] The most common origin of cancer metastatic to kidney is the lung (Figures 3.317 and 3.318), but other origins include colorectal, head and neck, female genital tract, breast, soft tissue, and thyroid.

PEARLS AND PIFTALLS: Metastases to the Kidney

- Often solitary/unilateral
- May be a long interval from primary cancer to metastasis (>10 years)
- May involve renal pelvis or veins, mimicking primary tumors
- Most common primary source: lung
- Organ-specific immunohistochemical markers and awareness of cancer history are most helpful

---

SPINDLE CELL TUMORS

Angiomyolipoma

Angiomyolipoma is a benign neoplasm and the most common mesenchymal tumor of the kidney.[289] Since most tumors that contain substantial fat can be recognized as such radiographically, those presenting to the surgical pathologist are usually spindle cell predominant, composed of myoid cells with a paucity of fat (Figure 3.319). However, the classic histology includes a mixture of myoid smooth muscle–like cells, lipid-laden cells, and abnormal blood vessels with thick walls (Figures 3.320-3.325). The constituent cells are referred to as perivascular epithelioid cells (PEC), an unusual tumor cell type that is not thought to have a normal counterpart.[130,235,236] PECs have a unique immunohistochemical phenotype with dual positivity for smooth muscle and melanocytic markers, such as smooth muscle actin, desmin, melan-A, and HMB45. For the pathologist evaluating renal specimens, especially biopsies, it is important to note that the labeling for melanocytic markers can be very focal (Figure 3.326). Staining for cathepsin K is usually more diffuse (Figure 3.327).[132] In most cases, diagnosis is straightforward upon seeing the H&E morphology alone; however, in biopsy specimens, evaluation may be more challenging. Multiple angiomyolipomas of the

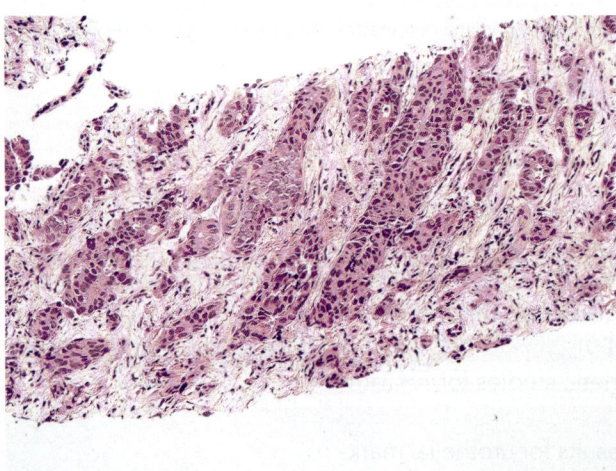

Figure 3.317. Lung cancer is the most common cancer to metastasize to the kidney. This patient had a known lung cancer and underwent renal mass biopsy, showing metastatic carcinoma involving the kidney.

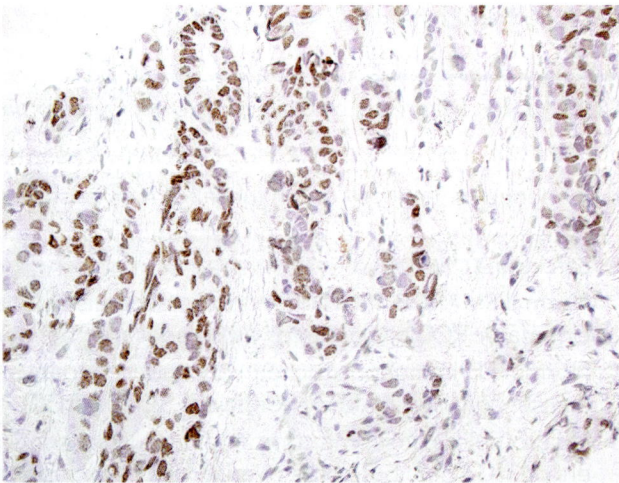

Figure 3.318. TTF1 immunohistochemical staining is positive, supporting lung origin, in the same case from Figure 3.317.

kidney can be encountered with tuberous sclerosis complex, although it is not clear that a certain number of angiomyolipoma lesions should suggest the diagnosis of tuberous sclerosis.[290] Focal epithelioid features are not unusual. However, since epithelioid angiomyolipoma is considered to have possible malignant potential, we would not recommend the terminology of epithelioid angiomyolipoma unless this is extensive, to the point that RCC is closely mimicked (see sections on epithelioid angiomyolipoma under clear cell and tubular/solid patterns). There is no current evidence that focal epithelioid features alter the benign nature of angiomyolipoma.

PEARLS AND PITFALLS: Angiomyolipoma

- Angiomyolipomas of the renal capsule are sometimes referred to as "capsuloma," although this term is nonspecific
- Tumors are often spindle cell predominant in surgical pathology practice, since fat-rich tumors can be recognized by radiology and not confused for RCC
- If melanocytic markers appear negative in suspected angiomyolipoma at low magnification, check at high magnification for rare positive cells
- Cathepsin K, if available, is usually more diffuse in angiomyolipoma
- Smooth muscle markers (smooth muscle actin, desmin) are also positive to a variable extent
- Focal epithelioid features do not appear to alter the benign behavior of angiomyolipoma

---

Sarcomatoid Renal Cell Carcinoma

Sarcomatoid RCC can evolve from any subtype of RCC. Therefore, it is not a specific variant per se, but a final common pathway of dedifferentiation that connotes increased aggressiveness. The optimal clinical treatment for sarcomatoid RCC in the metastatic setting is not entirely clear. Some studies have suggested the possibility of specific regimens that differ from conventional RCC.[16] Therefore, pathologists should make every effort to use this classification as accurately as possible. Our approach in general is to regard a tumor as sarcomatoid only if there are fields that would be readily mistaken for a sarcoma if viewed in isolation (Figures 3.328-3.331). However, a lesser degree of spindle cell change has been reported in clear cell RCC, the significance of which is less certain at present but currently thought not to be in the spectrum of sarcomatoid RCC (Figure 3.332).[291] For tumors that

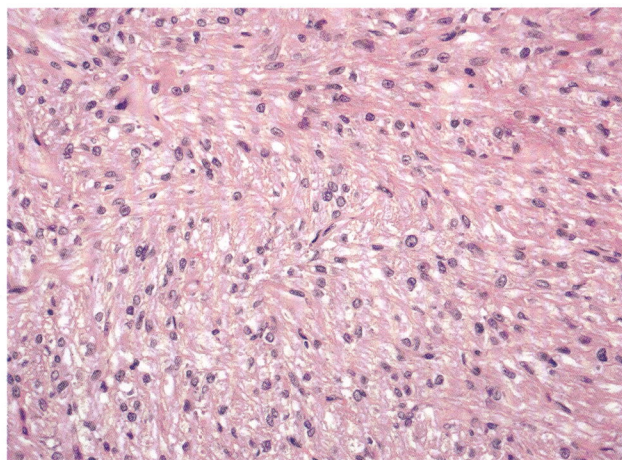

Figure 3.319. Often angiomyolipomas encountered in surgical pathology practice are myoid predominant, since those containing fat can be recognized by imaging. This example is composed of predominantly eosinophilic spindle-shaped cells.

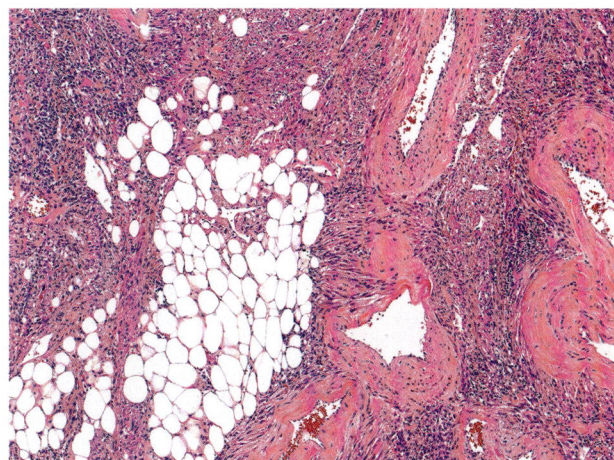

Figure 3.320. The classic angiomyolipoma contains spindle-shaped cells, lipid-laden cells resembling fat, and thick-walled blood vessels.

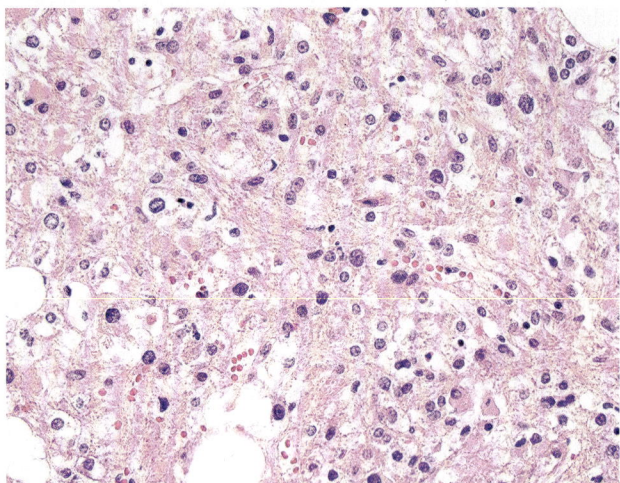

Figure 3.321. At high magnification, the eosinophilic spindle-shaped or epithelioid cells of angiomyolipoma may be mildly atypical; however, the diffuse growth pattern without discrete nests is helpful in discriminating from renal cell carcinoma.

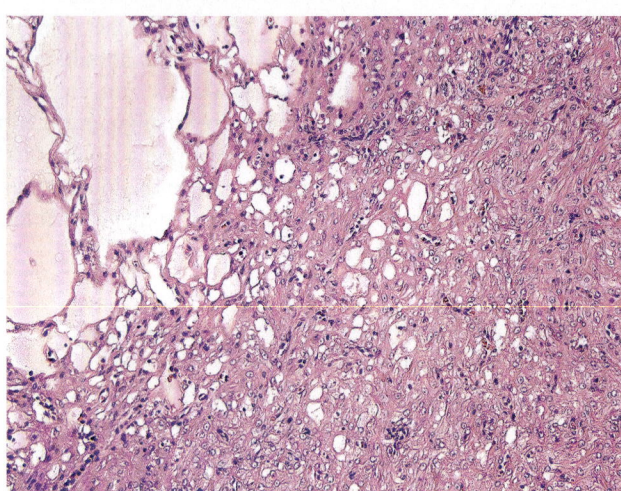

Figure 3.322. This renal angiomyolipoma demonstrates an unusual growth pattern with pseudocystic spaces and spindle-shaped epithelioid cells.

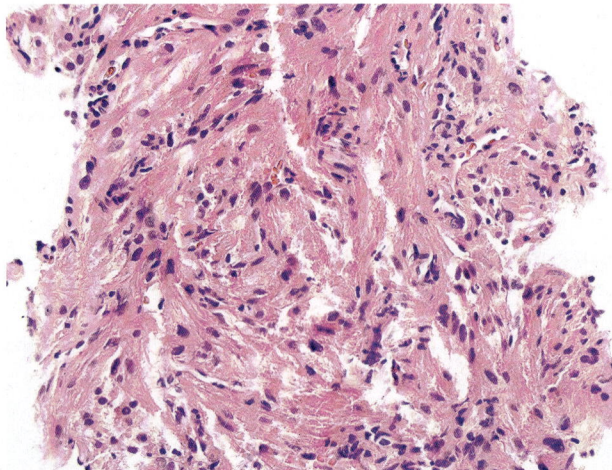

Figure 3.323. In renal mass biopsy, angiomyolipoma is a relevant diagnosis, being one of the few unequivocally benign renal tumors. This example shows predominantly spindle-shaped cells.

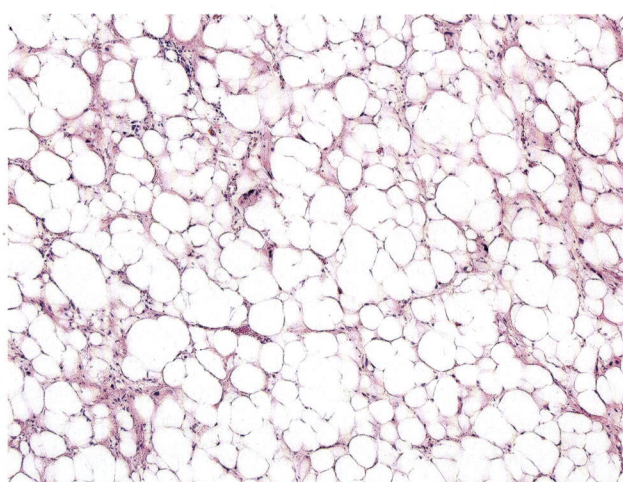

Figure 3.324. This large renal angiomyolipoma was composed of predominantly lipid cells, forming a huge intraabdominal mass that mimicked atypical lipomatous tumor/well-differentiated liposarcoma.

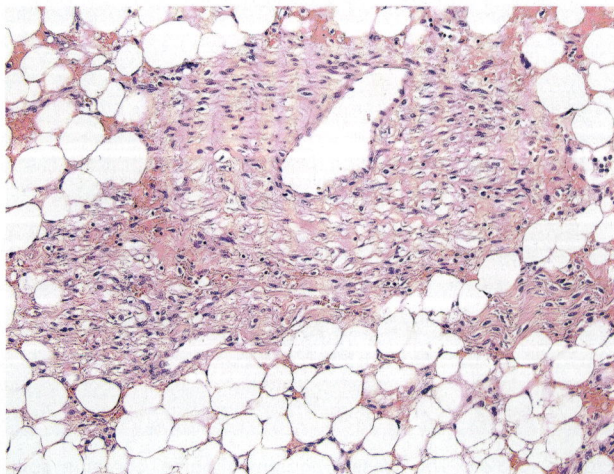

Figure 3.325. Focal blood vessels in the same tumor from Figure 3.324 are surrounded by epithelioid cells, a clue to the diagnosis of angiomyolipoma.

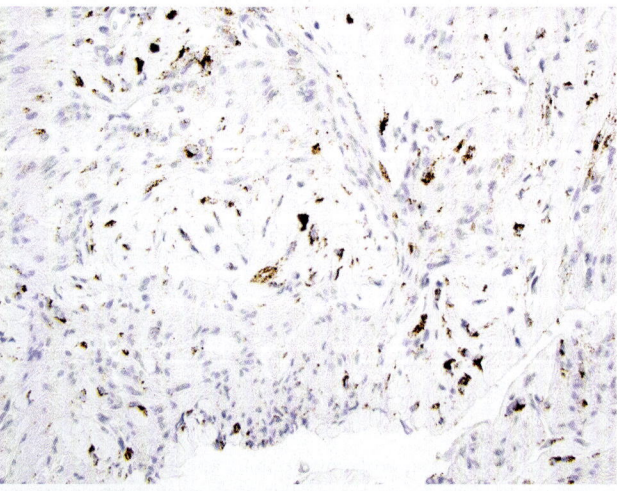

Figure 3.326. Labeling for melanocytic markers can be focal in renal angiomyolipoma. This field shows rare cells staining for HMB45, which is supportive of a diagnosis of angiomyolipoma.

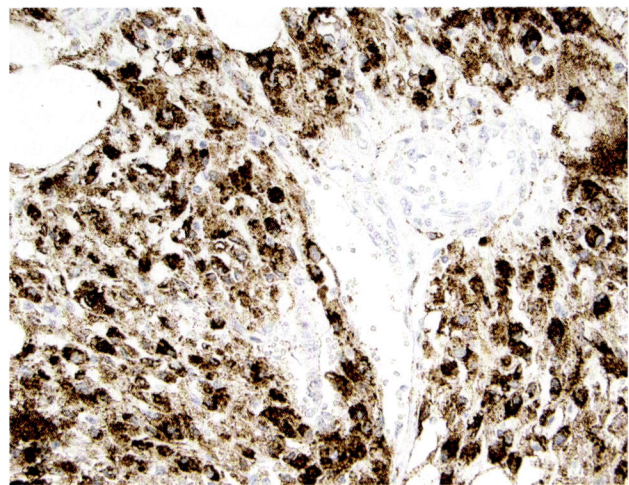

Figure 3.327. Staining for cathepsin K is usually more diffuse in angiomyolipoma.

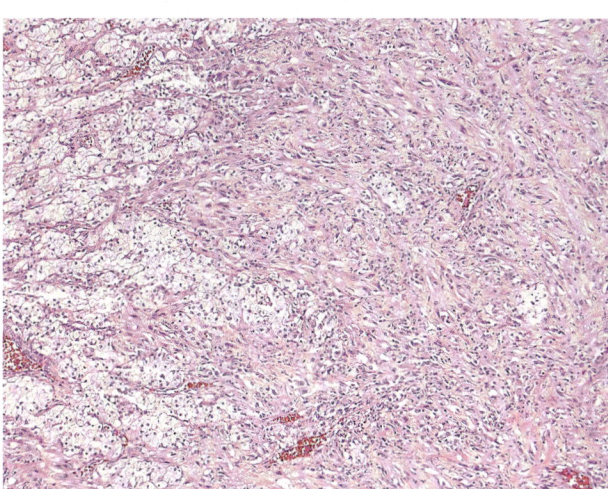

Figure 3.328. This sarcomatoid renal cell carcinoma (RCC) shows an abrupt transition from clear cell RCC (left) to malignant spindle cell proliferation (right).

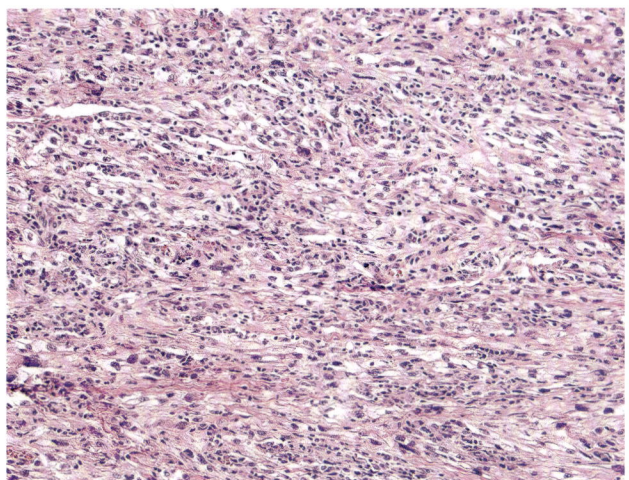

Figure 3.329. At high magnification, this sarcomatoid renal cell carcinoma shows a nonspecific spindle cell pattern that likely would be considered undifferentiated pleomorphic sarcoma.

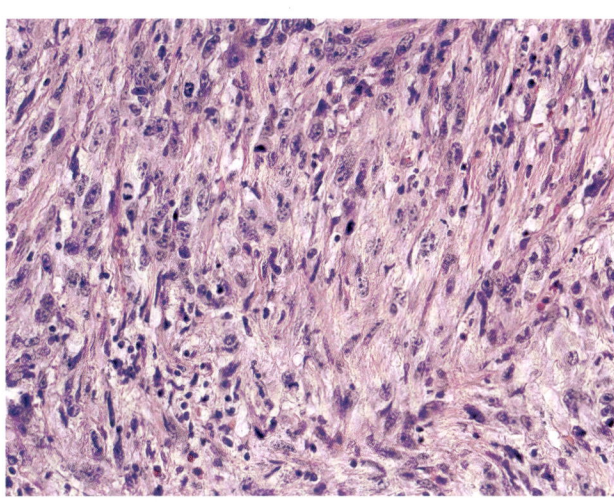

Figure 3.330. At high magnification, this sarcomatoid renal cell carcinoma is composed of pleomorphic cells without obvious epithelial differentiation.

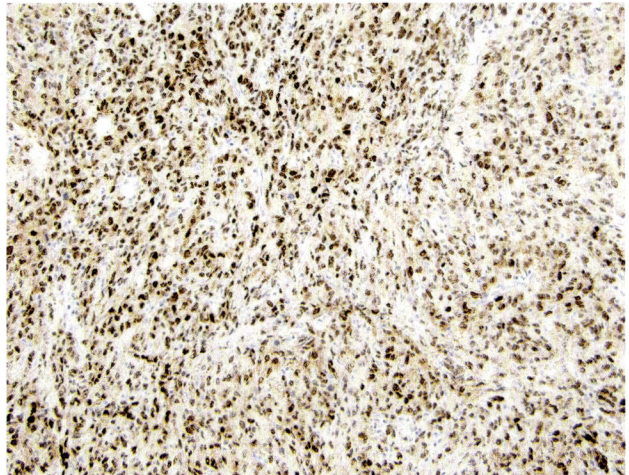

Figure 3.331. Immunohistochemistry shows PAX8 reactivity in sarcomatoid renal cell carcinoma, supporting epithelial origin.

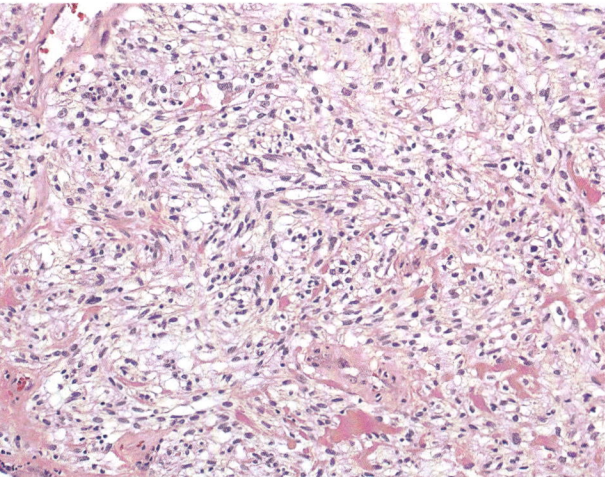

Figure 3.332. Spindle cell change has been reported in clear cell renal cell carcinoma. This example is still somewhat recognizable as epithelial, although the cells take on a spindle-shaped configuration rather than nests or tubules. It is currently debatable whether this represents a transition toward sarcomatoid change.

are purely sarcomatoid and the underlying subtype cannot be discerned, current recommendations are to regard as unclassified RCC. The histologic pattern of the sarcomatoid component usually is a nonspecific spindle cell pattern, resembling undifferentiated pleomorphic sarcoma[292]; however, other specific patterns have been reported, such as osteosarcoma-like, rhabdomyosarcoma-like, or liposarcoma-like.[293,294] Rarely, the spindle cell component may be relatively low grade (Figure 3.333).

Rhabdoid changes in RCC (Figures 3.334 and 3.335) have been increasingly recognized as indicating aggressive behavior.[295] This is referred to as rhabdoid rather than rhabdomyoblastic, since despite morphologic resemblance of the tumor cells to rhabdomyoblastic cells, they do not show evidence of skeletal muscle differentiation via immunohistochemistry. In current schemes, rhabdoid RCC is considered inherently grade 4.[62,63] However, there is some debate whether the prognosis is equally as poor as for spindle cell sarcomatoid RCC.[296-298] Therefore, it is reasonable to differentiate the two at present but to consider both inherently grade 4. This morphology is characterized by tumor cells having a globule of eosinophilic material in the cytoplasm that mimics the strap cells of rhabdomyosarcoma. Rhabdoid features are most commonly associated with clear cell RCC, but this has been reported in most RCC subtypes.[297]

Mucinous Tubular and Spindle Cell Carcinoma

Mucinous tubular and spindle cell carcinoma is discussed more extensively in the next section (tumors with spindle cell and epithelioid components); however, it has been rarely noted that these tumors can have a predominance of spindle-shaped cells, mimicking a mesenchymal neoplasm (Figures 3.336 and 3.337).[299] In this context, recognition that the spindle cell component is cytologically bland and uniform may be helpful in discriminating from sarcomatoid RCC. Immunohistochemical positivity for epithelial markers (cytokeratin, PAX8) may be helpful in distinguishing from a true mesenchymal neoplasm, and subtle morphologic clues to the diagnosis may be present, such as foamy macrophages, focal tubular formation, or mucin deposition. In general, mucinous tubular and spindle cell carcinoma has a similar immunohistochemical phenotype to papillary RCC (cytokeratin 7, AMACR).

Leiomyosarcoma

Although primary renal sarcomas are rare compared to carcinomas, leiomyosarcoma is among the most common to arise from the kidney or nearby structures, such as the renal vein or inferior vena cava. In fact, it is more likely for leiomyosarcoma to be extrarenal rather than parenchymal (such as arising from veins or the renal pelvis).[300] Like other sites in deep soft tissue, the threshold for diagnosis of leiomyosarcoma should be relatively low, such that even a mild degree of nuclear atypia, necrosis, or focal mitotic activity would favor leiomyosarcoma (Figures 3.338-3.340) over leiomyoma in renal/perirenal locations. For well-differentiated tumors, the features may closely mimic leiomyoma, with only slightly increased atypia or mitotic activity, whereas for high-grade tumors, immunohistochemistry may be necessary to confirm smooth muscle differentiation (ideally more than one smooth muscle marker positive, such as smooth muscle actin, desmin, or caldesmon, Figure 3.341).[300] For high-grade tumors, search for a RCC component may be helpful to exclude sarcomatoid RCC. Angiomyolipoma must also be considered in the differential diagnosis, which is relatively common. Angiomyolipomas typically have areas of pale to fibrillary cytoplasm, contrasting to the densely eosinophilic cytoplasm of true smooth muscle tumors. Likewise, the reactivity for melanocytic immunohistochemical markers will help to confirm a diagnosis of angiomyolipoma. As noted previously, positivity for melanocytic markers in angiomyolipoma can be very focal. Cathepsin K typically shows diffuse strong staining of angiomyolipoma.[132]

Leiomyoma

Until recently, it might have been reasonable to question the existence of renal leiomyoma, favoring that most of the historically reported examples likely represent angiomyolipoma with a myoid-predominant cell population. However, recent series have described well-characterized cohorts of renal leiomyomas, which appear to occur overwhelmingly in women and often arise from the renal capsule (Figures 3.342-3.344).[301,302] In keeping with

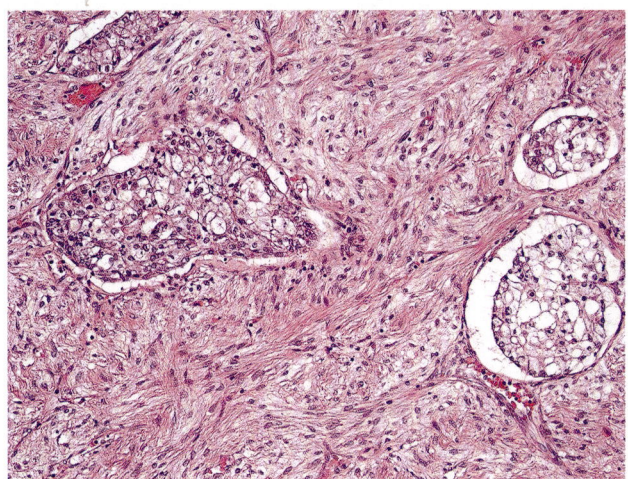

Figure 3.333. Rare sarcomatoid renal cell carcinomas (RCCs) have a deceptively low-grade sarcomatoid component. This example shows islands of clear cell RCC admixed with a bland spindle cell component that might be interpreted as myofibroblastic reaction. However, this patient later had a metastatic tumor composed of similar spindle cell proliferation with focal reactivity for epithelial markers.

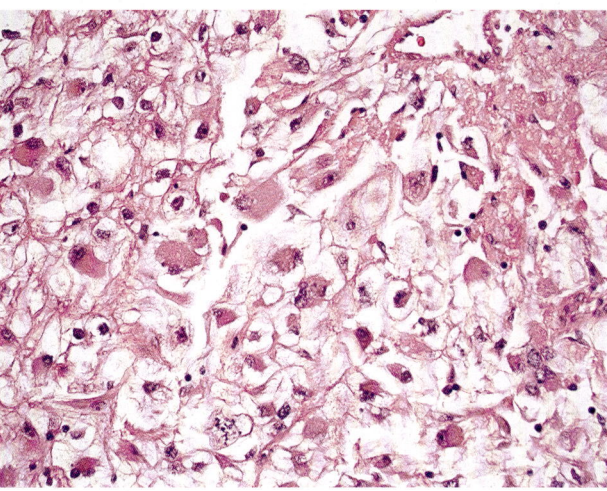

Figure 3.334. Rhabdoid features in renal cell carcinoma are characterized by cytoplasmic globules of eosinophilic material, mimicking rhabdomyoblastic "strap" cells.

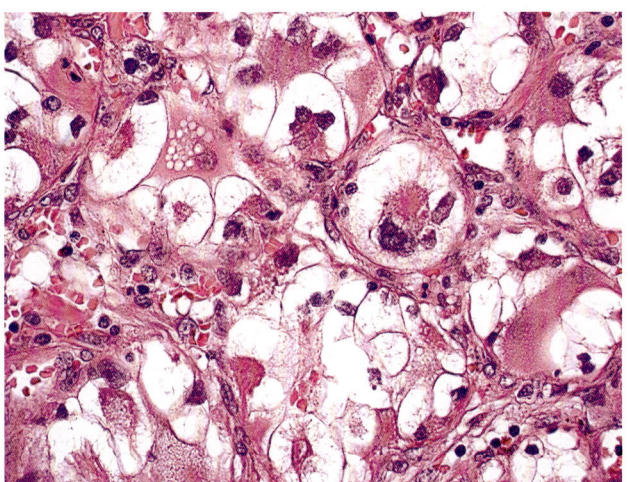

Figure 3.335. At high magnification, the tumor cells with clear cytoplasm contain globules of eosinophilic material in rhabdoid renal cell carcinoma.

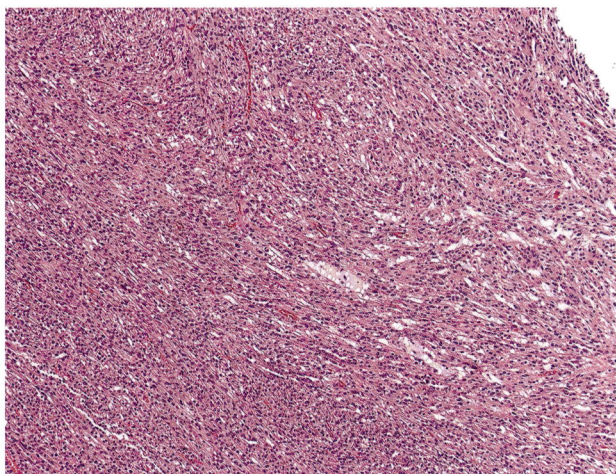

Figure 3.336. This mucinous tubular and spindle cell carcinoma is composed of predominantly spindle-shaped cells, which could lead to confusion with a mesenchymal tumor.

the marked predilection for women, these typically show immunohistochemical positivity for estrogen and progesterone receptors,[301] suggesting they are gynecologic-type leiomyomas arising at a site other than the uterus. Our approach would be to largely reserve this diagnosis for these characteristic scenarios (women, renal capsular location, estrogen or progesterone receptor positivity, and relatively small size). In contrast, larger tumors or those occurring in men with any atypical features (mitotic activity, necrosis, atypia) would be more concerning for leiomyosarcoma.

Renomedullary Interstitial Cell Tumor

Renomedullary interstitial cell tumor (formerly medullary fibroma) is a benign neoplasm that is usually an incidental finding when the kidney is resected for another reason or examined at autopsy (Figure 3.345).[303] These lesions are not thought to have any distinct clinical significance (although once thought to be possibly related to hypertension). However, rare tumors are large enough that they present as a clinical mass and are the indication for surgery of their own (Figure 3.346).[304] Most are 5 mm or less, composed of a variably

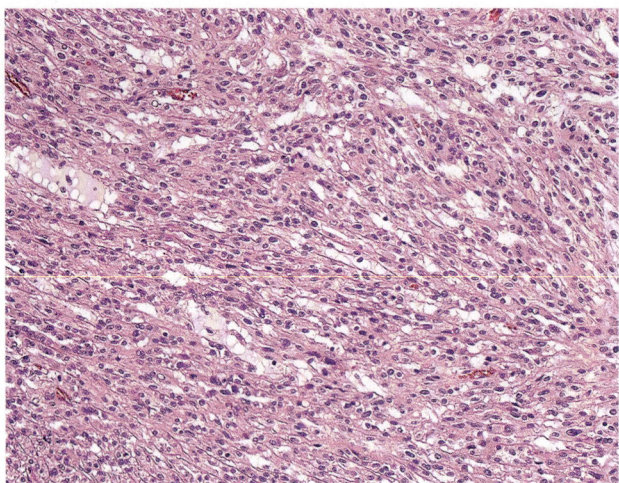

Figure 3.337. At higher magnification of the same tumor from Figure 3.336, focal glandular differentiation is evident, favoring mucinous tubular and spindle cell carcinoma.

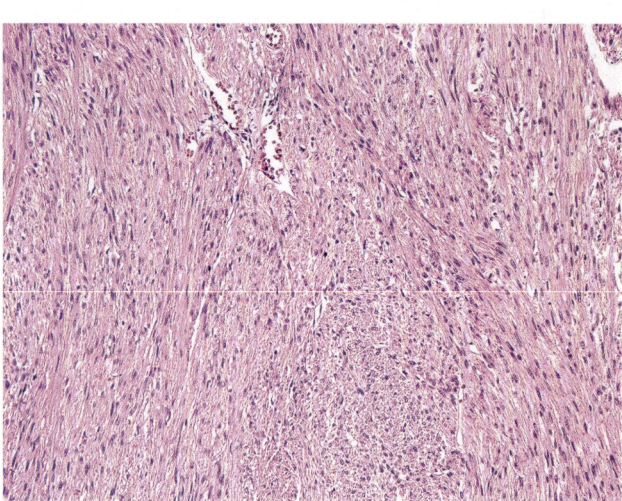

Figure 3.338. Leiomyosarcoma can occur in the kidney and at perirenal locations. This example shows fascicular architecture composed of eosinophilic smooth muscle cells.

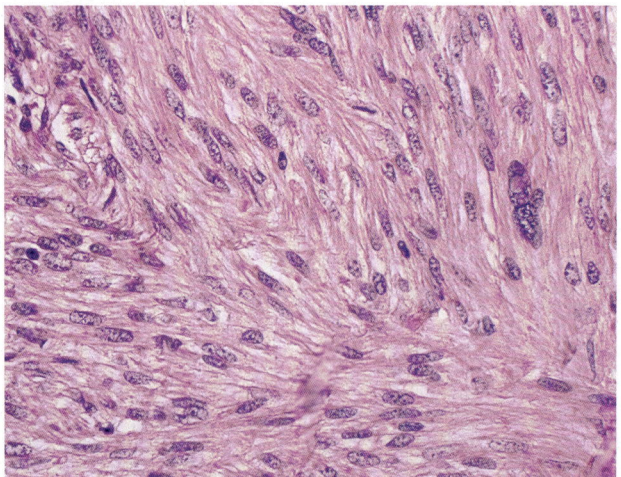

Figure 3.339. At higher magnification, even focal nuclear atypia would favor leiomyosarcoma over leiomyoma, once angiomyolipoma is excluded.

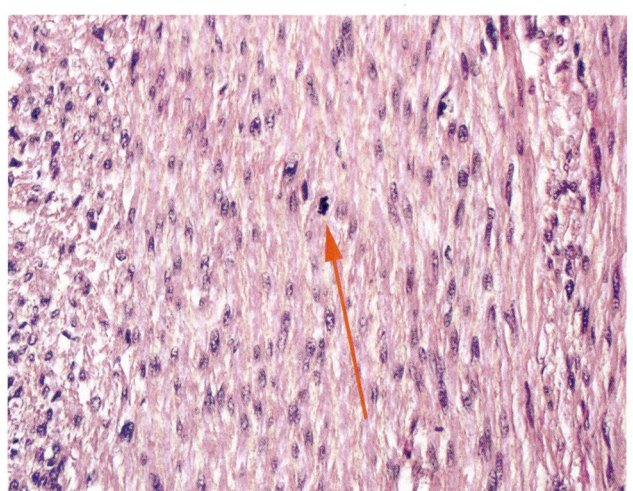

Figure 3.340. Mitotic activity of almost any extent (arrow) would favor renal leiomyosarcoma over leiomyoma.

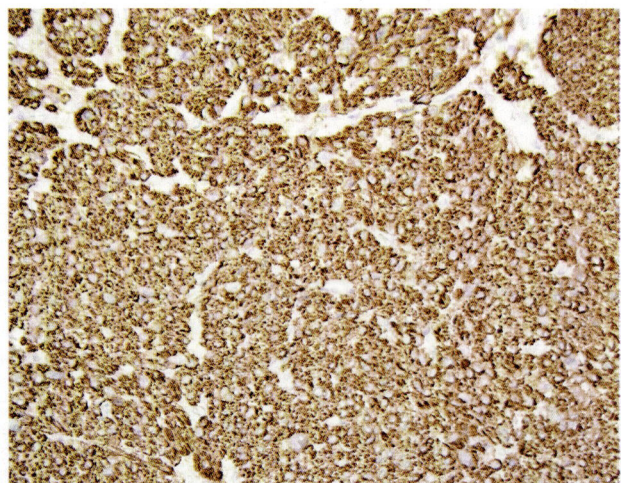

Figure 3.341. If smooth muscle differentiation is in doubt, preferably two smooth muscle markers with positive immunohistochemistry would be supportive of a diagnosis of renal leiomyosarcoma, assuming that angiomyolipoma is excluded. This example shows substantial positive caldesmon staining.

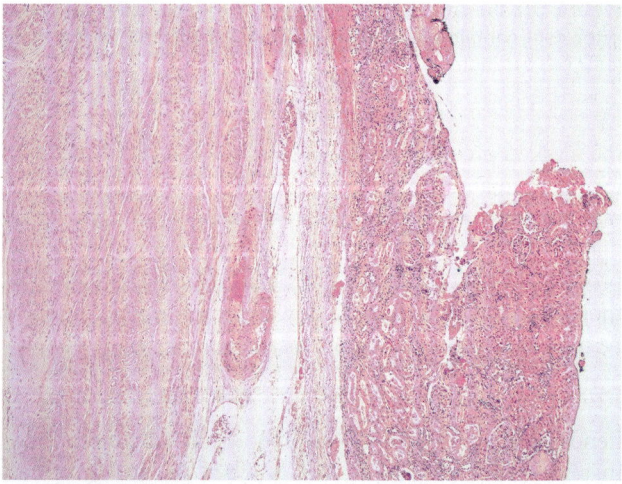

Figure 3.342. This renal leiomyoma appears to arise from the renal capsule, with a small amount of renal parenchyma at right removed via partial nephrectomy.

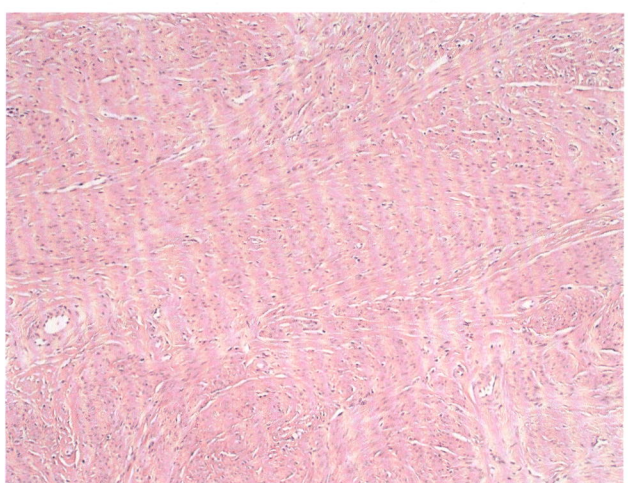

Figure 3.343. Higher magnification of the renal leiomyoma from Figure 3.342 shows fascicles of eosinophilic spindle-shaped cells, without the fat or thick-walled blood vessels of angiomyolipoma. Even focal labeling for melanocytic markers would favor angiomyolipoma over leiomyoma.

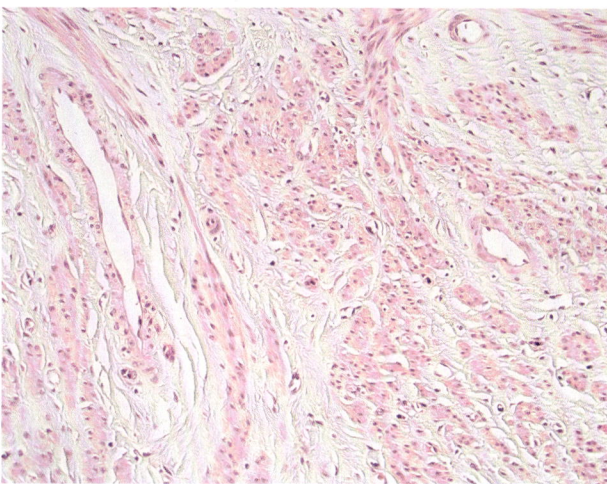

Figure 3.344. This renal leiomyoma has areas of loose fibrous stroma between the smooth muscle bundles, reminiscent of gynecologic-type leiomyomas, such as those of the uterus.

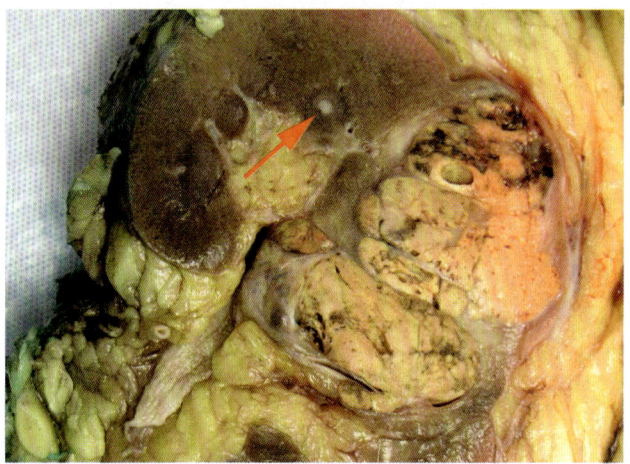

Figure 3.345. In this resection for clear cell renal cell carcinoma (right), a small renomedullary interstitial cell tumor is present in the medulla adjacent to the mass (arrow).

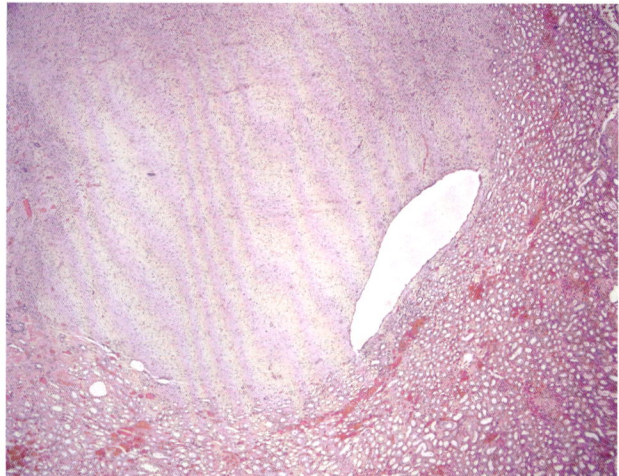

Figure 3.346. Rarely, renomedullary interstitial cell tumors are large enough that they come to clinical attention. This example raised a differential diagnosis of renomedullary interstitial cell tumor versus mixed epithelial and stromal tumor due to the large size and entrapped cystic tubules.

cellular proliferation of bland spindle-shaped cells with entrapment of medullary tubules (Figures 3.347-3.349). In most cases, no special evaluation or immunohistochemistry is necessary to arrive at the diagnosis, in view of the classic medullary location, small size, and morphology. However, for the rare cases that present as a larger, clinically evident mass, the immunohistochemical profile appears largely negative, with minor labeling for smooth muscle actin or calponin that is less than that of myofibroblastic or smooth muscle tumors. Estrogen receptor can be positive, raising consideration of mixed epithelial and stromal tumor; however, this is typically weak in renomedullary interstitial cell tumor. CD34 is usually negative, contrasting to solitary fibrous tumor.[305] Although it was previously thought that some of these may contain amyloid, more recent studies have found the pale eosinophilic material to be negative for Congo red, favoring it to be collagen.[303,305]

KEY FEATURES: Renomedullary Interstitial Cell Tumor

- Vast majority very small (<5 mm) and incidental finding
- Bland spindle-shaped cells

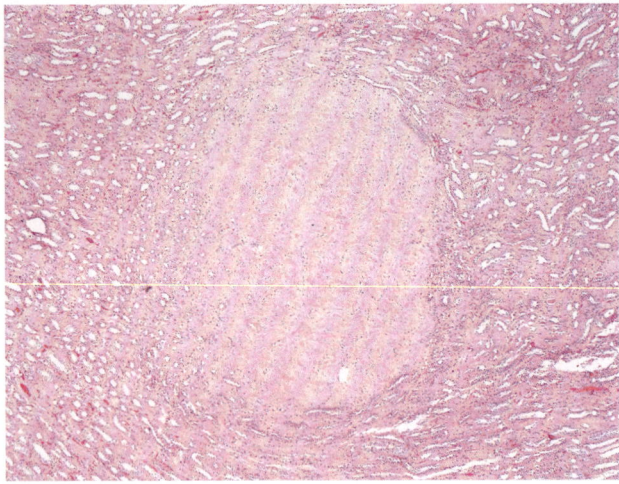

Figure 3.347. Most renomedullary interstitial cell tumors are less than 5 mm and incidental nodules. This example interrupts the monotonous pattern of the medullary tubules with a nodule of fibrous tissue.

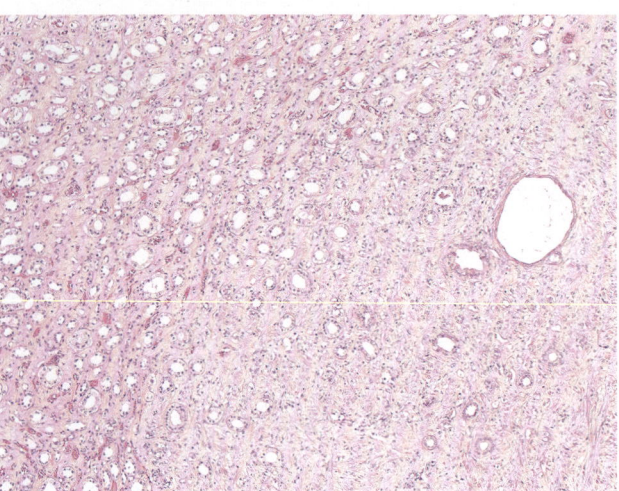

Figure 3.348. This renomedullary interstitial cell tumor is slightly more cellular, with a few entrapped renal tubules.

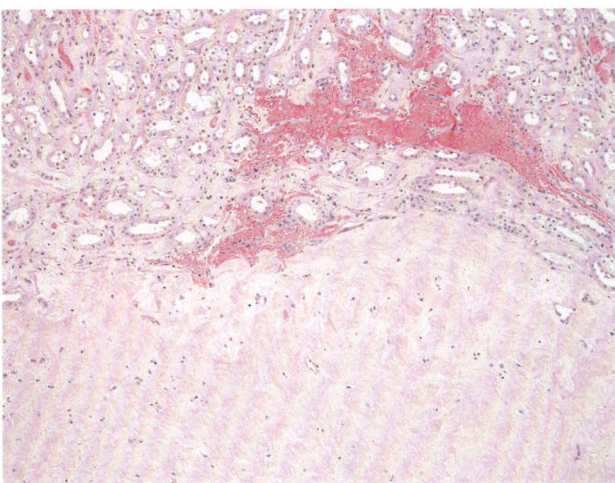

Figure 3.349. This renomedullary interstitial cell tumor is very paucicellular, mostly collagenous.

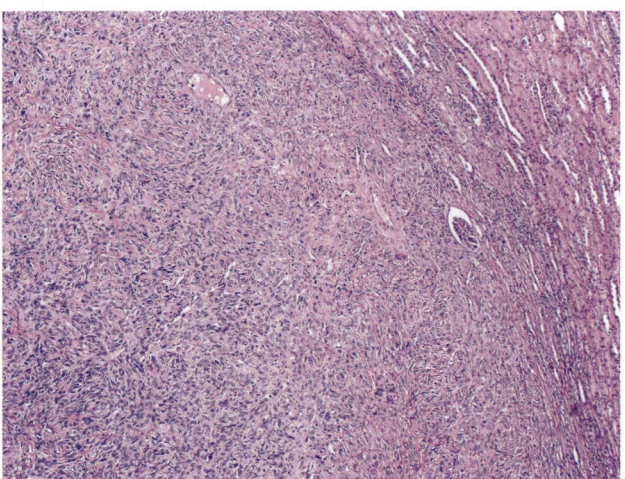

Figure 3.350. This renal solitary fibrous tumor demonstrates spindle cell proliferation partially replacing the kidney.

- Entrapped medullary tubules, sometimes cystic
- Sometimes eosinophilic collagen (negative for Congo red)
- Rare tumors larger presenting as clinical mass
- Immunohistochemistry: nonspecific
  - Relatively weak smooth muscle actin and calponin
  - Weak estrogen/progesterone receptor
  - Negative or minimal CD34

Solitary Fibrous Tumor

Solitary fibrous tumor can occur in the genitourinary tract, including the kidney. Its features are usually similar to those of other sites, including a spindle cell pattern varying from cellular to hypocellular, with intercellular collagen and a branching "staghorn" or "hemangiopericytoma-like" vasculature (Figures 3.350-3.352).[306,307] Similar to other sites, solitary fibrous tumor is thought to have malignant potential depending on some of its histologic and clinical features, such as mitotic activity and tumor size. A risk stratification system has recently been proposed, which considers the patient age, tumor size, mitotic activity, and

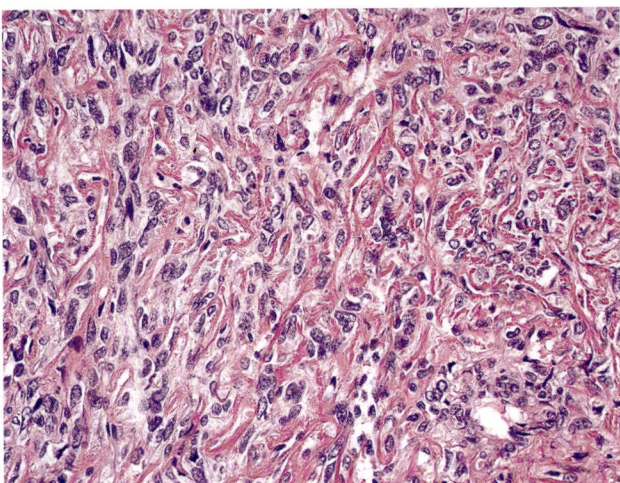

Figure 3.351. Solitary fibrous tumor can include areas of higher cellularity with prominent intercellular collagen.

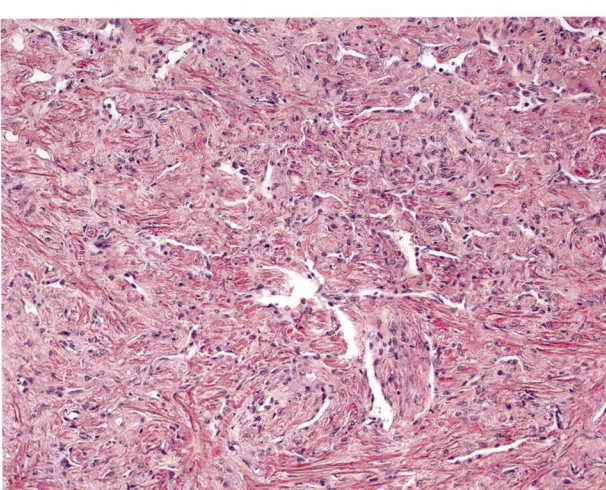

Figure 3.352. Solitary fibrous tumor can also include areas of lower cellularity, predominantly collagenous, with the branching vascular pattern.

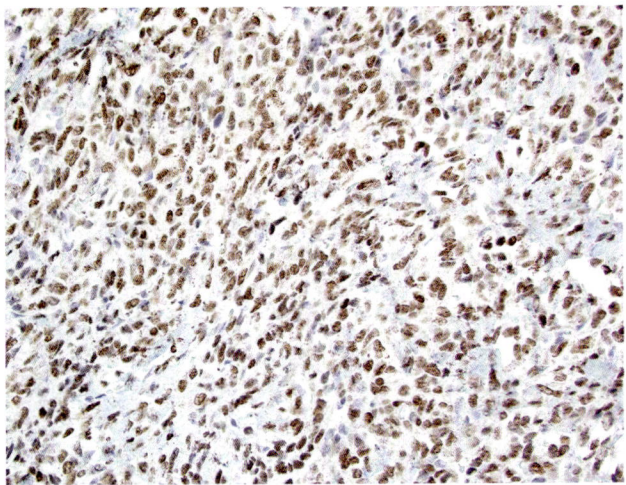

Figure 3.353. Immunohistochemistry for STAT6 is a helpful marker to confirm the diagnosis of solitary fibrous tumor.

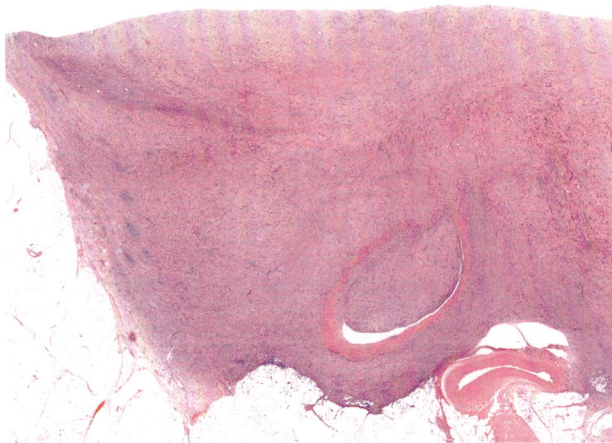

Figure 3.354. Rarely inflammatory myofibroblastic tumor may present as a renal mass. This example effaced much of the kidney and extends into the renal sinus at bottom. A vein is involved by tumor.

tumor necrosis to yield a risk class (Table 3.8).[308] As in other sites, CD34 positivity is common in solitary fibrous tumor, and immunohistochemical positivity for STAT6 (Figure 3.353) is a robust tool to confirm the diagnosis that correlates with the presence of the *NAB2-STAT6* fusion. Rarely solitary fibrous tumor of the kidney can be fat-forming, which may lead to difficulty distinguishing from liposarcoma or angiomyolipoma.[309] Of note, one study found occasional positivity for PAX8 in solitary fibrous tumors, which may lead to diagnostic difficulty if sarcomatoid RCC is a consideration.[310] Of note, this was using a polyclonal antibody, which may be less specific than monoclonal antibodies.

Inflammatory Myofibroblastic Tumor

Inflammatory myofibroblastic tumor occurs much more commonly in other sites but has been rarely described as a renal mass (Figures 3.354 and 3.355).[311] In general in soft tissue sites, inflammatory myofibroblastic tumor is considered a neoplasm of intermediate malignant potential with rare metastasis; however, relatively little is known for renal cases specifically. Inflammatory myofibroblastic tumors are composed of fusiform cells with long cytoplasmic processes. In keeping with the myofibroblastic phenotype, there are invariably positive for smooth muscle actin (often with a "tram-track" double linear staining pattern), and they may show positivity for desmin or cytokeratin.[312] Classically, inflammatory

TABLE 3.8: Risk Stratification for Solitary Fibrous Tumor

Age	Points
<55	0
≥55	1
Tumor size	
<5 cm	0
5-<10 cm	1
10-<15 cm	2
≥15 cm	3
Mitotic activity per 10 high-power fields	
0	0
1-3	1
≥4	2
Necrosis	
<10%	0
≥10	1
Overall risk score (sum of points)	
Low	0-3
Intermediate	4-5
High	6-7

From Demicco EG, Park MS, Araujo DM, et al. Solitary fibrous tumor: a clinicopathological study of 110 cases and proposed risk assessment model. *Mod Pathol.* 2012;25(9):1298-1306.

myofibroblastic tumors have rearrangement of *ALK*, which can be supported by positive ALK immunohistochemistry; however, many genitourinary tract examples of putative inflammatory myofibroblastic tumor have been found to be negative for ALK,[311,313] suggesting that they may be more accurately classified as pseudosarcomatous myofibroblastic proliferations rather than classic inflammatory myofibroblastic tumors.[314]

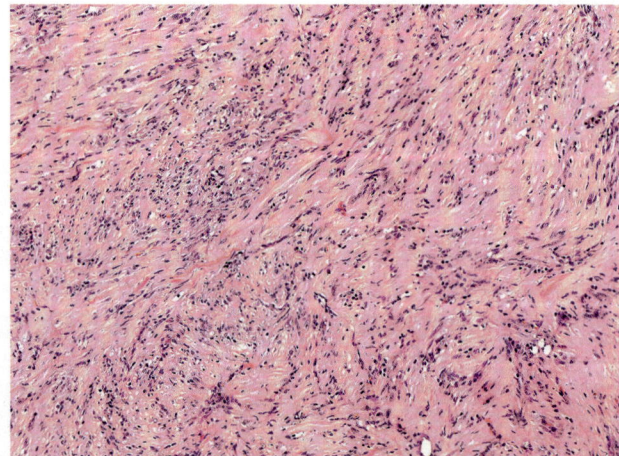

Figure 3.355. At high magnification, inflammatory myofibroblastic tumor is composed of spindle-shaped cells with a myofibroblastic phenotype and admixed inflammation. This tumor was positive for ALK immunohistochemistry, supporting the diagnosis.

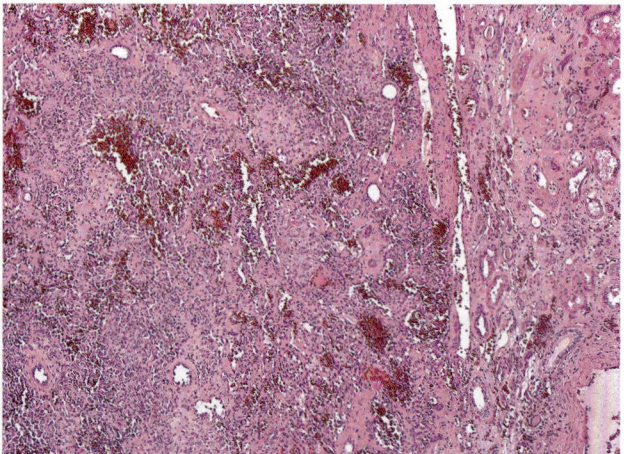

Figure 3.356. Hemangiomas have been increased recognized as renal masses, particularly with end-stage renal disease. A hemangioma with blood-filled spaces merges with the renal parenchyma (right).

Hemangioma

Hemangiomas have been increasingly recognized in the kidney, especially a novel variant termed anastomosing hemangioma (Figures 3.356-3.360).[315-320]

PEARLS AND PITFALLS: Anastomosing Hemangioma

- Predilection for genitourinary sites (kidney, ovary), paraspinal soft tissue, less frequently other sites
- Interconnecting vascular spaces may suggest abnormal architecture, i.e., angiosarcoma; however, no significant atypia or multilayering of the endothelial cells
- Often contains extramedullary hematopoiesis
- May be enriched in end-stage renal disease kidneys
- Often contains hyaline globules (Figure 3.359)
- Strongly consider using immunohistochemistry (Figure 3.360) to argue against RCC with sclerotic/regressive changes, which may have prominent vasculature and inconspicuous tumor cells[321,322]

Other Mesenchymal Tumors

A wide variety of other mesenchymal tumors have been reported in the kidney, including angiosarcoma, rhabdomyosarcoma, osteosarcoma, synovial sarcoma, Ewing sarcoma, lymphangioma, and schwannoma.[238] In general, these tumors are similar to their counterparts of other anatomic sites. Synovial sarcoma is discussed in the next section (tumors with spindle cell and epithelial components), as these often appear biphasic with entrapped tubular structures forming a cystic component.

TUMORS WITH SPINDLE CELL AND EPITHELIAL COMPONENTS

Mucinous Tubular and Spindle Cell Carcinoma

Mucinous tubular and spindle cell carcinoma is an unusual variant of RCC that contains a tubular component (usually resembling papillary RCC), a spindle cell component (formed by compressed, flatted tubules lacking the atypia of sarcomatoid change), and mucinous material (Figures 3.361-3.367).[299,323-331] Due to the similarity with papillary RCC, including typically strong AMACR staining, it has been hypothesized that it may be a variant of papillary

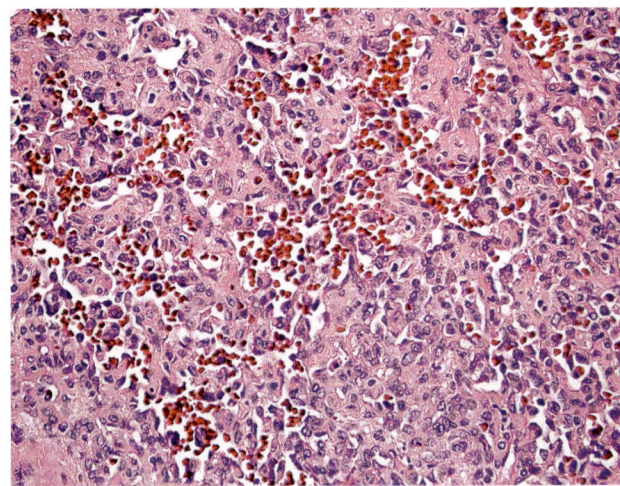

Figure 3.357. At higher magnification, there are multiple interconnecting vascular spaces in anastomosing hemangioma, which has led to potential confusion with angiosarcoma. However, the endothelial cells lack atypia and multilayering.

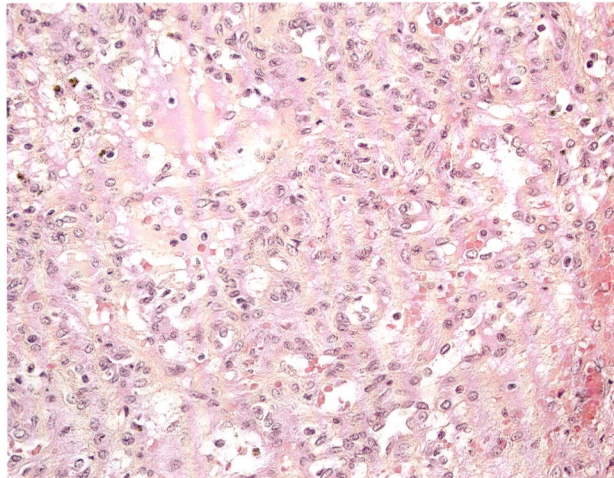

Figure 3.358. In this section of anastomosing hemangioma, there are bland endothelial cells lining vascular spaces.

RCC.[329] However, more recently it has been shown to have a unique genetic copy number pattern with multiple chromosomal losses involving chromosomes 1, 4, 6, 8, 9, 13, 14, 15, and 22,[323,327,328,332] and molecular alterations of genes in the Hippo pathway, supporting it as a distinct entity.[326,333] Unusual and potentially deceptive patterns of mucinous tubular and spindle cell carcinoma have been described, particularly mucin-poor and spindle cell predominant patterns (Figures 3.363 and 3.364, see also spindle cell tumors section).[299] Most cases have shown nonaggressive behavior; however, metastases and sarcomatoid transformation have been reported rarely.[69] Like most of the other uncommon subtypes of RCC discussed in this chapter, there are not necessarily specific treatment recommendations for this subtype, although RCC-directed therapies have been tested in the rare metastatic cases.

PEARLS AND PITFALLS: Mucinous Tubular and Spindle Cell Carcinoma

- Tubular component resembling papillary RCC, typically with strong AMACR staining
- Often cytokeratin 7 positive (Figure 3.368)
- Spindle cell component likely represents compressed, elongated tubular structures
- Lightly basophilic mucin
- Genetics: losses of multiple chromosomes, 1, 4, 6, 8, 9, 13, 14, 15, and 22
- Differential diagnosis: distinguishing from sarcomatoid RCC
  - Spindle cell component usually relatively monomorphic (lacks pleomorphism of sarcomatoid RCC)
  - Recognition of tubular and mucinous components can help avoid this pitfall

---

Angiomyolipoma With Epithelial Cysts

Angiomyolipoma and other PEComa tumors are discussed in other sections regarding spindle cell and epithelioid patterns; however, an unusual occurrence in the kidney is the formation of epithelial cysts within angiomyolipoma, termed angiomyolipoma with epithelial cysts or AMLEC (Figures 3.369-3.371).[334-336] This can form a biphasic-appearing neoplasm that mimics mixed epithelial and stromal tumor or other biphasic renal tumors. It has been noted in these tumors that the cellular spindle cell component is often denser under the epithelial lining of the cysts, resembling the cambium layer of rhabdomyosarcoma in the urinary bladder. Further compounding the similarity to mixed epithelial and stromal tumor, estrogen receptor, progesterone receptor, and CD10 are often positive in these areas as well.[334] Like other forms of angiomyolipoma, however, positive reactivity for melanocytic markers or cathepsin K can aid in recognition of this lesion. Another differential diagnosis that may be considered for this tumor pattern is synovial sarcoma, which is also covered in this section. Synovial sarcoma will have a greater degree of cytologic atypia and mitotic activity and lacks the labeling for melanocytic markers.

Mixed Epithelial and Stromal Tumor and Cystic Nephroma

There has been considerable debate as to whether mixed epithelial and stromal tumor and (adult) cystic nephroma are a spectrum of the same entity or two unrelated neoplasms.[337-339] For now, the WHO Classification regards these as a family of neoplasms.[340] Similarities between these two neoplasms include overwhelming predominance in perimenopausal women, positivity of the stromal cells for estrogen/progesterone receptors, and a resemblance of the spindle cell component to ovarian-type stroma. Importantly, cystic nephroma of children is now well accepted as an entirely unrelated neoplasm, characterized by *DICER1* gene mutations and predominantly occurring under age 2.[341] Although the estrogen and progesterone receptor positivity is a shared common feature of mixed epithelial and stromal tumor and cystic nephroma, it has been noted that this is not entirely specific, with positivity also occurring in angiomyolipoma, renomedullary interstitial cell tumor, and even in nontumor reactive areas of renal stroma.[305,334,342]

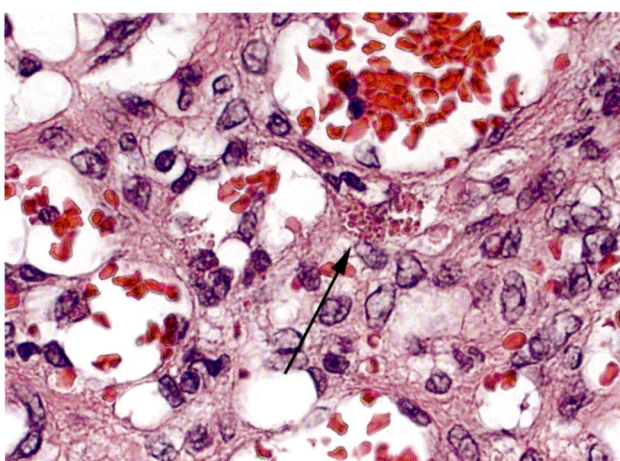

Figure 3.359. Anastomosing hemangiomas often contain hyaline globules (arrow).

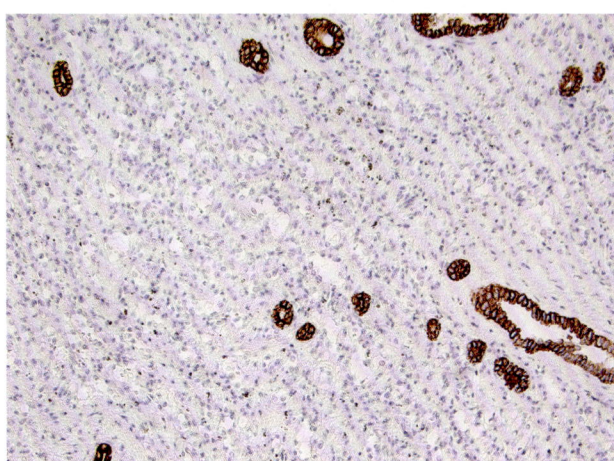

Figure 3.360. Before diagnosing a renal hemangioma, it is usually prudent to exclude renal cell carcinoma with regressive changes, such as by cytokeratin immunohistochemistry, as shown here, or with PAX8 or carbonic anhydrase IX staining.

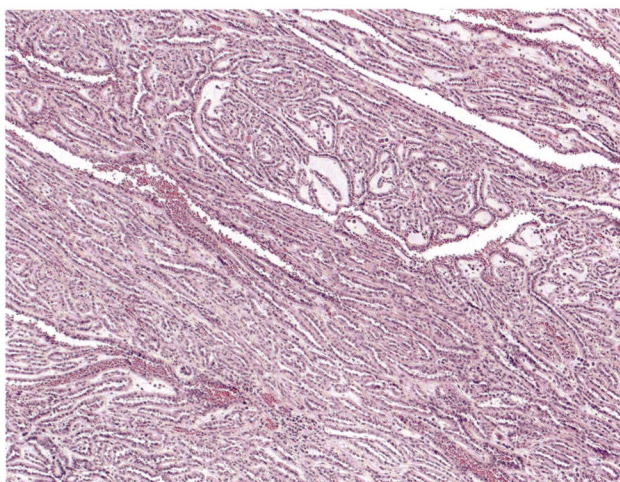

Figure 3.361. Mucinous tubular and spindle cell carcinoma is composed of tubular structures often forming compressed, elongated structures, with mucinous material.

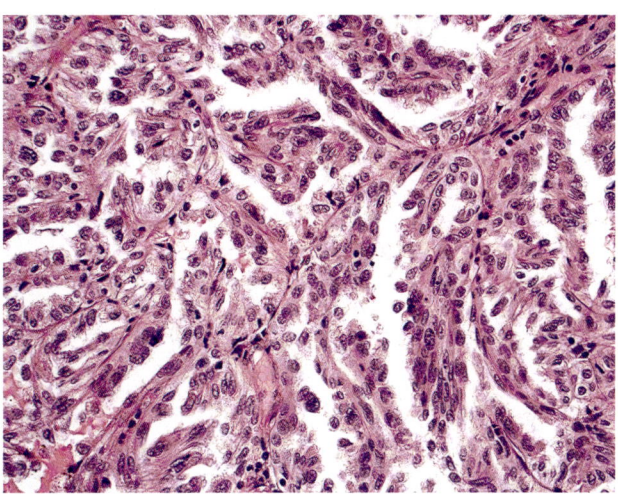

Figure 3.362. At higher magnification, this mucinous tubular and spindle cell carcinoma shows tubular formation with fusiform epithelial cells.

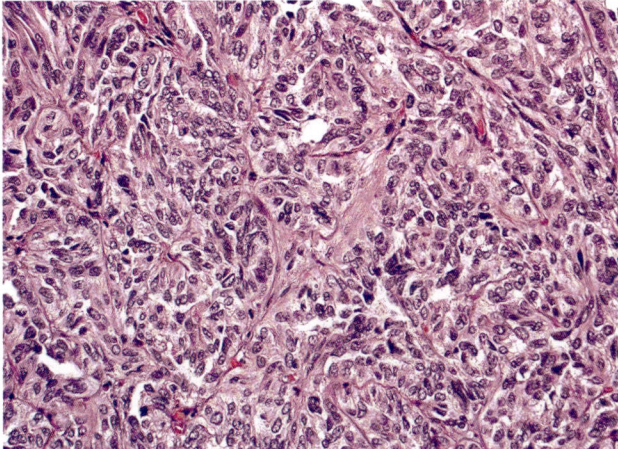

Figure 3.363. This field of mucinous tubular and spindle cell carcinoma shows fusiform cells arranged into packets. Although predominantly spindle-shaped morphology, there is a hint of epithelial differentiation based on the nested architecture.

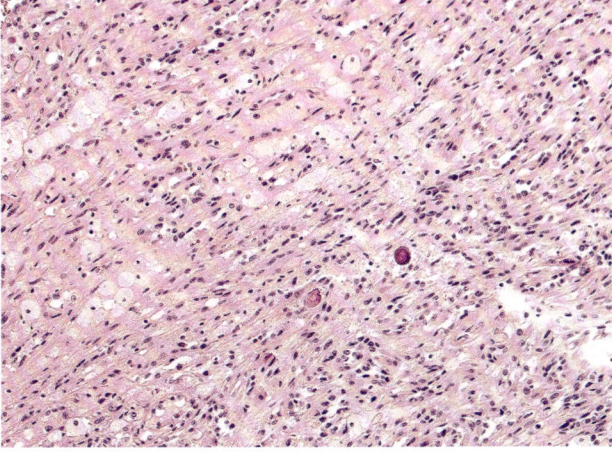

Figure 3.364. This field of mucinous tubular and spindle cell carcinoma predominantly mimics a spindle cell neoplasm; however, the foamy macrophages and psammoma bodies may be clues to the epithelial nature.

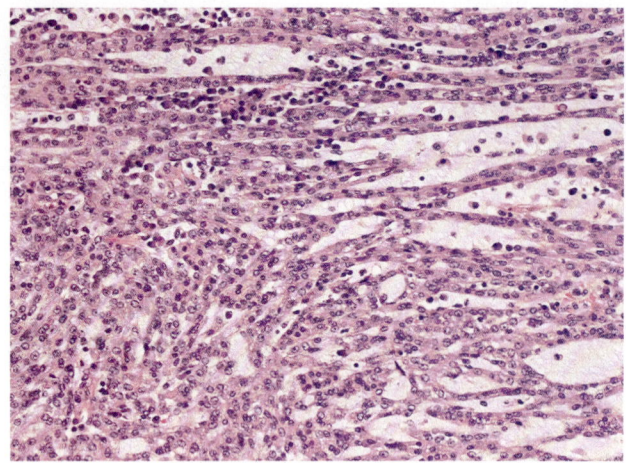

Figure 3.365. This field of mucinous tubular and spindle cell carcinoma shows elongated tubules with basophilic mucin between them.

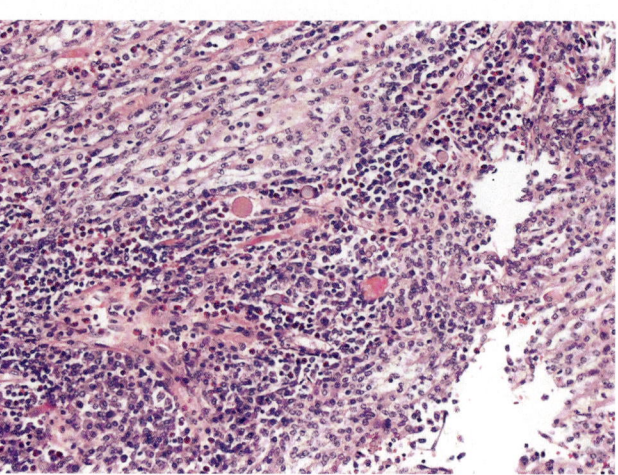

Figure 3.366. Mucinous tubular and spindle cell carcinoma often contains areas of chronic inflammation including plasma cells.

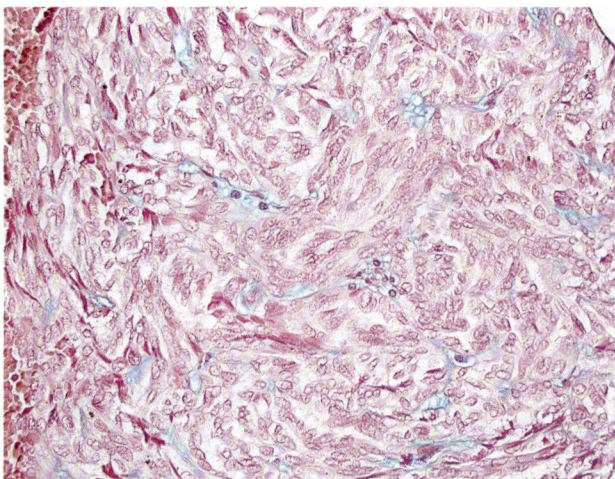

Figure 3.367. This Alcian blue stain highlights the mucinous material of a mucinous tubular and spindle cell carcinoma.

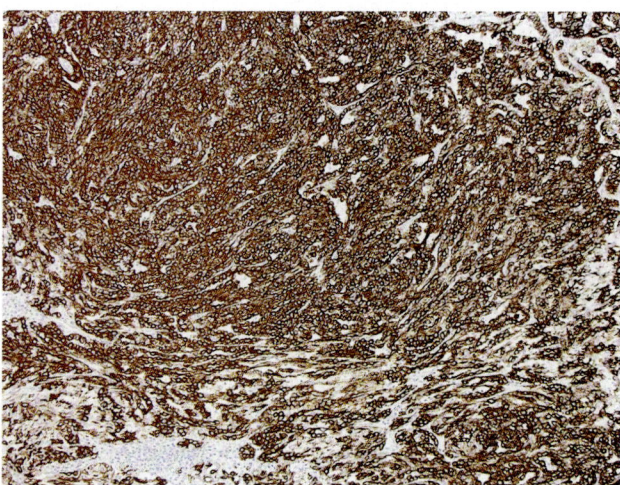

Figure 3.368. Mucinous tubular and spindle cell carcinoma is often positive for cytokeratin 7, like type 1 papillary renal cell carcinoma.

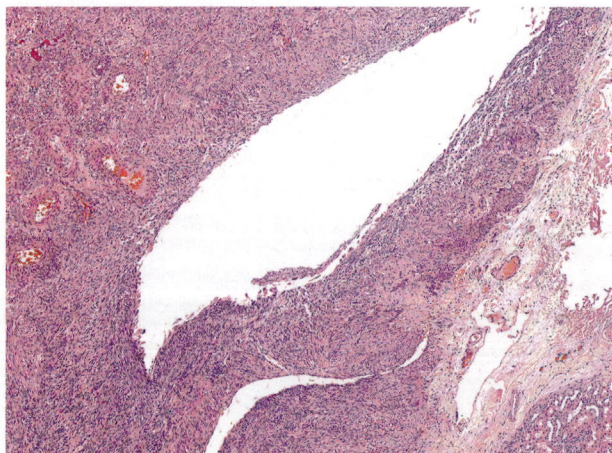

Figure 3.369. This angiomyolipoma contains large, dilated epithelial-lined cysts.

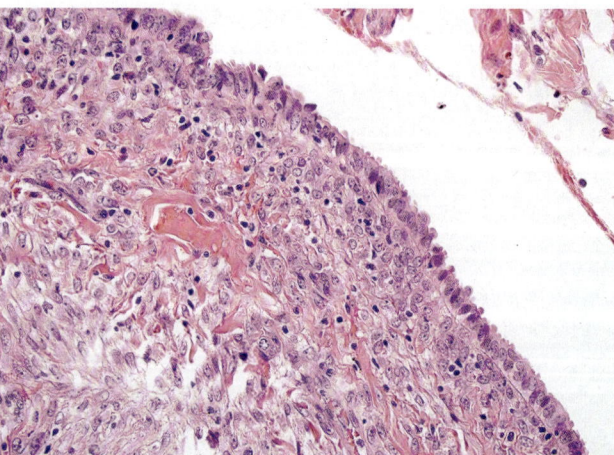

Figure 3.370. This angiomyolipoma contains epithelial cysts. There is some condensation with increased cellularity just under the cyst lining.

KEY FEATURES: Mixed Epithelial and Stromal Tumor Family

- Female predominance
- Solid and cystic architecture (Figure 3.372)
- Ovarian-like stroma (Figure 3.373)
- Hyalinized structures resembling corpora albicantia, likely representing hyalinized blood vessels (Figure 3.374)
- Condensation of spindle cell stroma around cystic structures
- Variable:
  - Phyllodes-like proliferation
  - Tubular proliferation
  - Adipose tissue
  - Papillae
  - Thyroid follicle–like tubules
- Immunohistochemistry:
  - Estrogen/progesterone receptor usually positive (Figure 3.375)
  - Smooth muscle actin (Figure 3.376), desmin, caldesmon often positive
  - CD34, CD10, WT1 variable
  - PAX8 positive in epithelial component

Synovial Sarcoma

Synovial sarcoma is much more common as a soft tissue tumor of the extremities; however, it can occur in the kidney and may show some peculiar features that are worth considering. The spindle cell component of renal synovial sarcoma is like that of soft tissue tumors; however, there may be an entrapped tubular component imparting a biphasic, multicystic appearance (Figures 3.377 and 3.378). Although the biphasic pattern of synovial sarcoma exists in soft tissue, the epithelial component of renal synovial sarcoma likely represents a different process, as the epithelial component has been found to be PAX8 positive and lack TLE1 staining, contrasting to the tumor cells of synovial sarcoma itself.[335,343] In other words, renal synovial sarcomas are predominantly of monophasic type with the epithelial component thought to be entrapped epithelium. Synovial sarcoma can be distinguished from mixed epithelial and stromal tumor and angiomyolipoma with epithelial cysts by the greater degree of cytologic atypia in synovial sarcoma as well as the estrogen/progesterone receptor positivity in mixed epithelial and stromal tumor and melanocytic marker positivity in angiomyolipoma. In challenging cases, molecular studies may be helpful, such as FISH to detect the *SS18* (formerly SYT) rearrangement of synovial sarcoma.[343]

Wilms Tumor/Nephroblastoma

Nephroblastoma is a malignant embryonal neoplasm composed of undifferentiated blastema cells with varying proportions of epithelial and stromal differentiation (Figures 3.379 and 3.380).[341] It occurs predominantly in children, overwhelmingly under 10 years of age; however, occurrence in adults is also possible (Figures 3.381 and 3.382). The classic example is triphasic, with blastema, tubules, and stromal cells; however, in some cases, two patterns, or rarely one (Figure 3.383), will predominate. Since this is predominantly a diagnosis for the pediatric pathologist and pediatric pathology textbooks, this section will focus briefly on discrimination from mimics in adults. Metanephric adenoma may be a consideration for a predominantly tubular neoplasm in adults. Importantly, the cells of metanephric adenoma are extremely bland, with small nuclei resembling those of lymphocytes. Larger nuclei with atypia or mitotic figures, in contrast, would raise concern for papillary RCC or nephroblastoma. Using a panel of markers proposed to distinguish papillary RCC from metanephric adenoma and epithelial predominant nephroblastoma, nephroblastoma typically shows diffuse staining for WT1, negative staining for AMACR, and minimal or negative staining for cytokeratin 7. In contrast, papillary RCC typically shows strong staining for AMACR and diffuse cytokeratin 7 (particularly for the latter in basophilic tumors

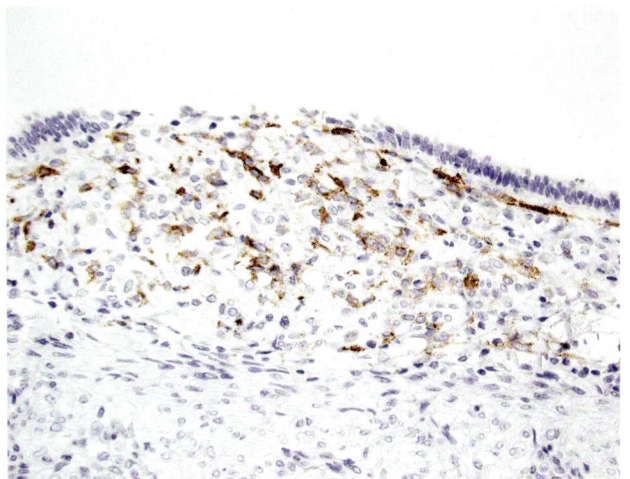

Figure 3.371. Melan-A staining in the same tumor from Figure 3.370 shows patchy staining in the cellular layer under the cyst, supporting angiomyolipoma.

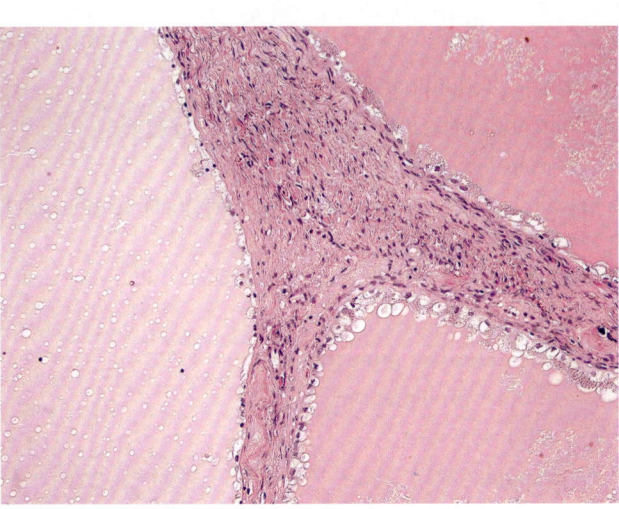

Figure 3.372. The mixed epithelial and stromal tumor family includes cystic nephroma and mixed epithelial and stromal tumor. This field is most in keeping with cystic nephroma, showing cysts lined by hobnail-shaped lining cells with spindle-shaped stromal cells in the wall.

that would be most likely to be considered in this differential diagnosis). Although both metanephric adenoma and nephroblastoma are diffusely positive for WT1 and may be positive for CD57, the extent of staining for CD57 is usually diffuse in metanephric adenoma and focal in nephroblastoma.[259]

Other Biphasic/Triphasic Neoplasms

Other renal neoplasms with biphasic or triphasic patterns are rare. One unusual pattern that has been increasingly recognized is RCC with angioleiomyoma-like stroma or RCC with smooth muscle stroma.[233,344,345] These tumors contain a renal epithelial component resembling clear cell RCC with a prominent smooth muscle proliferation (Figure 3.384). Interestingly, the epithelial component has a pattern resembling clear cell papillary RCC with positive immunohistochemistry for cytokeratin 7, high molecular weight cytokeratin, and carbonic anhydrase IX, although it differs slightly in its frequent positivity for CD10. This pattern seems to be enriched in patients with tuberous sclerosis, although it also appears to occur sporadically.[193,345-347] Recent work has found frequent mutations of *TSC1*, *TSC2*, and *MTOR* in these tumors, suggesting that like clear cell RCC, this tumor has a syndromic (tuberous sclerosis–associated) and sporadic form with molecular alterations of similar, related genes. Another subset of tumors with prominent stroma has been found to have mutations of *ELOC* (formerly TCEB1), the significance of which is less clear at present.[345,348]

SAMPLE NOTE: RCC With Smooth Muscle Stroma

RCC with smooth muscle or angioleiomyoma-like stroma has been recently recognized to contain a renal epithelial component resembling clear cell RCC, with prominent smooth muscle–rich stroma. This tumor lacks the usual molecular alterations of clear cell RCC and appears to occur both in the setting of tuberous sclerosis and sporadically. To date, the behavior appears mostly nonaggressive, although data are limited.

References:

Shah RB, Stohr BA, Tu ZJ, et al. "Renal cell carcinoma with leiomyomatous stroma" harbor somatic mutations of TSC1, TSC2, MTOR, and/or ELOC (TCEB1): clinicopathologic and molecular characterization of 18 sporadic tumors supports a distinct entity. *Am J Surg Pathol*. 2020;44:571-581.

Guo J, Tretiakova MS, Troxell ML, et al. Tuberous sclerosis-associated renal cell carcinoma: a clinicopathologic study of 57 separate carcinomas in 18 patients. *Am J Surg Pathol*. 2014;38:1457-1467.

Yang P, Cornejo KM, Sadow PM, et al. Renal cell carcinoma in tuberous sclerosis complex. *Am J Surg Pathol*. 2014;38:895-909.

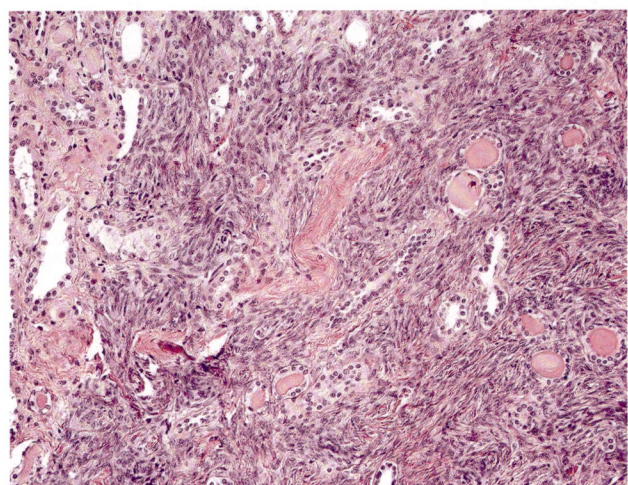

Figure 3.373. Solid areas in mixed epithelial and stromal tumor often resemble ovarian stroma. Renal tubules within the tumor may resemble thyroid-like follicles (right).

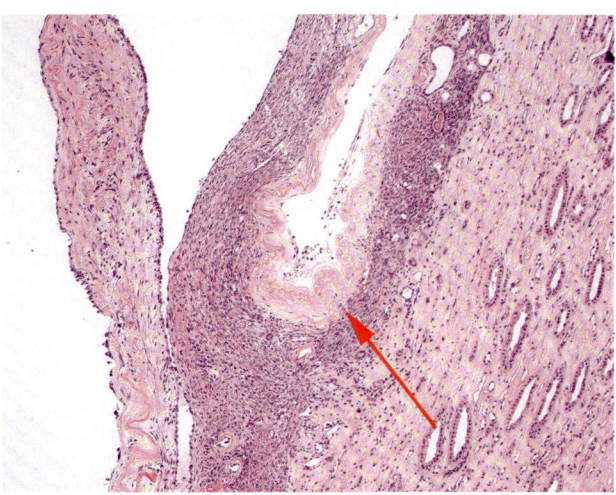

Figure 3.374. Structures resembling corpora albicantia have been reported in mixed epithelial and stromal tumor (arrow). It is thought that these actually are abnormal blood vessels. This field also shows cystic areas (left).

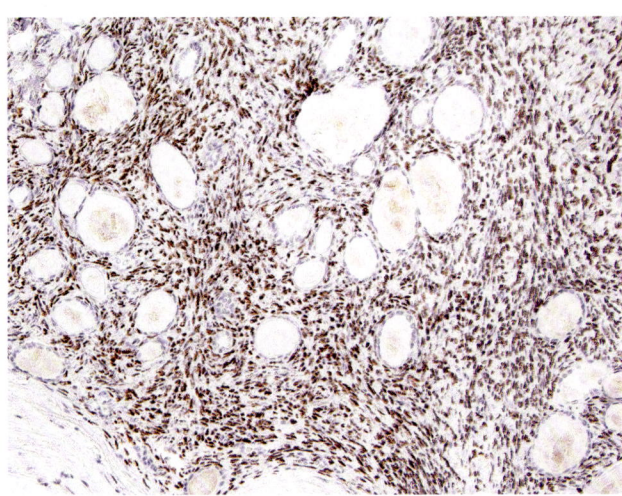

Figure 3.375. Immunohistochemistry typically shows reactivity for estrogen receptor in mixed epithelial and stromal tumor.

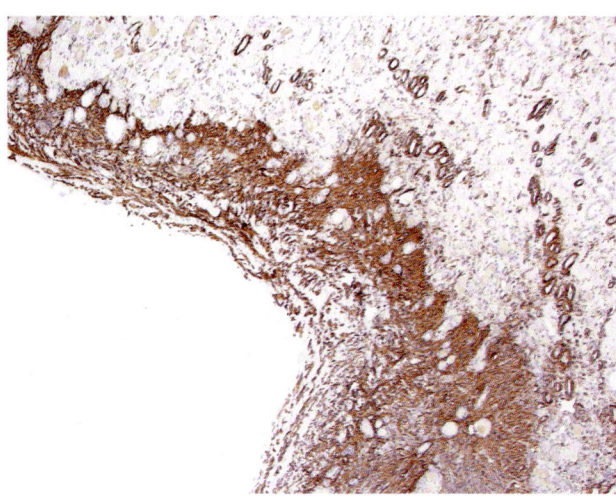

Figure 3.376. This smooth muscle actin immunohistochemical stain in mixed epithelial and stromal tumor shows increased staining adjacent to the cystic areas.

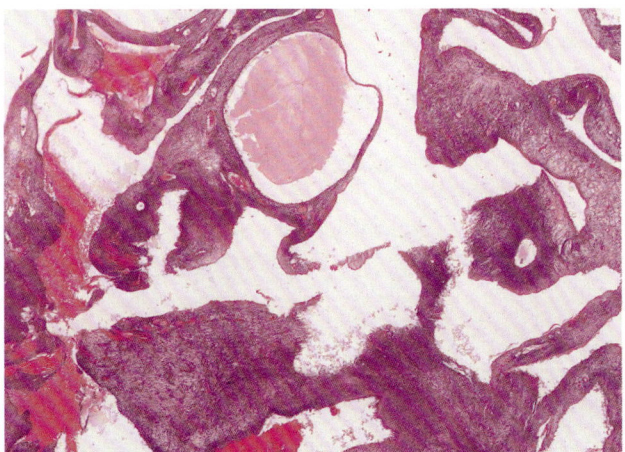

Figure 3.377. This renal synovial sarcoma deceptively mimics solid and cystic neoplasms of the kidney with numerous cystic spaces. (Courtesy Andres Matoso, MD, Johns Hopkins Medical Institutions.)

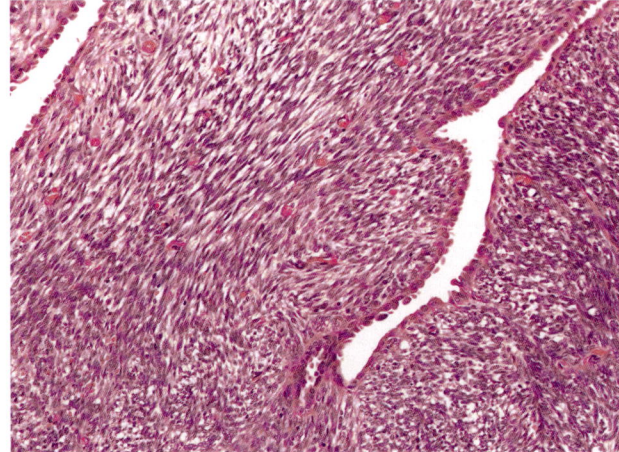

Figure 3.378. At higher magnification, this renal synovial sarcoma is more cellular than usual benign biphasic renal neoplasms, with mild atypia. (Courtesy Andres Matoso, MD, Johns Hopkins Medical Institutions.)

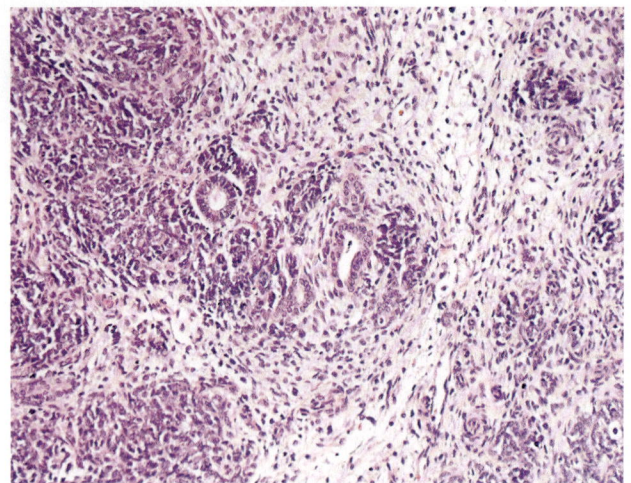

Figure 3.379. Nephroblastoma (Wilms tumor) classically contains three components: blastema, small crowded blue cells; stroma, spindle-shaped cells; and tubules, with evidence of epithelial formation.

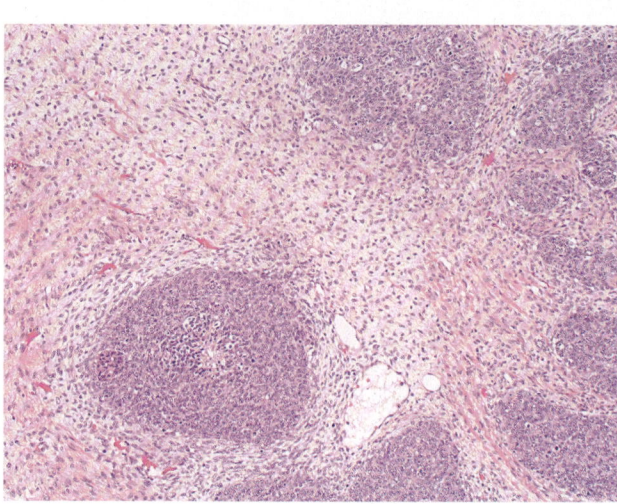

Figure 3.380. This field from nephroblastoma demonstrates islands of blastema in spindle cell stroma.

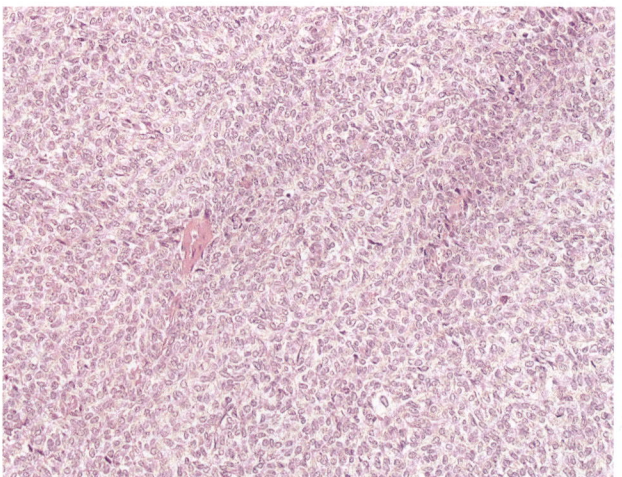

Figure 3.381. This nephroblastoma occurred in a 33-year-old man, containing blastema in this field.

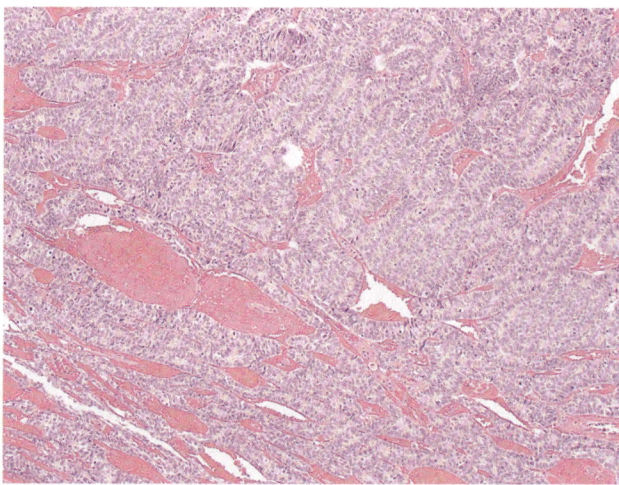

Figure 3.382. Other areas from the same tumor in Figure 3.381 show tubular differentiation.

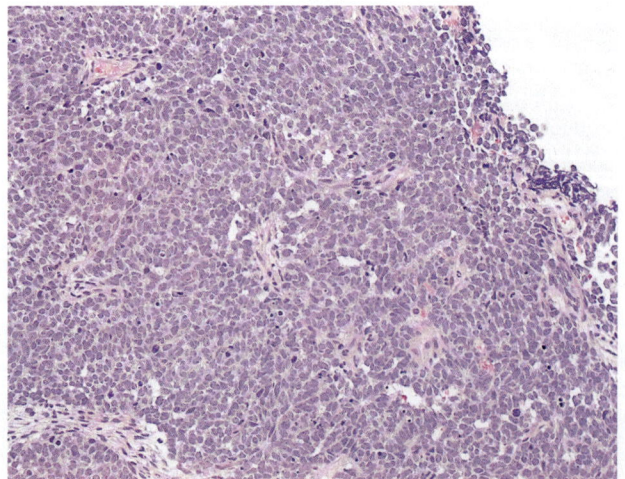

Figure 3.383. Nephroblastoma can be more deceptive when only one or two patterns are predominant. This example included mostly blastema.

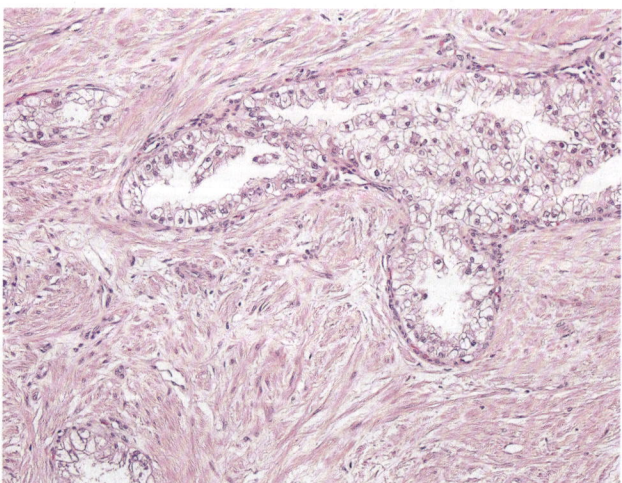

Figure 3.384. Renal cell carcinoma (RCC) with smooth muscle or leiomyoma-like stroma is a rare pattern of RCC with a biphasic pattern. The epithelium resembles clear cell RCC; however, there is abundant intervening stroma with a smooth muscle appearance.

Within the metanephric category of tumors, there are forms even rarer than metanephric adenoma, including metanephric stromal tumor, which is composed of spindle-shaped cells that form concentric rings around blood vessels and renal tubules, and metanephric adenofibroma, which has components resembling metanephric adenoma and metanephric stromal tumor.[258] As noted previously, rare examples of sarcomatoid RCC may have a pseudo-biphasic appearance due to a deceptively low-grade sarcomatoid component (see section on sarcomatoid RCC).[292] Finally, a rare pattern that has only been described in a single study as smooth muscle and adenoma-like renal tumor (SMART) contains an epithelial proliferation resembling papillary RCC and a smooth muscle stromal component. The authors raised the question of whether this neoplasm is a variant of mixed epithelial and stromal tumor or a distinct entity.[349]

RENAL CANCER STAGING

Renal cancer staging can be deceptive compared with staging of other cancers. While the classical carcinoma invades local structures destructively with desmoplastic response, a prototypical pattern of renal cancer invasion is for finger-like polypoid projections to extend into vein branches or the renal sinus tissue. This can easily be overlooked without careful attention to not only microscopy but also gross examination (Figures 3.385 and 3.386).[350,351]

KEY FEATURES: pT3a Stage Renal Cell Carcinoma

- Renal sinus invasion (may be vascular invasion within hilar soft tissue or direct invasion to hilar fat, Figures 3.387 and 3.388)
- Perinephric fat invasion (Figures 3.389 and 3.390)
- Extension into renal vein or branches of the renal vein (Figures 3.391-3.395)
- Extension into pelvicalyceal system (new for 2016 American Joint Commission on Cancer [AJCC] staging system, Figure 3.396)[9]

PEARLS AND PITFALLS: Renal Cancer Staging

- As tumor size increases over 5 cm, the likelihood of renal sinus invasion increases dramatically for clear cell RCC[10,11,352,353]
  - Additional sampling should be considered for clear cell RCC tumors over 5 to 6 cm that have no definite renal sinus invasion
  - Renal vein branches may have thin walls with scant or no muscle,[40] and therefore tumor involvement may be easily overlooked as multinodularity rather than vascular involvement (Figure 3.397)
  - Multiple nodules or a "snowman"-shaped tumor should be viewed with great suspicion as possible vein involvement, especially if there is one large tumor and multiple smaller nodules (Figure 3.398)

An interesting phenomenon that sometimes occurs with RCC, especially clear cell type, when it has invaded the main renal vein, is that multiple additional "satellite" nodules may form from backward spread of the tumor into vein branches, termed retrograde venous invasion (Figure 3.399).[41,353] This should be a major consideration whenever there is a main large mass (especially clear cell RCC) and multiple confluent or separate nodules elsewhere in the kidney. In our experience, it is actually quite rare for clear cell RCC to be multifocal outside of the setting of VHL disease.[353] Another consideration for multiple "clear cell" tumors is that they are actually clear cell papillary RCC, which is frequently multifocal.[72,353]

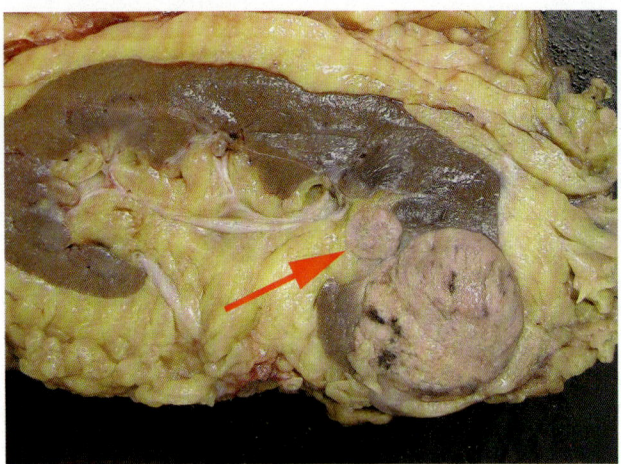

Figure 3.385. This renal cell carcinoma has a satellite nodule (arrow) bulging into the renal sinus. Any tumor that deviates from a circular or spherical shape with outpouchings should be viewed with great suspicion for renal vein or renal sinus invasion.

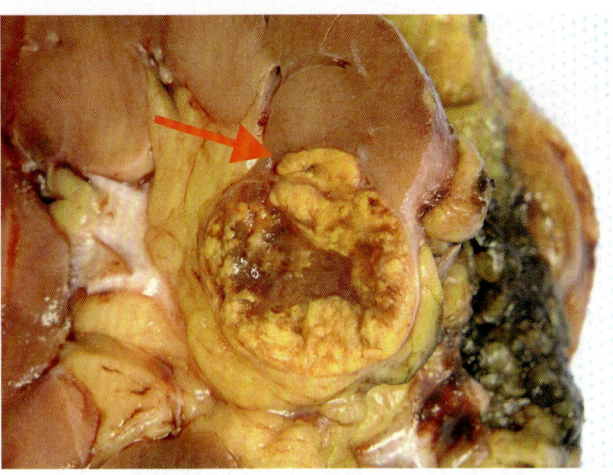

Figure 3.386. This clear cell renal cell carcinoma tumor has a small outpouching (arrow) that deviates slightly from the round shape of the mass overall. Areas like this should be carefully evaluated microscopically, as they may represent renal vein branch involvement.

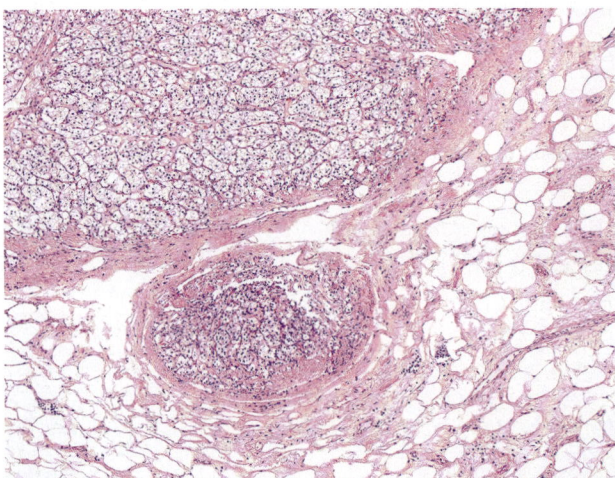

Figure 3.387. Renal sinus invasion can include involvement of small vascular spaces within the hilar fat.

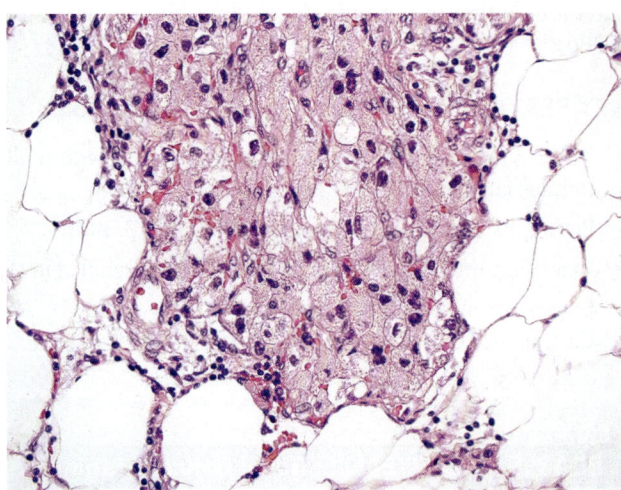

Figure 3.388. Direct invasion of fat is also regarded as renal sinus invasion.

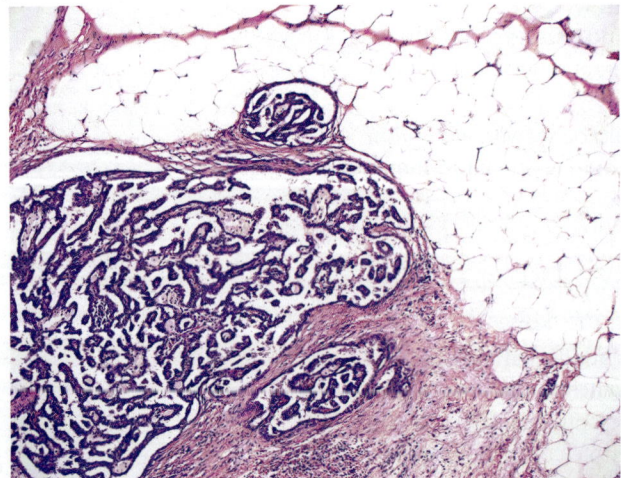

Figure 3.389. This papillary renal cell carcinoma shows multinodular outpouching into the perinephric fat, which we would consider perinephric fat invasion.

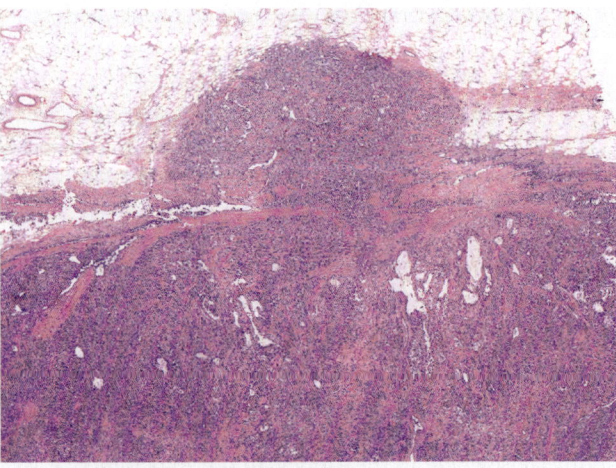

Figure 3.390. This high-grade renal cell carcinoma extends into the perinephric fat in a mushroom-shaped configuration.

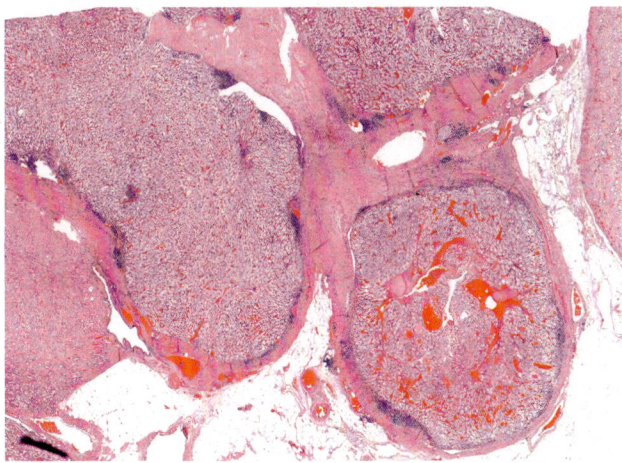

Figure 3.391. Multiple nodules of clear cell renal cell carcinoma in this case extend into renal vein branches in the renal sinus.

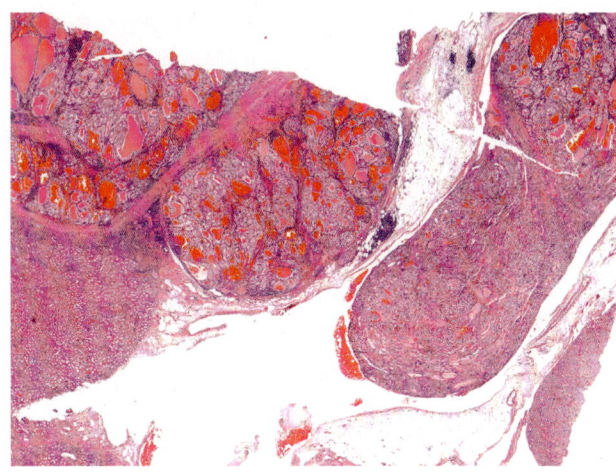

Figure 3.392. A large polypoid nodule of clear cell renal cell carcinoma involves a vein branch in the renal sinus, supporting pT3a.

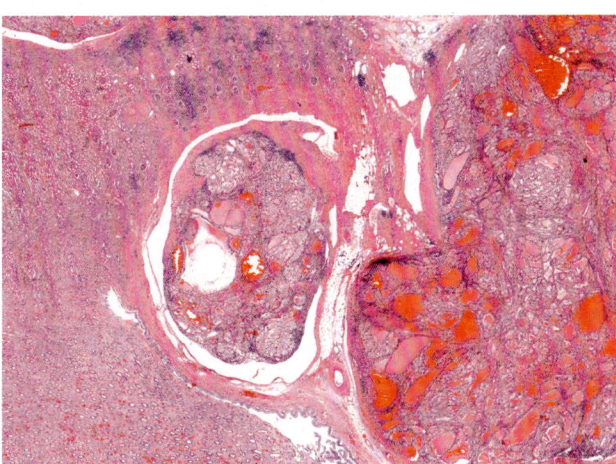

Figure 3.393. This clear cell renal cell carcinoma has a small outpouching into a small vein branch. Although it is surrounded by renal parenchyma, there is fat separating the main tumor from the vein involvement.

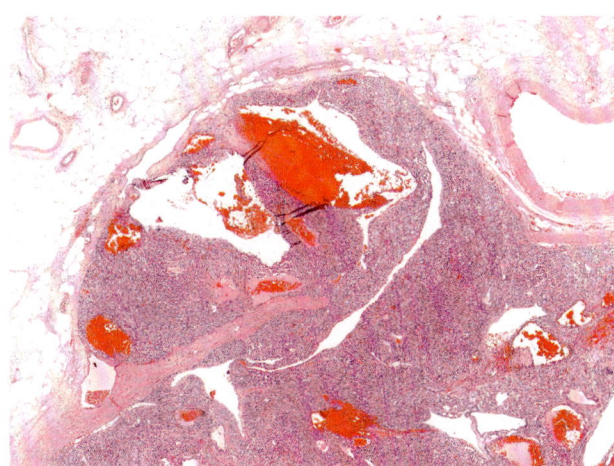

Figure 3.394. This clear cell renal cell carcinoma bulges into the renal sinus with a focally preserved vein lumen, suggesting vein branch invasion in the renal sinus.

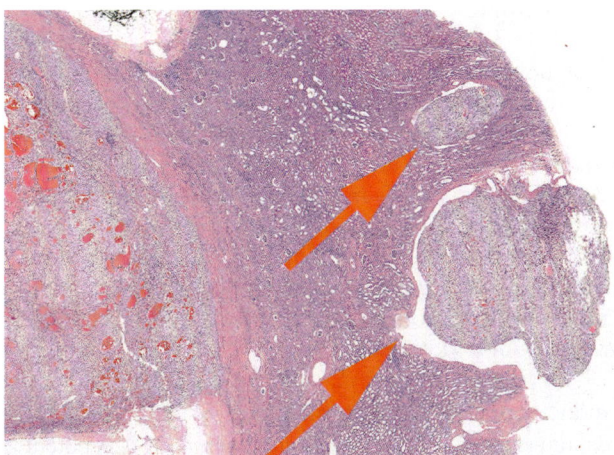

Figure 3.395. This partial nephrectomy shows small foci of vein branch invasion (arrows) with satellite nodules away from the main tumor.

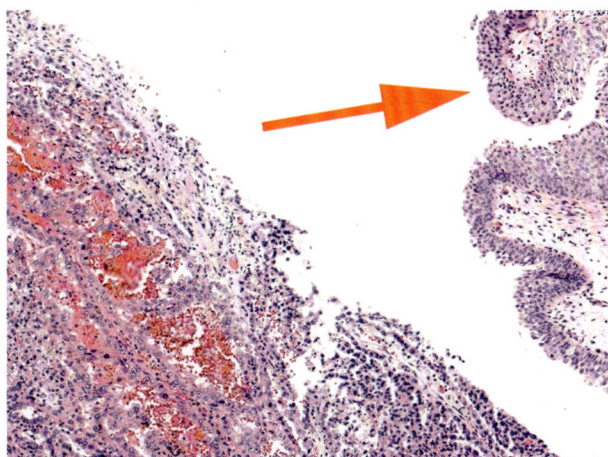

Figure 3.396. This papillary renal cell carcinoma extends into the renal pelvis (mucosa at arrow), which is now recognized as conferring pT3a stage in the 2016 AJCC staging system.

KEY FEATURES: Renal Cell Carcinoma Staging (AJCC 8th Edition)

- pT1a = size up to 4 cm, confined to the kidney
- pT1b = size > 4 cm, up to 7 cm, confined to the kidney
- pT2a = size >7 cm, up to 10 cm, confined to the kidney (Note: rare for clear cell RCC, consider additional sections!)
- pT2b = size >10 cm, confined to the kidney (Note: rare for clear cell RCC, consider additional sections!)
- pT3a = invasion of renal sinus, perinephric fat, renal vein or vein branches, or pelvicalyceal system
- pT3b = invasion to the vena cava below the diaphragm, without wall invasion
- pT3c = invasion to the vena cava above the diaphragm or wall invasion
- pT4 = direct invasion of the adrenal gland or invasion beyond Gerota fascia (rare)
- pN0 versus pN1 = involvement of one or more lymph nodes
- pM1 = distant metastasis or noncontiguous adrenal involvement

CHECKLIST: Reporting a Renal Cancer Specimen With a Large Clear Cell RCC Tumor (size >5 cm) But No Definite Extrarenal Extension

☐ Does the tumor abut the hilar fat at all? Consider submitting the entire interface for histologic sections to argue against invasion

☐ No polypoid or finger-like outpouchings (if yes, consider the possibility that these are vein involvement)

☐ No microscopic lymphovascular invasion within the renal sinus (which also constitutes invasion)

☐ No mushroom-shaped bulge into perinephric fat

In modern surgical practice, the adrenal gland is often spared when performing a radical nephrectomy. If the adrenal gland is present with the specimen, gross examination should attempt to discern whether there is direct invasion of RCC into the adrenal gland (pT4), discontinuous involvement (metastatic, pM1), or neither. Sometimes a separate vena cava specimen will be provided by the surgeon, which may consist of unoriented tumor fragments. We typically examine at least two to three blocks of such a specimen to attempt to discern whether there is muscular wall identifiable with adherent or invasive tumor (pT3b versus pT3c).

FAQ: Assessing the Renal Vein Margin

Since RCC can grow with a polypoid configuration into veins, a radical nephrectomy specimen will sometimes be received with a finger-like projection of tumor protruding from the vein at the margin of the specimen. Consensus is that this is not a positive margin unless tumor is adherent to, or invading, the wall of the vein at the margin.[351] If, conversely, the tumor is freely mobile within the vein lumen at the margin and not adherent, this is considered a negative margin (Figure 3.400). Sections can be chosen by either amputating the vein margin as a cross section, including the tumor, then histologically evaluating for adherence, or by trimming the vein wall free circumferentially with scissors as a strip and verifying histologic absence of adherent or invasive tumor (Figure 3.401).

Urothelial carcinoma of the kidney or ureter has its own staging system, based on the extent of invasion (lamina propria, muscularis propria, renal parenchyma, etc.). A potential pitfall when assessing urothelial carcinoma of the renal pelvis is that tumors may erode the renal medulla and spread noninvasively up medullary tubules without necessarily invading (Figure 3.402).

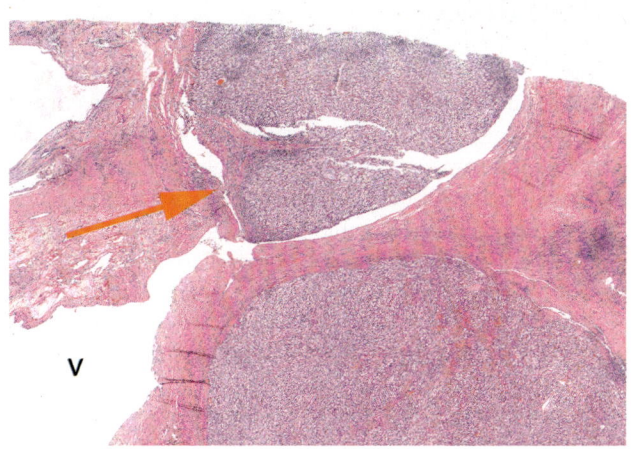

Figure 3.397. In some cases, renal vein branch invasion can be difficult to discriminate from multinodularity. Although this tumor had extensive hilar involvement grossly, it is less obvious microscopically. A tumor nodule (arrow) extends into a vein lumen (v).

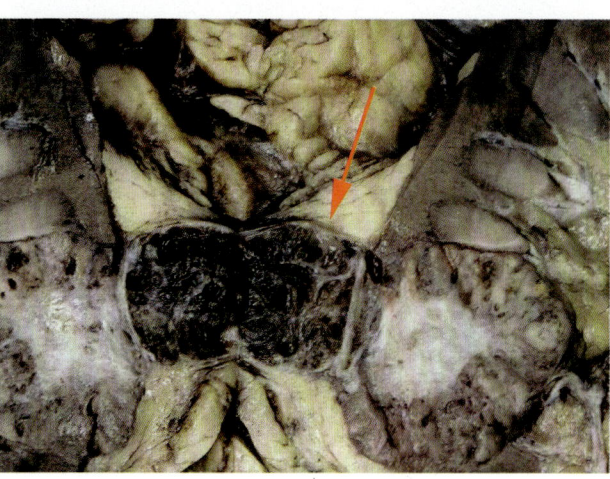

Figure 3.398. A renal cell carcinoma tumor with outpouchings resembling a snowman (arrow) should be considered very suspicious for vein or soft tissue invasion.

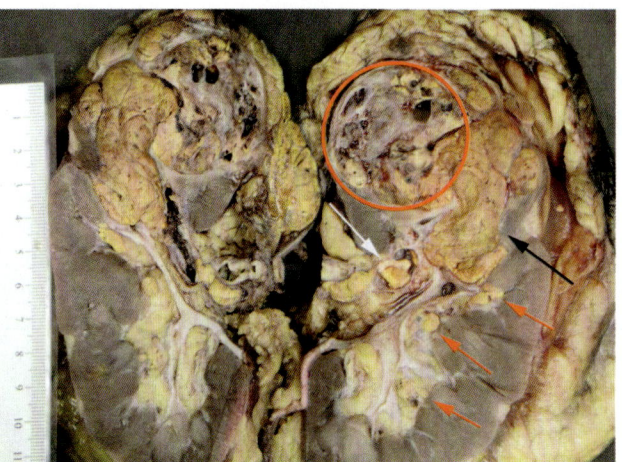

Figure 3.399. Retrograde venous invasion occurs when renal cell carcinoma extends into the main renal vein and spreads backward along other vein branches. In this example, the approximate location of the original tumor is marked with a circle. At the black arrow, tumor distends and fills intraparenchymal vein branches toward the main renal vein (white arrow). Several satellite nodules are formed distantly in the kidney via retrograde spread (red arrows).

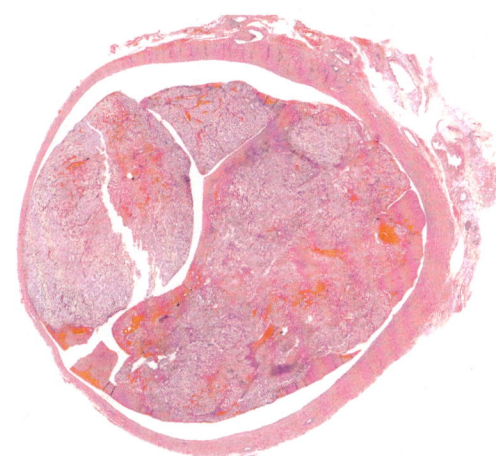

Figure 3.400. When sampling the renal vein margin, if tumor is present in the lumen but not adherent to the vein wall, this is typically considered a negative margin, as tumor has not necessarily been transected.

KEY FEATURES: Staging Urothelial Carcinoma of the Renal Pelvis or Ureter (AJCC 8th Edition)

- Noninvasive papillary tumor = pTa
- Noninvasive flat carcinoma in situ = pTis
- Lamina propria invasion = pT1
- Muscularis propria invasion (ureter or renal pelvis) = pT2 (Figure 3.403)
- Invades peripelvic or periureteric fat = pT3
- Invades renal parenchyma = pT3
- Invades adjacent organs = pT4
- Invades through kidney into perinephric fat = pT4 (Figure 3.404)

RENAL CANCER GRADING

Grading of RCC has been changed significantly in recent years, from the original Fuhrman system that utilized multiple nuclear morphometric parameters[354] to the current International Society of Urological Pathology (ISUP)/WHO system,[62,63,355] which uses the prominence of the nucleolus as the main parameter. This system is validated for clear cell and papillary RCC. Importantly, it is not helpful for chromophobe RCC, where inherently has more atypical nuclei yet which typically has a favorable prognosis.[62,65] Other types of RCC may be graded in this system, such as tubulocystic, clear cell papillary RCC, or others; however, this has not been validated to have prognostic implications in other tumor types.

KEY FEATURES: Nucleolar Grading of RCC (ISUP/WHO System, Figures 3.405-3.408)

- Nucleoli inconspicuous at high magnification (40× objective) = grade 1
- Nucleoli prominent at high magnification (40× objective) = grade 2
- Nucleoli prominent at intermediate magnification (10× objective) = grade 3
- Bizarre, multilobated nuclei or sarcomatoid/rhabdoid = grade 4
- Chromophobe RCC = grading not applicable

INFLAMMATORY PATTERN AND NONNEOPLASTIC PSEUDOTUMORS

LYMPHOMA

Various types of lymphoma can involve the kidney; however, primary renal lymphoma presenting without systemic involvement is extremely rare. Most renal lymphomas are B cell lymphomas.[356] We have occasionally encountered lymphoma in the tissue immediately surrounding a renal mass (Figure 3.409), which should be a consideration whenever peritumoral inflammation is unexpectedly brisk and monotonous.

XANTHOGRANULOMATOUS PYELONEPHRITIS

Xanthogranulomatous pyelonephritis is an infrequent pseudotumoral process affecting the kidney, usually resulting from obstruction (often due to stones) and subsequent infection (most commonly *Escherichia coli* or *Proteus mirabilis*).[357] Often the entire kidney is involved; however, segmental involvement may clinically mimic a renal malignancy (Figure 3.410). Other deceptive features that may be encountered clinically include involvement of adjacent structures, such as the psoas muscle or abdominal wall.[358,359] Histologic features include granulomatous inflammation with histiocytes, occasional giant cells or cholesterol clefts, and other inflammatory cells, including lymphocytes, neutrophils, and plasma cells (Figures 3.411-3.414).[357] As noted in the clear cell pattern section, prominent foamy histiocytes may lead to confusion with clear cell RCC, or a spindle cell pattern may mimic sarcomatoid RCC. Application of histiocytic versus epithelial immunohistochemical markers should resolve this distinction.

MALAKOPLAKIA

Malakoplakia is another histiocytic pseudotumoral process that more commonly is found in the urinary bladder but may affect the kidney.[289,360] It is thought that this occurs due to inability of macrophages to release lysosomal enzymes to degrade bacteria, most commonly *E. coli*.[361] The classic appearance of malakoplakia includes eosinophilic histiocytes (known as von Hansemann histiocytes) with targetoid basophilic structures in the cytoplasm (Michaelis-Gutmann bodies, Figure 3.416). The Michaelis-Gutmann bodies stain positively for calcium (von Kossa stain, Figure 3.417) or on periodic acid Schiff or iron stains. Although the classic pattern is of epithelioid eosinophilic histiocytes, a spindle cell

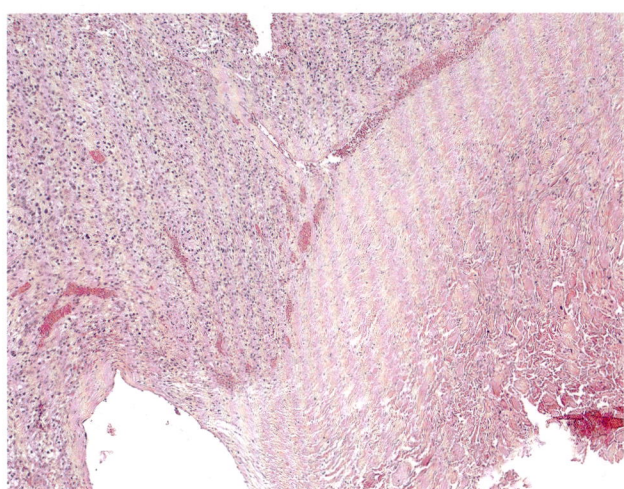

Figure 3.401. If renal cell carcinoma is adherent to the vein wall (right) at the vein margin of a nephrectomy specimen, this is interpreted as a positive margin.

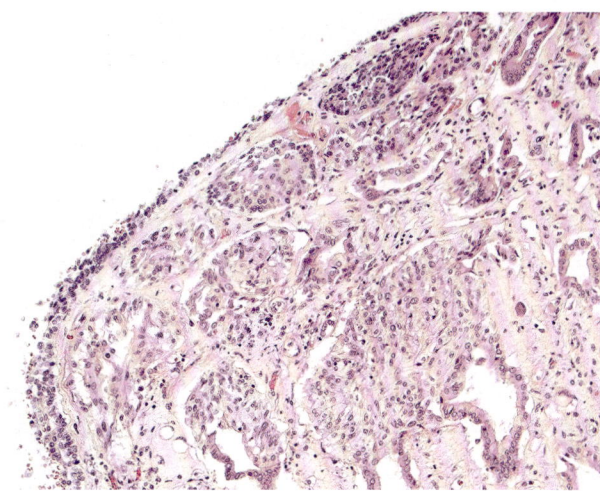

Figure 3.402. Urothelial carcinoma can extend noninvasively into medullary tubules. This does not constitute renal parenchyma invasion in isolation.

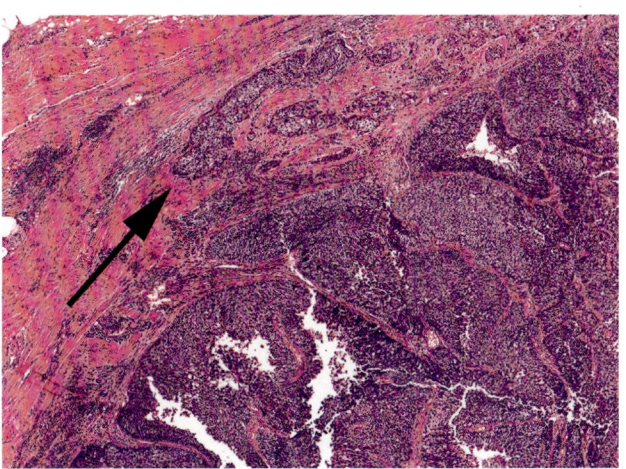

Figure 3.403. Invasion of the muscularis propria of the ureter or renal pelvis (arrow) constitutes pT2 urothelial carcinoma.

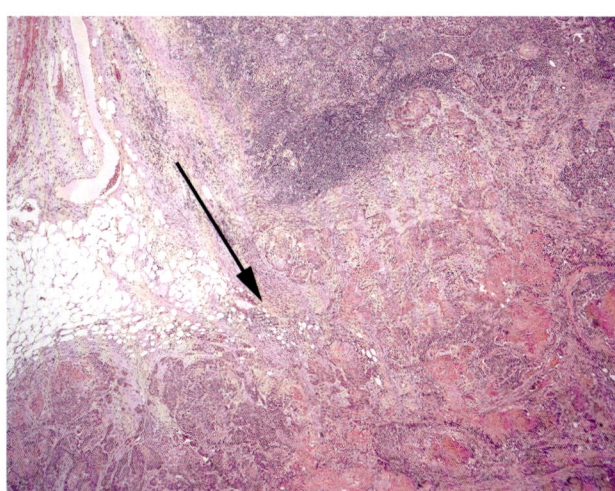

Figure 3.404. Urothelial carcinoma invading entirely through the kidney and into the perinephric fat (arrow) is staged as pT4.

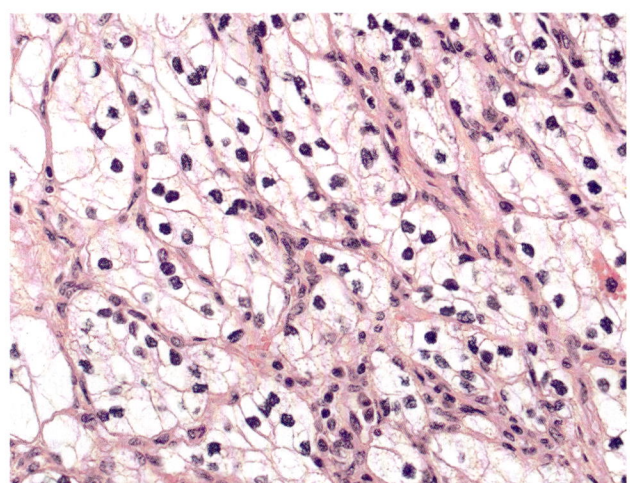

Figure 3.405. Grade 1 renal cell carcinoma demonstrates small nuclei, resembling those of lymphocytes, without conspicuous nucleoli, even at high magnification.

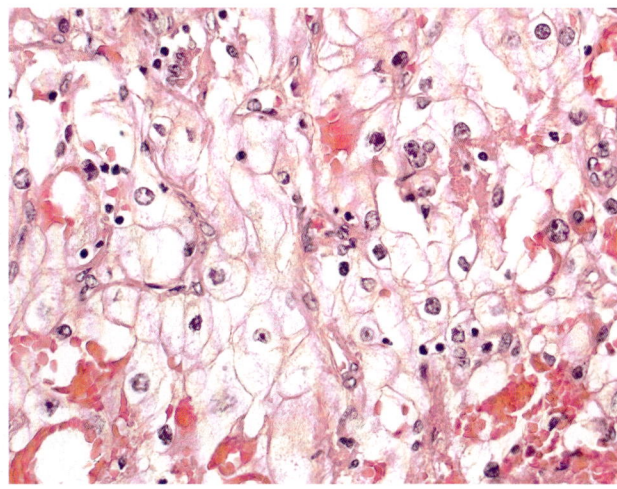

Figure 3.406. Grade 2 renal cell carcinoma demonstrates nucleoli visible at high magnification, but not conspicuous at 10× objective magnification.

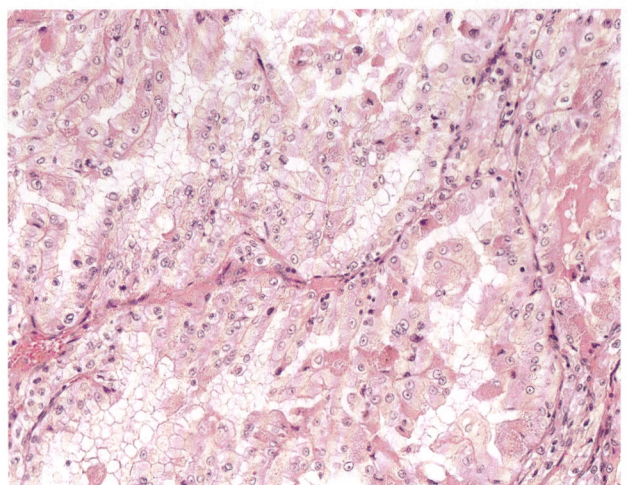

Figure 3.407. Grade 3 renal cell carcinoma contains nucleoli visible at 10× objective magnification.

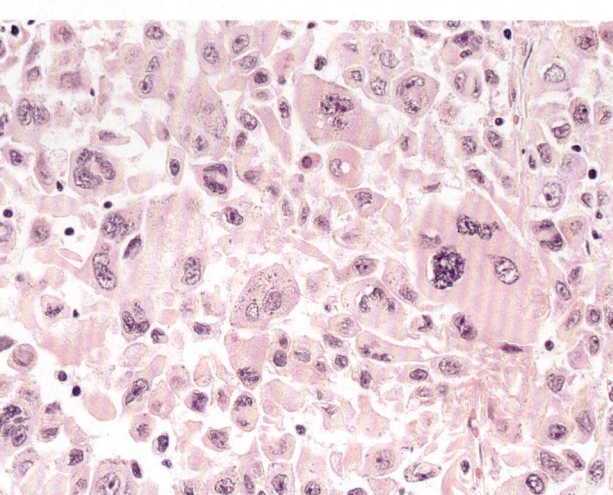

Figure 3.408. Grade 4 renal cell carcinoma exhibits markedly pleomorphic or multilobated nuclei. Sarcomatoid or rhabdoid features (not pictured) are also considered grade 4.

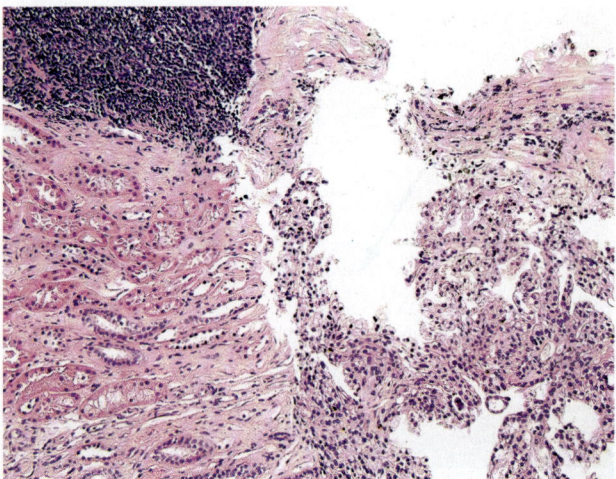

Figure 3.409. This renal mass biopsy shows papillary renal cell carcinoma (bottom right). The renal parenchyma is involved by small lymphocytic leukemia/chronic lymphocytic lymphoma (top left).

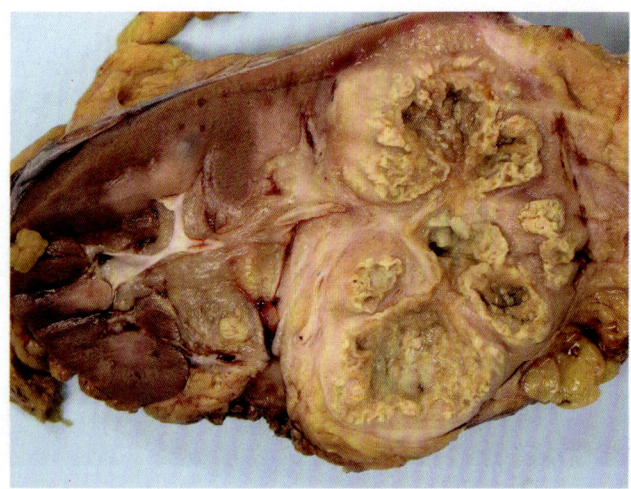

Figure 3.410. Xanthogranulomatous pyelonephritis may occasionally form a segmental mass, replacing only part of the kidney, which may clinically resemble renal cell carcinoma.

pattern can occasionally be present, mimicking a mesenchymal neoplasm or sarcomatoid RCC (Figure 3.418). Like xanthogranulomatous pyelonephritis, distinction from RCC can easily be achieved in difficult cases using immunohistochemistry for histiocytic and epithelial markers.

NEAR MISSES

HEMANGIOMA VERSUS RENAL CELL CARCINOMA

As noted in the spindle cell tumor section, hemangiomas are increasingly recognized in the kidney, especially the recently recognized variant known as anastomosing hemangioma.[315-318,320,362] However, before making this diagnosis, it is usually prudent to carefully consider the possibility of clear cell RCC in which the epithelial cells are inconspicuous or obscured by scar areas of the tumor (Figures 3.419-3.421).[321,363] Often immunohistochemistry would be prudent, to ensure lack of staining for RCC markers (keratin, PAX8, carbonic anhydrase IX, Figures 3.422 and 3.423). True anastomosing hemangiomas often contain hyaline globules and/or extramedullary hematopoiesis.

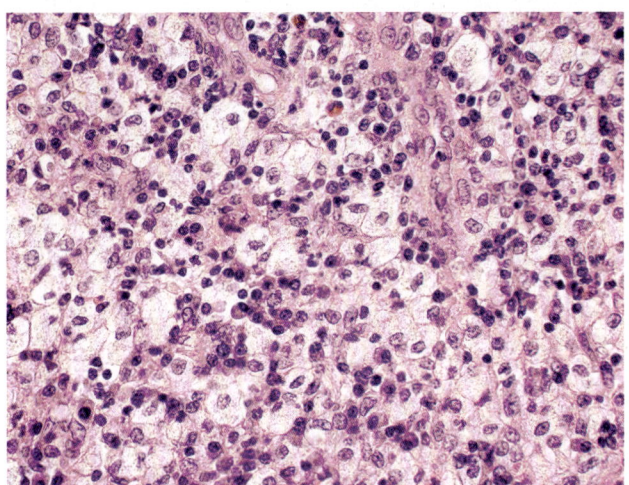

Figure 3.411. The classic pattern of xanthogranulomatous pyelonephritis is foamy histiocytes admixed with other inflammatory cells.

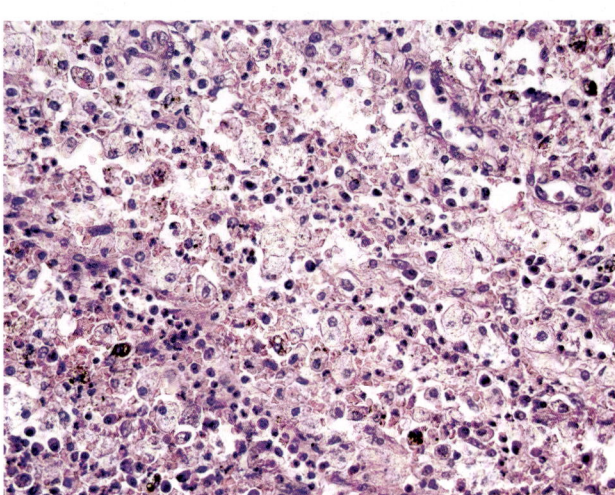

Figure 3.412. The presence of neutrophils may also help in discriminating xanthogranulomatous pyelonephritis from renal cell carcinoma or other neoplasms.

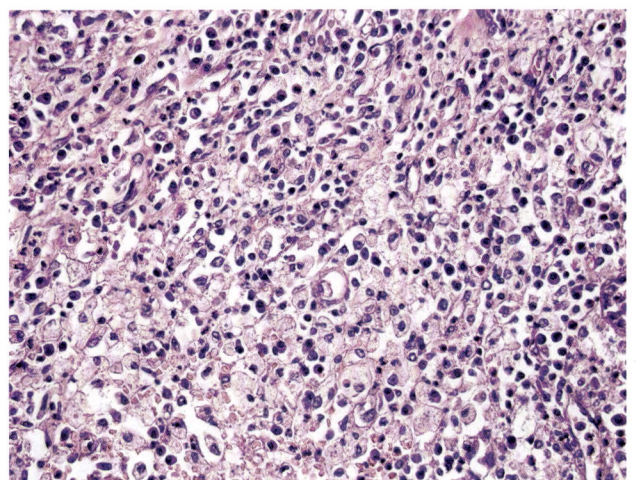

Figure 3.413. This example of xanthogranulomatous pyelonephritis shows a mixture of histiocytes and plasma cells.

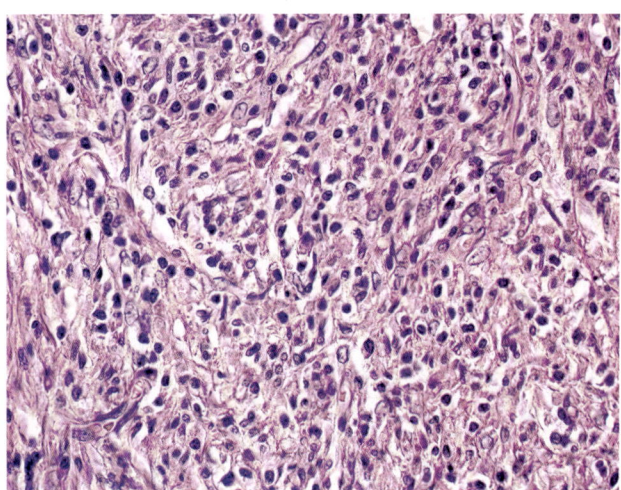

Figure 3.414. This field of xanthogranulomatous pyelonephritis may mimic a mesenchymal neoplasm, suggesting spindle-shaped cells.

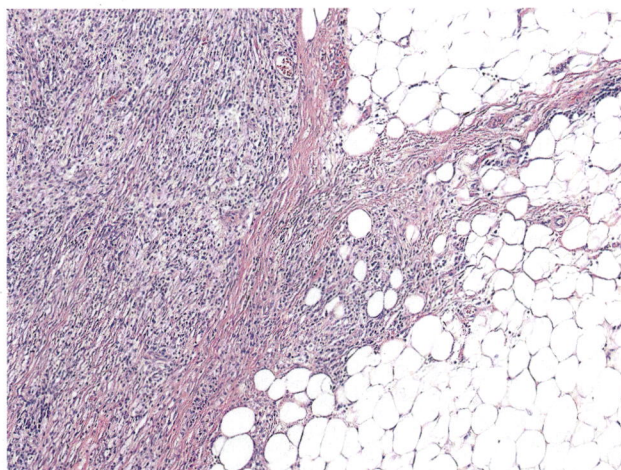

Figure 3.415. In this case of xanthogranulomatous pyelonephritis, the inflammatory process extends into perinephric tissue, which may clinically mimic an aggressive neoplasm.

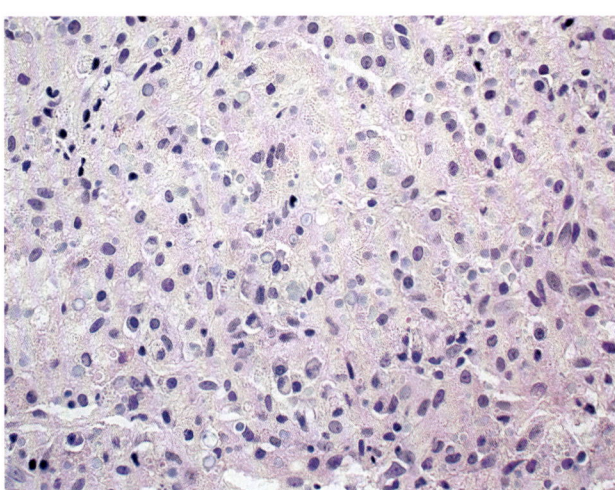

Figure 3.416. Malakoplakia is composed of numerous eosinophilic histiocytes with basophilic target-shaped structures in the cytoplasm (Michaelis-Gutmann bodies).

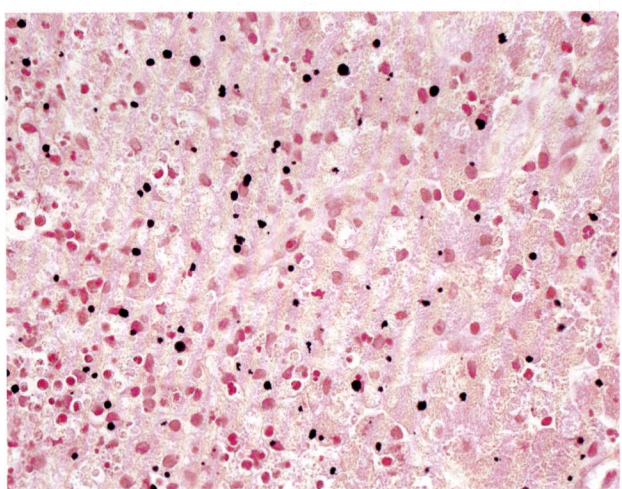

Figure 3.417. Michaelis-Gutmann bodies in malakoplakia stain positively (black) in the calcium (von Kossa) stain.

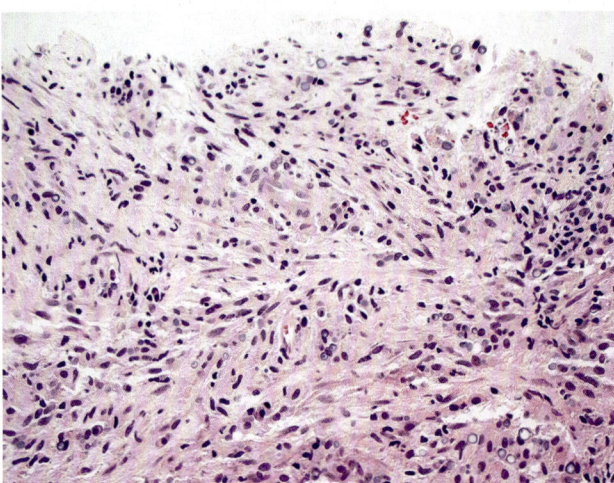

Figure 3.418. Rare cases of malakoplakia contain spindle-shaped cells. This renal case mimicked a neoplasm and was diagnosed in a core biopsy.

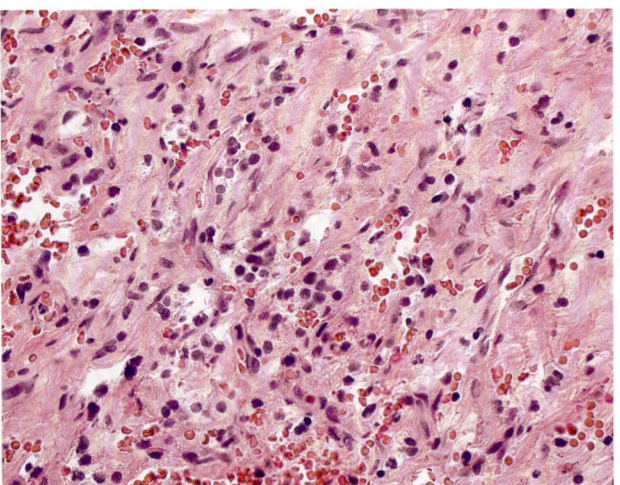

Figure 3.419. This renal cell carcinoma (RCC) in renal mass biopsy shows predominantly fibrous tissue with small vascular spaces, which could be mistaken for benign fibrous tissue or a mesenchymal lesion without awareness of this pattern in RCC.

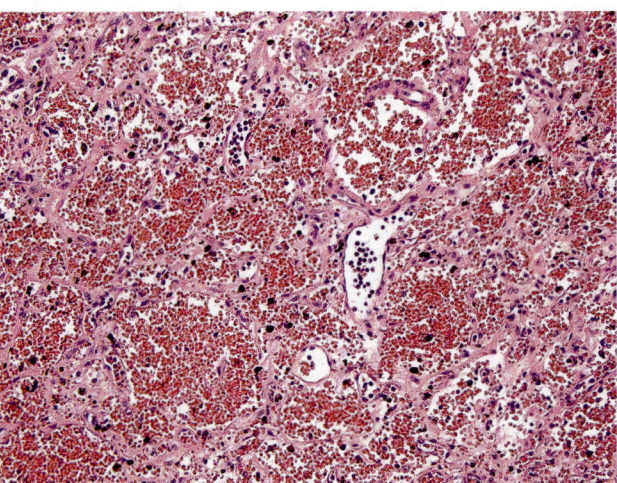

Figure 3.420. This renal cell carcinoma shows abundant blood-filled spaces, suggestive of a hemangioma; however, the slightly larger nuclei that represent the epithelial cells are a clue to the epithelial nature of the tumor.

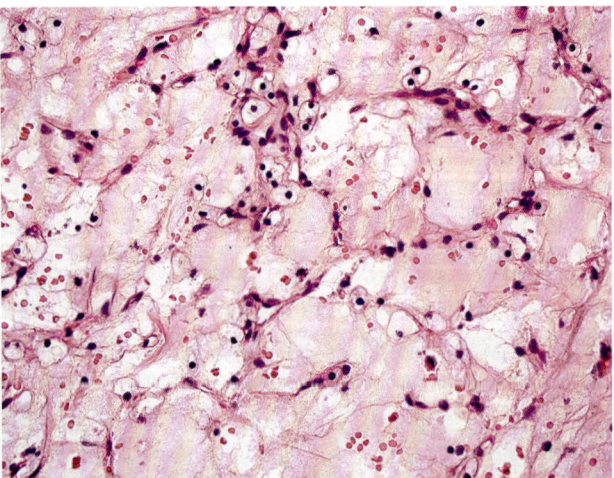

Figure 3.421. In this sclerotic area of clear cell renal cell carcinoma, there is edematous fibrous tissue with numerous capillaries. Epithelial tumor cells are present, but these could be easily mistaken for lymphocytes, histiocytes, or capillaries.

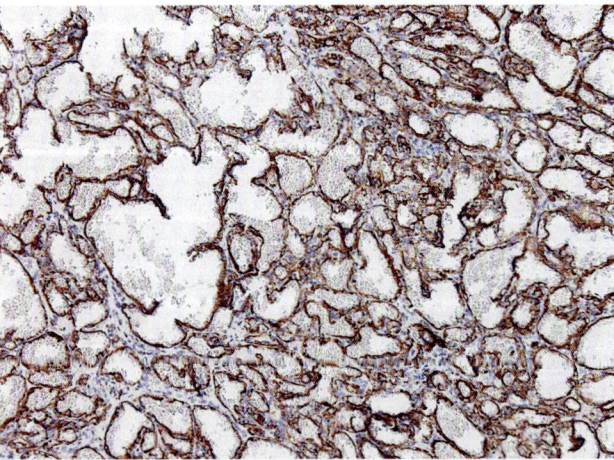

Figure 3.422. In this hemangioma-like renal cell carcinoma, keratin AE1/AE3 immunohistochemistry confirms the epithelial lining of the blood-filled spaces.

CLEAR CELL VERSUS CLEAR CELL PAPILLARY RENAL CELL CARCINOMA

Since clear cell papillary RCC has highly favorable behavior; it is likely worthwhile to ensure that restrictive criteria are used for its diagnosis. Although branched glandular structures and nuclear alignment are classic features of clear cell papillary tumors, these can occasionally be mimicked by clear cell RCC (Figure 3.424)[29,90] or even translocation RCC.[99] When the immunohistochemical findings are imperfect for clear cell papillary RCC, such as with positive staining for CD10 or AMACR or incomplete staining for cytokeratin 7 (Figures 3.425 and 3.426), it is typically prudent to diagnose clear cell RCC rather than clear cell papillary RCC.[29,90]

SUBTLE VEIN INVASION IN RENAL CANCER

As covered in the section on renal cancer staging, involvement of veins or renal sinus tissue can be easily missed at the gross level and certainly at the microscopic level, if sections are not specifically chosen to capture the nature of the tumor outpouchings. This near miss case (Figures 3.427 and 3.428) demonstrates a subtle example of early vein invasion that could be easily disregarded as part of the main tumor grossly.

UNCLASSIFIED ONCOCYTIC TUMOR

Oncocytoma is a benign renal neoplasm and eosinophilic chromophobe RCC is typically considered nonaggressive. Neoplasms with borderline features of these can be difficult to address in clinical practice. This near miss case shows a tumor with many features reminiscent of oncocytoma (Figure 3.429). However, on closer inspection, there are many single cells in the stroma and multiple readily identifiable mitotic figures (Figures 3.430 and 3.431). Most urologic pathologists would interpret multiple mitotic figures as incompatible with a diagnosis of oncocytoma.[162] Immunohistochemistry in this case also shows diffuse positivity for vimentin (Figure 3.432), which is highly unusual for oncocytoma or chromophobe RCC, except for focal staining that can occur in the "central scar" areas of the tumor.[175] Based on these incompatible features, we regarded this case as an unclassified RCC with oncocytic features. Although it is worthwhile to use the terminology of unclassified RCC relatively sparingly due to the clinical perception of aggressiveness,[178,179] we considered it necessary in this unusual case due to the very atypical findings of brisk mitotic activity and diffuse vimentin labeling, which would be odd even for eosinophilic chromophobe RCC.

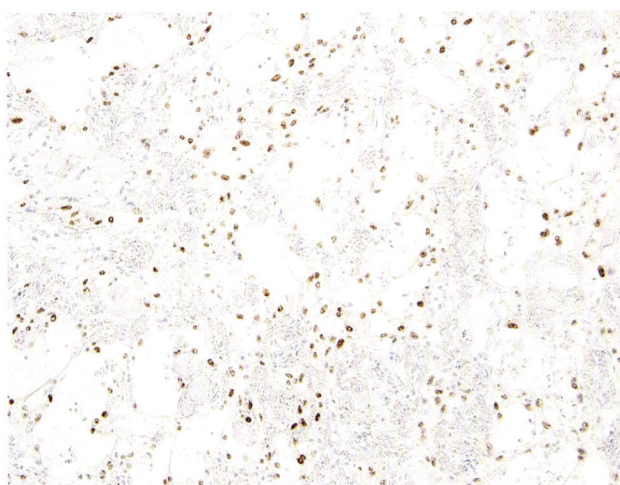

Figure 3.423. PAX8 can also help to confirm the presence of renal cell carcinoma (RCC) epithelial cells in hemangioma-like RCC.

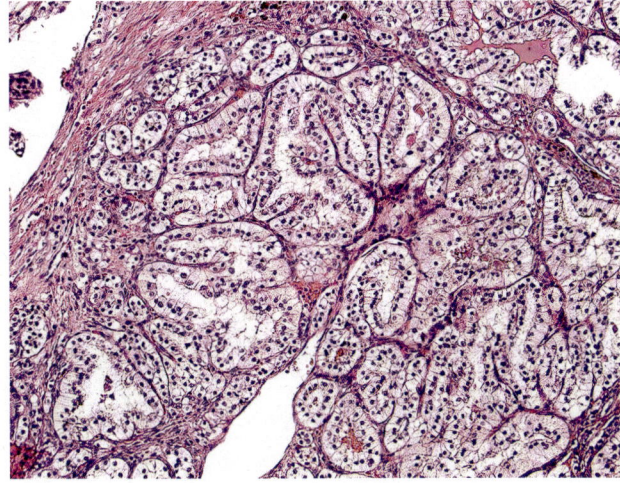

Figure 3.424. This tumor exhibits prominent nuclear alignment, reminiscent of clear cell papillary renal cell carcinoma. .

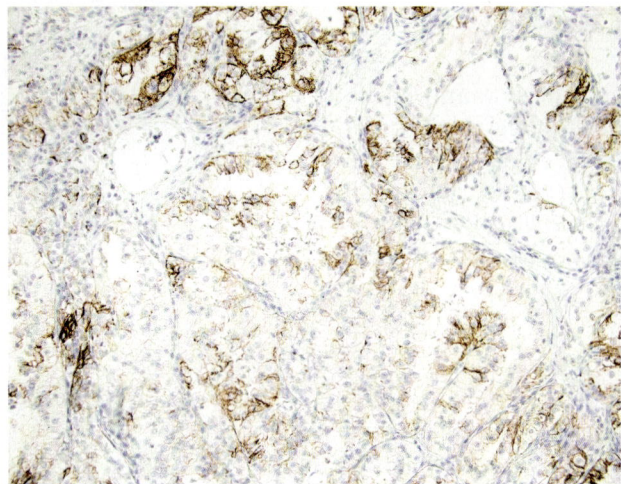

Figure 3.425. Immunohistochemistry for cytokeratin 7 shows patchy but not uniform, diffuse staining in the same tumor from Figures 3.424, which is atypical for clear cell papillary renal cell carcinoma.

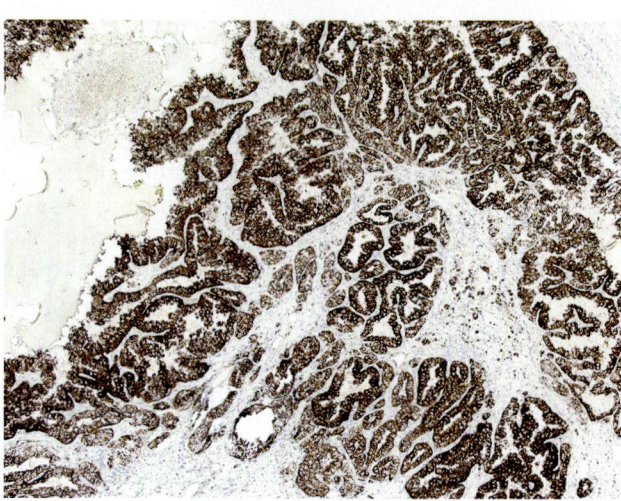

Figure 3.426. AMACR immunohistochemical staining is very strong in the tumor from Figures 3.424 and 3.425, which argues against clear cell papillary renal cell carcinoma (RCC). Our approach is to diagnose these tumors as clear cell RCC.

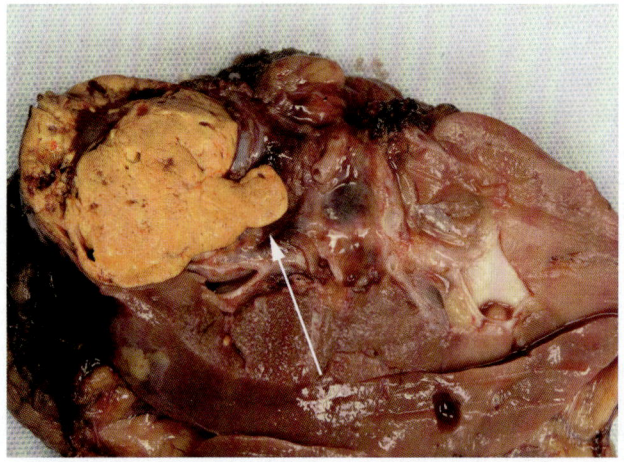

Figure 3.427. This clear cell renal cell carcinoma includes a small, finger-like outpouching (arrow) that might be assumed to be part of the tumor.

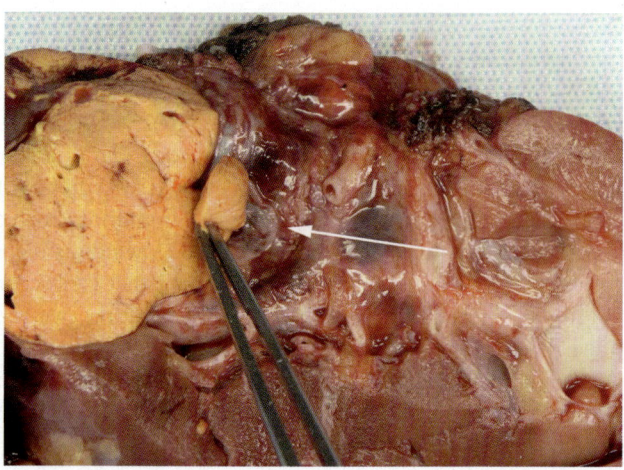

Figure 3.428. Careful gross inspection of the tumor from Figure 3.427 shows the outpouching to be a polypoid structure. When retracted, the smooth surface of the underlying vein can be visualized. Careful histologic sections should be taken to visualize the intravascular nature of such foci.

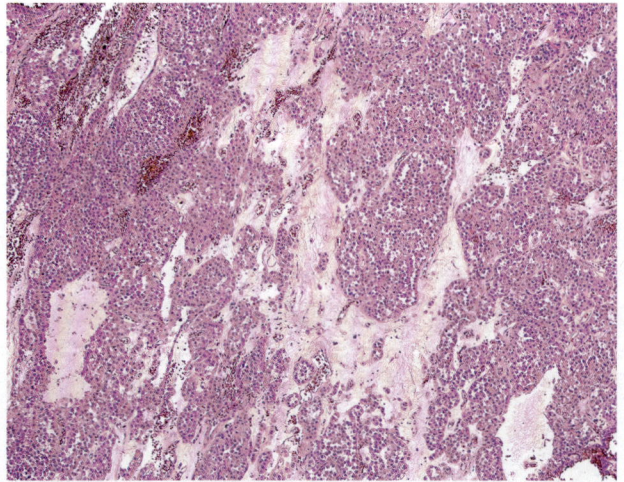

Figure 3.429. This neoplasm at low magnification shows features suggestive of oncocytoma.

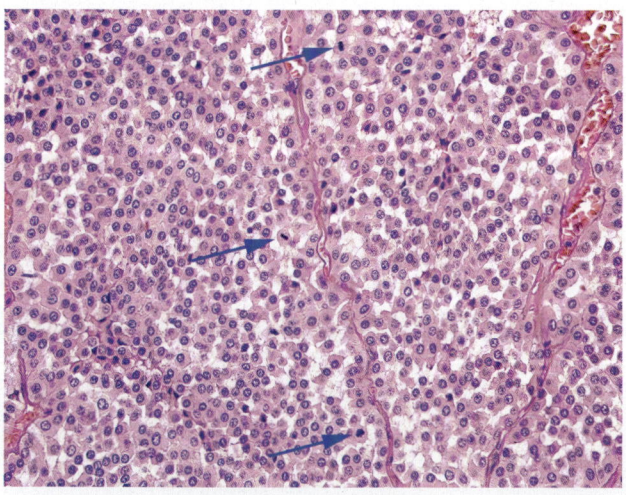

Figure 3.430. At higher magnification, the same tumor from Figure 3.429 has multiple appreciable mitotic figures (arrows).

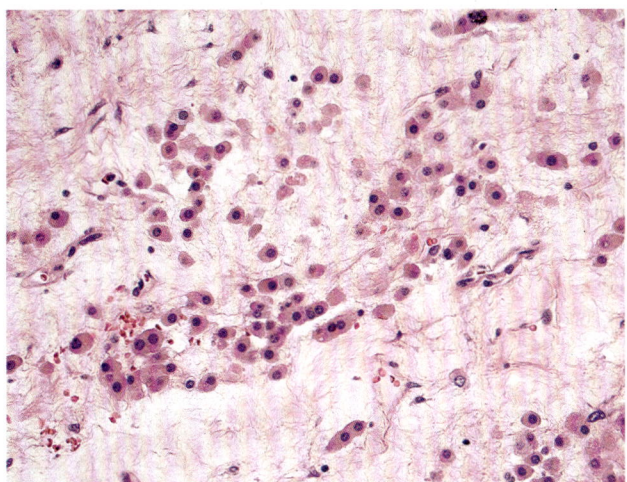

Figure 3.431. Numerous single cells are present in the stroma, which would be an unusual pattern for oncocytoma, in the same tumor from Figures 3.429 and 3.430.

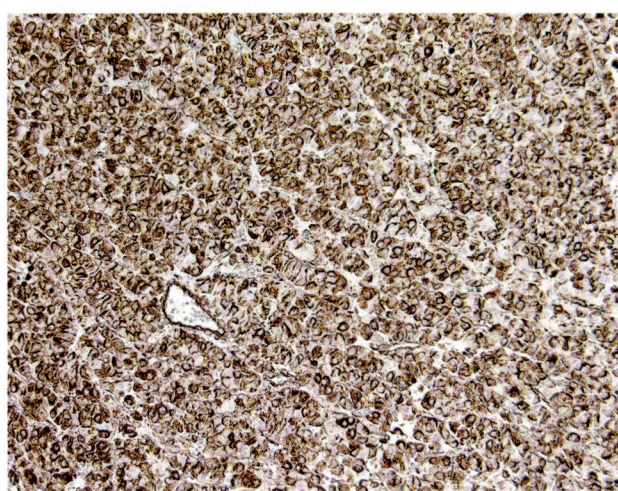

Figure 3.432. The tumor from Figures 3.429-3.431 shows diffuse immunohistochemical staining for vimentin, which is essentially incompatible with a diagnosis of oncocytoma.

References

1. Jennette JC, Olson JL, Silva FG, et al. *Heptinstall's Pathology of the Kidney*. Philadelphia, PA: Wolters Kluwer Health/Lippincott Williams & Wilkins; 2015.

2. Clapp WL, Croker BP. Kidney. In: Mills SE, ed. *Histology for Pathologists*. Philadelphia, PA: Wolters Kluwer Health/Lippincott Williams & Wilkins; 2012:891-970.

3. Henriksen KJ, Meehan SM, Chang A. Non-neoplastic renal diseases are often unrecognized in adult tumor nephrectomy specimens: a review of 246 cases. *Am J Surg Pathol*. 2007;31:1703-1708.

4. Truong LD, Shen SS, Park MH, et al. Diagnosing nonneoplastic lesions in nephrectomy specimens. *Arch Pathol Lab Med*. 2009;133:189-200.

5. Bonsib SM, Pei Y. The non-neoplastic kidney in tumor nephrectomy specimens: what can it show and what is important?. *Adv Anat Pathol*. 2010;17:235-250.

6. Bijol V, Mendez GP, Hurwitz S, et al. Evaluation of the nonneoplastic pathology in tumor nephrectomy specimens: predicting the risk of progressive renal failure. *Am J Surg Pathol*. 2006;30:575-584.

7. Fleming S. Distal nephron neoplasms. *Semin Diagn Pathol*. 2015;32:114-123.

8. Bonsib SM. Urologic diseases germane to the medical renal biopsy: review of a large diagnostic experience in the context of the renal architecture and its environs. *Adv Anat Pathol*. 2018;25:333-352.

9. Rini BI, McKiernan JM, Chang SS, et al. Kidney. In: Amin MB, Edge SB, Greene FL, et al, eds. *AJCC Cancer Staging Manual*. Switzerland: Springer; 2017:739-755.

10. Bonsib SM. T2 clear cell renal cell carcinoma is a rare entity: a study of 120 clear cell renal cell carcinomas. *J Urol*. 2005;174:1199-1202; discussion 1202.

11. Bonsib SM. The renal sinus is the principal invasive pathway: a prospective study of 100 renal cell carcinomas. *Am J Surg Pathol*. 2004;28:1594-1600.

12. Sarsik B, Simsir A, Yilmaz M, et al. Spectrum of nontumoral renal pathologies in tumor nephrectomies: nontumoral renal parenchyma changes. *Ann Diagn Pathol*. 2013;17:176-182.

13. Srigley JR, Zhou M, Allan R, et al. *Protocol for the Examination of Specimens From Patients With Invasive Carcinoma of Renal Tubular Origin*. 2017. Available at https://documents.cap.org/protocols/cp-kidney-17protocol-4011.pdf. Accessed November 27, 2019.

14. Moch H, Amin MB, Argani P, et al. Renal cell tumours. In: Moch H, Humphrey PA, Ulbright TM, et al, eds. *WHO Classification of Tumours of the Urinary System and Male Genital Organs*. Lyon: International Agency for Research on Cancer; 2016:14-17.

15. De Vriese AS, Sethi S, Nath KA, et al. Differentiating primary, genetic, and secondary FSGS in adults: a clinicopathologic approach. *J Am Soc Nephrol*. 2018;29:759-774.

16. Motzer RJ, Jonasch E, Agarwal N, et al. *NCCN Clinical Practice Guidelines in Oncology (NCCN Guidelines) Kidney Cancer.* 2019. Available at https://www.nccn.org/professionals/physician_gls/PDF/kidney.pdf. Accessed August 28, 2019.

17. Chang A, Brimo F, Montgomery EA, et al. Use of PAX8 and GATA3 in diagnosing sarcomatoid renal cell carcinoma and sarcomatoid urothelial carcinoma. *Hum Pathol.* 2013;44:1563-1568.

18. Higgins JP, Kaygusuz G, Wang L, et al. Placental S100 (S100P) and GATA3: markers for transitional epithelium and urothelial carcinoma discovered by complementary DNA microarray. *Am J Surg Pathol.* 2007;31:673-680.

19. Shen SS, Ro JY. Histologic diagnosis of renal mass biopsy. *Arch Pathol Lab Med.* 2019;143:705-710.

20. Merino MJ, Torres-Cabala C, Pinto P, et al. The morphologic spectrum of kidney tumors in hereditary leiomyomatosis and renal cell carcinoma (HLRCC) syndrome. *Am J Surg Pathol.* 2007;31:1578-1585.

21. Smith SC, Trpkov K, Chen YB, et al. Tubulocystic carcinoma of the kidney with poorly differentiated foci: a frequent morphologic pattern of fumarate hydratase-deficient renal cell carcinoma. *Am J Surg Pathol.* 2016;40:1457-1472.

22. Muller M, Guillaud-Bataille M, Salleron J, et al. Pattern multiplicity and fumarate hydratase (FH)/S-(2-succino)-cysteine (2SC) staining but not eosinophilic nucleoli with perinucleolar halos differentiate hereditary leiomyomatosis and renal cell carcinoma-associated renal cell carcinomas from kidney tumors without FH gene alteration. *Mod Pathol.* 2018;31:974-983.

23. Shuch B, Zhang J. Genetic predisposition to renal cell carcinoma: implications for counseling, testing, screening, and management. *J Clin Oncol.* 2018;36:JCO2018792523.

24. Moch H, Bonsib SM, Delahunt B, et al. Clear cell renal cell carcinoma. In: Moch H, Humphrey PA, Ulbright TM, et al, eds. *WHO Classification of Tumours of the Urinary System and Male Genital Organs.* Lyon: International Agency for Research on Cancer; 2016:18-21.

25. Reuter VE, Tickoo SK. Differential diagnosis of renal tumours with clear cell histology. *Pathology.* 2010;42:374-383.

26. Taneja K, Cheng L, Al-Obaidy K, et al. Clear cell renal cell carcinoma with a poorly-differentiated component: a novel variant causing potential diagnostic difficulty. *Mod Pathol.* 2019;32:147-148 (abstract).

27. Williamson SR, Kum JB, Goheen MP, et al. Clear cell renal cell carcinoma with a syncytial-type multinucleated giant tumor cell component: implications for differential diagnosis. *Hum Pathol.* 2014;4:735-744.

28. Williamson SR, MacLennan GT, Lopez-Beltran A, et al. Cystic partially regressed clear cell renal cell carcinoma: a potential mimic of multilocular cystic renal cell carcinoma. *Histopathology.* 2013;63:767-779.

29. Williamson SR, Gupta NS, Eble JN, et al. Clear cell renal cell carcinoma with borderline features of clear cell papillary renal cell carcinoma: combined morphologic, immunohistochemical, and cytogenetic analysis. *Am J Surg Pathol.* 2015;39:1502-1510.

30. Liu L, Qian J, Singh H, et al. Immunohistochemical analysis of chromophobe renal cell carcinoma, renal oncocytoma, and clear cell carcinoma: an optimal and practical panel for differential diagnosis. *Arch Pathol Lab Med.* 2007;131:1290-1297.

31. Laury AR, Perets R, Piao H, et al. A comprehensive analysis of PAX8 expression in human epithelial tumors. *Am J Surg Pathol.* 2011;35:816-826.

32. Tong GX, Yu WM, Beaubier NT, et al. Expression of PAX8 in normal and neoplastic renal tissues: an immunohistochemical study. *Mod Pathol.* 2009;22:1218-1227.

33. Tacha D, Zhou D, Cheng L. Expression of PAX8 in normal and neoplastic tissues: a comprehensive immunohistochemical study. *Appl Immunohistochem Mol Morphol.* 2011;19:293-299.

34. Favazza L, Chitale DA, Barod R, et al. Renal cell tumors with clear cell histology and intact VHL and chromosome 3p: a histological review of tumors from the Cancer Genome Atlas database. *Mod Pathol.* 2017;30:1603-1612.

35. Magers MJ, Cheng L. Practical molecular testing in a clinical genitourinary service. *Arch Pathol Lab Med.* 2020;144:277-289.

36. Chen YB, Xu J, Skanderup AJ, et al. Molecular analysis of aggressive renal cell carcinoma with unclassified histology reveals distinct subsets. *Nat Commun.* 2016;7:13131.

37. Klatte T, Said JW, Seligson DB, et al. Pathological, immunohistochemical and cytogenetic features of papillary renal cell carcinoma with clear cell features. *J Urol.* 2011;185:30-35.

38. Williamson SR, Grignon DJ, Cheng L, et al. Renal cell carcinoma with chromosome 6p amplification including the TFEB gene: a novel mechanism of tumor pathogenesis?. *Am J Surg Pathol.* 2017;41:287-298.

39. Bonsib SM. Renal lymphatics, and lymphatic involvement in sinus vein invasive (pT3b) clear cell renal cell carcinoma: a study of 40 cases. *Mod Pathol.* 2006;19:746-753.

40. Bonsib SM. Renal veins and venous extension in clear cell renal cell carcinoma. *Mod Pathol.* 2007;20:44-53.

41. Bonsib SM, Bhalodia A. Retrograde venous invasion in renal cell carcinoma: a complication of sinus vein and main renal vein invasion. *Mod Pathol.* 2011;24:1578-1585.

42. Trpkov K, Grignon DJ, Bonsib SM, et al. Handling and staging of renal cell carcinoma: the International Society of Urological Pathology consensus (ISUP) conference recommendations. *Am J Surg Pathol.* 2013;37:1505-1517.

43. Pagano S, Ruggeri P, Franzoso F, et al. Unusual renal cell carcinoma metastasis to the gallbladder. *Urology.* 1995;45:867-869.

44. Cheng SK, Chuah KL. Metastatic renal cell carcinoma to the pancreas: a review. *Arch Pathol Lab Med.* 2016;140:598-602.

45. Amin MB, Amin MB, Tamboli P, et al. Prognostic impact of histologic subtyping of adult renal epithelial neoplasms: an experience of 405 cases. *Am J Surg Pathol.* 2002;26:281-291.

46. Leibovich BC, Lohse CM, Crispen PL, et al. Histological subtype is an independent predictor of outcome for patients with renal cell carcinoma. *J Urol.* 2010;183:1309-1315.

47. Brugarolas J. Molecular genetics of clear-cell renal cell carcinoma. *J Clin Oncol.* 2014;32:1968-1976.

48. Reuter VE, Argani P, Zhou M, et al. Best practices recommendations in the application of immunohistochemistry in the kidney tumors: report from the International Society of Urologic Pathology consensus conference. *Am J Surg Pathol.* 2014;38:e35-e49.

49. Al-Ahmadie HA, Alden D, Fine SW, et al. Role of immunohistochemistry in the evaluation of needle core biopsies in adult renal cortical tumors: an ex vivo study. *Am J Surg Pathol.* 2011;35:949-961.

50. Al-Ahmadie HA, Alden D, Qin LX, et al. Carbonic anhydrase IX expression in clear cell renal cell carcinoma: an immunohistochemical study comparing 2 antibodies. *Am J Surg Pathol.* 2008;32:377-382.

51. Genega EM, Ghebremichael M, Najarian R, et al. Carbonic anhydrase IX expression in renal neoplasms: correlation with tumor type and grade. *Am J Clin Pathol.* 2010;134:873-879.

52. Stillebroer AB, Mulders PF, Boerman OC, et al. Carbonic anhydrase IX in renal cell carcinoma: implications for prognosis, diagnosis, and therapy. *Eur Urol.* 2010;58:75-83.

53. Donato DP, Johnson MT, Yang XJ, et al. Expression of carbonic anhydrase IX in genitourinary and adrenal tumours. *Histopathology.* 2011;59:1229-1239.

54. Gobbo S, Eble JN, Maclennan GT, et al. Renal cell carcinomas with papillary architecture and clear cell components: the utility of immunohistochemical and cytogenetical analyses in differential diagnosis. *Am J Surg Pathol.* 2008;32:1780-1786.

55. Deng FM, Kong MX, Zhou M. Papillary or pseudopapillary tumors of the kidney. *Semin Diagn Pathol.* 2015;32:124-139.

56. Paner G, Amin MB, Moch H, et al. Chromophobe renal cell carcinoma. In: Moch H, Humphrey PA, Ulbright TM, et al, eds. *WHO Classification of Tumours of the Urinary System and Male Genital Organs.* Lyon: International Agency for Research on Cancer; 2016:27-28.

57. Jacob JM, Williamson SR, Gondim DD, et al. Characteristics of the peritumoral pseudocapsule vary predictably with histologic subtype of T1 renal neoplasms. *Urology.* 2015;86:956-961.

58. Wobker SE, Williamson SR. Modern pathologic diagnosis of renal oncocytoma. *J Kidney Cancer VHL.* 2017;4:1-12.

59. Amin MB, Paner GP, Alvarado-Cabrero I, et al. Chromophobe renal cell carcinoma: histomorphologic characteristics and evaluation of conventional pathologic prognostic parameters in 145 cases. *Am J Surg Pathol.* 2008;32:1822-1834.

60. Przybycin CG, Cronin AM, Darvishian F, et al. Chromophobe renal cell carcinoma: a clinicopathologic study of 203 tumors in 200 patients with primary resection at a single institution. *Am J Surg Pathol.* 2011;35:962-970.

61. Akhtar M, Tulbah A, Kardar AH, et al. Sarcomatoid renal cell carcinoma: the chromophobe connection. *Am J Surg Pathol.* 1997;21:1188-1195.

62. Delahunt B, Cheville JC, Martignoni G, et al. The International Society of Urological Pathology (ISUP) grading system for renal cell carcinoma and other prognostic parameters. *Am J Surg Pathol*. 2013;37:1490-1504.

63. Delahunt B, Eble JN, Egevad L, et al. Grading of renal cell carcinoma. *Histopathology*. 2019;74:4-17.

64. Meskawi M, Sun M, Ismail S, et al. Fuhrman grade [corrected] has no added value in prediction of mortality after partial or [corrected] radical nephrectomy for chromophobe renal cell carcinoma patients. *Mod Pathol*. 2013;26:1144-1149.

65. Delahunt B, Sika-Paotonu D, Bethwaite PB, et al. Fuhrman grading is not appropriate for chromophobe renal cell carcinoma. *Am J Surg Pathol*. 2007;31:957-960.

66. Paner GP, Amin MB, Alvarado-Cabrero I, et al. A novel tumor grading scheme for chromophobe renal cell carcinoma: prognostic utility and comparison with Fuhrman nuclear grade. *Am J Surg Pathol*. 2010;34:1233-1240.

67. Davis CF, Ricketts CJ, Wang M, et al. The somatic genomic landscape of chromophobe renal cell carcinoma. *Cancer Cell*. 2014;26:319-330.

68. Sperga M, Martinek P, Vanecek T, et al. Chromophobe renal cell carcinoma–chromosomal aberration variability and its relation to Paner grading system: an array CGH and FISH analysis of 37 cases. *Virchows Arch*. 2013;463:563-573.

69. Srigley JR, Delahunt B, Eble JN, et al. The International Society of Urological Pathology (ISUP) vancouver classification of renal neoplasia. *Am J Surg Pathol*. 2013;37:1469-1489.

70. Srigley JR, Cheng L, Grignon DJ, et al. Clear cell papillary renal cell carcinoma. In: Moch H, Humphrey PA, Ulbright TM, et al, eds. *WHO Classification of Tumours of the Urinary System and Male Genital Organs*. Lyon: International Agency for Research on Cancer; 2016:40-41.

71. Tickoo SK, dePeralta-Venturina MN, Harik LR, et al. Spectrum of epithelial neoplasms in end-stage renal disease: an experience from 66 tumor-bearing kidneys with emphasis on histologic patterns distinct from those in sporadic adult renal neoplasia. *Am J Surg Pathol*. 2006;30:141-153.

72. Williamson SR, Eble JN, Cheng L, et al. Clear cell papillary renal cell carcinoma: differential diagnosis and extended immunohistochemical profile. *Mod Pathol*. 2013;26:697-708.

73. Zhou H, Zheng S, Truong LD, et al. Clear cell papillary renal cell carcinoma is the fourth most common histologic type of renal cell carcinoma in 290 consecutive nephrectomies for renal cell carcinoma. *Hum Pathol*. 2014;45:59-64.

74. Rohan SM, Xiao Y, Liang Y, et al. Clear-cell papillary renal cell carcinoma: molecular and immunohistochemical analysis with emphasis on the von Hippel-Lindau gene and hypoxia-inducible factor pathway-related proteins. *Mod Pathol*. 2011;24:1207-1220.

75. Brunelli M, Erdini F, Cima L, et al. Proximal CD13 versus distal GATA-3 expression in renal neoplasia according to WHO 2016 classification. *Appl Immunohistochem Mol Morphol*. 2018;26:316-323.

76. Mantilla JG, Antic T, Tretiakova M. GATA3 as a valuable marker to distinguish clear cell papillary renal cell carcinomas from morphologic mimics. *Hum Pathol*. 2017;66:152-158.

77. Aydin H, Chen L, Cheng L, et al. Clear cell tubulopapillary renal cell carcinoma: a study of 36 distinctive low-grade epithelial tumors of the kidney. *Am J Surg Pathol*. 2010;34:1608-1621.

78. Mantilla JG, Antic T, tretiakova MS. GATA-3 is a specific marker for clear cell papillary renal cell carcinoma. *Mod Pathol*. 2017;30:241A (abstract).

79. Martignoni G, Brunelli M, Segala D, et al. Validation of 34betaE12 immunoexpression in clear cell papillary renal cell carcinoma as a sensitive biomarker. *Pathology*. 2017;49:10-18.

80. Xu J, Reznik E, Lee HJ, et al. Abnormal oxidative metabolism in a quiet genomic background underlies clear cell papillary renal cell carcinoma. *eLife*. 2019;8:e38986.

81. Adam J, Couturier J, Molinie V, et al. Clear-cell papillary renal cell carcinoma: 24 cases of a distinct low-grade renal tumour and a comparative genomic hybridization array study of seven cases. *Histopathology*. 2011;58:1064-1071.

82. Fisher KE, Yin-Goen Q, Alexis D, et al. Gene expression profiling of clear cell papillary renal cell carcinoma: comparison with clear cell renal cell carcinoma and papillary renal cell carcinoma. *Mod Pathol*. 2014;27:222-230.

83. Inoue T, Matsuura K, Yoshimoto T, et al. Genomic profiling of renal cell carcinoma in patients with end-stage renal disease. *Cancer Sci*. 2012;103:569-576.

84. Munari E, Marchionni L, Chitre A, et al. Clear cell papillary renal cell carcinoma: micro-RNA expression profiling and comparison with clear cell renal cell carcinoma and papillary renal cell carcinoma. *Hum Pathol.* 2014;45:1130-1138.

85. Wolfe A, Dobin SM, Grossmann P, et al. Clonal trisomies 7,10 and 12, normal 3p and absence of VHL gene mutation in a clear cell tubulopapillary carcinoma of the kidney. *Virchows Arch.* 2011;459:457-463.

86. Morlote D, Rais-Bahrami S, Harada S, et al. A molecular profile of clear cell papillary renal cell carcinoma by next generation sequencing. *Mod Pathol.* 2018;31:370 (abstract).

87. Williamson SR, Cheng L. Clear cell renal cell tumors: not all that is "clear" is cancer. *Urol Oncol.* 2016;34:292.e217-292.e222.

88. Diolombi ML, Cheng L, Argani P, et al. Do clear cell papillary renal cell carcinomas have malignant potential?. *Am J Surg Pathol.* 2015;39:1621-1634.

89. Gupta S, Inwards CY, Van Dyke DL, et al. Defining clear cell papillary renal cell carcinoma in routine clinical practice. *Histopathology.* 2020;76:1093-1095.

90. Dhakal HP, McKenney JK, Khor LY, et al. Renal neoplasms with overlapping features of clear cell renal cell carcinoma and clear cell papillary renal cell carcinoma: a clinicopathologic study of 37 cases from a single institution. *Am J Surg Pathol.* 2016;40:141-154.

91. Williamson SR, Zhang S, Eble JN, et al. Clear cell papillary renal cell carcinoma-like tumors in patients with von Hippel-Lindau disease are unrelated to sporadic clear cell papillary renal cell carcinoma. *Am J Surg Path.* 2013;37:1131-1139.

92. Argani P. MiT family translocation renal cell carcinoma. *Semin Diagn Pathol.* 2015;32:103-113.

93. Gandhi JS, Malik F, Amin MB, et al. MiT family translocation renal cell carcinomas: a 15th anniversary update. *Histol Histopathol.* 2020;35:125-136.

94. Durinck S, Stawiski EW, Pavia-Jimenez A, et al. Spectrum of diverse genomic alterations define non-clear cell renal carcinoma subtypes. *Nat Genet.* 2015;47:13-21.

95. Xia QY, Wang XT, Ye SB, et al. Novel gene fusion of PRCC-MITF defines a new member of MiT family translocation renal cell carcinoma: clinicopathological analysis and detection of the gene fusion by RNA sequencing and FISH. *Histopathology.* 2018;72:786-794.

96. Camparo P, Vasiliu V, Molinie V, et al. Renal translocation carcinomas: clinicopathologic, immunohistochemical, and gene expression profiling analysis of 31 cases with a review of the literature. *Am J Surg Pathol.* 2008;32:656-670.

97. Martignoni G, Gobbo S, Camparo P, et al. Differential expression of cathepsin K in neoplasms harboring TFE3 gene fusions. *Mod Pathol.* 2011;24:1313-1319.

98. Martignoni G, Pea M, Gobbo S, et al. Cathepsin-K immunoreactivity distinguishes MiTF/TFE family renal translocation carcinomas from other renal carcinomas. *Mod Pathol.* 2009;22:1016-1022.

99. Xia QY, Wang Z, Chen N, et al. Xp11.2 translocation renal cell carcinoma with NONO-TFE3 gene fusion: morphology, prognosis, and potential pitfall in detecting TFE3 gene rearrangement. *Mod Pathol.* 2017;30:416-426.

100. Argani P, Zhang L, Reuter VE, et al. RBM10-TFE3 renal cell carcinoma: a potential diagnostic pitfall due to cryptic intrachromosomal Xp11.2 inversion resulting in false-negative TFE3 FISH. *Am J Surg Pathol.* 2017;41:655-662.

101. Just PA, Letourneur F, Pouliquen C, et al. Identification by FFPE RNA-Seq of a new recurrent inversion leading to RBM10-TFE3 fusion in renal cell carcinoma with subtle TFE3 break-apart FISH pattern. *Genes Chromosomes Cancer.* 2016;55:541-548.

102. Xia QY, Wang XT, Zhan XM, et al. Xp11 translocation renal cell carcinomas (RCCs) with RBM10-TFE3 gene fusion demonstrating melanotic features and overlapping morphology with t(6;11) RCC: interest and diagnostic pitfall in detecting a paracentric inversion of TFE3. *Am J Surg Pathol.* 2017;41:663-676.

103. Classe M, Malouf GG, Su X, et al. Incidence, clinicopathological features and fusion transcript landscape of translocation renal cell carcinomas. *Histopathology.* 2017;70:1089-1097.

104. Argani P, Zhang L, Sung YS, et al. A novel RBMX-TFE3 gene fusion in a highly aggressive pediatric renal perivascular epithelioid cell tumor. *Genes Chromosomes Cancer.* 2020;59:58-63.

105. Argani P, Hawkins A, Griffin CA, et al. A distinctive pediatric renal neoplasm characterized by epithelioid morphology, basement membrane production, focal HMB45 immunoreactivity, and t(6;11)(p21.1;q12) chromosome translocation. *Am J Pathol.* 2001;158:2089-2096.

106. Yousif MQ, Salih ZT, DeYoung BR, et al. Differentiating intrarenal ectopic adrenal tissue from renal cell carcinoma in the kidney. *Int J Surg Pathol*. 2018;26:588-592.

107. Sangoi AR, Fujiwara M, West RB, et al. Immunohistochemical distinction of primary adrenal cortical lesions from metastatic clear cell renal cell carcinoma: a study of 248 cases. *Am J Surg Pathol*. 2011;35:678-686.

108. Li H, Hes O, MacLennan GT, et al. Immunohistochemical distinction of metastases of renal cell carcinoma to the adrenal from primary adrenal nodules, including oncocytic tumor. *Virchows Arch*. 2015;466:581-588.

109. Doyle LA, Fletcher CD. Peripheral hemangioblastoma: clinicopathologic characterization in a series of 22 cases. *Am J Surg Pathol*. 2014;38:119-127.

110. Ip YT, Yuan JQ, Cheung H, et al. Sporadic hemangioblastoma of the kidney: an underrecognized pseudomalignant tumor?. *Am J Surg Pathol*. 2010;34:1695-1700.

111. Kuroda N, Agatsuma Y, Tamura M, et al. Sporadic renal hemangioblastoma with CA9, PAX2 and PAX8 expression: diagnostic pitfall in the differential diagnosis from clear cell renal cell carcinoma. *Int J Clin Exp Pathol*. 2015;8:2131-2138.

112. Liu Y, Qiu XS, Wang EH. Sporadic hemangioblastoma of the kidney: a rare renal tumor. *Diagn Pathol*. 2012;7:49.

113. Nonaka D, Rodriguez J, Rosai J. Extraneural hemangioblastoma: a report of 5 cases. *Am J Surg Pathol*. 2007;31:1545-1551.

114. Verine J, Sandid W, Miquel C, et al. Sporadic hemangioblastoma of the kidney: an underrecognized pseudomalignant tumor?. *Am J Surg Pathol*. 2011;35:623-624.

115. Wang CC, Wang SM, Liau JY. Sporadic hemangioblastoma of the kidney in a 29-year-old man. *Int J Surg Pathol*. 2012;20:519-522.

116. Yin WH, Li J, Chan JK. Sporadic haemangioblastoma of the kidney with rhabdoid features and focal CD10 expression: report of a case and literature review. *Diagn Pathol*. 2012;7:39.

117. Zhao M, Williamson SR, Yu J, et al. PAX8 expression in sporadic hemangioblastoma of the kidney supports a primary renal cell lineage: implications for differential diagnosis. *Hum Pathol*. 2013;44:2247-2255.

118. Carney EM, Banerjee P, Ellis CL, et al. PAX2(-)/PAX8(-)/inhibin A(+) immunoprofile in hemangioblastoma: a helpful combination in the differential diagnosis with metastatic clear cell renal cell carcinoma to the central nervous system. *Am J Surg Pathol*. 2011;35:262-267.

119. Ingold B, Wild PJ, Nocito A, et al. Renal cell carcinoma marker reliably discriminates central nervous system haemangioblastoma from brain metastases of renal cell carcinoma. *Histopathology*. 2008;52:674-681.

120. Jung SM, Kuo TT. Immunoreactivity of CD10 and inhibin alpha in differentiating hemangioblastoma of central nervous system from metastatic clear cell renal cell carcinoma. *Mod Pathol*. 2005;18:788-794.

121. Rivera AL, Takei H, Zhai J, et al. Useful immunohistochemical markers in differentiating hemangioblastoma versus metastatic renal cell carcinoma. *Neuropathology*. 2010;30:580-585.

122. Weinbreck N, Marie B, Bressenot A, et al. Immunohistochemical markers to distinguish between hemangioblastoma and metastatic clear-cell renal cell carcinoma in the brain: utility of aquaporin1 combined with cytokeratin AE1/AE3 immunostaining. *Am J Surg Pathol*. 2008;32:1051-1059.

123. Montironi R, Lopez-Beltran A, Cheng L, et al. Clear cell renal cell carcinoma (ccRCC) with hemangioblastoma-like features: a previously unreported pattern of ccRCC with possible clinical significance. *Eur Urol*. 2014;66:806-810.

124. Sancheti S, Menon S, Mukherjee S, et al. Clear cell renal cell carcinoma with hemangioblastoma-like features: a recently described pattern with unusual immunohistochemical profile. *Indian J Pathol Microbiol*. 2015;58:354-355.

125. Brimo F, Robinson B, Guo C, et al. Renal epithelioid angiomyolipoma with atypia: a series of 40 cases with emphasis on clinicopathologic prognostic indicators of malignancy. *Am J Surg Pathol*. 2010;34:715-722.

126. Eble JN, Amin MB, Young RH. Epithelioid angiomyolipoma of the kidney: a report of five cases with a prominent and diagnostically confusing epithelioid smooth muscle component. *Am J Surg Pathol*. 1997;21:1123-1130.

127. He W, Cheville JC, Sadow PM, et al. Epithelioid angiomyolipoma of the kidney: pathological features and clinical outcome in a series of consecutively resected tumors. *Mod Pathol*. 2013;26:1355-1364.

128. Kryvenko ON, Jorda M, Argani P, et al. Diagnostic approach to eosinophilic renal neoplasms. *Arch Pathol Lab Med.* 2014;138:1531-1541.

129. Martignoni G, Pea M, Reghellin D, et al. Perivascular epithelioid cell tumor (PEComa) in the genitourinary tract. *Adv Anat Pathol.* 2007;14:36-41.

130. Martignoni G, Pea M, Reghellin D, et al. PEComas: the past, the present and the future. *Virchows Arch.* 2008;452:119-132.

131. Nese N, Martignoni G, Fletcher CD, et al. Pure epithelioid PEComas (so-called epithelioid angiomyolipoma) of the kidney: a clinicopathologic study of 41 cases: detailed assessment of morphology and risk stratification. *Am J Surg Pathol.* 2011;35:161-176.

132. Martignoni G, Bonetti F, Chilosi M, et al. Cathepsin K expression in the spectrum of perivascular epithelioid cell (PEC) lesions of the kidney. *Mod Pathol.* 2012;25:100-111.

133. Argani P, Aulmann S, Illei PB, et al. A distinctive subset of PEComas harbors TFE3 gene fusions. *Am J Surg Pathol.* 2010;34:1395-1406.

134. Agaram NP, Sung YS, Zhang L, et al. Dichotomy of genetic abnormalities in PEComas with therapeutic implications. *Am J Surg Pathol.* 2015;39:813-825.

135. Eble JN, Moch H, Amin MB, et al. Papillary adenoma. In: Moch H, Humphrey PA, Ulbright TM, et al, eds. *WHO Classification of Tumours of the Urinary System and Male Genital Organs.* Lyon: International Agency for Research on Cancer; 2016:42-43.

136. Delahunt B, Algaba F, Eble J, et al. Papillary renal cell carcinoma. In: Moch H, Humphrey PA, Ulbright TM, et al, eds. *WHO Classification of Tumours of the Urinary System and Male Genital Organs.* Lyon: International Agency for Research on Cancer; 2016:23-25.

137. Skinnider BF, Folpe AL, Hennigar RA, et al. Distribution of cytokeratins and vimentin in adult renal neoplasms and normal renal tissue: potential utility of a cytokeratin antibody panel in the differential diagnosis of renal tumors. *Am J Surg Pathol.* 2005;29:747-754.

138. Skenderi F, Ulamec M, Vanecek T, et al. Warthin-like papillary renal cell carcinoma: clinico-pathologic, morphologic, immunohistochemical and molecular genetic analysis of 11 cases. *Ann Diagn Pathol.* 2017;27:48-56.

139. Ulamec M, Skenderi F, Trpkov K, et al. Solid papillary renal cell carcinoma: clinicopathologic, morphologic, and immunohistochemical analysis of 10 cases and review of the literature. *Ann Diagn Pathol.* 2016;23:51-57.

140. Hes O, Condom Mundo E, Peckova K, et al. Biphasic squamoid alveolar renal cell carcinoma: a distinctive subtype of papillary renal cell carcinoma?. *Am J Surg Pathol.* 2016;40:664-675.

141. Trpkov K, Athanazio D, Magi-Galluzzi C, et al. Biphasic papillary renal cell carcinoma is a rare mor-phological variant with frequent multifocality: a study of 28 cases. *Histopathology.* 2018;72:777-785.

142. Trpkov K, Hes O. New and emerging renal entities: a perspective post-WHO 2016 classification. *Histopathology.* 2019;74:31-59.

143. Pivovarcikova K, Peckova K, Martinek P, et al. "Mucin"-secreting papillary renal cell carcinoma: clinicopathological, immunohistochemical, and molecular genetic analysis of seven cases. *Virchows Arch.* 2016;469(1):71-80.

144. Cancer Genome Atlas Research Network, Linehan WM, Spellman PT, Ricketts CJ, et al. Comprehensive molecular characterization of papillary renal-cell carcinoma. *N Engl J Med.* 2016;374:135-145.

145. Delahunt B, Eble JN. Papillary renal cell carcinoma: a clinicopathologic and immunohistochem-ical study of 105 tumors. *Mod Pathol.* 1997;10:537-544.

146. Lefevre M, Couturier J, Sibony M, et al. Adult papillary renal tumor with oncocytic cells: clin-icopathologic, immunohistochemical, and cytogenetic features of 10 cases. *Am J Surg Pathol.* 2005;29:1576-1581.

147. Han G, Yu W, Chu J, et al. Oncocytic papillary renal cell carcinoma: a clinicopathological and genetic analysis and indolent clinical course in 14 cases. *Pathol Res Pract.* 2017;213:1-6.

148. Kunju LP, Wojno K, Wolf JS Jr, et al. Papillary renal cell carcinoma with oncocytic cells and nonoverlapping low grade nuclei: expanding the morphologic spectrum with emphasis on clinicopathologic, immunohistochemical and molecular features. *Hum Pathol.* 2008;39:96-101.

149. Hes O, Brunelli M, Michal M, et al. Oncocytic papillary renal cell carcinoma: a clinicopatho-logic, immunohistochemical, ultrastructural, and interphase cytogenetic study of 12 cases. *Ann Diagn Pathol.* 2006;10:133-139.

150. Saleeb RM, Brimo F, Farag M, et al. Toward biological subtyping of papillary renal cell carcinoma with clinical implications through histologic, immunohistochemical, and molecular analysis. *Am J Surg Pathol.* 2017;41:1618-1629.

151. Al-Obaidy KI, Eble JN, Nassiri M, et al. Recurrent KRAS mutations in papillary renal neoplasm with reverse polarity. *Mod Pathol*. 2020;33:1157-1164.

152. Al-Obaidy KI, Eble JN, Cheng L, et al. Papillary renal neoplasm with reverse polarity: a morphologic, immunohistochemical, and molecular study. *Am J Surg Pathol*. 2019;43:1099-1111.

153. Lau HD, Chan E, Fan AC, et al. A clinicopathologic and molecular analysis of fumarate hydratase-deficient renal cell carcinoma in 32 patients. *Am J Surg Pathol*. 2020;44:98-110.

154. Pivovarcikova K, Martinek P, Grossmann P, et al. Fumarate hydratase deficient renal cell carcinoma: chromosomal numerical aberration analysis of 12 cases. *Ann Diagn Pathol*. 2019;39:63-68.

155. Shyu I, Mirsadraei L, Wang X, et al. Clues to recognition of fumarate hydratase-deficient renal cell carcinoma: findings from cytologic and limited biopsy samples. *Cancer Cytopathol*. 2018;126:992-1002.

156. Trpkov K, Hes O, Agaimy A, et al. Fumarate hydratase-deficient renal cell carcinoma is strongly correlated with fumarate hydratase mutation and hereditary leiomyomatosis and renal cell carcinoma syndrome. *Am J Surg Pathol*. 2016;40:865-875.

157. Chen YB, Brannon AR, Toubaji A, et al. Hereditary leiomyomatosis and renal cell carcinoma syndrome-associated renal cancer: recognition of the syndrome by pathologic features and the utility of detecting aberrant succination by immunohistochemistry. *Am J Surg Pathol*. 2014;38:627-637.

158. Ohe C, Smith SC, Sirohi D, et al. Reappraisal of morphologic differences between renal medullary carcinoma, collecting duct carcinoma, and fumarate hydratase-deficient renal cell carcinoma. *Am J Surg Pathol*. 2018;42:279-292.

159. Grubb RL III, Franks ME, Toro J, et al. Hereditary leiomyomatosis and renal cell cancer: a syndrome associated with an aggressive form of inherited renal cancer. *J Urol*. 2007;177:2074-2079; discussion 2079-2080.

160. Smith SC, Sirohi D, Ohe C, et al. A distinctive, low-grade oncocytic fumarate hydratase-deficient renal cell carcinoma, morphologically reminiscent of succinate dehydrogenase-deficient renal cell carcinoma. *Histopathology*. 2017;71:42-52.

161. Klein MJ, Valensi QJ. Proximal tubular adenomas of kidney with so-called oncocytic features. A clinicopathologic study of 13 cases of a rarely reported neoplasm. *Cancer*. 1976;38:906-914.

162. Williamson SR, Gadde R, Trpkov K, et al. Diagnostic criteria for oncocytic renal neoplasms: a survey of urologic pathologists. *Hum Pathol*. 2017;63:149-156.

163. Trpkov K, Yilmaz A, Uzer D, et al. Renal oncocytoma revisited: a clinicopathological study of 109 cases with emphasis on problematic diagnostic features. *Histopathology*. 2010;57:893-906.

164. Perez-Ordonez B, Hamed G, Campbell S, et al. Renal oncocytoma: a clinicopathologic study of 70 cases. *Am J Surg Pathol*. 1997;21:871-883.

165. Amin MB, Crotty TB, Tickoo SK, et al. Renal oncocytoma: a reappraisal of morphologic features with clinicopathologic findings in 80 cases. *Am J Surg Pathol*. 1997;21:1-12.

166. Tickoo SK, Amin MB, Zarbo RJ. Colloidal iron staining in renal epithelial neoplasms, including chromophobe renal cell carcinoma: emphasis on technique and patterns of staining. *Am J Surg Pathol*. 1998;22:419-424.

167. Ng KL, Morais C, Bernard A, et al. A systematic review and meta-analysis of immunohistochemical biomarkers that differentiate chromophobe renal cell carcinoma from renal oncocytoma. *J Clin Pathol*. 2016;69:661-671.

168. Ng KL, Rajandram R, Morais C, et al. Differentiation of oncocytoma from chromophobe renal cell carcinoma (RCC): can novel molecular biomarkers help solve an old problem?. *J Clin Pathol*. 2014;67:97-104.

169. Trpkov K, Hes O, Bonert M, et al. Eosinophilic, solid, and cystic renal cell carcinoma: clinicopathologic study of 16 unique, sporadic neoplasms occurring in women. *Am J Surg Pathol*. 2016;40:60-71.

170. Sukov WR, Ketterling RP, Lager DJ, et al. CCND1 rearrangements and cyclin D1 overexpression in renal oncocytomas: frequency, clinicopathologic features, and utility in differentiation from chromophobe renal cell carcinoma. *Hum Pathol*. 2009;40:1296-1303.

171. Joshi S, Tolkunov D, Aviv H, et al. The genomic landscape of renal oncocytoma identifies a metabolic barrier to tumorigenesis. *Cell Rep*. 2015;13:1895-1908.

172. Williamson SR. Renal oncocytoma with perinephric fat invasion. *Int J Surg Pathol*. 2016;24:625-626.

173. Wobker SE, Przybycin CG, Sircar K, et al. Renal oncocytoma with vascular invasion: a series of 22 cases. *Hum Pathol*. 2016;58:1-6.

174. Hes O, Michal M, Sima R, et al. Renal oncocytoma with and without intravascular extension into the branches of renal vein have the same morphological, immunohistochemical, and genetic features. *Virchows Arch.* 2008;452:193-200.

175. Hes O, Michal M, Kuroda N, et al. Vimentin reactivity in renal oncocytoma: immunohistochemical study of 234 cases. *Arch Pathol Lab Med.* 2007;131:1782-1788.

176. Williamson SR, Cheng L, Gadde R, et al. Renal cell tumors with an entrapped papillary component: a collision with predilection for oncocytic tumors. *Virchows Arch.* 2020;476:399-407.

177. Richard PO, Jewett MA, Bhatt JR, et al. Active surveillance for renal neoplasms with oncocytic features is safe. *J Urol.* 2016;195:581-586.

178. Zisman A, Chao DH, Pantuck AJ, et al. Unclassified renal cell carcinoma: clinical features and prognostic impact of a new histological subtype. *J Urol.* 2002;168:950-955.

179. Karakiewicz PI, Hutterer GC, Trinh QD, et al. Unclassified renal cell carcinoma: an analysis of 85 cases. *BJU Int.* 2007;100:802-808.

180. Gobbo S, Eble JN, Delahunt B, et al. Renal cell neoplasms of oncocytosis have distinct morphologic, immunohistochemical, and cytogenetic profiles. *Am J Surg Pathol.* 2010;34:620-626.

181. Kuroda N, Tanaka A, Ohe C, et al. Review of renal oncocytosis (multiple oncocytic lesions) with focus on clinical and pathobiological aspects. *Histol Histopathol.* 2012;27:1407-1412.

182. Tickoo SK, Reuter VE, Amin MB, et al. Renal oncocytosis: a morphologic study of fourteen cases. *Am J Surg Pathol.* 1999;23:1094-1101.

183. Sabo E, Miselevich I, Bejar J, et al. The role of vimentin expression in predicting the long-term outcome of patients with localized renal cell carcinoma. *Br J Urol.* 1997;80:864-868.

184. Gill AJ, Amin MB, Smith S, et al. Succinate dehydrogenase-deficient renal carcinoma. In: Moch H, Humphrey PA, Ulbright TM, et al, eds. *WHO Classification of Tumours of the Urinary System and Male Genital Organs.* Lyon: International Agency for Research on Cancer; 2016:35-36.

185. Gill AJ, Hes O, Papathomas T, et al. Succinate dehydrogenase (SDH)-deficient renal carcinoma: a morphologically distinct entity: a clinicopathologic series of 36 tumors from 27 patients. *Am J Surg Pathol.* 2014;38:1588-1602.

186. Williamson SR, Eble JN, Amin MB, et al. Succinate dehydrogenase-deficient renal cell carcinoma: detailed characterization of 11 tumors defining a unique subtype of renal cell carcinoma. *Mod Pathol.* 2015;28:80-94.

187. Housley SL, Lindsay RS, Young B, et al. Renal carcinoma with giant mitochondria associated with germ-line mutation and somatic loss of the succinate dehydrogenase B gene. *Histopathology.* 2010;56:405-408.

188. Gill AJ, Benn DE, Chou A, et al. Immunohistochemistry for SDHB triages genetic testing of SDHB, SDHC, and SDHD in paraganglioma-pheochromocytoma syndromes. *Hum Pathol.* 2010;41:805-814.

189. Gill AJ. Succinate dehydrogenase (SDH) and mitochondrial driven neoplasia. *Pathology.* 2012;44:285-292.

190. Gill AJ. Succinate dehydrogenase (SDH)-deficient neoplasia. *Histopathology.* 2018;72:106-116.

191. Barletta JA, Hornick JL. Succinate dehydrogenase-deficient tumors: diagnostic advances and clinical implications. *Adv Anat Pathol.* 2012;19:193-203.

192. Doyle LA, Hornick JL. Gastrointestinal stromal tumours: from KIT to succinate dehydrogenase. *Histopathology.* 2014;64:53-67.

193. Guo J, Tretiakova MS, Troxell ML, et al. Tuberous sclerosis-associated renal cell carcinoma: a clinicopathologic study of 57 separate carcinomas in 18 patients. *Am J Surg Pathol.* 2014;38:1457-1467.

194. Trpkov K, Abou-Ouf H, Hes O, et al. Eosinophilic solid and cystic renal cell carcinoma (ESC RCC): further morphologic and molecular characterization of ESC RCC as a distinct entity. *Am J Surg Pathol.* 2017;41:1299-1308.

195. Li Y, Reuter VE, Matoso A, et al. Re-evaluation of 33 'unclassified' eosinophilic renal cell carcinomas in young patients. *Histopathology.* 2018;72:588-600.

196. Tretiakova MS. Eosinophilic solid and cystic renal cell carcinoma mimicking epithelioid angiomyolipoma: series of 4 primary tumors and 2 metastases. *Hum Pathol.* 2018;80:65-75.

197. McKenney JK, Przybycin CG, Trpkov K, et al. Eosinophilic solid and cystic renal cell carcinomas have metastatic potential. *Histopathology.* 2018;72:1066-1067.

198. Mehra R, Vats P, Cao X, et al. Somatic Bi-allelic loss of TSC genes in eosinophilic solid and cystic renal cell carcinoma. *Eur Urol*. 2018;74:483-486.

199. Palsgrove DN, Li Y, Pratilas CA, et al. Eosinophilic solid and cystic (ESC) renal cell carcinomas harbor TSC mutations: molecular analysis supports an expanding clinicopathologic spectrum. *Am J Surg Pathol*. 2018;42:1166-1181.

200. Parilla M, Kadri S, Patil SA, et al. Are sporadic eosinophilic solid and cystic renal cell carcinomas characterized by somatic tuberous sclerosis gene mutations?. *Am J Surg Pathol*. 2018;42:911-917.

201. Trpkov K, Williamson SR, Gao Y, et al. Low-grade oncocytic tumour of kidney (CD117-negative, cytokeratin 7-positive): a distinct entity?. *Histopathology*. 2019;75:174-184.

202. Chen YB, Mirsadraei L, Jayakumaran G, et al. Somatic mutations of TSC2 or MTOR characterize a morphologically distinct subset of sporadic renal cell carcinoma with eosinophilic and vacuolated cytoplasm. *Am J Surg Pathol*. 2019;43:121-131.

203. He H, Trpkov K, Martinek P, et al. "High-grade oncocytic renal tumor": morphologic, immunohistochemical, and molecular genetic study of 14 cases. *Virchows Arch*. 2018;473:725-738.

204. Trpkov K, Bonert M, Gao Y, et al. High-grade oncocytic tumour (HOT) of kidney in a patient with tuberous sclerosis complex. *Histopathology*. 2019;75:440-442.

205. Amin MB, MacLennan GT, Gupta R, et al. Tubulocystic carcinoma of the kidney: clinicopathologic analysis of 31 cases of a distinctive rare subtype of renal cell carcinoma. *Am J Surg Pathol*. 2009;33:384-392.

206. Zhou M, Yang XJ, Lopez JI, et al. Renal tubulocystic carcinoma is closely related to papillary renal cell carcinoma: implications for pathologic classification. *Am J Surg Pathol*. 2009;33:1840-1849.

207. Tran T, Jones CL, Williamson SR, et al. Tubulocystic renal cell carcinoma is an entity that is immunohistochemically and genetically distinct from papillary renal cell carcinoma. *Histopathology*. 2016;68:850-857.

208. Al-Hussain TO, Cheng L, Zhang S, et al. Tubulocystic carcinoma of the kidney with poorly differentiated foci: a series of 3 cases with fluorescence in situ hybridization analysis. *Hum Pathol*. 2013;44:1406-1411.

209. Skenderi F, Ulamec M, Vranic S, et al. Cystic renal oncocytoma and tubulocystic renal cell carcinoma: morphologic and immunohistochemical comparative study. *Appl Immunohistochem Mol Morphol*. 2016;24:112-119.

210. Kuroda N, Ohe C, Mikami S, et al. Review of acquired cystic disease-associated renal cell carcinoma with focus on pathobiological aspects. *Histol Histopathol*. 2011;26:1215-1218.

211. Cheuk W, Lo ES, Chan AK, et al. Atypical epithelial proliferations in acquired renal cystic disease harbor cytogenetic aberrations. *Hum Pathol*. 2002;33:761-765.

212. Matoso A, Chen YB, Rao V, et al. Atypical renal cysts: a morphologic, immunohistochemical, and molecular study. *Am J Surg Pathol*. 2016;40:202-211.

213. Amin MB, Gupta R, Ondrej H, et al. Primary thyroid-like follicular carcinoma of the kidney: report of 6 cases of a histologically distinctive adult renal epithelial neoplasm. *Am J Surg Pathol*. 2009;33:393-400.

214. Eble JN, Delahunt B. Emerging entities in renal cell neoplasia: thyroid-like follicular renal cell carcinoma and multifocal oncocytoma-like tumours associated with oncocytosis. *Pathology*. 2018;50:24-36.

215. Dhillon J, Tannir NM, Matin SF, et al. Thyroid-like follicular carcinoma of the kidney with metastases to the lungs and retroperitoneal lymph nodes. *Hum Pathol*. 2011;42:146-150.

216. Li C, Dong H, Fu W, et al. Thyroid-like follicular carcinoma of the kidney and papillary renal cell carcinoma with thyroid-like feature: comparison of two cases and literature review. *Ann Clin Lab Sci*. 2015;45:707-712.

217. Hes O, de Souza TG, Pivovarcikova K, et al. Distinctive renal cell tumor simulating atrophic kidney with 2 types of microcalcifications. Report of 3 cases. *Ann Diagn Pathol*. 2014;18:82-88.

218. Herlitz L, Hes O, Michal M, et al. "Atrophic kidney" -like lesion: clinicopathologic series of 8 cases supporting a benign entity distinct from thyroid-like follicular carcinoma. *Am J Surg Pathol*. 2018;42:1585-1595.

219. Argani P, Reuter VE, Zhang L, et al. TFEB-amplified renal cell carcinomas: an aggressive molecular subset demonstrating variable melanocytic marker expression and morphologic heterogeneity. *Am J Surg Pathol*. 2016;40:1484-1495.

220. Gupta S, Argani P, Jungbluth AA, et al. TFEB expression profiling in renal cell carcinomas: clinicopathologic correlations. *Am J Surg Pathol*. 2019;43:1445-1461.

221. Gupta S, Johnson SH, Vasmatzis G, et al. TFEB-VEGFA (6p21.1) co-amplified renal cell carcinoma: a distinct entity with potential implications for clinical management. *Mod Pathol*. 2017;30:998-1012.

222. Peckova K, Vanecek T, Martinek P, et al. Aggressive and nonaggressive translocation t(6;11) renal cell carcinoma: comparative study of 6 cases and review of the literature. *Ann Diagn Pathol*. 2014;18:351-357.

223. Skala SL, Xiao H, Udager AM, et al. Detection of 6 TFEB-amplified renal cell carcinomas and 25 renal cell carcinomas with MITF translocations: systematic morphologic analysis of 85 cases evaluated by clinical TFE3 and TFEB FISH assays. *Mod Pathol*. 2018;31:179-197.

224. Bodokh Y, Ambrosetti D, Kubiniek V, et al. ALK-TPM3 rearrangement in adult renal cell carcinoma: report of a new case showing loss of chromosome 3 and literature review. *Cancer Genet*. 2018;221:31-37.

225. Cajaiba MM, Jennings LJ, George D, et al. Expanding the spectrum of ALK-rearranged renal cell carcinomas in children: identification of a novel HOOK1-ALK fusion transcript. *Genes Chromosomes Cancer*. 2016;55:814-817.

226. Debelenko LV, Raimondi SC, Daw N, et al. Renal cell carcinoma with novel VCL-ALK fusion: new representative of ALK-associated tumor spectrum. *Mod Pathol*. 2011;24:430-442.

227. Hodge JC, Pearce KE, Sukov WR. Distinct ALK-rearranged and VCL-negative papillary renal cell carcinoma variant in two adults without sickle cell trait. *Mod Pathol*. 2013;26:604-605.

228. Kuroda N, Liu Y, Tretiakova M, et al. Clinicopathological study of seven cases of ALK-positive renal tumor identification of new fusion partners including CLIP1 and KIF5B genes. *Mod Pathol*. 2019;32:85.

229. Marino-Enriquez A, Ou WB, Weldon CB, et al. ALK rearrangement in sickle cell trait-associated renal medullary carcinoma. *Genes Chromosomes Cancer*. 2011;50:146-153.

230. Smith NE, Deyrup AT, Marino-Enriquez A, et al. VCL-ALK renal cell carcinoma in children with sickle-cell trait: the eighth sickle-cell nephropathy?. *Am J Surg Pathol*. 2014;38:858-863.

231. Sukov WR, Hodge JC, Lohse CM, et al. ALK alterations in adult renal cell carcinoma: frequency, clinicopathologic features and outcome in a large series of consecutively treated patients. *Mod Pathol*. 2012;25:1516-1525.

232. Yu W, Wang Y, Jiang Y, et al. Genetic analysis and clinicopathological features of ALK-rearranged renal cell carcinoma in a large series of resected Chinese renal cell carcinoma patients and literature review. *Histopathology*. 2017;71:53-62.

233. Williamson SR. Renal cell carcinomas with a mesenchymal stromal component: what do we know so far?. *Pathology*. 2019;51:453-462.

234. Pal SK, Bergerot P, Dizman N, et al. Responses to alectinib in ALK-rearranged papillary renal cell carcinoma. *Eur Urol*. 2018;74:124-128.

235. Hornick JL, Fletcher CD. PEComa: what do we know so far?. *Histopathology*. 2006;48:75-82.

236. Folpe AL, Kwiatkowski DJ. Perivascular epithelioid cell neoplasms: pathology and pathogenesis. *Hum Pathol*. 2010;41:1-15.

237. Martignoni G, Pea M, Bonetti F, et al. Oncocytoma-like angiomyolipoma. A clinicopathologic and immunohistochemical study of 2 cases. *Arch Pathol Lab Med*. 2002;126:610-612.

238. Martignoni G, Cheville J, Fletcher CDM, et al. Mesenchymal tumours occurring mainly in adults. In: Moch H, Humphrey PA, Ulbright TM, et al, eds. *WHO Classification of Tumours of the Urinary System and Male Genital Organs*. Lyon: International Agency for Research on Cancer; 2016:59-69.

239. Kuroda N, Gotoda H, Ohe C, et al. Review of juxtaglomerular cell tumor with focus on pathobiological aspect. *Diagn Pathol*. 2011;6:80.

240. Kuroda N, Maris S, Monzon FA, et al. Juxtaglomerular cell tumor: a morphological, immunohistochemical and genetic study of six cases. *Hum Pathol*. 2013;44:47-54.

241. Duan X, Bruneval P, Hammadeh R, et al. Metastatic juxtaglomerular cell tumor in a 52-year-old man. *Am J Surg Pathol*. 2004;28:1098-1102.

242. Sirohi D, Smith SC, Epstein JI, et al. Pericytic tumors of the kidney-a clinicopathologic analysis of 17 cases. *Hum Pathol*. 2017;64:106-117.

243. Zhao M, Williamson SR, Sun K, et al. Benign perivascular myoid cell tumor (myopericytoma) of the urinary tract: a report of 2 cases with an emphasis on differential diagnosis. *Hum Pathol*. 2014;45:1115-1121.

244. Al-Ahmadie HA, Yilmaz A, Olgac S, et al. Glomus tumor of the kidney: a report of 3 cases involving renal parenchyma and review of the literature. *Am J Surg Pathol*. 2007;31:585-591.

245. Herawi M, Parwani AV, Edlow D, et al. Glomus tumor of renal pelvis: a case report and review of the literature. *Hum Pathol*. 2005;36:299-302.

246. Li J, Zhao M, Chen Z, et al. Renal myopericytoma: a clinicopathologic study of six cases and review of the literature. *Int J Clin Exp Pathol*. 2015;8:4307-4320.

247. Lamba G, Rafiyath SM, Kaur H, et al. Malignant glomus tumor of kidney: the first reported case and review of literature. *Hum Pathol*. 2011;42:1200-1203.

248. Hansel DE, Epstein JI, Berbescu E, et al. Renal carcinoid tumor: a clinicopathologic study of 21 cases. *Am J Surg Pathol*. 2007;31:1539-1544.

249. Kuroda N, Alvarado-Cabrero I, Sima R, et al. Renal carcinoid tumor: an immunohistochemical and molecular genetic study of four cases. *Oncol Lett*. 2010;1:87-90.

250. Kuroda N, Tanaka A, Ohe C, et al. Review of renal carcinoid tumor with focus on clinical and pathobiological aspects. *Histol Histopathol*. 2013;28:15-21.

251. Pivovarcikova K, Agaimy A, Martinek P, et al. Primary renal well-differentiated neuroendocrine tumour (carcinoid): next-generation sequencing study of 11 cases. *Histopathology*. 2019;75:104-117.

252. Lane BR, Chery F, Jour G, et al. Renal neuroendocrine tumours: a clinicopathological study. *BJU Int*. 2007;100:1030-1035.

253. Raslan WF, Ro JY, Ordonez NG, et al. Primary carcinoid of the kidney. Immunohistochemical and ultrastructural studies of five patients. *Cancer*. 1993;72:2660-2666.

254. Aung PP, Killian K, Poropatich CO, et al. Primary neuroendocrine tumors of the kidney: morphological and molecular alterations of an uncommon malignancy. *Hum Pathol*. 2013;44:873-880.

255. Jeung JA, Cao D, Selli BW, et al. Primary renal carcinoid tumors: clinicopathologic features of 9 cases with emphasis on novel immunohistochemical findings. *Hum Pathol*. 2011;42:1554-1561.

256. Liau JY, Tsai JH, Jeng YM, et al. The diagnostic utility of PAX8 for neuroendocrine tumors: an immunohistochemical reappraisal. *Appl Immunohistochem Mol Morphol*. 2016;24:57-63.

257. Moch H, Cheville J. Neuroendocrine tumours. In: Moch H, Humphrey PA, Ulbright TM, et al, eds. *WHO Classification of Tumours of the Urinary System and Male Genital Organs*. Lyon: International Agency for Research on Cancer; 2016:72-73.

258. Grignon DJ, Eble JN, Argani P, et al. Metanephric tumours. In: Moch H, Humphrey PA, Ulbright TM, et al, eds. *WHO Classification of Tumours of the Urinary System and Male Genital Organs*. Lyon: International Agency for Research on Cancer; 2016:45-47.

259. Kinney SN, Eble JN, Hes O, et al. Metanephric adenoma: the utility of immunohistochemical and cytogenetic analyses in differential diagnosis, including solid variant papillary renal cell carcinoma and epithelial-predominant nephroblastoma. *Mod Pathol*. 2015;28:1236-1248.

260. Montironi R, Cheng L, Lopez-Beltran A, et al. Multilocular cystic renal neoplasm of low malignant potential. In: Moch H, Humphrey PA, Ulbright TM, et al, eds. *WHO Classification of Tumours of the Urinary System and Male Genital Organs*. Lyon: International Agency for Research on Cancer; 2016:22.

261. Corica FA, Iczkowski KA, Cheng L, et al. Cystic renal cell carcinoma is cured by resection: a study of 24 cases with long-term follow-up. *J Urol*. 1999;161:408-411.

262. Park JJ, Jeong BC, Kim CK, et al. Postoperative outcome of cystic renal cell carcinoma defined on preoperative imaging: a retrospective study. *J Urol*. 2017;197:991-997.

263. Williamson SR, Halat S, Eble JN, et al. Multilocular cystic renal cell carcinoma: similarities and differences in immunoprofile compared with clear cell renal cell carcinoma. *Am J Surg Pathol*. 2012;36:1425-1433.

264. Brimo F, Atallah C, Li G, et al. Cystic clear cell papillary renal cell carcinoma: is it related to multilocular clear cell cystic neoplasm of low malignant potential?. *Histopathology*. 2016;68:666-672.

265. von Teichman A, Comperat E, Behnke S, et al. VHL mutations and dysregulation of pVHL- and PTEN-controlled pathways in multilocular cystic renal cell carcinoma. *Mod Pathol*. 2011;24:571-578.

266. Halat S, Eble JN, Grignon DJ, et al. Multilocular cystic renal cell carcinoma is a subtype of clear cell renal cell carcinoma. *Mod Pathol*. 2010;23:931-936.

267. Liapis H, Winyard PJD. Cystic diseases and developmental kidney defects. In: Jennette JC, Olson JL, Silva FG, et al, eds. *Heptinstall's Pathology of the Kidney*. Philadelphia, PA: Wolters Kluwer Health/Lippincott Williams & Wilkins; 2015:119-171.

268. Smith SC, Mohanty SK, Kunju LP, et al. Uroplakin II outperforms uroplakin III in diagnostically challenging settings. *Histopathology*. 2014;65:132-138.

269. Leivo MZ, Elson PJ, Tacha DE, et al. A combination of p40, GATA-3 and uroplakin II shows utility in the diagnosis and prognosis of muscle-invasive urothelial carcinoma. *Pathology*. 2016;48:543-549.

270. Miettinen M, McCue PA, Sarlomo-Rikala M, et al. GATA3: a multispecific but potentially useful marker in surgical pathology: a systematic analysis of 2500 epithelial and nonepithelial tumors. *Am J Surg Pathol*. 2014;38:13-22.

271. Gonzalez-Roibon N, Albadine R, Sharma R, et al. The role of GATA binding protein 3 in the differential diagnosis of collecting duct and upper tract urothelial carcinomas. *Hum Pathol*. 2013;44:2651-2657.

272. Albadine R, Schultz L, Illei P, et al. PAX8 (+)/p63 (-) immunostaining pattern in renal collecting duct carcinoma (CDC): a useful immunoprofile in the differential diagnosis of CDC versus urothelial carcinoma of upper urinary tract. *Am J Surg Pathol*. 2010;34:965-969.

273. Amin MB, Smith SC, Agaimy A, et al. Collecting duct carcinoma versus renal medullary carcinoma: an appeal for nosologic and biological clarity. *Am J Surg Pathol*. 2014;38:871-874.

274. Liu Q, Galli S, Srinivasan R, et al. Renal medullary carcinoma: molecular, immunohistochemistry, and morphologic correlation. *Am J Surg Pathol*. 2013;37:368-374.

275. Calderaro J, Masliah-Planchon J, Richer W, et al. Balanced translocations disrupting SMARCB1 are hallmark recurrent genetic alterations in renal medullary carcinomas. *Eur Urol*. 2016;69:1055-1061.

276. Calderaro J, Moroch J, Pierron G, et al. SMARCB1/INI1 inactivation in renal medullary carcinoma. *Histopathology*. 2012;61:428-435.

277. Carlo MI, Chaim J, Patil S, et al. Genomic characterization of renal medullary carcinoma and treatment outcomes. *Clin Genitourin Cancer*. 2017;15:e987-e994.

278. Cheng JX, Tretiakova M, Gong C, et al. Renal medullary carcinoma: rhabdoid features and the absence of INI1 expression as markers of aggressive behavior. *Mod Pathol*. 2008;21:647-652.

279. Jia L, Carlo MI, Khan H, et al. Distinctive mechanisms underlie the loss of SMARCB1 protein expression in renal medullary carcinoma: morphologic and molecular analysis of 20 cases. *Mod Pathol*. 2019;32:1329-1343.

280. Rao P, Tannir NM, Tamboli P. Expression of OCT3/4 in renal medullary carcinoma represents a potential diagnostic pitfall. *Am J Surg Pathol*. 2012;36:583-588.

281. Colombo P, Smith SC, Massa S, et al. Unclassified renal cell carcinoma with medullary phenotype versus renal medullary carcinoma: lessons from diagnosis in an Italian man found to harbor sickle cell trait. *Urol Case Rep*. 2015;3:215-218.

282. Sirohi D, Smith SC, Ohe C, et al. Renal cell carcinoma, unclassified with medullary phenotype: poorly differentiated adenocarcinomas overlapping with renal medullary carcinoma. *Hum Pathol*. 2017;67:134-145.

283. Folpe AL. "Hey! Whatever happened to hemangiopericytoma and fibrosarcoma?" an update on selected conceptual advances in soft tissue pathology which have occurred over the past 50 years. *Hum Pathol*. 2020;95:113-136.

284. Gupta R, Billis A, Shah RB, et al. Carcinoma of the collecting ducts of Bellini and renal medullary carcinoma: clinicopathologic analysis of 52 cases of rare aggressive subtypes of renal cell carcinoma with a focus on their interrelationship. *Am J Surg Pathol*. 2012;36:1265-1278.

285. Pal SK, Choueiri TK, Wang K, et al. Characterization of clinical cases of collecting duct carcinoma of the kidney assessed by comprehensive genomic profiling. *Eur Urol*. 2016;70:516-521.

286. Huang H, Tamboli P, Karam JA, et al. Secondary malignancies diagnosed using kidney needle core biopsies: a clinical and pathological study of 75 cases. *Hum Pathol*. 2016;52:55-60.

287. Wu AJ, Mehra R, Hafez K, et al. Metastases to the kidney: a clinicopathological study of 43 cases with an emphasis on deceptive features. *Histopathology*. 2015;66:587-597.

288. Zhou C, Urbauer DL, Fellman BM, et al. Metastases to the kidney: a comprehensive analysis of 151 patients from a tertiary referral centre. *BJU Int*. 2016;117:775-782.

289. Tamboli P, Ro JY, Amin MB, et al. Benign tumors and tumor-like lesions of the adult kidney. Part II: benign mesenchymal and mixed neoplasms, and tumor-like lesions. *Adv Anat Pathol*. 2000;7:47-66.

290. Calio A, Warfel KA, Eble JN. Pathological features and clinical associations of 58 small incidental angiomyolipomas of the kidney. *Hum Pathol*. 2016;58:41-46.

291. Tanas Isikci O, He H, Grossmann P, et al. Low-grade spindle cell proliferation in clear cell renal cell carcinoma is unlikely to be an initial step in sarcomatoid differentiation. *Histopathology*. 2018;72:804-813.

292. de Peralta-Venturina M, Moch H, Amin M, et al. Sarcomatoid differentiation in renal cell carcinoma: a study of 101 cases. *Am J Surg Pathol*. 2001;25:275-284.

293. Delahunt B. Sarcomatoid renal carcinoma: the final common dedifferentiation pathway of renal epithelial malignancies. *Pathology*. 1999;31:185-190.

294. Petersson F, Michal M, Franco M, et al. Chromophobe renal cell carcinoma with liposarcomatous dedifferentiation – report of a unique case. *Int J Clin Exp Pathol*. 2010;3:534-540.

295. Przybycin CG, McKenney JK, Reynolds JP, et al. Rhabdoid differentiation is associated with aggressive behavior in renal cell carcinoma: a clinicopathologic analysis of 76 cases with clinical follow-up. *Am J Surg Pathol*. 2014;38:1260-1265.

296. Chapman-Fredricks JR, Herrera L, Bracho J, et al. Adult renal cell carcinoma with rhabdoid morphology represents a neoplastic dedifferentiation analogous to sarcomatoid carcinoma. *Ann Diagn Pathol*. 2011;15:333-337.

297. Kuroda N, Karashima T, Inoue K, et al. Review of renal cell carcinoma with rhabdoid features with focus on clinical and pathobiological aspects. *Pol J Pathol*. 2015;66:3-8.

298. Zhang BY, Cheville JC, Thompson RH, et al. Impact of rhabdoid differentiation on prognosis for patients with grade 4 renal cell carcinoma. *Eur Urol*. 2015;68:5-7.

299. Fine SW, Argani P, DeMarzo AM, et al. Expanding the histologic spectrum of mucinous tubular and spindle cell carcinoma of the kidney. *Am J Surg Pathol*. 2006;30:1554-1560.

300. Samaratunga H, Delahunt B. Mesenchymal tumors of adult kidney. *Semin Diagn Pathol*. 2015;32:160-171.

301. Patil PA, McKenney JK, Trpkov K, et al. Renal leiomyoma: a contemporary multi-institution study of an infrequent and frequently misclassified neoplasm. *Am J Surg Pathol*. 2015;39:349-356.

302. Gupta S, Jimenez RE, Folpe AL, et al. Renal leiomyoma and leiomyosarcoma: a study of 57 cases. *Am J Surg Pathol*. 2016;40:1557-1563.

303. Calio A, Warfel KA, Eble JN. Renomedullary interstitial cell tumors: pathologic features and clinical correlations. *Am J Surg Pathol*. 2016;40:1693-1701.

304. Bazzi WM, Huang H, Al-Ahmadie H, et al. Clinicopathologic features of renomedullary interstitial cell tumor presenting as the main solid renal mass. *Urology*. 2014;83:1104-1106.

305. Lu Z, Al-Obaidy K, Cheng L, et al. Immunohistochemical characteristics of renomedullary interstitial cell tumor: a study of 41 tumors with emphasis on differential diagnosis of mesenchymal neoplasms. *Hum Pathol*. 2018;82:46-50.

306. Kouba E, Simper NB, Chen S, et al. Solitary fibrous tumour of the genitourinary tract: a clinicopathological study of 11 cases and their association with the NAB2-STAT6 fusion gene. *J Clin Pathol*. 2017;70:508-514.

307. Kuroda N, Ohe C, Sakaida N, et al. Solitary fibrous tumor of the kidney with focus on clinical and pathobiological aspects. *Int J Clin Exp Pathol*. 2014;7:2737-2742.

308. Demicco EG, Park MS, Araujo DM, et al. Solitary fibrous tumor: a clinicopathological study of 110 cases and proposed risk assessment model. *Mod Pathol*. 2012;25:1298-1306.

309. Cortes LG, Caserta NM, Billis A. Fat-forming solitary fibrous tumor of the kidney: a case report. *Anal Quant Cytopathol Histpathol*. 2014;36:295-298.

310. McDaniel AS, Palanisamy N, Smith SC, et al. A subset of solitary fibrous tumors express nuclear PAX8 and PAX2: a potential diagnostic pitfall. *Histol Histopathol*. 2016;31:223-230.

311. Kapusta LR, Weiss MA, Ramsay J, et al. Inflammatory myofibroblastic tumors of the kidney: a clinicopathologic and immunohistochemical study of 12 cases. *Am J Surg Pathol*. 2003;27:658-666.

312. Montgomery EA, Shuster DD, Burkart AL, et al. Inflammatory myofibroblastic tumors of the urinary tract: a clinicopathologic study of 46 cases, including a malignant example inflammatory fibrosarcoma and a subset associated with high-grade urothelial carcinoma. *Am J Surg Pathol*. 2006;30:1502-1512.

313. Hirsch MS, Dal Cin P, Fletcher CD. ALK expression in pseudosarcomatous myofibroblastic proliferations of the genitourinary tract. *Histopathology*. 2006;48:569-578.

314. Jebastin JAS, Smith SC, Perry KD, et al. Pseudosarcomatous myofibroblastic proliferations of the genitourinary tract are genetically different from nodular fasciitis and lack USP6, ROS1 and ETV6 gene rearrangements. *Histopathology*. 2018;73:321-326.

315. Brown JG, Folpe AL, Rao P, et al. Primary vascular tumors and tumor-like lesions of the kidney: a clinicopathologic analysis of 25 cases. *Am J Surg Pathol*. 2010;34:942-949.

316. Kryvenko ON, Gupta NS, Meier FA, et al. Anastomosing hemangioma of the genitourinary system: eight cases in the kidney and ovary with immunohistochemical and ultrastructural analysis. *Am J Clin Pathol*. 2011;136:450-457.

317. Kryvenko ON, Haley SL, Smith SC, et al. Haemangiomas in kidneys with end-stage renal disease: a novel clinicopathological association. *Histopathology*. 2014;65:309-318.

318. Kuroda N, Ohe C, Deepika S, et al. Review of renal anastomosing hemangioma with focus on clinical and pathological aspects. *Pol J Pathol*. 2016;67:97-101.

319. Mehta V, Ananthanarayanan V, Antic T, et al. Primary benign vascular tumors and tumorlike lesions of the kidney: a clinicopathologic analysis of 15 cases. *Virchows Arch*. 2012;461:669-676.

320. Montgomery E, Epstein JI. Anastomosing hemangioma of the genitourinary tract: a lesion mimicking angiosarcoma. *Am J Surg Pathol*. 2009;33:1364-1369.

321. Kryvenko ON, Roquero L, Gupta NS, et al. Low-grade clear cell renal cell carcinoma mimicking hemangioma of the kidney: a series of 4 cases. *Arch Pathol Lab Med*. 2013;137:251-254.

322. Verine J. Differential diagnosis of primary benign vascular tumors and/or tumor-like lesions of the kidney: immunohistochemical stains should not be restricted to vascular and pan cytokeratin markers. *Virchows Arch*. 2013;462:365-367.

323. Cossu-Rocca P, Eble JN, Delahunt B, et al. Renal mucinous tubular and spindle carcinoma lacks the gains of chromosomes 7 and 17 and losses of chromosome Y that are prevalent in papillary renal cell carcinoma. *Mod Pathol*. 2006;19:488-493.

324. Eble JN. Mucinous tubular and spindle cell carcinoma and post-neuroblastoma carcinoma: newly recognised entities in the renal cell carcinoma family. *Pathology*. 2003;35:499-504.

325. Kenney PA, Vikram R, Prasad SR, et al. Mucinous tubular and spindle cell carcinoma (MTSCC) of the kidney: a detailed study of radiological, pathological and clinical outcomes. *BJU Int*. 2015;116:85-92.

326. Mehra R, Vats P, Cieslik M, et al. Biallelic alteration and dysregulation of the hippo pathway in mucinous tubular and spindle cell carcinoma of the kidney. *Cancer Discov*. 2016;6:1258-1266.

327. Peckova K, Martinek P, Sperga M, et al. Mucinous spindle and tubular renal cell carcinoma: analysis of chromosomal aberration pattern of low-grade, high-grade, and overlapping morphologic variant with papillary renal cell carcinoma. *Ann Diagn Pathol*. 2015;19:226-231.

328. Ren Q, Wang L, Al-Ahmadie HA, et al. Distinct genomic copy number alterations distinguish mucinous tubular and spindle cell carcinoma of the kidney from papillary renal cell carcinoma with overlapping histologic features. *Am J Surg Pathol*. 2018;42:767-777.

329. Shen SS, Ro JY, Tamboli P, et al. Mucinous tubular and spindle cell carcinoma of kidney is probably a variant of papillary renal cell carcinoma with spindle cell features. *Ann Diagn Pathol*. 2007;11:13-21.

330. Thway K, du Parcq J, Larkin JM, et al. Metastatic renal mucinous tubular and spindle cell carcinoma. Atypical behavior of a rare, morphologically bland tumor. *Ann Diagn Pathol*. 2012;16:407-410.

331. Wang L, Zhang Y, Chen YB, et al. VSTM2A overexpression is a sensitive and specific biomarker for mucinous tubular and spindle cell carcinoma (MTSCC) of the kidney. *Am J Surg Pathol*. 2018;42:1571-1584.

332. Sadimin ET, Chen YB, Wang L, et al. Chromosomal abnormalities of high-grade mucinous tubular and spindle cell carcinoma of the kidney. *Histopathology*. 2017;71:719-724.

333. Ged Y, Chen YB, Knezevic A, et al. Mucinous tubular and spindle-cell carcinoma of the kidney: clinical features, genomic profiles, and treatment outcomes. *Clin Genitourin Cancer*. 2019;17:268-274.e1.

334. Fine SW, Reuter VE, Epstein JI, et al. Angiomyolipoma with epithelial cysts (AMLEC): a distinct cystic variant of angiomyolipoma. *Am J Surg Pathol*. 2006;30:593-599.

335. Karafin M, Parwani AV, Netto GJ, et al. Diffuse expression of PAX2 and PAX8 in the cystic epithelium of mixed epithelial stromal tumor, angiomyolipoma with epithelial cysts, and primary renal synovial sarcoma: evidence supporting renal tubular differentiation. *Am J Surg Pathol*. 2011;35:1264-1273.

336. Davis CJ, Barton JH, Sesterhenn IA. Cystic angiomyolipoma of the kidney: a clinicopathologic description of 11 cases. *Mod Pathol*. 2006;19:669-674.

337. Turbiner J, Amin MB, Humphrey PA, et al. Cystic nephroma and mixed epithelial and stromal tumor of kidney: a detailed clinicopathologic analysis of 34 cases and proposal for renal epithelial and stromal tumor (REST) as a unifying term. *Am J Surg Pathol.* 2007;31:489-500.

338. Calio A, Eble JN, Grignon DJ, et al. Mixed epithelial and stromal tumor of the kidney: a clinicopathologic study of 53 cases. *Am J Surg Pathol.* 2016;40:1538-1549.

339. Calio A, Eble JN, Grignon DJ, et al. Cystic nephroma in adults: a clinicopathologic study of 46 cases. *Am J Surg Pathol.* 2016;40:1591-1600.

340. Michal M, Amin MB, Delahunt B, et al. Mixed epithelial and stromal tumour family. In: Moch H, Humphrey PA, Ulbright TM, et al, eds. *WHO Classification of Tumours of the Urinary System and Male Genital Organs.* Lyon: International Agency for Research on Cancer; 2016:70-71.

341. Argani P, Bruder E, Dehner L, et al. Nephroblastic and cystic tumours occurring mainly in children. In: Moch H, Humphrey PA, Ulbright TM, et al, eds. *WHO Classification of Tumours of the Urinary System and Male Genital Organs.* Lyon: International Agency for Research on Cancer; 2016:48-58.

342. Tickoo SK, Gopalan A, Tu JJ, et al. Estrogen and progesterone-receptor-positive stroma as a non-tumorous proliferation in kidneys: a possible metaplastic response to obstruction. *Mod Pathol.* 2008;21:60-65.

343. Schoolmeester JK, Cheville JC, Folpe AL. Synovial sarcoma of the kidney: a clinicopathologic, immunohistochemical, and molecular genetic study of 16 cases. *Am J Surg Pathol.* 2014;38:60-65.

344. Williamson SR, Cheng L, Eble JN, et al. Renal cell carcinoma with angioleiomyoma-like stroma: clinicopathological, immunohistochemical, and molecular features supporting classification as a distinct entity. *Mod Pathol.* 2015;28:279-294.

345. Shah RB, Stohr BA, Tu ZJ, et al. "Renal cell carcinoma with leiomyomatous stroma" harbor somatic mutations of TSC1, TSC2, MTOR, and/or ELOC (TCEB1): clinicopathologic and molecular characterization of 18 sporadic tumors supports a distinct entity. *Am J Surg Pathol.* 2020;44:571-581.

346. Williamson SR, Hornick JL, Eble JN, et al. Renal cell carcinoma with angioleiomyoma-like stroma and clear cell papillary renal cell carcinoma: exploring SDHB protein immunohistochemistry and the relationship to tuberous sclerosis complex. *Hum Pathol.* 2018;75:10-15.

347. Yang P, Cornejo KM, Sadow PM, et al. Renal cell carcinoma in tuberous sclerosis complex. *Am J Surg Pathol.* 2014;38:895-909.

348. Parilla M, Alikhan M, Al-Kawaaz M, et al. Genetic underpinnings of renal cell carcinoma with leiomyomatous stroma. *Am J Surg Pathol.* 2019;43:1135-1144.

349. Smith NE, Epstein JI, Parwani AV, et al. Smooth muscle and adenoma-like renal tumor: a previously unreported variant of mixed epithelial stromal tumor or a distinctive renal neoplasm?. *Hum Pathol.* 2015;46:894-905.

350. Williamson SR, Rao P, Hes O, et al. Challenges in pathologic staging of renal cell carcinoma: a study of interobserver variability among urologic pathologists. *Am J Surg Pathol.* 2018;42:1253-1261.

351. Williamson SR, Taneja K, Cheng L. Renal cell carcinoma staging: pitfalls, challenges, and updates. *Histopathology.* 2019;74:18-30.

352. Bonsib SM, Gibson D, Mhoon M, et al. Renal sinus involvement in renal cell carcinomas. *Am J Surg Pathol.* 2000;24:451-458.

353. Taneja K, Arora S, Rogers CG, et al. Pathologic staging of renal cell carcinoma: a review of 300 consecutive cases with emphasis on retrograde venous invasion. *Histopathology.* 2018 73:681-691.

354. Fuhrman SA, Lasky LC, Limas C. Prognostic significance of morphologic parameters in renal cell carcinoma. *Am J Surg Pathol.* 1982;6:655-663.

355. Delahunt B, Sika-Paotonu D, Bethwaite PB, et al. Grading of clear cell renal cell carcinoma should be based on nucleolar prominence. *Am J Surg Pathol.* 2011;35:1134-1139.

356. Amin MB, Moch H, Alkan S, et al. Renal haematopoietic neoplasms. In: Moch H, Humphrey PA, Ulbright TM, et al, eds. *WHO Classification of Tumours of the Urinary System and Male Genital Organs.* Lyon: International Agency for Research on Cancer; 2016:73-75.

357. Li L, Parwani AV. Xanthogranulomatous pyelonephritis. *Arch Pathol Lab Med.* 2011;135:671-674.

358. Kuo CC, Wu CF, Huang CC, et al. Xanthogranulomatous pyelonephritis: critical analysis of 30 patients. *Int Urol Nephrol.* 2011;43:15-22.

359. Rajesh A, Jakanani G, Mayer N, et al. Computed tomography findings in xanthogranulomatous pyelonephritis. *J Clin Imaging Sci.* 2011;1:45.

360. Esparza AR, McKay DB, Cronan JJ, et al. Renal parenchymal malakoplakia. Histologic spectrum and its relationship to megalocytic interstitial nephritis and xanthogranulomatous pyelonephritis. *Am J Surg Pathol*. 1989;13:225-236.

361. Lusco MA, Fogo AB, Najafian B, et al. AJKD atlas of renal pathology: malakoplakia. *Am J Kidney Dis*. 2016;68:e27-e28.

362. Buttner M, Kufer V, Brunner K, et al. Benign mesenchymal tumours and tumour-like lesions in end-stage renal disease. *Histopathology*. 2013;62:229-236.

363. Taneja K, Arora S, Rogers CG, et al. Unclassified hemangioma-like renal cell carcinoma: a potential diagnostic pitfall. *Hum Pathol*. 2018;75:132-136.

CHAPTER OUTLINE

THE UNREMARKABLE TESTIS

ANATOMY AND HISTOLOGY

The testicles are paired organs that normally descend into the scrotum, attached to the spermatic cord. Their embryologic development begins high in the abdomen and follows the path of the gubernaculum through the inguinal canal and into the scrotum as their final destination. The vascular and lymphatic supply of the testis are linked to the embryologic development. The scrotal skin is the outermost layer, below which is the dartos muscle, Colles fascia, and then the parietal layer of tunica vaginalis surrounds the testis. The testicles are invested within three layers of thin tissue: the tunica vaginalis that is in direct continuity with the peritoneum, the tunica albuginea, which provides a protective fibrous covering, and the tunica vasculosa which interdigitates within the parenchyma. Within the testicular parenchyma, seminiferous tubules convolute into around 250 tightly packed lobules, separated by fibrous septa[1] (Figure 4.1).

The interstitial component between tubules is loose and contains blood vessels, lymphatic vessels, nerves, and Leydig cells (Figure 4.2). Leydig cells are granular eosinophilic cells that produce testicular androgens in response to luteinizing hormone (LH) (Figure 4.3). The tunica vasculosa is in close approximation with Leydig cells to facilitate delivery of hormones between the tubules and interstitium.

The seminiferous tubules converge into the rete testis in the testicular hilum, then enter the epididymis and ultimately into the ductus deferentia. The rete testis functions as an intermediate between the seminiferous tubules and the epididymis and allows various substances to mix with seminal fluid or resorb back into the epithelium (Figure 4.4).

The epididymis is a paratesticular structure attached to the posterosuperior aspect of the testis (Figure 4.5). The tubules exiting the rete testis enter the head of the epididymis at the superior aspect of the testis, continue through the body and tail, and then exit the epididymis at the inferior aspect into the vas deferens.

The types of germ cells and their supporting cellular elements are listed in Table 4.1.[1] The testicular tubular architecture, relative amounts, and types of these cells change over time based on the influence of the sex hormones. A general overview of testicular maturation is described in Table 4.2 and demonstrated in Figures 4.6-4.15.

THE NEAR NORMAL TESTIS

Cryptorchidism

Cryptorchidism refers to the absence of one or both testes, usually due to failure of the testis to descend completely into the scrotum. The testis is usually identified along the path of testicular descent in the upper scrotum, inguinal region, or abdomen. Testicular

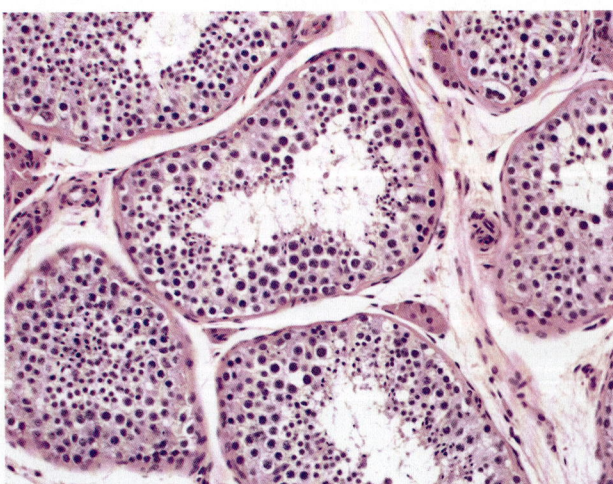

Figure 4.1. Low power image of multiple normal spermatic tubules demonstrating intact spermatogenesis. Leydig cell clusters are present in the interstitium along with small blood vessels.

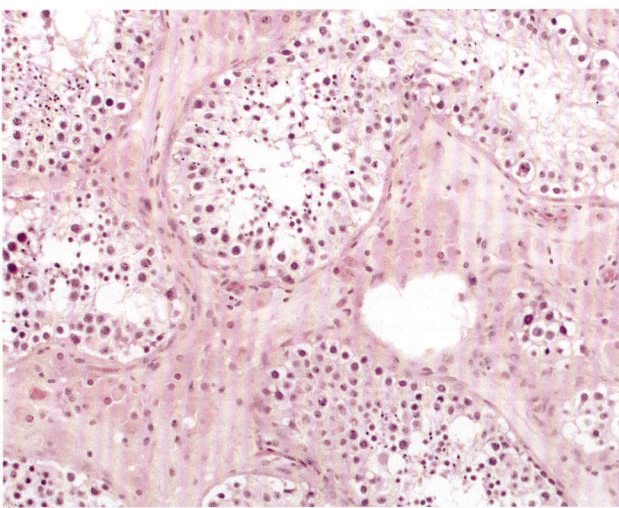

Figure 4.2. The interstitium of the testis contains blood vessels, lymphatic vessels, nerves, and Leydig cells within loose fibrous stroma.

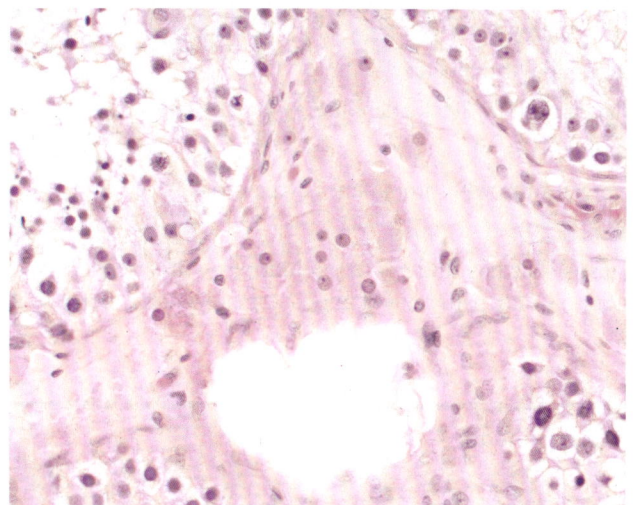

Figure 4.3. Leydig cells are found within the interstitium of the testis and produce androgens to support germ cell development.

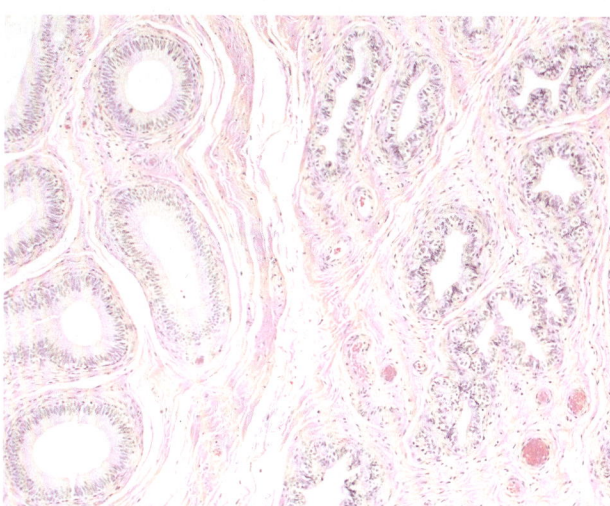

Figure 4.4. The rete testis is located in the hilum or mediastinum of the testis and comprises slitlike, complex glands that act as a conduit between the spermatic tubules and the epididymis.

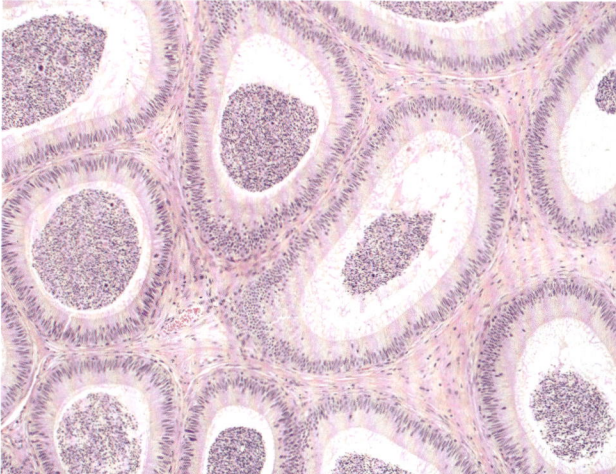

Figure 4.5. The epididymis is located within the scrotum on the posterior aspect of the testis. The tubules in the epididymis show a distinct straight luminal border lined with pseudostratified, ciliated epithelial cells. In this image, the lumens are filled with sperm.

descent normally begins around 8 to 15 weeks of gestation and is normally completed by the 35th week of gestation. This is a common condition affecting approximately 2% to 8% of male children. Risk factors for cryptorchidism include low birth weight, being small for gestational age, and prematurity.[2]

The cryptorchid testis is at increased risk of developing germ cell tumors (GCTs), with approximately 5% of GCTs arising in the setting of cryptorchidism. The risk of germ cell neoplasia is even higher in patients with bilateral cryptorchidism. As a result, prompt surgical correction is recommended in the form of orchidopexy. This procedure involves the identification of the undescended testis within the inguinal canal or abdomen, placement of the testis into the scrotum, and tacking it into place. In addition to the risk of neoplasia, infertility is more common in patients with cryptorchidism. Torsion is also more common in cryptorchid testes when compared to normally descended testes.

Vanishing testis or testicular regression occurs when testicular development halts around the seventh month of gestation, so the testicular remnant is often present along with an epididymis and vas deferens. In testicular regression, both testes fail to form or completely disappear. The testicular remnant may be identified with fibrosis, hemosiderin deposition, and calcifications[3] (Figures 4.16 and 4.17).

KEY FEATURES: Histologic Findings in Cryptorchid Testis

- Tubular atrophy with decreased tubular diameter
- Sertoli-only pattern or Sertoli cell nodules "Pick adenoma" (Figure 4.18)
- Microlithiasis within tubules (Figure 4.19)
- Peritubular fibrosis, fibrotic interstitium with prominent Leydig cells
- Hemosiderin deposition (Figure 4.20)
- In adults with cryptorchid testis that has undergone orchidopexy, may see a mixed pattern of maturation arrest, Sertoli-only pattern, and hypospermatogenesis, along with Leydig cell hyperplasia

TABLE 4.1: Normal Testicular Cellular Components

	Histologic Appearance	Location	Function
Germ cells			
• Spermatogonium Figure 4.6	Round cells with clear to lightly eosinophilic cytoplasm, central round nuclei with prominent nucleoli	Intratubular, basal compartment	Most undifferentiated germ-cell type
• Primary spermatocyte Figure 4.7	Similar to spermatogonia with more condensed, filamentous chromatin pattern	Intratubular, intermediate location between basal and luminal aspects—"adluminal" compartment	Chromosomal duplication in preparation for meiosis I
• Secondary spermatocyte Figure 4.8	Smaller round nuclei compared to primary spermatocytes with dispersed, granular chromatin	Intratubular, adluminal compartment	Chromosome complement divided in half with meiosis II to become spermatid
• Spermatid Figure 4.9	Oval to elongated nuclear shape, condensed chromatin	Intratubular, luminal surface; remains in contact with Sertoli cells	Final maturation step before detaching from Sertoli cells and becoming a spermatozoa
• Spermatozoa Figure 4.10	Fully mature sperm with acrosome and motile tail	Detached from Sertoli cells and present in lumen	Fully motile cells capable of fertilization
Sertoli cell Figure 4.11	Tall, pyramidal-shaped with ill-defined cellular borders, abundant pale eosinophilic cytoplasm, round nucleus with prominent central nucleolus	Intratubular basal location	Supports spermatogenesis by surrounding germ cells with cytoplasm during their maturation; phagocytoses excess cytoplasm in maturing spermatid
Leydig cell Figure 4.12	Round cell with abundant granular eosinophilic cytoplasm, round nucleus with prominent nucleolus; often contain cytoplasmic lipid, lipofuscin pigment, and may demonstrate Reinke crystalloids in adults	Interstitium, however, may also be encountered in spermatic cord and hilum, often associated with nerves	Produce androgens and insulin-like factor 3

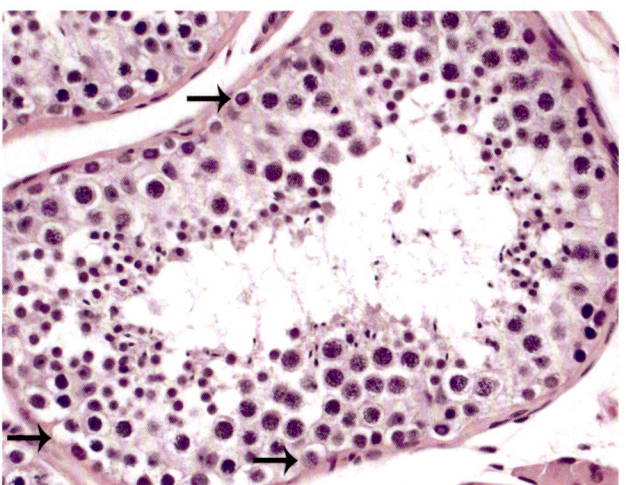

Figure 4.6. In Table 4.1: Spermatogonium. Arrows point to the basally oriented spermatogonia. These are the most primitive germ cell within the spermatic tubule.

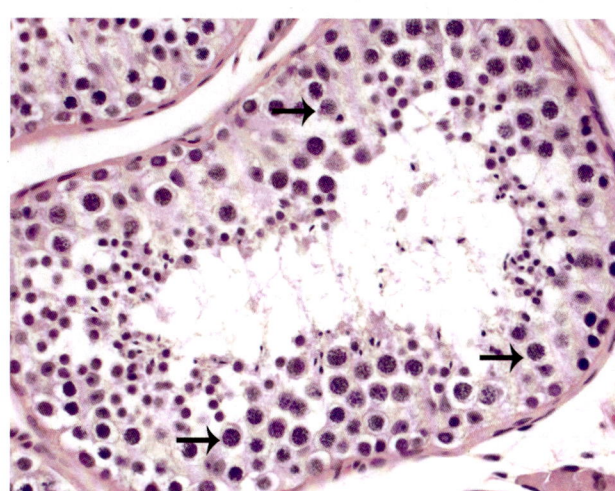

Figure 4.7. In Table 4.1: Primary spermatocyte. Arrows point to primary spermatocytes, which are present just above the basal aspect of the tubule, but not yet to the luminal surface.

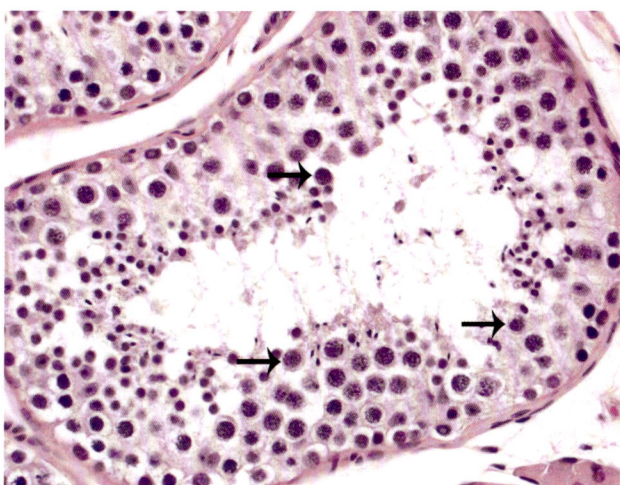

Figure 4.8. In Table 4.1: Secondary spermatocyte. Arrows point to secondary spermatocytes. These cells are located more towards the luminal aspect when compared to primary spermatocytes. In reality, they are incredibly difficult to differentiate from primary spermatocytes on H&E alone.

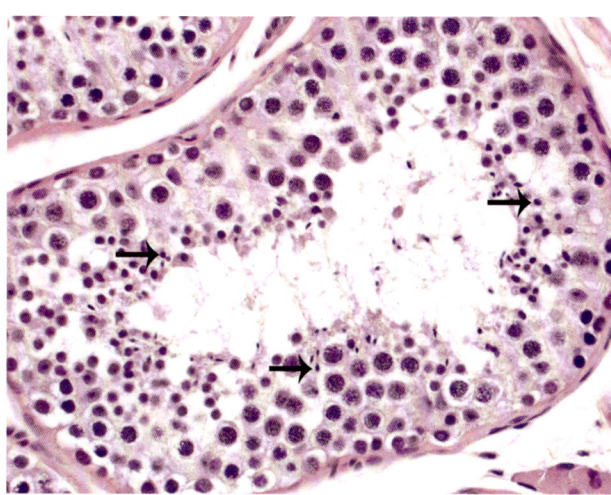

Figure 4.9. In Table 4.1: Spermatid. Arrows point to spermatids, which still show attachment to the Sertoli cells within the tubule.

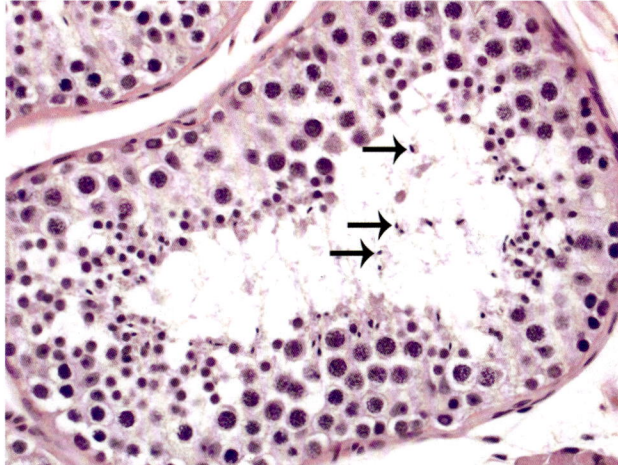

Figure 4.10. In Table 4.1: Spermatozoa. Arrows point to spermatozoa, which have been released into the lumen and will be carried out of the testis via the vas deferens.

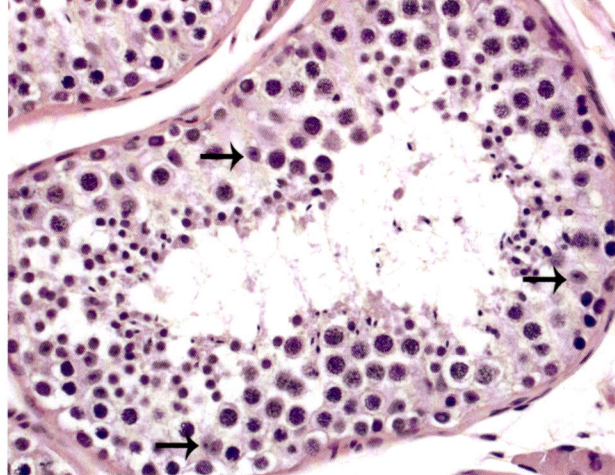

Figure 4.11. In Table 4.1: Sertoli cell. Arrows point to Sertoli cells, which are pyramidal shaped cells with prominent nucleoli. They have indistinct cell borders as they interdigitate between the germ cells of the tubule.

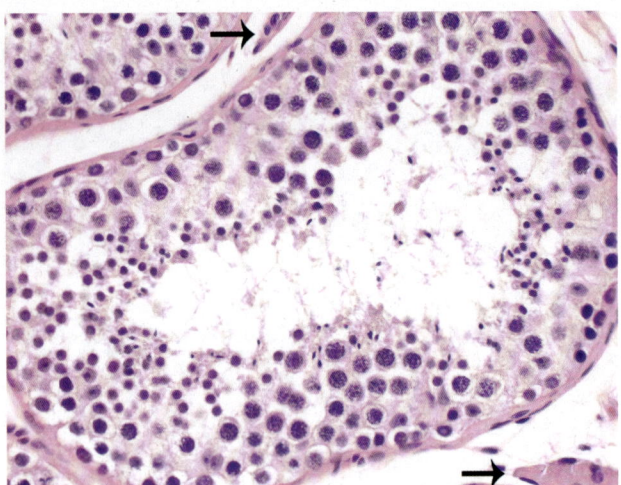

Figure 4.12. In Table 4.1: Leydig cell. Arrows point to Leydig cells present in the interstitium surrounding the tubule.

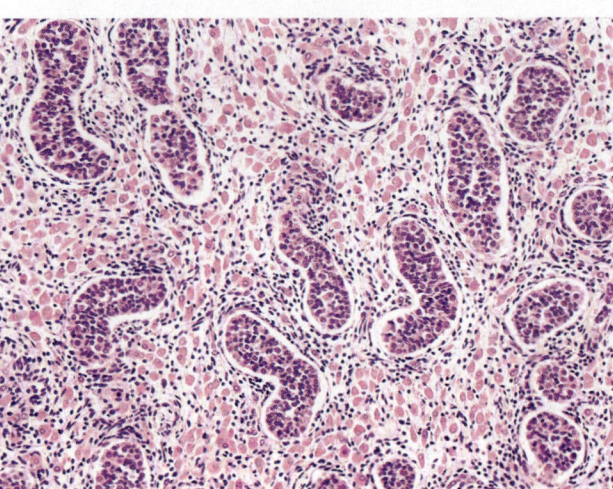

Figure 4.13. The fetal testis comprises immature seminiferous tubules without lumens. The tubules are lined by immature, cuboidal Sertoli cells. Immature Leydig cells are present in the interstitium.

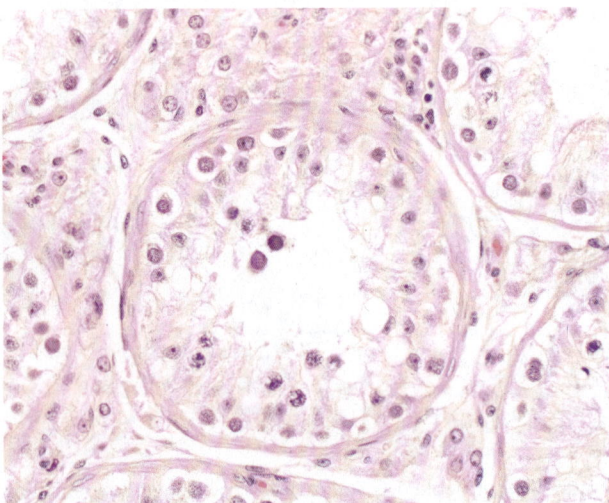

Figure 4.14. Prepubertal seminiferous tubules showing incomplete maturation lacking spermatozoa. Sertoli cells are prominent.

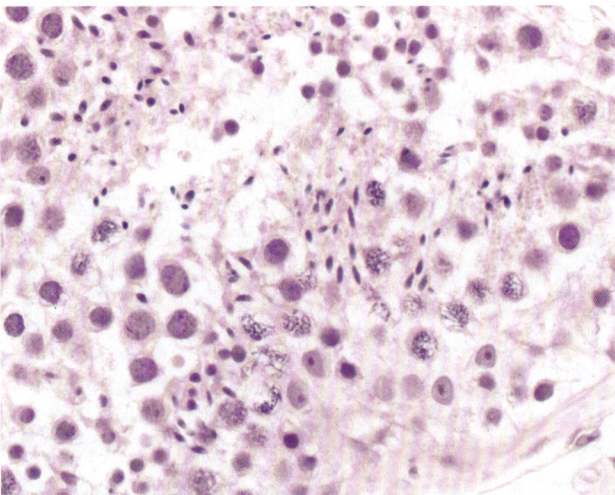

Figure 4.15. Complete spermatogenesis in the adult male. All stages of germ cell maturation are present, with spermatozoa identified in the tubular lumen. Sertoli cells, with prominent nucleoli, are admixed between germ cells to provide necessary factors for germ cell development.

Disorders of Sexual Development

"Disorders of sexual development" is a broad category of conditions that include gonadal dysgenesis, agonadism, and ovotesticular disorder. This term was chosen by a consensus group in 2006 to encompass "congenital conditions in which development of chromosomal, gonadal, or anatomic sex is atypical."[4] The underlying physiology of these conditions varies and may be related to chromosomal abnormalities (Turner syndrome and Klinefelter syndrome), disorders of testicular or ovarian development (ovotesticular syndrome), or alterations in androgen signaling (5-alpha reductase deficiency and congenital adrenal hyperplasia [CAH]).

Ovotesticular Disorder

Ovotestis is the most common anatomical finding in the setting of disordered sexual differentiation. The most common chromosomal karyotype in these patients is 46,XX, although mosaic phenotypes with combinations of XY and XXY are also seen. Patients usually present with ambiguous genitalia. Grossly, the mixed ovotestis will show an end-to-end arrangement of ovarian tissue and testicular tissue (Figure 4.21). Histologically, a combination

TABLE 4.2: Testicular Development and Histology by Developmental Age Group

Developmental Age	Histologic Features
Fetal testis	Tubules contain numerous Sertoli cells and gonocytes (primordial germ cells) and lack open lumina. Interstitium contains numerous Leydig cells. Formation of interlobular septa begins (Figure 4.13).
Testis at birth	Tubules are solid and contain numerous Sertoli cells and germ cells, including gonocytes, and spermatogonia. Leydig cells are present in lesser numbers than fetal testis and lack Reinke crystalloids. Interlobular septation is complete, forming approximately 250 lobules.
Prepubertal testis	Tubules are growing in length, width, and diameter and contain Sertoli cells, which are increasing in number. Spermatogonia of all types are also proliferating with variation between tubules. No mature spermatozoa are present. Interstitial Leydig cells are rare and represent remaining fetal Leydig cells (Figure 4.14).
Pubertal testis	Under hormonal influence, mature Leydig cells proliferate and secrete androgens that stimulate Sertoli cell and germ cell development. The tubules develop open lumina. Overall testicular volume increases as a result of puberty.
Postpubertal/adult testis	Tubules are highly convoluted within lobules, making up the vast majority of the parenchymal volume. Mature Sertoli cells are present at the basal aspect of the tubules, supporting the maturing germ cells. Complete spermatogenesis is present, culminating in spermatozoa within the tubular lumen. Mature Leydig cells are present in small clusters or as single cells in the interstitium (Figure 4.15).
Senescent testis	Scattered sclerotic tubules and decreased spermatogenesis.

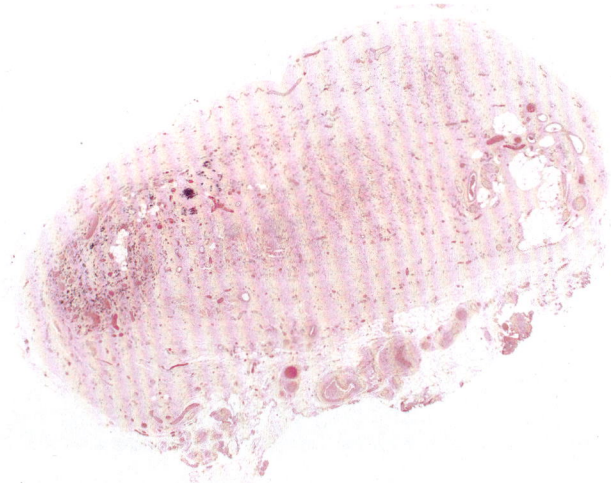

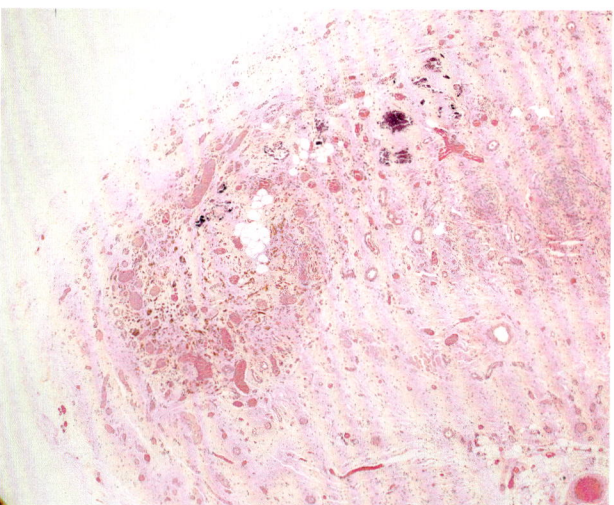

Figure 4.16. In cryptorchid testes, the testicle is often identified in the inguinal canal or even in the abdomen. The testicle is small and fibrotic.

Figure 4.17. At medium power, numerous vessels, hemosiderin deposition, and calcifications are present and well-formed spermatic tubules are absent.

of the ovarian parenchyma with the fallopian tube is present in close association with immature spermatic tubules (Figure 4.22). The seminiferous tubules are lined by immature Sertoli cells, lack open lumens, and germ cells are absent (Figure 4.23). Ovarian fibrous stroma is indicative of the ovarian component, along with the serous-epithelium-lined fallopian tube (Figure 4.24).

FAQ: Features of Gonadoblastoma

- Gonadoblastoma usually arises in the setting of disordered sexual development
- Most commonly identified in gonadal dysgenesis involving the Y chromosome
- Tumors comprise of a mixture of GCT and sex cord stromal tumor
- Areas that resemble seminoma/dysgerminoma with annular tubules surrounded by ovarian stroma (Figure 4.25)
- Calcifications are common (Figure 4.26)

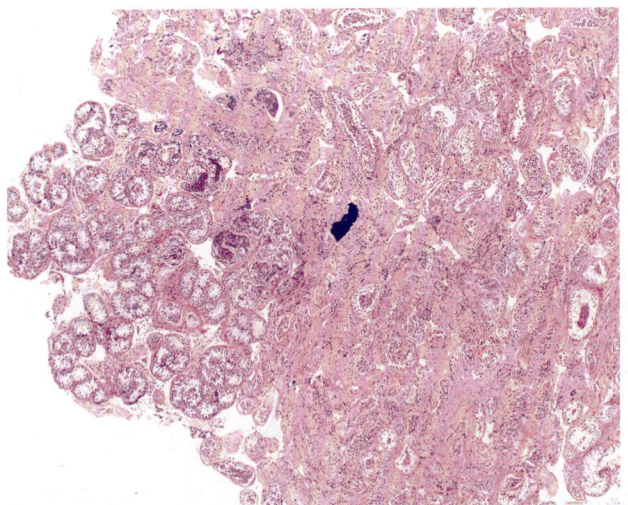

Figure 4.18. The finding of Sertoli cell–only pattern, discussed below, is common in cryptorchid testis. A discrete nodule of Sertoli cells, the so-called Pick adenoma, is also associated with cryptorchidism.

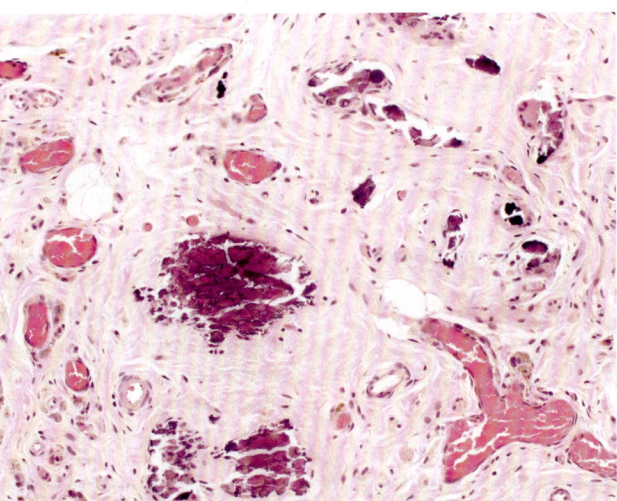

Figure 4.19. Microlithiasis within the remnant of spermatic tubules is another feature of cryptorchid testis.

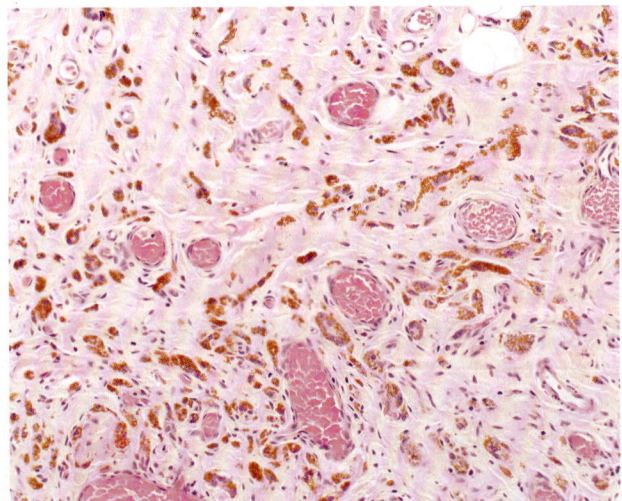

Figure 4.20. Hemosiderin deposition is a common feature of cryptorchid testis, along with prominent vessels.

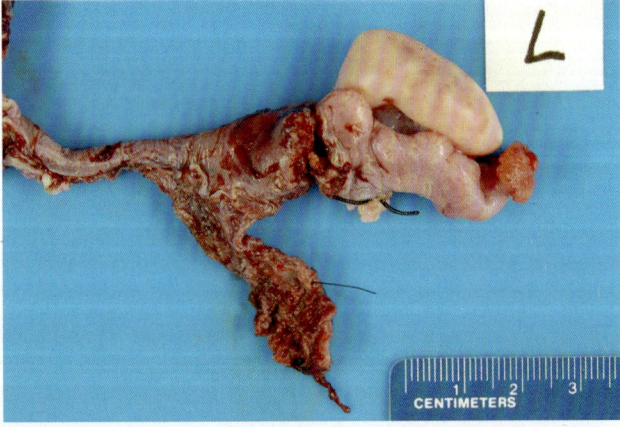

Figure 4.21. Gross photograph of an ovotestis demonstrates the intact fallopian tube on the left, leading to a combined ovary and testis. The fimbriated end of the fallopian tube is present at the right side of the image.

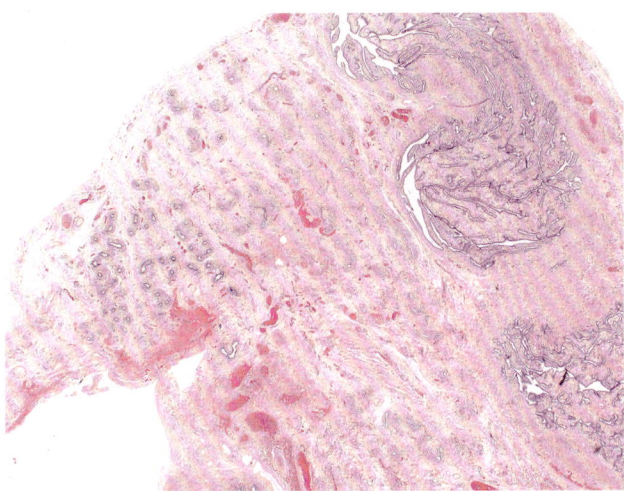

Figure 4.22. Low-power image of an ovotestis with the fallopian tube coursing along the right and top of the image and immature spermatic tubules on the left.

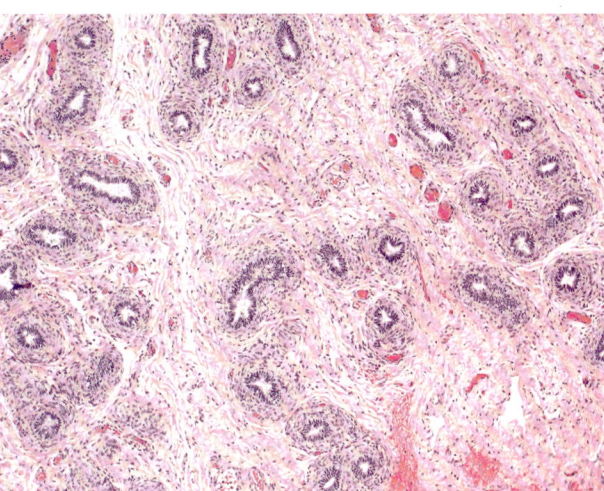

Figure 4.23. At higher power, the spermatic tubules in the ovotestis show fetal-type immature Sertoli cells, without any germ cells present.

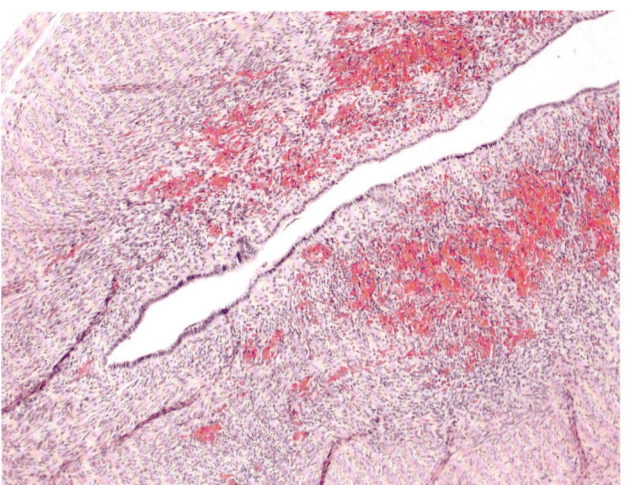

Figure 4.24. Ovarian fibrous stroma is present in ovotestis, surrounding the fallopian tube with serous-type epithelium.

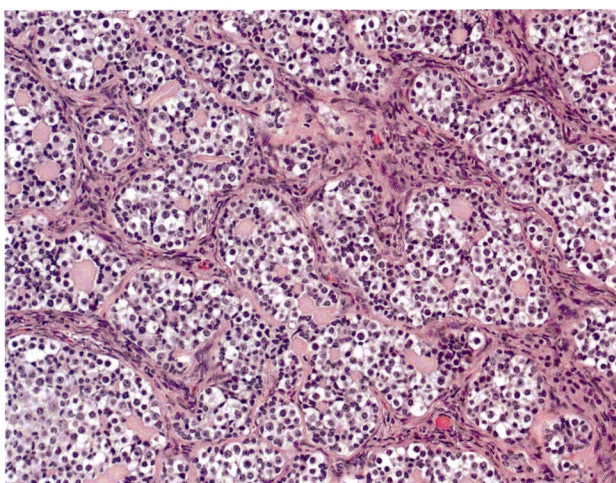

Figure 4.25. Gonadoblastomas are mixed germ cell and sex cord stromal tumors that occur in the setting of gonadal dysgenesis. Microscopically, they resemble seminoma/dysgerminoma in the germ cell component but also show foci of eosinophilic material similar to sex cord tumor with annular tubules.

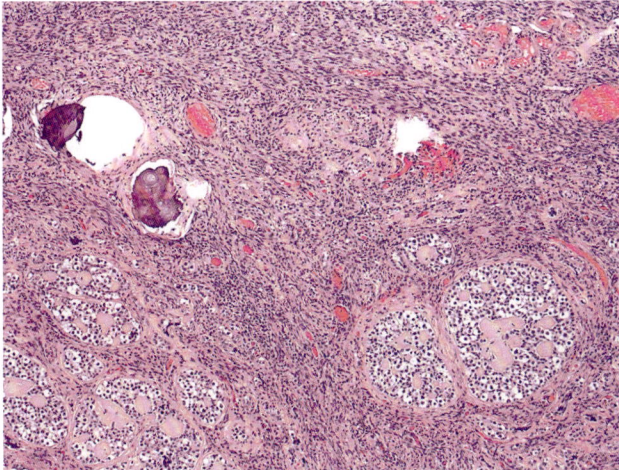

Figure 4.26. In gonadoblastoma, tubules are surrounded by ovarian-type stroma. Calcifications and hyalinization are common in these tumors.

Congenital Adrenal Hyperplasia

Congenital adrenal hyperplasia is an autosomal recessive syndrome in which specific enzyme deficiencies cause lack of production of sex hormones. Depending on which enzyme is deficient, the clinical presentation can vary. Because sex hormones are impacted, these syndromes often present with virilization and hirsutism associated with androgen excess.

The most common type of CAH is 21-Hydroxylase deficiency, which is responsible for over 95% of cases. 21-hydroxylase deficiency is the syndrome most closely associated with testicular "tumor" of the adrenogenital syndrome (TTAGS). These proliferations of steroid cells are usually located in the testicular hilum and are thought to arise from excess hormonal stimulation of preexisting cells. These tumors have also been referred to as "testicular adrenal rest tumors (TARTs)" though this term is less favored given the hypothesis that the steroid cells are a normal component of the testicular hilum, rather than an ectopic location of the adrenal tissue.

TTAGS is often nodular and comprises of round cells with abundant eosinophilic cytoplasm, morphologically similar to Leydig cells (Figure 4.27). Bilaterality is common in this entity, a finding that should immediately raise the possibility of CAH, rather than Leydig cell tumor. Consistent with their endocrine origin, random nuclear atypia is commonly identified, and rare mitotic figures are acceptable (Figure 4.28). Given the histologic overlap with Leydig cells, Leydig cell tumor is leading differential diagnosis for TTAGS. Clues to the correct diagnosis include the clinical presentation of other signs of CAH, bilaterality and the presence of fibrous bands, adipose metaplasia, and nuclear pleomorphism. Immunohistochemically, TTAGS strongly expresses CD56 and is negative for androgen receptor (AR), whereas Leydig cell tumors are positive for androgen receptor.[5] Of note, Leydig cell tumor may have some expression of both CD56 and synaptophysin, so AR positivity strongly supports Leydig cell tumor.

Androgen Insensitivity Syndrome

Androgen insensitivity syndrome (AIS) is a type of disordered sexual development where the presence of a Y chromosome leads to formation of testicles, which may occur in otherwise phenotypically female patients. The testicles produce androgens and luteinizing hormone; however, patients lack functional androgen receptors and therefore virilization does not occur. Clinically, the most common presentation is a 46X,Y chromosomal compliment in a patient who appears phenotypically female, often with tall stature, and lack of development of gynecologic organs. These patients have an increased risk of developing GCTs, and gonadectomy is generally recommended. Gonads are often located in the abdomen, inguinal canal, or may be within labia. Histologically, AIS gonads show small tubules lacking lumina lined by immature Sertoli cells (Figure 4.29). Leydig cell hyperplasia is common because of persistent LH elevation.

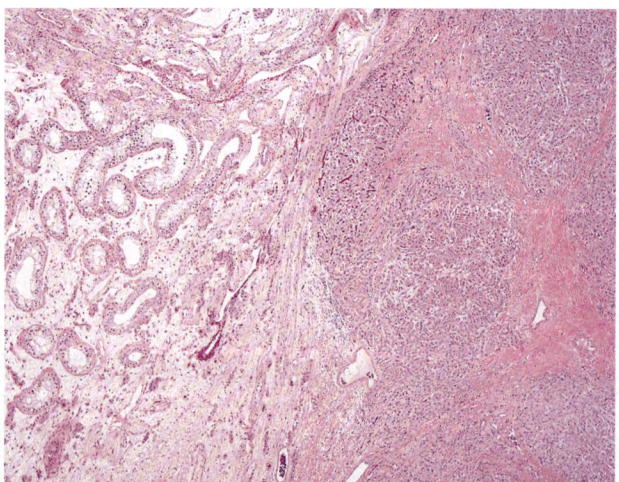

Figure 4.27. Testicular tumors of the adrenogenital syndrome (TTAGSs) are associated with adrenogenital syndrome and result from hyperplasia of existing steroid cells in the testis. They arise within the testis and comprise eosinophilic nests of cells that are morphologically similar to Leydig cells.

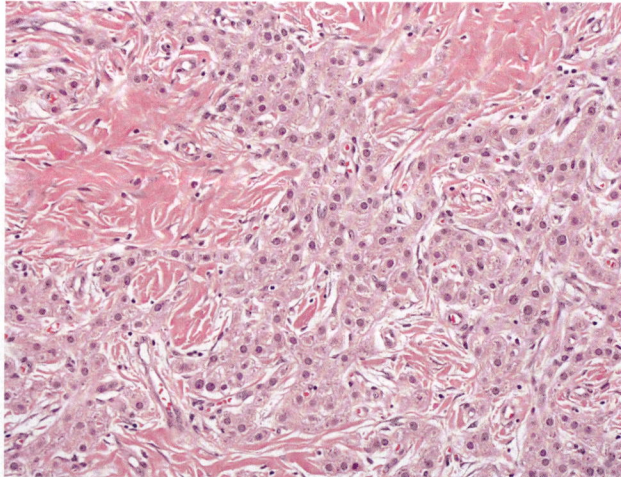

Figure 4.28. A higher power image of testicular tumor of the adrenogenital syndrome (TTAGS) shows their granular eosinophilic cytoplasm, round nuclei with random atypia—consistent with their endocrine origin.

PEARLS AND PITFALLS: Adrenocortical Rests

- Nodules of benign adrenal cortical tissue found in the paratesticular soft tissue, as well as along the spermatic cord and epididymis
- Exceedingly rare instances of adrenal tissue within testicular tissue reported
- May be more common in cryptorchid males
- Occurs when adrenal tissue follows testis from abdomen into the inguinal region during development
- Rests are well circumscribed, contain only adrenal cortical tissue, and lack a medullary component (Figure 4.30)

FAQ: What Ectopic Tissues May Be Identified in Testis and Paratestis?

- Spleen: Splenogonadal fusion occurs when the embryonic gonad fuses with ectopic spleen and migrates to the scrotum. The left testicle is exclusively involved, consistent with the usual anatomic location of the spleen.[6]
- Liver: Hepatotesticular fusion has been reported in hernia specimens and in undescended testis.[7]
- Kidney: Ectopic renal tissue associated with undescended testis.[8]
- Various metaplastic tissues may be seen in testes including fat, cartilage, and bone.[9]

NONNEOPLASTIC TESTIS AND EPIDIDYMIS

TESTIS BIOPSY FOR INFERTILITY

Organic azoospermia is the clinical term for the absence of sperm within semen. In the workup of azoospermia, testis biopsy may be employed for histologic confirmation of the cause of azoospermia (Figure 4.31). Azoospermia can be caused by obstruction within the vas deferens (as seen in cystic fibrosis) or nonobstructive causes stemming from abnormal spermatogenesis. The five main categories of findings for testicular biopsy for fertility include normal, hypospermatogenesis, maturation arrest, Sertoli cell–only pattern, and atrophy.[10] A description of the common patterns identified on testicular biopsies for infertility is provided in Table 4.3. When the patterns co-occur, it is useful to give percentages of each pattern seen in the sampled tubules.

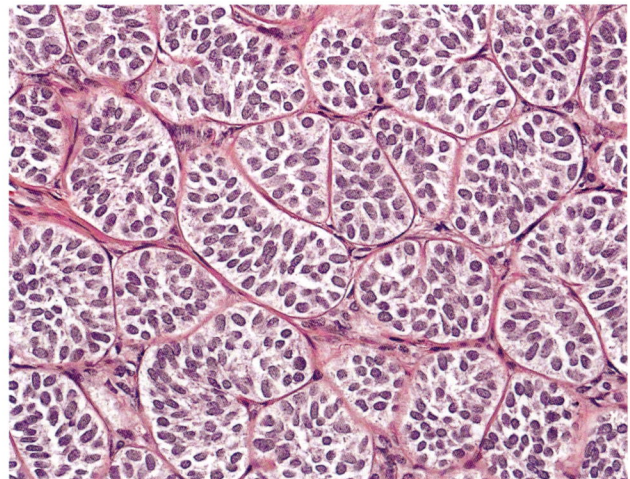

Figure 4.29. Histologic examination of androgen insensitivity syndrome showing small, packed seminiferous tubules lined by immature Sertoli cells. Germ cells are largely absent.

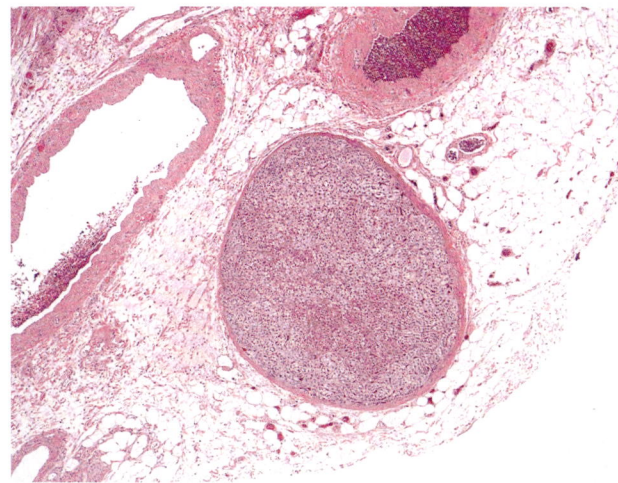

Figure 4.30. Adrenocortical rests are benign nodules of adrenal cortical cells most commonly identified in the paratesticular soft tissue.

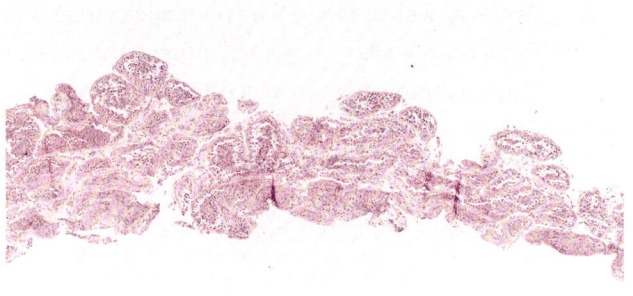

Figure 4.31. Testicular biopsies performed for fertility workup are challenging specimens due to frequent architectural and cytologic distortion. At low power, it is helpful to scan the specimen to get a sense for the degree of crush artifact and number of intact and evaluable tubules. Providing an estimated number of evaluable tubules may provide an idea of adequacy of the specimen.

TABLE 4.3: Common Patterns for Testicular Biopsy for Infertility

	Sperm?	Germ Cells?	Suggested Diagnostic Line	Clinical Implications
Normal spermatogenesis (Figures 4.32-4.34)	Yes, normal numbers	Yes, with appropriate maturation pattern	Intact spermatogenesis, appropriate for age	Associated with extraductal obstruction, fertility usually possible
Hypospermatogenesis (Figure 4.35)	Yes, decreased numbers and not identified in all tubules (heterogeneous pattern)	Yes, with appropriate maturation pattern in some tubules	Intact spermatogenesis (50%), decreased for age (hypospermatogenesis) with heterogeneous pattern including Sertoli cell only (50%)	Fertility often possible with testicular sperm extraction (TESE)
Maturation arrest (Figures 4.36 and 4.37)	No	Yes, but only to early or late stage of maturation	Maturation arrest with no intact spermatogenesis identified	Fertility more likely in men with late compared with early maturation arrest
Sertoli cell only (Figures 4.38 and 4.39)	No	No	Sertoli cell–only pattern (germ cell aplasia), no intact spermatogenesis identified	Fertility possible with TESE
Atrophy/hyalinized tubules (Figures 4.40 and 4.41)	No (in pure form)	No (in pure form)	Atrophic tubules present (comment on any other patterns seen and presence or absence of spermatogenesis if mixed pattern)	In pure form, fertility usually not possible

A recent study highlighted the use of select immunomarkers for detection of germ cells and spermatogonia. DOG1 was expressed in spermatocytes and spermatids, and MAGE-A4 was expressed preferentially in spermatogonia, helping to distinguish maturation arrest from Sertoli-only syndrome (Figures 4.32-4.41).[11]

PEARLS AND PITFALLS: Klinefelter Syndrome

- Klinefelter syndrome occurs in males with an extra X chromosome (47,XXY)
- Findings include infertility and small testicular volume with decreased testosterone production
- Testicular biopsy demonstrates numerous sclerotic tubules and Leydig cell hyperplasia, with overall reduction in the number of germ cells
- When sperms are present, microtesticular sperm extraction (TESE) may be successful for assisted reproduction

CHECKLIST: Approach to Testicular Biopsy for Fertility[10]

☐ Look for intact spermatogenesis in all tubules; if absent in any tubules, consider diagnostic entities in Table 4.3

☐ Determine if the process involves all tubules versus heterogeneous, mixed pattern

☐ If heterogeneous, give approximate percentage of tubules involved by each pattern

☐ Comment on presence or absence of germ cell neoplasia in situ (GCNIS)

☐ Assess interstitium for presence of Leydig cells and other findings such as fibrosis, inflammation, or granulomas

☐ Report the number of tubular cross sections present as a biopsy-quality indicator

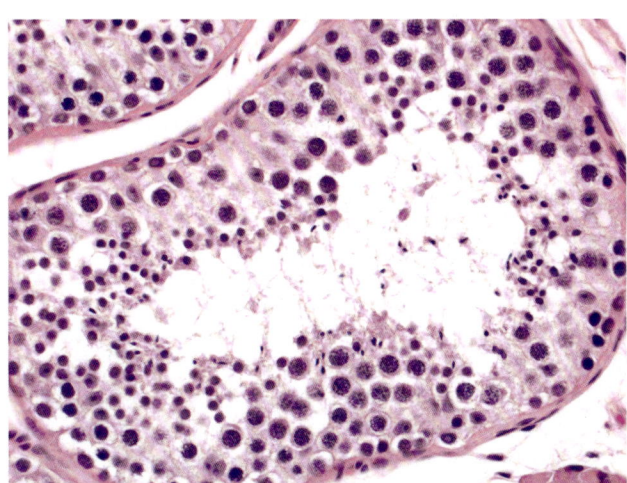

Figure 4.32. A reference image of complete spermatogenesis in a well-oriented seminiferous tubule showing all stages of germ cell maturation from spermatogonia to spermatozoa. Sertoli cells are admixed within the adluminal space providing nutrients to the developing germ cells. A few Leydig cells are present in the interstitium surrounding the tubule.

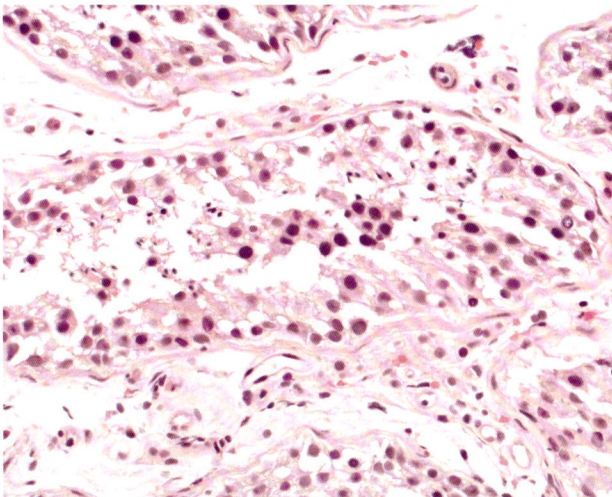

Figure 4.33. Testis biopsy showing typical distortion of seminiferous tubules due to handling of small specimens. Despite the artifactual changes, mature spermatozoa are present in the lumen of this tubule, consistent with intact spermatogenesis. Sloughed maturing germ cells are commonly identified in the lumen and are also likely due to rough handling of the specimen.

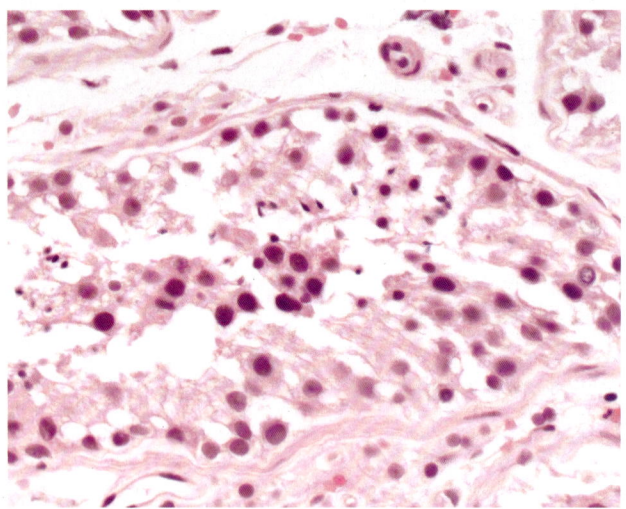

Figure 4.34. Higher power image of tubular lumen showing mature spermatozoa with tapered nuclei and no appreciable cytoplasm. The presence of spermatozoa is consistent with intact spermatogenesis.

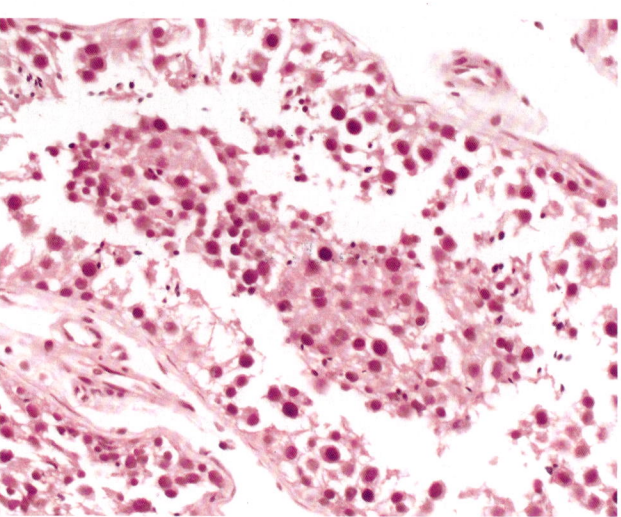

Figure 4.35. When spermatozoa are only identified in some tubules with other tubules showing maturation arrest or Sertoli cell–only pattern, the recommended diagnosis is hypospermatogenesis and including the other patterns and the approximate percentage of those patterns.

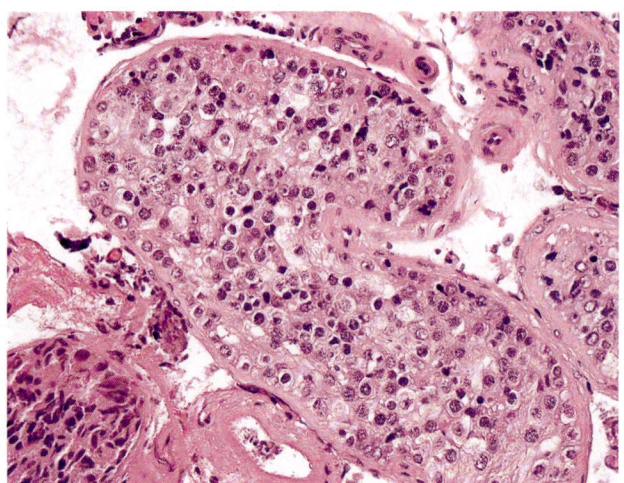

Figure 4.36. In maturation arrest, germ cells are present and show maturation to the secondary spermatocyte stage in this tubule. The tubular lumen is obscured and no spermatids or spermatozoa are identified.

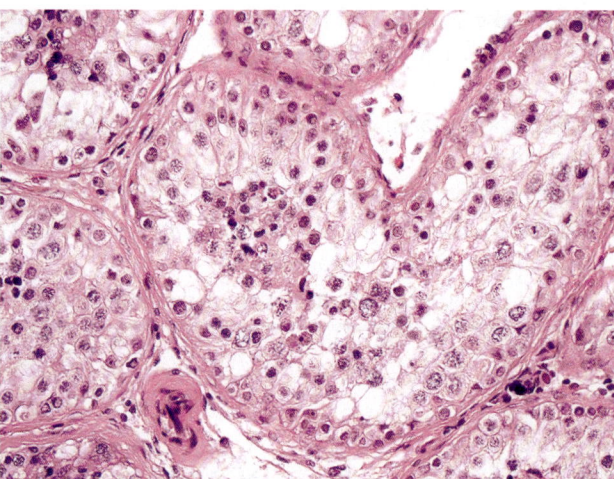

Figure 4.37. At higher power, the cytologic features of secondary spermatocytes are evident by the filamentous chromatin pattern and presence of the cells away from the adluminal compartment. Again, no spermatids or spermatozoa are present in the tubule.

INFECTIOUS/INFLAMMATORY
Orchitis and Epididymitis

Inflammation of the testis or epididymis is referred to as orchitis and epididymitis, respectively; however, they often occur together. These are usually clinical rather than histologic diagnoses, made when a patient presents with testicular pain and swelling. If a mass persists after appropriate antibiotic treatment, or the pain does not resolve, an orchiectomy may be performed for symptom relief. Categories that are more specific include acute, chronic, and granulomatous orchitis. Histologically, the inflammatory component may be either acute (neutrophilic) or chronic (lymphoplasmacytic or granulomatous), which can provide information about possible etiologies.

Acute infectious orchitis often occurs along with epididymitis, and common infectious agents include the usual urinary tract bacteria *Escherichia coli*, Pseudomonas, Klebsiella, Staphylococcus, Streptococcus, and Actinomyces species. *Neisseria gonorrhea* and *Chlamydia trachomatis* may be causative organisms in sexually active men. In acute epididymo-orchitis,

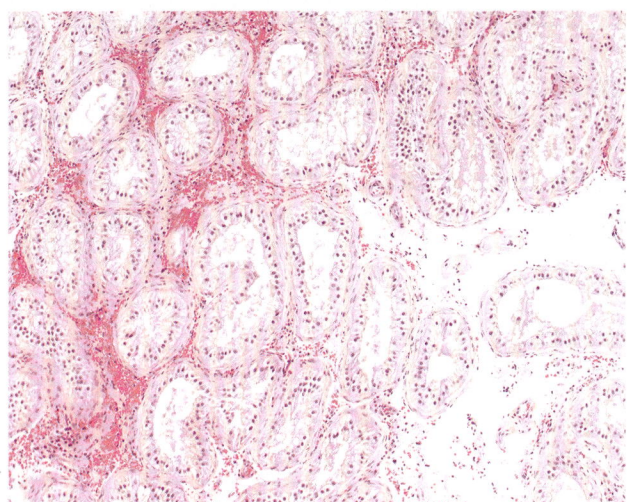

Figure 4.38. Sertoli cell–only pattern at low power, the tubules show a single cell type and lack mature spermatozoa in the lumens.

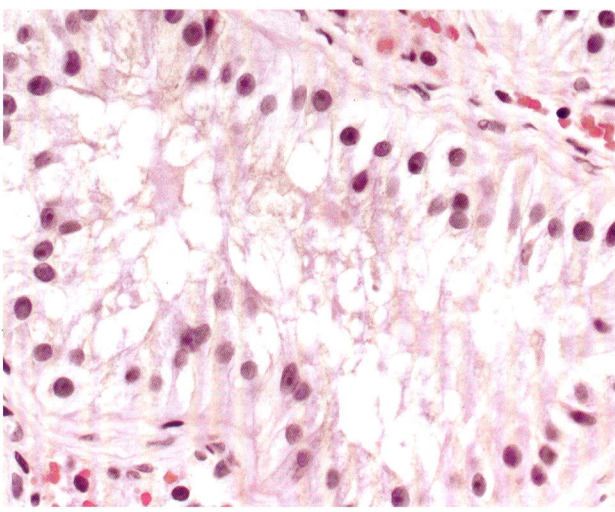

Figure 4.39. At high power, the classic cytologic features of Sertoli cells are present—pyramidal cells with wispy eosinophilic cytoplasm and ill-defined cell borders. Nuclei are round with prominent nucleoli.

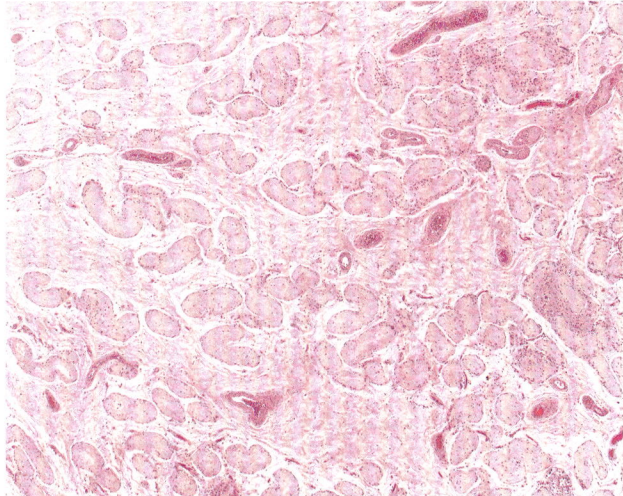

Figure 4.40. Atrophic testis showing hyalinized tubules with small diameters. The interstitium appears fibrotic with loss of Leydig cells.

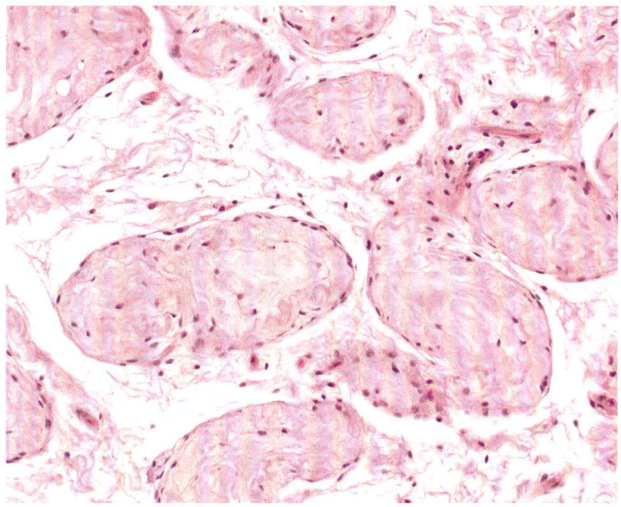

Figure 4.41. At high power, atrophic testis showing obliteration of tubular lumens and loose collagen occupying the majority of the surface area. No germ cells or Sertoli cells are present within the tubule.

a prominent neutrophilic infiltrate is expected, with a dominant abscess or microabscesses commonly identified. Chronic epididymo-orchitis may result from a long-standing bacterial infection, with a transition to more lymphoplasmacytic inflammatory cells and associated fibrosis and tubular destruction. This fibrotic stage is more likely to be confused for a possible malignancy as the tissues become fixed to surrounding soft tissue.

PEARLS AND PITFALLS: Mumps

- Orchitis and epididymitis usually co-occur, and isolated epididymitis is rare
- In a patient with isolated epididymitis, mumps should be the primary clinical consideration as epididymitis often occurs prior to orchitis
- Mumps epididymo-orchitis is an important diagnosis to make as it can often lead to infertility

Specific etiologies of granulomatous orchitis include fungal infection, tuberculosis, and sarcoidosis. Rarely, brucellosis can cause orchitis in men who handle livestock. A fungal organism known to cause epididymo-orchitis is Histoplasma, characterized by granulomas and small yeast forms with narrow-based budding. The yeast forms are highlighted on silver staining. Tuberculous epididymo-orchitis demonstrates findings similar to tubercular infections elsewhere, with caseating granulomas surrounded by multinucleated Langhans-type giant cells and histiocytes (Figure 4.42). Acid-fast bacilli can be demonstrated by Ziehl-Neelsen staining. In contrast to the caseating granulomas seen in tuberculosis, sarcoidosis involving the testis and epididymis demonstrates well-defined noncaseating granulomas.[12]

CHECKLIST: Differential Diagnosis of Granulomatous Processes in the Testis and Paratestis[13]

☐ Fungal infection
☐ Tuberculosis
☐ Sarcoidosis
☐ Vasculitis
☐ Malakoplakia
☐ Sperm granuloma
☐ Sclerosing lipogranuloma
☐ Seminoma with brisk granulomatous response

Malakoplakia

Malakoplakia can involve the testis and epididymis similar to other anatomic regions in continuity with the urinary tract. It involves the testis alone in more than two-thirds of cases and the testis and epididymis in a smaller percentage. Similar to other genitourinary cases, it is associated with chronic *E. coli* infections. It has a similar appearance of sheets of histiocytes, some of which contain targetoid inclusions (Michaelis-Gutmann bodies) (Figures 4.43 and 4.44). The process can be mass forming and lead to a concern for malignancy. Leydig cell tumor shares similar morphologic features of numerous cells with abundant eosinophilic cytoplasm; however, this differential is easily resolved with immunohistochemistry (Figure 4.45). Malakoplakia will show diffuse positivity for CD68 with an iron stain highlighting Michaelis-Gutmann bodies, and Leydig cell tumor will not express CD68 and show diffuse staining for inhibin and calretinin.[12]

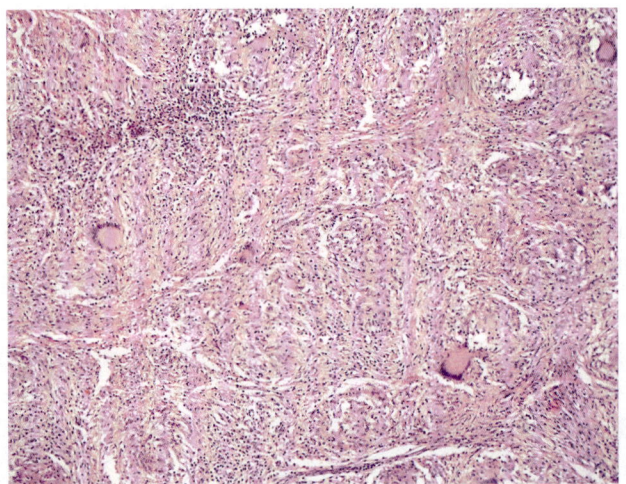

Figure 4.42. Granulomatous inflammation within the testis presents a broad differential diagnosis. In this image, the giant cells are of Langhans type, raising the possibility of tuberculous epididymo-orchitis.

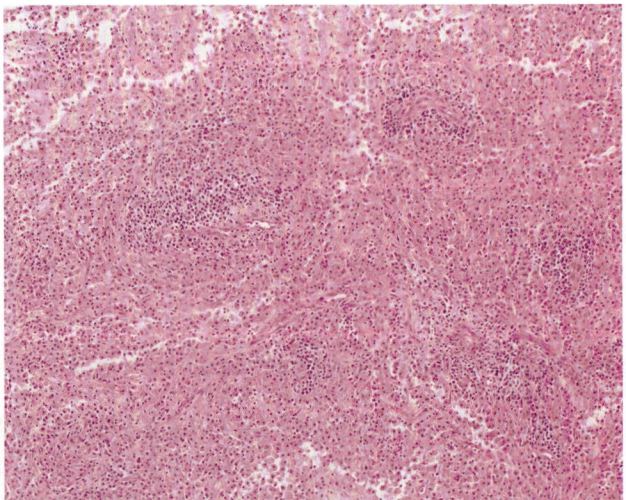

Figure 4.43. At low power, malakoplakia appears as sheets of eosinophilic histiocytes with scattered chronic inflammation.

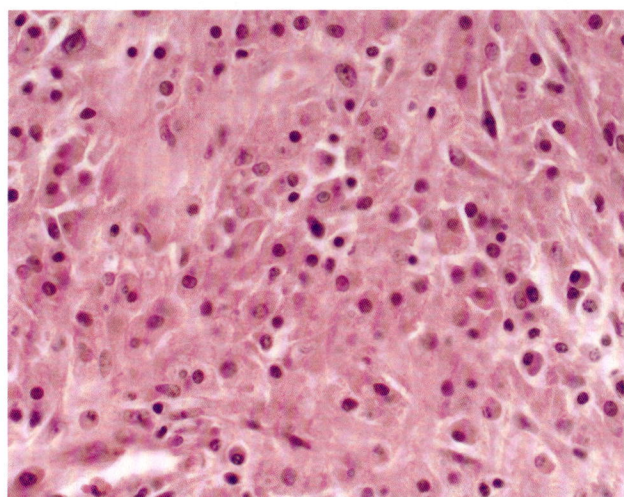

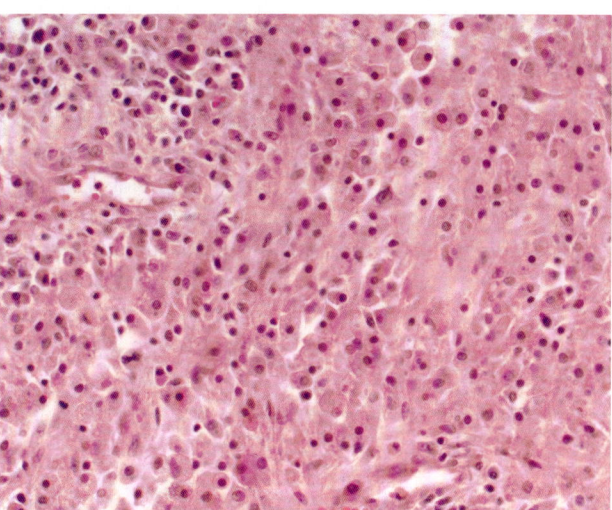

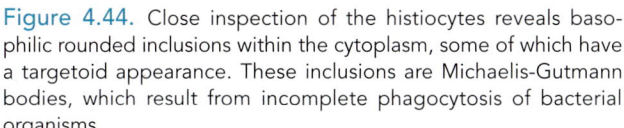

Figure 4.44. Close inspection of the histiocytes reveals basophilic rounded inclusions within the cytoplasm, some of which have a targetoid appearance. These inclusions are Michaelis-Gutmann bodies, which result from incomplete phagocytosis of bacterial organisms.

Figure 4.45. The epithelioid nature of the histiocytes with their abundant eosinophilic cytoplasm leads to some morphologic overlap with Leydig cell tumors.

Sperm Granuloma

Sperm granulomas form in reaction to extravasated sperm, which may occur after trauma or vasectomy. The resultant mass is painful and may mimic malignancy. These lesions are centered in the epididymis, with an initial neutrophilic response to sperm which evolves to granulomatous inflammation and fibrosis.[12]

TORSION AND VASCULITIS

Altered blood supply to the testis results in areas of infarction. The blood supply may be disrupted as a result of torsion, where the spermatic cord twists and cuts off the afferent blood supply, or vasculitis, where damaged blood vessels deliver insufficient blood to the testis. The clinical presentation of either type of the infarct is severe pain, which usually prompts a clinical examination and testicular ultrasound.

If torsion is suspected clinically, the urologist may first attempt a gentle twist of the testicle to see if blood flow can be quickly restored. Complete occlusion of blood supply to the testis can result in loss of a testicle, so this is treated as a urologic emergency. If the scrotal ultrasound shows no blood flow after the attempt to untwist the testis and the testicle is considered nonviable, an orchiectomy is performed. Depending on the time interval between initial torsion and orchiectomy, different histologic appearances are seen. Because the blood supply to the entire testis is affected in torsion, all of the parenchyma is infarcted. In the acute phase, there is hemorrhagic infarct with dilated vessels and extravasated red blood cells surrounding relatively normal tubules (Figure 4.46). As the time interval increases, the tubules begin to show necrosis, and fibrinoid vascular necrosis may predominate.

Isolated acute torsion is the primary cause of testicular torsion and has been associated with the bell-clapper deformity, which permits the testis to rotate within the tunica vaginalis. Given this association and the possibility of a bilateral deformity, orchidopexy is performed on the contralateral testis to ensure it does not torse in the future. There is also some evidence that torsion may be intermittent; histologic findings in these cases show vasculitis manifested by chronic vasculitis and fibrinoid necrosis of vessels, without any history or future development of systemic vasculitis.[14]

The differential diagnosis of an ischemic testis includes vasculitis. Testicular vasculitis is often a manifestation of a systemic process. Obtaining the patient's clinical history may reveal signs and symptoms of vasculitis affecting other organs. Polyarteritis nodosa (PAN)-like vasculitis is the most common type of vasculitis to affect the testis. Less commonly, granulomatosis with polyangiitis is responsible for testicular vasculitis.[15] The full differential diagnosis of the specific type of vasculitis depends on the size of vessels involved and is beyond the scope of this chapter. Regardless, recognition of a vasculitic process in the testis should prompt additional clinical workup.

The most important clue to the diagnosis of vasculitis is the presence of a segmental, rather than global, infarct (Figures 4.47 and 4.48). In the area of infarct, tubules may be completely necrotic, and only the outlines of "ghost tubules" remain (Figure 4.49). This often will involve only one lobule of the testis, with the remainder staying perfused and viable. In cases of segmental infarct, close inspection of the vessels is necessary to identify features of vasculitis: leukocytoclasis, red cell extravasation, fibrinoid necrosis, and granulomatous or nongranulomatous inflammation (Figures 4.50 and 4.51).

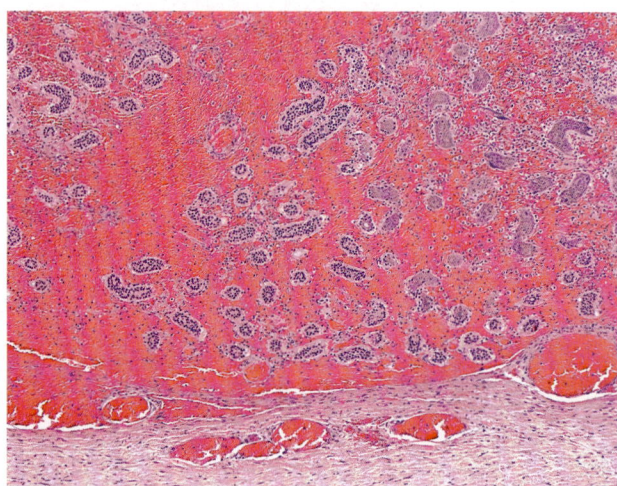

Figure 4.46. Acute testicular torsion in a pediatric patient showing diffuse hemorrhage within the interstitium. A subset of the tubules appears necrotic in the upper right corner, while others remain viable. If vascular occlusion persists, all of the tubules will become necrotic.

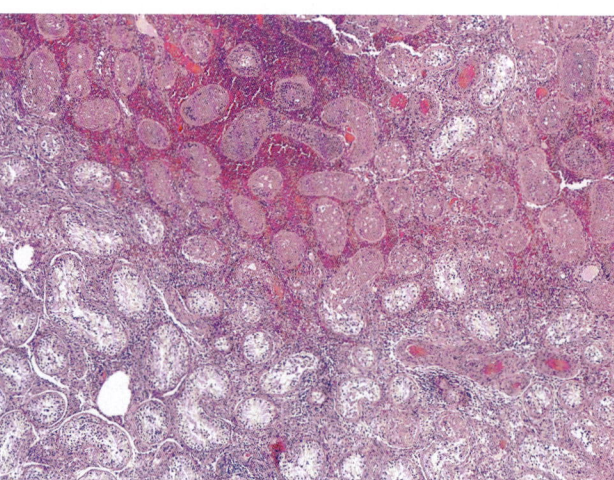

Figure 4.47. A segmental infarct of the testis resulting in focal necrosis of tubules, surrounded by viable tubules. This finding should prompt close examination of the vessels both adjacent and remote from the infarct.

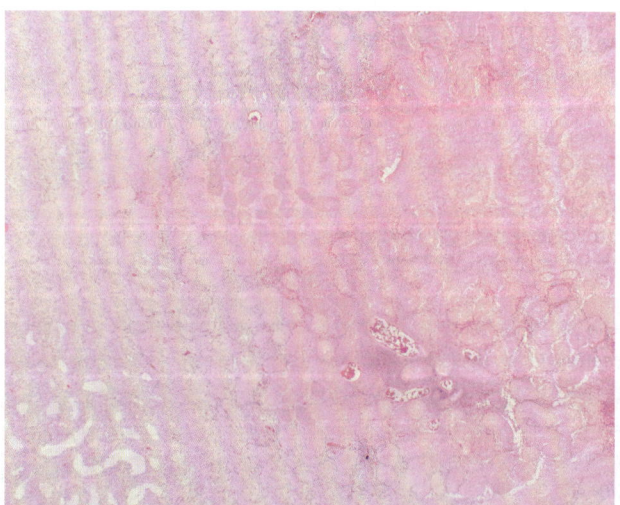

Figure 4.48. Another low-power image demonstrating the focal necrosis of a segmental infarct, with necrotic tubules immediately adjacent to viable tubules.

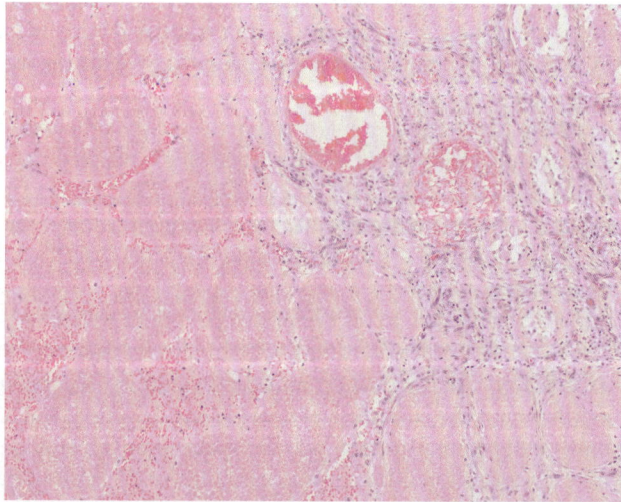

Figure 4.49. Area of remote infarction showing outlines of necrotic tubules with surrounding inflammation.

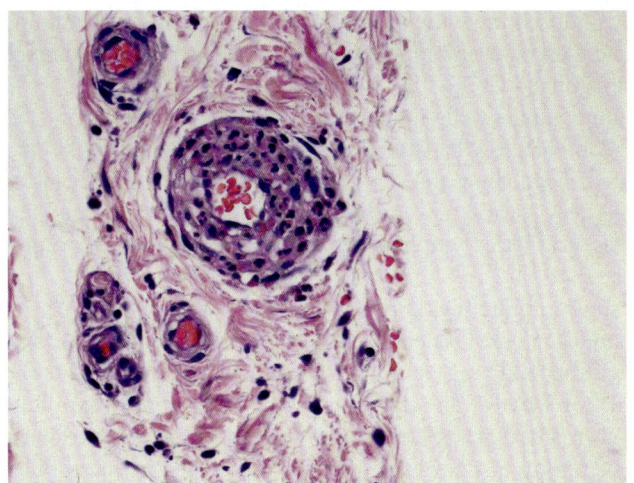

Figure 4.50. Close examination of the vessels of the testis should be undertaken for signs of vasculitis. At high power, leukocytoclasis—neutrophils transgressing the vessel wall—is identified in this specimen.

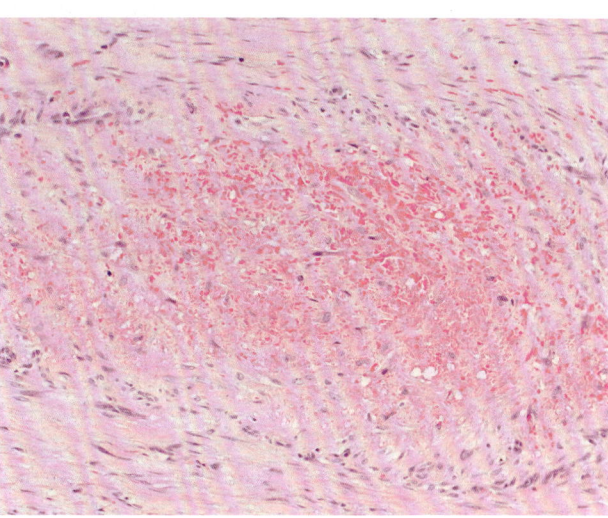

Figure 4.51. This vessel has been obliterated with fibrinoid necrosis evident in the vessel wall. Extravasated red blood cells are present surrounding the vessel, consistent with damaged, leaky vessels.

TESTICULAR TUMORS

Testicular tumors include all of the benign and malignant neoplasms arising in the testicular parenchyma, located within the tunica albuginea. The most common category of tumors within the testis is GCTs, those tumors that originate from the primordial germ cell.[16] These tumors can have a vast array of differing morphologies and will be discussed based on their general patterns below. It is important to know that while GCTs can arise in pure forms, especially in children, they are most commonly encountered as mixed GCTs comprised of multiple tumor types. The second most common category of testicular tumors is sex cord stromal tumors, which arise from the supporting cells within the testicular interstitium. The last category of testicular tumors is those that involve the testis secondarily in the form of metastatic disease or direct extension. The classic categorization of testicular tumors by cell of origin as designated in the 2016 WHO monograph is included in Table 4.4.[17]

When evaluating a testicular tumor, it is useful to start with a pattern-based approach. Specifically, recognizing whether you are dealing with a pure or mixed pattern can help direct you to a category—sex cord stromal tumors are generally a pure population of cells, whereas GCTs are often mixtures of different tumor types. Pure GCTs do occur, more commonly in children than in young adults. Once a general category of tumor is favored, or a focused differential diagnosis is formed, immunohistochemistry can be employed to confirm your impression.

The discussion on testicular tumors will be organized based on overall pattern recognition, with monomorphic or "pure" cell populations discussed first, followed by pleomorphic and organoid (forming organized cellular structures.)

MONOMORPHIC

Tumors in this category show a generally monomorphic pattern of growth. At scanning magnification, this group of neoplasms typically demonstrates solid or diffuse architecture. The cells are largely monotonous, with each individual cell looking quite similar to its neighboring cells in most cases. By pattern, the tumors included in monomorphic category include seminoma, lymphoma, Leydig cell tumor, granulosa cell tumor, and carcinoid/neuroendocrine tumor.

Seminoma

Seminoma is the most common GCT of the testis, comprising almost 50% of testicular GCTs. Seminoma is also the most common pure GCT, though it is also commonly identified in mixed GCTs. In clinical terms, a mixed GCT that contains any component other than seminoma would be considered "nonseminomatous," despite the presence of a seminoma component. This can be confusing as "nonseminomatous" does not exclude the presence of some amount of seminoma in a mixed GCT.

The gross appearance of seminoma is a well-circumscribed, white-tan fleshy lobulated mass (Figure 4.52). The gross lobular growth pattern is derived from the fibrous septa found within the tumor (Figure 4.53). Along the septa and scattered with the sheets of tumor are lymphocytes (Figure 4.54). At low power, the pattern of a white or cleared out area interrupted by pink (fibrosis) and blue (lymphocytes) is a useful pattern to recognize for seminoma.

Microscopically, the tumors show monotonous sheets of large cells with clear cytoplasm, polygonal nuclei (often with rounded square corners), and prominent central nucleoli. The classic description of these cells is the "fried egg" appearance, of a yolk in the middle of the cooked white (Figures 4.55 and 4.56). However, seminoma may exhibit more eosinophilic cytoplasm or even very scant cytoplasm. It is also common to see a granulomatous reaction within the tumor with numerous plump histiocytes, which may be located within tubules (Figure 4.57). The presence of a granulomatous reaction within the testis should prompt a careful search for possible seminoma or GCNIS (Figures 4.58 and 4.59). Likewise, clusters of lymphocytes are a helpful clue for possible intertubular seminoma, small tumors which may be grossly undetectable.[12]

TABLE 4.4: Malignant Testicular Tumors, Organized by Cell of Origin

Tumor Category	Tumors	Pattern	Page Reference
Germ cell tumors (GCTs) derived from germ cell neoplasia in situ	Germ cell neoplasia in situ	Organoid	371
	Seminomatous GCT		
	Seminoma	Monomorphic	351
	Nonseminomatous GCT		
	Embryonal carcinoma	Pleomorphic	363
	Yolk sac tumor	Pleomorphic	364
	Choriocarcinoma	Pleomorphic	368
	Teratoma (postpubertal)	Organoid	374
	Mixed germ cell tumor	Mixed	
	Regressed germ cell tumor	Spindle	377
Germ cell tumors unrelated to germ cell neoplasia in situ	Spermatocytic tumor	Pleomorphic	369
	Teratoma (prepubertal)	Organoid	372
	Dermoid and epidermoid cyst	Organoid	372
	Well-differentiated neuroendocrine tumor	Monomorphic	361
	Yolk sac tumor (prepubertal)	Pleomorphic	364
Sex cord stromal tumors	Leydig cell tumor	Monomorphic	357
	Sertoli cell tumor	Monomorphic	355
	Granulosa cell tumor	Monomorphic	360
	Fibroma-thecoma	Spindle	376
Secondary/metastatic tumors	Lymphoma	Monomorphic	354
	PNET/Ewing sarcoma	Monomorphic	362

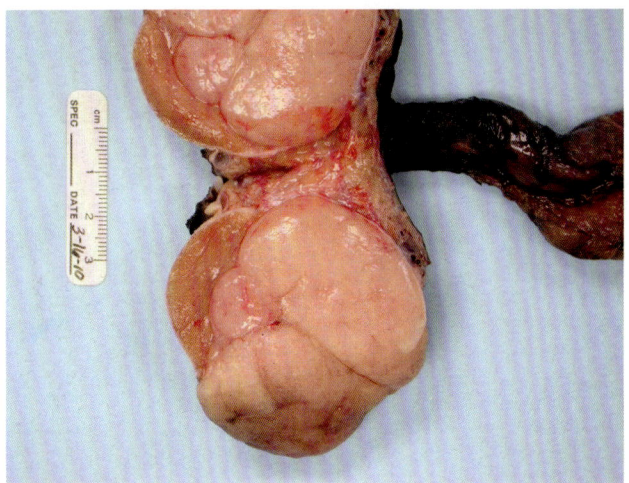

Figure 4.52. Gross photograph of a testis with seminoma. The gross appearance shows a white-tan, lobulated mass that bulges on cut section.

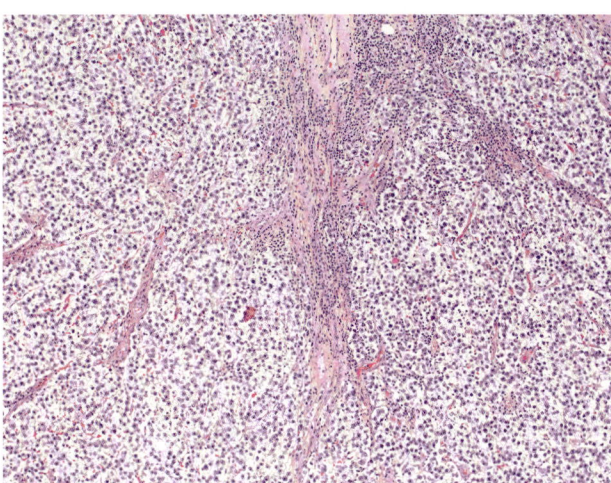

Figure 4.53. At low power, fibrous septa are evident as pink bands intersecting lobules of tumor. These bands correspond to the gross lobulated appearance.

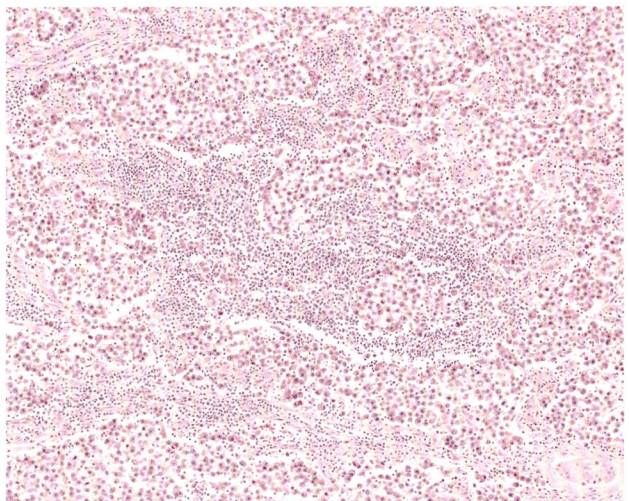

Figure 4.54. Lymphocytes are often closely associated with seminoma and often congregate along the fibrous septa.

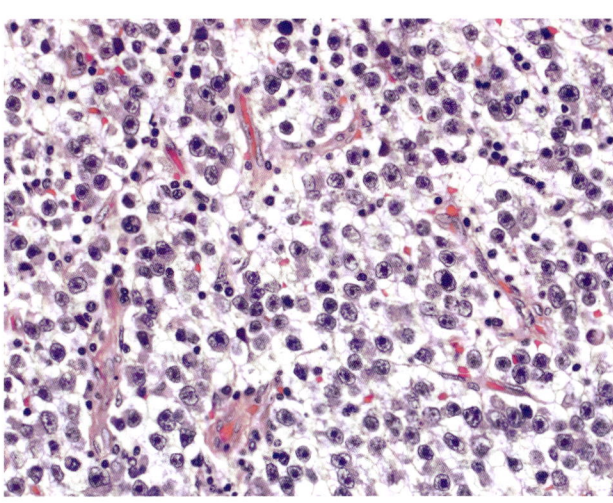

Figure 4.55. Cytologically, seminomas are often described as "fried egg" cells with abundant clear cytoplasm, polygonal nuclei, and prominent nucleoli. The clear cytoplasm and relatively low nuclear-to-cytoplasmic ratio give the tumor an overall white appearance.

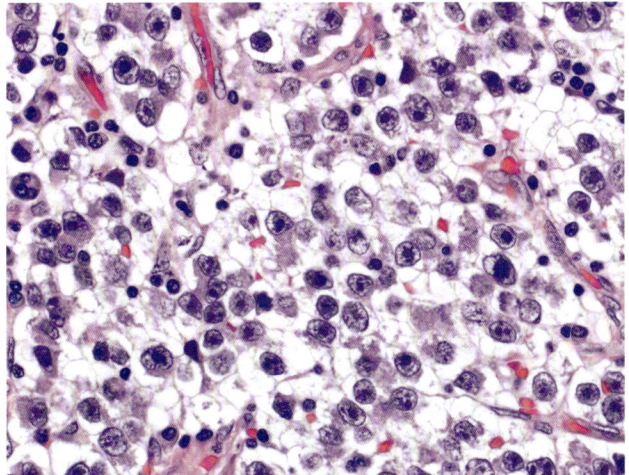

Figure 4.56. Nuclear features of seminoma are demonstrated in this image with the polygonal, squared-off nuclei and prominent macronucleoli.

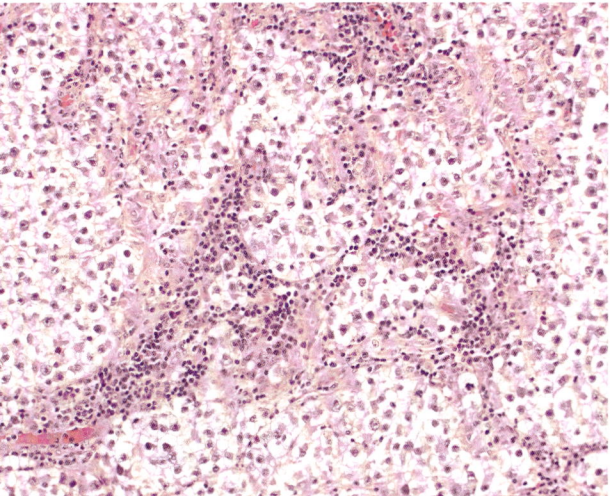

Figure 4.57. A granulomatous reaction is frequently present in seminomas. Plump eosinophilic histiocytes are present along with lymphocytes and seminoma cells. The finding of histiocytic reaction in a testis should prompt a close examination for possible seminoma cells.

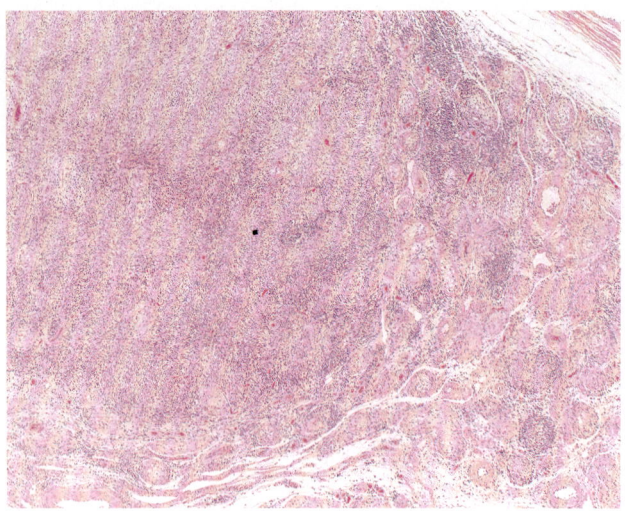

Figure 4.58. A brisk histiocytic response and numerous admixed lymphocytes in this image should raise suspicion for a possible seminoma.

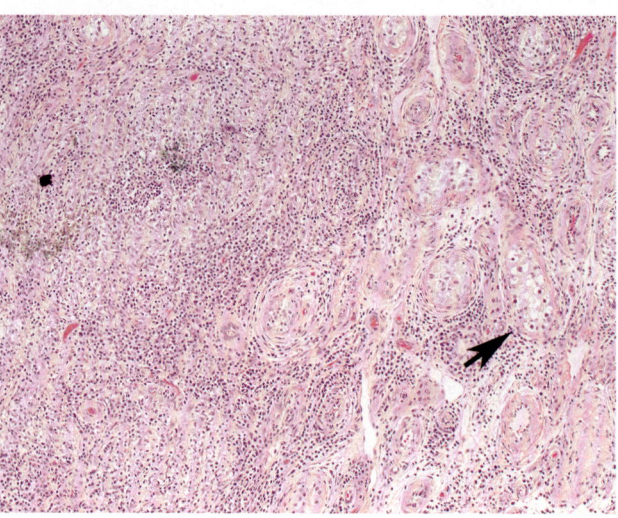

Figure 4.59. The presence of germ cell neoplasia in situ (GCNIS) (arrow) within the tubules also suggests a germ cell tumor is present.

Syncytiotrophoblastic cells may also be present in classic seminoma and do not represent a component of choriocarcinoma. These cells are large and multinucleated with abundant cytoplasm, morphologically identical to their counterparts in choriocarcinoma (Figures 4.60 and 4.61). Syncytiotrophoblastic cells can produce beta–human chorionic gonadotropin (bHCG) in measurable quantities—usually in the hundreds, rather than the thousands, which is more commonly seen when a choriocarcinoma is present. Presence of syncytiotrophoblastic cells and mild elevations in bHCG in an otherwise pure seminoma are not sufficient evidence of a choriocarcinoma.

Seminoma classically expresses OCT3/4, placental alkaline phosphatase (PLAP), and KIT, with OCT3/4 being the most specific stain for this entity. OCT3/4 also stains embryonal carcinoma, however. In seminomas with syncytiotrophoblastic cells, these multinucleated cells will stain for bHCG and should not be confused with a choriocarcinoma component.

> **PEARLS AND PITFALLS: Uncommon Architectural Patterns of Seminoma**
>
> - While classically solid, less common patterns of seminoma have been described and may cause confusion with other GCTs
> - Unusual morphologic variants and their nonseminomatous mimickers include:
>   - Microcystic → yolk sac tumor (YST)[18]
>   - Pseudoglandular → embryonal carcinoma (Figures 4.62 and 4.63)
>   - Tubular → Sertoli cell tumor
>   - Signet ringlike → other adenocarcinomas
> - Interstitial/intertubular pattern of seminoma occurs when single cells are found infiltrating within the interstitium without forming a solid mass[19] (Figure 4.64)

Lymphoma

Lymphoma may involve the testis secondarily as part of a more systemic presentation or rarely arises as a primary testicular lymphoma. The most common subtype of lymphoma is diffuse large B cell and as such, older men are more likely to present with testicular lymphoma. High-grade lymphomas comprise of pleomorphic malignant B lymphocytes, with high mitotic rates. The differential diagnosis of primary testicular lymphoma includes seminoma and spermatocytic tumor, which can be distinguished with immunohistochemistry.[20] When lymphoma involves the testis, it presents as sheets of cells with a relatively monotonous appearance, which spares the seminiferous tubules and expands the interstitium (Figure 4.65).

PEARLS AND PITFALLS: Distinguishing Seminoma From Lymphoma in the Testis

- Morphologic overlap of seminoma and lymphoma based on the relatively monotonous cytology and numerous lymphocytes (Figure 4.66)
- Clinically, lymphoma often occurs in older adults, whereas seminoma occurs in younger males; however, some pure seminomas occur in older men
- Most common lymphoma to involve testis in adults is diffuse large B-cell lymphoma, which is highly pleomorphic
- Seminoma usually is more monotonous than lymphoma (Figure 4.67)
- Lymphoma spares the tubules and proliferates within the interstitium
- No GCNIS identified in lymphoma
- Seminoma positive for OCT3/4, SALL4, and PLAP
- Lymphoma positive for lymphoid markers (CD45, CD20)
- Occasionally, lymphomas can express OCT3/4 or SALL4, so these markers should be applied as part of a panel[21]

Sertoli Cell Tumor

Sertoli cell tumors are the second most common type of stromal tumors in the testis. They comprise of nodules of Sertoli cells, which may have varying morphologic features depending on the clinical scenario. The most common morphologic pattern seen across all patients would be Sertoli cell tumor, not otherwise specified. In special patient populations, such as Carney syndrome and Peutz-Jeghers syndrome (specifically the large cell calcifying type) and AISs, variant histology may be the rule. Syndromic cases are more likely to present as bilateral tumors. Like Leydig cell tumors, the overwhelming majority of cases are benign. Malignant features are similar to those listed below for Leydig cell tumors. (Page 358 for **Key Features: Features of malignancy in Leydig cell tumors**).

Sertoli cell tumors demonstrate a number of growth patterns, but generally, some degree of tubule formation is present, which is the most reliable feature for recognizing Sertoli cell differentiation. Intervening myxoid or sclerotic stroma is frequently identified (Figures 4.68-4.70). The cytologic features of Sertoli cell tumors include pale eosinophilic to cleared out cytoplasm, resulting from the presence of lipid within the cells (Figure 4.71). The other patterns observed in this tumor type include solid, nodular, trabecular, and nested (Figures 4.72 and 4.73). Because of the abundance of growth patterns, the differential diagnosis of this tumor is broad (see Pearls and Pitfalls below).

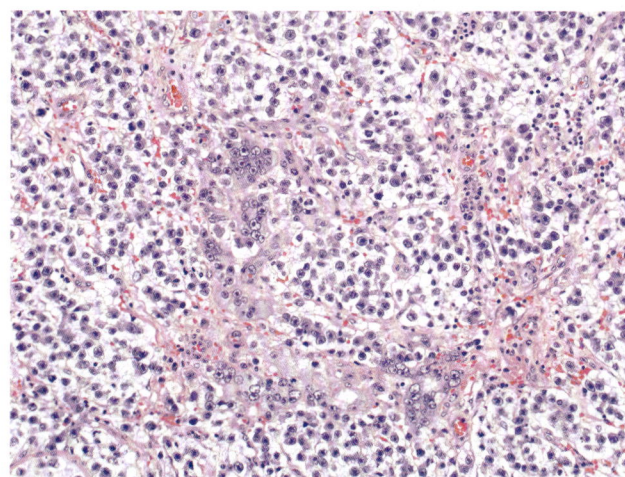

Figure 4.60. Syncytiotrophoblastic cells may be present in otherwise pure seminomas. They do not signify a component of choriocarcinoma by themselves.

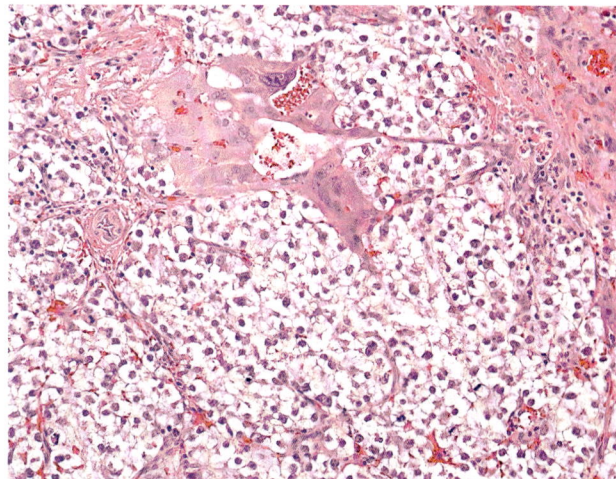

Figure 4.61. Multinucleated cells with abundant cytoplasm are present in a background of classic seminoma cells. These syncytiotrophoblastic cells secrete beta human chorionic gonadotropin (bHCG) and can lead to a minimal elevation in serum bHCG.

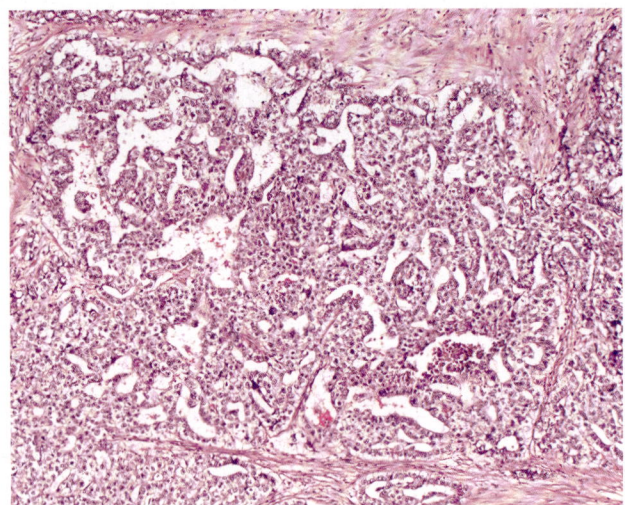

Figure 4.62. At low power, this tumor shows a glandular pattern that may suggest an embryonal carcinoma. However, the cytologic features are too monotonous for embryonal carcinoma, which shows marked pleomorphism and frequent mitotic figures. This image demonstrates a pseudoglandular pattern of seminoma, which can mimic embryonal carcinoma.

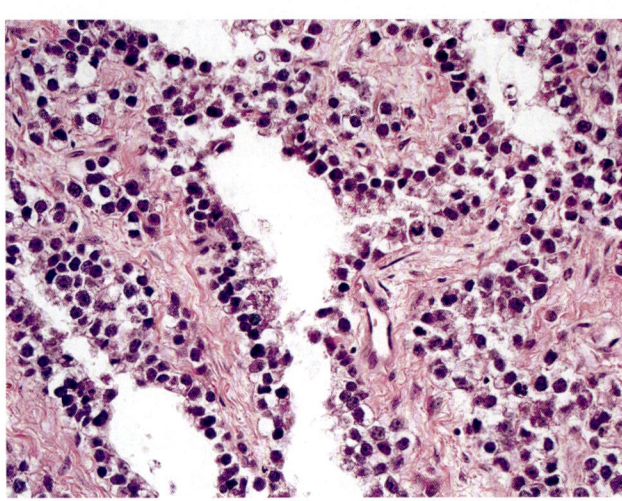

Figure 4.63. In this image, a focus of the pseudoglandular pattern arising in seminoma shows open glandular areas. However, the cytoplasm of this case is less abundant than classic seminoma, the nuclear shape (polygonal) and prominent nucleoli are consistent with seminoma. Immunohistochemistry can help resolve this differential, with seminoma expressing CD117 (KIT) and D2-40, and embryonal carcinoma expressing keratin and CD30.

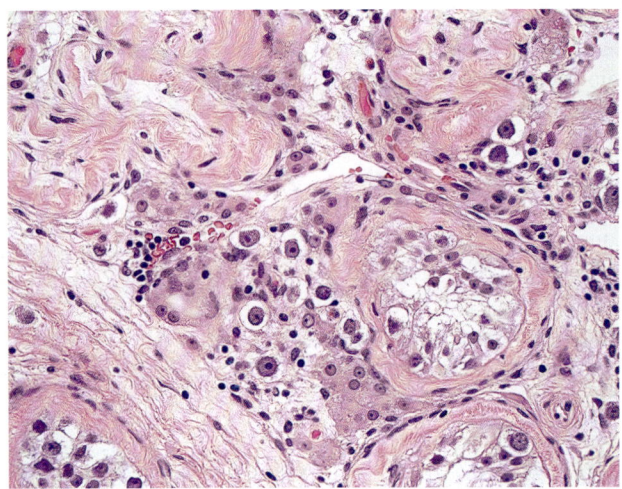

Figure 4.64. In interstitial/intertubular seminoma, malignant cells percolate between seminiferous tubules without forming an obvious mass.

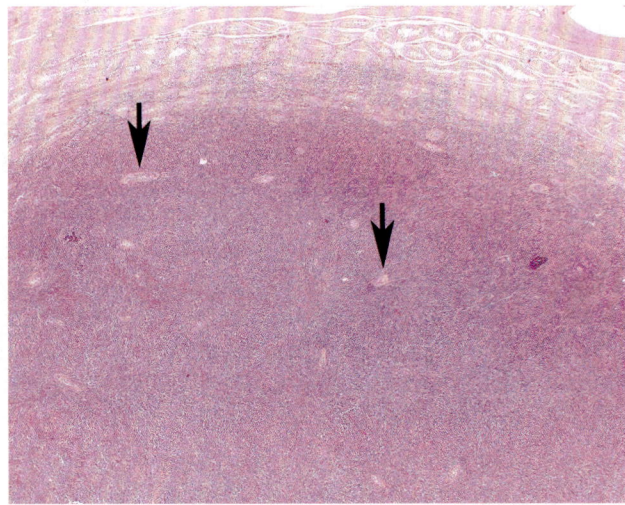

Figure 4.65. Low-power image of testicular lymphoma forming a sheet of monotonous cells surrounding and entrapping the seminiferous tubules (arrows). Uninvolved tubules are present at the periphery and should be evaluated for the presence of germ cell neoplasia in situ (GCNIS), which would support a diagnosis of seminoma when identified.

Immunohistochemistry may assist in the differential diagnosis of these tumor types. Sertoli cell tumors are strongly and diffusely positive for inhibin, calretinin, and SF1. Carcinoid tumor would be positive for neuroendocrine markers, YST would stain for alpha-fetoprotein (AFP) and glypican 3, and seminoma would be positive for PLAP and OCT3/4. There is immunohistochemical overlap with Leydig cell tumors, with both tumors expressing inhibin and calretinin. Melan A is more likely to be expressed in Leydig cell tumors.

PEARLS AND PITFALLS: Growth Patterns of Sertoli Cell Tumors and the Associated Differential Diagnosis

- Trabecular/nested → carcinoid tumor
- Retiform → yolk sac tumor
- Solid with clear cytoplasm → seminoma[22]
- Solid with eosinophilic cytoplasm → Leydig cell tumor (Figure 4.74)
- Cords → granulosa cell tumor

FAQ: What are the Genetic and Clinical Features of Carney Syndrome?

- Autosomal dominant germline mutation in *PRKAR1A* at 17q23-24
- Skin manifestations are often first clue to syndrome: lentigines and blue nevi[23]
- Strongly associated with large cell calcifying Sertoli cell tumor (Figure 4.75)
- Multiple organs affected including CAH and various tumor types including pituitary adenomas, myxomas, myxoid fibroadenomas, and schwannomas

Leydig Cell Tumor

In the category of stromal cell tumors of the testis, Leydig cell tumors are the most common subtype. Because they comprise of functional Leydig cells, they may produce androgens, which lead to clinical signs such as gynecomastia or precocious puberty.

Histologically, Leydig cell tumors are usually well-circumscribed, monotonous proliferations of rounded cells with abundant granular eosinophilic cytoplasm and round nuclei (Figure 4.76). The neoplastic cells are morphologically similar to normal Leydig cells, and lipofuscin pigment and Reinke crystals are commonly identified within the cytoplasm (Figure 4.77). Expression of alpha-inhibin, calretinin, Melan A, steroidogenic factor 1 (SF1), and androgen receptor antibodies is found in Leydig cell tumors.[24] Neuroendocrine markers may show patchy expression. This immunoprofile is relatively nonspecific and overlaps with other sex cord stromal tumors, though Melan A may be helpful.

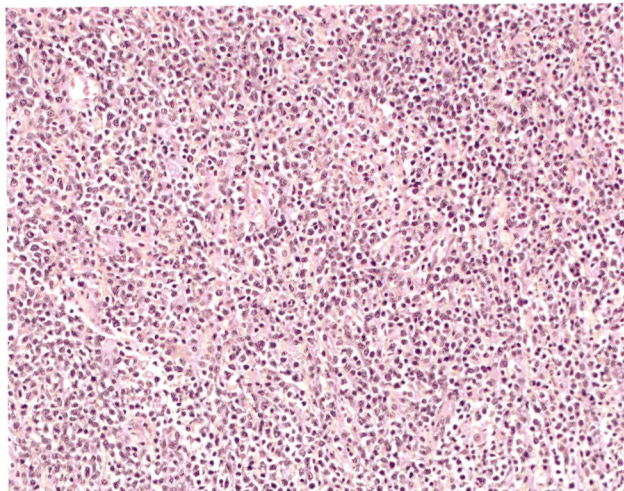

Figure 4.66. Lymphoma demonstrating sheets of relatively small, monotonous cells with a lymphoid appearance. Although diffuse large B-cell lymphoma is the most common lymphoma to involve the testis, small to intermediate cell lymphomas are more likely to be confused with seminoma due to lesser degree of pleomorphism.

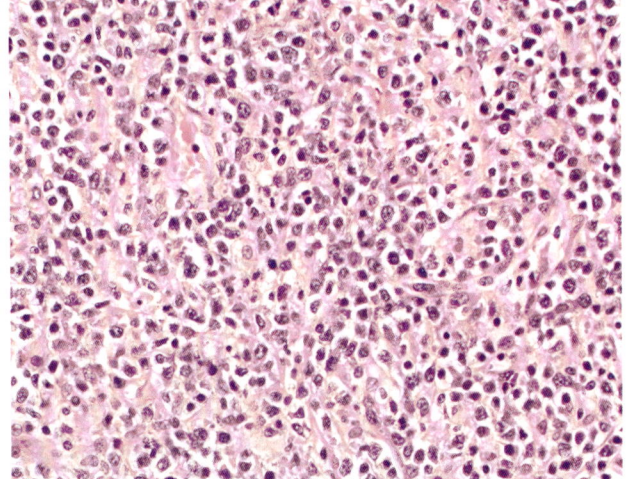

Figure 4.67. Lymphoma cells at high power show more nuclear pleomorphism with crinkled and pyknotic cells throughout the mass. While the cytoplasm is clumped in areas, large distinct nucleoli are not identified, which would be expected in seminoma.

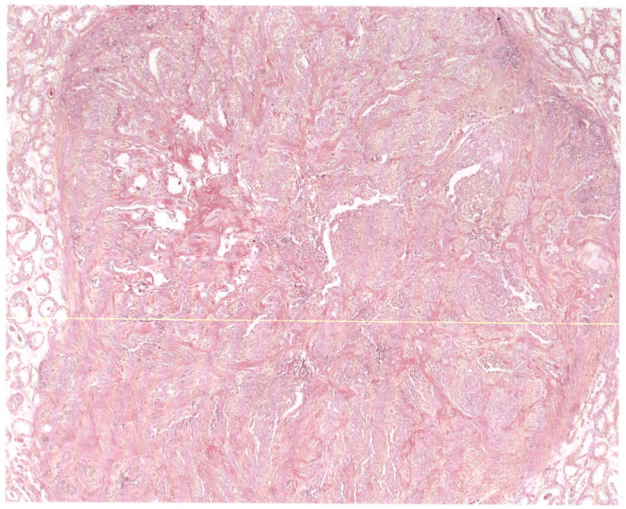

Figure 4.68. Low-power image of Sertoli cell tumor, not otherwise specified (NOS) showing relative circumscription and a nested to tubular appearance with intervening fibrous septa.

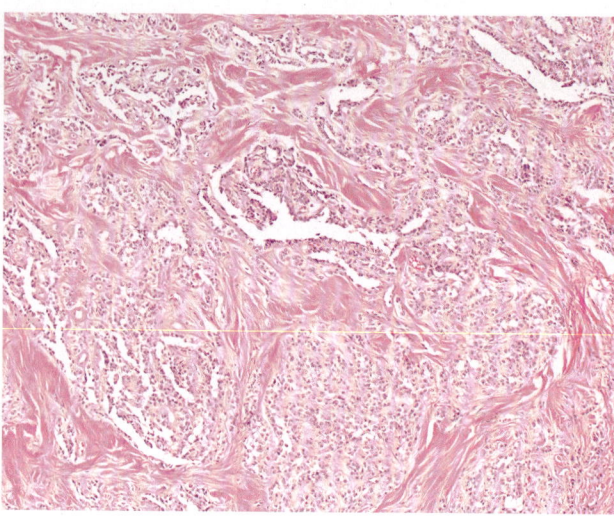

Figure 4.69. Dense fibrous bands are a low-power clue to the diagnosis of Sertoli cell tumor, as seen in this image.

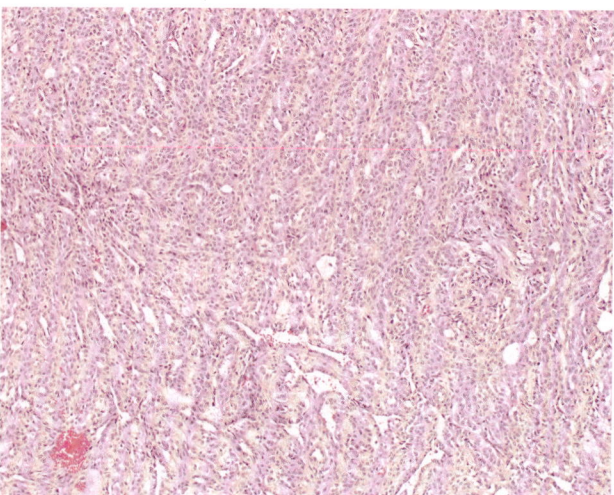

Figure 4.70. Some degree of tubule formation is found in the vast majority of Sertoli cell tumors and is one of the immediate clues to the diagnosis.

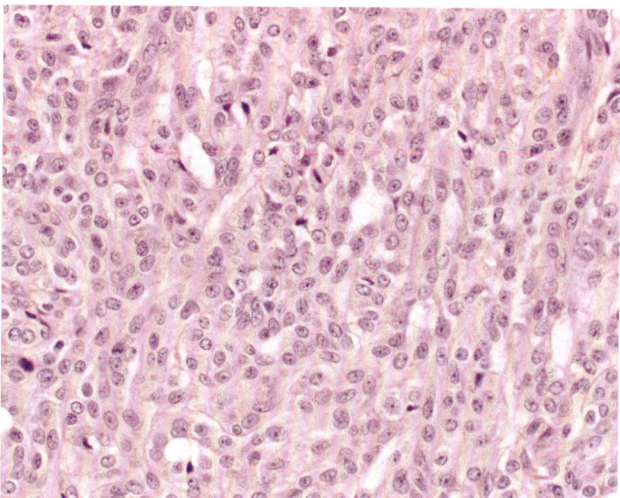

Figure 4.71. The cytologic features of Sertoli cell tumor are monotonous rounded cells with pale, eosinophilic to cleared-out cytoplasm, resulting from the presence of lipid within the cells. There is morphologic overlap with the carcinoid tumor, given the bland appearance of the cells and somewhat stippled chromatin; immunohistochemistry can be useful to distinguish the two entities.

These tumors usually have an indolent course, without only 10% exhibiting malignant behavior. Metastatic disease is the only definitive sign of malignancy; however, specific features suggestive of malignancy have been described (see FAQ).

KEY FEATURES: Features of Malignancy in Leydig Cell Tumors[25,26]

- Large size (>5 cm)
- Infiltrative margins
- Extratesticular extension (Figure 4.78)
- Cytologic atypia (Figure 4.79)
- Increased or atypical mitotic figures
- Lymphovascular invasion (LVI) (Figure 4.80)
- Necrosis (Figures 4.81 and 4.82)
- Increased Ki-67 proliferation index

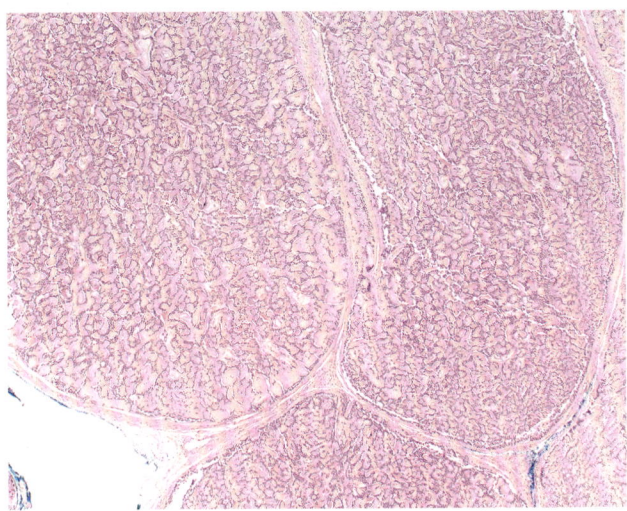

Figure 4.72. A more trabecular arrangement of cells is seen in this Sertoli cell tumor, another morphologic mimic of the carcinoid tumor.

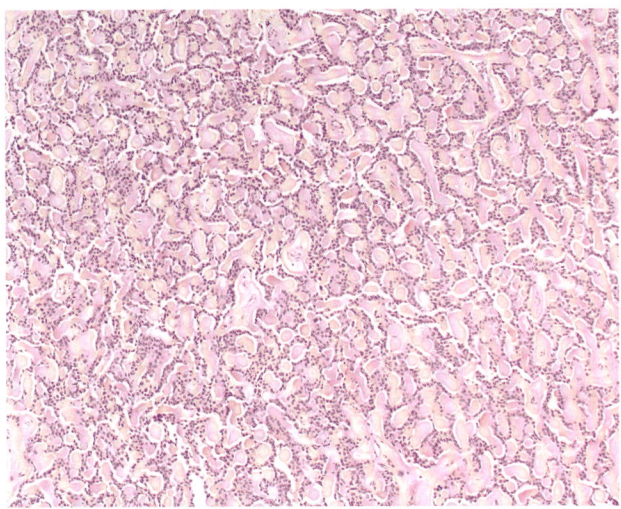

Figure 4.73. At higher power, dense hyaline material is present between the trabeculae. This material recapitulates the seminiferous tubule basement membrane.

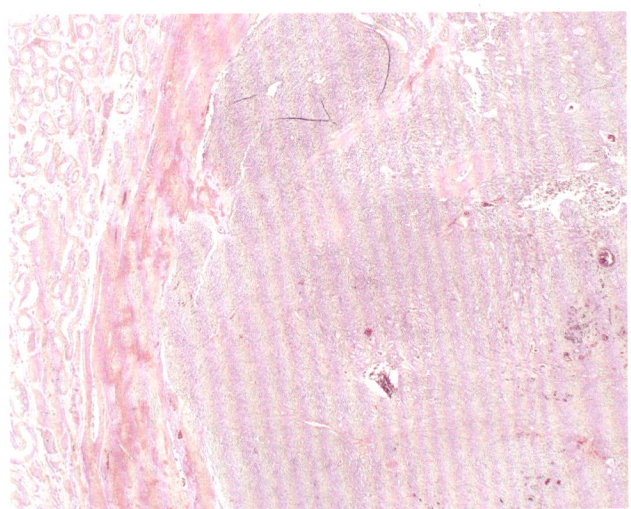

Figure 4.74. This well-circumscribed eosinophilic neoplasm may raise the possibility of Leydig cell tumor at low power. Sertoli cell tumors have overlapping histologic features, but typically, some tubular growth pattern and fibrous septa are evident to assist in the diagnosis.

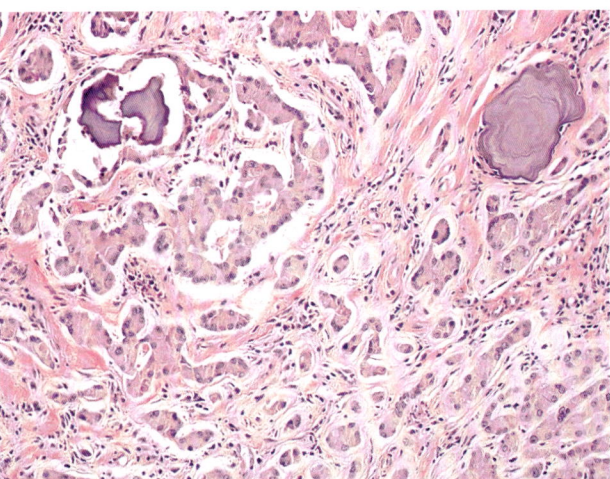

Figure 4.75. Large-cell calcifying Sertoli cell tumor is a very specific histologic variant associated with Carney syndrome. This tumor demonstrates cords of Sertoli cells with abundant eosinophilic cytoplasm (as compared with the smaller cells of Sertoli cell tumor not otherwise specified [NOS]) and large calcifications.

SAMPLE NOTE: Leydig Cell Tumors

Testis, left, radical orchiectomy:
Leydig cell tumor, 2.0 cm
Tumor lacks features associated with aggressive behavior (see Note)

Note: The majority of Leydig cell tumors exhibit indolent behavior. Features associated with potential for aggressive behavior include size >5 cm, infiltrative margins, extratesticular extension, cytologic atypia, increased or atypical mitotic figures, LVI, necrosis, and increased Ki-67 proliferation index. These features are not identified in this tumor.

PEARLS AND PITFALLS: Ectopic Leydig Cells in Spermatic Cord

- Finding Leydig cells outside of the testicular parenchyma does not mean they are malignant!
- Benign Leydig cells have the propensity to grow along nerves and may be identified in the spermatic cord, testicular mediastinum, tunica albuginea, and epididymis

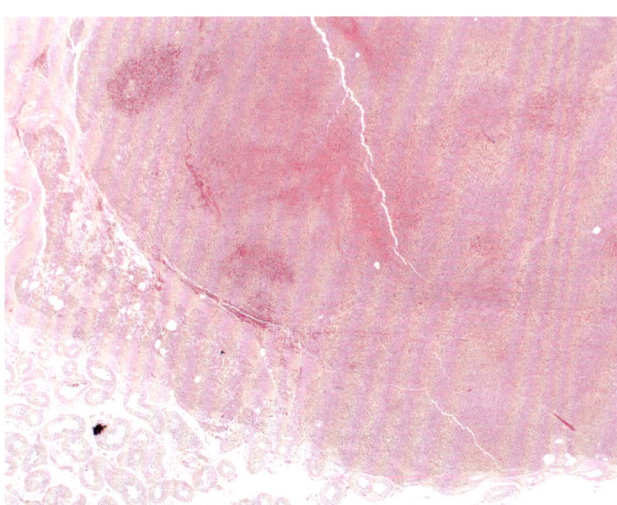

Figure 4.76. Benign Leydig cell tumors are well-circumscribed tumors with an eosinophilic appearance at low power.

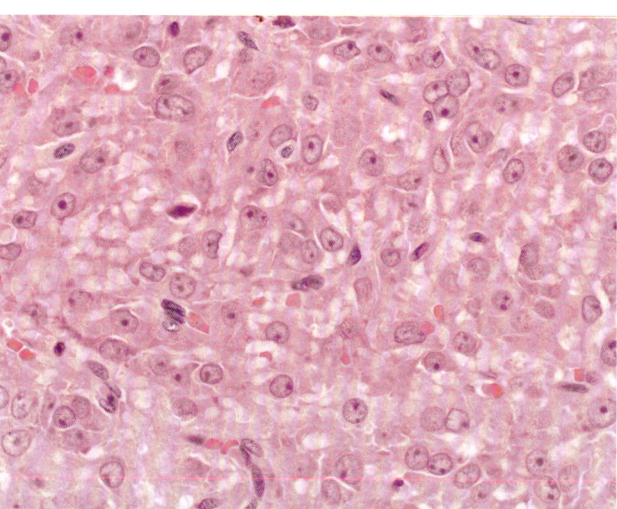

Figure 4.77. Cytologically, Leydig cell tumors have the same cytologic features as benign Leydig cells with ample eosinophilic cytoplasm, often containing lipofuscin pigment. Crystalline material is present within the cytoplasm.

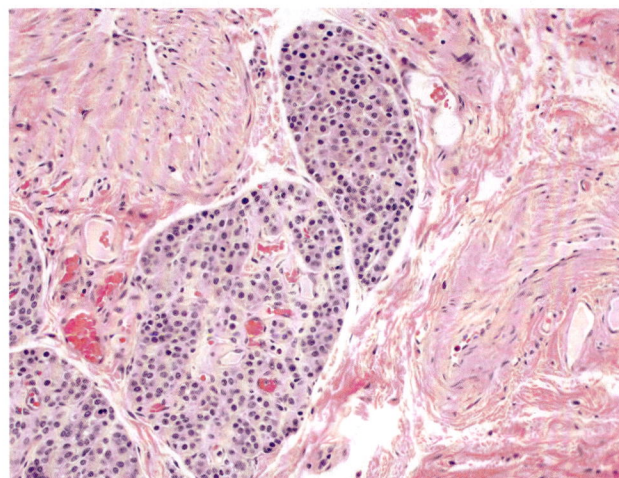

Figure 4.78. Leydig cell tumor with positive spermatic cord margin, consistent with extratesticular extension. Infiltrative margins and extension beyond the testis are features of potential malignant behavior in sex cord stromal tumors.

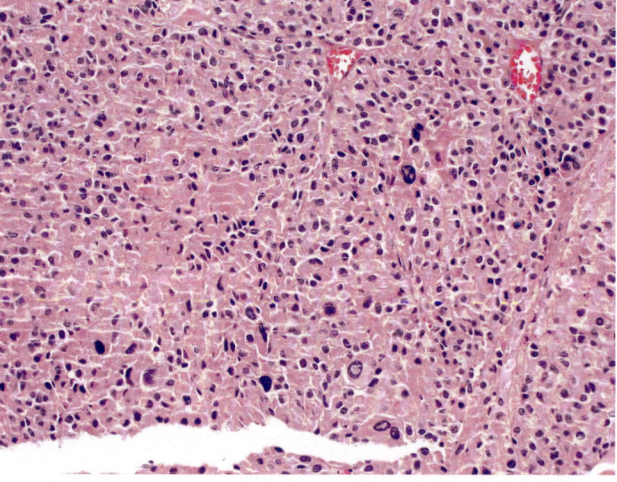

Figure 4.79. High-grade nuclear atypia arising in a Leydig cell tumor is another finding suggestive of potential aggressive behavior.

Granulosa Cell Tumor

Granulosa cell tumors are a rare sex cord tumor occurring more commonly in the ovary, but also in the testis. These tumors are derived from the FSH-responsive granulosa cells, which in turn secrete estrogens and can lead to clinical signs of gynecomastia. Serum levels of inhibin are often elevated in these patients. Like the other tumors in the sex cord stromal category, the majority of granulosa cell tumors have a benign course. Granulosa cell tumors are divided into two subtypes: juvenile and adult type.

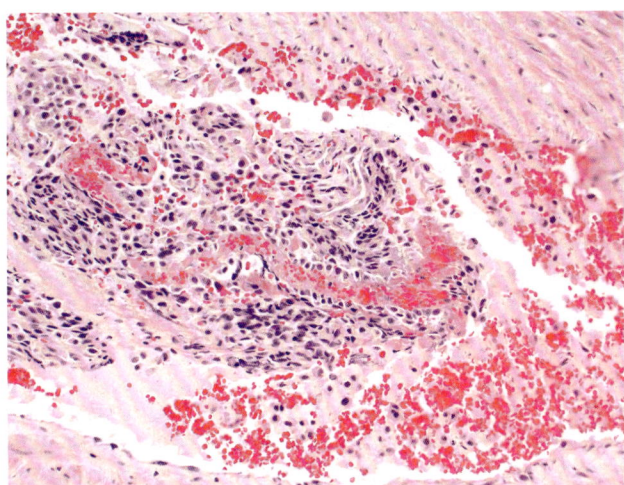

Figure 4.80. Leydig cell tumor with lymphovascular invasion raises suspicion for malignant behavior.

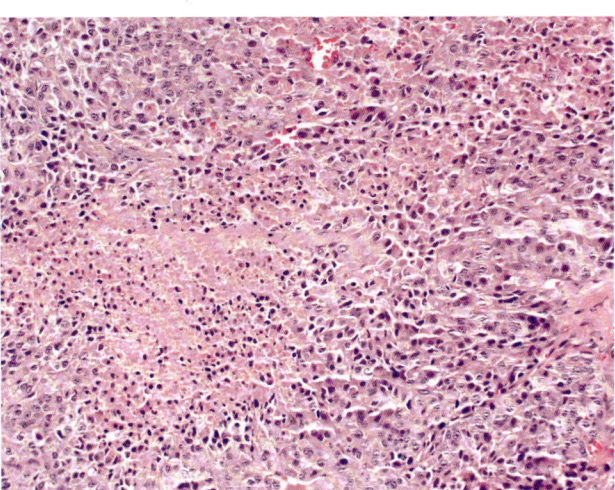

Figure 4.81. Another finding supporting the possibility of malignant behavior in Leydig cell and other sex cord stromal tumors is necrosis.

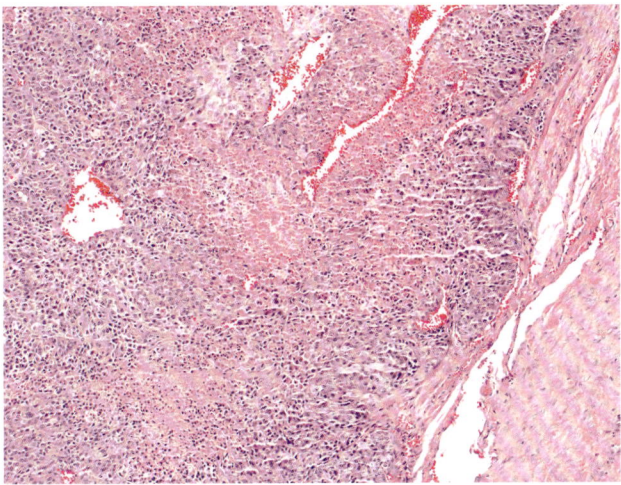

Figure 4.82. Geographic necrosis is present in this Leydig cell tumor, a finding that would not be expected in a benign tumor.

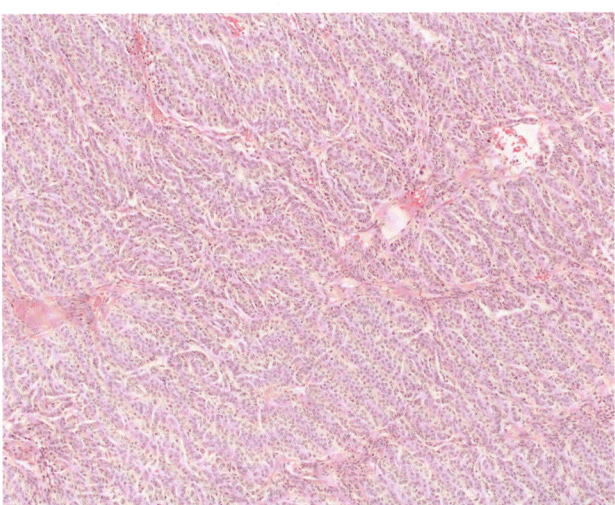

Figure 4.83. Granulosa cell tumor demonstrating a solid, nodular pattern of growth and relatively bland appearance at low power.

Histologically, adult-type granulosa cell tumors show a solid/diffuse to nodular growth pattern, often with areas displaying the classic Call-Exner bodies (Figures 4.83 and 4.84). Call-Exner bodies are small follicular arrangements of granulosa cells surrounding acellular eosinophilic material. Cytologically, the tumor cells are classically described as showing "coffee bean" morphology with a grooved nucleus (Figure 4.85). Inhibin is the most commonly positive IHC marker in granulosa cell tumors, along with other nonspecific markers of sex cord stromal derivation like SF1 and calretinin.[17]

Juvenile granulosa cell tumors occur in boys younger than 1 year. These tumors are distinguished from their adult counterparts by a mixture of architectural patterns, with prominent large follicles frequently identified. A nodular growth pattern is common, containing the variably sized follicles and intervening cellular stroma. Within the follicular spaces, basophilic material is frequently present.

Carcinoid/Well-Differentiated Neuroendocrine Tumor

Like carcinoid tumor in other locations, testicular carcinoid tumors are well-differentiated neuroendocrine neoplasms. Primary pure testicular carcinoids are rare, comprising less than 1% of testicular tumors. Carcinoid tumors have been found associated with teratoma, epidermoid, and dermoid cysts.[27] These tumors are felt to represent a monodermal teratoma of the testis. Due to the rarity of primary testicular carcinoid, one must exclude secondary involvement of the testis from a carcinoid tumor in another primary location.

The classic architectural pattern of the carcinoid tumor is nested or trabecular growth and rosettes may be present (Figures 4.86-4.88). Cytologically, the nuclear features of carcinoid tumor are finely stippled chromatin without apparent nucleoli (Figure 4.89). Neuroendocrine markers are positive in these tumors, including synaptophysin, chromogranin, and CD56.

Overall, testicular carcinoid tumors have a favorable outcome and benign course following orchiectomy. However, "atypical" carcinoid tumors with increased mitotic figures (2-10 mitotic figures per high-power field) or coagulative necrosis have metastatic potential. Additionally, larger tumors are more likely to metastasize than smaller tumors.

Primitive Neuroectodermal Tumors

Primitive neuroectodermal tumors (PNETs) in their pure form are rare in the testis and the subject of case reports only.[28,29] More commonly, they arise as secondary somatic-type malignancy in a teratoma as overgrowth of immature neural tissues.[30] The morphology of a primary PNET is similar to that seen in the central nervous system (CNS): primitive small round blue cells forming tubules and true rosettes and solid sheets of tumor (Figure 4.90). Neurofibrillary-type stroma may be present. These tumors will express CD99 in a strong, membranous pattern like their CNS counterparts.

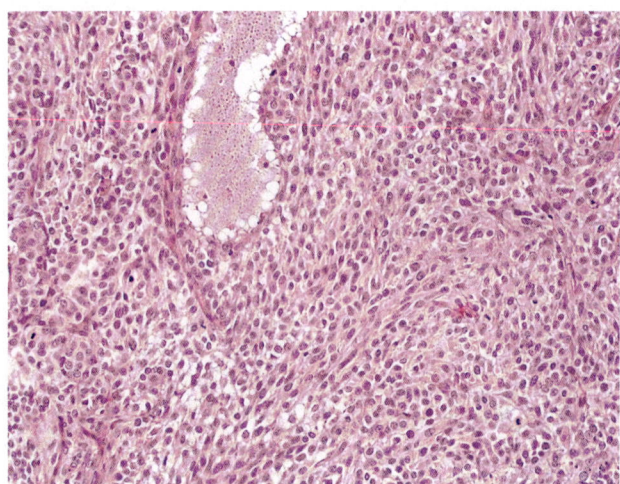

Figure 4.84. Granulosa cell tumors are hypercellular and can be highly mitotically active, which does not necessarily reflect their potential for aggressive behavior.

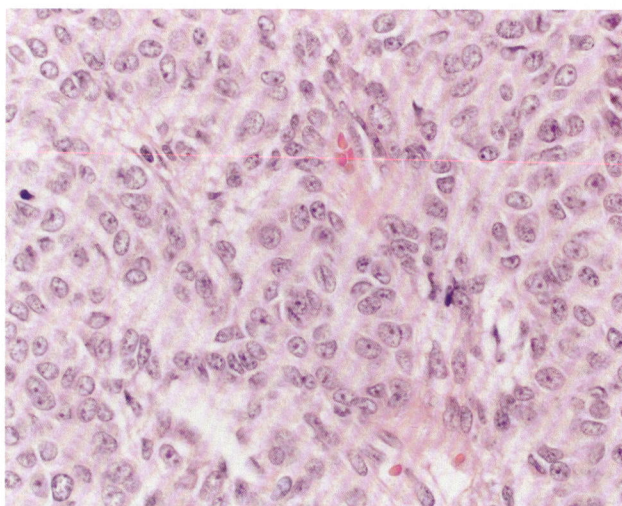

Figure 4.85. The classic cytologic features of granulosa cells include finely granular chromatin with nuclear grooves, leading to the comparison with "coffee beans."

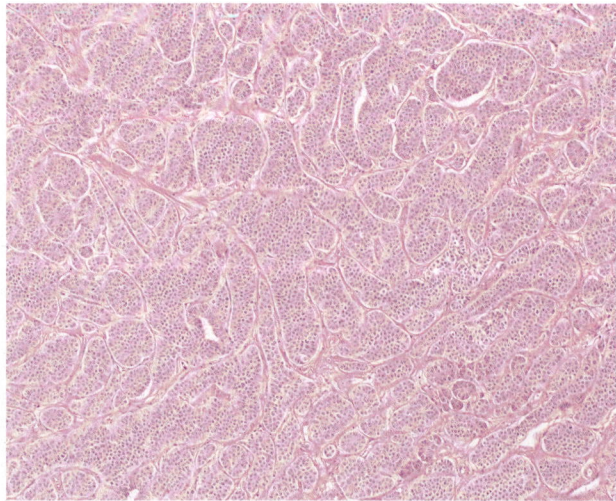

Figure 4.86. Low-power view of carcinoid tumor demonstrating the classic architectural growth pattern of trabecular cords and nests.

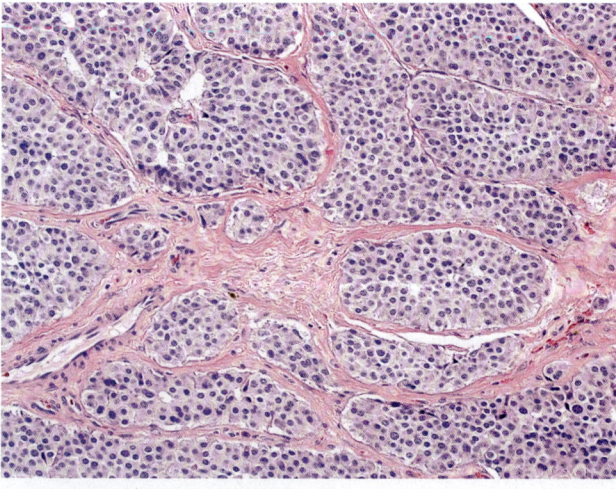

Figure 4.87. Medium-sized nests of monotonous rounded cells are present in this carcinoid tumor.

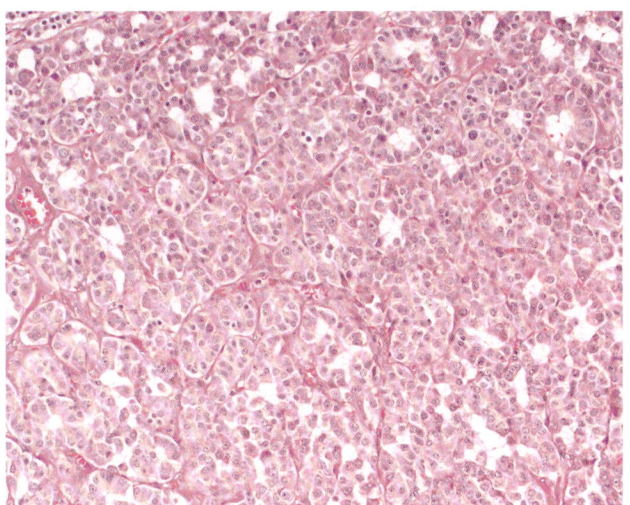

Figure 4.88. Rosettes are also frequently identified in carcinoid tumors and may mimic tubular growth in Sertoli cell tumors.

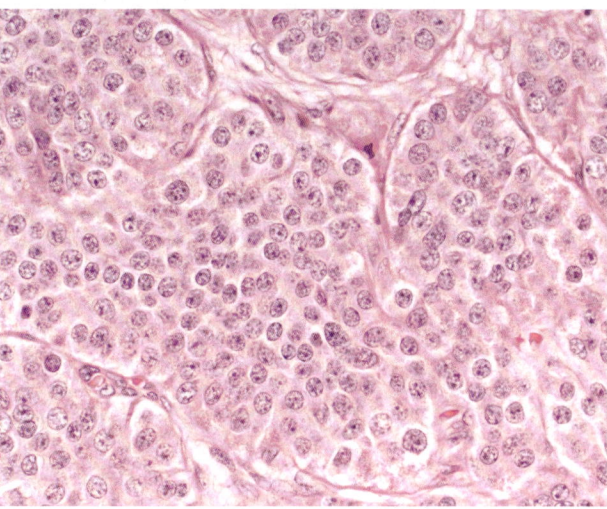

Figure 4.89. Neuroendocrine cytologic features are present in carcinoid tumors, demonstrated by round nuclei with finely stippled "salt and pepper" chromatin, lacking discrete nucleoli.

PLEOMORPHIC

Embryonal Carcinoma

Embryonal carcinoma is a highly primitive GCT. The cells of origin recapitulate primordial embryonic tissue. Pure embryonal carcinoma is the second most common pure form of GCT, preceded by pure seminoma. However, it is still quite rare—estimates of frequency of pure embryonal carcinoma are between 2% and 20%, with experts settling on 5% as the best estimate. Unlike some other pure forms of GCTs, embryonal carcinoma is exceedingly rare in prepubertal children. Conversely, an embryonal component is identified in the vast majority of mixed GCTs. In mixed GCTs, a large component of embryonal carcinoma is considered an adverse feature associated with risk of recurrence.

The gross appearance of these tumors is of a soft gray mass with frequent hemorrhage and necrosis present. Histologically, embryonal carcinomas are markedly pleomorphic and primitive tumors with numerous patterns of growth. In order of decreasing frequency, the described patterns include solid, papillary/tubular, and pseudoendodermal sinus (Figure 4.91). Glandular areas are commonly identified and a useful feature to suggest embryonal carcinoma (Figure 4.92). When closely admixed with YST, the diffuse embryoma pattern is also common. The hallmark features of embryonal carcinoma are its highly pleomorphic and atypical cytologic features. The tumor cells are large round to columnar cells with abundant cytoplasm. The nuclei are angular and show clumped hyperchromatic chromatin, prominent nucleoli, and irregular nuclear membranes. Abutting and overlapping nuclei are more commonly seen in embryonal carcinoma than in seminoma. Mitotic figures are easily identified, in addition to frequent necrosis (Figures 4.93 and 4.94). At the periphery of the tumor, intratubular embryonal carcinoma may be easily recognized by the intensely pink necrotic material and degenerating tumor cells (Figure 4.95).[12]

The most common diagnostic difficulty surrounding embryonal carcinoma is distinguishing it from the more pleomorphic forms of seminoma. When seminoma cells become more atypical, embryonal carcinoma may be considered. A simple immunohistochemistry panel can help sort out the diagnosis: KIT, AE1/3, CD30 should be employed. Seminoma will show diffuse positivity for KIT with only patchy or negative AE1/3 and negative CD30. Embryonal carcinoma will show diffuse AE1/3 and CD30 positivity with no expression of KIT. Sometimes embryonal carcinomas include smudged cells at the periphery of intact tumor cells, which has been referred to as the "applique" pattern. This may lead to consideration of choriocarcinoma, with the smudged cells mimicking syncytiotrophoblastic cells; however, the consistent diffuse OCT3/4 labeling in embryonal carcinoma should resolve this distinction easily.[31]

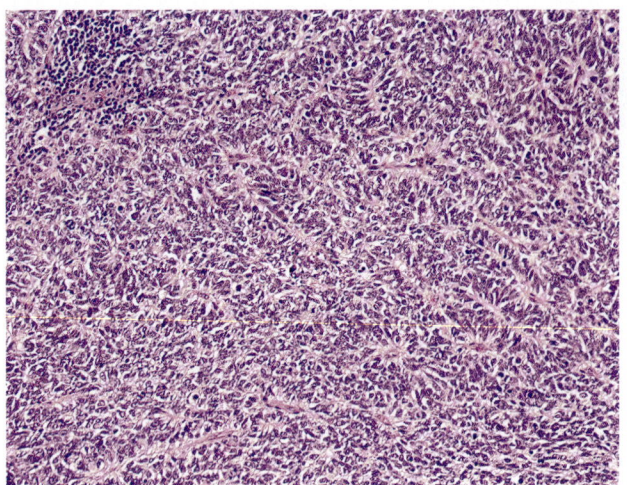

Figure 4.90. Primitive neuroectodermal tumor (PNET) arising in the testis has the same morphologic features as tumors arising in the central nervous system (CNS) with small round blue cells forming rosettes and tubules, along with solid sheets of tumor cells.

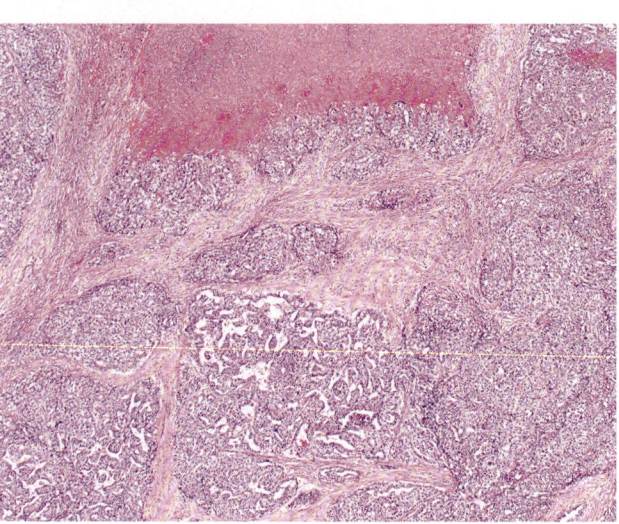

Figure 4.91. Embryonal carcinoma shows high-grade pleomorphism with marked atypia recognizable at low power. Glandular features and necrosis are also commonly identified.

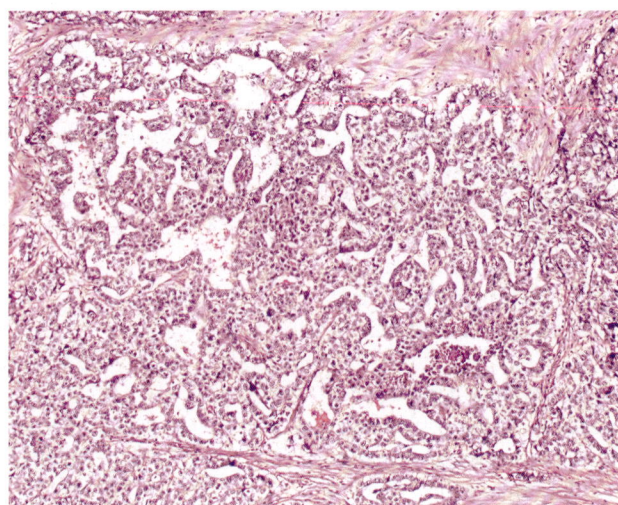

Figure 4.92. Glandular areas of embryonal carcinoma demonstrating marked nuclear pleomorphism and frequent mitoses. Other germ cell tumors can have a glandular pattern including seminoma and yolk sac tumor; however, the nuclear features of embryonal carcinoma can be used to distinguish it from the more monotonous cells of other tumor types.

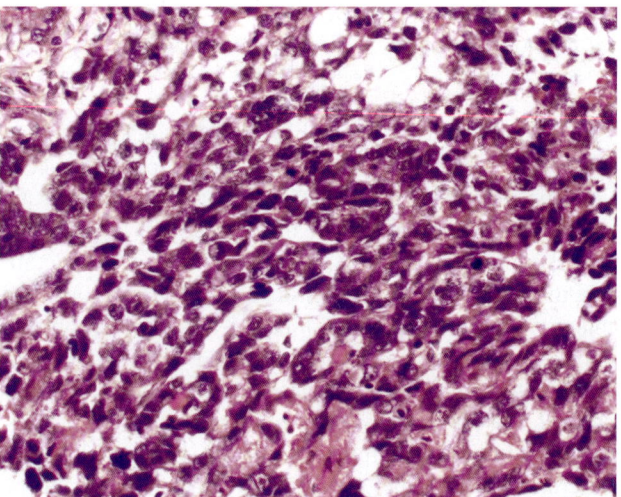

Figure 4.93. High-grade cytologic features, with frequent mitotic figures, overlapping, and pleomorphic nuclei, are identified in a high-power image of embryonal carcinoma. These tumors have a greater degree of nuclear atypia than other germ cell tumors.

Yolk Sac Tumor

Yolk sac tumor derives its name from the morphologic recapitulation of the structures of a developing embryo. These tumors have been historically referred to as endodermal sinus tumors. In adults, YST almost always occurs as one component of a mixed GCT. Clinically, a yolk sac component is supported by the finding of elevated serum AFP, usually greater than 100 ng/mL. Although YST is not necessarily considered an adverse histology in current practice like embryonal carcinoma, some data do indicate tumors with a yolk sac component are prone to late relapse with unusual tumors that are resistant to conventional GCT chemotherapy.[32]

YSTs demonstrate a wide variety of morphologies, making diagnosis more complicated. These tumors often associate closely with embryonal carcinomas, which may be a helpful starting point for a search (Figure 4.96). Common patterns include microcystic,

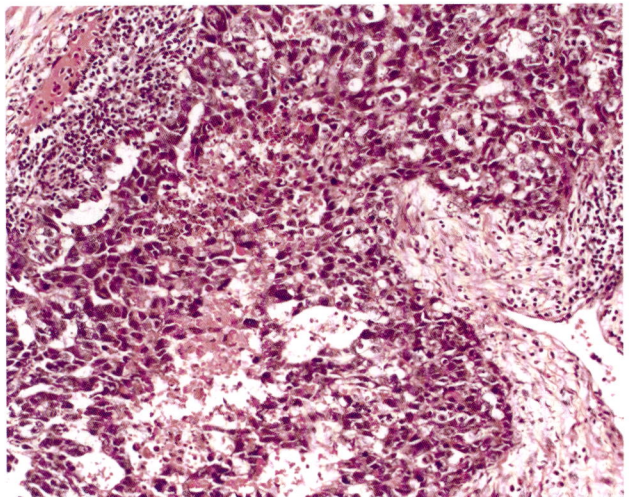

Figure 4.94. Geographic necrosis is frequently present in embryonal carcinoma.

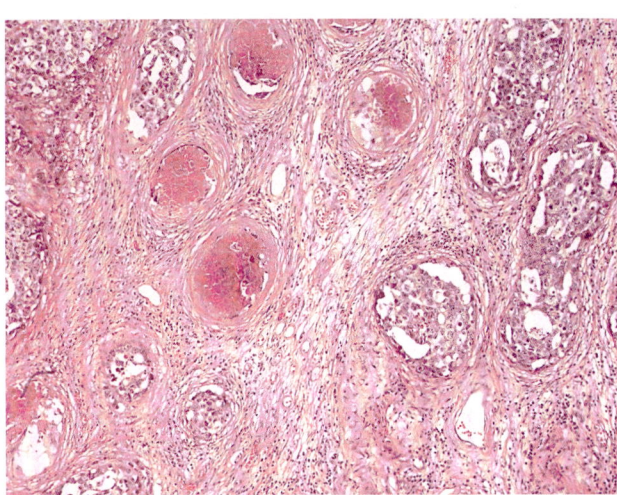

Figure 4.95. Embryonal carcinoma may grow into seminiferous tubules in an intratubular pattern. When necrotic tumor is present within tubules, they show intense pink amorphous material secondary to the cellular necrosis.

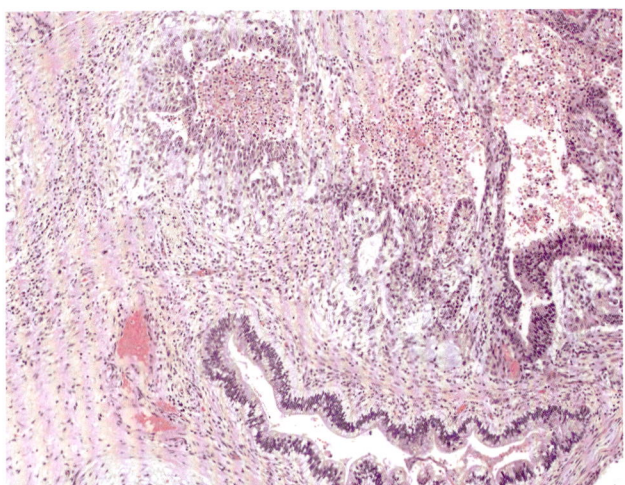

Figure 4.96. Yolk sac tumor and embryonal carcinoma are often contiguous patterns in mixed germ cell tumors. The loose myxoid stroma surrounding the highly pleomorphic tumor cells of embryonal carcinoma should be evaluated for yolk sac tumor features when present.

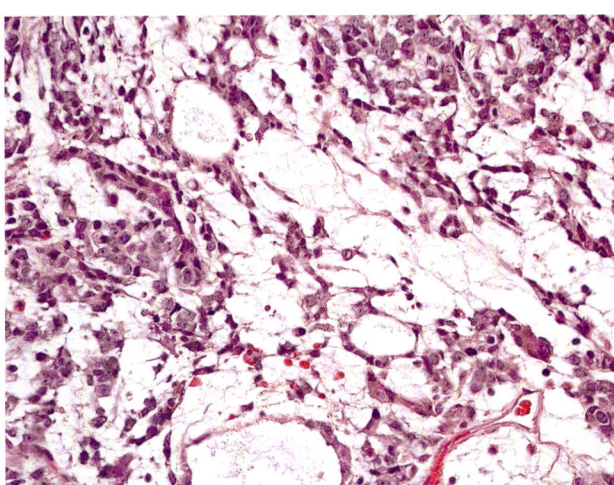

Figure 4.97. Myxoid substance is frequently identified in yolk sac tumors and is a helpful low-power clue for the diagnosis. Myxoid substance may be more diffuse with tumor cells dispersed within it, or form pools as in this case, lending a macrocystic appearance to the tumor.

macrocystic, solid, glandular, endodermal sinus with Schiller-Duval bodies, parietal pattern with basement membrane material, hepatoid, papillary, and sarcomatoid patterns (Figures 4.97-4.105). The glandular pattern often shows subnuclear vacuoles, akin to the "piano keys" of secretory endometrium. Myxoid matrix is often identified in areas of YST, sometimes as diffuse ground substance or discrete pools. Within all patterns, common cytologic features include intracytoplasmic and extracellular hyaline globules and basement membrane substance (Figure 4.106).[12]

Sarcomatoid differentiation is especially common in metastatic sites, sometimes long after the primary tumor diagnosis, leading to diagnostic difficulty.[33] Sarcomatoid YST should be considered any time a spindle neoplasm (low or high grade) is identified in a patient at risk for GCT (Figure 4.107). Helpful features to diagnose sarcomatoid YST in the setting of spindle cell neoplasm of unknown origin include formation of ringlet structures and immunohistochemical staining for cytokeratin AE1/AE3 and glypican 3 in the spindle cells. Prior history of GCT of any type and location within a usual metastatic site are also helpful clinical clues.

PEARLS AND PITFALLS: Rete Testis Hyperplasia

- Rete testis hyperplasia may exhibit hyaline globules, similar to those seen in YST[34]
- Hyperplastic rete may show a florid proliferation of solid and microcystic nests of epithelial cells containing hyaline globules (Figure 4.108)
- Rete hyperplasia will be limited to the area of normal rete testis, expanding usual slitlike glands
- Rete hyperplasia lacks cytologic atypia and mitotic activity expected in YST

Immunohistochemistry may be useful when H&E is not diagnostic. YSTs are positive for SALL4 and pan-keratin, which are not entirely specific. In contrast to seminoma and embryonal carcinoma, they are negative for OCT3/4. AFP is usually positive in these tumors; however, a high serum AFP level may cause high background staining, and one should confirm the histologic features are consistent with YST when using this stain. Additionally, glypican 3 is a highly specific marker for YST, staining all tumors in one series of 39 YST cases.[35] If some of these specialized GCT markers are not available, it may be helpful to note that CDX2 is often positive in YST.[36]

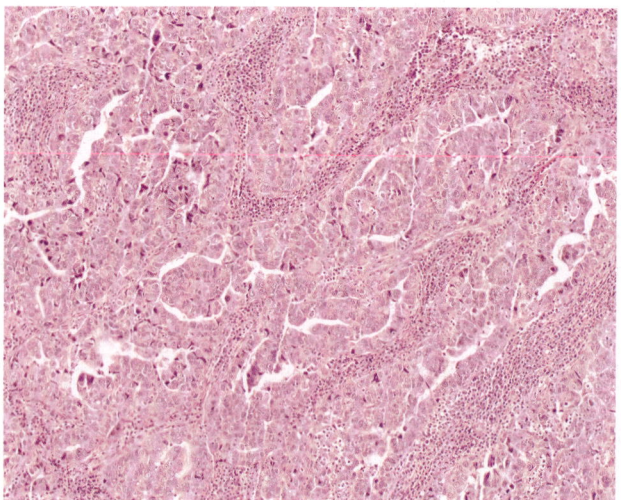

Figure 4.98. Glandular pattern of yolk sac tumor may show closely packed glandular structures with slitlike lumens.

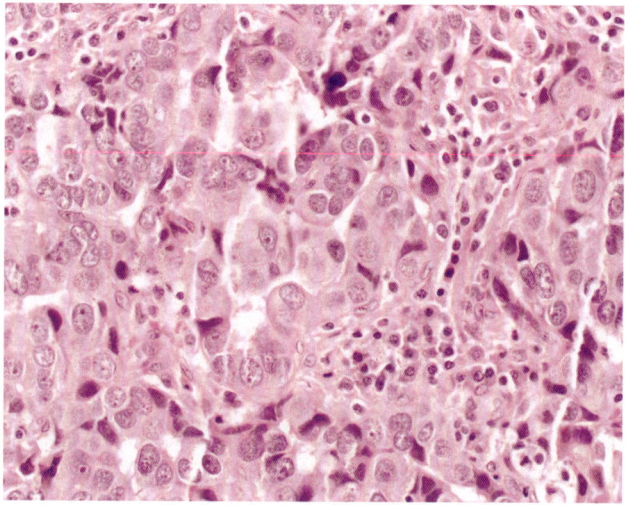

Figure 4.99. At higher power, the abundant eosinophilic cytoplasm in this yolk sac tumor raises the possibility of some degree of hepatoid differentiation.

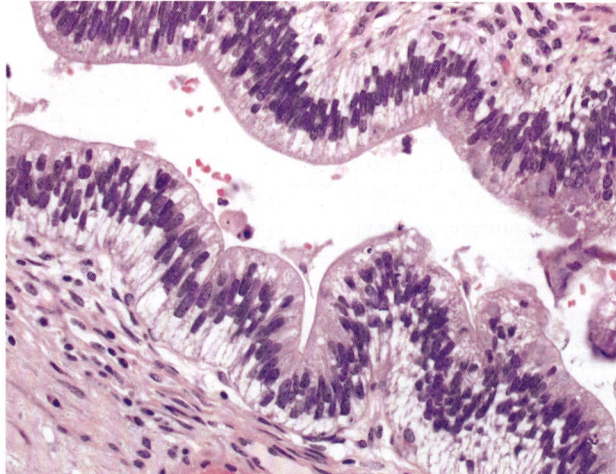

Figure 4.100. The classic finding of subnuclear vacuoles is a very helpful clue to the diagnosis of glandular yolk sac tumor, giving it a "piano-key" appearance.

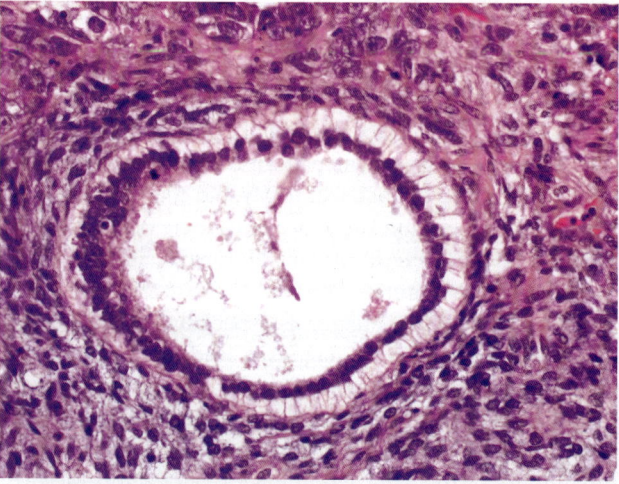

Figure 4.101. Perfectly arranged subnuclear vacuoles are present in a small focus of yolk sac tumor. This morphologic finding may mimic other teratomatous glandular elements.

PEARLS AND PITFALLS: Identifying Small Foci of Yolk Sac Tumor

- Yolk sac tumor can be difficult to identify
- Elevated AFP should prompt a thorough investigation for a component of YST, including additional sections as needed
- Recognize multiple architectural patterns of growth
- Often closely associated with embryonal carcinoma
- Strands of basement membrane material (parietal pattern) and/or hyaline globules
- "Diffuse embryoma pattern" of central embryonal carcinoma with amnionlike space and surrounding YST[37] (Figure 4.109)

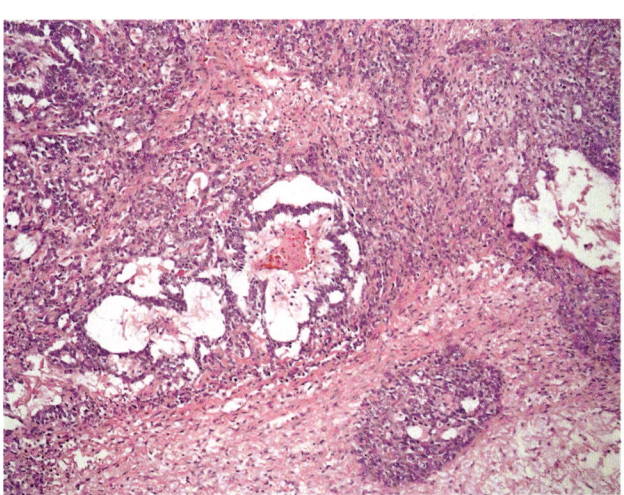

Figure 4.102. Schiller-Duval bodies are condensation of yolk sac tumor cells around vessels, known as the endodermal sinus pattern.

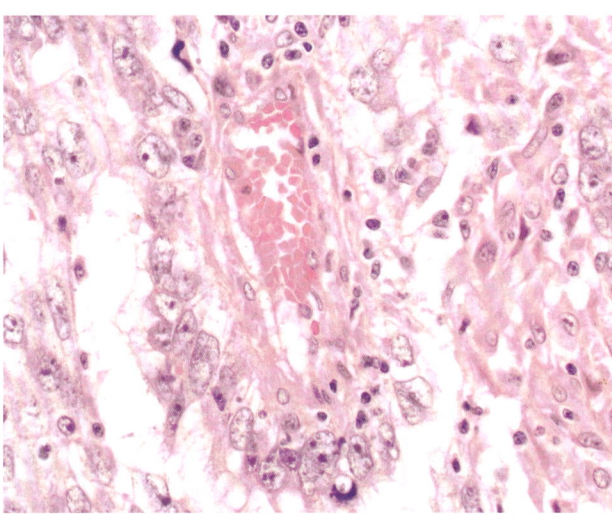

Figure 4.103. Although considered a hallmark of yolk sac tumor, Schiller-Duval bodies are found in a minority of cases.

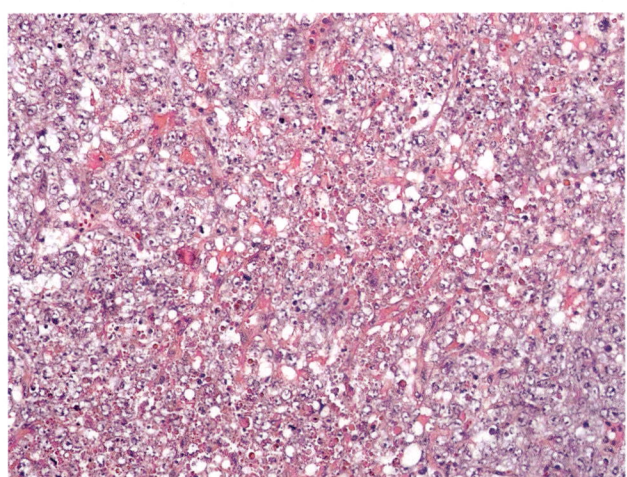

Figure 4.104. This example of solid variant of yolk sac tumor mimics other solid germ cell tumors including seminoma and embryonal carcinoma. The presence of extracellular hyaline globules is strongly suggestive of a yolk sac tumor.

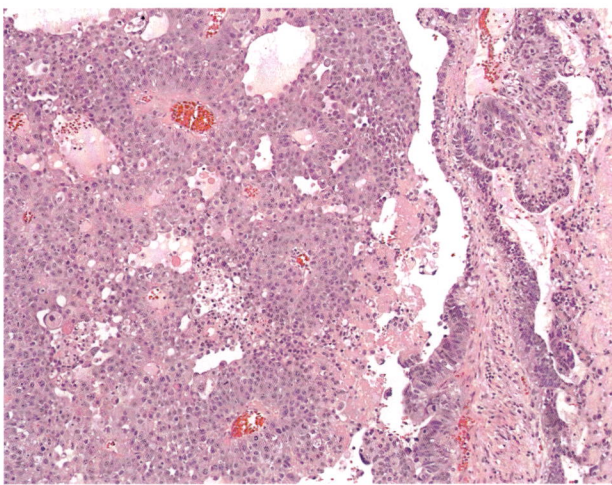

Figure 4.105. Hepatoid yolk sac tumor demonstrating abundant dense eosinophilic cytoplasm.

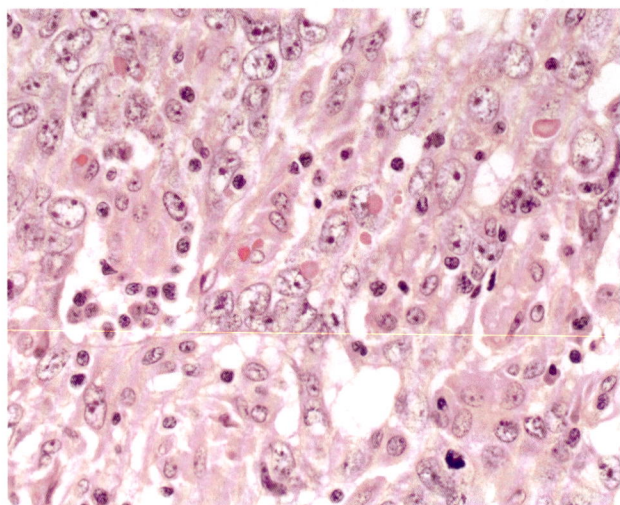

Figure 4.106. Extracellular hyaline globules are a useful feature for the identification of yolk sac tumor, especially when the tumor comprises an unusual pattern. Similarly, the identification of basement membrane material strongly supports the parietal pattern of yolk sac tumor.

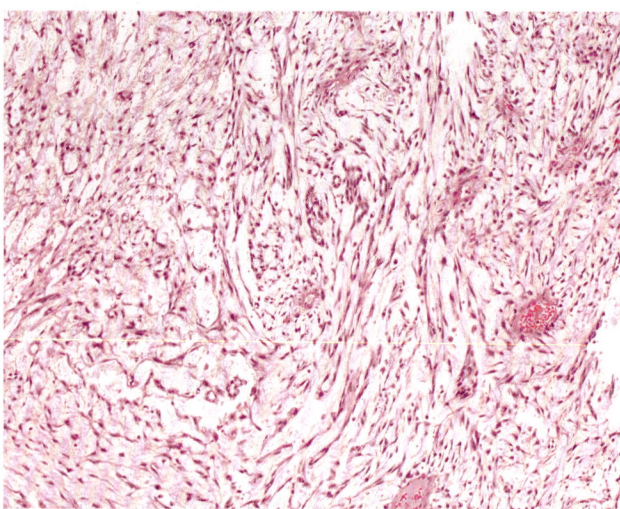

Figure 4.107. Sarcomatoid yolk sac tumor is a pattern frequently identified in metastatic sites and can lead to diagnostic difficulty. It should be considered in any patient with a risk of germ cell tumor, and diagnosis is aided by the use of AE1/3 and glypican 3 immunohistochemistry.

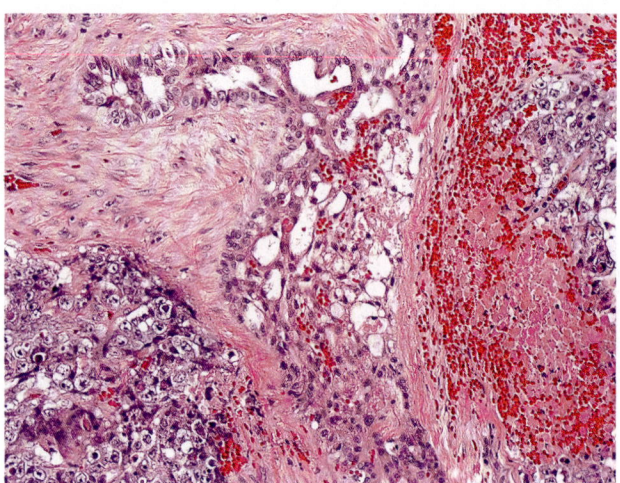

Figure 4.108. Rete testis hyperplasia may mimic yolk sac tumor by the presence of hyaline globules. Clues that argue against a yolk sac tumor are the bland nature of the surrounding cells and being centered in the rete testis.

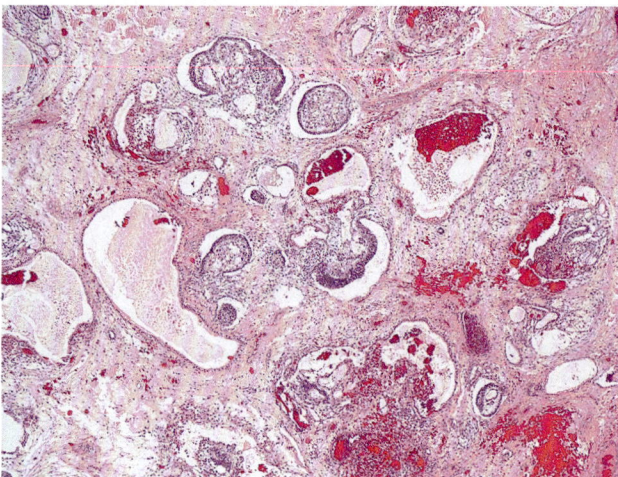

Figure 4.109. The diffuse embryoma or polyembryoma pattern is a specific morphologic pattern of closely intermingled embryonal carcinoma and yolk sac tumor. A proliferation of yolk sac tumor protrudes into an empty space and is lined by embryonal carcinoma, recapitulating the developing embryo.

Choriocarcinoma

Choriocarcinoma is a GCT with trophoblast-type differentiation, comprising cytotrophoblastic cells, intermediate trophoblastic cells, and syncytiotrophoblastic cells. They are most commonly a component of a mixed GCT, though pure tumors are documented. Unfortunately, these tumors may also present with metastatic disease, particularly with pulmonary metastasis manifesting as hemoptysis. Like YST, serum tumor markers are useful in the diagnosis of choriocarcinoma, with bHCG elevated into the tens of thousands.

Identifying choriocarcinoma in a mixed GCT often starts with a low-power scan and focus on areas of hemorrhage (Figure 4.110). For this reason, gross specimens should be sampled carefully in any areas of hemorrhage. Cytologically, choriocarcinomas usually demonstrate at least two cell types: mononucleated cytotrophoblastic cells and multinucleated syncytiotrophoblastic cells. The mononuclear cells show clear to pale pink cytoplasm and irregular nuclei with prominent nucleoli (Figure 4.111). Mitotic figures are easily identifiable. Syncytiotrophoblastic cells have abundant dark pink cytoplasm with indistinct borders. Some clusters of syncytiotrophoblastic cells will form lumens with hemorrhage (Figure 4.112). The quantity of syncytiotrophoblastic cells may be quite low, though occasionally clusters of these cells are evident (Figure 4.113). Well-formed areas resembling villi may occasionally be identified, though small foci often lack organized arrangement of the two cell types.

Choriocarcinomas express SALL4 and GATA3, specifically in the cytotrophoblastic cells.[36,38] These tumors are negative for OCT3/4, contrasting to seminoma and embryonal carcinoma. Syncytiotrophoblastic cells express beta-HCG and human placental lactogen (HPL), along with inhibin and glypican 3.[39]

FAQ: Why is Leydig Cell Hyperplasia Frequently Identified in Patients With Choriocarcinoma?

- Elevated beta-HCG from the choriocarcinoma leads to a direct stimulatory effect on Leydig cells, resulting in Leydig cell hyperplasia

---

Spermatocytic Tumor

Formerly known as "spermatocytic seminoma," this primary testicular tumor demonstrates three distinct cell types. Although included in the GCT category, these tumors differ from other GCTs, in that they do not occur at other extragonadal midline sites in the same way that extragonadal GCTs occur in mediastinum or brain. Other distinctions from seminoma include a lack of fine fibrous septa, associated lymphocytes, or granulomatous inflammation. The presence of GCNIS is not consistent with this diagnosis, as spermatocytic tumor is a non–GCNIS-derived neoplasm. Another difference between the spermatocytic tumor and seminoma is the patient demographics—seminoma has a median age of around 40 years, whereas spermatocytic tumor predominantly occurs in older patients in their 50s and above. However, both seminoma and spermatocytic tumor can overlap in their age ranges, so neither diagnosis should be discounted based on age.

Histologically, these tumors grow in sheets and solid nests, similar to seminoma and lymphoma (Figure 4.114). Higher power evaluation is necessary to identify the "tripartite" cytologic appearance of these tumors (Figure 4.115). The cytologic features prompted the term "spermatocytic" because the three cell types—small, intermediate, and giant

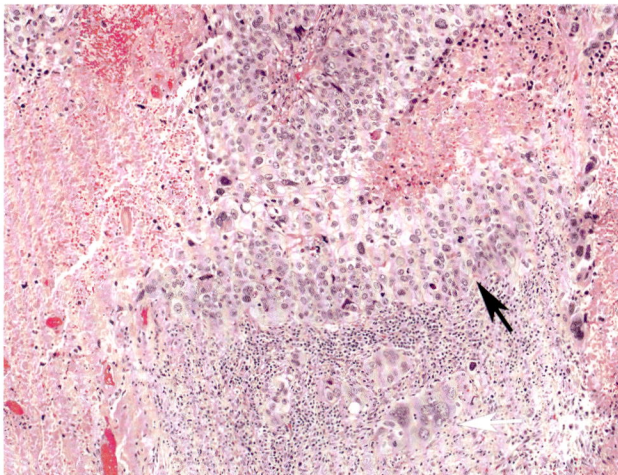

Figure 4.110. At low power, scanning for areas of hemorrhage can be a useful way to identify foci of choriocarcinoma. The mononuclear cytotrophoblastic cells (black arrow) make up the majority of the tumor cells, with scattered syncytiotrophoblastic cells (white arrow) also identified.

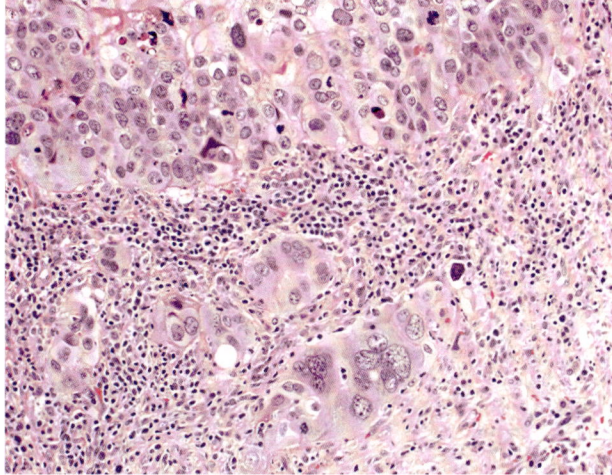

Figure 4.111. Cytotrophoblastic cells in the upper half of the image showing abundant clear to pink cytoplasm with vesicular chromatin and moderate pleomorphism. A syncytiotrophoblast is present in the lower half the image, recognizable by its multinucleation.

cells—appeared to resemble the various stages of maturing spermatogonia. The small cells are small round blue cells that resemble lymphocytes. The intermediate cells are round with moderate amounts of cytoplasm and more open, pale chromatin. The giant cells have unique spiremelike filamentous chromatin, connoting the primary spermatocytes undergoing meiosis (Figure 4.116). These tumors are very mitotically active, and necrosis may be present. Rarely, these tumors may undergo sarcomatoid differentiation.[40] Intratubular growth can also occur.

This diagnosis can generally be made on H&E alone by recognition of the three cell types; however, the most likely differential diagnosis is seminoma. Spermatocytic tumors are negative for PLAP and OCT3/4, in contrast to their diffuse expression in seminoma.[41]

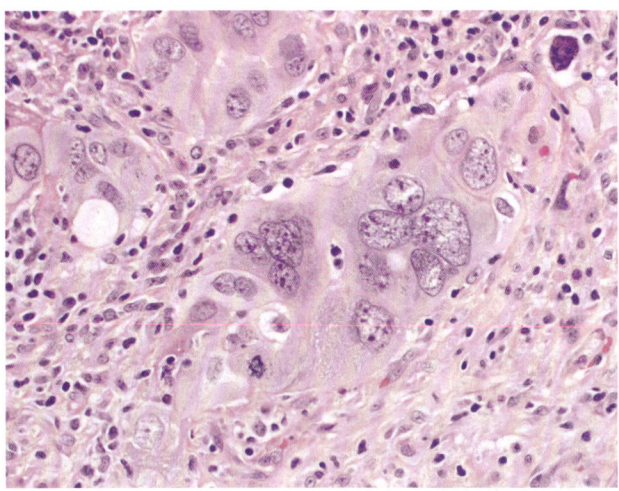

Figure 4.112. Syncytiotrophoblast at high power, showing multiple enlarged and atypical nuclei surrounded by abundant dark pink cytoplasm. These are the cells responsible for producing beta human chorionic gonadotropin (bHCG) and will mark strongly with immunohistochemistry for bHCG.

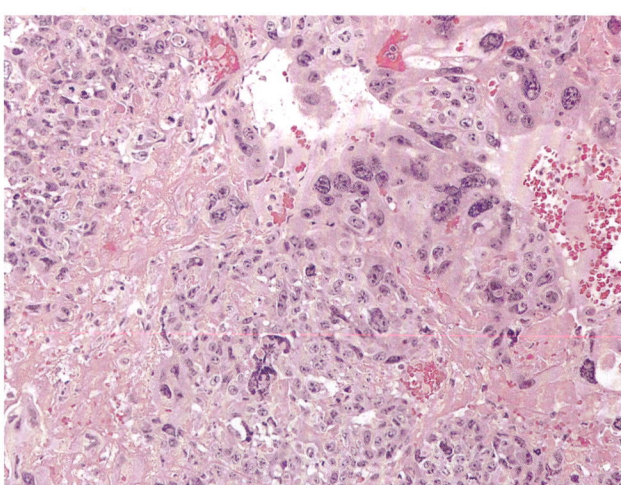

Figure 4.113. A cluster of syncytiotrophoblastic cells in this choriocarcinoma is a useful feature, but many cases only demonstrate a minority population of syncytiotrophoblastic cells.

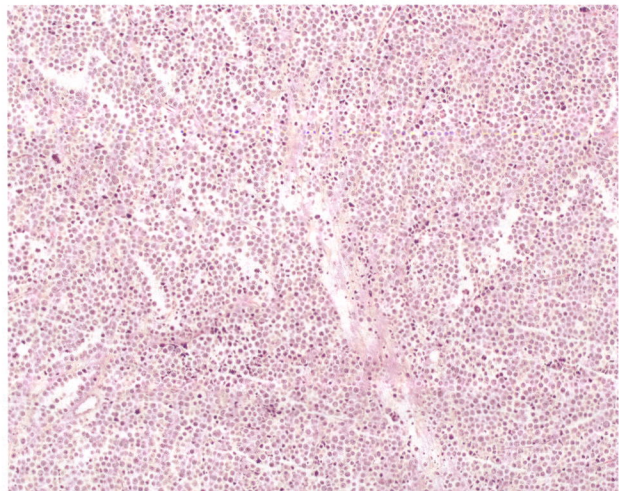

Figure 4.114. Spermatocytic tumor grows in a solid pattern, with areas of edema pushing cells apart to form empty spaces within the tumor.

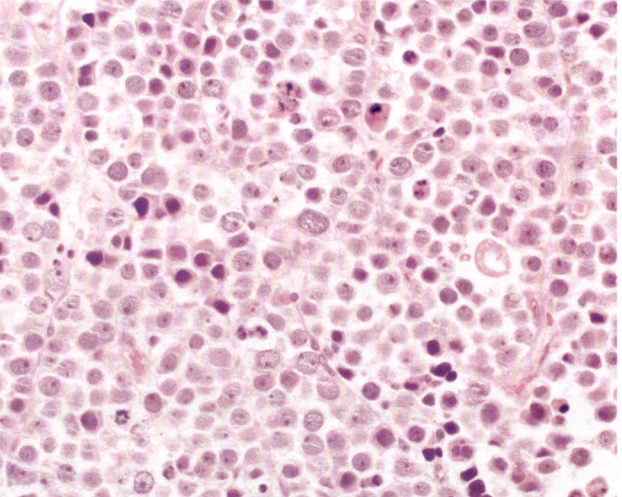

Figure 4.115. At higher power, the classic "tripartite" or three cell population becomes evident and helps distinguish spermatocytic tumor from seminoma.

ORGANOID

Germ Cell Neoplasia In Situ

Germ cell neoplasia in situ, formerly intratubular germ cell neoplasia, is a proliferation of malignant germ cells confined to the spermatogonial niche (adjacent to the basement membrane) of the seminiferous tubules. GCNIS is identified in the majority of cases of mixed GCTs and many seminomas. The malignant cells are thought to arise from primordial germ cells that do not appropriately mature into spermatogonia.

A helpful clue for identifying GCNIS is to look in tubules that lack intact spermatogenesis, although the malignant cells may spread in a Pagetoid fashion into tubules with sperm present (Figures 4.117-4.119). GCNIS is often found in a patchy distribution throughout the testis. The malignant cells resemble seminoma cells, are located at the basal aspect of the tubule, and show hyperchromatic enlarged nuclei with prominent nucleoli and abundant clear cytoplasm.

GCNIS stains similarly to seminoma, expressing OCT3/4, PLAP, KIT, and D2-40.[42] The differential diagnosis of this intratubular process includes intratubular seminoma, which is often associated with a mass or intertubular seminoma elsewhere, and immature/maturation-delayed germ cells. Unlike immature germ cells that are located centrally and diffusely within tubules, GCNIS should be located at the basal aspect of the tubules in a patchy distribution.[17] When mildly atypical nuclei are present in basally located germ cells without prominent nucleoli, immunohistochemistry for OCT3/4 can be helpful to distinguish mild atypia of germ cells from true GCNIS.

FAQ: Conditions Leading to an Increased Risk of GCNIS or Germ Cell Tumor

1. Cryptorchidism—the higher the testis is in the abdomen, the higher the risk of malignancy
2. Disorders of sexual development—due to presence of GBY region on Y chromosome[43]
3. Subfertility/infertility

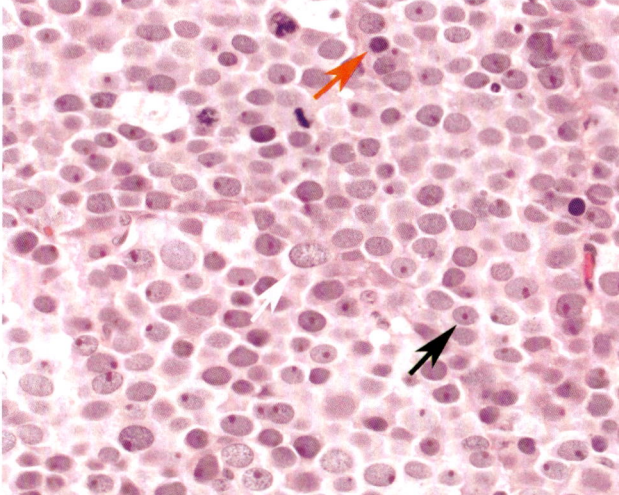

Figure 4.116. The cytologic features of the three cell types include small cells (red arrow) resembling lymphocytes, intermediate cells (black arrow) with smooth chromatin and single nucleolus, and the giant cells (white arrow) with large nuclear size and filamentous chromatin. This filamentous chromatin resembles spermatocytes undergoing meiosis and prompted the naming of these tumors as "spermatocytic."

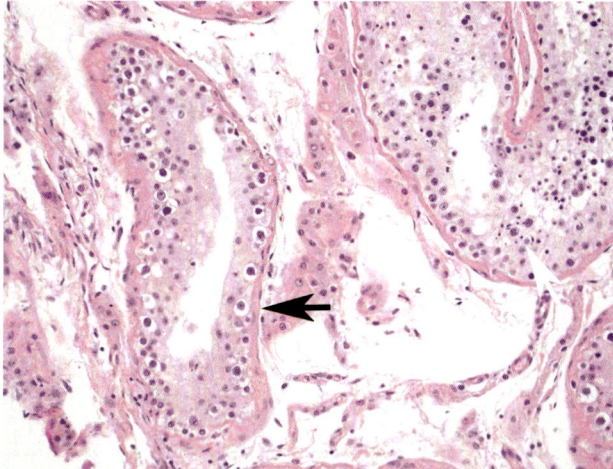

Figure 4.117. Germ cell neoplasia in situ (GCNIS) (black arrow) is often present in a patchy distribution within the testis and commonly identified in mixed germ cell tumors and seminoma. At scanning magnification, a helpful feature is the lack of intact spermatogenesis in tubules containing GCNIS. Indicative of the patchy nature of this process, an adjacent tubule (white arrow) shows intact spermatogenesis.

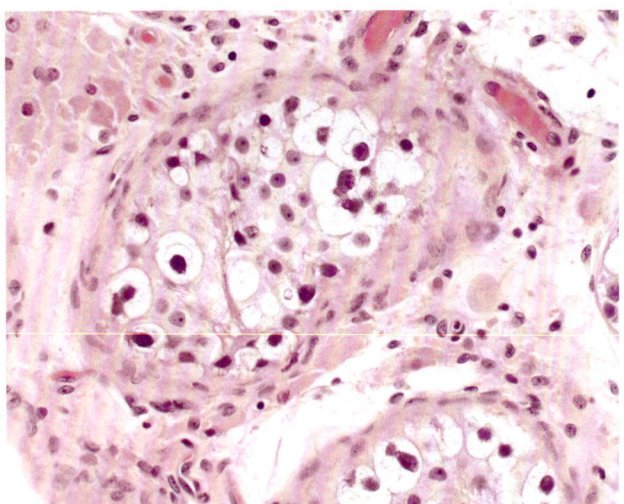

Figure 4.118. Germ cell neoplasia in situ (GCNIS) cells should show marked enlargement and nuclear atypia that stands out at medium power.

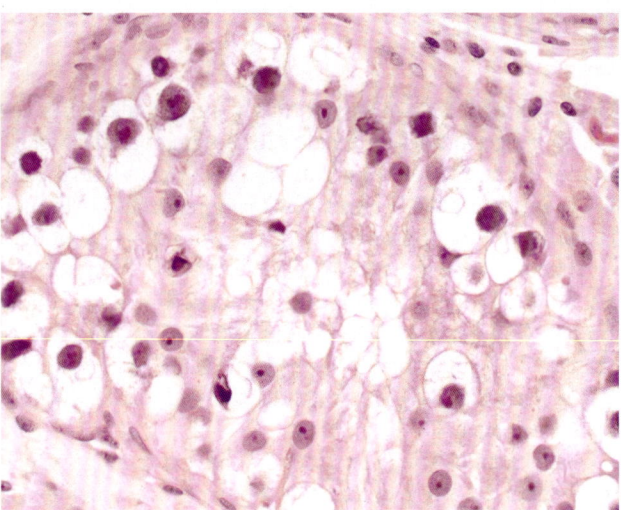

Figure 4.119. Cytologically, germ cell neoplasia in situ (GCNIS) resembles malignant seminoma cells with abundant clear cytoplasm and enlarged nuclei with prominent nucleoli. The GCNIS cells are confined to the adluminal compartment of the tubule, unlike germ cells that are distributed more centrally in the tubule.

Teratoma

Broadly speaking, teratomas are neoplasms comprising a variety of tissue types in the same mass, of endodermal, mesodermal, and ectodermal origin.[16] In the testis, teratomas usually demonstrate at least two of the tissue types; rare monodermal teratomas occur as carcinoid tumors (discussed in section on Monomorphic Pattern). Teratomas arising within the testis may be benign or malignant. Benign teratomas originate from nontransformed germ cells and include dermoid cysts, epidermoid cysts, and prepubertal mature teratomas. Malignant postpubertal teratoma originates from another malignant GCT. In general, teratomas of the postpubertal testis should be presumed malignant unless carefully proven to meet criteria for a benign (prepubertal type) teratoma, as discussed later. In addition to histology, clinical demographics are important in distinguishing these tumors into pre- and postpubertal forms, which have different capacity for malignant behavior.

Epidermoid Cyst

These rare benign tumors are morphologically similar to epidermoid cysts elsewhere in the body. They form a well-circumscribed cyst lined by bland keratinizing squamous epithelium without adnexal structures[44] (Figures 4.120 and 4.121). They have a benign course, and testis sparing surgery is an option when the diagnosis is suspected.

Dermoid Cyst

Dermoid cysts are another type of benign mature teratoma. They are well-circumscribed cysts with keratinizing squamous epithelial lining; however, they also contain the skin adnexal structures such as sebaceous glands and hair follicles. Hair is grossly present within the cyst, similar to its ovarian counterpart.[45]

Prepubertal Type Mature Teratomas

Prepubertal teratomas are benign and develop from nontransformed germ cells. These tumors represent almost one-third of testicular GCTs occurring in children, the second most common pure GCT in children after YST. They are almost always pure tumors and must not have associated GCNIS. Histologically, they comprise of varying tissue types that maintain their normal organoid arrangement, hence the inclusion of this entity in the organoid section. Common tissue types include neural tissue, cartilage, intestinal epithelium, or epidermis (Figure 4.122). The teratomatous elements lack significant cytologic atypia or increased mitotic figures[37] (Figure 4.123). It is important to be extremely cautious

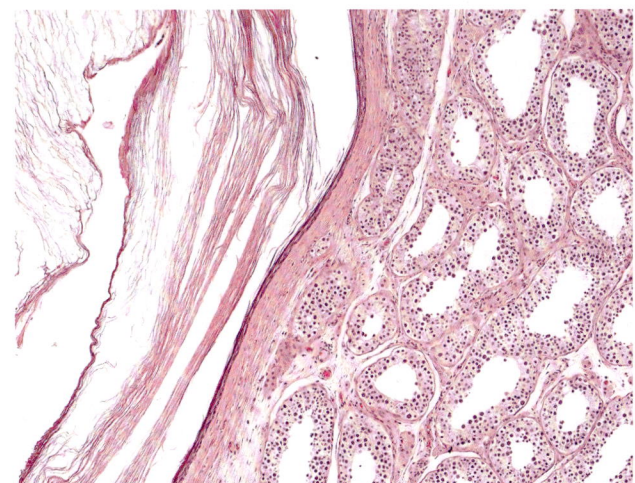

Figure 4.120. Epidermoid cysts arising in the testis are one type of benign teratoma. These neoplasms are morphologically identical to epidermoid cysts in other locations.

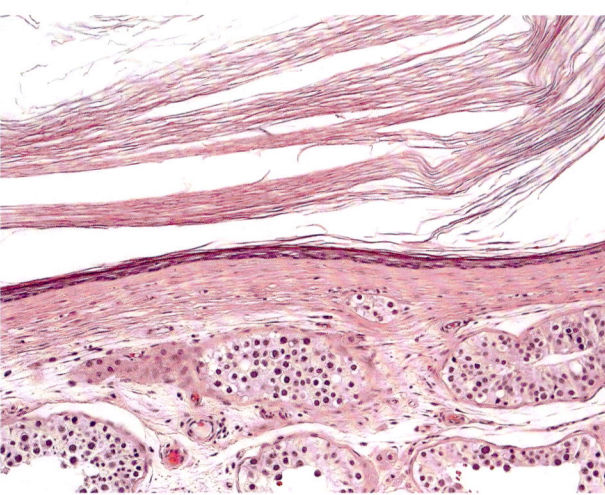

Figure 4.121. Epidermoid cysts are lined by bland, keratinizing squamous epithelium and lack adnexal structures.

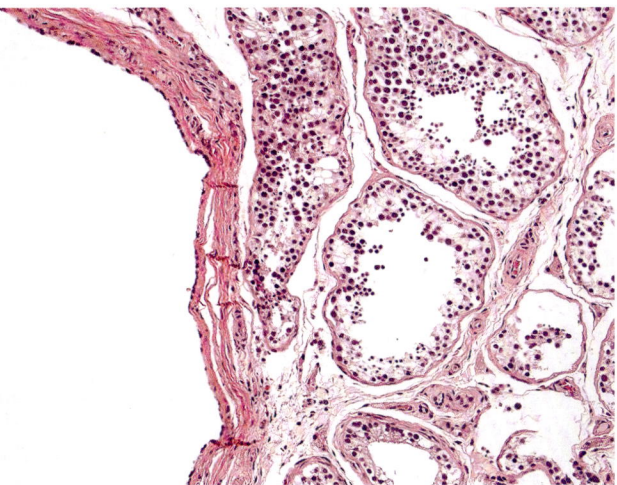

Figure 4.122. A benign prepubertal mature teratoma lined by bland, low cuboidal epithelium. The key difference between an epidermoid/dermoid cyst of the testis and prepubertal teratomas is the admixture of different mature epithelial, neural, and mesenchymal components.

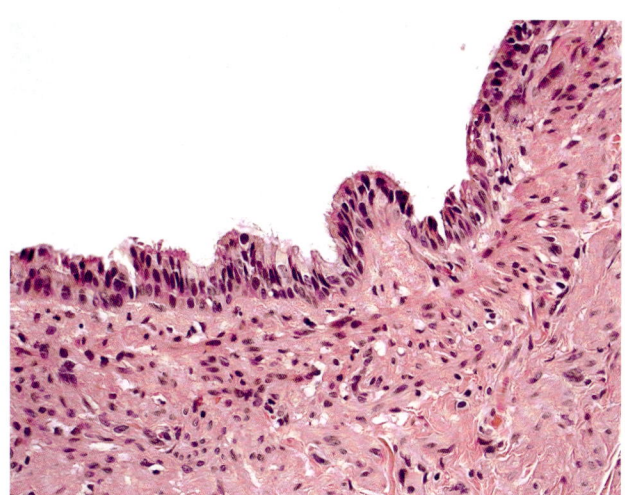

Figure 4.123. At higher power, the lining of this area of prepubertal teratoma shows ciliated pseudostratified columnar epithelium, consistent with respiratory-type mucosa. No significant cellular atypia or mitotic figures are permitted in the teratomatous elements in a prepubertal teratoma.

before diagnosing a "benign" teratoma (ie, prepubertal type) in an adult (see Checklist), as the majority of adult testicular teratomas are derived from GCNIS and other malignant GCT elements. Therefore, even patients with apparently pure testicular teratomas can have metastases of other nonteratomatous components of malignant GCT.

CHECKLIST: Diagnostic Criteria for a Benign Prepubertal Type Teratoma in an Adult[46]

Lack of cytologic atypia
No GCNIS
Lack of tubular atrophy/scar
Spermatogenesis normal
Lack of microlithiasis
Lack of isochromosome 12p/12p gain
Organoid morphology
Prominent ciliated epithelium
Prominent smooth muscle

Postpubertal Mature Teratomas

In contrast, postpubertal mature teratomas occur in older patients with a range of 20 to 40 years. These are malignant tumors hypothesized to originate from other GCTs, such as YST. A study of 16 patients with a component of mature teratoma in mixed GCT showed that allelic loss patterns were similar between the teratoma component and germ cell components in 71% of cases.[47] The identification of isochromosome 12p in many postpubertal teratomas also supports their derivation from other GCTs. Another phenomenon that supports the origin of teratoma from other GCTs is the finding of metastatic tumors with other germ cell components, despite the testicular tumor demonstrating only pure teratoma. This is thought to occur when the other germ cell elements have differentiated into teratoma in the primary tumor after already having given rise to metastases.

Histologically, postpubertal mature teratomas have a similar appearance to prepubertal teratomas with a few exceptions. The usual organoid architecture of prepubertal teratomas is less evident in postpubertal teratomas; varying elements of tissue types may be intermingled (Figures 4.124 and 4.125). Tissue types that are commonly present include neural tissue, cartilage, intestinal epithelium, or epidermis (Figures 4.126 and 4.127). Cytologic atypia and increased mitotic figures are common in postpubertal teratomas, along with the capacity for transformation to somatic (non–germ cell type) malignancy (Figure 4.128). In keeping with their malignant GCT status, GCNIS is frequently identified in background spermatic tubules. They are often a component of mixed GCTs.

SAMPLE NOTE: Postpubertal Mature Teratomas

Testis, right, radical orchiectomy:
- Teratoma, postpubertal type (1.5 cm)
- See Note

Note: The tumor comprises entirely of mature teratomatous components and lacks other GCT components. However, postpubertal teratomas arise from malignant GCT precursors and have metastatic potential. Other germ cell components may be present in metastatic sites. Germ cell neoplasia is present, which also supports derivation from a malignant GCT. (*Helpful when present, does not need to be included when absent.*)

PEARLS AND PITFALLS: Somatic Malignancy Arising in Teratoma

- Somatic malignancy arising in a teratoma is the transformation of mature teratomatous elements into their malignant counterparts (ie, sarcoma, carcinoma) (Figure 4.129)
- Diagnostic criteria for somatic malignancy are a pure population of malignant cells occupying an entire low-power (4× objective) field, approximately 5 mm diameter
- The most common types of somatic malignancy in testis are derived from primitive elements: most commonly PNET, rhabdomyosarcoma (embryonal type), and rarely other forms such as nephroblastoma (Figures 4.130 and 4.131)
- Less commonly, epithelial carcinomas, adenocarcinomas, and squamous cell carcinomas are identified (Figure 4.132)
- Some experts favor that a subset of somatic malignancies arise from YSTs, rather than teratoma, especially myxoid sarcomatous neoplasms[48]

FAQ: What are the Differences Between a Prepubertal Teratoma and Postpubertal Teratoma?[30,46]

- Prepubertal teratomas are benign, exhibit organized tissue architecture with little atypia or mitotic activity present; these tumors arise from nontransformed germ cells and lack isochromosome 12p
- Postpubertal teratomas are malignant, have less organized architecture with cellular atypia, and increased mitotic figures; these tumors arise from other GCTs and demonstrate isochromosome 12p

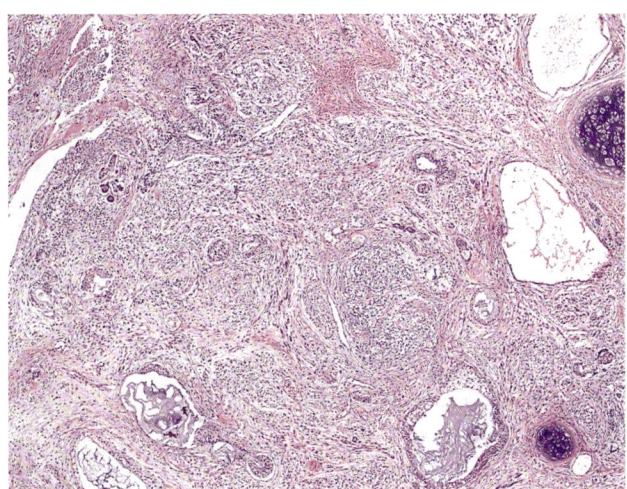

Figure 4.124. In postpubertal teratomas, different tissue types are frequently intermingled. In this field, cartilage- and intestinal-type glands are present within a dense myomatous stroma.

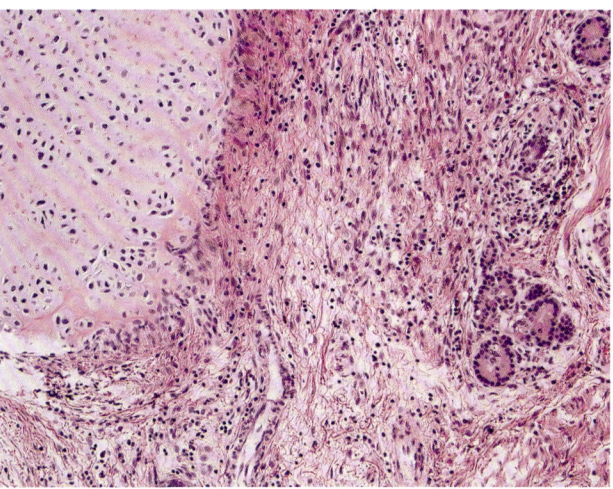

Figure 4.125. Postpubertal teratomas show less organization to their differing tissue types, though still have an overall organoid pattern. Demonstrated in this field are pancreatic acini adjacent to cartilage.

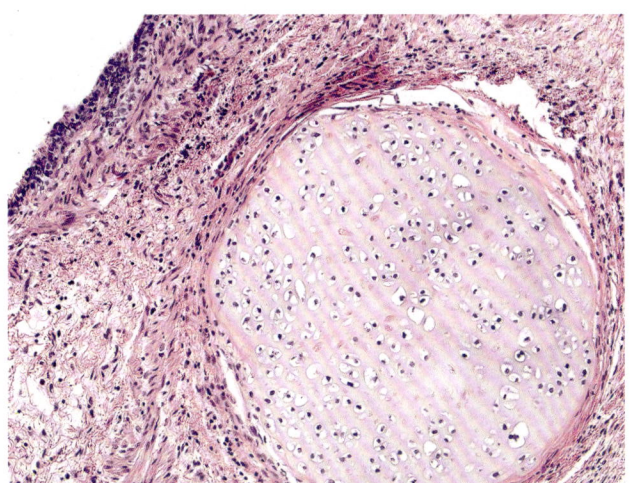

Figure 4.126. Cartilage is frequently identified in postpubertal teratomas. Its proximity to ciliated epithelium in the left hand corner of the image is unusual for a prepubertal teratoma.

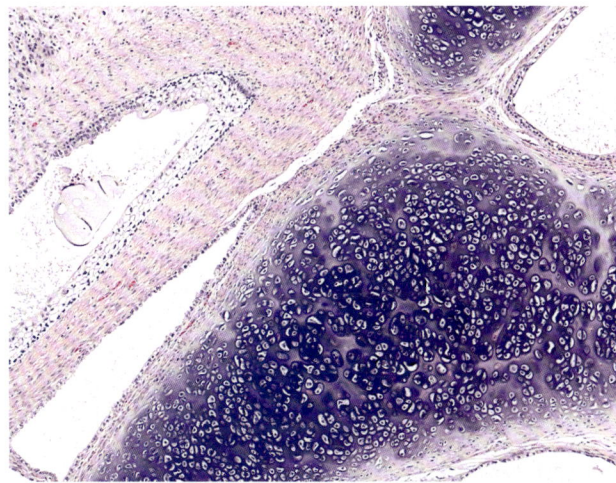

Figure 4.127. Hypercellular cartilage is identified in this postpubertal teratoma. This degree of atypia and hypercellularity would be inconsistent with a diagnosis of prepubertal teratoma. Postpubertal teratomas frequently demonstrate more nuclear atypia and mitotic figures than their benign counterparts.

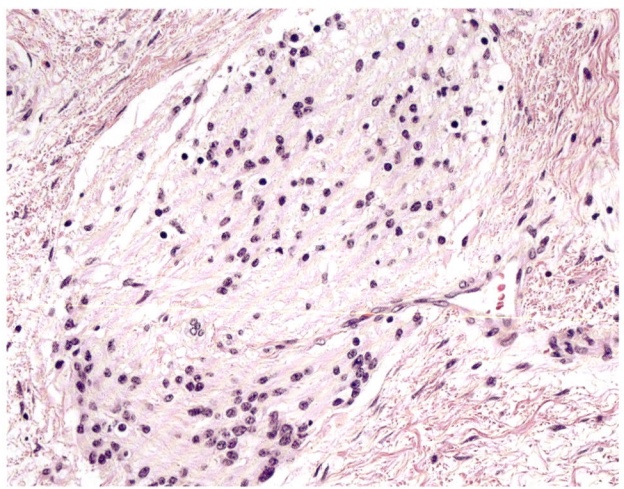

Figure 4.128. Neural tissue is another frequent component of postpubertal teratomas. Neural tissue may give rise to primitive neuroectodermal tumor (PNET) if it undergoes transformation to somatic malignancy.

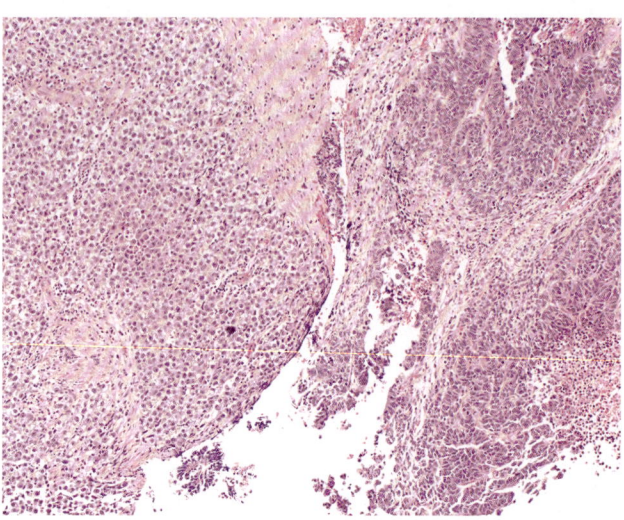

Figure 4.129. Somatic malignancy arising in a germ cell tumor results from the transformation of teratomatous elements into their malignant counterparts. This image shows seminoma with adjacent primitive small round blue cells, consistent with somatic malignancy.

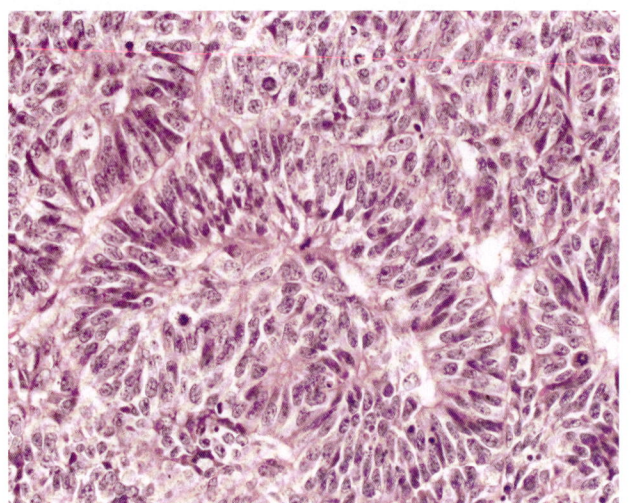

Figure 4.130. Somatic transformation to malignant primitive neuroectodermal tumor (PNET) is one of the most common types of somatic malignancy arising in germ cell tumors. The morphology is identical to PNET in other settings, with primitive small round blue cells forming tubules and rosettes.

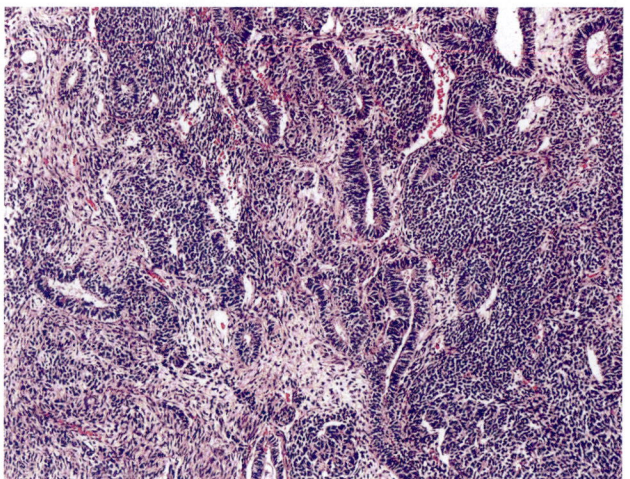

Figure 4.131. Less common types of somatic malignancy include nephroblastoma (Wilms tumor) arising in germ cell tumor. The morphology of a triphasic neoplasm with epithelial, blastemal, and stromal elements is similar to nephroblastoma arising in the kidney.

SPINDLE CELL PATTERN
Fibroma-Thecoma

The fibroma-thecoma group of tumors are relatively rare sex cord stromal tumors occurring in the testis. The vast majority of these tumors are morphologically comparable to ovarian fibromas, and thecomatous features are almost never encountered in the testis. The neoplastic cells resemble ovarian stromal cells—spindle-shaped with scant cytoplasm—which are arranged in a vaguely storiform pattern with intervening collagenous stroma (Figures 4.133 and 4.134). As the tumors become more cellular, the mitotic rate may be increased with up to 2 mitotic figures per 10 high-power fields.[12]

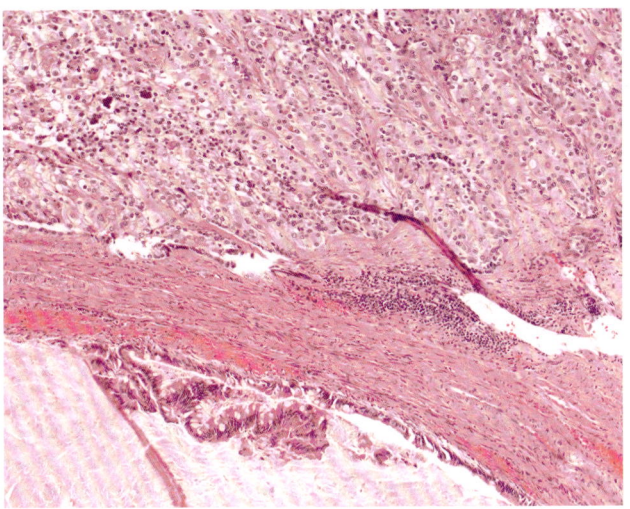

Figure 4.132. An even less common phenomenon is somatic transformation to malignant carcinomas. This teratoma shows intestinal-type epithelium in the lower half of the image, with a nested carcinoma with abundant eosinophilic cytoplasm above. This somatic malignancy was positive for PAX-8 and represented a renal cell carcinoma arising in a teratoma.

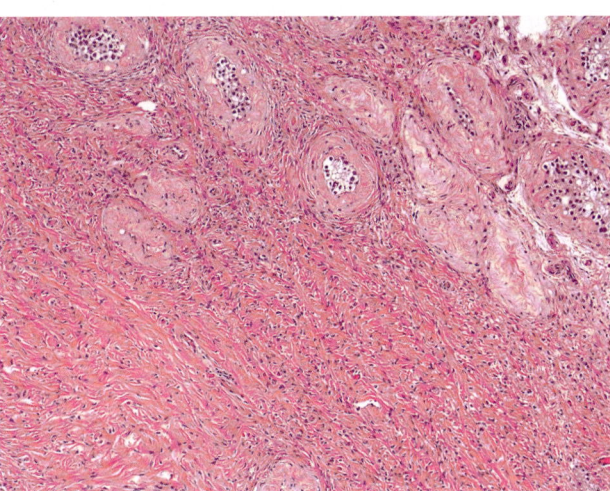

Figure 4.133. The fibroma-thecoma group of sex cord stromal tumors are less common in the testis than in the ovary. Morphologically, they comprise a proliferation of ovarian-type stromal spindle cells. In this case, the proliferation is entrapping a few seminiferous tubules at the edge of the field.

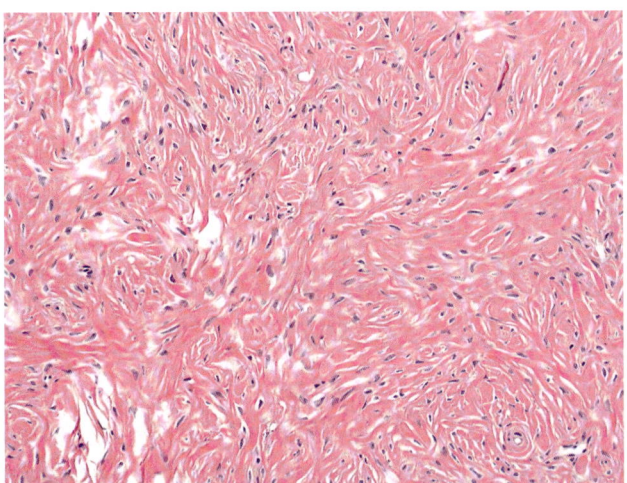

Figure 4.134. The dense collagenous stroma between spindle cells is prominent in this fibroma. In the testis, these tumors rarely show thecomatous change.

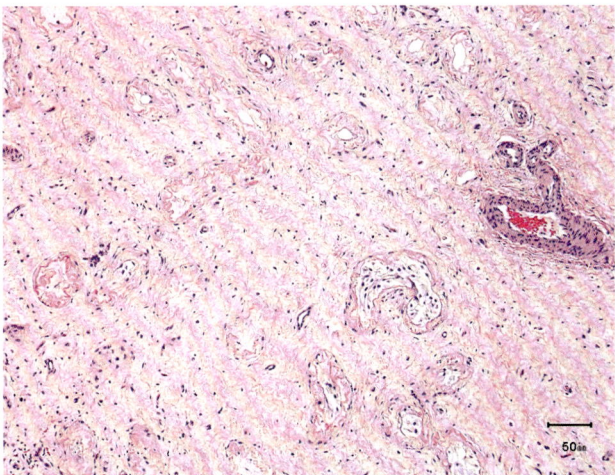

Figure 4.135. Regressed germ cell tumors are effectively scars left behind from the involution of a germ cell tumor. As such, the general features include fibrotic nodules of bland spindle cells and vessels, as seen in this image.

Regressed Germ Cell Tumor

Regression, or "burn out," of GCTs of the testis is not an uncommon occurrence and is most closely associated with seminoma. Clinically, these often are suspected after metastasis from an unknown primary is confirmed to be of germ cell origin and no testicular mass is identified. Histologically, regressed GCTs are discrete nodules of fibrosis that may contain hemosiderin-laden macrophages, calcifications, hyalinized/atrophic tubules, and chronic inflammation (Figures 4.135-4.137). The most specific finding for a regressed GCT is large coarse calcifications within tubules, which are thought to result from intratubular growth of embryonal carcinoma, followed by necrosis and subsequent calcification (Figure 4.138). Adjacent tubules containing GCNIS are also considered highly supportive of a regressed GCT over other causes of scarring.[49] Even if neither of these features is identified, it is worth communicating to clinicians that a "scar" in the testis may represent a regressed GCT, and clinical staging may be warranted (imaging and serum tumor markers, see Sample Note).

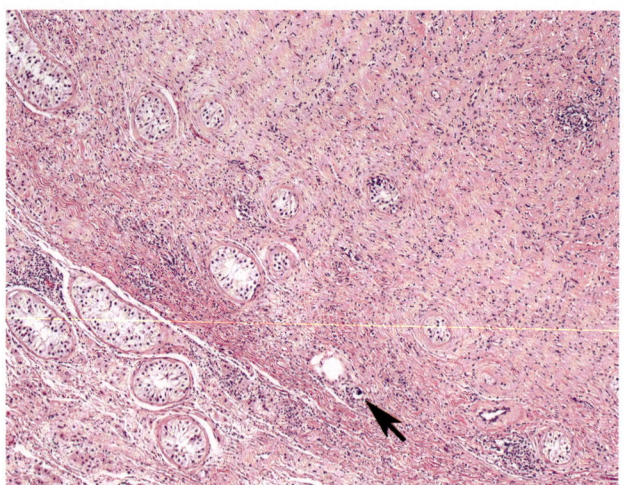

Figure 4.136. Features that help support regression over other causes of testicular scar include microliths (arrow) and the background Sertoli cell–only pattern in this patient. Although not present in this image, the finding of germ cell neoplasia in situ (GCNIS) within the testis is essentially diagnostic of regressed germ cell tumor.

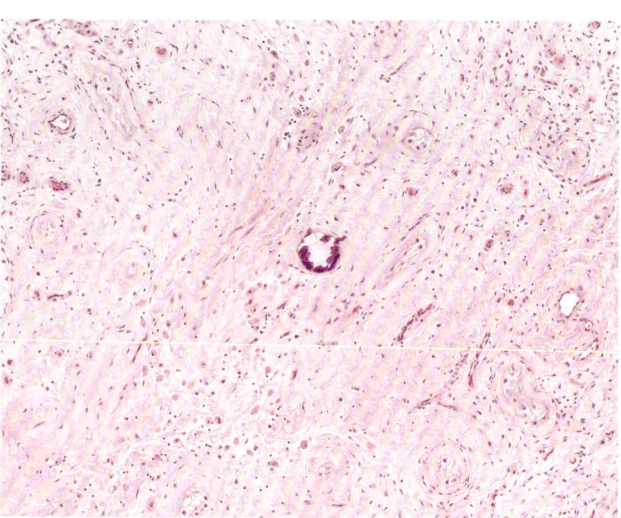

Figure 4.137. In addition to fibrosis and a microlith, this field shows numerous hemosiderin-laden macrophages indicative of the cleanup of a prior tumor.

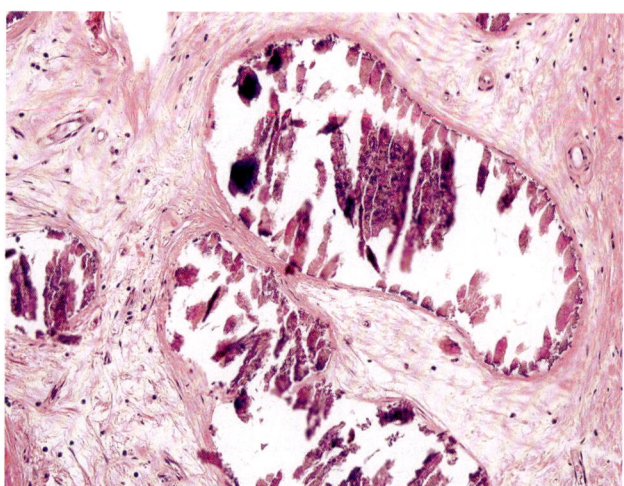

Figure 4.138. Large, course intertubular calcifications are considered the most specific finding for regressed germ cell tumor. They are hypothesized to be the remnant of necrotic embryonal carcinoma. When identified in a testicular scar, regressed germ cell tumor should be favored and staged as a pT0 tumor.

SAMPLE NOTE: Testicular Scar Without GCNIS or Coarse Calcification

Testis, left, orchiectomy:
• Scar, 1.5 cm greatest dimension—see Comment

Comment: The clinical mass represents an area of scarring in the testicular parenchyma. Although no viable GCT is identified, the possibility of spontaneous regression of a GCT is difficult to exclude. Clinical evaluation (imaging, serum tumor markers) for the possibility of a regressed tumor may be considered.

Reference:
Balzer BL, Ulbright TM. Spontaneous regression of testicular germ cell tumors: an analysis of 42 cases. *Am J Surg Pathol.* 2006;30(7):858-865.

SAMPLE NOTE: Testicular Scar With GCNIS or Coarse Calcification

Testis, left, orchiectomy:
- Scar, consistent with regressed GCT—see Comment
- 1.5 cm gross greatest dimension
- GCNIS is present (pTis) and/or large coarse calcifications are present (pT0)

Comment: The clinical mass represents an area of scarring in the testicular parenchyma. The adjacent testis shows GCNIS ([pTis] and/or coarse calcification [pT0]), which is considered diagnostic for spontaneous regression of a GCT (reference below). (Coarse calcifications are thought to typically result from necrosis and calcification of embryonal carcinoma.)

Reference:
Balzer BL, Ulbright TM. Spontaneous regression of testicular germ cell tumors: an analysis of 42 cases. *Am J Surg Pathol.* 2006;30(7):858-865.

SERUM TUMOR MARKERS IN TESTICULAR CANCER

Laboratory studies for tumor markers produced by GCTs are an essential component of clinical diagnosis, staging, and surveillance of testicular tumors. The AJCC includes an additional "S" stage in testicular tumors based on the degree of elevation in these markers. Higher levels of AFP and bHCG are associated with worse prognosis and incorporated into the International Germ Cell Consensus Classification risk groups. Chemotherapy decisions are based on these risk groups. The role of these serum tumor markers is summarized in Table 4.5.

LDH, AFP, and bHCG should be obtained prior to orchiectomy and serially after treatment until levels have normalized. Following normalization, increasing levels of any of these markers are indicative of residual/recurrent disease.

TABLE 4.5: Serum Tumor Markers in the Diagnosis and Clinical Treatment of Germ Cell Tumors (GCTs)[50]

Hormone	Primary Associated Tumor	Other GCT which May Elevate	Non-GCT Reasons for Elevation	Clinical Utility
LDH (lactate dehydrogenase)	Seminoma	Nonspecific marker, frequently elevated in all germ cell tumors	Leukemia, rhabdomyolysis, hemolysis, pulmonary embolism, myocardial infarction	• Marked elevations in LDH are associated with higher disease burden • Rising LDH following treatment indicates recurrence
AFP (alpha-fetoprotein)	Yolk sac tumor	Rarely elevated in embryonal carcinoma and teratoma	Hepatocellular carcinoma, pancreaticobiliary tumors, liver disease	• Finding of AFP elevation in pure seminoma indicates an unsampled nonseminomatous component • AFP levels normalize within 1 mo following curative surgery
bHCG (human chorionic gonadotropin)	Choriocarcinoma (markedly elevated into the thousands)	Mild elevations in seminoma and embryonal carcinoma (<500 mIU/mL)	Numerous cancers which contain syncytiotrophoblastic cells, hypogonadism, marijuana use, pituitary adenomas	• bHCG levels normalize within 1 wk of curative surgery • Persistent elevation indicates residual/recurrent disease

IMMUNOHISTOCHEMISTRY IN TESTICULAR TUMORS

Recognizing the classic morphologic features of the various germ cell and sex cord stromal tumors is the first step in accurate diagnosis; however, as mentioned in the above discussion, many of these tumors have unusual patterns that may lead to confusion. A thoughtful and H&E-guided immunohistochemical workup can usually resolve the diagnosis.

General markers for GCTs include SALL4, PLAP, and OCT4. SALL4 and OCT3/4 are both markers of pluripotent stem and germ cells. SALL4 is a nuclear marker which showed strong positive staining in 100% of GCNIS, seminoma, embryonal carcinoma, and YST in one study.[51] Choriocarcinoma showed weaker staining, but all had some degree of expression. SALL4 is a useful marker for distinguishing between GCTs and sex cord stromal tumors or in the setting of a metastatic tumor of unknown origin when GCT is in the differential diagnosis. OCT4 is relatively specific for GCTs, but somewhat less sensitive, as it marks GCNIS, seminoma, and embryonal carcinomas only.[52] PLAP is expressed in the majority of GCNIS, seminoma, and embryonal carcinomas, with a subset of cases of YST and choriocarcinoma demonstrating reactivity.[53]

The most common general markers for sex cord stromal tumors are steroid factor 1 (SF1), inhibin, and calretinin. Importantly, as mentioned above, sex cord stromal tumors are negative for SALL4. SF1 is the most specific marker for sex cord stromal tumors, with positive expression in all of the sex cord stromal tumors in one study and no staining of the GCTs.[54]

There are a range of markers that can be used to determine subtypes of GCTs, but they must be used in the context of the H&E-based differential diagnosis because of the overlap in expression between various tumor types. For example, embryonal carcinoma and pleomorphic seminoma may have morphologic similarities requiring IHC for resolution. In this differential, OCT3/4 is not helpful as it is expressed in both. A panel of AE1/3, CD30, KIT, and D2-40 would be useful, with embryonal carcinoma expressing AE1/3 and CD30 and lacking KIT and D2-40 expression. Seminoma has the opposite immunoprofile with KIT and D2-40 positivity.[55] OCT3/4 is also useful for the distinction of GCNIS from germ cells (Figures 4.139 and 4.140).

YST and embryonal carcinoma may also be closely admixed and difficult to distinguish the relative percentages of these germ cell types. In this instance, a panel including glypican and CD30 can highlight the individual components (Figures 4.141-4.143). Table 4.6 lists immunohistochemical stains that are most useful in the diagnosis of testicular tumors (Figures 4.144-4.161).

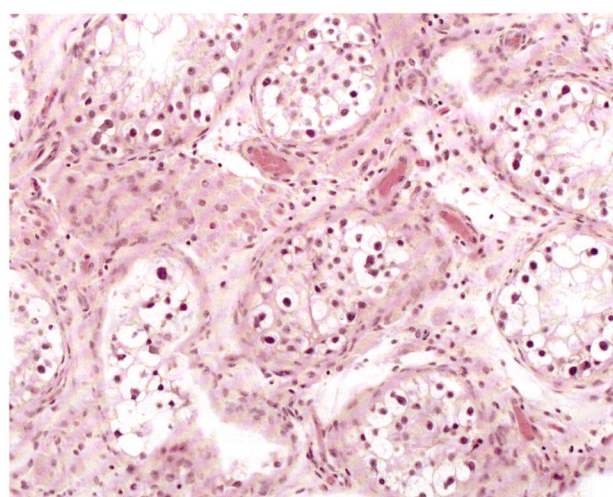

Figure 4.139. In this H&E stained section, large atypical cells with abundant cytoplasm are present in the adluminal compartment of this seminiferous tubule. If there is any doubt as to the nature of the cells, OCT3/4 staining can be used to support a diagnosis of germ cell neoplasia in situ (GCNIS).

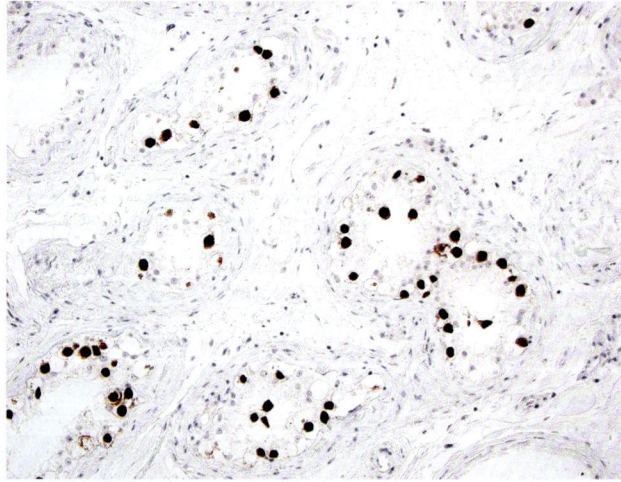

Figure 4.140. OCT3/4 shows strong nuclear expression in the atypical cells, consistent with germ cell neoplasia in situ (GCNIS).

FAQ: What is the Utility of Isochromosome 12p in the Diagnosis of Germ Cell Tumors?

- Duplication of the short arm of chromosome 12, yielding two copies of the short arm on each side of the centromere = i(12p)
- Other gains of 12p other than isochromosome also occasionally reported
- Frequently identified in GCTs of testis, ovary, and CNS
- Detection of i(12p) by fluorescence in situ hybridization (FISH) can be useful in metastatic or primary tumors lacking classic histologic or immunohistochemical features of GCT
- Lack of i(12p) does not exclude the possibility of a GCT

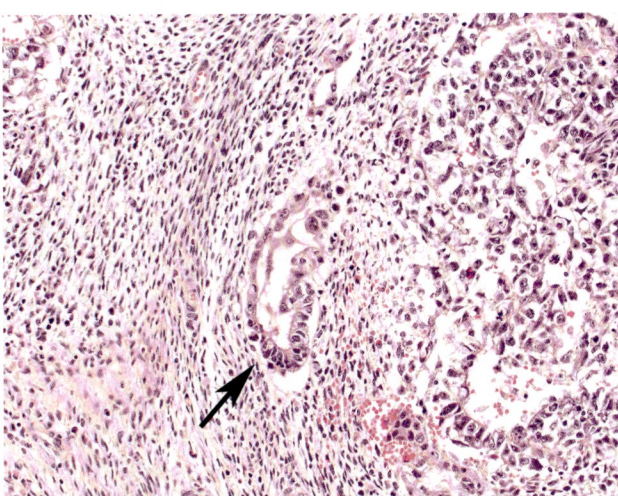

Figure 4.141. H&E-stained section of a mixed germ cell tumor demonstrating two glandular proliferations with slightly different cytologic features. The arrow is pointing to a gland with somewhat smaller, less pleomorphic nuclear features when compared to the highly atypical glandular proliferation on the right. By H&E alone, it is unclear if this represents a focus of glandular yolk sac tumor or if it could all represent embryonal carcinoma.

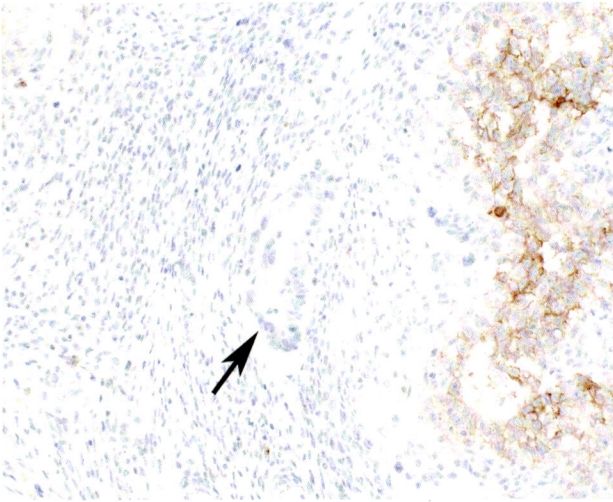

Figure 4.142. Immunohistochemistry for CD30 is performed and shows diffuse positivity in the more atypical cells on the right side of the image, consistent with embryonal carcinoma. The arrow points to the smaller gland, which is negative for CD30 and supports a diagnosis of yolk sac tumor.

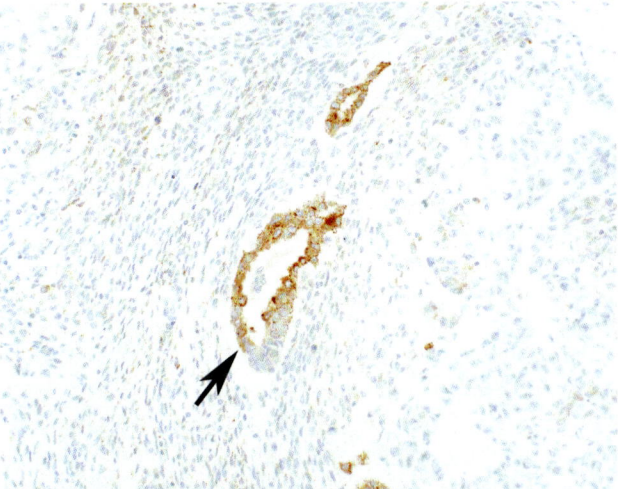

Figure 4.143. The converse is true for glypican staining, which shows diffuse positivity in the single gland marked by the arrow. Glypican is negative in the embryonal carcinoma. A panel of stains is more reliable than a single stain, and immunohistochemical markers should be chosen careful with a thoughtful differential diagnosis in mind based on H&E features.

TABLE 4.6: Commonly Used Immunohistochemical Markers in Testicular Tumors With Expected Results and Common Pitfalls

Immunohistochemical Marker	Staining Pattern	Expected Positive Staining	Expected Negative Staining	Pitfalls
OCT3/4	Nuclear	Seminoma Embryonal carcinoma Germ cell neoplasia in situ (GCNIS)	Yolk sac tumor Choriocarcinoma Spermatocytic tumor Sex cord stromal tumors	Rarely, EC can lose OCT3/4 expression after chemotherapy May stain large B-cell lymphomas
SALL4 (Figure 4.144)	Nuclear	All germ cell tumors[a] Spermatocytic tumor GCNIS	All sex cord stromal tumors	[a]Choriocarcinoma may show variable staining Some lymphomas, carcinomas, and sarcomas of other origins can be positive
Placental alkaline phosphatase (PLAP) (Figure 4.145)	Cytoplasmic	Seminoma Embryonal carcinoma Yolk sac tumor Choriocarcinoma GCNIS	Spermatocytic tumor[b]	[b]Rare patchy staining has been reported in spermatocytic tumor
D2-40/podoplanin (Figure 4.146)	Cytoplasmic	Seminoma	Embryonal carcinoma Yolk sac tumor Choriocarcinoma[c] Spermatocytic tumor	[c]Focal staining observed in some choriocarcinomas[56]
KIT (c-KIT or CD117) (Figure 4.147)	Circumferential membranous cytoplasmic	Seminoma Spermatocytic tumor (var) GCNIS	Embryonal carcinoma Yolk sac tumor (var)[d] Choriocarcinoma Spermatocytic tumor (var)	[d]Positivity has been reported in yolk sac tumor, especially solid pattern which may mimic seminoma
AE1/3 (Figure 4.148)	Cytoplasmic	Embryonal carcinoma Yolk sac tumor Choriocarcinoma	Seminoma (var) GCNIS Spermatocytic tumor	
CD30 (Figure 4.149)	Cytoplasmic membranous/golgi pattern	Embryonal carcinoma[e]	Seminoma Yolk sac tumor Choriocarcinoma Spermatocytic tumor GCNIS	[e]Rarely, EC can lose CD30 expression after chemotherapy[57] Positive in some lymphomas Focal staining in some apparently pure seminomas, which does not necessarily indicate embryonal carcinoma unless there is a morphologic correlate
Glypican 3 (Figures 4.150 and 4.151)	Diffuse cytoplasmic membranous	Yolk sac tumor Choriocarcinoma	Seminoma Embryonal carcinoma (var)	
Alpha-fetoprotein (AFP) (Figure 4.152)	Cytoplasmic, patchy	Yolk sac tumor	Seminoma Embryonal carcinoma (var) Choriocarcinoma Spermatocytic tumor GCNIS	Staining may be very patchy High background staining when serum AFP is elevated (Figure 4.153)

TABLE 4.6: Commonly Used Immunohistochemical Markers in Testicular Tumors With Expected Results and Common Pitfalls   (Continued)

Immunohistochemical Marker	Staining Pattern	Expected Positive Staining	Expected Negative Staining	Pitfalls
Beta–human chorionic growth (bHCG) (Figures 4.154 and 4.155)	Cytoplasmic	Choriocarcinoma (primarily stains syncytiotrophoblastic cells)	Yolk sac tumor Seminoma[f] Embryonal carcinoma Spermatocytic tumor GCNIS	[f]Can be positive in seminomas (or non-GCT tumors) with syncytiotrophoblastic cells High background staining when serum HCG is elevated (Figure 4.156)
Gata-binding protein 3 (GATA3) (Figure 4.157)	Nuclear	Choriocarcinoma Yolk sac tumor (var)	Seminoma Embryonal carcinoma Spermatocytic tumor GCNIS	
Steroidogenic factor 1 (SF1) (Figure 4.158)	Nuclear	Sex cord stromal tumors	All germ cell tumors	Also expressed in adrenal cortical tumors
Calretinin (Figures 4.159 and 4.160)	Cytoplasmic	Sex cord stromal tumors	All germ cell tumors	Nonspecific for these tumors, must be used in context with appropriate differential
Inhibin (Figure 4.161)	Cytoplasmic	Sex cord stromal tumors	All germ cell tumors	Nonspecific for these tumors, must be used in context with appropriate differential

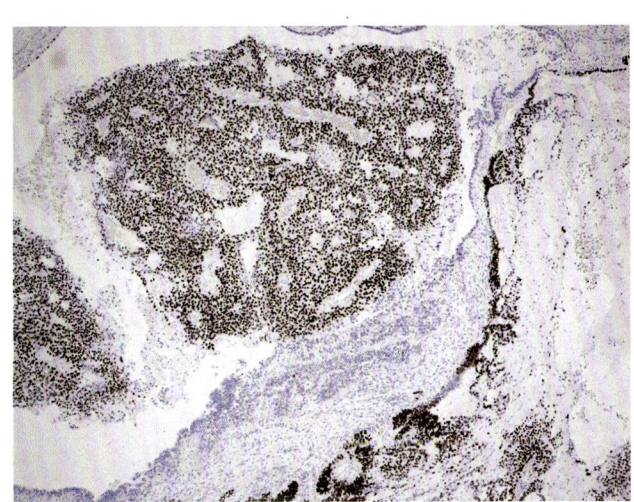

Figure 4.144. SALL4 is a specific and broad immunomarker for germ cell tumors, with expected nuclear positivity in all types of germ cell tumors, though choriocarcinoma may demonstrate variable staining.

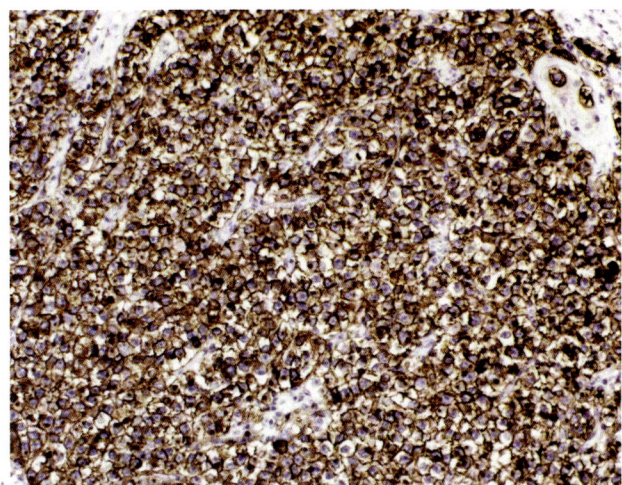

Figure 4.145. Placental alkaline phosphatase (PLAP) is another widely expressed marker for germ cell tumors. In this image, it shows strong membranous staining of a seminoma. It can be useful in the distinction of seminoma from spermatocytic tumor, although rare positivity has been reported in the latter.

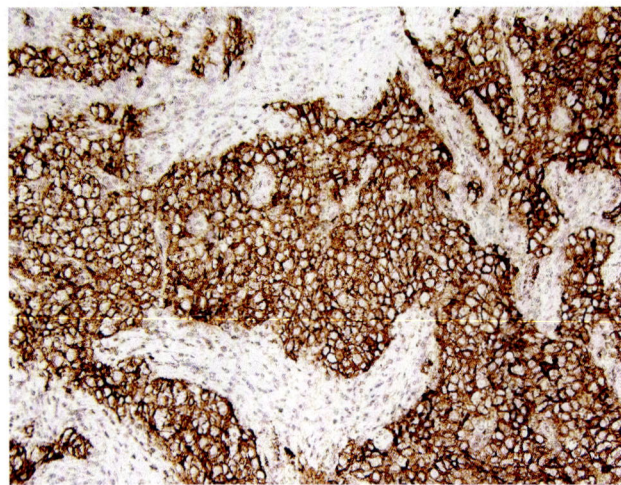

Figure 4.146. D2-40, also known as podoplanin, is diffusely expressed in seminoma. It demonstrates a membranous cytoplasmic pattern similar to placental alkaline phosphatase (PLAP) in this seminoma.

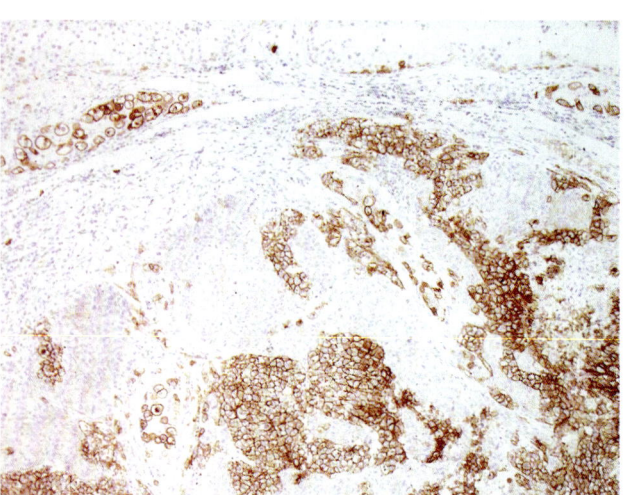

Figure 4.147. KIT (c-KIT or CD117) is expressed diffusely in a membranous fashion in seminomas and should be used as part of the panel to distinguish seminoma from embryonal carcinoma.

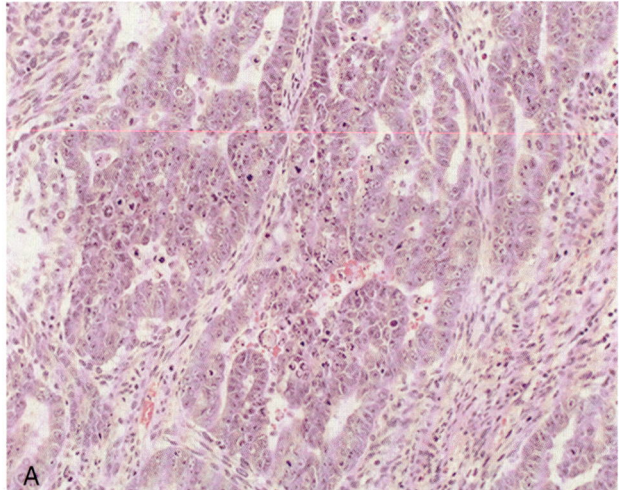

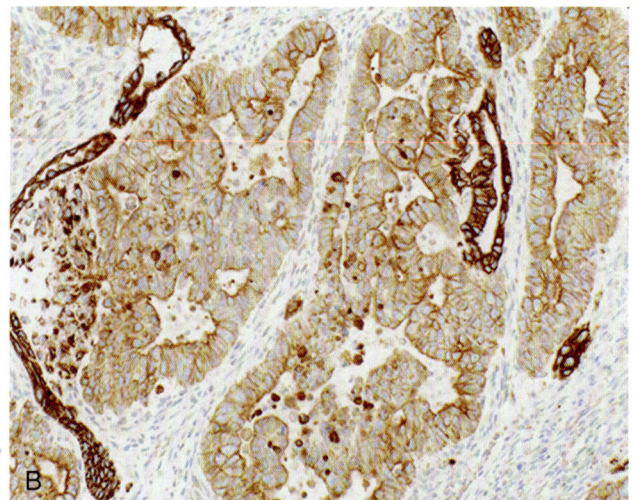

Figure 4.148. A, High-grade pleomorphic cells in a glandular pattern consistent with embryonal carcinoma. B, AE1/3 is not a specific marker for embryonal carcinoma; however, it will also mark yolk sac tumor and choriocarcinoma. Keratin can be useful in the distinction of embryonal carcinoma from seminoma.

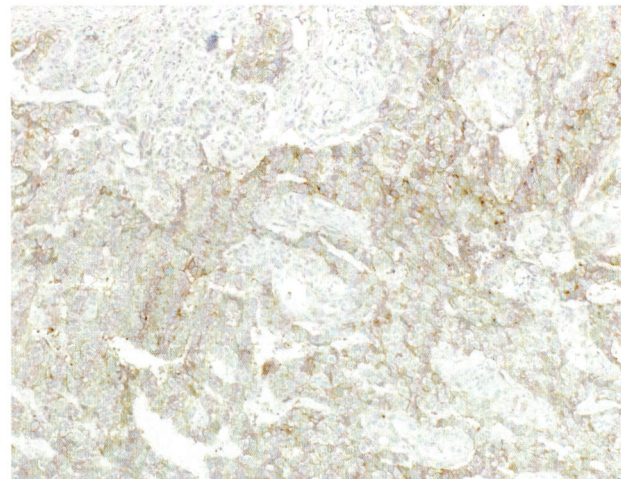

Figure 4.149. CD30 is a more specific marker for embryonal carcinoma and is often employed as part of a panel of stains for the differentiation of embryonal carcinoma and seminoma.

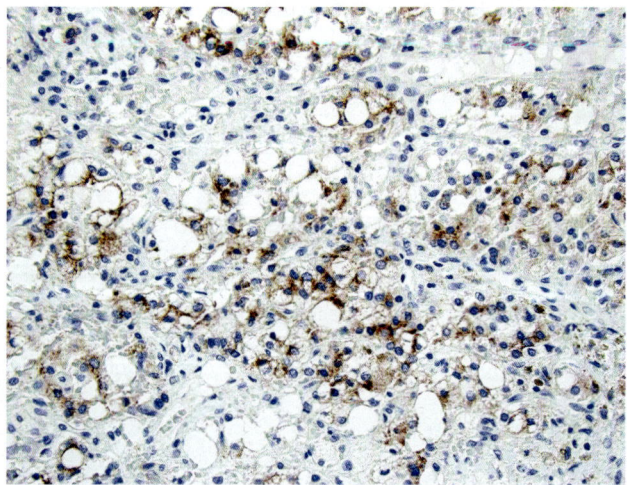

Figure 4.150. Glypican 3 is the most specific marker for yolk sac tumor when considering a germ cell tumor. It stains in a diffuse cytoplasmic and membranous fashion.

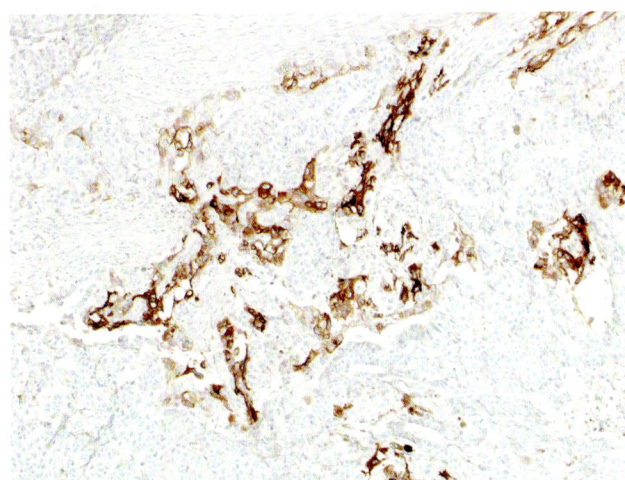

Figure 4.151. When yolk sac tumor is admixed with embryonal carcinoma, glypican 3 is useful to highlight the yolk sac component.

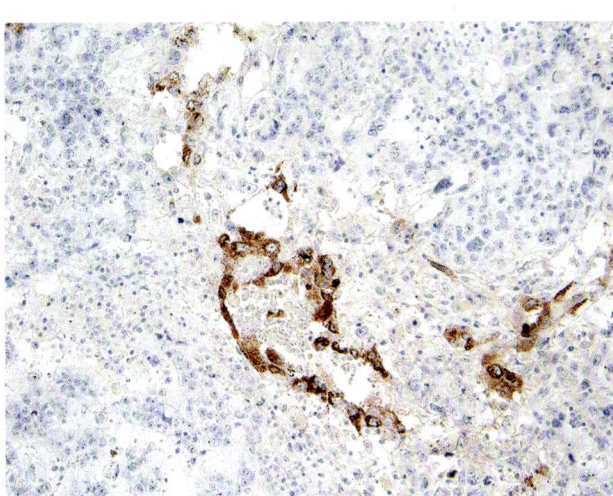

Figure 4.152. Alpha-fetoprotein (AFP) is a relatively specific marker for yolk sac tumor, though it may only have patchy expression.

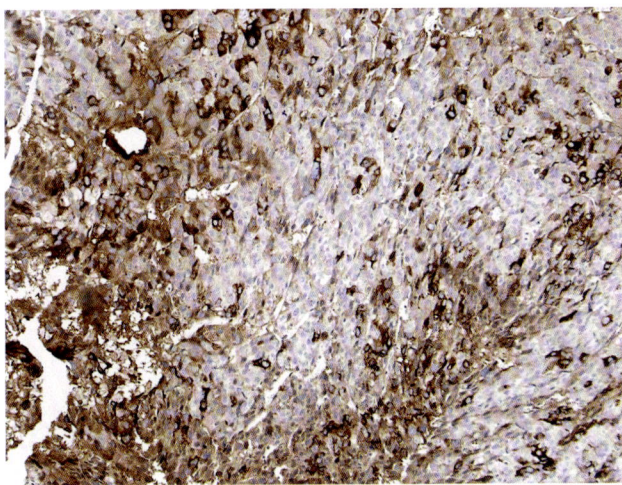

Figure 4.153. Another pitfall with alpha-fetoprotein (AFP) staining is that in the setting of a high serum AFP, there can be nonspecific background staining of areas with blood and serum present that do not correspond to actual yolk sac tumor areas. While much of this image represents real tumor staining, be aware that areas of necrosis and hemorrhage may stain due to the presence of serum alpha-fetoprotein (AFP).

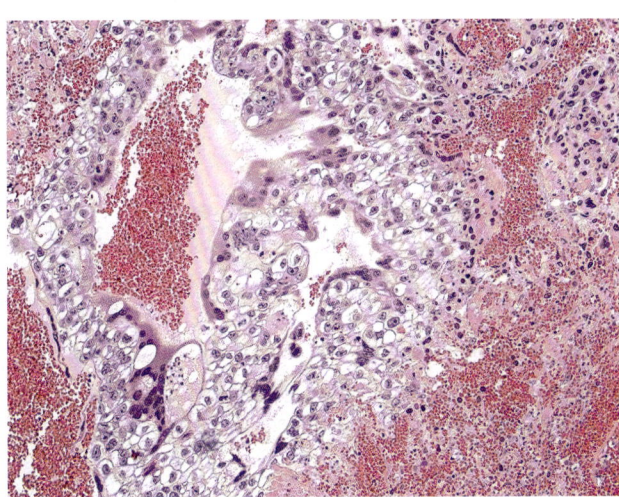

Figure 4.154. Beta human chorionic gonadotropin (bHCG) is a useful marker for choriocarcinoma, where it primarily stains the syncytiotrophoblastic cells. H&E-stained section showing a choriocarcinoma largely comprises cytotrophoblastic cells and rare syncytiotrophoblastic cell.

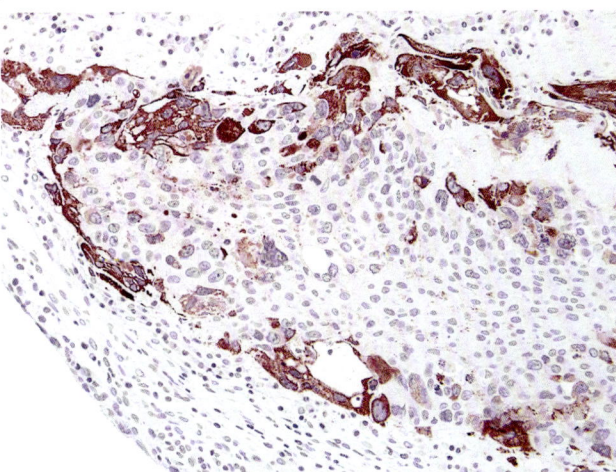

Figure 4.155. Beta human chorionic gonadotropin (bHCG) marking only the large multinucleated syncytiotrophoblastic cells in this choriocarcinoma.

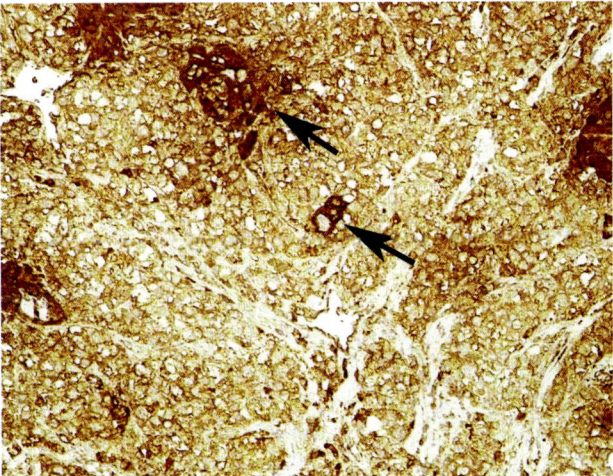

Figure 4.156. Similar to alpha-fetoprotein (AFP), beta human chorionic gonadotropin (bHCG) can have high nonspecific background staining when serum bHCG is elevated. Expression in the syncytiotrophoblastic cells (arrows) is much stronger than the background staining.

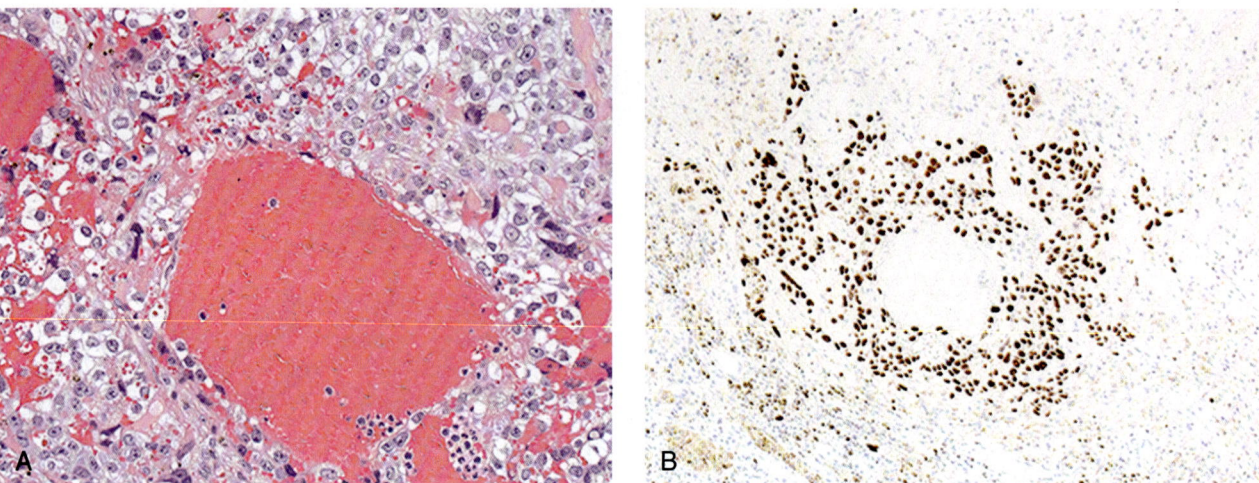

Figure 4.157. A, Metastatic choriocarcinoma with unusual morphology following chemotherapy. The abundant clear cytoplasm may be confused with seminoma, and immunohistochemistry is useful to prove the tumor is residual choriocarcinoma. B, GATA3 is expressed in the overwhelming majority of choriocarcinomas and is a useful marker of trophoblastic tissues. (Images provided by Dr Chia-Sui Kao.)

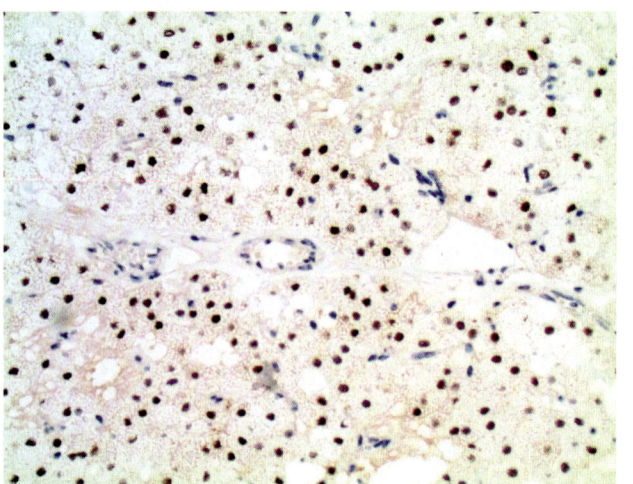

Figure 4.158. SF1 is a general marker for sex cord stromal tumors and is useful in their distinction from germ cell tumors. Here it shows diffuse nuclear positivity in a Leydig cell tumor. (Image provided by Dr Ankur Sangoi.)

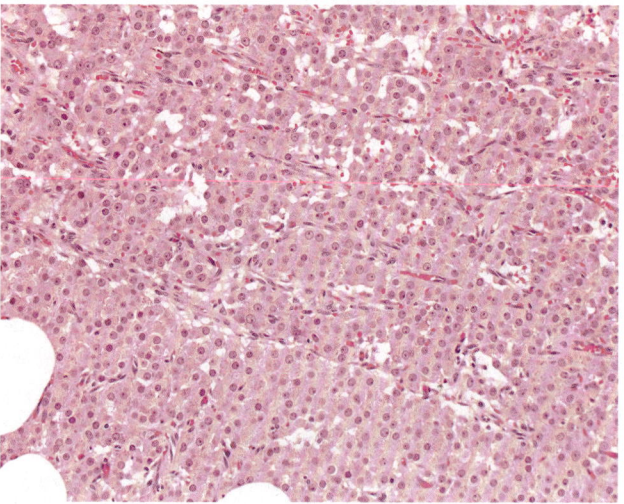

Figure 4.159. H&E section of Leydig cell tumor demonstrating classic cytomorphology with plump eosinophilic cells with rounded nuclei.

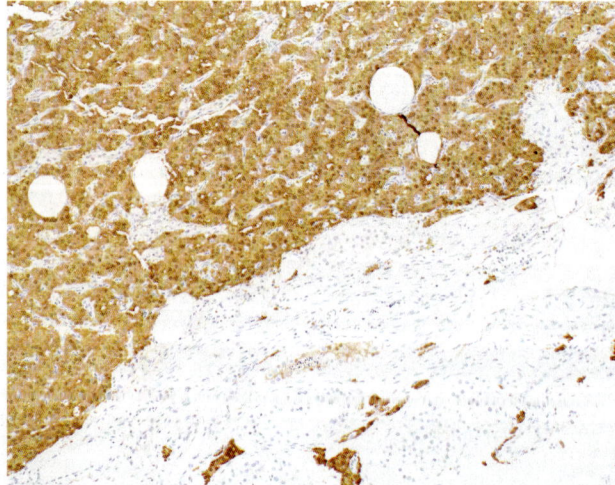

Figure 4.160. Calretinin showing diffuse cytoplasmic positivity in a Leydig cell tumor. The spermatic tubules are negative, though residual clusters of normal Leydig cells are highlighted. Calretinin marks many other tumor types (mesothelial, adrenal) and should be used with an appropriate panel of markers.

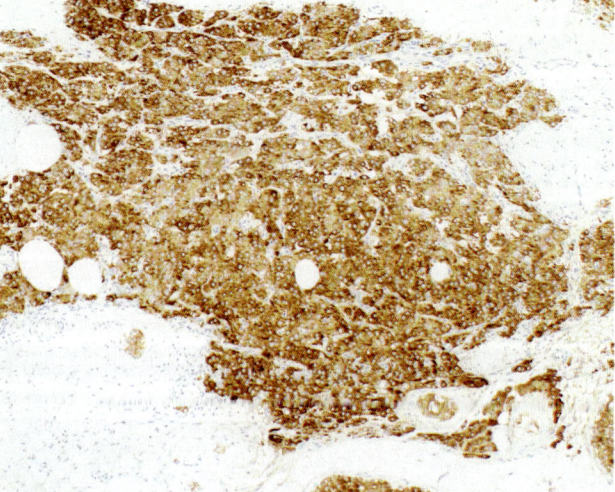

Figure 4.161. Similarly, inhibin marks this Leydig cell tumor and is negative in the surrounding tubules.

TESTICULAR CANCER REPORTING AND STAGING

Testicular cancer staging can be challenging based on the complex anatomy of the testis and surrounding structures. Gross examination technique is essential to accurate staging and is dependent on thorough sampling of the tumor and adjacent tunica, epididymis, and spermatic cord. (See Checklist: CAP and International Society of Urologic Pathology [ISUP] recommendations for gross examination, reporting, and staging of testicular tumors below.)

CHECKLIST: CAP and International Society of Urologic Pathology Recommendations for Grossing, Reporting, and Staging of Testicular Tumors[58-60]

- ☐ Entirely submit tumors 2 cm or less
- ☐ For tumors greater than 2 cm, submit whichever is greater: 10 blocks or 1 to 2 blocks per centimeter
- ☐ Thorough sampling of all grossly different-appearing areas of tumor with adjacent testicular parenchyma and tunica albuginea
- ☐ Sections of testicular hilum/mediastinum, epididymis, spermatic cord base, and spermatic cord margin
- ☐ In mixed GCTs, report percentages of each component (see sample note below)
- ☐ Evaluate extent of tumor
  - o Rete testis involvement does not increase stage but should be reported as it is prognostic
  - o Hilar soft-tissue involvement is staged as pT2
  - o Invasive tumor present in section of epididymis/spermatic cord base is staged as pT3
- ☐ Identify presence or absence of LVI
  - o Presence of LVI makes a tumor pT2 regardless of tumor size
  - o Beware artifactual tumor displacement; if no definitive LVI identified, report as negative
  - o LVI in the spermatic cord should be staged as pT2, not pT3 which requires soft-tissue invasion
- ☐ Comment on presence of GCNIS
  - o If intact spermatogenesis is present in a tubule, it usually does not contain GCNIS

Based on the WHO 2016 recommendations, tumors should be assigned a histologic subtype, which fall into the broad categories of "Germ Cell Tumors Derived From Germ Cell Neoplasia In Situ," "Germ Cell Tumors Unrelated to Germ Cell Neoplasia In Situ," and "Sex Cord Stromal Tumors." Much rarer tumors may also be encountered and are discussed with staging considerations in the WHO monograph. Reporting the percentages of varying types of GCTs in non-seminomatous GCTs is useful for clinicians and yields important details for decision-making. Cancer synoptic templates should provide a guide for reporting these tumors, but attention to the unique challenges of testicular tumors is incumbent on the sign-out pathologist.

Staging is by the AJCC TNM system and based on tumor size, confinement or non-confinement to the testis, and LVI. Pathologic T1 disease is completely confined to the testis without LVI, and substaging for pure seminoma only is dependent on the cutoff of less than (pT1a) or greater than or equal to 3 cm in size (pT1b). The finding of any LVI or involvement of hilar soft tissue, epididymis, or tunica albuginea results in upstaging to pT2, regardless of tumor size. The importance of accurate diagnosis of LVI is essential to avoid falsely upstaging the patient to pT2. (See Pearls and Pitfalls: Artifactual displacement mimics LVI in testicular tumors.)

GCTs are especially prone to dyscohesion, and gross technical artifact may lead to tumor displacement within vessels, mimicking LVI. Fastidious gross examination technique may help; for example, rinsing cutting blade between sections and then rinsing sections before submitting in cassette. When this artifact is present, it is prudent to avoid calling LVI definitively and add a note describing the findings. (See Sample Note below.)

FAQ: What are the Diagnostic Features of LVI Versus Artifactual Displacement in Testicular Germ Cell Tumors?[59]

Features That Favor Diagnostic LVI	Features That Favor Artifactual Displacement of Tumor
Clean surfaces that lack obvious artifactual displacement of tumor	Finding tumor "buttered" on the tunica or other cut surfaces (Figure 4.166)
Tumor in vessels at tumor periphery and near tunica albuginea	Tumor deposits scattered throughout a specimen
Intravascular tumor within fibrin thrombus	Dyscohesive tumor cells "floating" in vascular space (Figure 4.167)
Rounded outline and cohesive tumor implant (Figures 4.162 and 4.163)	Irregular, angulated tumor deposits with dyscohesive edges (Figure 4.168)
Frank invasion of vessel or attachment to vascular endothelial lining (Figures 4.164 and 4.165)	Lack of attachment to vascular wall (Figure 4.169)

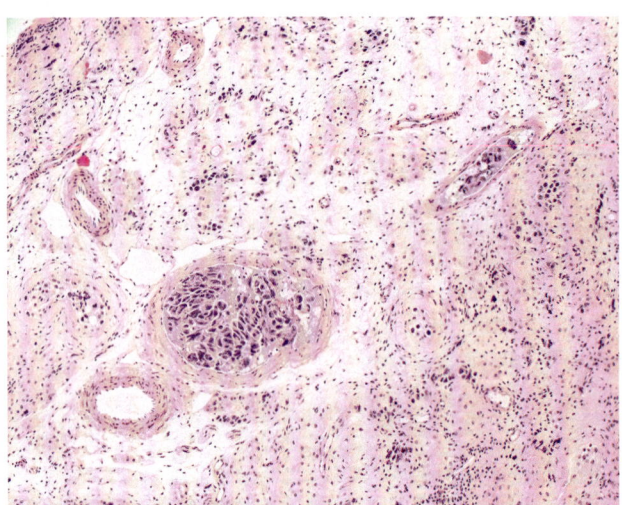

Figure 4.162. At scanning magnification, the finding of rounded foci of tumor is suggestive of possible lymphovascular invasion.

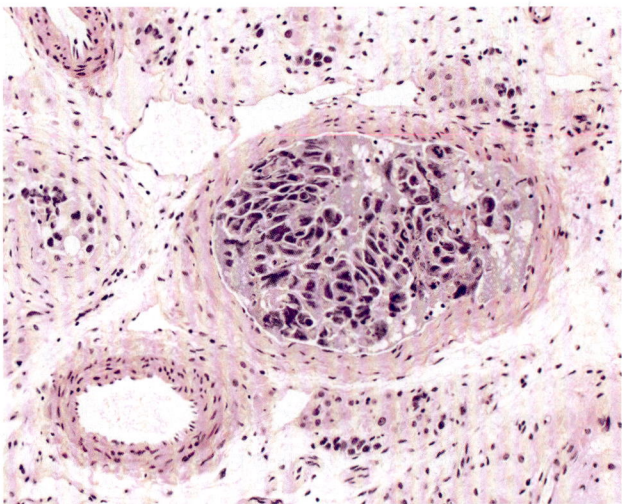

Figure 4.163. A higher power examination shows a vessel distended by a rounded, cohesive cluster of tumor cells, consistent with lymphovascular invasion.

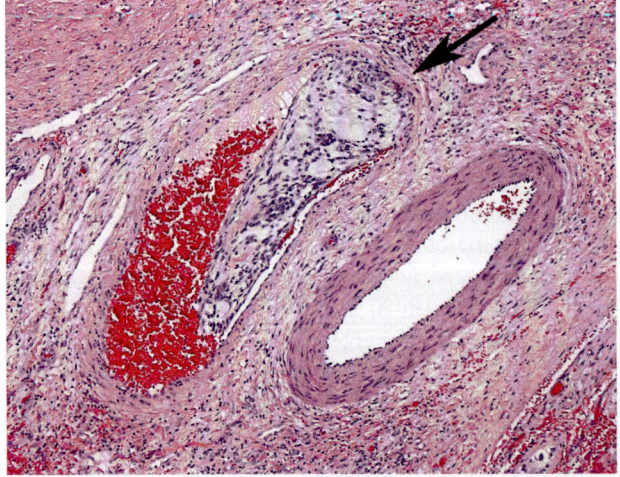

Figure 4.164. In this example of diagnostic lymphovascular invasion, the tumor cells are adherent to the vessel wall (arrow).

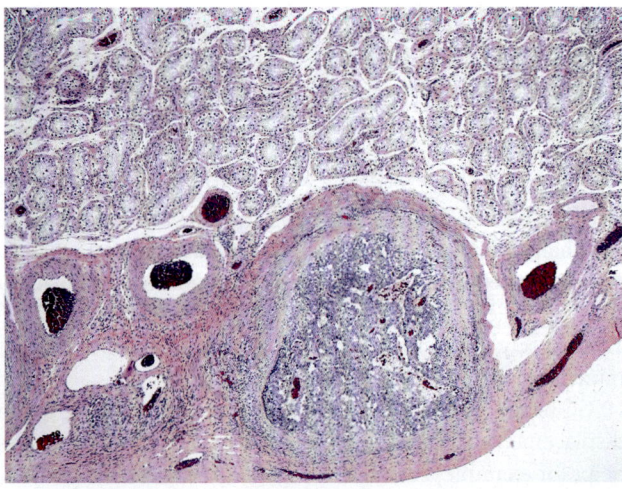

Figure 4.165. Another example of densely adherent tumor involving the vessel wall, diagnostic for lymphovascular invasion.

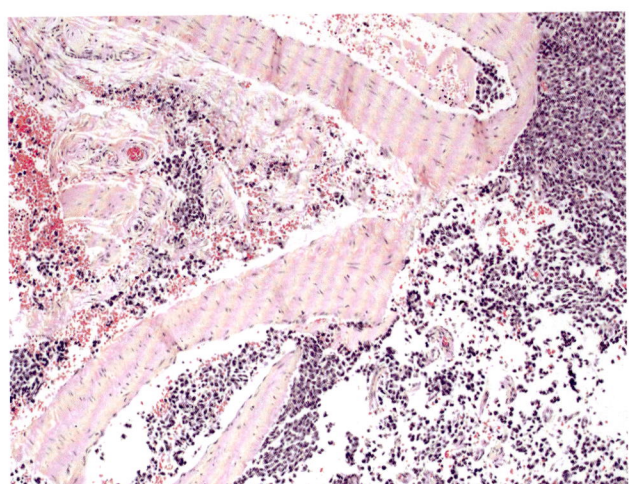

Figure 4.166. An example of "buttering" or extensive artifactual tumor carryover in a testicular germ cell tumor. The tumor is displaced into many potential spaces, some of which are large vessels; however, this does not represent diagnostic lymphovascular invasion (LVI). When this amount of carryover is identified in a specimen, caution is warranted in calling LVI.

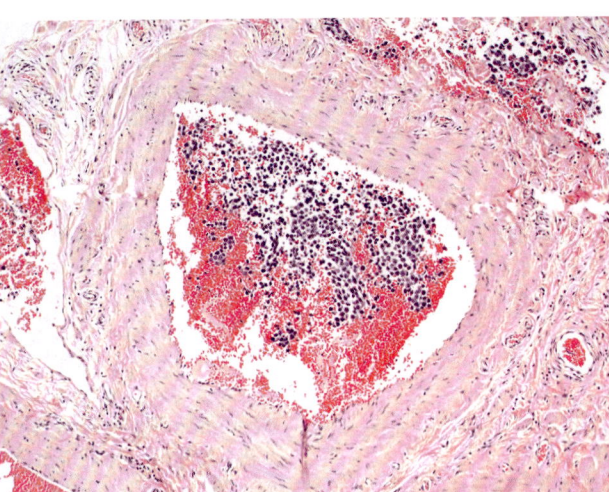

Figure 4.167. Tumor cells floating within a vessel lumen; cells are dyscohesive and not tightly clustered in a rounded shape. This finding is not diagnostic of lymphovascular invasion (LVI).

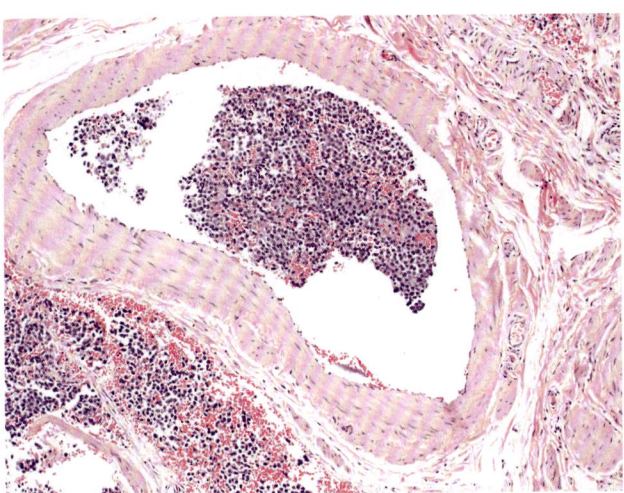

Figure 4.168. A representative image of dyscohesive, non-rounded collection of tumor cells within a vessel, also supports carryover rather than being diagnostic of lymphovascular invasion (LVI).

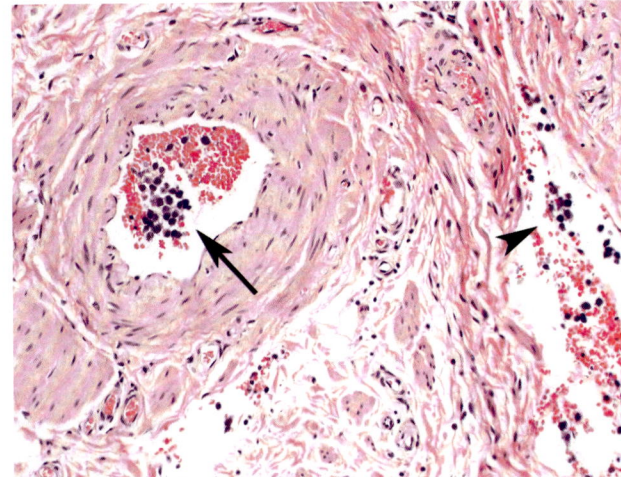

Figure 4.169. Few dyscohesive tumor cells in a vessel (arrow) that lack any attachment to the vessel wall and also are not tightly clustered or rounded into a smooth outline. There are adjacent loose tumor cells suggestive of artifact (arrowhead). This finding is not sufficient for a diagnosis of lymphovascular invasion (LVI).

SAMPLE NOTE: Artifactual Displacement of Tumor-Mimicking Lymphovascular Invasion

Testis, left, orchiectomy:
- Seminoma, 2.0 cm
- Tumor confined to testis (pT1a)
- No definitive LVI identified (see Note)

Note: Dyscohesive tumor is present within vessels and identified on cut surfaces, consistent with artifactual displacement. In order to make a definitive diagnosis of LVI, the tumor must show invasion or attachment to vessel wall, association with fibrin thrombus, or show a compact, rounded profile within vessel. In the absence of these definitive features, the specimen should be interpreted as negative for LVI.

Reference:
Verrill C, Yilmaz A, Srigley JR, et al. Reporting and staging of testicular germ cell tumors: the International Society of Urological Pathology (ISUP) testicular cancer consultation conference recommendations. *Am J Surg Pathol*. 2017;41(6):e22-e32.

Stage 3 testicular tumors directly invade the spermatic cord soft tissue, with or without LVI. However, it should be noted that LVI alone in the spermatic cord does not count as pT3 disease, unless there is frank invasion of the soft tissue of the cord (Figures 4.170-4.172). Stage 4 tumors invade the scrotum, regardless of presence or absence of LVI.

Involvement of the rete testis occurs when tumor invades the stroma between the rete testis tubules (Figure 4.173). This finding does not increase the stage itself, but it should be reported as it may have prognostic importance.[61] Pagetoid spread of GCNIS into the rete epithelium is a common occurrence; however, it does not constitute rete testis involvement (Figures 4.174 and 4.175). Involvement of the testicular hilar soft tissue is handled in a similar manner, given that this is likely the path of least resistance for tumors to grow beyond the testis. Although hilar soft-tissue involvement currently does not result in upstaging the tumor, there is evidence that it is associated with a worse prognosis and it should be reported when present[61] (Figure 4.176).

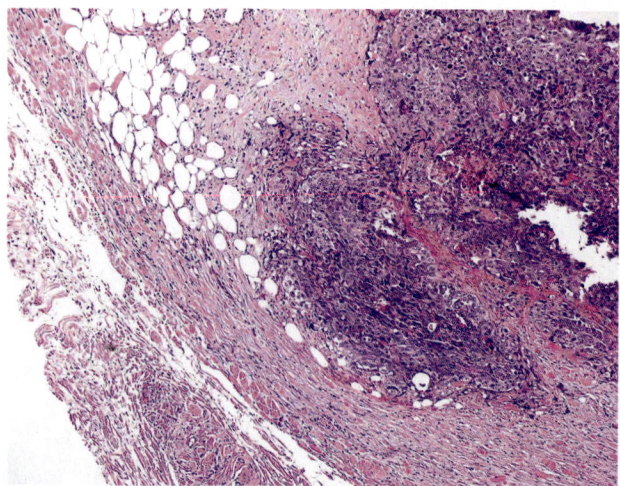

Figure 4.170. A cross section of the spermatic cord demonstrating tumor present in the soft tissue and fat of the cord, diagnostic of pT3 disease.

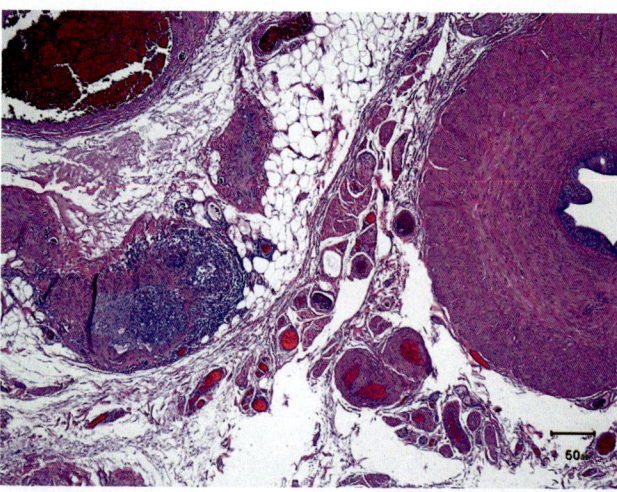

Figure 4.171. At scanning magnification, tumor is present within the fat of this spermatic cord section; however, it appears to be partly involving lymphovascular spaces. Lymphovascular invasion (LVI) in the spermatic cord does not upstage the patient to pT3.

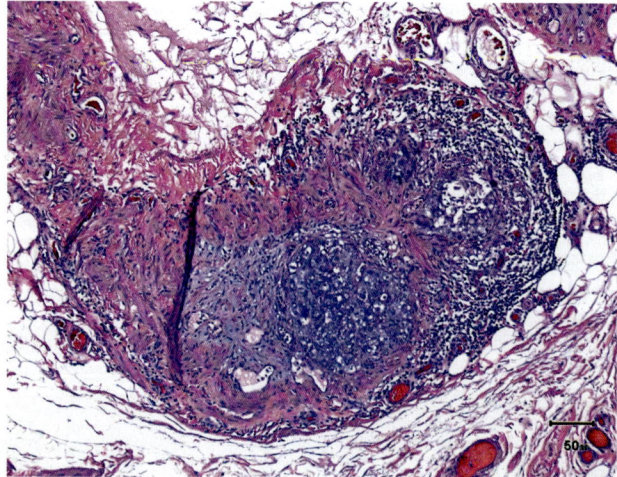

Figure 4.172. At higher power, the tumor is seen extending beyond the vessel wall and into soft tissue, so in this instance, there is both lymphovascular invasion (LVI) and spermatic cord soft-tissue invasion resulting in pT3 disease.

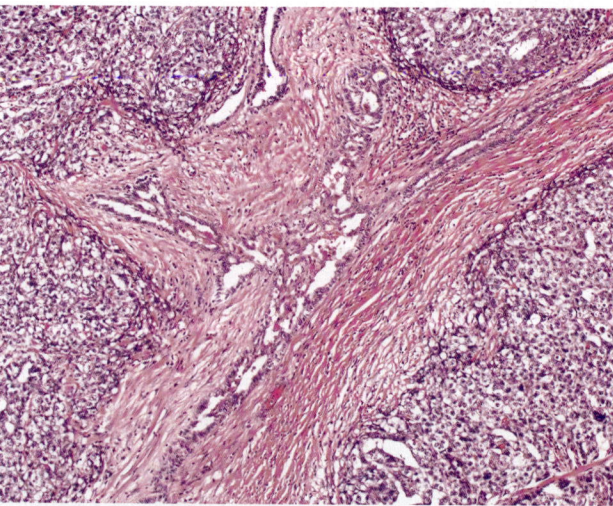

Figure 4.173. Diagnostic rete testis involvement with tumor infiltrating on both sides of rete glands. This finding does not currently change pathologic stage but is associated with worse prognosis and should be reported.

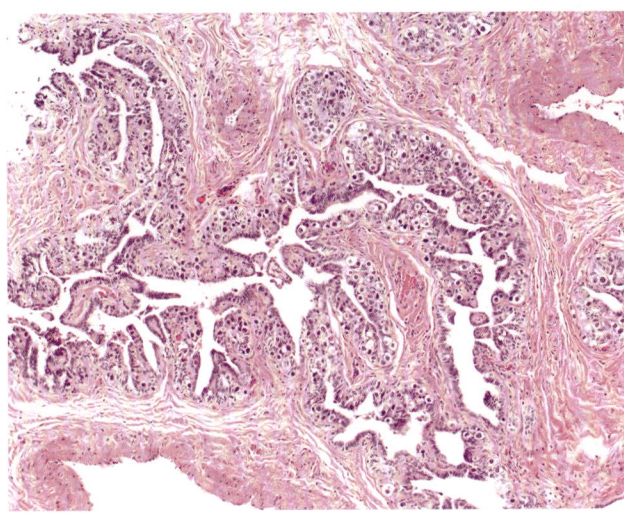

Figure 4.174. Pagetoid spread of germ cell neoplasia in situ (GCNIS) in the rete epithelium is a common occurrence and does not qualify as rete testis involvement. In this image, numerous GCNIS cells distend into the lumen of the rete gland but are not seen within the stroma around the glands.

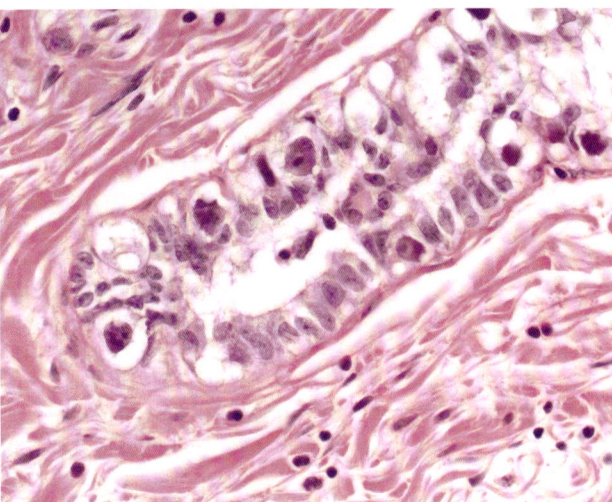

Figure 4.175. At high power, the classic cytologic features of germ cell neoplasia in situ (GCNIS)—abundant clear cytoplasm and enlarged, atypical nucleus—are demonstrated within the rete epithelium.

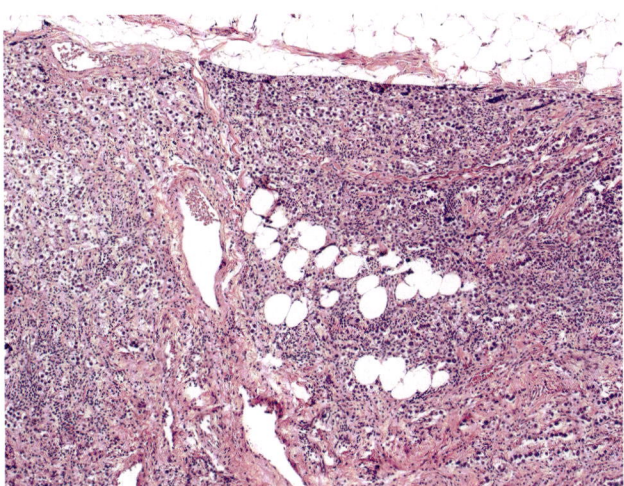

Figure 4.176. Similar to rete testis involvement, the presence of invasive tumor within hilar soft tissue should be reported. This finding does not lead to an increase in stage but is associated with a worse prognosis.

In summary, testicular tumors present many challenges to accurate staging and understanding the anatomy, staging guidelines and potential pitfalls are important for accurate reporting.

FAQ: What are the Most Common Tumors to Metastasize to the Testis?[62]

1. Prostate
2. Kidney
3. Colon
4. Urinary tract
5. Lung
6. Esophagus

NEAR MISSES

TESTICULAR INFARCT

An adult male presents with testicular pain and swelling. Serum tumor markers are performed and are within normal range, but clinical concern for a tumor prompts radical orchiectomy.

Sections show a well-demarcated region of infarcted spermatic tubules with necrosis and acute inflammation. The surrounding testicular parenchyma appears normal, without evidence of infarction (Figure 4.177). The first clue to the diagnosis is the focal nature of the infarct, supporting a single segmental vessel was involved. The classic "segmental infarct" often in a wedge-shape is consistent with vasculitis (Figures 4.178 and 4.179). When a segmental infarct is identified, close inspection of the surrounding vessels is warranted to look for signs of vasculitis (Figure 4.180). The main differential diagnosis is with testicular torsion, which results in global infarction of the entire testicular parenchyma due to the obstruction of venous return at the level of the main spermatic vessels. Interstitial hemorrhage is often prominent throughout the testicle in torsion (Figure 4.181).

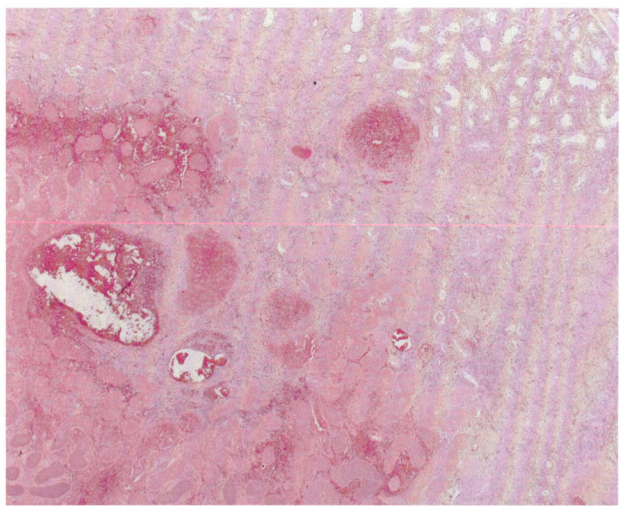

Figure 4.177. A low-power image of segmental infarct showing preserved, viable seminiferous tubules in the upper right of the image, with a wedge-shape infarction present in the remainder of the specimen. This appearance strongly favors a vasculitic process over torsion and should prompt close inspection for damaged vessels.

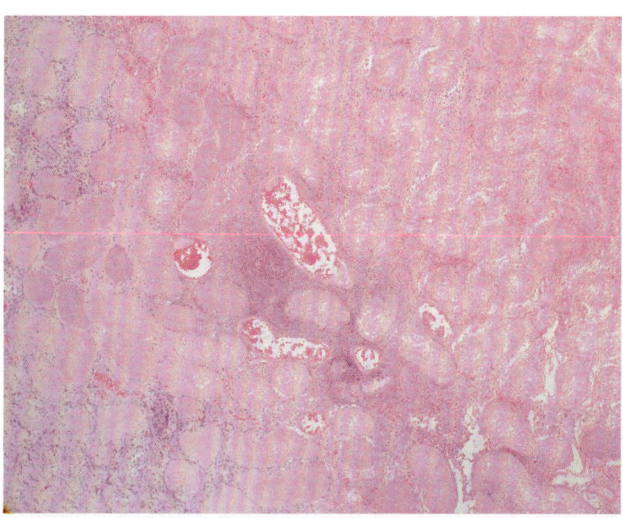

Figure 4.178. At higher power, the ghosts of seminiferous tubules are evident in the area of infarction.

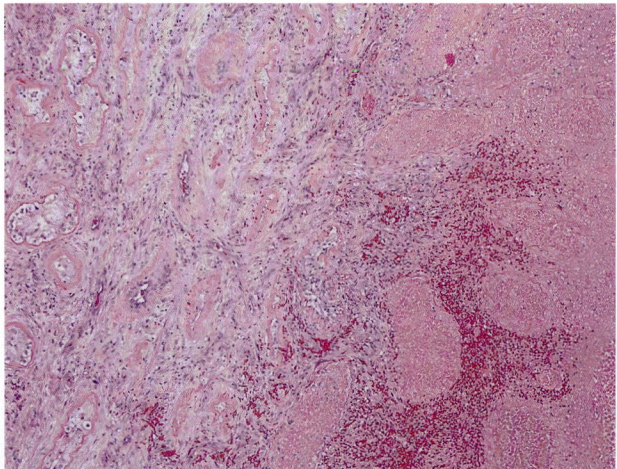

Figure 4.179. Another image demonstrating a combination of viable tubules in the upper left of the image, with necrotic ghost tubules in the remainder of the field. A few slitlike vessels are present in this field and should be examined at high power for signs of vasculitis; however, the affected vessels may also be found away from the infarct.

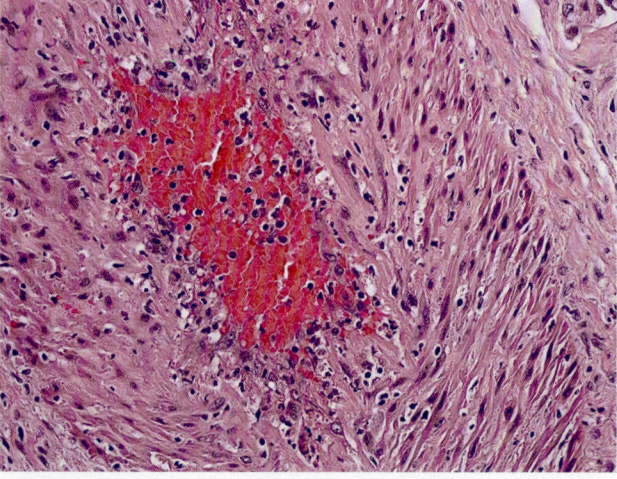

Figure 4.180. Representative image of a vessel with leukocytoclasis, neutrophils within the vessel wall. When in doubt, elastin stain is useful to demonstrate the destruction of the elastic lamina.

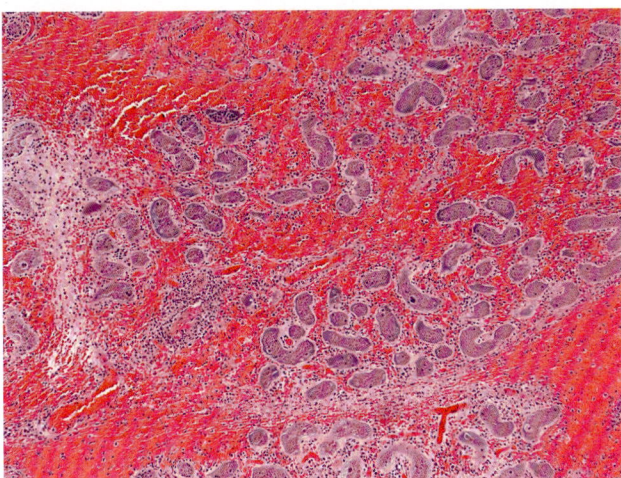

Figure 4.181. In contrast to the segmental infarct, global infarction with involvement of the entire testis is most consistent with torsion. All blood flow to the testis is stopped, and backpressure in the veins results in interstitial hemorrhage as seen here.

While isolated testicular vasculitis is reported, it is often a systemic process, and clinical history may reveal other signs and symptoms of vasculitis. Clinical features include musculoskeletal complaints, elevated erythrocyte sedimentation rate (ESR), and anemia. The most common type of vasculitis to affect the testis is PAN-like vasculitis, with granulomatosis with polyangiitis identified in a minority of cases.[15] Once vasculitis is suspected based on the recognition of the focal nature of the infarct, a close inspection of vessels will often demonstrate features of vasculitis: leukocytoclasis, red cell extravasation, fibrinoid necrosis, granulomatous, or nongranulomatous inflammation. The differential diagnosis of the specific type of vasculitis depends on the size of vessels involved. A full discussion of vasculitides is beyond the scope of this chapter, but recognition of this common pattern in testicular infarct is important for insuring the patient receives full clinical workup.

Conversely, recent work has suggested that "isolated" testicular vasculitis may often represent a phenomenon of chronic intermittent torsion that yields only a segmental infarct rather than the classic hemorrhagic infarct of the entire testis in typical torsion. Therefore, if no clinical evidence of systemic symptoms is present, a comment regarding the possibility of intermittent torsion versus true vasculitis can be given.[14]

REGRESSED GERM CELL TUMOR

A young male presents with abdominal pain, prompting a CT scan that demonstrates severe retroperitoneal lymphadenopathy. A core needle biopsy is performed which demonstrates involvement by seminoma. A scrotal ultrasound is performed which demonstrates a subcentimeter hypoechoic area and a few microcalcifications. Given the biopsy findings, the clinical diagnosis is a regressed GCT, and a radical orchiectomy is performed.

The first element of this case to recognize is that a young male with retroperitoneal lymphadenopathy or other midline mass should raise the suspicion for GCT. Appropriate immunohistochemical workup of the biopsy of an involved lymph node should include germ cell markers. Serum tumor markers should also be performed in this setting, as they may guide treatment decisions. The lack of a definitive testicular mass on scrotal ultrasound does not rule out a testicular primary, and radical orchiectomy is appropriate in these patients. Paradoxically, the testis harboring the tumor is often the smaller one, and the laterality can sometimes be predicted based on the distribution of the metastases.

Regression of GCTs is thought to occur either by ischemic changes—when the blood supply of the mass is disrupted—or cytotoxic effects of antitumor T lymphocytes attacking the tumor cells.[63] Histologically, supportive features for the diagnosis of regressed GCT include a fibrotic scar with adjacent tubules involved by GCNIS, intratubular large coarse calcifications, and hemosiderin-laden macrophages (Figures 4.182-4.184). The finding of intertubular calcifications is considered the strongest evidence of regressed GCT (Figure 4.185). Chronic inflammation and microliths are also commonly identified.

The main differential diagnosis of regressed GCT is simply a scar from a prior trauma or infarct. A testicular scar does not have any specific features; instead, it lacks the key features suggestive of a regressed GCT. No associated intratubular coarse calcifications or GCNIS are identified, although some degree of tubular atrophy is acceptable. Due to role of trauma and vasculitis in some testicular scars, chronic inflammation and hemosiderin-laden macrophages may be present, so these findings are not specific for either entity.

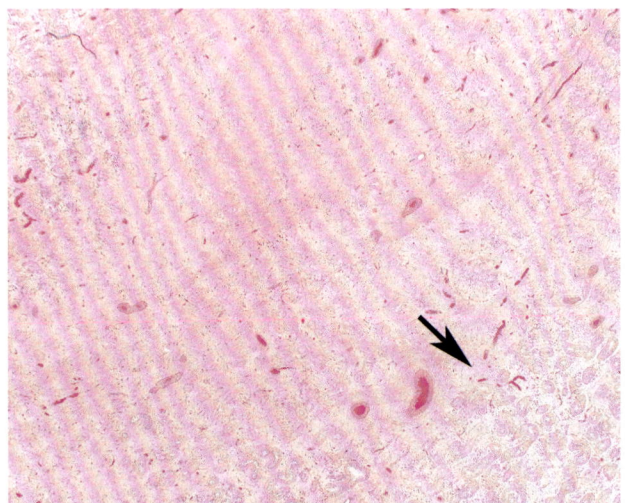

Figure 4.182. A fibrotic scar with adjacent seminiferous tubules in a patient with metastatic seminoma. The tubules (arrow) should be closely examined for the presence of germ cell neoplasia in situ (GCNIS), which is frequently identified in cases of regressed germ cell tumor and strongly supports the diagnosis.

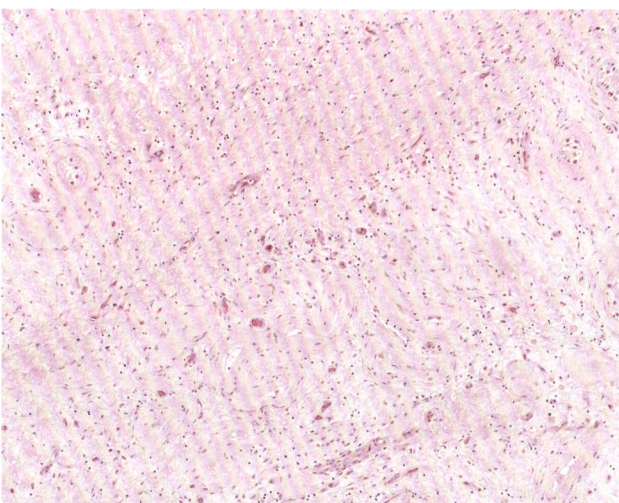

Figure 4.183. At low power, the testis shows a fibrotic scar with foci of hemosiderin deposition and rare atrophic seminiferous tubules. These findings alone are not diagnostic of regressed germ cell tumor; however, the clinical findings of metastatic seminoma with a testicular scar are strongly suggestive of the diagnosis.

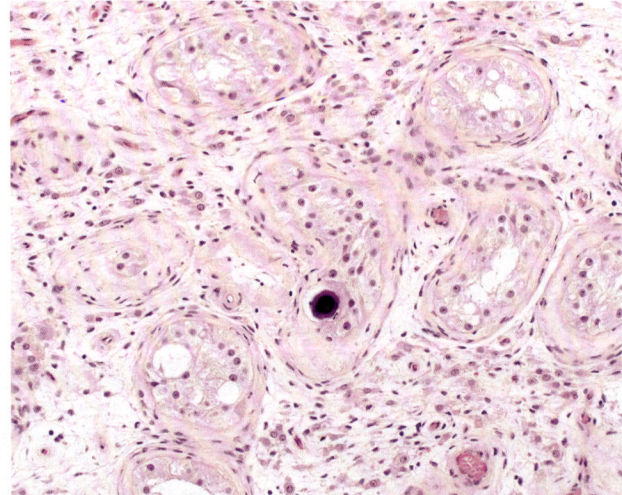

Figure 4.184. In this field, the background of Sertoli-only pattern is suggestive of a gonad with some form of dysgenesis, a soft finding for the possibility of regressed germ cell tumor. Microliths are another characteristic finding in regressed germ cell tumors.

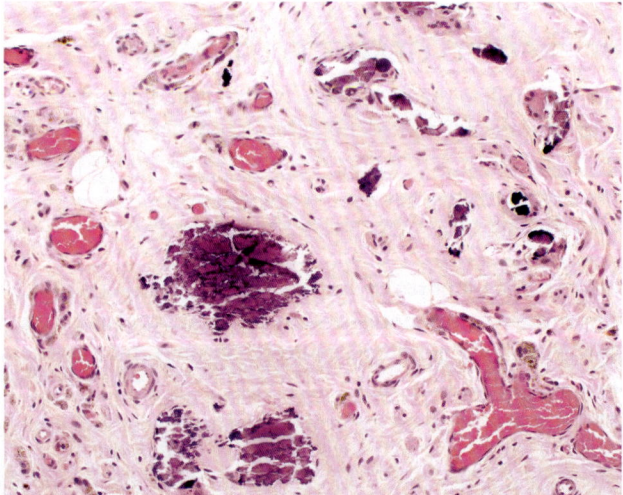

Figure 4.185. The most useful feature for the diagnosis of regressed germ cell tumor is intratubular large coarse calcifications, as pictured here. These calcifications are thought to arise from necrotic embryonal carcinoma within the tubules.

IDENTIFYING LYMPHOVASCULAR INVASION IN GERM CELL TUMOR

An orchiectomy is performed for a testicular mass in a young adult male. The tumor is a mixed GCT with components of seminoma, teratoma, and YST. On evaluation of the case, numerous sections show detached tumor cells present on the cut surfaces away from the tumor (Figure 4.186). Small collections of tumor cells are identified within rounded spaces in multiple areas, suspicious for LVI.

Diagnosis of LVI in GCTs, especially those with a seminoma component, is challenging. Seminoma cells are particularly prone to dyscohesion and artifactually dispersed onto surfaces and sometimes into vessels. One of the first things to confirm is that a rounded area with tumor is in fact a vessel; endothelial markers such as CD34, CD31, and D2-40 are useful to highlight surrounding endothelium. If the space is confirmed to be vascular, strict criteria should be applied to diagnose LVI. These include rounded cluster of tumor cells, associated fibrous clot, attachment to vessel wall, and lack of dyscohesive cells elsewhere (Figures 4.187 and 4.188). Barring definitive evidence of LVI, it is recommended that you avoid diagnosis of LVI because of the staging and prognostic implications (Figure 4.189).

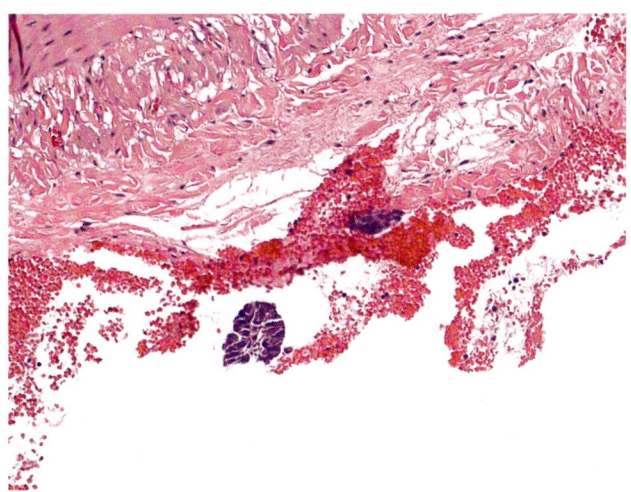

Figure 4.186. When detached clusters of tumor are seen "buttered" on the surface of multiple sections of tumor, artifactual carryover during the gross examination has occurred. In light of this finding, the diagnosis of lymphovascular invasion (LVI) should be made with caution as artifactual displacement into vessels can closely mimic LVI.

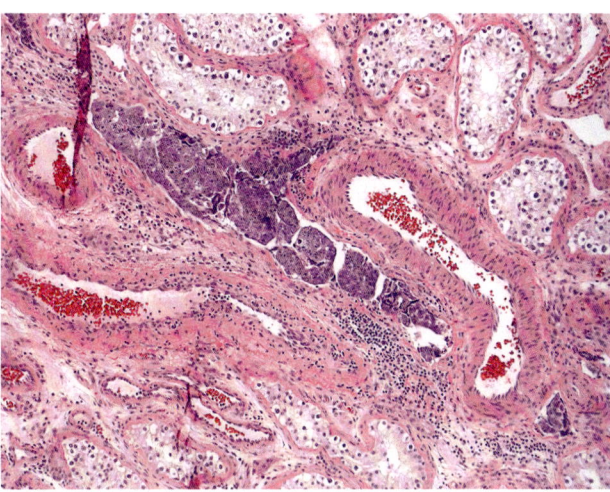

Figure 4.187. Features supporting a diagnosis of lymphovascular invasion (LVI) include rounded, cohesive clusters of tumor and attachment to the vessel wall, as seen here.

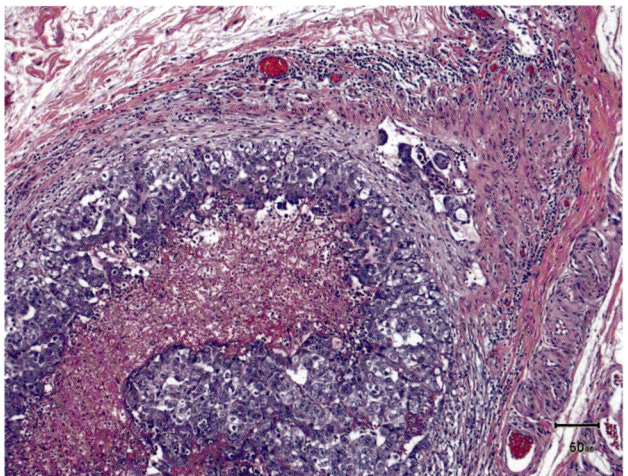

Figure 4.188. At higher power, definite attachment to the vessel wall along with extension through the vessel is diagnostic of lymphovascular invasion (LVI).

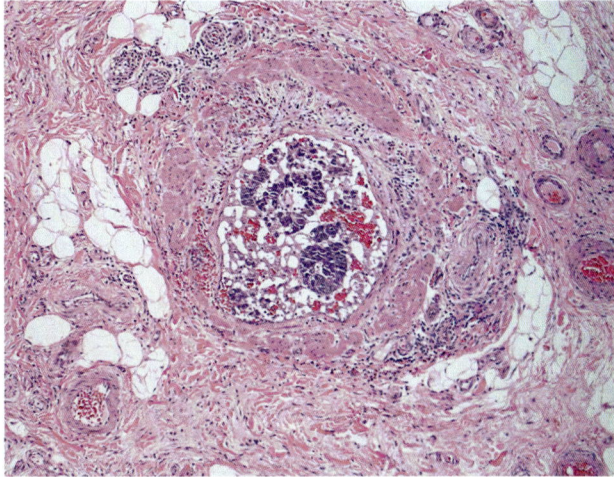

Figure 4.189. In this image, small, dyscohesive collections of tumor are present within the vessel. No definitive attachment to the wall, tumor-fibrin clot, or the rounded and smooth contours of the cells is present. This finding would be considered indefinite for lymphovascular invasion (LVI), and the tumor should not be upstaged to pT2 based on this finding in isolation.

References

1. Reuter VE, Al-ahmadie H, Tickoo SK. Urinary bladder, ureter and renal pelvis. In: Mills SE, ed. *Histology for Pathologists*. 4th ed. Philadelphia, PA: Lippincott Williams and Wilkins; 2012.

2. Virtanen HE, Bjerknes R, Cortes D, et al. Cryptorchidism: classification, prevalence and long-term consequences. *Acta Paediatr*. 2007;96(5):611-616. doi:10.1111/j.1651-2227.2007.00241.x.

3. Antic T, Hyjek EM, Taxy JB. The vanishing testis: a histomorphologic and clinical assessment. *Am J Clin Pathol*. 2011;136(6):872-880. doi:10.1309/AJCPWPSJSK58RFUI.

4. Lee PA, Houk CP, Ahmed SF, et al. Consensus statement on management of intersex disorders. *Pediatrics*. 2006;118:e488-e500. doi:10.1542/peds.2006-0738.

5. Wang Z, Yang S, Shi H, et al. Histopathological and immunophenotypic features of testicular tumour of the adrenogenital syndrome. *Histopathology*. 2011;58(7):1013-1018. doi:10.1111/j.1365-2559.2011.03861.x.

6. Preece J, Phillips S, Sorokin V, Herz D. Splenogonadal fusion in an 18-month-old. *J Pediatr Urol*. 2017;13(2):214-215. doi:10.1016/j.jpurol.2016.06.005.

7. Lund JM, Bouhadiba N, Sams V, Tsang T. Hepato-testicular fusion: an unusual case of undescended testes. *BJU Int*. 2001;88(4):439-440. doi:10.1046/j.1464-410X.2001.02359.x.

8. McDougall EM, Mikhael BR, Carpenter B. Ectopic renal tissue associated with an undescended testis: a case report. *J Urol*. 1986;135(5):1018-1019. doi:10.1016/s0022-5347(17)45965-9.

9. Cheng L, MacLennan GT, Bostwick DG. *Urologic Surgical Pathology*. 4th ed. Philadelphia, PA: Elsevier; 2019.

10. Cerilli LA, Kuang W, Rogers D. A practical approach to testicular biopsy interpretation for male infertility. *Arch Pathol Lab Med*. 2010;134(8):1197-1204. doi:10.1043/2009-0379-RA.1.

11. Salama R, Al-Obaidy KI, Perrino CM, Grignon DJ, Ulbright TM, Idrees MT. DOG1 immunohisto-chemical staining of testicular biopsies is a reliable tool for objective assessment of infertility. *Ann Diagn Pathol*. 2019;40:18-22. doi:10.1016/j.anndiagpath.2019.02.015.

12. Ulbright TM, Young RH, Robert H; Armed Forces Institute of Pathology (U.S.); American Registry of Pathology. *Tumors of the Testis and Adjacent Structures*. Silver Spring, MD: American Registry of Pathology; 2013.

13. Oliva E, Young RH. Paratesticular tumor-like lesions. *Semin Diagn Pathol*. 2000;17(4):340-358. Available at http://www.ncbi.nlm.nih.gov/pubmed/11202549. Accessed December 9, 2019.

14. Kao CS, Zhang C, Ulbright TM. Testicular hemorrhage, necrosis, and vasculopathy: likely manifestations of intermittent torsion that clinically mimic a neoplasm. *Am J Surg Pathol*. 2014;38(1):34-44. doi:10.1097/PAS.0b013e31829c0206.

15. Hernández-Rodríguez J, Tan CD, Koening CL, Khasnis A, Rodríguez ER, Hoffman GS. Testicular vasculitis: findings differentiating isolated disease from systemic disease in 72 patients. *Medicine (Baltimore)*. 2012;91(2):75-85. doi:10.1097/MD.0b013e31824156a7.

16. Bahrami A, Ro JY, Ayala AG. An overview of testicular germ cell tumors. *Arch Pathol Lab Med*. 2007;131(8):1267-1280. doi:10.1043/1543-2165(2007)131[1267:AOOTGC]2.0.CO;2.

17. Moch H, Humphrey PA, Ulbright T, Reuter VE. *WHO Classification of Tumours of the Urinary System and Male Genital Organs*. 4th ed. Lyon, France: International Agency for Research on Cancer; 2016.

18. Ulbright TM, Young RH. Seminoma with tubular, microcystic, and related patterns: a study of 28 cases of unusual morphologic variants that often cause confusion with yolk sac tumor. *Am J Surg Pathol*. 2005;29(4):500-505. doi:10.1097/01.pas.0000155146.60670.3f.

19. Henley JD, Young RH, Wade CL, Ulbright TM. Seminomas with exclusive intertubular growth: a report of 12 clinically and grossly inconspicuous tumors. *Am J Surg Pathol*. 2004;28(9):1163-1168. doi:10.1097/01.pas.0000132742.12221.82.

20. Al-Abbadi MA, Hattab EM, Tarawneh M, Orazi A, Ulbright TM. Primary testicular and paratesticular lymphoma: a retrospective clinicopathologic study of 34 cases with emphasis on differential diagnosis. *Arch Pathol Lab Med*. 2007;131(7):1040-1046. doi:10.1043/1543-2165(2007)131[1040:PTAPLA]2.0.CO;2.

21. Williams AS, Shawwa A, Merrimen J, Haché KD. Expression of OCT4 and SALL4 in diffuse large B-cell lymphoma. *Am J Surg Pathol*. 2016;40(7):950-957. doi:10.1097/PAS.0000000000000648.

22. Henley JD, Young RH, Ulbright TM. Malignant Sertoli cell tumors of the testis: a study of 13 examples of a neoplasm frequently misinterpreted as seminoma. *Am J Surg Pathol*. 2002;26(5):541-550. doi:10.1097/00000478-200205000-00001.

23. Carney JA. The Carney complex (myxomas, spotty pigmentation, endocrine overactivity, and schwannomas). *Dermatol Clin*. 1995;13(1):19-26.

24. Al-Agha OM, Axiotis CA. An in-depth look at leydig cell tumor of the testis. *Arch Pathol Lab Med.* 2007;131(2):311-317. doi:10.1043/1543-2165(2007)131[311:AILALC]2.0.CO;2.

25. Cheville JC, Sebo TJ, Lager DJ, Bostwick DG, Farrow GM. Leydig cell tumor of the testis: a clinicopathologic, DNA content, and MIB-1 comparison of nonmetastasizing and metastasizing tumors. *Am J Surg Pathol.* 1998;22(11):1361-1367. doi:10.1097/00000478-199811000-00006.

26. Kim I, Young RH, Scully RE. Leydig cell tumors of the testis. A clinicopathological analysis of 40 cases and review of the literature. *Am J Surg Pathol.* 1985;9(3):177-192. doi:10.1097/00000478-198503000-00002.

27. Wang WP, Guo C, Berney DM, et al. Primary carcinoid tumors of the testis: a clinicopathologic study of 29 cases. *Am J Surg Pathol.* 2010;34(4):519-524. doi:10.1097/PAS.0b013e3181d31f33.

28. Nocks BN, Dann JA. Primitive neuroectodermal tumor (immature teratoma) of testis. *Urology.* 1983;22(5):543-544. doi:10.1016/0090-4295(83)90239-x.

29. Aguirre P, Scully RE. Primitive neuroectodermal tumor of the testis. Report of a case. *Arch Pathol Lab Med.* 1983;107(12):643-645. Available at http://www.ncbi.nlm.nih.gov/pubmed/6314925. Accessed January 22, 2020.

30. Kao CS, Bangs CD, Aldrete G, Cherry AM, Ulbright TM. A clinicopathologic and molecular analysis of 34 mediastinal germ cell tumors suggesting different modes of teratoma development. *Am J Surg Pathol.* 2018;42(12):1662-1673. doi:10.1097/PAS.0000000000001164.

31. Kao CS, Ulbright TM, Young RH, Idrees MT. Testicular embryonal carcinoma: a morphologic study of 180 cases highlighting unusual and unemphasized aspects. *Am J Surg Pathol.* 2014;38(5):689-697. doi:10.1097/PAS.0000000000000171.

32. Michael H, Lucia J, Foster RS, Ulbright TM. The pathology of late recurrence of testicular germ cell tumors. *Am J Surg Pathol.* 2000;24(2):257-273. doi:10.1097/00000478-200002000-00012.

33. Howitt BE, Magers MJ, Rice KR, Cole CD, Ulbright TM. Many postchemotherapy sarcomatous tumors in patients with testicular germ cell tumors are sarcomatoid yolk sac tumors: a study of 33 cases. *Am J Surg Pathol.* 2015;39:251-259. doi:10.1097/PAS.0000000000000322.

34. Ulbright TM, Gersell DJ. Rete testis hyperplasia with hyaline globule formation: a lesion simulating yolk sac tumor. *Am J Surg Pathol.* 1991;15(1):66-74. doi:10.1097/00000478-199101000-00008.

35. Zynger DL, McCallum JC, Luan C, Chou PM, Yang XJ. Glypican 3 has a higher sensitivity than alpha-fetoprotein for testicular and ovarian yolk sac tumour: immunohistochemical investigation with analysis of histological growth patterns. *Histopathology.* 2010;56(6):750-757. doi:10.1111/j.1365-2559.2010.03553.x.

36. Osman H, Cheng L, Ulbright TM, Idrees MT. The utility of CDX2, GATA3, and DOG1 in the diagnosis of testicular neoplasms: an immunohistochemical study of 109 cases. *Hum Pathol.* 2016;48:18-24. doi:10.1016/j.humpath.2015.09.028.

37. Ulbright TM. Germ cell tumors of the gonads: a selective review emphasizing problems in differential diagnosis, newly appreciated, and controversial issues. *Mod Pathol.* 2005;18:S61-S79. doi:10.1038/modpathol.3800310.

38. Banet N, Gown AM, Shih IM, et al. GATA-3 expression in trophoblastic tissues: an immunohistochemical study of 445 cases, including diagnostic utility. *Am J Surg Pathol.* 2015;39(1):101-108. doi:10.1097/PAS.0000000000000315.

39. Zynger DL, Dimov ND, Luan C, Tean Teh B, Yang XJ. Glypican 3: a novel marker in testicular germ cell tumors. *Am J Surg Pathol.* 2006;30(12):1570-1575. doi:10.1097/01.pas.0000213322.89670.48.

40. True LD, Otis CN, Delprado W, Scully RE, Rosai J. Spermatocytic seminoma of testis with sarcomatous transformation. A report of five cases. *Am J Surg Pathol.* 1988;12(2):75-82. doi:10.1097/00000478-198802000-00001.

41. Cummings OW, Ulbright TM, Eble JN, Roth LM. Spermatocytic seminoma: an immunohistochemical study. *Hum Pathol.* 1994;25(1):54-59. doi:10.1016/0046-8177(94)90171-6.

42. Ulbright TM. Recently described and clinically important entities in testis tumors: a selective review of changes incorporated into the 2016 classification of the world health organization. *Arch Pathol Lab Med.* 2019;143(6):711-721. doi:10.5858/arpa.2017-0478-RA.

43. Looijenga LHJ, Kao CS, Idrees MT. Predicting gonadal germ cell cancer in people with disorders of sex development; insights from developmental biology. *Int J Mol Sci.* 2019;20(20):5017. doi:10.3390/ijms20205017.

44. Umar SA, MacLennan GT. Epidermoid cyst of the testis. *J Urol.* 2008;180(1):335. doi:10.1016/j.juro.2008.03.170.

45. Ulbright TM, Srigley JR. Dermoid cyst of the testis: a study of five postpubertal cases, including a pilomatrixoma-like variant, with evidence supporting its separate classification from mature testicular teratoma. *Am J Surg Pathol*. 2001;25(6):788-793. doi:10.1097/00000478-200106000-00011.

46. Zhang C, Berney DM, Hirsch MS, Cheng L, Ulbright TM. Evidence supporting the existence of benign teratomas of the postpubertal testis: a clinical, histopathologic, and molecular genetic analysis of 25 cases. *Am J Surg Pathol*. 2013;37(6):827-835. doi:10.1097/PAS.0b013e31827dcc4c.

47. Kernek KM, Ulbright TM, Zhang S, et al. Identical allelic losses in mature teratoma and other histologic components of malignant mixed germ cell tumors of the testis. *Am J Pathol*. 2003;163(6):2477-2484. doi:10.1016/S0002-9440(10)63602-4.

48. Magers MJ, Kao CS, Cole CD, et al. "Somatic-type" malignancies arising from testicular germ cell tumors: a clinicopathologic study of 124 cases with emphasis on glandular tumors supporting frequent yolk sac tumor origin. *Am J Surg Pathol*. 2014;38(10):1396-1409. doi:10.1097/PAS.0000000000000262.

49. Balzer BL, Ulbright TM. Spontaneous regression of testicular germ cell tumors: an analysis of 42 cases. *Am J Surg Pathol*. 2006;30(7):858-865. doi:10.1097/01.pas.0000209831.24230.56.

50. Milose JC, Filson CP, Weizer AZ, Hafez KS, Montgomery JS. Role of biochemical markers in testicular cancer: diagnosis, staging, and surveillance. *Open Access J Urol*. 2011;4(1):1-8. doi:10.2147/OAJU.S15063.

51. Cao D, Li J, Guo CC, Allan RW, Humphrey PA. SALL4 is a novel diagnostic marker for testicular germ cell tumors. *Am J Surg Pathol*. 2009;33(7):1065-1077. doi:10.1097/PAS.0b013e3181a13eef.

52. Cheng L, Sung MT, Cossu-Rocca P, et al. OCT4: biological functions and clinical applications marker of germ cell neoplasia. *J Pathol*. 2007;211(1):1-9. doi:10.1002/path.2105.

53. Manivel JC, Jessurun J, Wick MR, Dehner LP. Placental alkaline phosphatase immunoreactivity in testicular germ-cell neoplasms. *Am J Surg Pathol*. 1987;11(1):21-29. doi:10.1097/00000478-198701000-00003.

54. Sangoi AR, McKenney JK, Brooks JD, Higgins JP. Evaluation of SF-1 expression in testicular germ cell tumors: a tissue microarray study of 127 cases. *Appl Immunohistochem Mol Morphol*. 2013;21(4):318-321. doi:10.1097/PAI.0b013e318277cf5a.

55. Ulbright TM, Tickoo SK, Berney DM, et al. Best practices recommendations in the application of immunohistochemistry in testicular tumors: report from the International Society of Urological Pathology Consensus Conference. *Am J Surg Pathol*. 2014;38(8):e50-e59. doi:10.1097/PAS.0000000000000233.

56. Idrees M, Saxena R, Cheng L, Ulbright TM, Badve S. Podoplanin, a novel marker for seminoma: a comparison study evaluating immunohistochemical expression of podoplanin and OCT3/4. *Ann Diagn Pathol*. 2010;14(5):331-336. doi:10.1016/j.anndiagpath.2010.05.008.

57. Berney DM, Shamash J, Pieroni K, Oliver RTD. Loss of CD30 expression in metastatic embryonal carcinoma: the effects of chemotherapy? *Histopathology*. 2001;39(4):382-385. doi:10.1046/j.1365-2559.2001.01226.x.

58. Verrill C, Perry-keene J, Srigley JR, et al. Intraoperative consultation and macroscopic handling: the International Society of Urological Pathology (ISUP) testicular cancer consultation conference recommendations. *Am J Surg Pathol*. 2018;42(6):e33-e43. doi:10.1097/PAS.0000000000001049.

59. Verrill C, Yilmaz A, Srigley JR, et al. Reporting and staging of testicular germ cell tumors: the International Society of Urological Pathology (ISUP) testicular cancer consultation conference recommendations. *Am J Surg Pathol*. 2017;41(6):e22-e32. doi:10.1097/PAS.0000000000000844.

60. of American Pathologists C. *Protocol for the Examination of Specimens From Patients With Malignant Germ Cell and Sex Cord-Stromal Tumors of the Testis*.; 2017. Available at www.cap.org/cancerprotocols. Accessed February 10, 2020.

61. Yilmaz A, Cheng T, Zhang J, Trpkov K. Testicular hilum and vascular invasion predict advanced clinical stage in nonseminomatous germ cell tumors. *Mod Pathol*. 2013;26(4):579-586. doi:10.1038/modpathol.2012.189.

62. Ulbright TM, Young RH. Metastatic carcinoma to the testis: a clinicopathologic analysis of 26 nonincidental cases with emphasis on deceptive features. *Am J Surg Pathol*. 2008;32(11):1683-1693. doi:10.1097/PAS.0b013e3181788516.

63. Lehmann D, Muller H. Analysis of the autoimmune response in an "in situ" carcinoma of the testis. *Int J Androl*. 1987;10(1):163-168. doi:10.1111/j.1365-2605.1987.tb00178.x.

CHAPTER OUTLINE

PARATESTIS

THE UNREMARKABLE PARATESTIS

The paratestis and external genitalia include a number of anatomic locations and entities that are seen by genitourinary pathologists, but also encompass a number of lesions that cross over into dermatopathology and soft tissue pathology. As such, this chapter will provide a relatively broad overview of these topics to ensure the reader's familiarity with the various entities. Specific references and specialized texts are referenced for in-depth reading on the more esoteric topics.

The "paratestis" or "paratesticular adnexa" are general terms that encompass the testicular tunics, efferent ductules, epididymis, rete testis, spermatic cord, and vas deferens. It covers essentially all of the structures outside of the testicular parenchyma, but within the scrotal skin. The tunica vaginalis arises from the parietal peritoneum and lined by mesothelium, which serves as the origin of mesothelial neoplasms in this area. The tunica albuginea is a dense connective tissue lining that may give rise to fibrous proliferations. The rete testis and epididymis arise as the spermatic tubules converge and exit the testicular parenchyma (Figures 5.1-5.3). The efferent ductules are lined by tall columnar cells. These ductules terminate in the vas deferens, which is located within the spermatic cord (Figures 5.4-5.6). Along with the vas deferens, the spermatic cord contains the testicular artery, pampiniform vascular plexus, nerves, and lymphatics.

"CELES" AND CYSTIC LESIONS

This category of paratesticular lesions are related in that they often present with scrotal swelling or a paratesticular mass that is painless. They vary in what anatomic location they arise from, and as a result, their histology is related to the normal lining of those anatomic locations. These are very common specimens seen in both specialty and general surgical pathology practices. Although they do not often present a diagnostic dilemma, a few possible pitfalls and unusual findings are noted here.

Hydrocele

When serous fluid accumulates between the visceral and parietal layers of the tunica albuginea, a hydrocele develops. These cystic lesions are associated with a history of trauma and obstruction. Hydroceles are lined by mesothelium, though they may become denuded over time (Figures 5.7 and 5.8). In chronic hydrocele, the lining may become thickened and fibrotic with chronic inflammation and mesothelial hyperplasia (Figure 5.9). There is a low, but measurable risk of development of malignant mesothelioma in long-standing hydroceles, and any thickened or papillary areas of a hydrocele should be sampled extensively.

PEARLS AND PITFALLS: Mesothelial Hyperplasia

- Mesothelial hyperplasia is frequently encountered in hydrocele specimens
- More common in long-standing hydroceles, may be traumatized or inflamed
- In hyperplasia, the mesothelial clusters are confined to the superficial fibrous tissue and respect an imaginary line without deep infiltration (Figure 5.10)
- Mesothelial cells are present in small clusters or nests, but do not form an obvious mass lesion (Figures 5.11 and 5.12)

Spermatocele

Spermatoceles occur when efferent ductules of the head of epididymis become dilated, often due to obstruction. These lesions can reach large sizes and are more commonly identified on the right side. Histologically, they comprise a dilated cystic lesion with a fibromuscular wall lined by cuboidal to pseudostratified epithelium, which may demonstrate cilia (Figures 5.13-5.15). The key diagnostic feature of spermatoceles is the identification of sperm within the cyst lumen; however, the sperm are commonly absent in opened specimens (Figure 5.16).

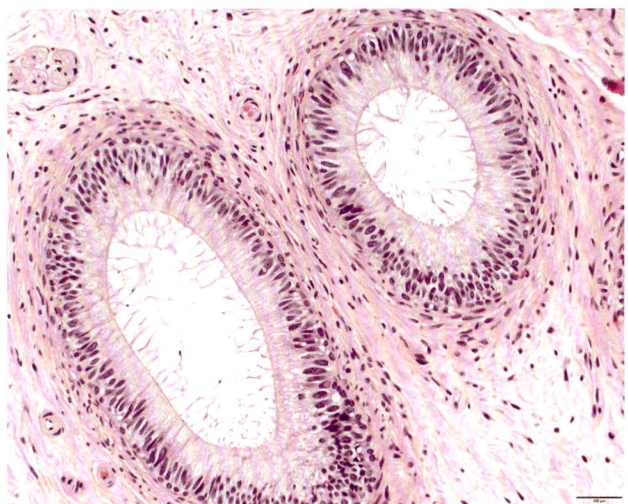

Figure 5.1. The normal epididymis demonstrates multiple cross-sectional profiles of convoluted ductules lined by columnar epithelium.

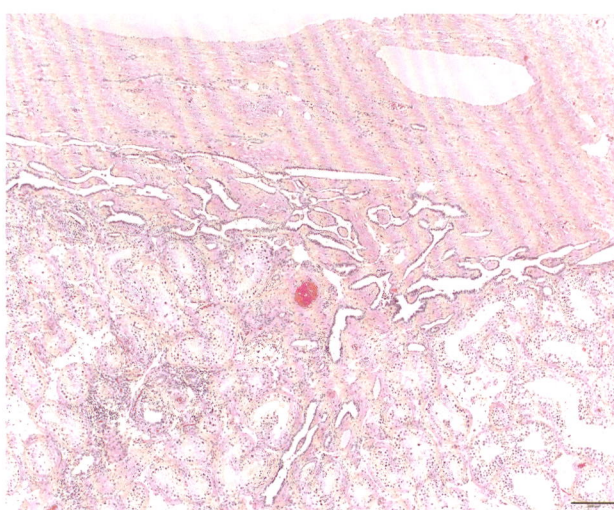

Figure 5.2. The rete testis is formed by the confluence of the spermatic tubules into large, slit-like ducts that exit through the tunica vaginalis and enter the epididymis.

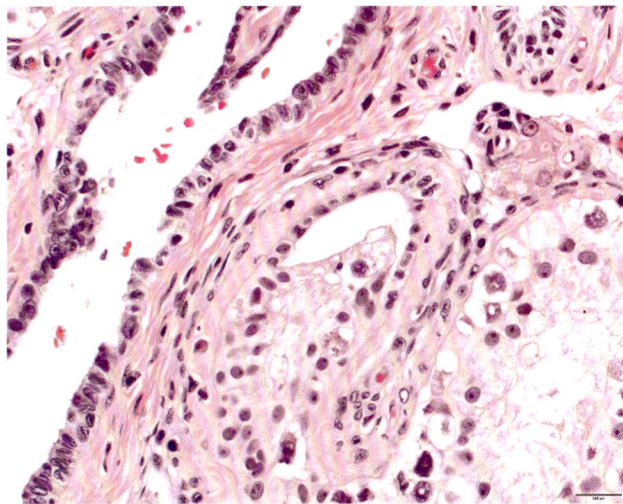

Figure 5.3. At high power, the transition from spermatic tubules with germ cells into the rete testis is demonstrated in the middle ductule profile.

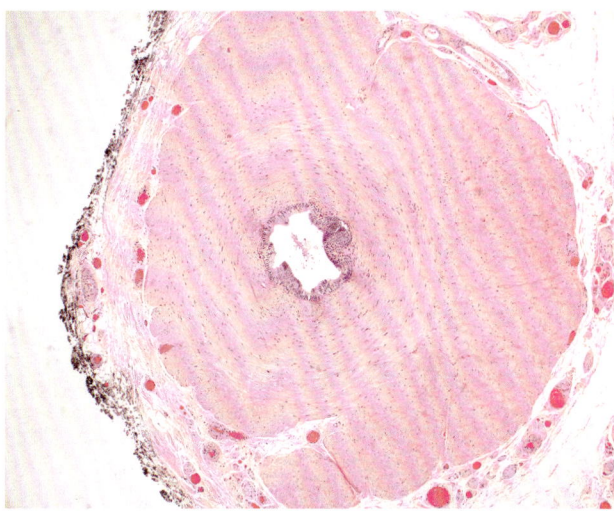

Figure 5.4. The vas deferens is a thick muscular tube that is located within the spermatic cord, connecting the tail of the epididymis to the ejaculatory ducts.

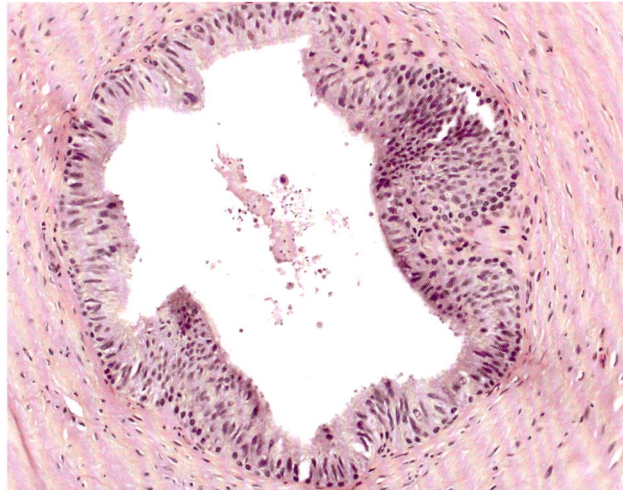

Figure 5.5. The epithelium of the vas deferens demonstrates an undulating appearance protruding into the lumen.

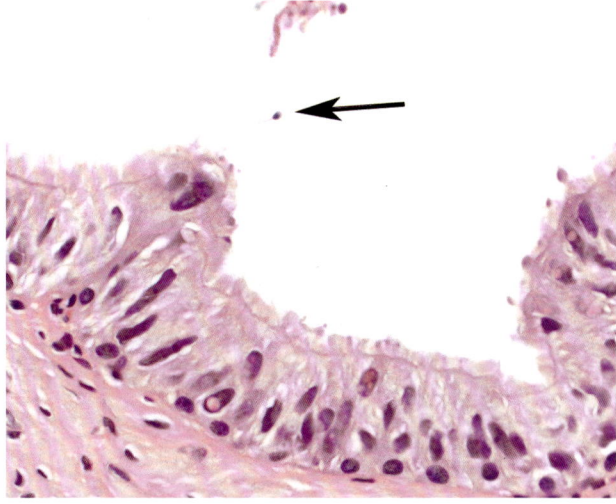

Figure 5.6. The cytologic features of vas deferens include pseudostratified columnar cells with cilia. A single spermatozoon is present in the lumen (arrow).

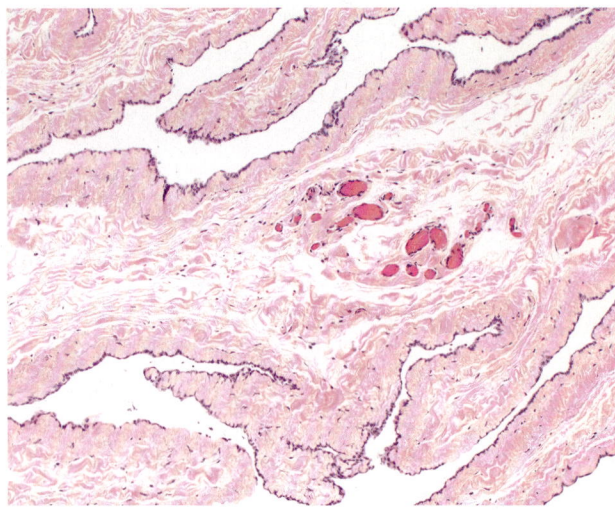

Figure 5.7. Hydroceles are collections of fluid within the tunica vaginalis. Surgical resection results in a collapsed cystic wall lined by mesothelium.

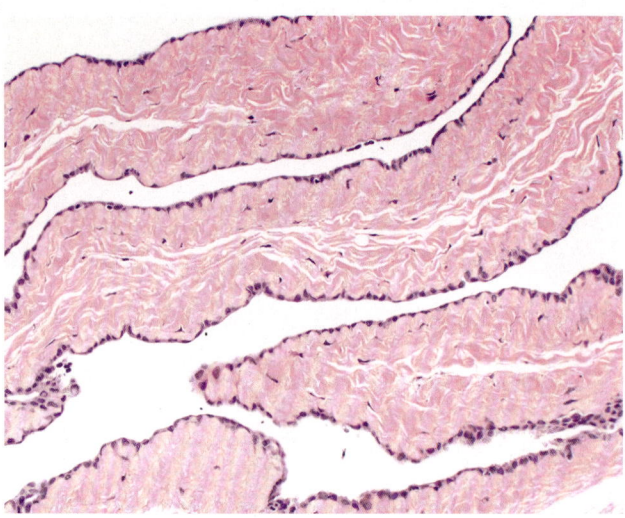

Figure 5.8. At higher power, a hydrocele specimen demonstrates a single layer of flattened to cuboidal mesothelial cells. The underlying fibrous tissue shows a corrugated appearance and can be a useful feature in a denuded specimen.

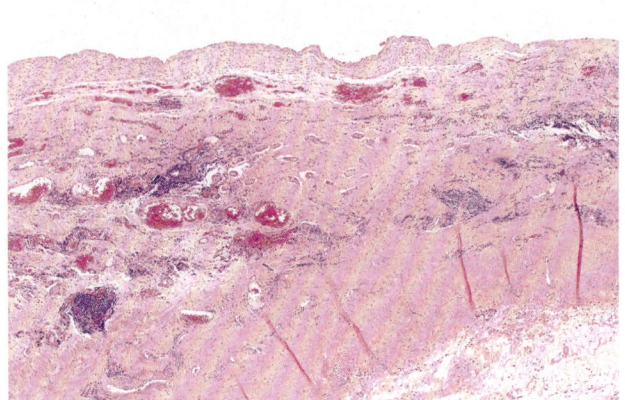

Figure 5.9. Mesothelial hyperplasia is a common occurrence in long-standing hydrocele specimens. Thickened and chronically inflamed fibrous tissue is evident at low power, with small nests of entrapped mesothelial cells present.

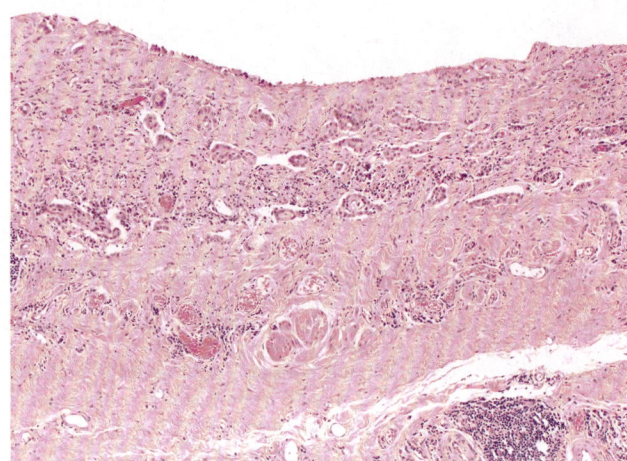

Figure 5.10. Features of mesothelial hyperplasia used to distinguish it from malignant mesothelioma include scattered nests of mesothelial cells, rather than a mass-forming lesion.

SAMPLE NOTE: Spermatocele

- Spermatocele, left, excision: Bland epithelial lined cyst, consistent with the clinical impression of a spermatocele. No evidence of malignancy.

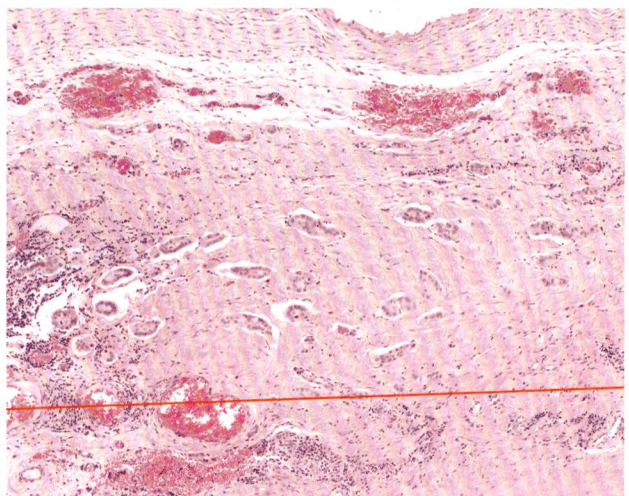

Figure 5.11. In this image, a red line demarcates the limit of the mesothelial nests. Irregular infiltration beyond a line parallel with the surface should raise suspicion for a malignant process. Involvement of adipose tissue is not consistent with mesothelial hyperplasia.

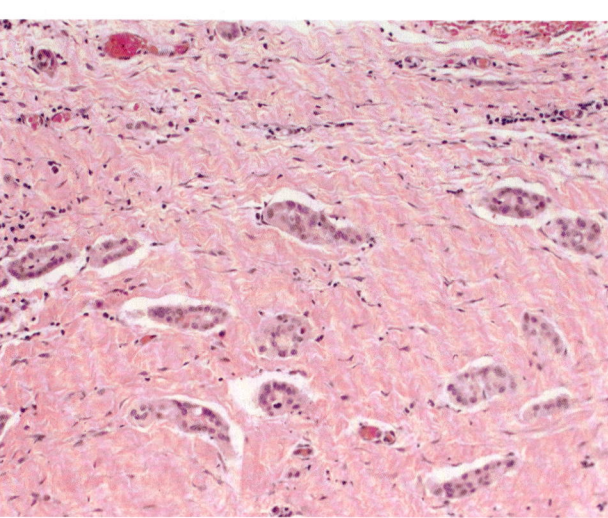

Figure 5.12. Cytologically bland mesothelial nests without atypical features are consistent with a diagnosis of mesothelial hyperplasia.

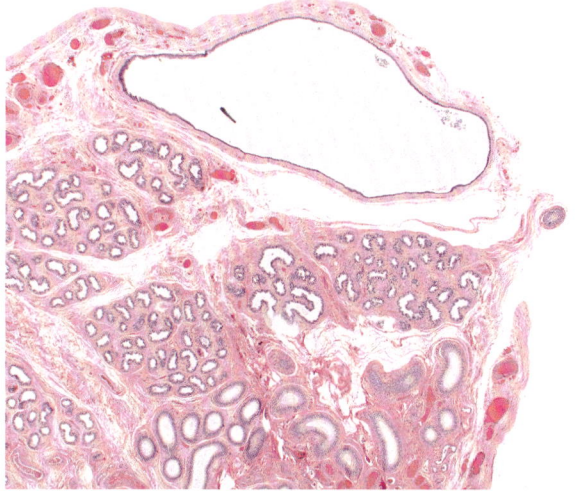

Figure 5.13. Spermatoceles arise from dilated epididymal or rete ducts. Here, a spermatocele is seen centered in the epididymis.

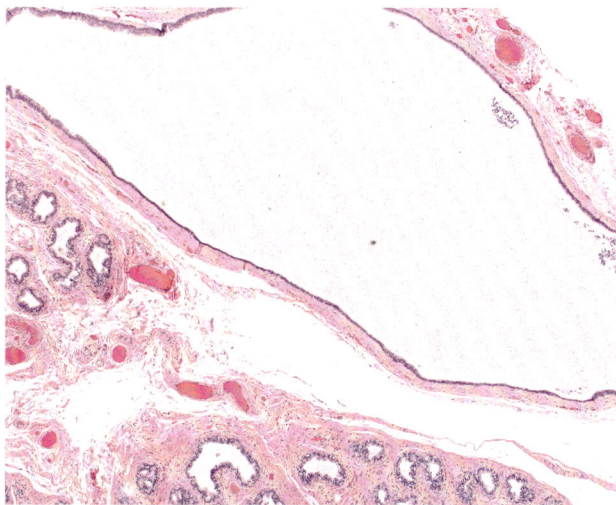

Figure 5.14. Spermatoceles are usually unilocular, although they may be multilocular. The classic feature of a spermatocele is the presence of spermatozoa, a finding rarely encountered in excised specimens due to their being opened.

PEARLS AND PITFALLS: Small Blue Cells in Spermatocele and Hydrocele Specimens

- An uncommon finding of detached clusters of cohesive cells in a hydrocele specimen
- Cellular clusters show high nuclear to cytoplasmic ratio, smooth to smudgy chromatin, and suggestion of nuclear molding, raising the possibility of a high-grade neuroendocrine tumor (small cell carcinoma) (Figures 5.17 and 5.18)
- The immunoprofile of these cells shows diffuse staining for CD56, also suggestive of a small cell carcinoma (Figure 5.19 and 5.20)
- However, the cells are negative for synaptophysin and chromogranin and demonstrate a low Ki-67
- These small blue cells are felt to represent shed rete testis cells with degenerative changes that have exfoliated into the hydrocele specimen and are benign![1]

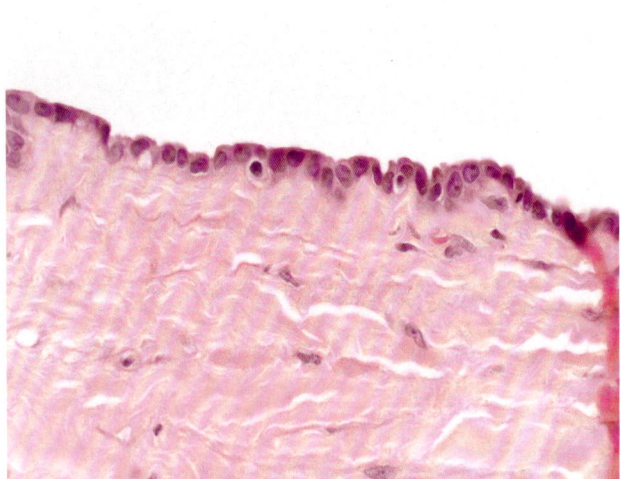

Figure 5.15. The epithelial lining of a spermatocele is low cuboidal to flat, and cilia may be present.

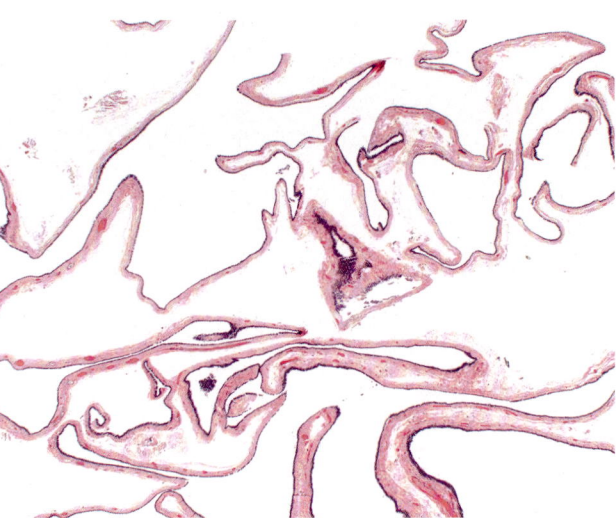

Figure 5.16. An example of a large spermatocele that collapsed into folds once excised. The location and clinical impression during the excisional procedure are often useful to confirming the diagnosis of spermatocele.

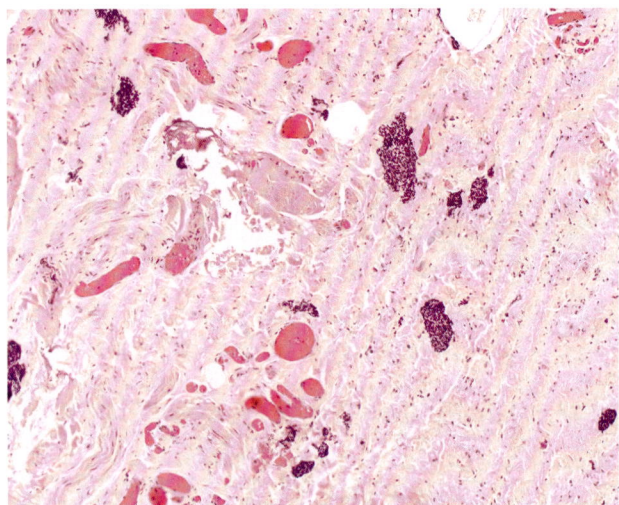

Figure 5.17. The rare finding of clusters of detached small blue cells in a hydrocele specimen may result in confusion as to the origin of the cells. The small blue cells are thought to represent benign sloughed rete testis epithelial cells with degenerative-type changes.

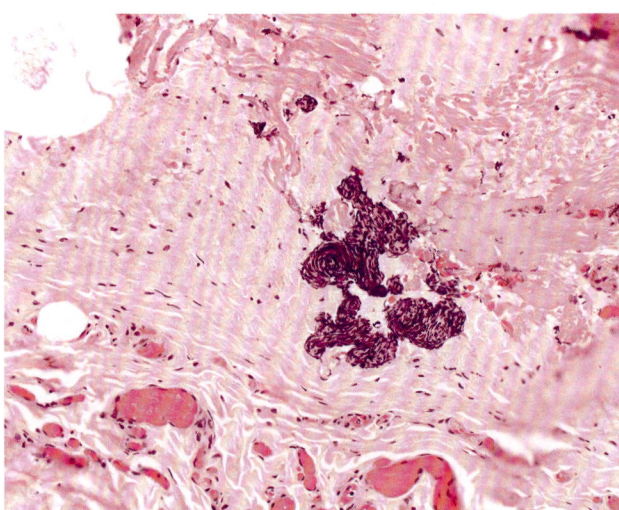

Figure 5.18. Same case as Figure 5.17 at higher power, the clusters demonstrate tightly cohesive groups of cells of high nuclear to cytoplasmic ratio, with smudgy dark chromatin. The morphology is similar to that of small cell carcinoma; however, these cells are benign.

Varicocele

Dilation of the venous pampiniform plexus and internal testicular veins due to incompetent valves, or obstruction from tumor, leads to the formation of a varicocele. Physical examination of the mass reveals a tortuous tangle of vessels, the "bag of worms." The mass may enlarge with the Valsalva maneuver. Unlike spermatoceles, varicoceles are more commonly identified on the left side that has more valves, due to the drainage of the right internal spermatic vein directly into the inferior vena cava. These vascular lesions are located above the testis and may be large enough to extend through the inguinal ring. The vessels in a varicocele show numerous thickened veins with hypertrophic smooth muscle (Figure 5.21). These lesions are not frequently submitted for pathologic evaluation in our experience, as they are routinely treated by vessel ligation.

Other Cystic Lesions

Numerous benign cystic lesions occur in the paratesticular region, all of which are benign. Some "cysts" are actually dilations of normal structures, like a cystic change of the rete testis. Determining the precise origin of a cyst or cystic process is dependent largely on the presence and type of epithelial lining of the cyst wall.

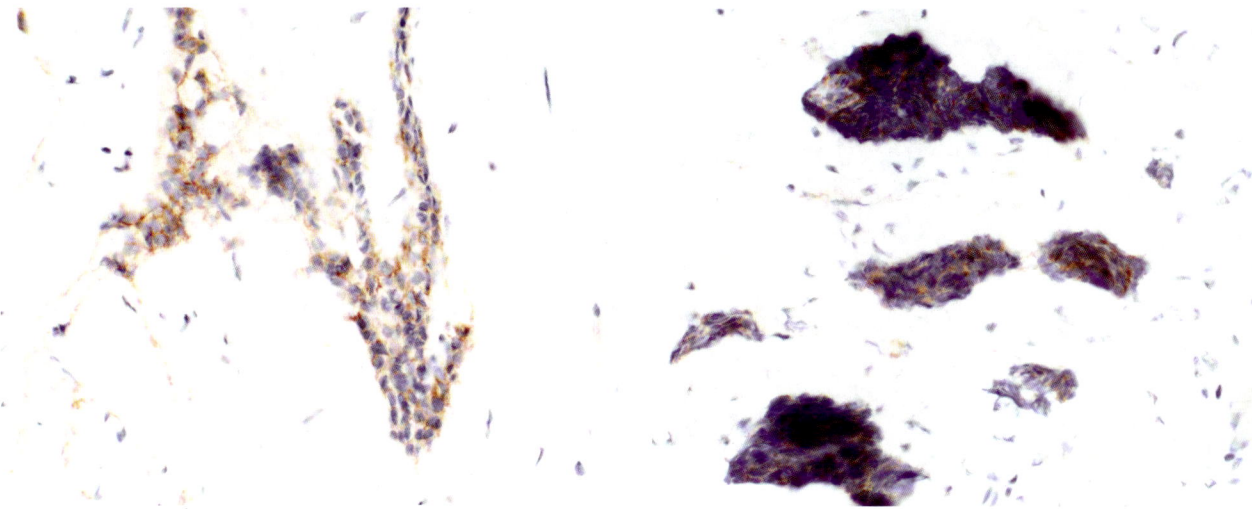

Figure 5.19. Confusing the issue is the finding that the shed rete testis cells express CD56 as demonstrated in this cluster.

Figure 5.20. Another image showing clusters of shed rete testis cells with expression of CD56. Unlike a small cell carcinoma, these cells are negative for synaptophysin and chromogranin.

Cystic changes in the rete testis have various etiologies (Figure 5.22). *Cystic dysplasia of the rete testis* occurs in children and is associated with renal malformations. There are multiple cysts lined by rete testis epithelium, which may be flattened. *Acquired cystic transformation of the rete testis* is a similar lesion, associated with renal dialysis. The cysts are lined by rete testis epithelium that is columnar to pseudostratified, and the luminal spaces contain proteinaceous fluid, spermatozoa, and calcium oxalate crystals.

Other cysts of the paratesticular region include tunica albuginea cysts, isolated rete cysts, cystic Walthard nests, epididymal cysts, multilocular cysts of paradidymal origin, and mesothelial cysts. As with rete testis cystic lesions, these entities are all defined by their anatomic location and lining cells.

FAQ: What Are the Common Mesothelial Proliferations Identified in Nontumor Specimens?

- Numerous common specimens contain mesothelial lining—hydroceles, hernia sacs
- Mesothelium may become irritated and reactive in chronic setting or incarceration
- Florid mesothelial proliferations are a reactive process marked by a linear row of mesothelial lined tubules that do not infiltrate fat
- Benign proliferations are cytologically bland without mitotic figures, often in association with chronic inflammation
- Well-differentiated papillary mesotheliomas are exophytic, bland papillary proliferations of mesothelial cells without invasion
- Malignant mesothelial proliferations are rarely detected incidentally; however, they show more complex tubular structures with architectural crowding, complex papillary formations, and infiltration of fat

---

GLANDULAR LESIONS

Vasitis Nodosa

Vasitis nodosa is a reactive proliferation of ductular cells arising from the damaged vas deferens, usually following vasectomy procedure. The condition may also arise after damage leading to obstruction or transection from a hernia repair or trauma. Small reactive ducts proliferate, and the epithelial lining may demonstrate mild reactive atypia with nucleoli (Figures 5.23 and 5.24). The reactive ducts can extend far beyond the intact vas lumen with surrounding smooth muscle proliferation resulting in a mass mimicking adenocarcinoma.

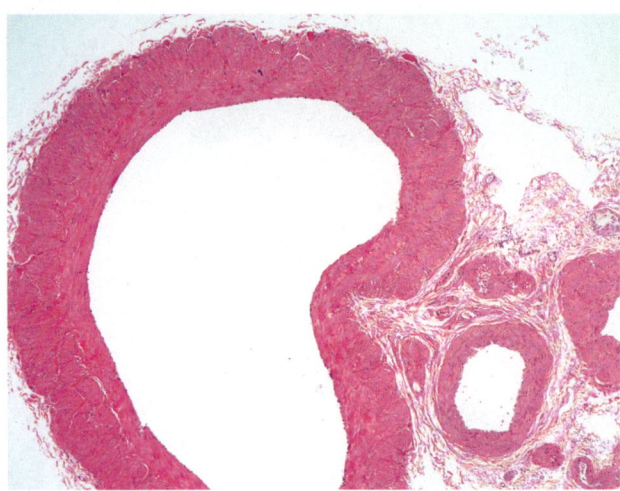

Figure 5.21. Varicoceles are collections of tortuous and dilated veins in the spermatic cord, leading to the clinical impression of a "bag of worms." Vessels are dilated and thickened with hypertrophic smooth muscle.

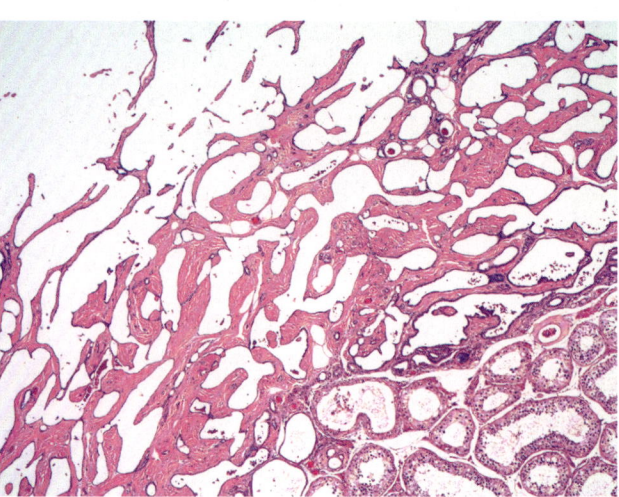

Figure 5.22. Cystic dilation of the rete testis is demonstrated in this image by increased diameter of the rete ducts. It is associated with hemodialysis, obstruction of epididymis, and ischemia.

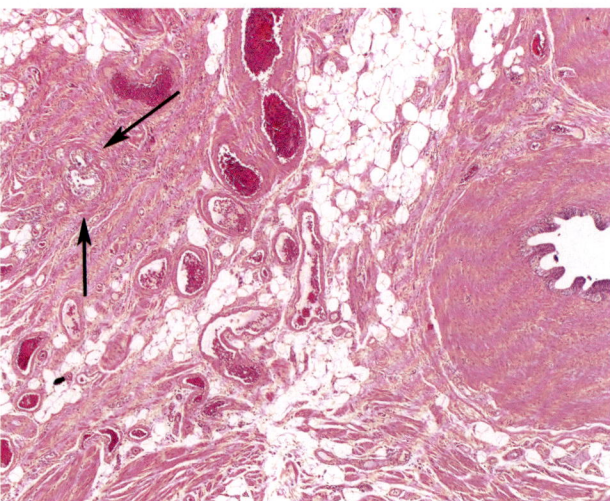

Figure 5.23. At low power, vasitis nodosa demonstrates infiltrating tubules (arrows) that may occur far beyond the muscular wall of the vas deferens. The infiltrating growth pattern can mimic adenocarcinoma.

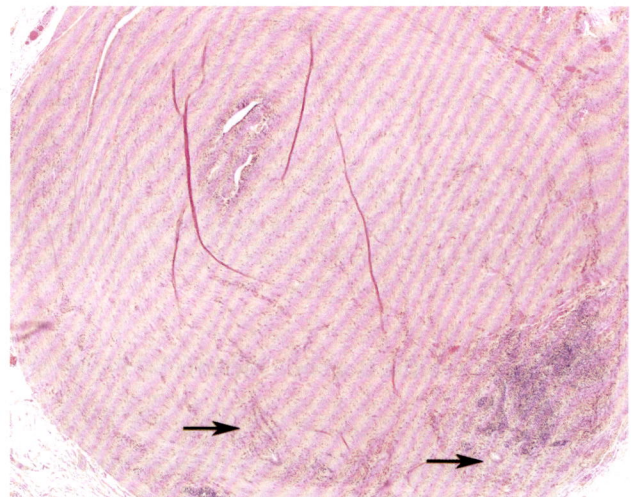

Figure 5.24. Small tubules (arrows) located away from the vas lumen and within the muscular wall are consistent with vasitis nodosa. Despite the apparent separation of the tubules from the lumen, vasitis nodosa is thought to be in continuity with the lumen.

The infiltrative growth pattern is suggestive of a malignant process; however, the cytologic features are very bland and similar to the vas epithelium (Figure 5.25). The proliferative ducts often contain sperm, demonstrating a continuity with the intact vas (Figures 5.26 and 5.27). Compounding this pitfall is that the ducts may intimately involve nerves and vessels.[2] Usually the diagnosis is straightforward due to the location and clinical scenario (post vasectomy); however, when the differential diagnosis includes urothelial or prostatic carcinoma, immunohistochemistry may be helpful. The proliferative glands diffusely express PAX8 and patchy GATA3, but are negative for PSA and NKX3.1.[3]

PEARLS AND PITFALLS: Vasitis Nodosa Involving the Prostate

- Vasitis nodosa may occur in the ampulla of the prostate
- At low power, the bland simple glands can mimic invasive prostatic carcinoma
- Immunohistochemistry can be useful in this setting, as the vasitis nodosa glands are negative for PSA and NKX3.1 and express PAX8

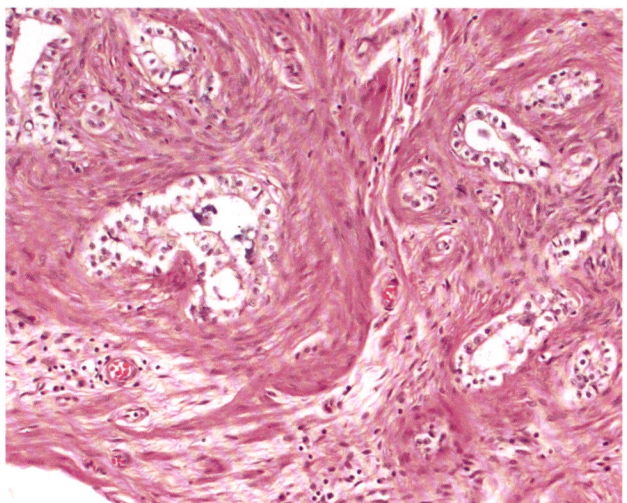

Figure 5.25. The cytologic features of vasitis nodosa include bland, columnar to cuboidal cells ample clear cytoplasm. Nuclei are small, lack significant pleomorphism, and are not mitotically active.

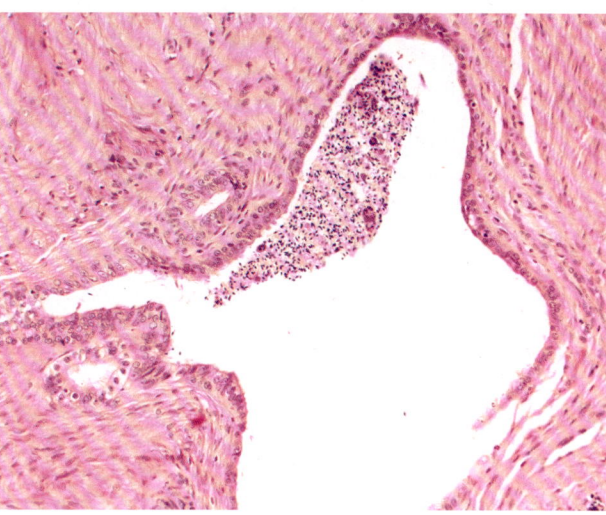

Figure 5.26. A helpful feature in the diagnosis of vasitis nodosa is the presence of sperm within the tubules. This phenomenon occurs due to the continuity of the tubules with the vas lumen.

Adenomatoid Tumor

Adenomatoid tumor is a benign mesothelial neoplasm involving the paratesticular region that can mimic adenocarcinoma. These tumors are common, usually identified in men in the fourth to sixth decade of life. They should be truly paratesticular in location, although rarely an adenomatoid tumor can involve the testicular parenchyma. The tumors are usually small and well circumscribed, with a firm, white to gray cut surface. The classic architectural pattern of these tumors demonstrates gland-like structures with flattened mesothelial lining (Figure 5.28). The identification of thread-like strands that bridge across the lumen is a helpful feature.[4] Because of the numerous patterns (see Pearls and Pitfalls below) and the possibility of testicular involvement, the differential diagnosis of adenomatoid tumor is broad. Depending on the pattern, consideration of germ cell tumors (yolk sac tumor in particular), sex cord-stromal tumors, adenocarcinoma, and mesothelioma may be entertained (Figure 5.29). In these instances, the classic immunoprofile of adenomatoid tumors is helpful with the expression of D2-40, calretinin, and WT-1 (Figures 5.30 and 5.31). However, this pattern does not serve to exclude malignant mesothelioma, but mesotheliomas would be expected to be larger and have more cytologic atypia with possible necrosis present.

PEARLS AND PITFALLS: Patterns of Growth in Adenomatoid Tumors[5,6]

- Classically, adenomatoid tumors show a glandular architecture with occasional signet ring-like vacuoles (tubular pattern)
- Angiomatoid pattern shows a canalicular pattern with glands lined by flattened mesothelial cells
- The plexiform pattern demonstrates a solid growth pattern of epithelioid cells
- A rare cystic pattern comprises cysts lined by flattened mesothelial cells
- Rarely, infarction may lead to central necrosis, which does not necessarily indicate malignancy[7]

Adenomatous Hyperplasia of the Rete Testis

Adenomatous hyperplasia is a rare benign process in the rete testis, comprising tubular and papillary epithelium proliferating into rete lumen (Figures 5.32-5.34). The lining shows bland low cuboidal cells without significant atypia. A clue to the diagnosis is the identification of hyaline globules, resembling those found in yolk sac tumors (Figure 5.35).[8] A confounding issue is that rete hyperplasia may also occur as a reaction to germ cell tumor invasion (Figure 5.36).[9]

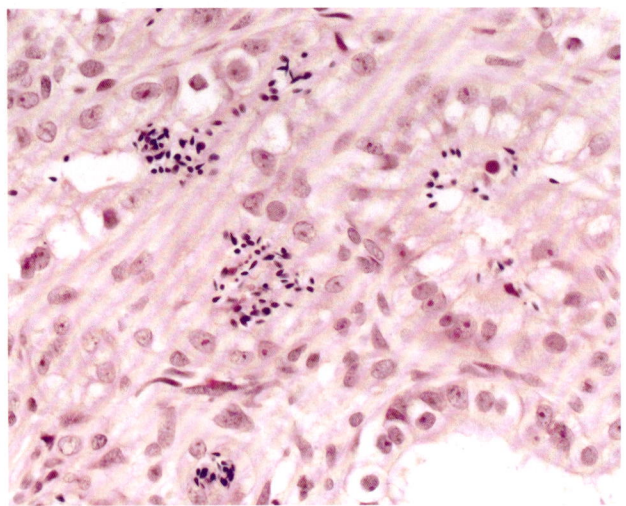

Figure 5.27. At higher power, sperm within the tubules are recognized by their tapered heads and their tails are often imperceptible. Referring back to Figure 5.24, there are collections of sperm in the lower right hand of the image that can be a low-power clue for vasitis nodosa.

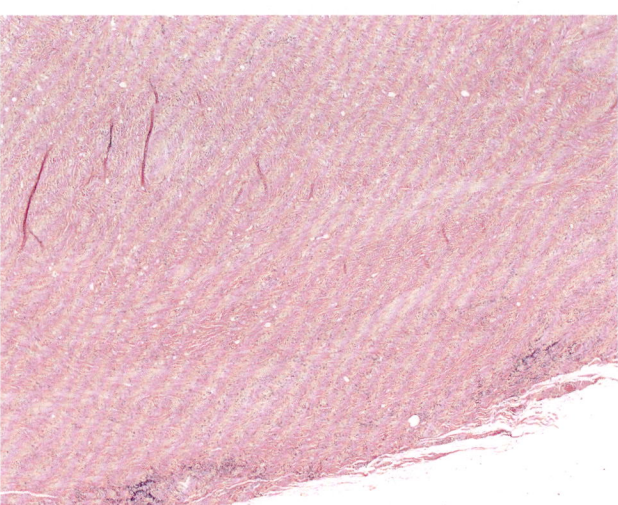

Figure 5.28. Adenomatoid tumors are common paratesticular masses and are generally well-circumscribed, gray-white nodules on gross examination. Histologically, they comprise variable amounts of smooth muscle and fibrous tissue containing gland-like structures lined by flattened mesothelial cells.

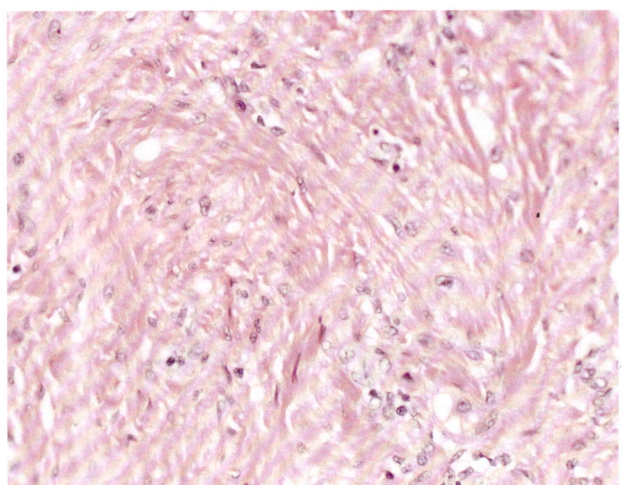

Figure 5.29. The tubules in adenomatoid tumor may be compressed, be angulated, or mimic signet-ring cells. The tubules appear infiltrative, mimicking adenocarcinoma. However, they lack nuclear atypia, mitotic activity, or extensive necrosis (rarely infarcted adenomatoid tumors may show necrosis).

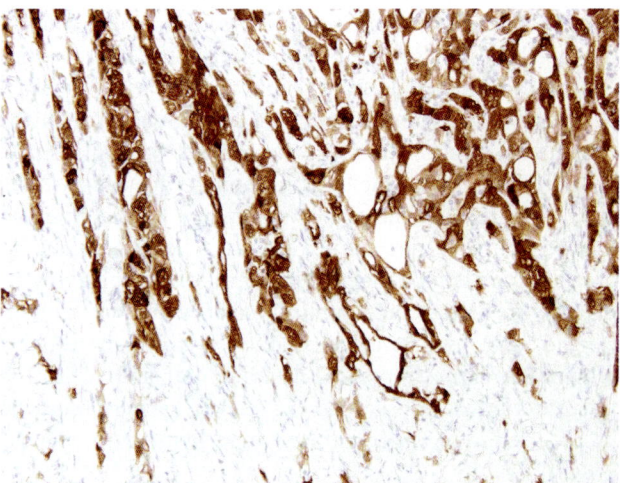

Figure 5.30. When adenomatoid tumor is suspected, immunohistochemical staining for mesothelial markers will highlight the tubule lining. This image depicts strong diffuse staining of the tubules with calretinin.

Rete Testis Adenocarcinoma

This is an exceedingly rare adenocarcinoma located in the testicular hilum and derived from the rete epithelium. The location of the tumor and identification of intrarete growth can help support this diagnosis, although specific criteria have been proposed for this entity (see FAQ). Because of its rarity, it is important to exclude other more common entities before diagnosing a primary rete testis adenocarcinoma. Architecturally, rete testis adenocarcinoma classically shows infiltrative glandular growth with slit-like spaces, which may merge into more solid or spindle-shaped areas (Figures 5.37 and 5.38). Other architectural patterns have been reported, including papillary, tubulopapillary, cribriform, and nested. Necrosis is a helpful feature to distinguish from benign rete testis hyperplasia (Figure 5.39).

There is no specific immunohistochemical profile for these tumors; however, one study found positivity of AE1/AE3 cytokeratin, CK7, epithelial membrane antigen (EMA), and vimentin in the majority of cases. A subset of these cases shows nuclear positivity for

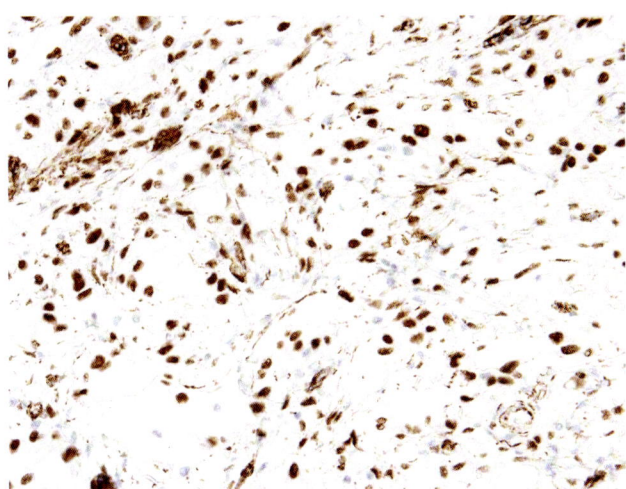

Figure 5.31. Another mesothelial marker, WT-1 also demonstrates strong nuclear positivity in the mesothelial cells lining the tubules of adenomatoid tumor.

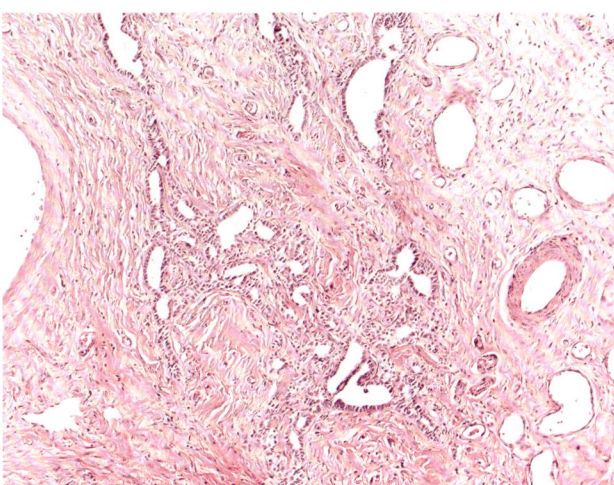

Figure 5.32. Hyperplasia of the rete testis is a benign, likely reactive, process that leads to the proliferation of ducts of the rete testis. It may occur in association with germ cell tumors as a reaction to invasion.

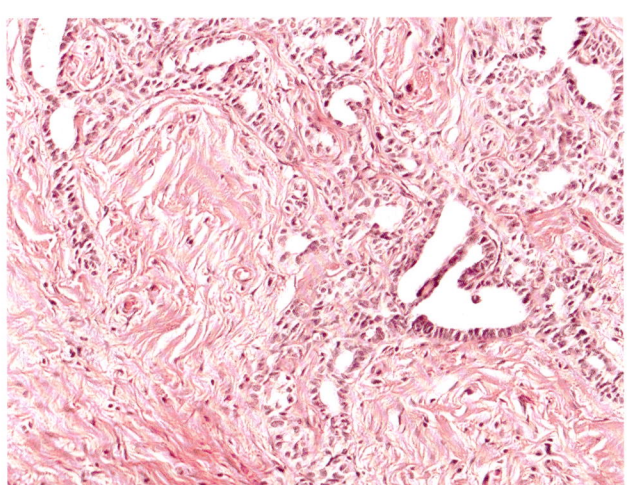

Figure 5.33. Higher power image of rete testis hyperplasia showing numerous ducts growing side by side, with a more cellular appearance than usual rete testis. The finding can resemble rete testis adenocarcinoma; however, carcinoma is very rare.

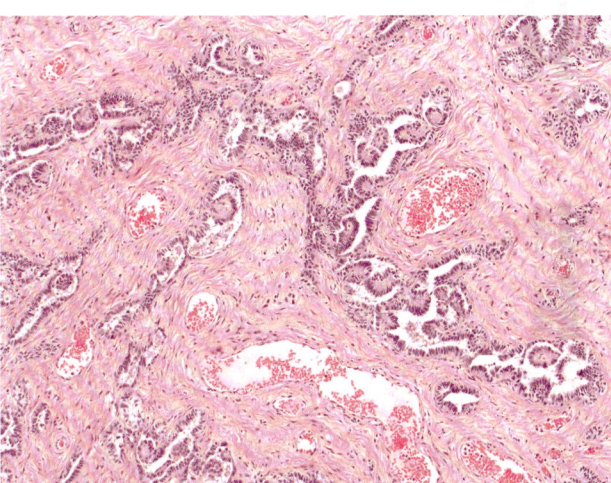

Figure 5.34. Papillary proliferation within the rete testis lumen is another pattern of rete testis hyperplasia as demonstrated in this image. The lack of nuclear atypia, frank invasive growth, or necrosis supports a benign diagnosis.

WT-1 and PAX-8.[10] These tumors have poor outcomes, with a high frequency of retroperitoneal lymph node metastasis. The main differential diagnosis in these tumors is secondary involvement by another metastatic adenocarcinoma, serous tumors, and malignant mesothelioma.

CHECKLIST: Diagnostic Criteria for Rete Testis Adenocarcinoma[11]

1. Tumor centered on the testicular hilum with intrarete growth
2. Morphology differs from all other testicular or paratesticular tumors
3. Lack of another extrascrotal tumor that could represent the primary site
4. Exclusion of all other paratesticular tumors, including malignant mesothelioma and papillary serous carcinoma

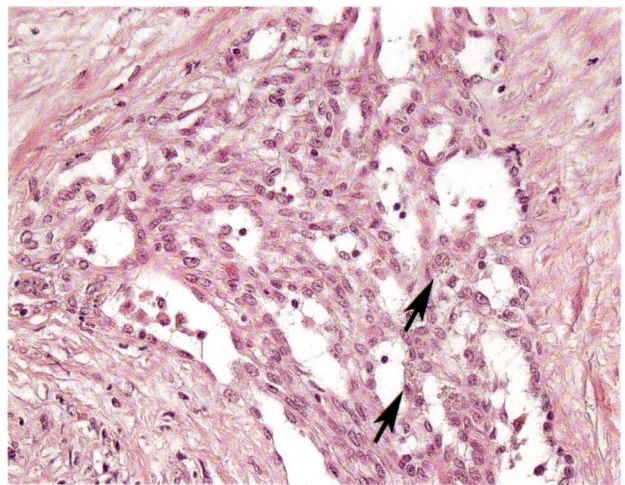

Figure 5.35. A pitfall for the misdiagnosis of rete testis hyperplasia as yolk sac tumor is the presence of hyaline globules (arrows) within rete testis hyperplasia.

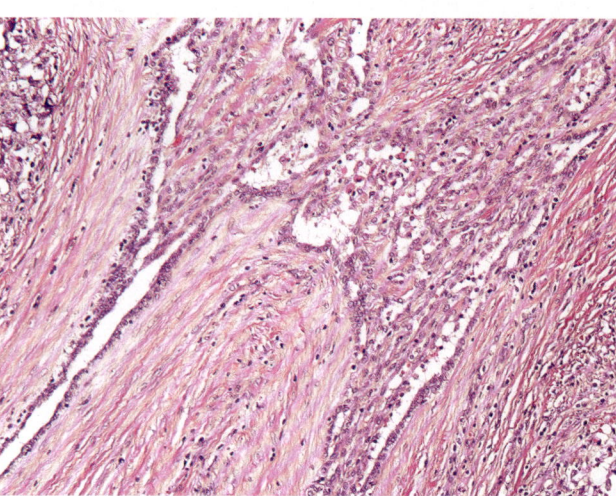

Figure 5.36. In this image, rete testis hyperplasia is present in association with invasion by germ cell tumor. The germ cell tumor component is present in the upper left and lower right corner, with proliferation rete testis epithelium in the middle.

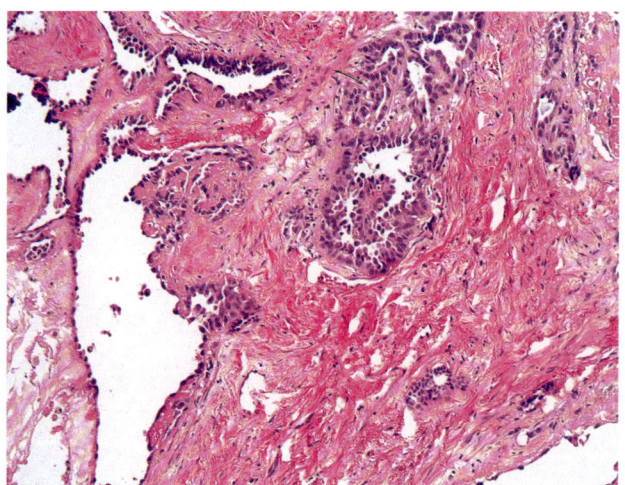

Figure 5.37. Rete testis adenocarcinoma is extremely rare and is diagnosed when centered in the testicular hilum, and there is evidence of intrarete growth, as depicted here.

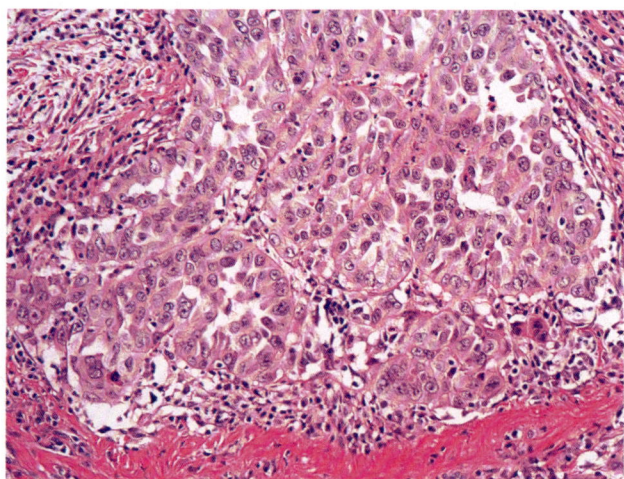

Figure 5.38. Overt malignant nuclear features are present in this high-power image of rete testis adenocarcinoma, with marked pleomorphism, vesicular chromatin, and prominent nuclei. Mitotic figures are easily identified.

Primary Epididymal Adenocarcinoma

Another exceedingly rare tumor, primary epididymal adenocarcinoma is the malignant counterpart of papillary cystadenoma. Centered in the epididymis, these tumors show frank invasive growth. The patterns of growth described in these tumors include tubular, tubulocystic, or tubulopapillary. Cytologically, the malignant cells show abundant clear cytoplasm containing glycogen.[12] Similar to adenocarcinoma of the rete testis, it is critical to exclude other primary sites of adenocarcinoma before making this diagnosis.

Malignant Mesothelioma

The tunica vaginalis may give rise to malignant mesothelioma centered in the paratesticular region. However, paratesticular mesotheliomas make up only 1% of all mesotheliomas, which are far more common in the pleura and peritoneum.[13] The tunica vaginalis is in continuity with the abdominal peritoneal lining, and in many ways, this lesion is similar to primary peritoneal mesothelioma, including a poor prognosis. These tumors show a lower association with asbestos exposure when compared to pleural mesothelioma.[14] Chronic hydroceles are linked with mesothelioma, and any hydrocele specimen with thickened or roughened areas should be sampled carefully (Figures 5.40 and 5.41).

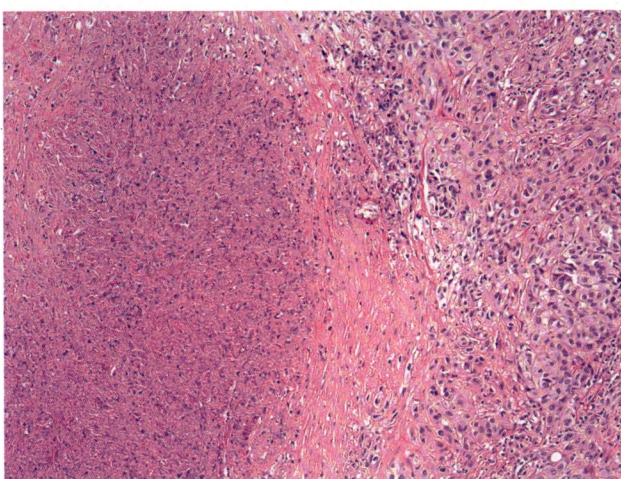

Figure 5.39. Solid growth and the presence of geographic necrosis are not consistent with a benign process. Once other possible secondary malignancies are excluded, rete testis adenocarcinoma may be considered.

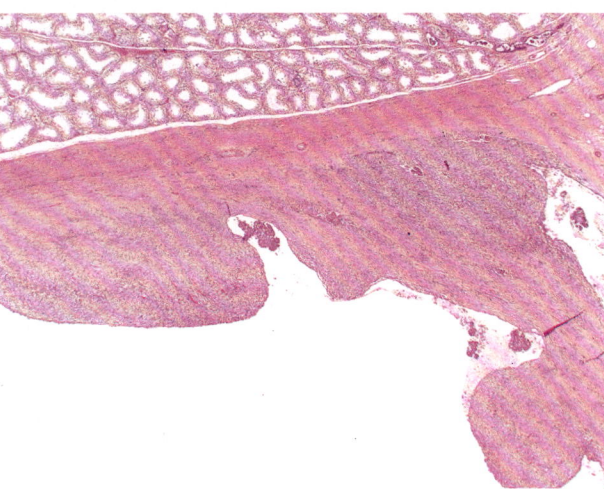

Figure 5.40. Long-standing hydroceles are associated with malignant mesothelioma and should be carefully sampled if nodules or areas of thickening are present. In this image, the mesothelial lining of the hydrocele sac is thickened, with multiple foci of epithelial proliferation present.

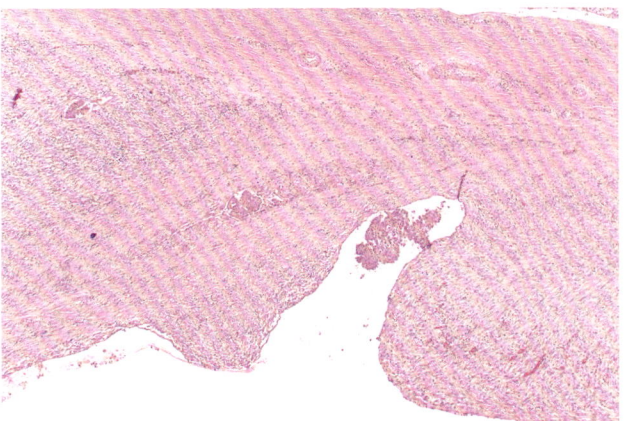

Figure 5.41. At higher power, the infiltrative nature of the malignant mesothelial nests is evident as it extends irregularly into the hydrocele sac and surrounding fibrous tissue.

Similar to malignant mesothelioma in other anatomic locations, in paratesticular mesothelioma, the mesothelial lining is grossly thickened and studded with tumor nodules. On sectioning, the malignant mesothelial cells infiltrate deeply into fat and other structures with a truly invasive pattern of growth. One should be aware that mesothelial hyperplasia may involve superficial clusters of mesothelial cells below the surface, a reactive pattern.

FAQ: What Are the Histologic Features That Favor Malignant Mesothelial Proliferations?

- Grossly identifiable mass (i.e., not incidental microscopic finding)
- Stromal invasion (Figure 5.42)
- Hypercellularity (Figure 5.43)
- Cytologic atypia (Figure 5.44)
- Stromal desmoplasia
- Necrosis

Architectural patterns in epithelioid mesotheliomas (which are most common) include papillary, tubulopapillary, tubular, and solid.[15] Biphasic or sarcomatoid mesothelioma is discussed later in the section on spindle cell pattern. Psammoma bodies may be present (Figure 5.45). The less common biphasic malignant mesotheliomas show both epithelial and sarcomatous components. The malignant epithelioid cells are plump with abundant, dense eosinophilic cytoplasm with pleomorphic nuclei and large nucleoli. Mesothelial markers (calretinin, D2-40, WT-1) are positive and may be used to distinguish these tumors from invasive adenocarcinomas.

PAPILLARY LESIONS

Papillary Cystadenoma

Papillary cystadenoma arises from the epididymis as a papillary and cystic neoplasm lined by bland cells with ample clear cytoplasm. These benign tumors are associated with von Hippel Lindau syndrome.[16,17] An underlying genetic syndrome is more likely when tumors are present bilaterally. Histologically, it is nearly identical to clear cell papillary renal cell carcinoma. The architectural pattern shows blunt papillary cores and numerous cystic spaces, with intervening fibrous stroma (Figures 5.46-5.48). Cytologically, the cells demonstrate cleared out cytoplasm and nuclei may align themselves at the luminal aspect of the cell leading to subnuclear vacuoles (Figures 5.49 and 5.50). Benign cytology is essential for this diagnosis—no increased atypia, mitotic figures, or necrosis is permitted. The immunoprofile is also identical to that of clear cell papillary renal cell carcinoma, with positive expression of PAX8, carbonic anhydrase IX in a cup-shaped pattern, and CK7 and lack of expression of CD10, RCC marker, and α-methylacyl-CoA racemase.[18]

The main differential diagnosis for these lesions includes metastatic conventional clear cell renal cell carcinoma, which should exhibit some atypia, a more nested growth pattern, and should lack true papillary fronds. The immunoprofile should also differ, with the expression of CD10 and RCC in a metastatic clear cell renal cell carcinoma. A second differential diagnosis includes tumors of Mullerian origin—serous borderline tumor and papillary serous carcinoma. Both of these lesions exhibit more architectural complexity and cytologic atypia than expected in papillary cystadenoma.

Well-Differentiated Papillary Mesothelioma

Well-differentiated papillary mesotheliomas are associated with hydroceles and often occur in younger men when compared to malignant mesotheliomas. These tumors are noninvasive, exophytic proliferations of mesothelial cells that stud the peritoneal/tunical surface. The papillary fronds are simple, without complex branching architecture and lined by a single layer of bland cuboidal mesothelial cells (Figures 5.51 and 5.52).[19] Mitotic figures should be minimal to absent, and no necrosis or invasive growth is permitted. Classic well-differentiated papillary mesotheliomas are considered benign entities and can be treated with hydrocelectomy.

Occasionally, there is more cytologic atypia or complex architecture identified in these lesions that appear to exist on a morphologic spectrum with malignant mesothelioma. The term "well-differentiated papillary mesothelioma with borderline malignant potential" has been applied to lesions with any of the following features identified in focal areas: atypia or stratification of lining mesothelial cells, increased mitotic figures, tubular or cribriform pattern, or fused papillary fronds (Figures 5.53 and 5.54).[20] If these features are extensive, then a close search for an invasive component is warranted to rule out the possibility of a frankly malignant mesothelioma.

Ovarian-type Epithelial Tumors

Ovarian-type epithelial tumors are named after their ovarian counterparts and include serous cystadenomas, serous tumors of borderline malignant potential, serous carcinomas, and both benign and malignant mucinous cystic tumors.[13] These tumors are hypothesized to arise from the tunica vaginalis with Mullerian metaplasia or other Mullerian remnants within the paratesticular region.[21,22] Although extremely rare, serous tumors are slightly more common than mucinous tumors. They are morphologically identical to the ovarian tumors of the same name.

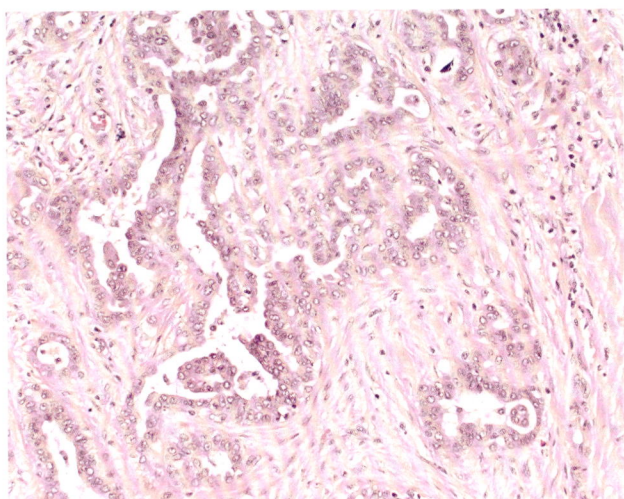

Figure 5.42. Stromal invasion by irregular glands and tubules identified in an epithelial malignant mesothelioma.

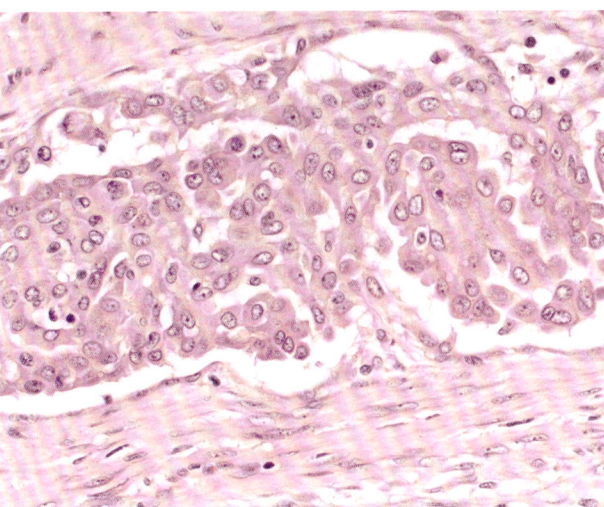

Figure 5.43. Malignant mesotheliomas show a greater degree of hypercellularity when compared to benign mesothelial proliferations, forming expansile nests.

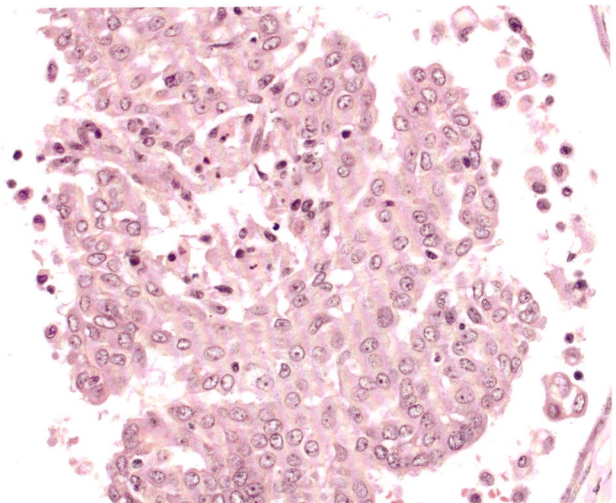

Figure 5.44. Cytologic atypia is a requirement for the diagnosis of malignant mesothelioma, demonstrated in this image of malignant cells with abundant, dense eosinophilic cytoplasm with pleomorphic nuclei and large nucleoli.

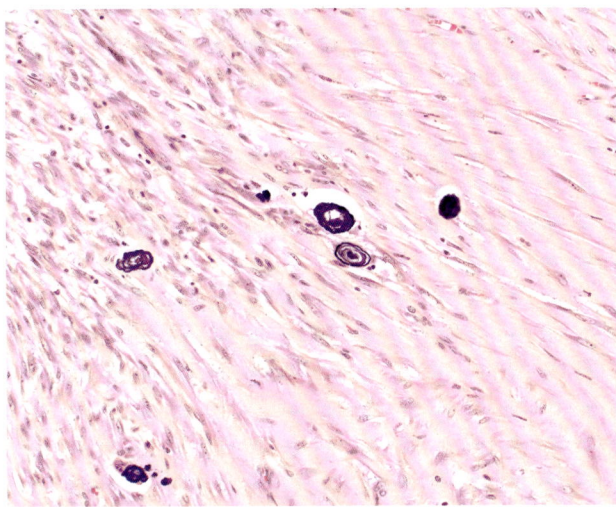

Figure 5.45. Psammoma bodies, concentric lamellated calcifications, are commonly identified in malignant mesothelioma.

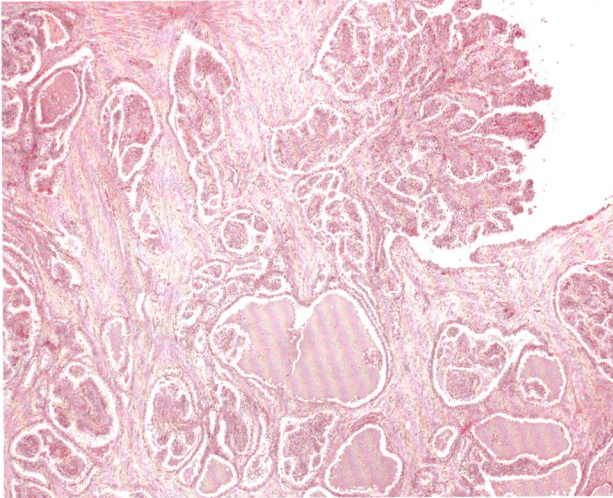

Figure 5.46. Papillary cystadenoma of the paratestis is a papillary and cystic neoplasm with intervening fibrous bands.

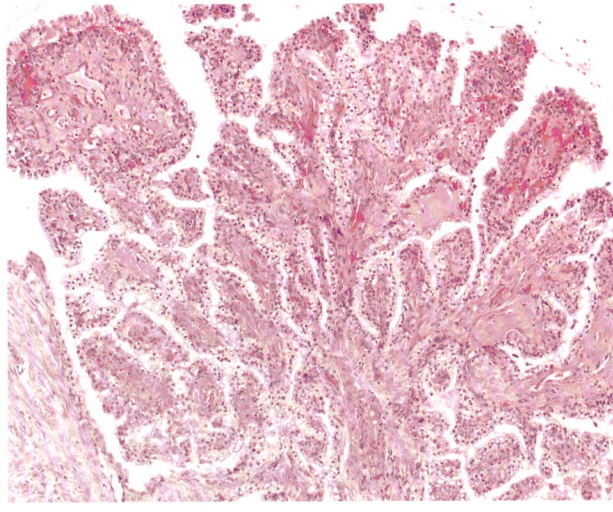

Figure 5.47. The papillary cores are often short and blunt, rather than long and delicate, as demonstrated in this image.

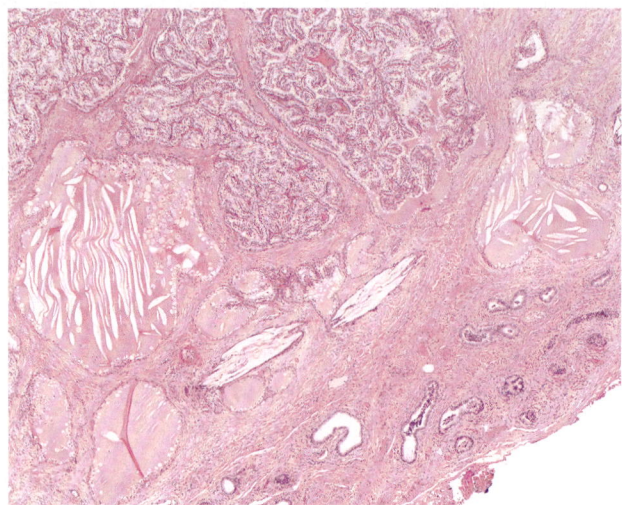

Figure 5.48. Cystically dilated spaces are common in papillary cystadenoma, and the majority of the tumor may be cystic in some cases. Intervening dense fibrous bands are another helpful feature for the diagnosis.

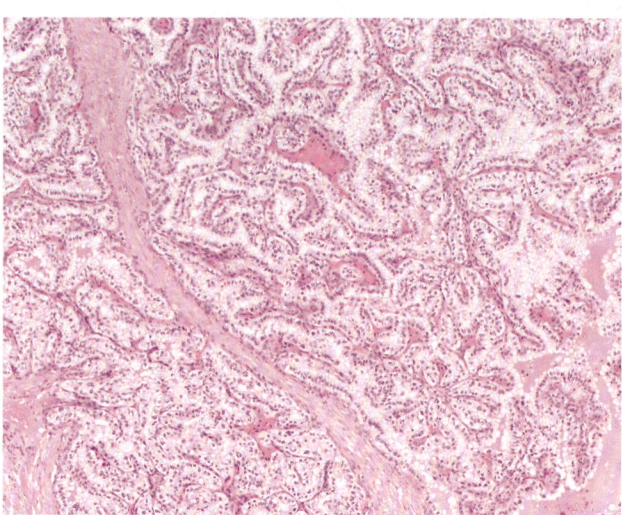

Figure 5.49. The cytologic features of papillary cystadenoma include ample clear cytoplasm with small, monotonous nuclei.

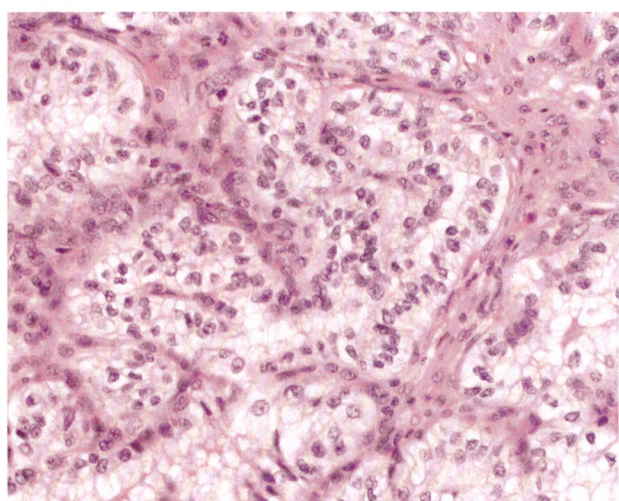

Figure 5.50. Nuclei are frequently located closer to the luminal aspect of the cell, leading to the impression of subnuclear vacuoles or "piano keys."

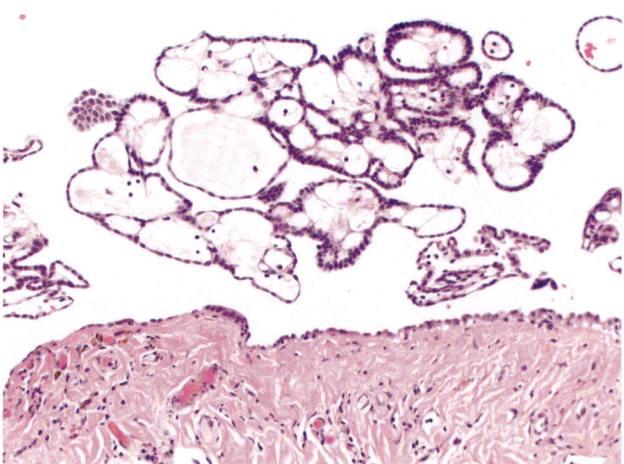

Figure 5.51. Well-differentiated papillary mesothelioma may arise in the setting of hydrocele or otherwise present in the paratestis region. These proliferations comprise simple papillary fronds lined by bland mesothelial cells. Invasive growth is not acceptable in this entity.

Serous tumors of borderline malignant potential are usually cystic lesions lined by stratified tubal-type epithelial cells with minimal cytologic atypia, negligible mitotic activity, and architectural complexity in the form of branching, complex papillary fronds (Figures 5.55-5.57). Consistent with their Mullerian origin, these tumors strongly express PAX-8 (Figure 5.58). In a series of seven cases of serous borderline tumor of the paratestis, there were no recurrences or metastases reported after radical orchiectomy.[23] In contrast, serous carcinomas show invasive growth of tumor cells with high-grade nuclear atypia, frequent mitotic figures, and necrosis and are often associated with psammoma bodies.

Similar to the ovary, mucinous tumors of the paratestis occur on a spectrum of benign (mucinous cystadenoma) to malignant (mucinous carcinoma). In the middle are mucinous borderline tumors, which show atypical mucinous epithelium without invasive growth, whereas mucinous carcinoma shows invasion. Tumors can show either intestinal-type or endocervical-like epithelium. With mucinous tumors of this area considered so rare, it is critical to exclude metastasis from other sites before making the diagnosis of a primary mucinous neoplasm of the paratestis.[24]

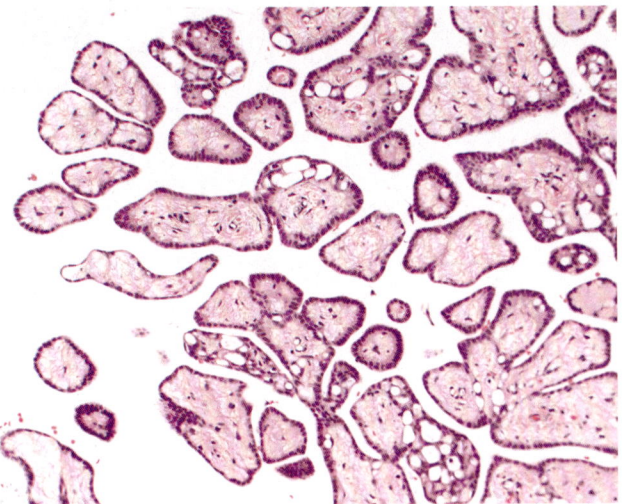

Figure 5.52. In well-differentiated papillary mesothelioma, there is no cytologic atypia or marked architectural complexity to the fronds.

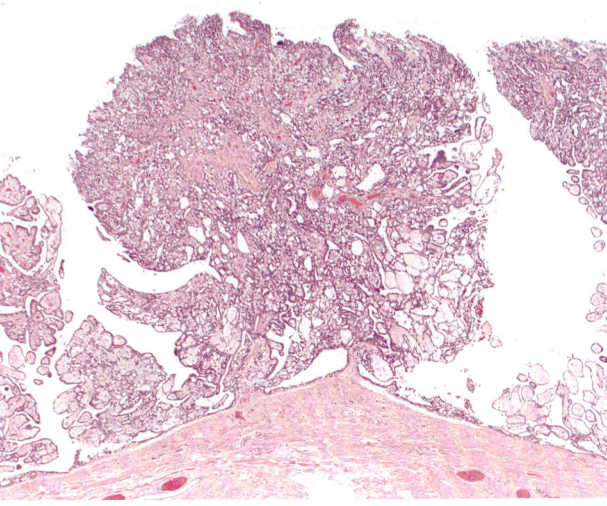

Figure 5.53. If increasing architectural complexity is identified, a separate category of "well-differentiated papillary mesothelioma with borderline malignant potential" is applied. These tumors show the fusion of papillary fronds or tubular/cribriform growth pattern, but lack invasive growth.

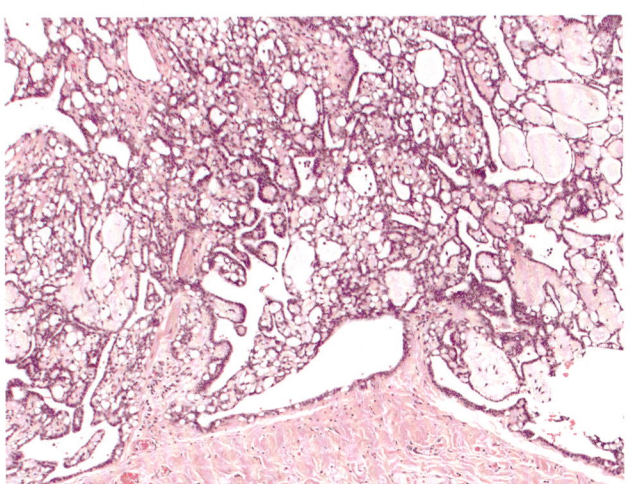

Figure 5.54. At higher power, the tubular growth and back-to-back pattern with fused glands of this well-differentiated papillary mesothelioma with borderline malignant potential is contrasted with the simple fronds of well-differentiated papillary mesothelioma in Figure 5.52. Additionally, well-differentiated papillary mesothelioma with borderline malignant potential may show cytologic atypia or stratification with occasional mitotic figures.

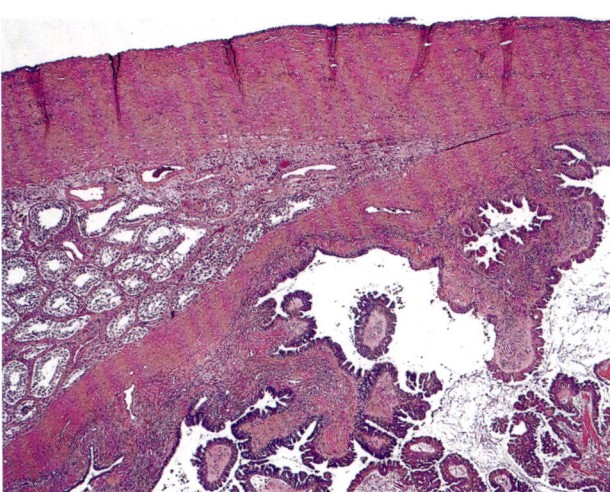

Figure 5.55. Serous tumors of borderline malignant potential are cystic and papillary lesions of ovarian-type, favored to arise from Mullerian remnants within the paratesticular region.

Other less common ovarian-type malignancies include Brenner tumor of testis, endometrioid adenocarcinoma, and clear cell adenocarcinoma.

ADIPOCYTIC LESIONS

Lipoma

The most common paratesticular mesenchymal tumor is lipoma. Despite their benign nature, these are controversial lesions in the genitourinary and surgical literature. Many authors consider these fatty accumulations about the cord to represent retroperitoneal fat that has tracked down the cord, rather than a true neoplasm. For those that consider it a discrete entity, "cord lipomas" are discrete, encapsulated masses attached to the spermatic

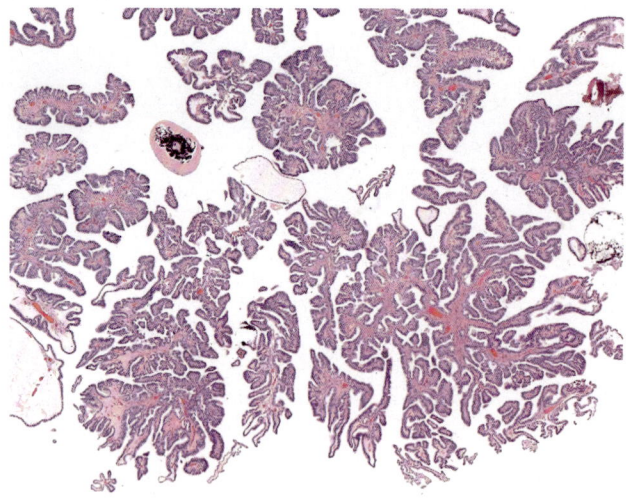

Figure 5.56. These tumors demonstrate complex branching papillary fronds with mild cytologic atypia and rare to no mitotic figures identified.

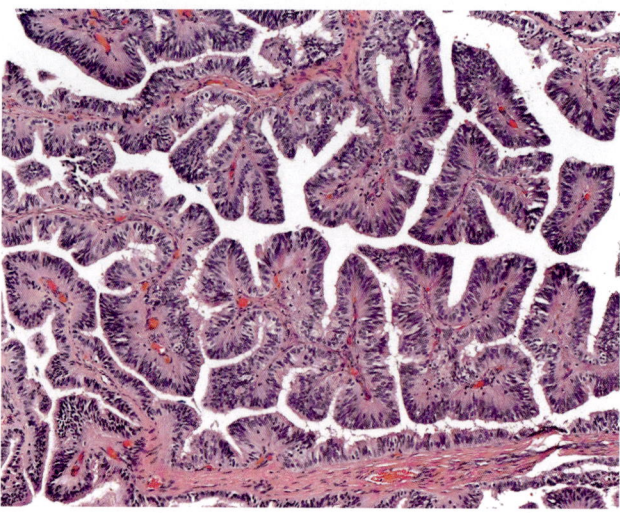

Figure 5.57. Cytologic features of serous tumor of borderline malignant potential include serous-type epithelium with pseudostratification and minimal atypia.

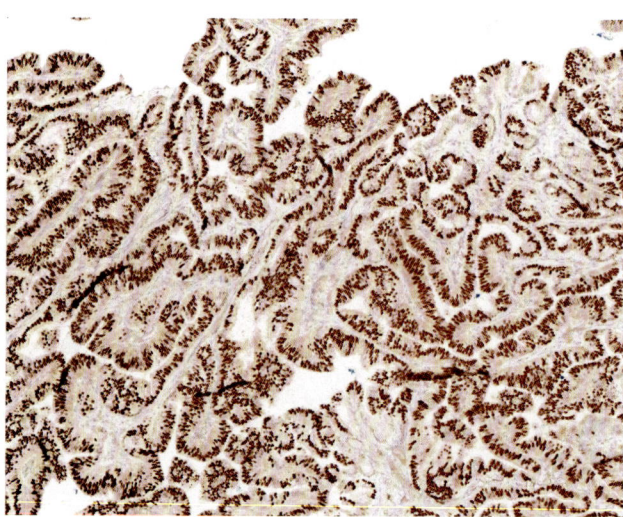

Figure 5.58. Strong and diffuse nuclear positivity for PAX-8 is seen in serous tumors of the paratestis, consistent with their Mullerian origin.

cord rather than an indistinct aggregate of adipose tissue present in the inguinal canal. Regardless, these lesions comprise mature adipose tissue without atypia, similar to lipomas occurring in the other regions (Figures 5.59-5.61). Large true lipomatous neoplasms of the spermatic cord (>10 cm) are "deep" lipomatous tumors and should be evaluated for the possibility of atypical lipomatous tumor/well-differentiated liposarcoma, such as with fluorescence in situ hybridization (FISH) for *MDM2* amplification.[25]

Liposarcoma

Liposarcomas are malignant adipocytic tumors primarily occurring in older individuals. Similar to lipomas in this area, they may arise as true paratesticular/spermatic cord lesions or extension from a retroperitoneal liposarcoma. In the latter case, radiographic imaging would be necessary to determine the tumor extent. Well-differentiated liposarcomas are readily identifiable as lipomatous neoplasms, with an abundance of adipocytes and morphologic overlap with lipoma; however, there is nuclear atypia. Atypical features include enlarged, hyperchromatic nuclei, frequently present within fibrous septa (Figures 5.62 and 5.63). Dedifferentiation in a liposarcoma may confound the diagnosis, especially in small biopsy specimens. Amplification of *MDM2*, best assessed by FISH studies, is useful in the distinction of lipoma from liposarcoma.

> **PEARLS AND PITFALLS: Dedifferentiated Liposarcoma**
>
> - Important to sample any residual fatty areas in a gross specimen with concern for dedifferentiated liposarcoma, as these areas may contain the well-differentiated liposarcoma component to assist with the diagnosis (Figure 5.64)
> - A dedifferentiated component in a well-differentiated liposarcoma may entirely lack adipocytes with undifferentiated pleomorphic sarcoma or features of another high-grade sarcoma (Figure 5.65)
> - Always consider the possibility of a dedifferentiated liposarcoma in an otherwise nonspecific malignant spindle cell neoplasm, especially in a retroperitoneal location (Figure 5.66)
> - *MDM2* FISH is useful in the diagnosis and will be amplified in both the well-differentiated and dedifferentiated components. *MDM2* FISH is more sensitive and specific than MDM2 immunohistochemistry (Figure 5.67)

SPINDLE PATTERN

Fibrous Pseudotumor

Fibrous pseudotumors of the paratestis are uncommon mass-forming lesions that occur within the scrotum and are often associated with hydroceles or a history of trauma. The masses may be plaque-like or nodular and are frequently multifocal, leading to an alternate terminology "nodular periorchitis."[13] Histologically, the masses comprise dense fibrous tissue with hyalinization and some degree of inflammation, usually lymphoplasmacytic (Figures 5.68 and 5.69). The differential diagnosis of this entity includes inflammatory myofibroblastic tumor and fibromatosis. By immunohistochemistry, fibrous pseudotumors lack ALK and β-catenin expression, which distinguishes them from inflammatory myofibroblastic tumors and fibromatosis.[26] These lesions behave indolently and are cured with conservative excision.

> **PEARLS AND PITFALLS: Adenomatoid Tumor With Smooth Muscle Predominance**
>
> - Adenomatoid tumors infrequently present with a spindle cell pattern due to smooth muscle predominance (Figure 5.70)
> - May be referred to as "leiomyoadenomatoid tumors" due to the overlap in appearance with benign leiomyomas.
> - While the smooth muscle stroma may predominate, the mesothelial cells are generally identifiable on H&E stain
> - Immunohistochemistry for mesothelial markers (WT-1, calretinin, D2-40) may be useful if the epithelial component is not readily identifiable
> - Once excised, these tumors behave in a benign fashion

Smooth Muscle Hyperplasia of the Testicular Adnexa

A rare bland smooth muscle proliferation encircling ducts of the epididymis is one of the typical patterns of smooth muscle hyperplasia of the testicular adnexa (SMH-TA), which is a benign process of unknown etiology. These lesions are not true neoplasms, rather they are made up of a benign excess of the patient's usual smooth muscle component of the paratestis or spermatic cord. In one series, the mean age of patients with SMH-TA was 51 years, and the majority presented with testicular pain or mass.[27] The smooth muscle proliferates within the interstitium, between vessels, or interdigitates with or "cuffs" the efferent ducts of the epididymis. Histologically, SMH-TA demonstrates fascicular growth of smooth muscle that lacks the interlacing pattern of leiomyoma.[28]

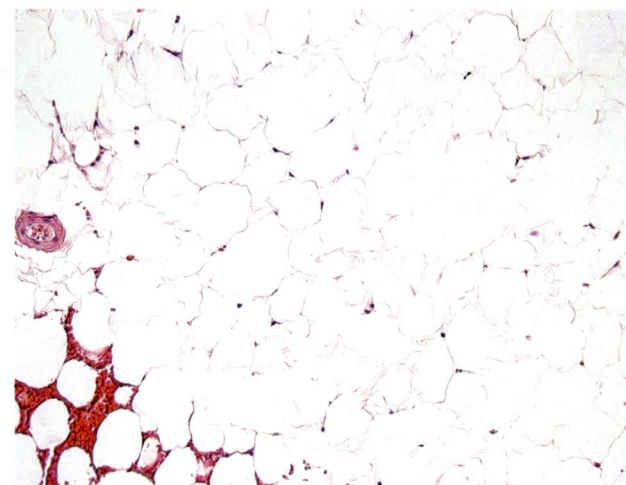

Figure 5.59. Lipomas occurring in the paratesticular region may represent herniated retroperitoneal fat, or if a discrete, encapsulated nodule of fat is adherent to the spermatic cord, the term "spermatic cord lipoma" is appropriate.

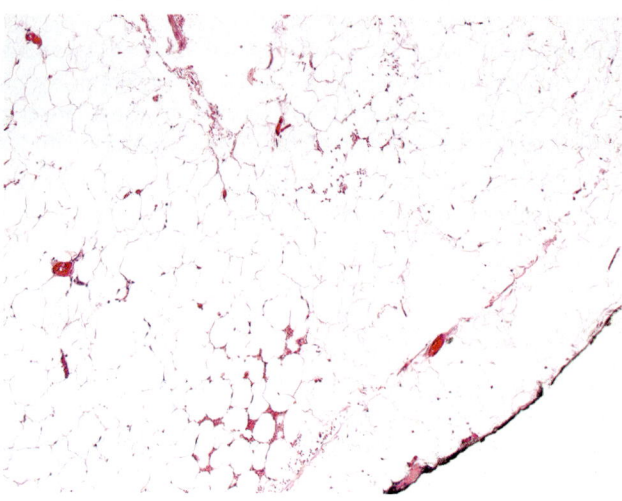

Figure 5.60. Like lipomas elsewhere, they comprise mature adipose tissue without atypia. While a thin capsule is often evident at the time of surgery, it is not easily identifiable on microscopic evaluation.

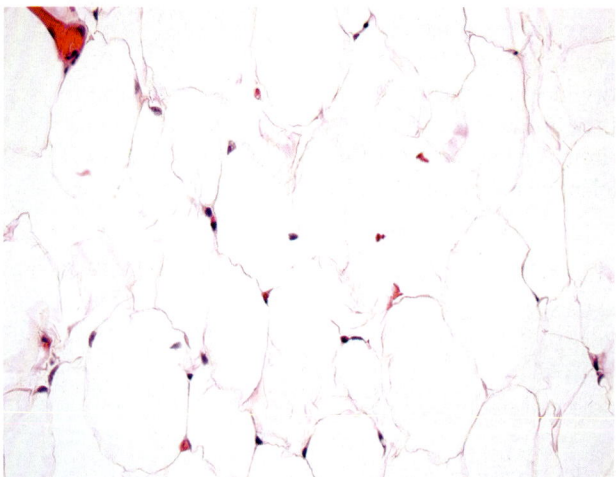

Figure 5.61. High-power examination shows mature fat with thin cell membranes and small monotonous nuclei. No atypia or mitotic figures are seen in lipoma, although fat necrosis may occur in the setting of a traumatized lesion.

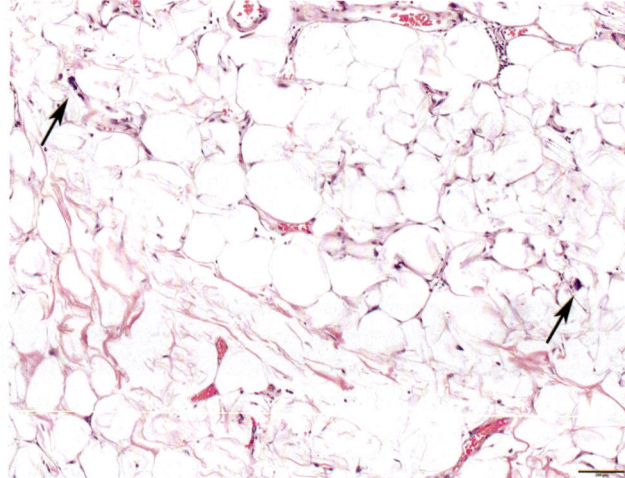

Figure 5.62. Well-differentiated liposarcoma resembles lipoma at low power, comprising abundant adipocytes. Close examination reveals nuclear atypia (arrows) in the form of hyperchromasia and irregular elongated shapes.

Leiomyosarcoma

Leiomyosarcomas rarely arise in the paratesticular area, presenting as a scrotal mass. They may arise from the tunica vaginalis, spermatic cord, scrotal subcutaneous soft tissue, dartos muscle, or epididymis.[29] Like leiomyosarcomas elsewhere, these tumors comprise a fascicular arrangement of malignant spindle cells with cigar-shaped nuclei (Figure 5.71). Frank malignant features such as nuclear pleomorphism, increased mitotic rate, and necrosis are present, which distinguishes these tumors from their benign leiomyoma counterpart. In poorly differentiated leiomyosarcomas, other sarcomas may enter the differential diagnosis including dedifferentiated liposarcoma and spindle cell rhabdomyosarcoma. In this instance, immunohistochemistry and FISH can help confirm the diagnosis with leiomyosarcoma expressing the usually smooth muscle markers desmin, muscle-specific actin, and smooth muscle actin. The lack of *MDM2* amplification makes a liposarcoma less likely, and rhabdomyosarcoma is discussed more below.

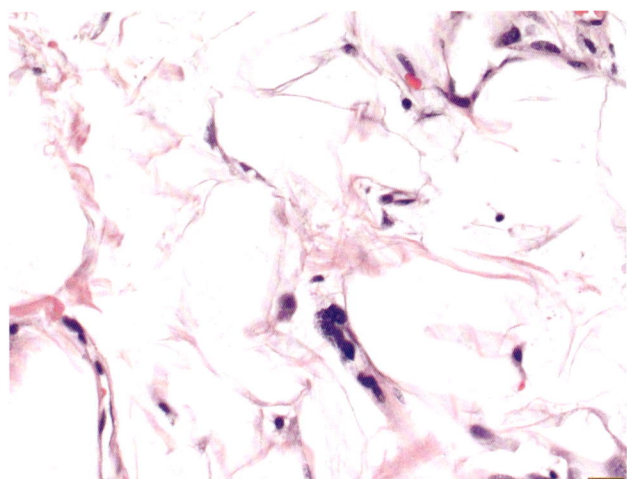

Figure 5.63. At higher power, the nuclear atypia within well-differentiated liposarcoma is impressive. It should be noted that the atypia may be relatively scant and scattered throughout the lesion, and some high-power scanning is worthwhile in large fatty lesions.

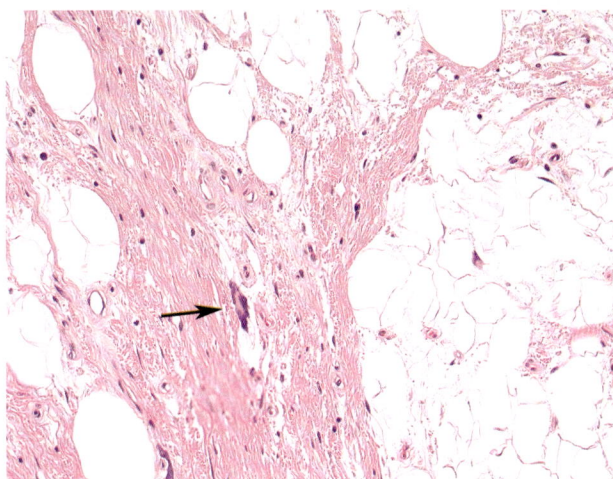

Figure 5.64. Dedifferentiated component can occur in otherwise usual well-differentiated liposarcoma and appears as more solid, often spindle cell components with marked nuclear atypia (arrow). When a background of adipocytic neoplasm is present, it is relatively straightforward to recognize the dedifferentiated component.

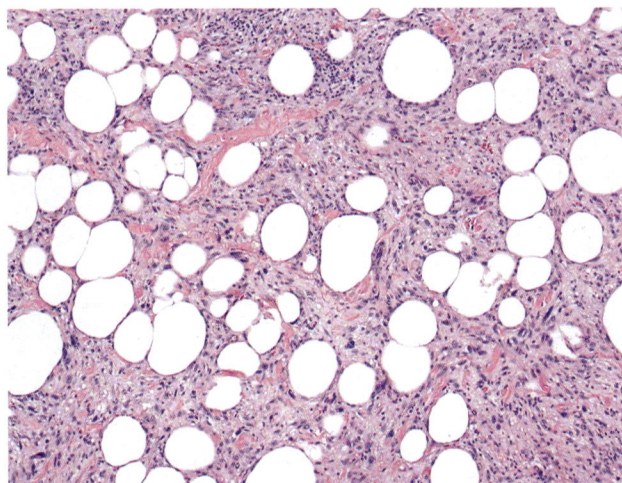

Figure 5.65. Depending on what area is sampled, the relative amounts of adipocytes to dedifferentiation may change. Here, an admixture of fat cells and spindle cell neoplasm is consistent with a dedifferentiated liposarcoma.

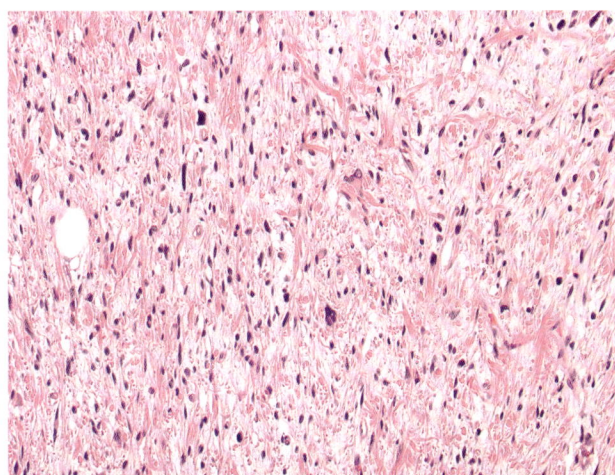

Figure 5.66. Occasionally, only the malignant spindle cell component is sampled—this is a particularly dangerous pitfall in biopsy specimens. One must consider the possibility of a dedifferentiated liposarcoma despite the lack of adipocytes.

Biphasic/Sarcomatoid Mesothelioma

Malignant mesotheliomas often show a biphasic growth pattern with a combination of epithelial component (often papillary) and sarcomatoid component. Biphasic mesotheliomas occur about one-third as frequently as epithelial mesotheliomas in this anatomic location. No pure sarcomatoid mesotheliomas have been described in the paratestis region.[13] These tumors frequently exhibit local recurrence and lymph node metastasis, with overall poor prognosis. Histologically, the epithelial component may show any of the patterns described above in the papillary pattern section. The sarcomatoid component shows a spectrum of fascicles of low-grade-appearing spindle cells to high-grade pleomorphic nuclei (Figures 5.72-5.75).

If the sarcomatoid component predominates in a small sampling, the differential diagnosis is broad and includes most of the spindle lesions discussed in this chapter (Figure 5.76). However, the identification of calretinin, D2-40, and WT-1 expression supports a mesothelial origin.

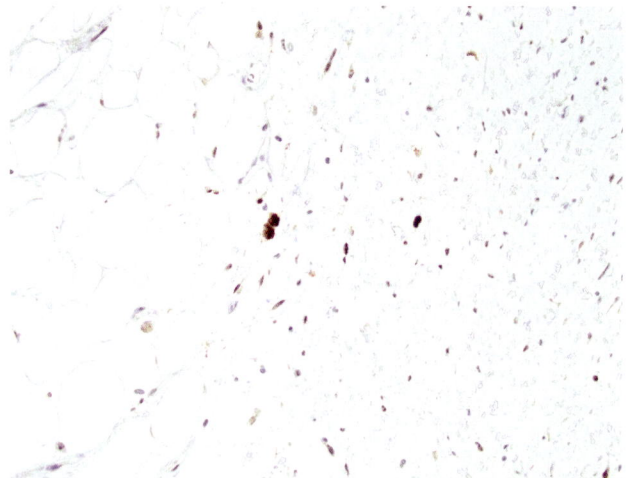

Figure 5.67. A recognizable well-differentiated component is present in the left upper part, whereas a more solid dedifferentiated component is present in the lower right. Both components show the nuclear expression of MDM2 by immunohistochemistry. Immunohistochemistry for MDM2 can assist in the diagnosis of dedifferentiated liposarcoma, although FISH for *MDM2* amplification is much more sensitive.

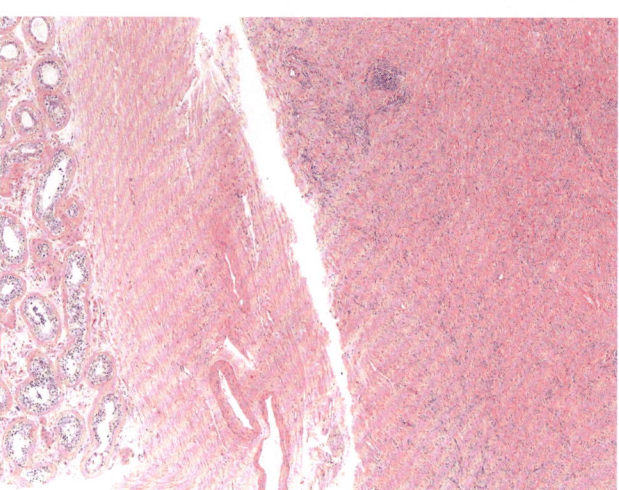

Figure 5.68. Fibrous pseudotumor of the paratestis may form a mass or multiple nodules within the scrotum and is frequently associated with hydrocele or trauma. Histologically, the nodules comprise dense fibrous tissue with hyalinization.

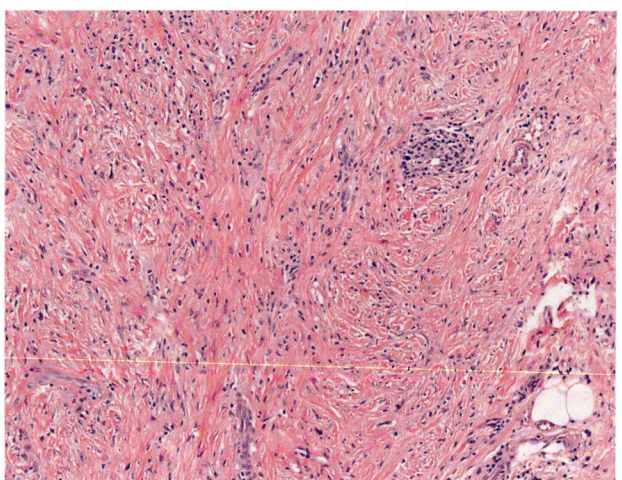

Figure 5.69. At higher power, this image of fibrous pseudotumor of the paratestis shows dense hyalinized fibrous tissue with scattered chronic inflammatory cells, mostly lymphocytes and rare plasma cells. These lesions are distinct from inflammatory myofibroblastic tumor and are ALK negative.

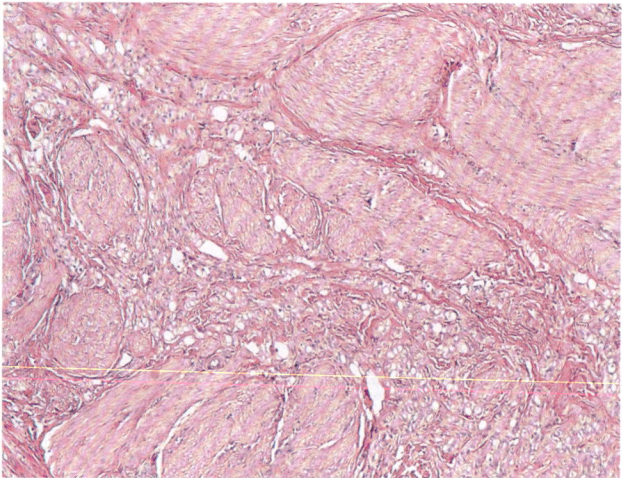

Figure 5.70. Adenomatoid tumors can demonstrate smooth muscle predominance that obscures the glandular and tubular elements classically associated with adenomatoid tumors. When the diagnosis is confounded by smooth muscle predominance and a spindle cell lesion is considered, mesothelial markers will highlight the mesothelial elements in the background.

Rhabdomyosarcoma

Over 90% of rhabdomyosarcomas arising in the paratesticular area are of the embryonal subtype, and the spindle cell variant of embryonal rhabdomyosarcoma is overrepresented in this region. About 25% are spindle cell type, with the majority being conventional embryonal type and a smaller percentage a mixture of spindle and nonspindle types.[13] In this location, the spindle cell variant has an overall better prognosis when compared to other sites.[30] Histologically, the spindle cell variant demonstrates a storiform architectural pattern of spindle cells with intervening collagen (Figures 5.77 and 5.78). A helpful pattern to recognize possible rhabdomyosarcomatous differentiation is the presence of "tails" or "comets"—cytoplasmic extensions off one side of the cell (Figure 5.79). Immunohistochemistry for these tumors shows evidence of skeletal muscle differentiation with the expression of myogenin and myo-D1 (Figure 5.80).

FAQ: Differential Diagnosis and Prevalence of Paratesticular Soft Tissue Masses[31]

- Most symptomatic paratesticular masses are malignant
- Overall: rhabdomyosarcoma, liposarcoma, leiomyosarcoma, undifferentiated pleomorphic sarcoma
- Rhabdomyosarcoma should be a primary consideration in children (younger than 18 years)
- In the adult, the differential diagnosis for this anatomic location begins with the most common entity, liposarcoma
- The next most common tumors are rhabdomyosarcoma, leiomyosarcoma, and undifferentiated pleomorphic sarcoma
- Benign neoplastic entities: spermatic cord lipoma and leiomyoma
- Nonneoplastic entities: adrenal cortical rest and inflammatory pseudotumor

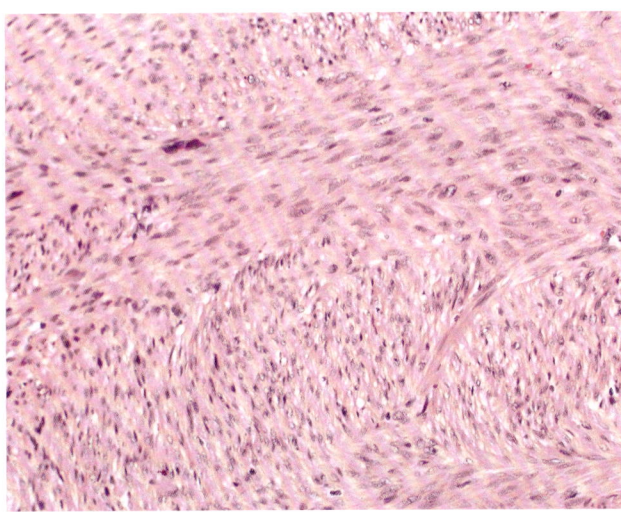

Figure 5.71. Leiomyosarcoma is exceedingly rare in the paratesticular region, but has the same morphologic features as those identified elsewhere. The tumor comprises fascicles of atypical spindle cells with cigar-shaped nuclei and overt nuclear atypia.

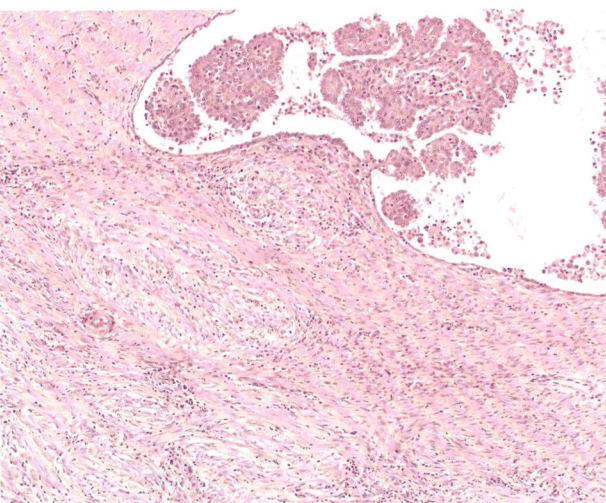

Figure 5.72. Biphasic malignant mesothelioma comprises a component of usual epithelial mesothelioma and sarcomatoid areas. The epithelioid portions will demonstrate the usual cytologic features of mesothelioma.

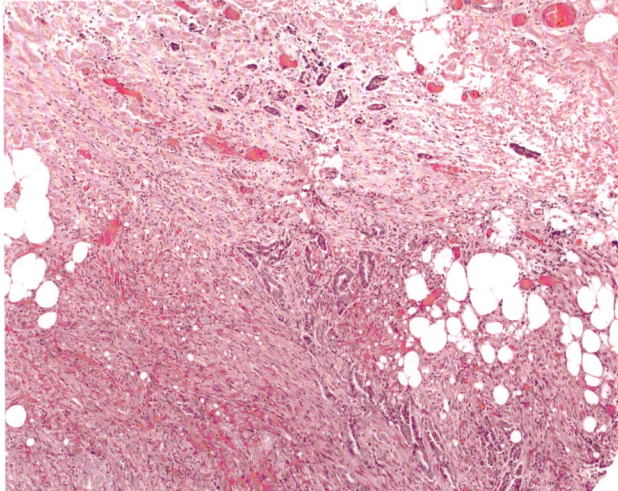

Figure 5.73. Infiltration into fat is a diagnostic feature of malignant mesothelioma. In this image, the epithelial component is glandular, whereas the sarcomatoid component has a nonspecific spindle cell appearance.

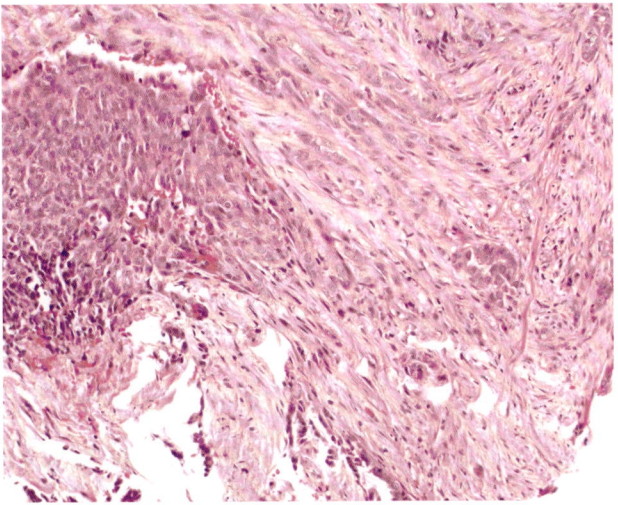

Figure 5.74. In this high-power image, the solid epithelial areas (left) blend into the sarcomatoid areas with small epithelioid nests infiltrating within the lesion. The spindle cell component may show a spectrum of low- to high-grade cytologic features.

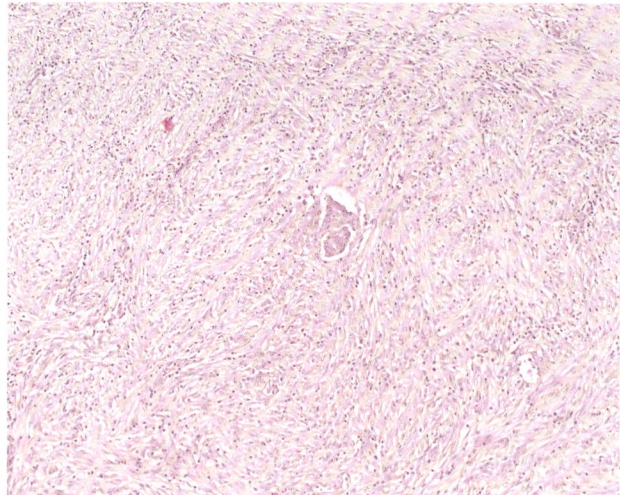

Figure 5.75. Occasionally, the sarcomatoid component predominates and only rare epithelial components are identified. In this image, a lone nest of epithelioid cells is present in a background of spindle cells.

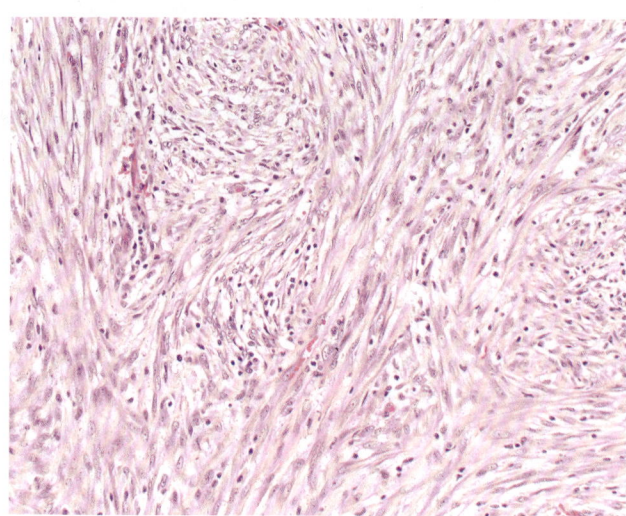

Figure 5.76. A higher power image showing areas of high-grade cytology within the sarcomatoid component. In a limited sampling, the finding of only sarcomatoid features may raise a broad differential of other sarcomas.

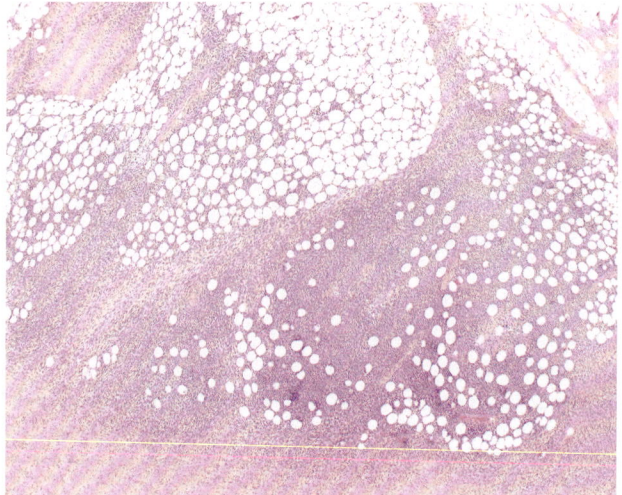

Figure 5.77. Rhabdomyosarcoma is the most common malignant paratesticular mass in children. The majority are of the embryonal subtype, and spindle cell subtype is overrepresented in this region.

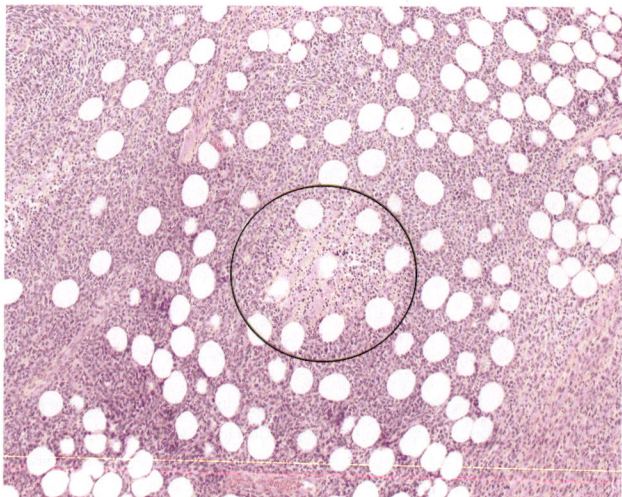

Figure 5.78. In addition to infiltrating within fat, necrosis is a helpful feature in recognizing malignant spindle cell proliferations, although it is not frequently identified in the embryonal subtype of rhabdomyosarcoma. A central area of necrosis is highlighted in the circle.

SCROTUM AND PENIS

Pathologic lesions of the scrotum and penis largely comprise soft tissue and skin-based entities. Although frequently encountered by the genitourinary pathologist because of their anatomic location and involvement of urologists, these disease processes are often more familiar to the dermatopathology or soft tissue specialist. A brief overview of relatively common entities occurring in the inguinal, scrotal, and penile skin and soft tissue is included for completeness, with a caveat that there is no shame in sharing these cases with the appropriate subspecialized consultant!

THE UNREMARKABLE EXTERNAL GENITALIA

Penile anatomy is quite complex and has important staging implications, so is worth reviewing in this chapter. Broadly, the penis is divided from the region nearest the abdomen into the root, shaft, and glans distally. The root (or bulb) of the penis is not actually external to the body; instead, it is located deep within the perineal tissue. It comprises erectile tissue and surrounded by dense connective tissue.[32]

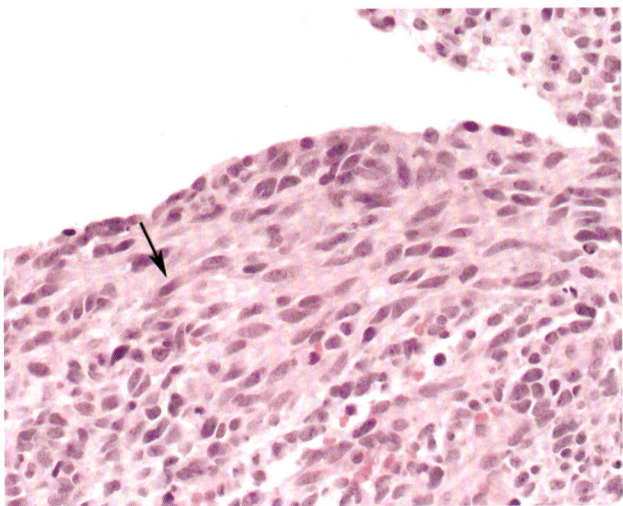

Figure 5.79. At high power, the "comet" shape of these cells (arrow) are supportive of a rhabdomyomatous origin. In the spindle cell type of embryonal rhabdomyosarcoma, there is usually some component of the primitive, round cells of usual embryonal cytology.

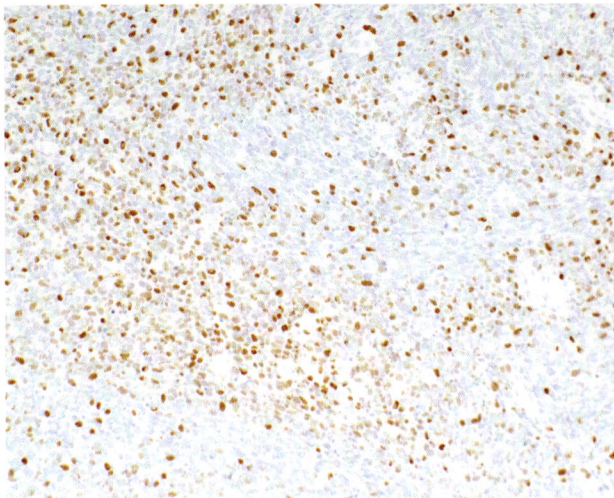

Figure 5.80. Immunohistochemistry for myogenin highlights the majority of cells in this rhabdomyosarcoma and is often patchy in the embryonal subtype of rhabdomyosarcoma. Conversely, myogenin usually demonstrates diffuse positivity in the alveolar subtype of rhabdomyosarcoma.

The shaft (also referred to as body or corpus) of the penis begins the external portion of the penis. The surface that is contiguous with the pubis area is considered dorsal, whereas the surface that is contiguous with the perineum is considered ventral. The shaft comprises a complex arrangement of tissues that are described in the FAQ below. Corpora cavernosa are two cylindrical masses of erectile tissue that are located dorsally in the penis ("dual and dorsal"). In the proximal penis, these two cylinders diverge laterally to form the crura and attach to the pubis via dense connective tissue. Histologically, corpora cavernosa are vascular tissues with irregular, dilated vascular channels invested in thick muscular stroma. The corpora spongiosum is a single mass of erectile tissue, is located ventrally, and surrounds the urethra. It also comprises vascular channels; however, the intervening stroma is more loose fibrous tissue without the thick muscles of the corpora cavernosum. It also surrounds the urothelium of the urethra, which can be a useful landmark.[32]

The distal end of the penis is highly complex, and anatomic variations are not uncommon. The glans forms the distal conical tip of the penis, and the urethral meatus is present slightly ventrally within the glans. The glans corona is the circumferential rim of the glans, which is delineated by the coronal sulcus at the border with the shaft. Typically, the dartos muscle and Buck fascia insert at the coronal sulcus. In uncircumcised males, the foreskin can cover the majority of the glans or only part of the glans. Cross-sectional diagrams are helpful references for accurate staging of tumors in the glans, as the various underlying tissues may vary depending on where a section is taken.[32]

FAQ: **What Are the Layers of the Penile Shaft From External to Internal?**

- Epidermis and dermis
- Dartos muscle—discontinuous smooth muscle layer immediately below the skin, surrounds entire shaft
- Adipose tissue—contains vessels and nerves
- Buck fascia—loose connective tissue that invests the erectile tissue and urethra
- Tunica albuginea—dense hyalinized connective tissue covering the corpora cavernosum
- Erectile tissues—corpora cavernosa ("dual and dorsal") and spongiosum (ventral)
- Urethra—located ventrally and surrounded by corpora spongiosum; divided into three regions: prostatic or proximal, membranous, and penile or distal urethra

The scrotum is made up of skin and underlying fibromuscular tissues that form the sac holding the testes and paratesticular structures. Along the midline of the scrotum lies the median raphe, which is the remnant of the fused genital fold. The layers of the scrotum are similar to those of the penis, traversing from the skin inward to dartos muscle, external spermatic fascia, cremasteric muscle, and internal spermatic fascia that interdigitates with the tunica vaginalis.[32]

INFLAMMATORY PATTERN

Scrotal Calcinosis

The finding of single, or often multiple, calcified nodules in the scrotal skin is called scrotal calcinosis. It is a benign condition that is thought to arise in the setting of resolved epidermal cysts that rupture or are otherwise traumatized and begin to calcify (Figures 5.81 and 5.82).[33] The calcific deposits are commonly surrounded by foreign-body giant cells, also suggesting a reparative/reactive process following epidermal cyst disruption (Figures 5.83 and 5.84). Not infrequently, intact remnants of epidermal inclusion cysts that remain are identifiable in the specimen.

Balanitis

> **FAQ: What Is Balanitis?**
>
> - Balanitis is a general clinical term used to describe inflammation of the penis, commonly associated with phimosis or the inability to retract the foreskin over the glans penis.
> - Two histopathologic entities associated with the clinical finding of balanitis are lichen sclerosus et atrophicus/balanitis xerotica obliterans and plasma cell balanitis (Zoon balanitis).

Lichen Sclerosus et Atrophicus/Balanitis Xerotica Obliterans

Lichen sclerosus et atrophicus (LSA), also known as balanitis xerotica obliterans (BXO), is a chronic dermatologic condition affecting the skin of the penis, most commonly the foreskin, glands, and meatal region. It is a relatively common condition affecting mostly older uncircumcised men, but also identified in children when associated with phimosis. Grossly, the early lesions are often multifocal pink or purple macules (flat lesions) that become raised papules. Over time, chronic lesions become white-gray smooth or irregular patches and may demonstrate erosion or ulceration.

The microscopic appearance of the early lesions shows vacuolar interface change with dyskeratosis, a variably thickened basement, and an associated lichenoid lymphocytic

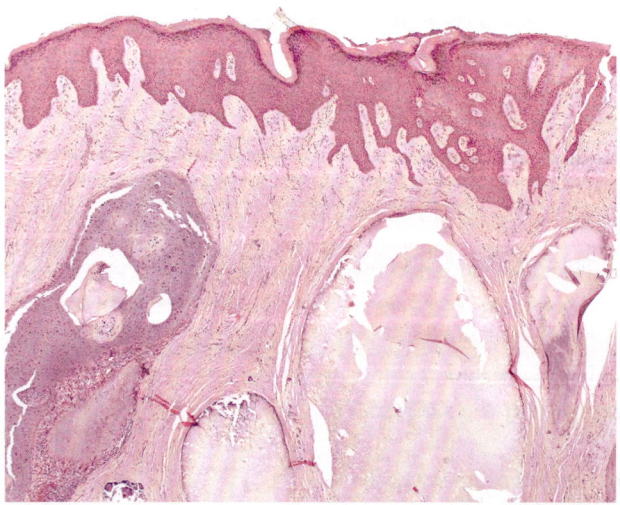

Figure 5.81. Scrotal calcinosis presents as firm nodules below the scrotal skin, which are freely mobile over the tunica. Histologically, the nodules are calcific deposits within the dermis and dartos muscle.

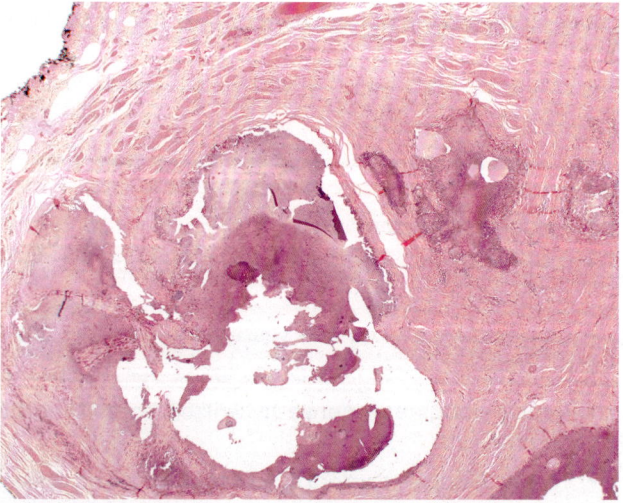

Figure 5.82. The basophilic nodules of scrotal calcinosis can vary in size from millimeters to many centimeters in greatest dimension. Although not pictured here, occasionally the remnants of epidermal inclusion cyst or other adnexal cystic structures can be appreciated.

infiltrate with variable papillary dermal edema (Figures 5.85-5.88). As the disease progresses, epidermal atrophy develops and the papillary dermis becomes fibrotic and homogenized, forming a pale band beneath the epithelium. The inflammatory infiltrate is displaced beneath the zone of fibrosis and is of variable intensity.

LSA is associated with the development of squamous cell dysplasia, usually well-differentiated penile intraepithelial neoplasia (PeIN) and non–HPV-related invasive squamous cell carcinoma (similar to the etiology of differentiated vulvar squamous cell carcinomas).[34,35] Penile LSA was associated with malignant proliferations in 5.8% of patients in a series of 86 men with genital LSA.[36]

FAQ: What Is the Preferred Terminology—Balanitis Xerotica Obliterans or Lichen Sclerosus et Atrophicus?

- The term balanitis xerotica obliterans (BXO) was first used to describe an inflammatory dermatosis of the penis
- However, to be consistent across tissue types, the term *lichen sclerosus et atrophicus* is preferred, as it encompasses both urologic and gynecologic lesions
- BXO is commonly used by urologists to describe the clinical appearance of these lesions; therefore, the term persists, and it may be useful to include BXO in diagnostic lines for familiarity

Plasma Cell Balanitis

Plasma cell balanitis, also known as Zoon balanitis or balanitis circumscripta plasmacellularis, occurs in uncircumcised older men and appears as shiny red-orange plaques on the glans or foreskin.[37] It is a chronic inflammatory condition, possibly due to localized irritation, although the exact underlying etiology is unknown. The gross lesions are nonspecific and raise the differential of benign processes like allergic contact dermatitis, psoriasis, and lichen planus. However, squamous cell carcinoma/Bowen disease can also have a similar gross appearance. The nature of the lesion can typically be sorted out on routine histology. The most consistent finding is the presence of a lichenoid infiltrate composed of lymphocytes and plasma cells. Early lesions may also show acanthosis, spongiosis, and parakeratosis. As the disease progresses, the epidermis becomes atrophic, sometimes with erosions and/or neutrophils in the epithelium. Later stages also show dermal fibrosis, and there may be subepidermal cleft formation (Figures 5.89-5.91).[37] The epithelium may demonstrate mild reactive atypia, which should not be overinterpreted as dysplastic or neoplastic. Treatment includes circumcision, laser therapy, or topical ointments.

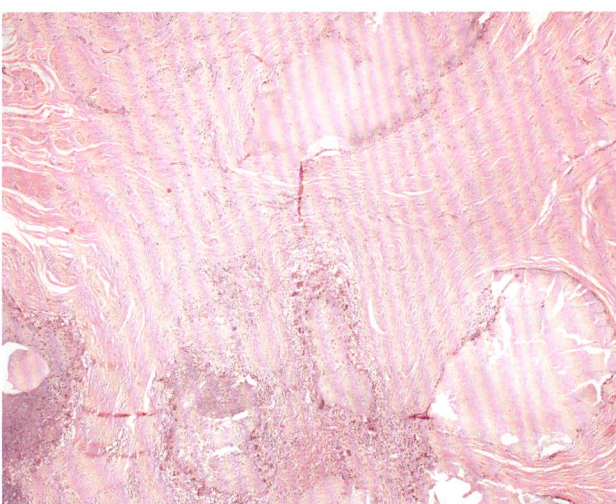

Figure 5.83. An inflammatory reaction is commonly identified surrounding the calcified material. In this image, both chronic inflammation and foreign-body giant cells are present.

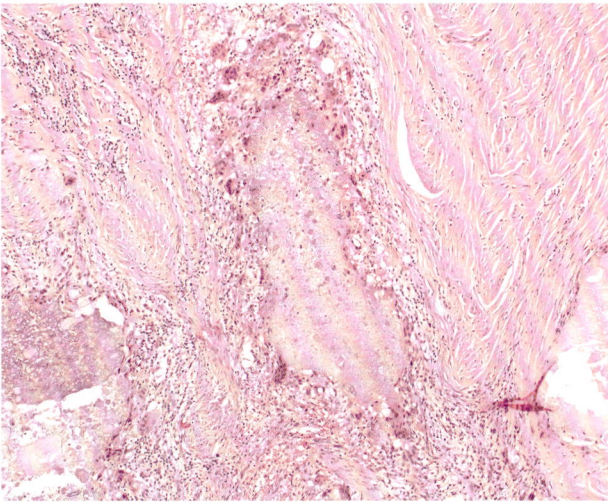

Figure 5.84. Robust histiocytic and foreign-body giant cell reaction is seen surrounding this nodule of scrotal calcinosis.

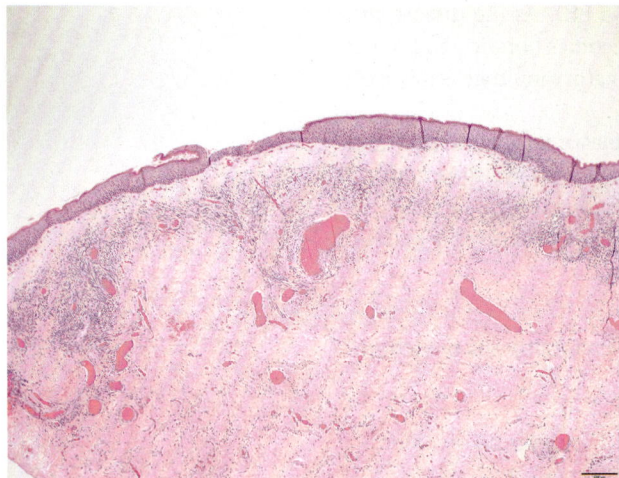

Figure 5.85. Lichen sclerosus et atrophicus (LSA)/balanitis xerotica obliterans (BXO), a synonym for lichen sclerosus et atrophicus, may show surface erosion or thinning of the epithelium.

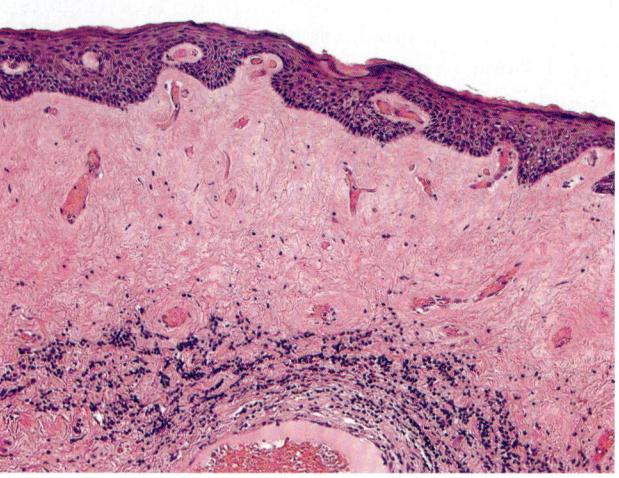

Figure 5.86. The classic diagnostic feature of LSA/BXO is the finding of a cleared out zone below the surface epithelium, and a band-like infiltrate of chronic inflammatory cells immediately below.

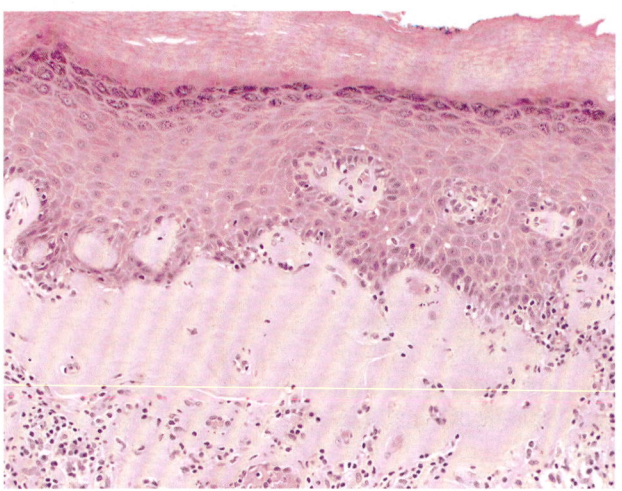

Figure 5.87. High-power examination of LSA/BXO highlights basal layer spongiosis and the densely hyalinized fibrosis below the epithelium.

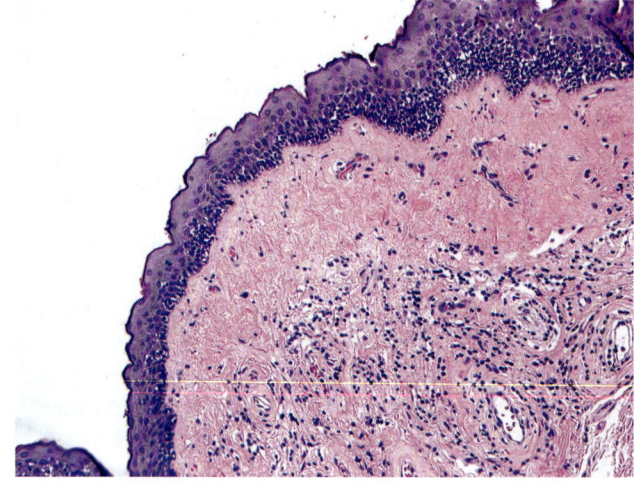

Figure 5.88. Another high-power image of LSA/BXO demonstrating cleared out an area of hyalinization and chronic inflammation. Another feature of this entity is the presence of dilated capillary vessels, present in the lower right of the image.

PEARLS AND PITFALLS: Plasma Cell–Rich Inflammation in the Genitourinary Tract

- The finding of a plasma cell–rich inflammatory infiltrate anywhere in the GU tract should raise the possibility of syphilis (Figures 5.92 and 5.93)
- Special stains for spirochetes should be employed in this differential diagnosis. The immunohistochemical stain for *Treponema pallidum* is more sensitive than the traditional Warthin-Starry and Steiner stains
- Immunohistochemistry for *Treponema pallidum* is not entirely specific, as it can cross-react with other spirochetes (Figure 5.94)
- Laboratory serologic testing with both nontreponemal and treponemal test is necessary for confirming the diagnosis of syphilis

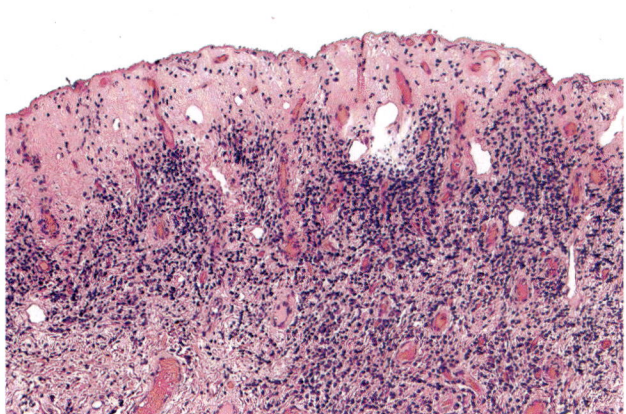

Figure 5.89. In this example of plasma cell balanitis, the surface epithelium is entirely eroded. A robust chronic inflammatory infiltrate is present in the lamina propria, comprising almost entirely of plasma cells. The differential diagnosis of a plasma cell–rich inflammatory dermatosis includes plasma cell balanitis and syphilis.

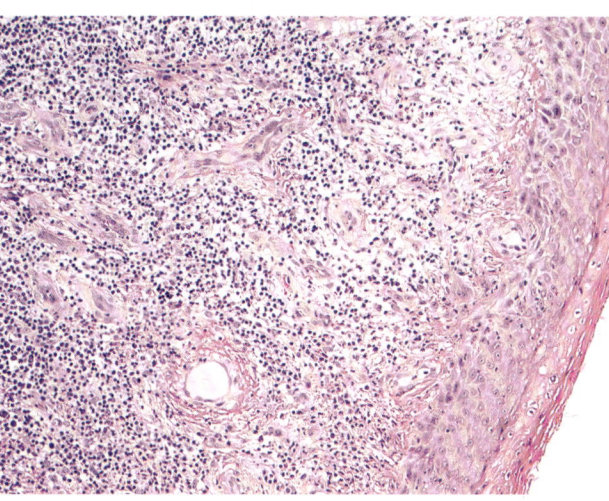

Figure 5.90. Another example of plasma cell balanitis at higher power, demonstrating diffuse infiltrating plasma cells. Spongiosis and parakeratosis of the epithelium are also present.

FAQ: What Are the Cystic Lesions of the Penis and Scrotum?

- Median raphe cyst—common; located ventrally on the penis ("parameatal cyst") or along the median line of the scrotum/perineum as a result of failed closure of the genital fold; epithelial lining may be squamous, columnar, urothelial, mucinous, ciliated, or some combination of these types (Figures 5.95-5.97)[38]

- Epidermal inclusion cyst—common; morphologically identical to EIC in other locations[39]

- Mucoid cyst—rare; located in distal penis, thought to arise from ectopic urethral mucosa and demonstrate columnar mucinous epithelium[40]

- Dermoid cyst—rare; morphologically similar to dermoid cysts located elsewhere, contains adnexal structures[41]

- Lymphatic cyst—exceedingly rare; one case described of a multilocular cyst containing thin fluid (Table 5.1)[42]

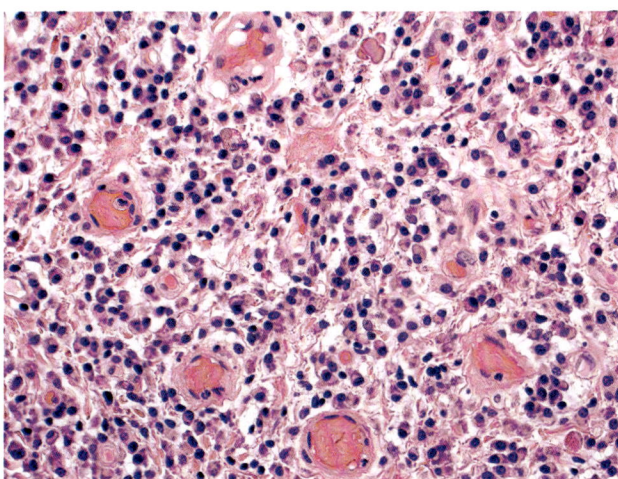

Figure 5.91. High-power image highlighting the near-complete prevalence of plasma cells in the inflammatory infiltrate. Before making a diagnosis of plasma cell balanitis, the diagnosis of syphilis should be considered.

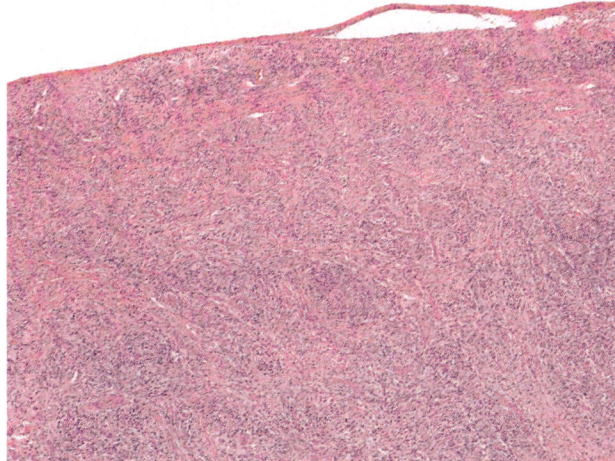

Figure 5.92. Deep and diffuse chronic inflammatory infiltrate is seen in this image, and in combination with the clinical history and gross appearance, syphilis was the leading differential diagnosis.

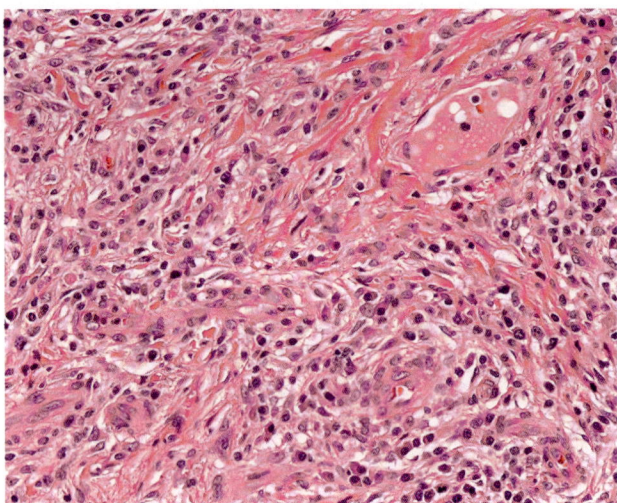

Figure 5.93. At higher power, the inflammatory infiltrate comprises predominantly plasma cells, which also suggests syphilis as a possible underlying cause.

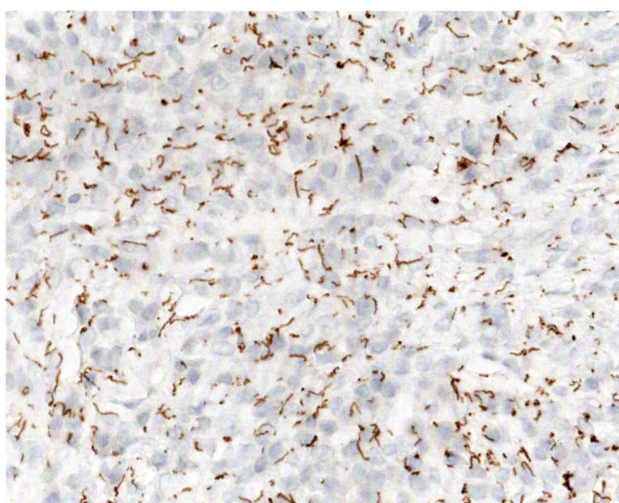

Figure 5.94. Immunohistochemistry for *Treponema pallidum* can be used to support the diagnosis; however, caution is warranted as the antibody can cross-react with other spirochetes. Confirmatory serologic testing is necessary for a definitive diagnosis of syphilis.

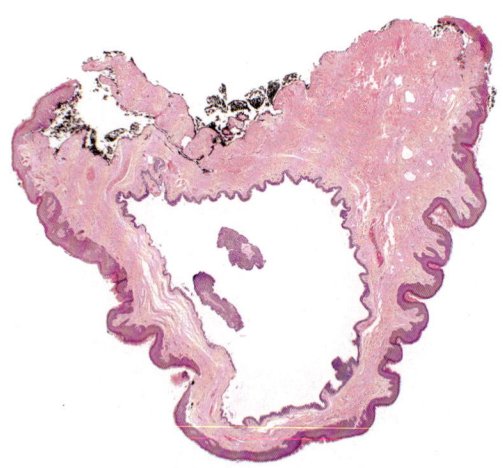

Figure 5.95. Median raphe cysts are located superficially and ventrally on the penis or along the median line of the scrotum and perineum. In this example of a median raphe cyst, a simple unilocular cyst is present within the dermis. These cysts may also be multilocular.

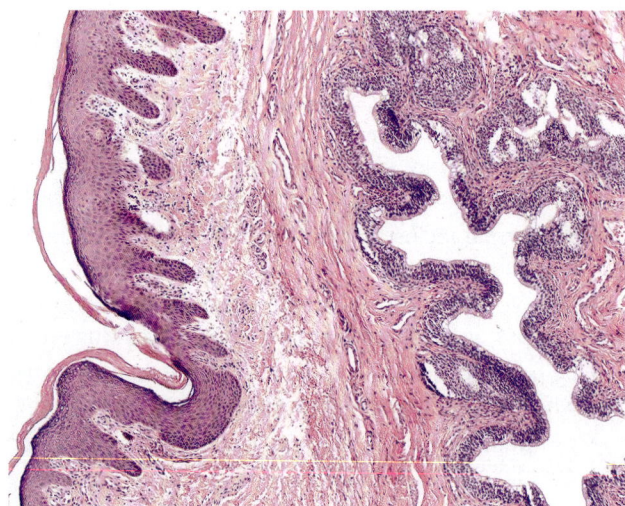

Figure 5.96. Median raphe cysts can have a variety of epithelial linings; this image depicts a median raphe cyst with mucinous epithelium. Other types of epithelium described in these cysts include urothelial, squamous, pseudostratified columnar, and ciliated.

SPINDLE PATTERN

Peyronie Disease

Peyronie disease is a form of superficial fibromatosis affecting the penile shaft, in the same family of lesions as palmar fibromatosis (Dupuytren contracture) and plantar fibromatosis. Trauma has been proposed as a possible etiology, but frequently men do not recall a specific injury. The lesions are usually recognized by the patient as a nodule that may lead to a curvature of the penis. It is a relatively common occurrence, identified in 8.9% of men screened for prostate cancer presenting without specific complaints related to penile functions.[43] The process involves abnormal fibrosis and thickening of the tunica albuginea surrounding the penile shaft. Histologically, the lesions comprise nodules of disorganized collagenous fibers, which may undergo ossification in the later stages.[44] A less common feature is the presence of a perivascular lymphoid infiltrate, particularly in early lesions.[45] Hemosiderin deposition is a common finding, which may be related to prior trauma (Figures 5.98 and 5.99).

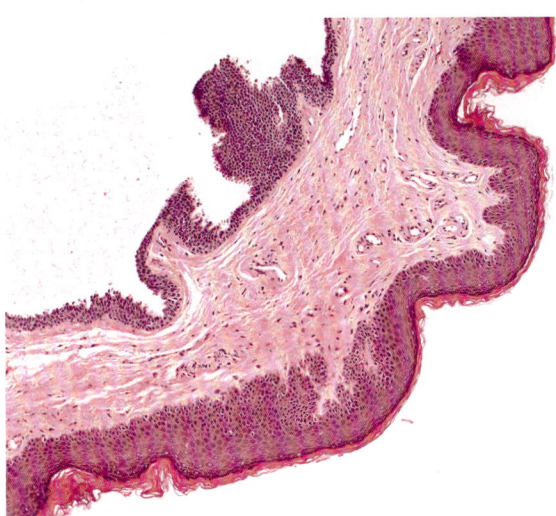

Figure 5.97. At higher power, the squamous epithelium of the penis is present on the right side of the image and the median raphe cyst shows urothelial epithelium.

Massive Localized Lymphedema

Massive localized lymphedema is a reactive pseudotumor arising in the setting of morbid obesity. It is most commonly associated with masses of the lower limbs, usually arising from the inner thigh.[46] However, this process has also been recognized to involve the external genitalia as well.[47] In a series of six patients, the masses involved the scrotum most

TABLE 5.1: Common Infectious Lesions of the Penis[92]

Disease	Infectious Agent	Clinical Presentation	Histologic Findings	Differential Diagnosis
Genital herpes	Herpes simplex virus, type 2 (most common)	Viral-like illness followed by genital vesicles that progress to pustules	Three M's: Multinucleation, Molding of nuclei, Marginated chromatin,	Lichen nitidus
Condyloma acuminata	Human papillomavirus	Exophytic, cauliflower-like growths	Papillary growth with hyperkeratosis and koilocytes (may be infrequent/absent)	Specific subtypes of PeIN and squamous cell carcinoma
Syphilis	*Treponema pallidum*	Chancre, ulcerated lesion	Prominent plasma cell reaction in early lesions. Late lesions include condyloma lata and gummas	Plasma cell balanitis
Fungal balanitis	*Candida albicans* (most common)	Mild burning and pruritis with erythema and thick discharge	Rarely biopsied. Fungal organisms with both hyphal and yeast forms present	Other infectious agents such as HSV, STI, allergic contact dermatitis

HSV, herpes simplex virus; PeIN, penile intraepithelial neoplasia commonly as diffuse edematous change. These masses can be massive, up to 55 cm in the genital cases and 71 cm in the lower limb. The histologic features include thickened, indurated skin overlying adipose tissue with edematous interlobular fibrous septa. Within the septa were fibroblasts that showed occasional multi- or binucleation. Chronic inflammation and dilated lymphatics were frequently identified. In the cases involving the scrotum and penis, hyperplasia and hypertrophy of the dartos muscle were identified in some cases.

Sclerosing Lipogranuloma

Sclerosing lipogranuloma, also referred to as "paraffinoma" or "Tancho nodule," is a pseudotumor occurring as a reaction to the injection of exogenous material under the skin. The penis is most commonly involved, but lesions of the scrotum, spermatic cord, and perineum have also been reported.[48] Mineral oil, paraffin, silicone, and wax are most commonly used. The lesions present as a deformity of the penis with associated pain with intercourse. Grossly, the nodules are located in the subcutis and the penile skin may be fixed to the nodule.[49] The key histologic features of sclerosing lipogranuloma are the identification of intact fat globules and fat necrosis surrounded by histiocytic reaction, often with giant cells (Figures 5.100-5.102). Spindle-shaped fibrosis makes up the sclerosing portion of the lesion. Associated chronic inflammation is common. Depending on the location, the differential diagnosis of sclerosing lipogranuloma includes adenomatoid tumor (in a paratesticular mass), liposarcoma (spermatic cord), or lymphangioma.

Cellular Angiofibroma

Cellular angiofibromas are painless, circumscribed nodules usually identified in the subcutaneous tissue of the scrotum or inguinal area of older men. They comprise spindle cells within a fibrous or edematous stroma with wispy collagen. A key feature is the presence of numerous small to medium-sized thick-walled vessels. Fibrin thrombi, fibrinoid changes, and hyalinization are commonly identified in the vessel, a classic feature of this entity (Figures 5.103-5.105). Mitotic figures are generally infrequent. Atypical mitotic figures and necrosis are not acceptable features for this diagnosis. Although they are relatively circumscribed, infiltrative pattern may be demonstrated with entrapped fat present at the peripheral edges of the mass. Once completely excised, these tumors do not tend to recur.[50]

Cellular angiofibromas can often be diagnosed by H&E alone with the classic features of a well-circumscribed nodule with bland spindle cells and thick-walled vessels. However, if there is uncertainty about the diagnosis, a limited panel of immunohistochemical stains may be helpful. These lesions are usually positive for CD34 and also commonly express estrogen and progesterone receptors (Figures 5.106 and 5.107). They are desmin negative, which helps distinguish them from aggressive angiomyxoma that can also occur in this area.[51]

KEY FEATURES: Cellular Angiofibroma

- Occurs in inguinal/scrotal region of older men
- Painless, well-circumscribed nodule in superficial subcutaneous tissue
- Hypercellular bland, spindle-shaped lesion with wispy collagen
- Small to medium-sized thick-walled vessels
- Vessels may have fibrin thrombi, hyalinization, or fibrinoid change
- Mitotic figures are rare
- Usually express CD34, ER, and PR; desmin negative
- Indolent behavior, do not recur after complete excision

Aggressive Angiomyxoma

In contrast to cellular angiofibroma, aggressive angiomyxomas are usually large, occur in deep locations, and are not well circumscribed. Given their large size and inguinoscrotal location, the bulging mass may mimic a hernia. Histologically, these are hypocellular, infiltrative masses with bland spindle and stellate cells present within a true myxoid stroma. A key feature in this entity is the presence of a haphazard arrangement of small to medium-sized blood vessels, some of which demonstrate thickened walls or hyalinization.[52]

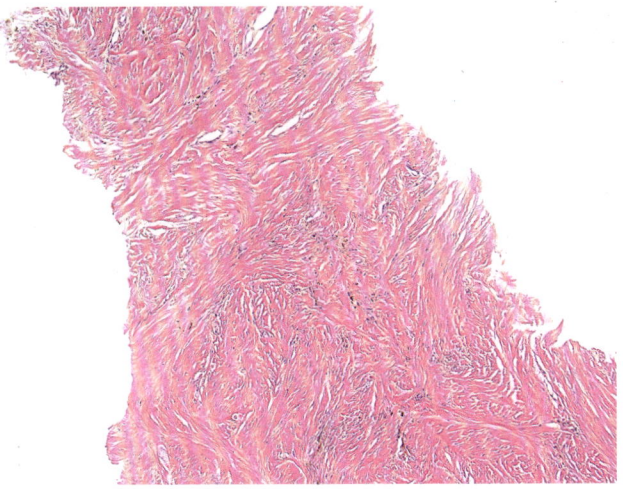

Figure 5.98. Superficial fibromatosis of the penis (Peyronie disease) is demonstrated here with abnormal fibrosis of the tunica albuginea. These lesions comprise haphazardly arranged collagen fibers and are usually very hypocellular. Scattered hemosiderin deposition is considered evidence of prior trauma.

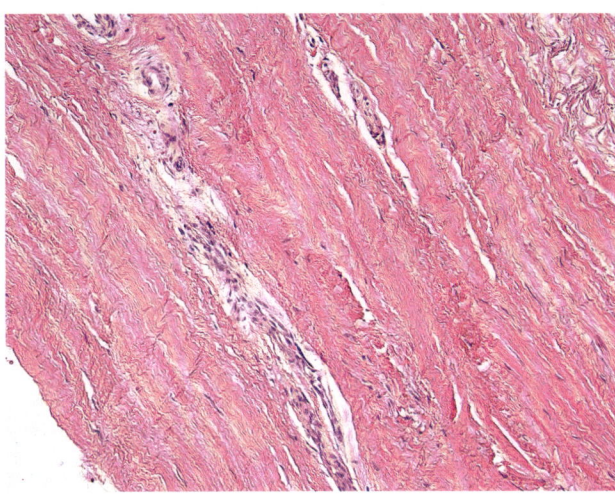

Figure 5.99. Higher power image demonstrating the hypocellular collagen fibers and areas of lymphocytic perivascular infiltrate seen in Peyronie disease.

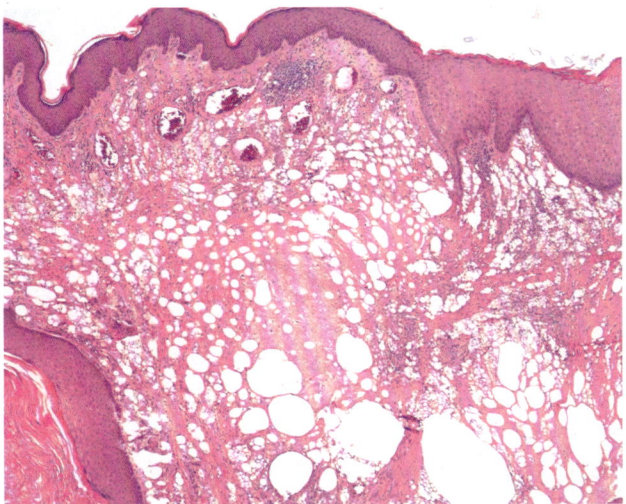

Figure 5.100. Sclerosing lipogranuloma results from the injection of exogenous material, such as paraffin, mineral oil, silicone, or wax, under the skin. The resulting histologic findings are subcutaneous vacuoles of varying sizes with surrounding fat necrosis and foreign-body giant cell reaction.

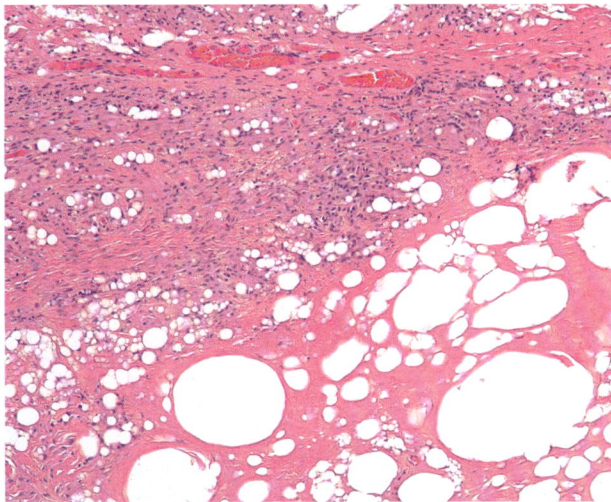

Figure 5.101. In this example of sclerosing lipogranuloma, fat necrosis is evident in the lower right-hand corner and surrounding histiocytic reaction with intracytoplasmic fat vacuoles throughout the rest of the field. The "sclerosing" component of the lesion comprises spindle-shaped fibroblasts within the mass.

Scattered chronic inflammatory cells, including mast cells, may be present[13] (Figure 5.108). In contrast to cellular angiofibromas, the spindle cells are consistently desmin positive; however, one must use caution as ER and PR show variable positivity and can confound the diagnosis. Establishing the correct diagnosis of aggressive angiomyxoma is important, because these lesions have locally aggressive behavior and may recur.

Angiomyofibroblastoma

First described in the vulva, angiomyofibroblastomas are less commonly identified in males but may occur in the superficial perineal soft tissue. These are usually less than 5 cm, well-circumscribed nodules with a thin pseudocapsule. Histologically, they demonstrate areas of hyper- and hypocellularity within an edematous background. The stromal cells are spindle-shaped to rounded and may aggregate around vessels. Thin-walled capillary-sized vessels (in contrast to the thickened, hyalinized vessels in the two lesions above) are a key feature of this entity. While circumscription is the rule in this lesion, fat may be identified within the mass. Desmin and actin expression is common in this lesion, unlike cellular angiofibroma in which these markers are only rarely positive.

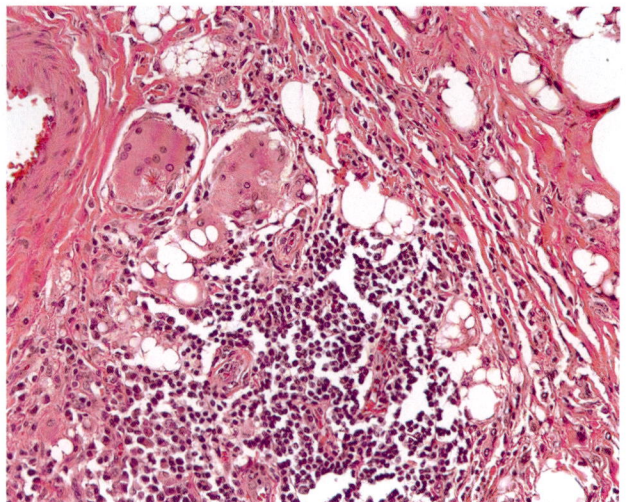

Figure 5.102. Chronic inflammation and foreign-body giant cells are commonly identified in sclerosing lipogranuloma as a reaction to exogenous material.

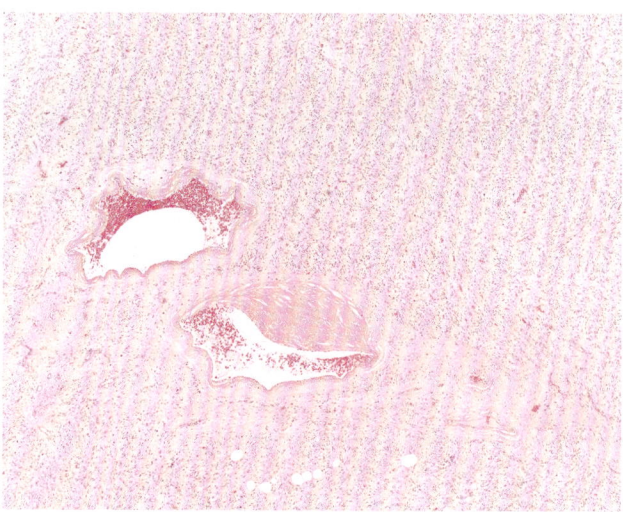

Figure 5.103. Cellular angiofibromas are well-circumscribed myofibroblastic neoplasms with a prominent vascular component. Medium-sized vessels with fibrinoid change are common features, with numerous small vessels in the background of a bland spindle cell proliferation. Mature adipose tissue may be seen at the peripheral edge of the lesion.

FAQ: What Are the Defining Features of Scrotal Leiomyoma?

- Scrotal leiomyomas are very rare benign smooth muscle neoplasms involving scrotal skin or dartos muscle
- Leiomyomas arising in the skin are classified as leiomyoma cutis and may be further divided into pilar leiomyoma (adnexal smooth muscle) and angioleiomyoma (vascular smooth muscle)[32]
- Those arising in the dartos are called dartoic leiomyoma
- Most common features are that of leiomyoma elsewhere—circumscribed lesion with fascicular growth of smooth muscle
- Cytologic features include cigar-shaped nuclei with abundant eosinophilic cytoplasm
- While no hypercellularity, necrosis, increased mitotic figures, or infiltrative growth is accepted in this lesion, there may be symplastic features with bizarre nuclei[53]
- Symplastic features include hyperchromasia, pleomorphic nuclei, and macronucleoli
- Differential diagnosis includes leiomyosarcoma, and this diagnosis is favored if there is increased mitotic activity or tumor cell necrosis

Myointimoma

Myointimomas are rare lesions but discussed here because they occur almost exclusively in the corpus spongiosum of the penis. They are benign lesions arising from the myointimal layer of blood vessels that grow intravascularly. Histologically, the tumors comprise bland spindle cell proliferations growing in a plexiform pattern within vessels.[54,55] The cells demonstrate abundant eosinophilic cytoplasm, consistent with a myofibroblastic appearance (Figures 5.109 and 5.110). Myxoid stroma is frequently identified. Because the corpus spongiosum is so highly vascular, the lesion can grow within the entire vascular network forming a nodular growth pattern. Smooth muscle actin is diffusely expressed in the myofibroblastic cells, whereas desmin will highlight the residual native vessel wall (Figure 5.111). Consistent with their indolent and benign nature, these masses do not recur, even with incomplete excision.

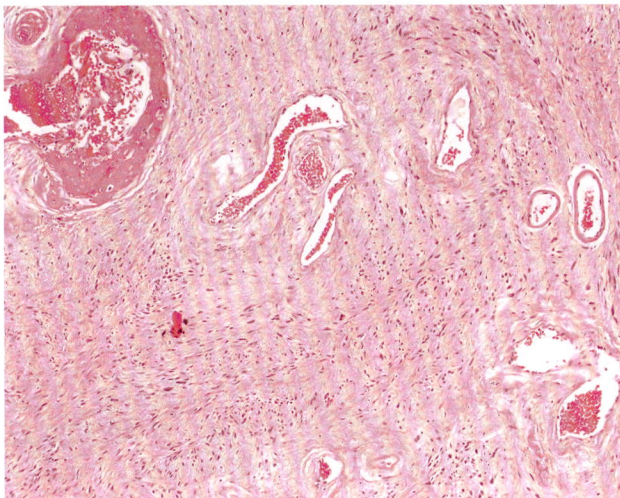

Figure 5.104. At higher power, the numerous and variably sized vessels in this cellular angiofibroma are helpful diagnostic features.

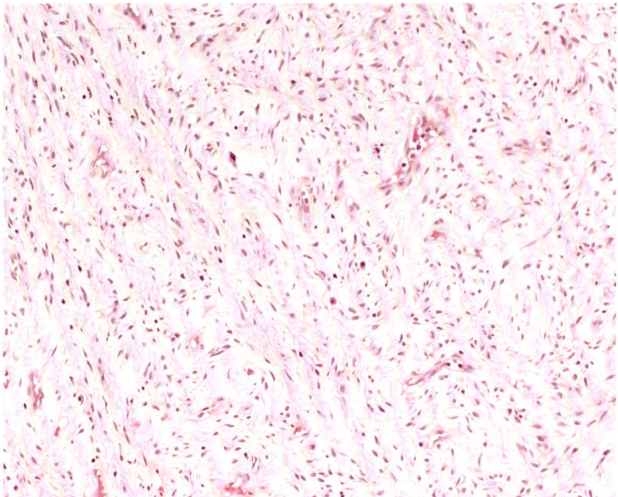

Figure 5.105. Cytologic features of the myofibromatous component in a cellular angiofibroma include monotonous spindle cells with tapered nuclei, without increased mitotic figures or necrosis. These cells are arranged haphazardly within a loose fibrous stroma.

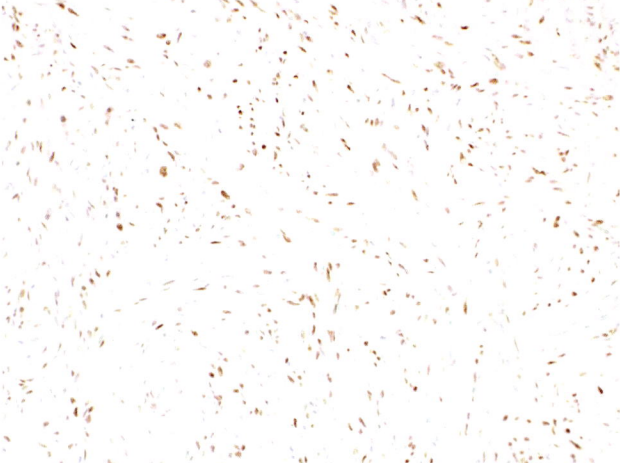

Figure 5.106. In addition to marking with CD34 as indication of their myofibroblastic origin, approximately one-third of cellular angiofibromas also express estrogen receptor.

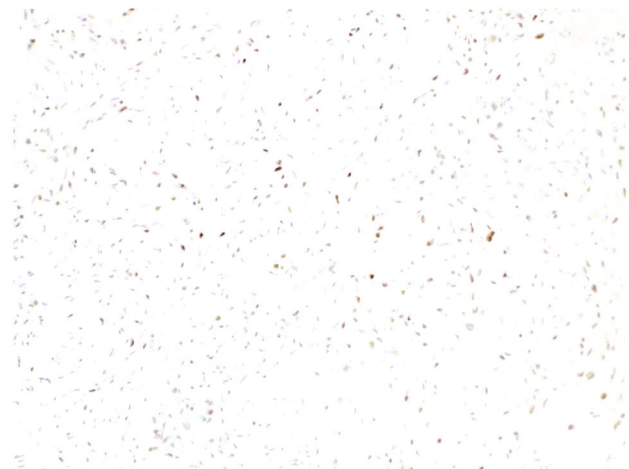

Figure 5.107. Progesterone receptor expression is identified in about half of cellular angiofibromas.

Sarcomatoid Carcinoma

In the penis or external genitalia, a malignant spindle cell neoplasm arising in a superficial location may represent a primary sarcoma or a sarcomatoid carcinoma. Malignant biphasic mesothelioma is also in the differential but has been discussed in the prior section and is usually more paratesticular in location. Although some locations may favor one or the other (for example, in the bladder a sarcomatoid carcinoma is much more likely than a primary sarcoma), sarcomatoid carcinoma arising as a subtype of squamous cell carcinoma may be favored if the lesion appears to be centered in the skin. In a series of 15 sarcomatoid squamous cell carcinomas, gross features included large, polypoid tumors that were frequently ulcerated.[56] Cytologic features include a predominant population of high-grade spindle cells arranged in fascicles. Increased mitotic figures and necrosis were common in the tumors (Figures 5.112-5.114). By immunohistochemistry, the majority of spindled cells expressed high-molecular-weight cytokeratin and p63, consistent with a carcinoma of squamous origin (Figure 5.115). The diffuse expression of vimentin is also consistent with the mesenchymal transformation of this tumor and should not be used to support a diagnosis of primary sarcoma given its lack of specificity. Inguinal metastases are common, and the prognosis of these tumors is uniformly bad.

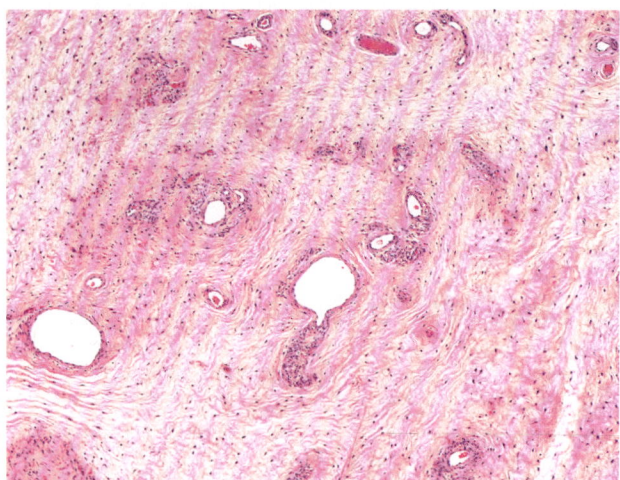

Figure 5.108. Aggressive angiomyxomas are usually large, infiltrative, poorly circumscribed neoplasms rarely identified in the scrotum or deep perineum, and similar in appearance to its gynecologic counterpart. Bland spindle to stellate with minimal atypia are present within a variably myxoid stroma. Small to medium-sized vessels are prominent throughout the lesion.

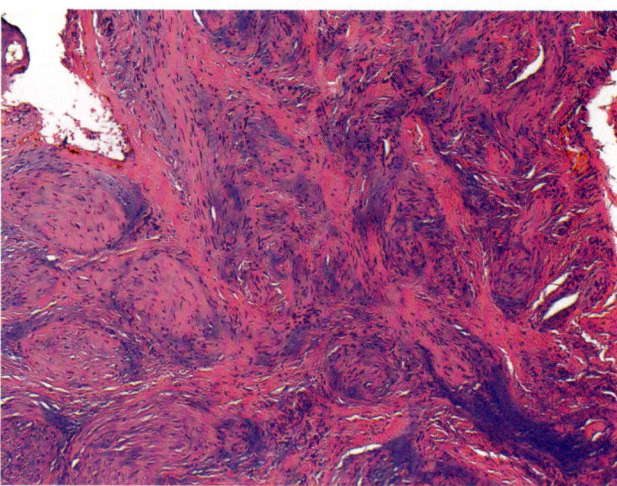

Figure 5.109. Myointimoma demonstrating a plexiform growth pattern of bland spindle cells and myxoid stroma.

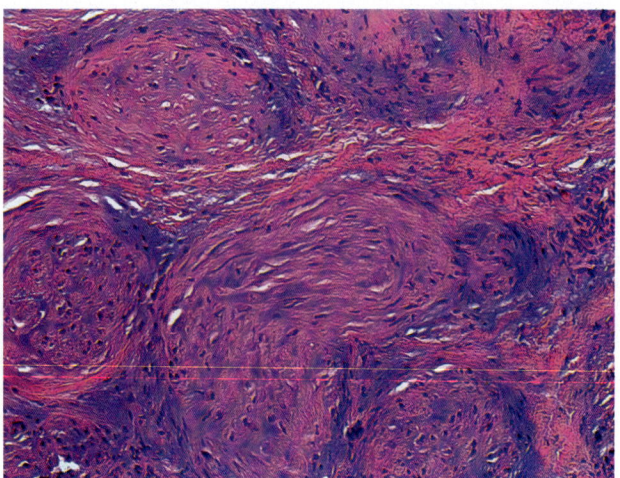

Figure 5.110. At higher power, the bland cytologic features of the myofibroblastic proliferation of myointimoma are evident within the vascular network of the corpus spongiosum of the penis.

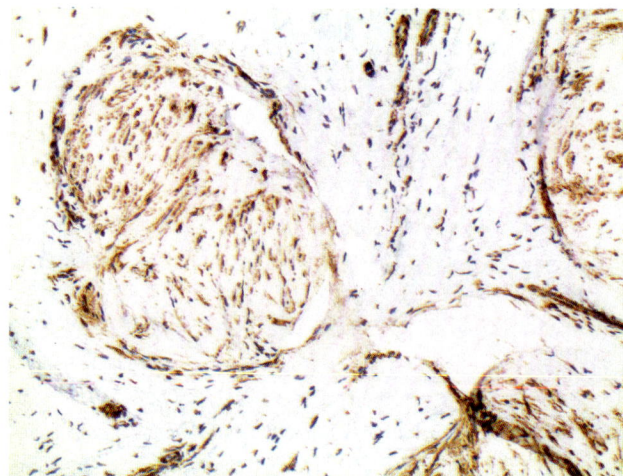

Figure 5.111. Smooth muscle actin highlights the myofibroblastic cells in this myointimoma.

PAPILLARY/EXOPHYTIC PATTERN

Fibroepithelial Polyp/Acrochordon

Often referred to as skin tags, fibroepithelial polyps may occur on any area of the skin but are frequently identified in areas with skin folds, including the groin. These are benign skin lesions, although they are frequently excised for cosmetic reasons due to irritation from clothing or rubbing. Both grossly and microscopically fibroepithelial polyps show fibrovascular cores lined by flattened squamous epithelium. The stroma is often collagenized and vascular, and possibly contain adipose tissue. If they have been irritated or picked by the patient, ischemic necrosis or surface ulceration may be apparent. They can grow to multiple centimeters in greatest dimension, sometimes associated with condom catheters; the large size may raise concern for a condyloma or possibly squamous cell carcinoma.[57,58] However, once excised, they rarely recur.

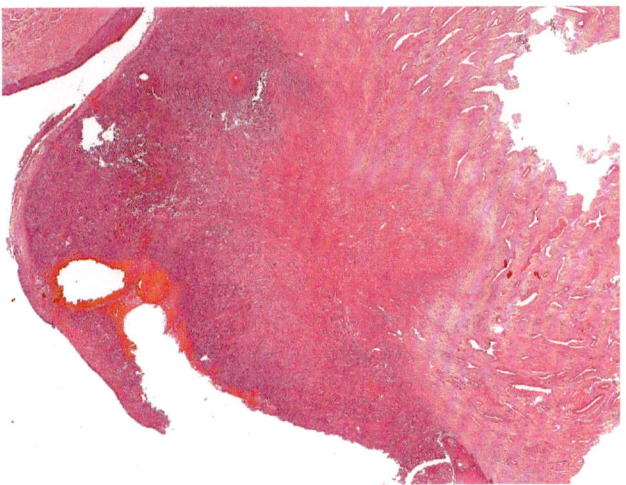

Figure 5.112. Low-power image of sarcomatoid carcinoma of the penis, which shows both a superficial and deep component, involving the corpora cavernosum.

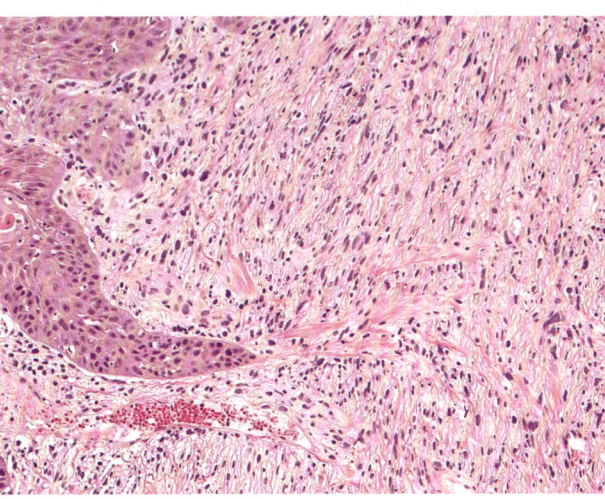

Figure 5.113. In this example of sarcomatoid carcinoma, a focus of usual squamous cell carcinoma is present (upper left) in a background of malignant spindle cells. When both components are present, the diagnosis of sarcomatoid carcinoma is relatively straightforward. However, when only the sarcomatoid component is sampled, the astute pathologist must consider sarcomatoid carcinoma in addition to sarcoma.

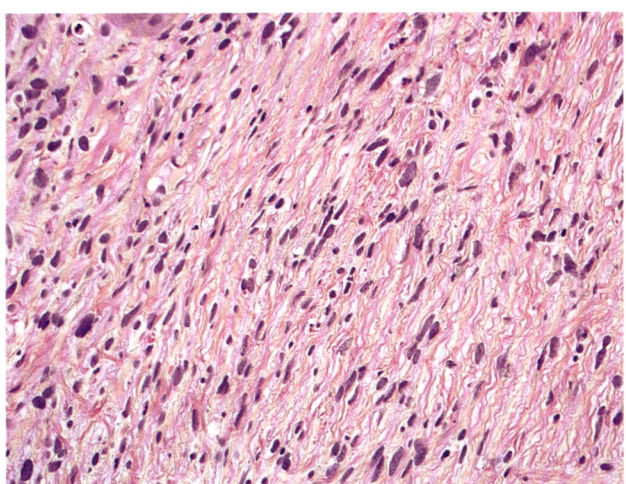

Figure 5.114. High-power image of malignant spindle cells in a sarcomatoid carcinoma. Cells are spindle-shaped to epithelioid, with marked nuclear pleomorphism.

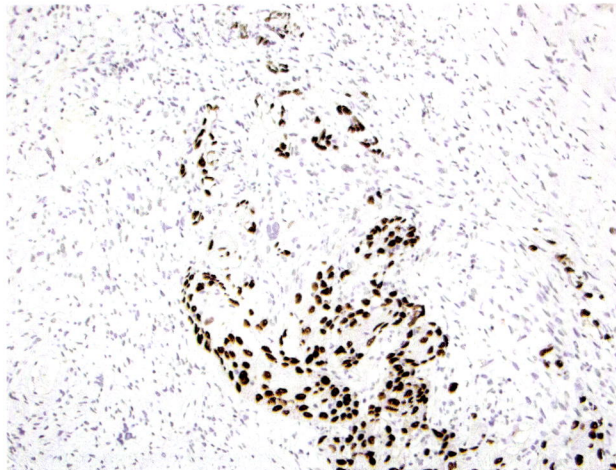

Figure 5.115. Nuclear expression of p63 in this sarcomatoid carcinoma supports a squamous origin for the tumor.

Angiokeratoma

Angiokeratomas of the scrotum arise in two clinical scenarios: angiokeratoma corporis diffusum, associated with genetic enzyme abnormalities, and angiokeratomas of Fordyce. Angiokeratomas of Fordyce are sporadic lesions localized to the scrotum.[59] Conversely, angiokeratoma corporis diffusum the lesions can occur diffusely, most commonly involving the lower trunk, buttocks, and thighs, and are associated with an inborn metabolic error.[60] Grossly, angiokeratomas present as multiple dark blue or red papules stuck on the skin, which may bleed easily. Both lesions are histologically similar and comprise benign vascular proliferations of dilated, ectatic vessels with overlying hyperkeratosis (Figures 5.116 and 5.117).

Condyloma Acuminatum

Condyloma acuminatum is a human papillomavirus (HPV)–related squamous proliferation, most closely associated with HPV types 6 and 11. Infection of the squamous epithelium by HPV results in warty growths, commonly arising in a multifocal manner in the anogenital region. They frequently involve the penile shaft, foreskin, glans, and coronal sulcus.

Histologically, these growths are recognized by their complex papillomatous growth pattern and hyperplastic squamous epithelium (Figures 5.118-5.121). The cytologic hallmark of condyloma acuminatum is the koilocyte, a virally infected cell with a large, cavitary perinuclear halo and hyperchromatic raisinoid nucleus. Koilocytes may be binucleated. Importantly, the base of the lesion is sharply defined without evidence of irregular infiltrative growth. Occasionally, seborrheic keratosis-like lesions are identified as plaque-like lesions and surface epithelium containing horn pseudocysts and acanthosis.[61] A subset of these lesions has been associated with low-risk HPV subtypes.[62]

CHECKLIST: Condyloma Acuminatum Versus Giant Condyloma[63]

	Condyloma Acuminatum	Giant Condyloma
Demographics	Younger, sexually active males (third decade of life)	Older men (third to fifth decades of life)
Location	Any anogenital site	Penis and anorectum
Pattern of growth	Exophytic	Endophytic and exophytic
HPV association	Low-risk subtypes (HPV 6, 11)	Low-risk subtypes (HPV 6, 11)
Size	Usually less than 2-3 cm	5-10 cm
Histologic features	Verrucous growth with fibrovascular cores lined by mild hyperkeratosis	Downward endophytic growth of fibrovascular cores with rounded, pushing deep border
Cytologic features	Koilocytes in a background of maturing squamous epithelium (may be absent in seborrheic keratosis-like lesions)	Numerous koilocytes present; malignant foci may be present in deeper areas
Prognosis	Good; negligible risk of malignancy	Tends to recur, is locally destructive, and may progress to invasive carcinoma

PEARLS AND PITFALLS: Differential Diagnosis of "Warty" Lesions of the External Genitalia[63]

- Condyloma acuminatum
- Giant condyloma
- Verruca vulgaris
- Verruciform xanthoma
- Seborrheic keratosis
- Angiokeratoma
- Fibroepithelial polyp
- Papillary squamous cell carcinoma
- Verrucous carcinoma
- Warty/Warty-basaloid PeIN
- Invasive Warty/Warty-basaloid squamous cell carcinoma

FAQ: What Is the Definition of and Best Terminology for Precursor Squamous Lesions of the External Genitalia?

- There are a variety of terms to describe full-thickness dysplasia of the squamous epithelium in the absence of invasive carcinoma
- The terminology has evolved over time, and references in the literature may be confusing
- The WHO-accepted terminology for these precancerous lesions is penile intraepithelial neoplasia (PeIN), with subtypes based on the morphology described below
- Older terms include squamous cell carcinoma in situ, high-grade dysplasia, squamous intraepithelial lesion, Bowen disease, erythroplasia of Queyrat
- For consistency, it is recommended to use the PeIN system

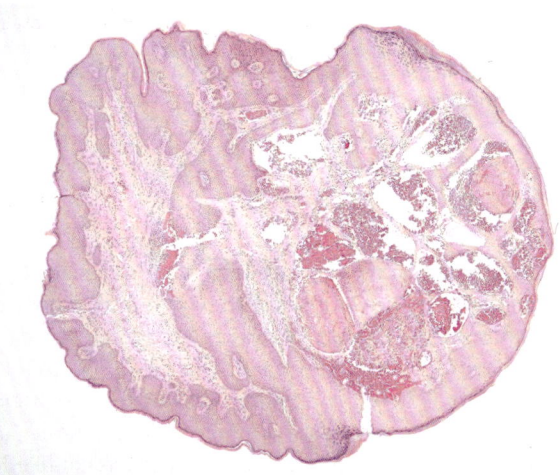

Figure 5.116. Angiokeratomas occur on the scrotum as dark blue or red papules and often present with bleeding. They are polypoid to papillary in architecture as shown in this low-power image.

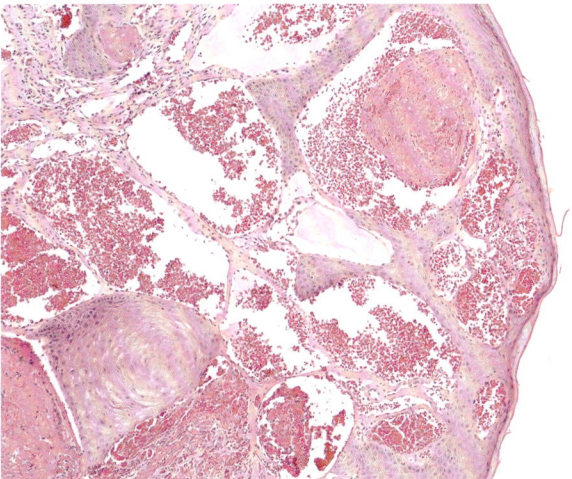

Figure 5.117. Angiokeratomas comprise dilated blood vessels that may contain fibrin thrombi and invaginations of squamous epithelium with hyperkeratosis.

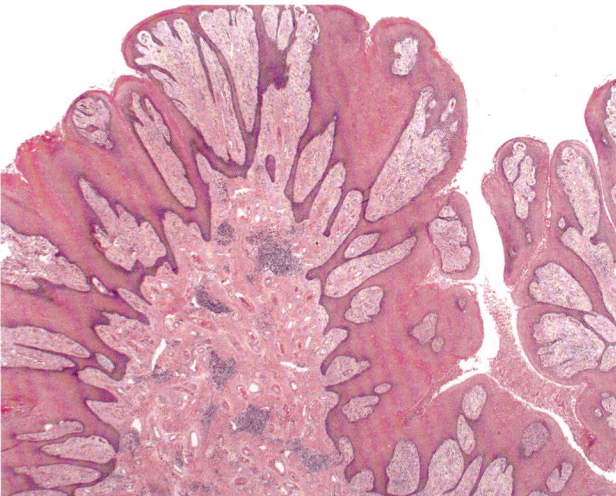

Figure 5.118. Condylomas are common papillary/verrucous lesions of the genital region associated with HPV. The finding of complex, spiky papillary projections and overlying hyperkeratosis is classic for this lesion.

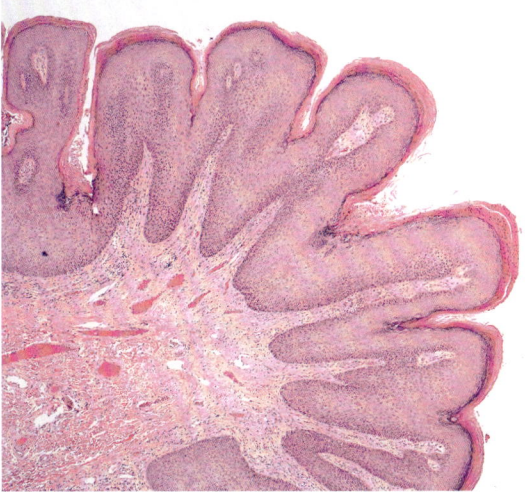

Figure 5.119. Another example of condyloma demonstrating the papillomatous architecture. There are hyperkeratosis and a prominent granular layer evident in this image. The base of the papillae is smooth and continuous, with no evidence of invasion.

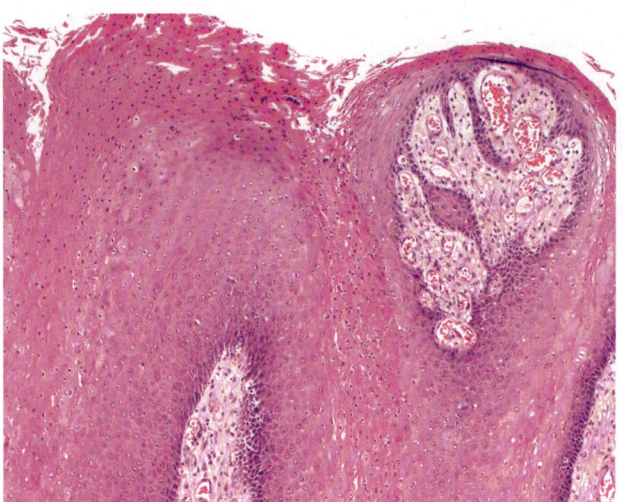

Figure 5.120. At high power, several features of condyloma are identified in this image—epithelium that matures to the surface with hyperkeratosis, and acanthosis, with scattered koilocytes.

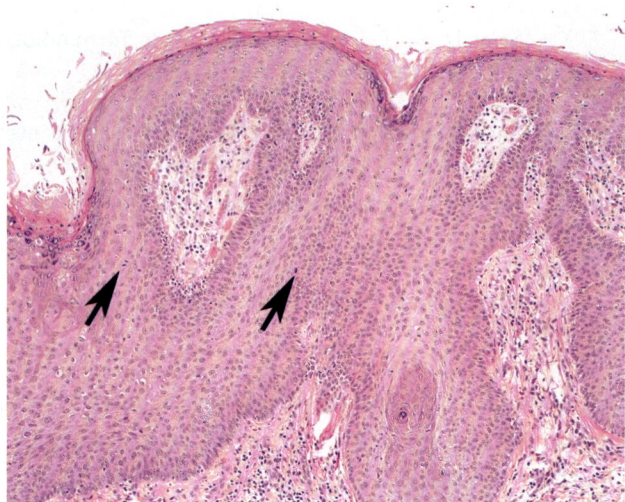

Figure 5.121. In this example of condyloma, scattered mitotic figures are present, which is permissible given that they are basally oriented. With tangential sectioning, it is important to orient to the base of the epithelium lining the papillary core, which may mimic a higher level mitosis.

Bowenoid Papulosis

Bowenoid papulosis is a multifocal HPV-associated disease involving the anogenital region. The disease most commonly occurs in sexually active young adults, and high-risk HPV subtypes are most prevalent. The terminology may be confused with Bowen disease, which is another term for PeIN. Bowenoid lesions rarely progress to invasive carcinoma and may regress on their own; at the most, local therapy or topical treatments are used.[64] Given that the overall prognosis of Bowenoid papulosis is good, it is important to use the correct terminology and ensure the clinical impression is consistent with Bowenoid papulosis. To confuse the issue, the histologic features of Bowenoid papulosis overlap with basaloid PeIN (Bowen disease). In one series, the most useful feature for distinguishing the two entities was the finding of maturation and sparing of the follicular epithelium from atypia.[64]

The penile shaft is the most frequently involved site, but any anogenital skin may be involved. Grossly, Bowenoid papulosis demonstrates multiple red or flesh-colored papules. This multifocality is one of the most useful clinical features to distinguish between Bowenoid papulosis and PeIN. On microscopic examination, the epithelium is dysplastic. However, the dysplastic foci may be limited to scattered single cells with high nuclear to cytoplasmic ratio to full-thickness atypia similar to squamous cell carcinoma in situ (Figures 5.122 and 5.123).[65] The presence of koilocytosis is a helpful feature and is identified in the majority of cases. There may be a deposition of melanin throughout the epithelium in some cases. If morphologic features alone are not diagnostic of Bowenoid papulosis, immunohistochemistry for p16 may be useful. The finding of diffuse, strong p16 expression supports a diagnosis of Bowenoid papulosis versus a reactive, nondysplastic process.[66] p16 immunohistochemistry does not help to distinguish Bowenoid papulosis from HPV-related PeIN, which requires clinical correlation and assessment of the gross lesion for an accurate diagnosis.

Verrucous Carcinoma

Another exophytic lesion identified in the penile and scrotal skin is verrucous carcinoma. This is a very well-differentiated squamous cell carcinoma with a broad-based, warty or verrucous growth pattern closely resembling condyloma. Despite their invasive nature, these tumors have a good prognosis and rarely metastasize. Recurrences are not uncommon, especially with incomplete excision. These tumors are not considered to be HPV related and are categorized as such in the latest World Health Organization monograph.[67]

The histologic features of verrucous carcinoma include a combination of both exophytic papillomatous architecture and endophytic, pushing borders with sharp demarcation

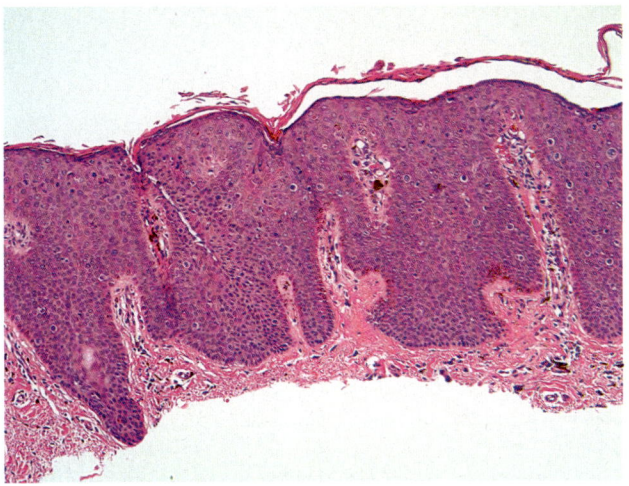

Figure 5.122. Bowenoid papulosis demonstrates dysplastic epithelium that is morphologically similar to basaloid PeIN/squamous cell carcinoma in situ. The epithelium shows a lack of maturation and full-thickness atypia. Clinical correlation is necessary to exclude the possibility of basaloid PeIN.

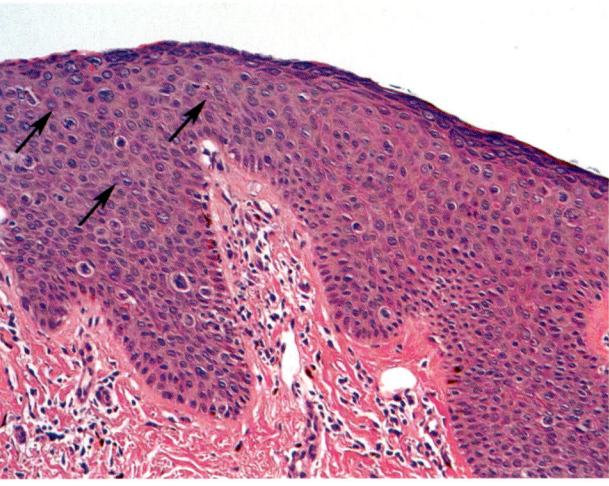

Figure 5.123. At high power, this example of Bowenoid papulosis shows dysplastic epithelium with numerous large atypical cells and several mitotic figures. Melanin may be deposited throughout the epithelium as seen here (arrows).

between tumor and stroma. The surface often demonstrates a spiky "church-spire" appearance with hyperkeratosis and acanthosis (Figure 5.124). The squamous cells have abundant glassy cytoplasm with minimal nuclear atypia, giving an overall low nuclear to cytoplasmic ratio (Figures 5.125 and 5.126).[68] The prognosis of verrucous carcinoma is related to the depth of invasion, which is measured from the nucleated surface of the tumor to the deepest point of invasion.

The well-differentiated epithelium and lack of irregular, infiltrating borders in verrucous carcinoma lead to considerable morphologic overlap with condyloma. However, verrucous carcinoma will lack the koilocytosis seen in condyloma.[63] Consistent with their lack of association with HPV, these tumors do not express p16 or show evidence of low-risk HPV infection.[69,70]

Papillary Squamous Cell Carcinoma

One of the non–HPV-related variants of invasive squamous cell carcinoma is papillary squamous cell carcinoma. It is also well differentiated and lacks koilocytosis, similar to verrucous carcinoma. Consistent with their lack of HPV association, these tumors are frequently

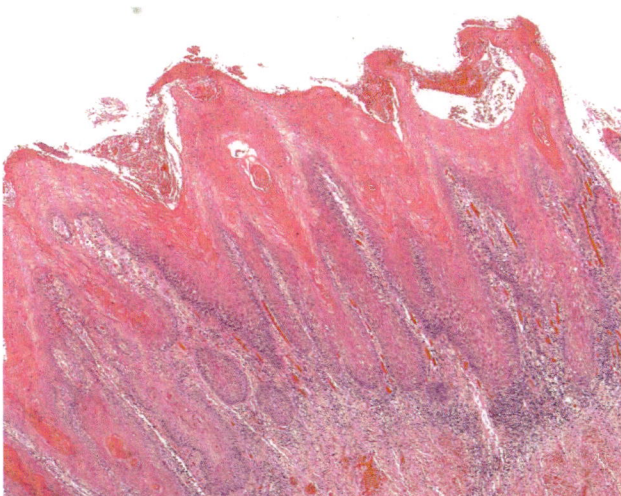

Figure 5.124. Verrucous carcinoma is a diagnostically difficult lesion that can mimic condyloma. Key features to identify verrucous carcinoma are a combination of both exophytic and endophytic growth, with pushing borders.

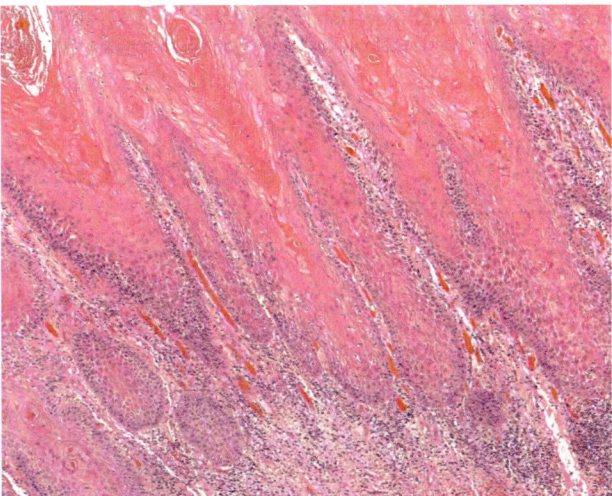

Figure 5.125. At higher power, the downward endophytic growth pattern of this verrucous carcinoma is evident. Compare with condyloma (Figures 5.118 and 5.119), which has a smoother epithelial–stromal interface without downward growth.

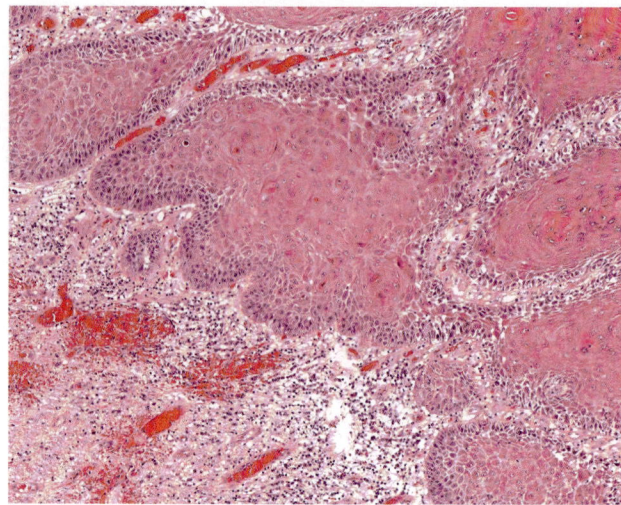

Figure 5.126. The epithelium in verrucous carcinoma is remarkably well differentiated and lacks overt atypia. Nests of the epithelium at the base of this verrucous carcinoma are consistent with a pushing border and infiltrative nature of the lesion. Chronic inflammation is a common finding at the base of the lesion.

identified in patients with lichen sclerosus. The behavior of these tumors is generally indolent; they may recur, but metastasis is rarely reported.[71]

Papillary squamous carcinomas usually involve the penile glans and demonstrate exophytic, papillary growths that can be quite large. The surface is irregular, as well as the tumor base that will demonstrate a more irregular, invasive interface when compared to verrucous carcinoma. The histologic features include irregular papillae of varying heights and some fibrovascular cores.[35,72] The squamous epithelium is hyperkeratotic, well differentiated with maturation, and lacks koilocytes, distinguishing it from condyloma acuminatum. Adjacent surface epithelium may demonstrate differentiated PeIN or lichen sclerosus.[72]

KEY FEATURES: HPV-Related Exophytic Subtypes of Invasive Squamous Cell Carcinoma

- Warty carcinomas have spiky, cauliflower-like projections similar to condyloma lined by well- to moderately differentiated squamous cells with koilocytic change
- Warty-basaloid carcinomas usually demonstrate both an endophytic and exophytic component, with the exophytic component showing papillary fronds lined by a mixture of basaloid cells and clear cells[73]
- Papillary-basaloid carcinoma shows prominent fibrovascular cores lined by uniform cells with high nuclear to cytoplasmic ratios[74]

SQUAMOUS EPITHELIAL IN SITU PROCESSES

Penile Intraepithelial Neoplasia

Penile intraepithelial neoplasia is defined as dysplasia of the squamous epithelium of the penis with an intact basement membrane.[67] It is synonymous with squamous cell carcinoma in situ and considered a precursor lesion for invasive squamous cell carcinoma. PeIN tends to arise most commonly on the glans or foreskin.

Subtypes of PeIN are divided by their association with HPV infection. A hallmark feature of HPV-related lesions is the presence of basaloid cells, undifferentiated squamous cells with high nuclear to cytoplasmic ratio and nuclear pleomorphism (Table 5.2).[75]

HPV-Associated PeIN Subtypes

As stated earlier, the most helpful pattern to recognize an HPV-related intraepithelial neoplasm is the basaloid cell. Basaloid cells are small- to intermediate-sized round cells that, by definition, are immature with high nuclear to cytoplasmic ratios. The most apparent

TABLE 5.2: Subtypes of Penile Intraepithelial Neoplasia (PeIN) and Their Association With Human Papillomavirus (HPV)

HPV Associated	Non-HPV Associated
Basaloid	Differentiated (Simplex)
Warty	
Warty-basaloid	

example of this appearance is the basaloid subtype of PeIN, which comprises immature basaloid cells throughout the full thickness of the epithelium (Figures 5.127-5.129). The low-power evaluation will demonstrate a monotonous, dark blue epithelium with minimal to no keratinization, although overlying parakeratosis may be seen. Nuclei show moderate pleomorphism with prominent nucleoli and clumped chromatin. Mitotic figures and apoptotic bodies are readily identified throughout the epithelium. Irregular and elongated rete ridges are commonly identified.

Warty PeIN is recognized by its surface pattern of papillary projections with a spiky appearance. Parakeratosis with atypia is also a prominent feature of the surface epithelium. The squamous cells are relatively large, with abundant eosinophilic cytoplasm conveying a pinker appearance when compared to basaloid PeIN (Figure 5.130). Koilocytes are frequently identified in this subtype, demonstrating multinucleation, raisinoid nuclei with perinuclear halos. Mitotic figures are frequent.

Warty-basaloid PeIN is the final subtype in the HPV-associated group. It is recognized by the combination of both papillomatous architecture with basaloid cytology. Unlike basaloid PeIN, which tends to have a flat surface, warty-basaloid PeIN shows a spiky, undulating surface with parakeratosis. Well-formed papillary cores are present. Koilocytic features are most likely to be identified in the upper half of the epithelium, while the lower half of the epithelium demonstrates the most pronounced basaloid features (Figures 5.131-5.134).

As with other HPV-associated malignancies, the subtypes of PeIN associated with HPV also demonstrate diffuse p16 positivity (Figure 5.135).[76] Additionally, the use of p53 and Ki-67 has been advocated for the distinction between squamous hyperplasia, differentiated PeIN, and HPV-associated subtypes. In a cohort of 74 cases of penile lesions including squamous hyperplasia, differentiated PeIN, basaloid, and warty PeIN, the authors found that negative p16 and p53 with patchy Ki-67 was seen in squamous hyperplasia. The warty and basaloid subtypes demonstrated diffuse expression of p16, increased Ki-67, and variable p53.[77]

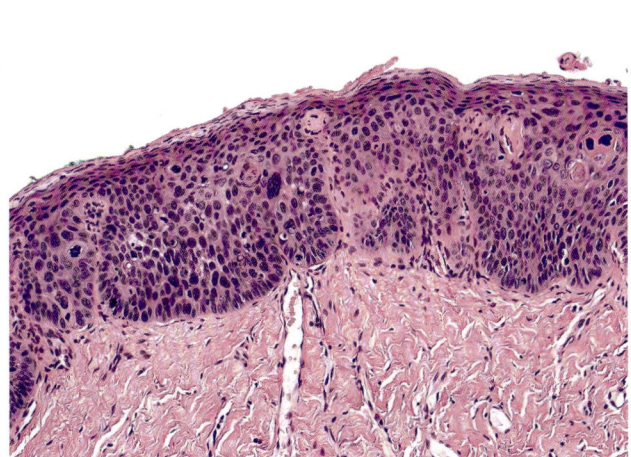

Figure 5.127. Basaloid penile intraepithelial neoplasia (PeIN) is recognized at low power by the uniformly dark blue appearance to the epithelium. This finding is due to high-grade, very poorly differentiated squamous cells involving the full thickness of the epithelium.

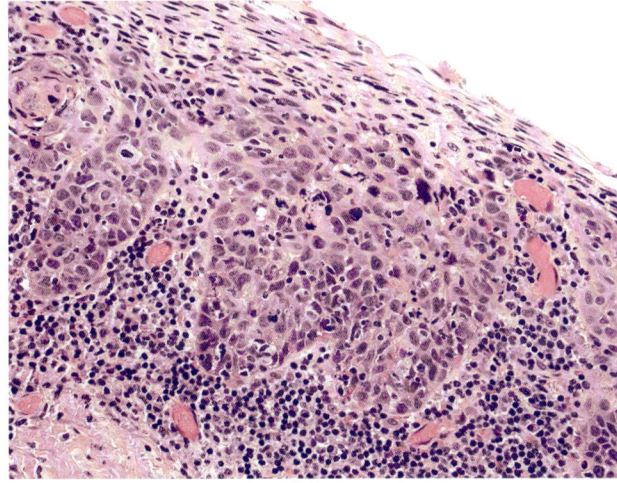

Figure 5.128. At high power, frequent mitotic figures are readily apparent within a background of high-grade poorly differentiated basaloid cells in this basaloid PeIN.

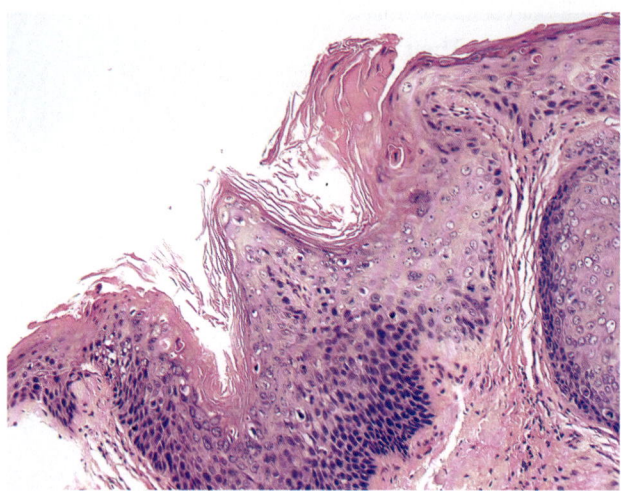

Figure 5.129. Warty PeIN demonstrates spiky papillary architecture with epithelial maturation and overlying parakeratosis. Scattered koilocytes may be present. Individual squamous cells contain abundant glassy eosinophilic cytoplasm, making this type of PeIN pinker than its basaloid counterparts. However, atypia is prominent and mitotic figures present at all levels of epithelium.

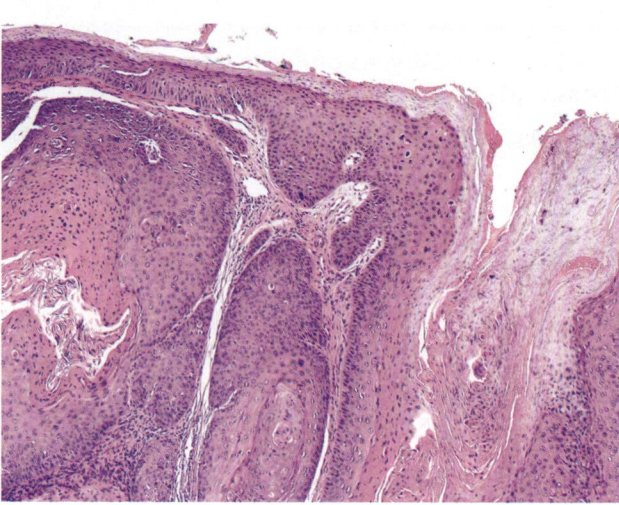

Figure 5.130. Warty-basaloid PeIN combines features of both warty and basaloid PeIN. The architectural pattern demonstrates more of a papillomatous appearance, whereas the cytology is more basaloid, especially in the lower levels of the epithelium.

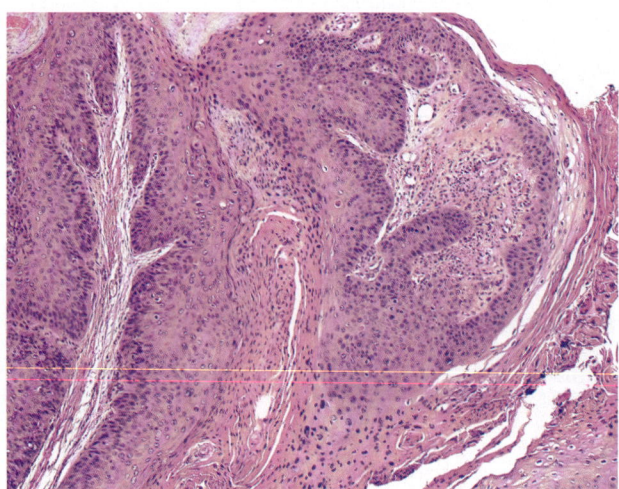

Figure 5.131. At higher power, the surface of the papillary cores shows more mature, parakeratosis squamous features. The poorly differentiated basaloid features are mostly confined to the lower half of the epithelium.

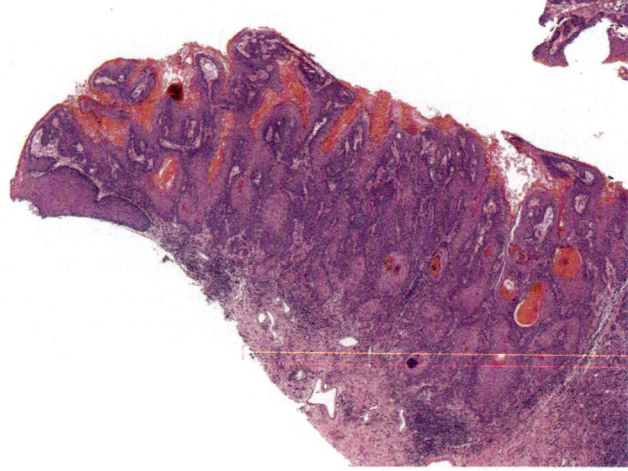

Figure 5.132. In this example of warty-basaloid PeIN demonstrating the overall papillomatous appearance with surface parakeratosis. The alternation of pink and blue areas is consistent with the combination of more differentiated areas (warty) along with the poorly differentiated (basaloid) areas.

Non–HPV-Associated PeIN/Differentiated PeIN

Differentiated PeIN is not associated with HPV, rather it frequently occurs in an older group of men with lichen sclerosus. It is the most common subtype of PeIN. Differentiated PeIN is the result of chronic inflammation of the penile squamous epithelium and most frequently involves the foreskin. These differentiated lesions are recognized by their thickened, keratinized appearance and lack high-grade basaloid features (Figures 5.135 and 5.136). Cells contain abundant glassy, eosinophilic cytoplasm giving the lesions an overall pink appearance (Figure 5.137). Nuclear atypia is readily identifiable and may be more evident at the base of the epithelium. Because of their well-differentiated appearance, it can be difficult to recognize these precursor lesions (Checklist: Identifying Differentiated PeIN). If differentiated PeIN gives rise to invasive carcinoma, it is most frequently of the "usual" type with keratinization.

CHECKLIST: Identifying Differentiated Penile Intraepithelial Neoplasia

☐ Checking the notes for a history of lichen sclerosus, clinical description of the lesion and its location can be helpful

☐ Differentiated PeIN usually occurs on the mucosal surface of the foreskin of older men

☐ Usually solitary white or pink macules with sharp to irregular borders

☐ Thickened epithelium with parakeratosis

☐ Elongated and irregular rete ridges

☐ Histologic features of enlarged, mature keratinizing cells with keratin pearls

☐ Lack of koilocytes

☐ Lack of basaloid features; may see subtle dysplasia of basal cells with mitotic figures

☐ Negative p16 with increased Ki-67 and variable p53 expression (Figure 5.138)

Extramammary Paget Disease

Extramammary Paget disease (EMPD) is a malignant intraepithelial process characterized by scattered large, round cells with abundant pale cytoplasm that may show obvious mucinous features. When EMPD arises independent of an invasive tumor, so-called primary EMPD, the malignant cells originate from apocrine sweat glands. Conversely, secondary EPMD occurs when an underlying carcinoma such as colorectal, prostate, or bladder involves the epithelium in a pagetoid fashion. As a result, it is critical to evaluate for the possibility of other malignancies when EMPD is identified. Grossly, the lesions are red and plaque-like, which may mimic eczema, and can ooze thin fluid.

The diagnosis of EMPD relies on inspection of the epithelium for abnormal single cells or small clusters of cells, which are often much larger and paler than the surrounding keratinocytes. The malignant cells are commonly identified at the basal aspect of the epithelium but may be identified at all levels. Cytologically, the cells have abundant clear to vacuolated cytoplasm and may show overt mucinous features. Nuclei are large and vesicular with prominent nucleoli (Figure 5.139). Importantly, the cells lack squamous features of intracellular bridges or keratinization and stand out as cytologically dissimilar to the surrounding keratinocytes.

In primary EMPD, special stains for mucin including mucicarmine (MUC) and Alcian blue highlight the mucin within the malignant cells. Because of the possibility of secondary involvement from another primary adenocarcinoma, an immunohistochemical panel may be useful to confirm primary EMPD. EMPD shows an expression of CK7, EMA, carcinoembryonic antigen, and gross cystic disease fluid protein (GCDFP-15) (Figure 5.140).[78,79] MUC5AC is a specific apocrine mucin that is expressed in most EMPD, but is not expressed in mammary Paget disease. With a differential diagnosis that includes squamous cell carcinoma in situ, spread from colorectal, urothelial, prostate primaries, and melanoma, a tailored immunohistochemical panel would include specific markers for each of these. However, it should be noted that GATA3 may be positive in EMPD, leading to confusion with the intraepithelial spread of urothelial carcinoma.[80]

FAQ: What Are the Most Useful Stains to Distinguish Primary EMPD From Secondary EMPD?[81]

- GCDFP-15 is positive in the vast majority of primary EMPD and only a minority of secondary EMPD

- CK20 expression is seen in the majority of secondary EMPD and less frequently expressed in primary EMPD

- Specific markers may help confirm secondary EMPD site of origin such as p40/p63 for squamous, CDX-2 for colorectal, and NKX3.1 for prostate

- GATA3 is not useful in this differential, as it may be positive in primary EPMD

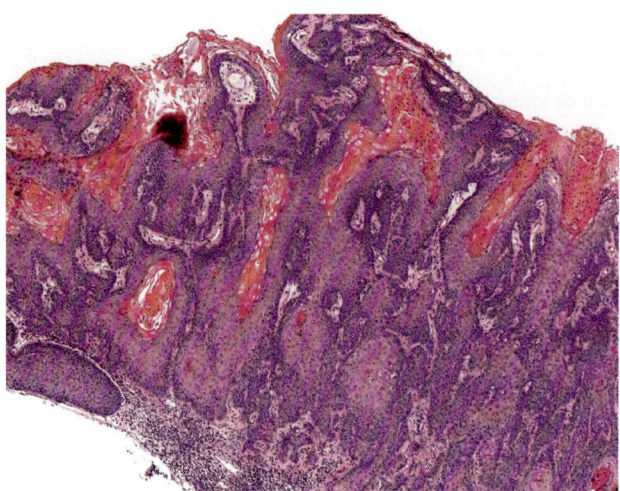

Figure 5.133. The cytologic features of both areas of this warty-basaloid PeIN include mature squamous cells with abundant pink cytoplasm and immature basaloid cells with scant cytoplasm, enlarged and pleomorphic nuclei with frequent mitoses.

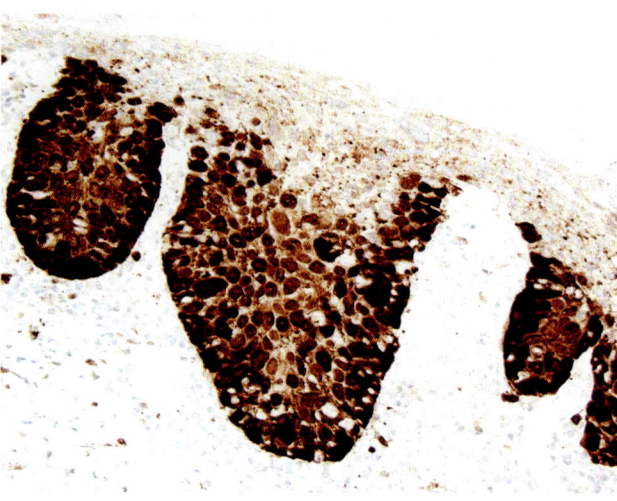

Figure 5.134. Strong and diffuse p16 positivity, demonstrated here, is an expected finding in HPV-related PeIN.

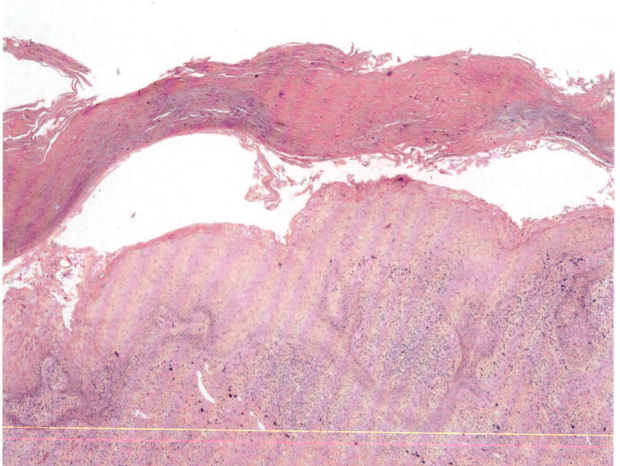

Figure 5.135. Differentiated PeIN is associated with chronic inflammatory conditions such as lichen sclerosus et atrophicus and is not HPV related. As such, it lacks basaloid features and instead shows well-differentiated squamous cells with abundant glassy eosinophilic cytoplasm. Parakeratosis, as seen here, is a helpful feature.

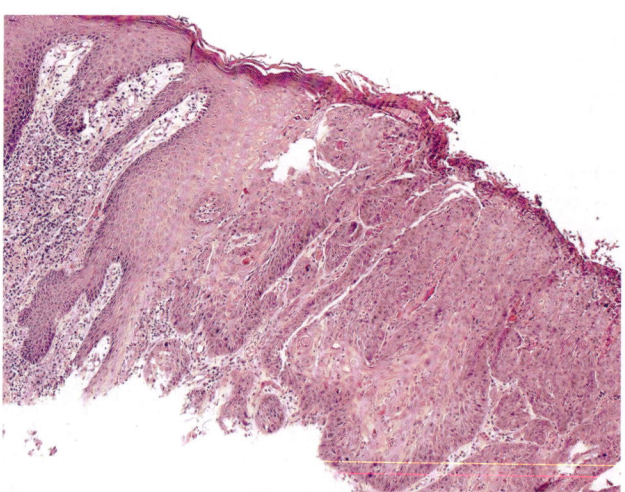

Figure 5.136. In this overtly keratinizing lesions, differentiated PeIN has an overall pink appearance due to the mature nature of the squamous cells with abundant pink cytoplasm. Cellular atypia is evident at scanning magnification and is especially prominent at the basal aspect of the epithelium.

WELL-DIFFERENTIATED/KERATINIZING PATTERN

Invasive Usual Squamous Cell Carcinoma

Invasive squamous cell carcinomas involving the penis usually arise in males in their 40s to 50s. Risk factors for developing invasive squamous cell carcinoma include any chronic infection or irritant such as phimosis, lichen sclerosus, or HPV. As is the case with precursor lesions, HPV-related squamous cell carcinomas are associated with unique morphologic features and will be discussed later. Anatomically, penile squamous cell carcinomas most commonly involve the glans, foreskin, coronal sulcus, and shaft in decreasing order of frequency.

FAQ: Where Is the Most Common Site of Nodal Metastasis for Penile SCC?

- Penile squamous cell carcinoma preferentially metastasizes to the inguinal lymph nodes
- Inguinal node metastasis may be the first presentation of penile SCC

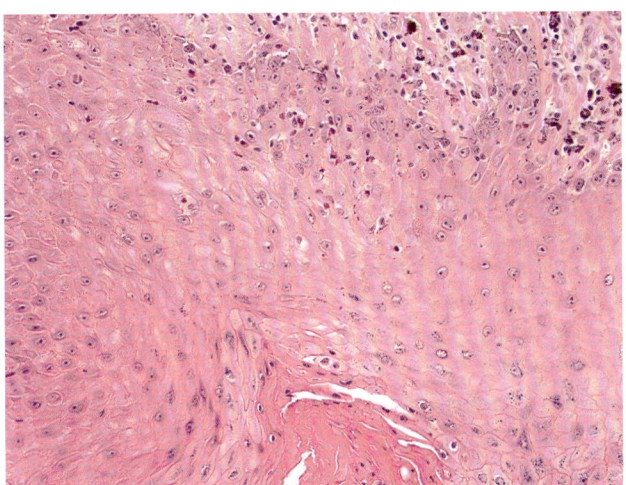

Figure 5.137. Cytologic features of differentiated PeIN include abundant eosinophilic glassy cytoplasm, prominent intercellular bridges, and nuclear atypia with vesicular chromatin and prominent nucleoli.

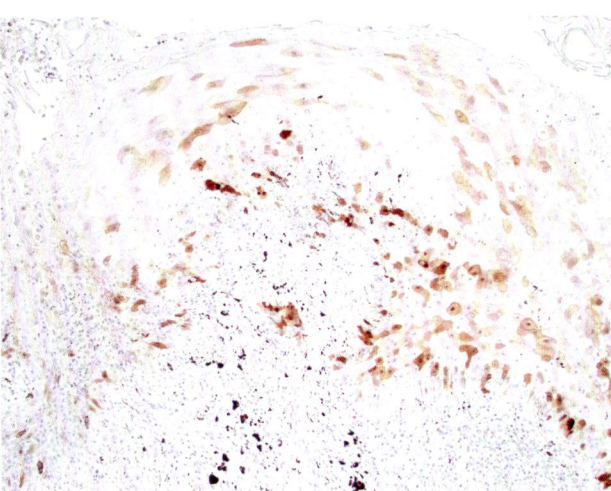

Figure 5.138. In contrast to HPV-associated forms of PeIN, differentiated PeIN is not associated with HPV. Hence, a p16 stain will show only weak, patchy staining that should be interpreted as negative.

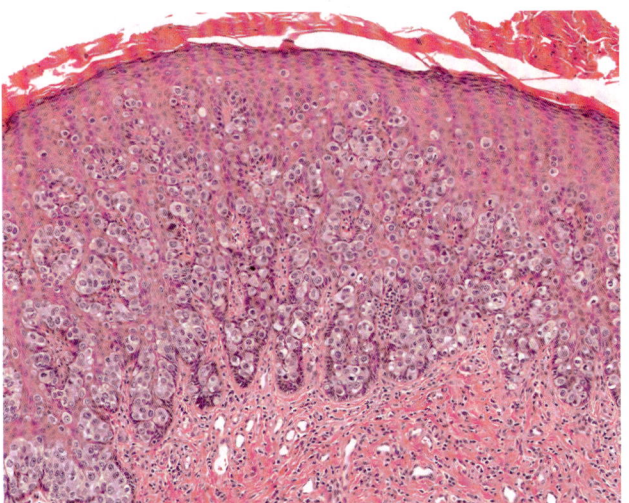

Figure 5.139. Extramammary Paget disease showing scattered atypical cells throughout the squamous epithelium. The Paget cells have abundant, lightly eosinophilic cytoplasm that makes them stand out from the surrounding squamous cells. Nuclei are obviously atypical, and mitotic figures are easily identified.

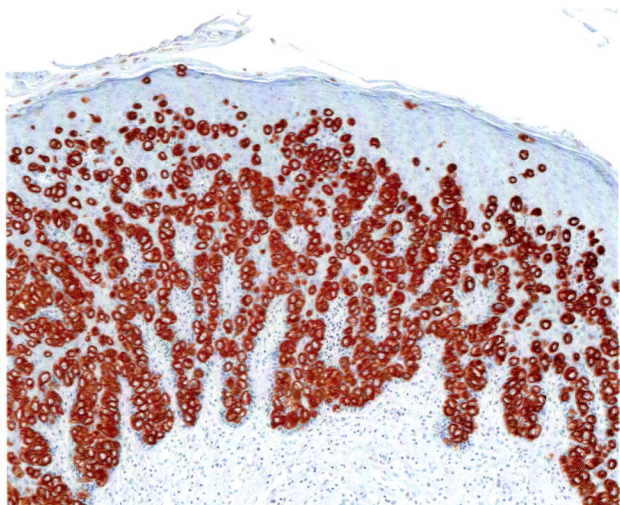

Figure 5.140. Immunohistochemistry for CK7 highlights the Paget cells throughout the epithelium.

The most frequently identified subtype of penile SCC is the usual type. These are relatively well-differentiated carcinomas with apparent squamous features and often keratinization. Architecturally, these tumors tend to grow as nests with irregular infiltrative borders (Figure 5.141). The tumor cells have ample dense eosinophilic cytoplasm consistent with squamous differentiation. Intercellular bridges are present, consistent with their squamous origin.

The WHO/ISUP consensus paper recommends that usual squamous cell carcinomas be graded using a three-tiered system.[82] Well-differentiated tumors (grade I) are the most recognizably "squamous" tumors with obvious keratinization and keratin pearls. Moderately differentiated (grade II) tumors demonstrate smaller, irregular nests of tumor invested in the desmoplastic stroma (Figure 5.142). Cells demonstrate less obvious keratinization, increasing cytologic atypia, and readily identifiable mitotic figures. Poorly differentiated (grade III) squamous cell carcinomas are high-grade, pleomorphic tumors that show few obvious squamous features, although individual keratinized cells may be identified (Figure 5.143).

Usual squamous cell carcinoma does not show a strong association with HPV, although up to 20% were shown to have HPV positivity in one study[83] (Table 5.3).

FAQ: What Are the Common Features of Squamous Neoplasia in the Scrotum?

- Classically associated with chimney sweeps due to direct contact of carcinogens with scrotal skin
- In the modern era, squamous neoplasia involving the scrotum is associated with HPV infection, immune compromise, and inflammatory conditions[84]
- Most cases of scrotal squamous cell carcinoma showed usual squamous features (usually, but not always HPV negative)
- The remainder of cases were either basaloid or warty pattern (consistently HPV-related)
- Approximately half of HPV-related squamous cell carcinomas of the scrotum in one series were not associated with HPV16/18, presenting a potential pitfall with the use of high-risk HPV in situ hybridization[85]

CHECKLIST: Staging of Penile Carcinoma

☐ Penile squamous cell carcinomas are staged using the American Joint Committee on Cancer pTNM system[86]

☐ Stage is determined by the depth of invasion and involvement of penile tissues including corpora spongiosum and cavernosa

☐ Depth of invasion is measured from the epithelial-stromal junction of the adjacent normal epithelium to the deepest area of invasion

☐ In the pT1 category, staging varies based on the anatomic region of the primary lesion

  o Glans: tumor infiltrates into the lamina propria

  o Foreskin: tumor infiltrates into the dermis, lamina propria, or dartos fascia

  o Shaft: tumor infiltrates connective tissue beyond dermis, but without the involvement of the corpora

  o To be staged pT1a, there must be low-grade cytology, no perineural invasion, and absence of lymphovascular invasion

  o If any of these features (high-grade cytology, perineural invasion, or lymphovascular invasion) are present, the tumor is staged as pT1b

☐ In the pT2 category, there is the involvement of the corpus spongiosum

☐ pT3 tumors involve the corpus cavernosum or tunica albuginea

☐ Involvement of scrotum, prostate, pubic bone, or other adjacent structures is staged as pT4

BASALOID/UNDIFFERENTIATED PATTERN
Basaloid Squamous Cell Carcinoma

Basaloid squamous cell carcinoma is the archetypal HPV-driven invasive squamous cell carcinoma.[75] It is highly aggressive with a tendency to recur and frequently presents with regional metastasis.[71] These tumors demonstrate a solid, nested pattern of growth that may show comedonecrosis[87] (Figure 5.148). The cytologic features are that of a classic basaloid neoplasm, monotonous sheets of small- to medium-sized cells with high nuclear to cytoplasmic ratio, imparting an overall dark blue appearance to the tumor (Figure 5.149). Mitotic figures, apoptotic bodies, and karyorrhexis are easily identified (Figure 5.150). The abrupt transition to keratinization located centrally in the nest of the tumor is rarely observed and may be associated with a better outcome.[88] These tumors are HPV driven and therefore show strong and diffuse p16 expression (Figure 5.151).

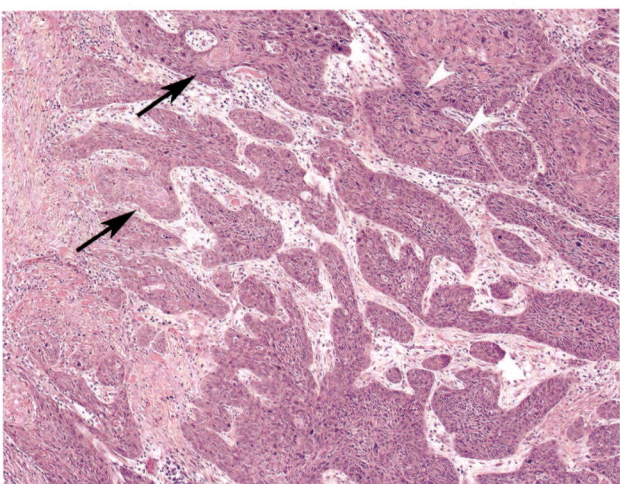

Figure 5.141. Invasive usual squamous cell carcinoma is a non-HPV-associated tumor that is well differentiated, and typically shows some degree of keratinization. In this example, keratin pears are present (black arrows) in addition to individual keratinized cells (white arrowheads). Evidence of invasion includes irregular and jagged nests within a desmoplastic stroma.

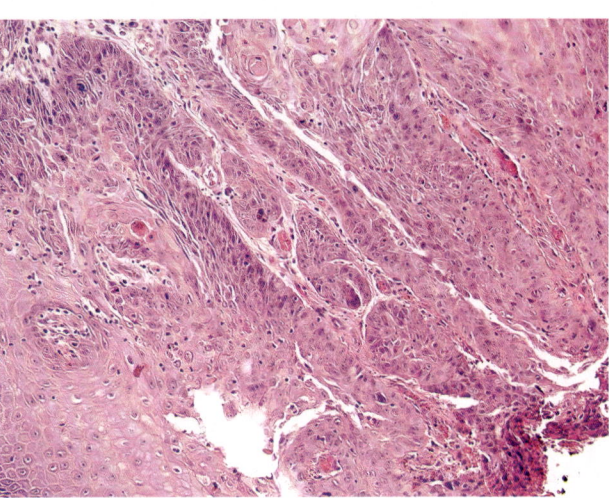

Figure 5.142. At higher power, the mature squamous cells are evident with abundant glassy cytoplasm and prominent intercellular bridges consistent with invasive usual squamous cell carcinoma.

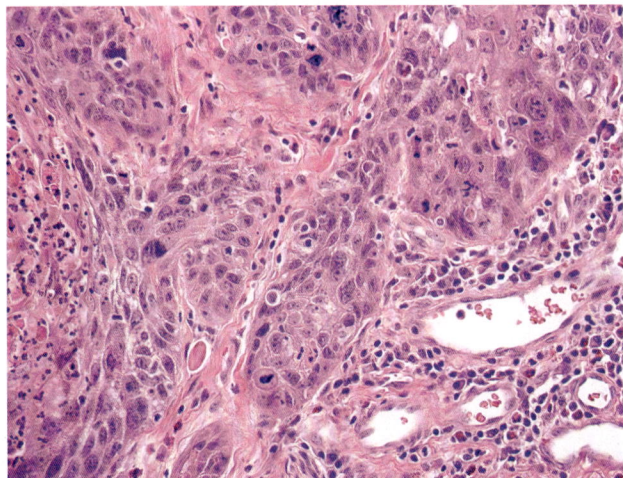

Figure 5.143. Invasive usual squamous cell carcinoma is graded in a three-tier system. This example shows high-grade features, without diffuse keratinization, and represents a poorly differentiated (grade III) squamous cell carcinoma.

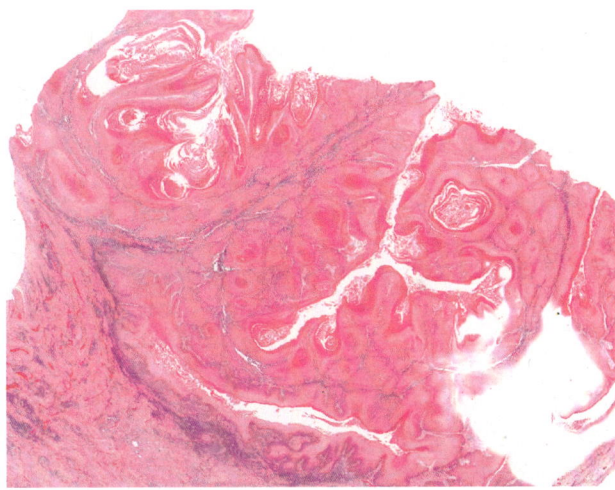

Figure 5.144. Carcinoma cuniculatum is a highly differentiated subtype of squamous cell carcinoma with a unique pattern of growth and overall good prognosis. The surface shows verrucous growth and hyperkeratosis, with the formation of cysts containing keratin debris.

Given the relatively undifferentiated appearance of basaloid squamous cell carcinoma, the differential diagnosis includes urothelial carcinoma, small cell carcinoma, and basal cell carcinoma.

Basal Cell Carcinoma

Basal cell carcinoma of the penile skin is included in this category given the morphologic overlap with other basaloid neoplasms. Although this is the most common tumor of skin, it is still very rare in the penis. As a primary skin neoplasm, it is more likely to be identified on the shaft of the penis, rather than the glans where the squamous cell carcinomas arising in the mucosa are centered.[89] The classic features of basal cell carcinoma with peripheral palisading, clefting, and myxoid stroma are helpful in distinguishing these tumors from basaloid squamous cell carcinoma.

Lymphoma

Lymphoma can involve the penis either as a primary disease or secondarily as part of disseminated lymphoma. Primary penile lymphoma is exceptionally rare and is a diagnosis

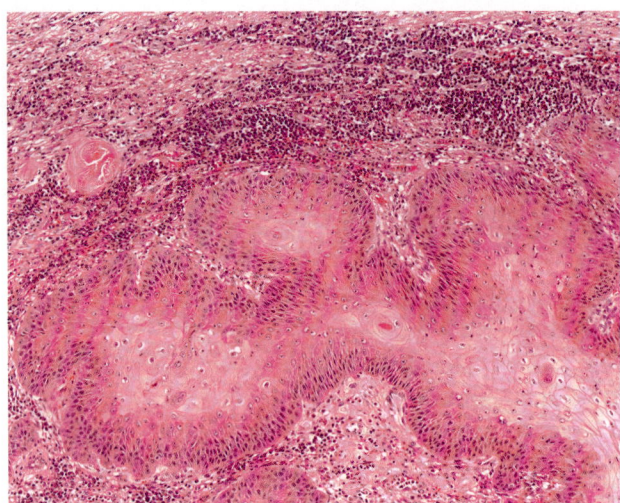

Figure 5.145. Higher power image demonstrating the burrowing pattern of infiltration in this carcinoma cuniculatum. Cytologic features include very well-differentiated squamous cells with abundant pink cytoplasm.

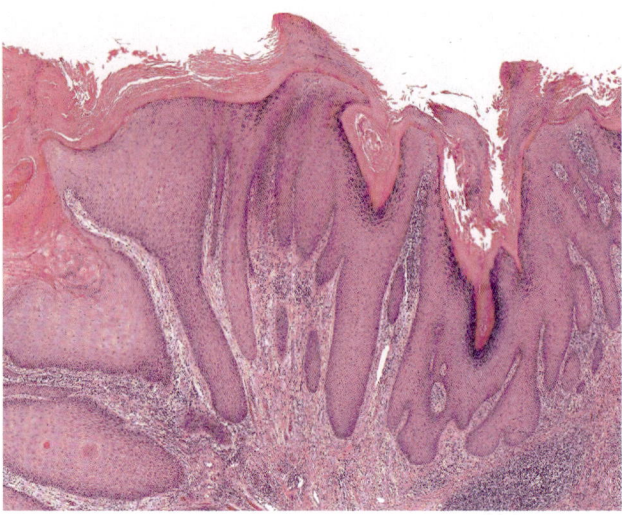

Figure 5.146. Pseudohyperplastic carcinoma is another subtype of non-HPV-related squamous cell carcinoma that is well differentiated. Keratinization is prominent.

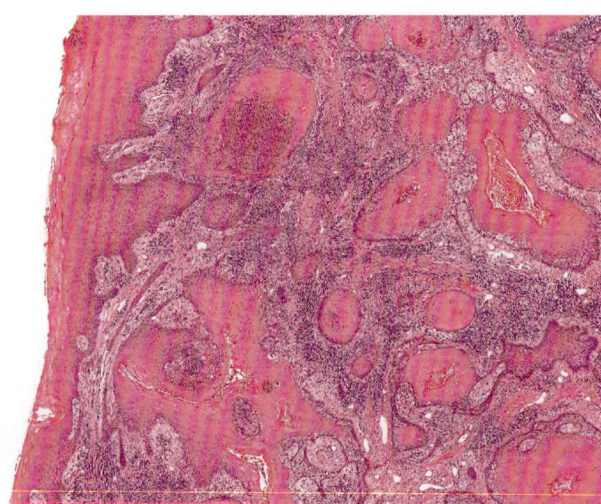

Figure 5.147. Pseudohyperplastic carcinoma grows downward with irregular squamous nests and does not elicit a prominent desmoplastic response. In this image, the nests comprise well-differentiated squamous cells, invade as irregular nests, and lack desmoplastic response.

of exclusion. Most primary penile lymphomas are diffuse large B cell lymphomas (Figure 5.152). Any area of the penis can be involved, although mucosal sites are more likely to harbor a mucosa-associated lymphoid tissue lymphoma.[90] When encountering an undifferentiated tumor in the penis, lymphoma should be included in the differential diagnosis and appropriate immunohistochemical stains performed.

Melanoma

Primary penile malignant melanoma is a rare occurrence, representing only about 1.5% of penile cancers. Most melanomas are located on the glans but may also involve the foreskin or shaft. The lesions are flat and often show ulceration and irregular borders. The architectural growth patterns are similar to those found in skin, with superficial spreading, nodule, and lentiginous patterns described. Histologically, penile melanomas comprise atypical melanocytes that may have both intraepithelial and invasive components. The cells are large and pleomorphic and may contain melanin pigment, and mitotic figures are readily identified.[32] The classic cytologic features associated with melanoma include extreme nuclear pleomorphism, prominent nucleoli, intranuclear inclusions, and bi- and multinucleation (Figures 5.153-5.155).

TABLE 5.3: WHO 2016 Classification of Penile Squamous Cell Carcinoma (SCC)[82]

Non-HPV related	SCC, usual type
	Pseudoglandular carcinoma
	Verrucous carcinoma
	Pure verrucous carcinoma
	Carcinoma Cuniculatum (Figures 5.144 and 5.145)
	Pseudohyperplastic carcinoma (Figures 5.146 and 5.147)
	Papillary carcinoma, NOS
	Adenosquamous carcinoma
	Sarcomatoid SCC
	Mixed carcinoma
HPV related	Basaloid carcinoma
	Papillary-basaloid carcinoma
	Warty carcinoma
	Warty-basaloid carcinoma
	Clear cell carcinoma
	Lymphoepithelioma-like carcinoma
Other rare carcinomas	Neuroendocrine carcinoma
	Basal cell carcinoma
	Sebaceous carcinoma

Note: Human papillomavirus (HPV) status is a clinically significant prognostic factor.

METASTATIC DISEASE

Although rare, metastatic tumors may involve the penis. Urothelial and prostate carcinomas are the most common tumors to metastasize to the penis (Figures 5.156-5.158). Other less common tumors reported to involve the penis include kidney, testicular germ cell tumors, and gastrointestinal adenocarcinoma.[32] Secondary involvement of the penis is generally identified in a patient with widely metastatic disease and rarely presents as the initial site of metastasis, such that clinical history is often the most helpful clue to making the diagnosis. Clinically, patients may present with either a palpable mass or less commonly with priapism.[91]

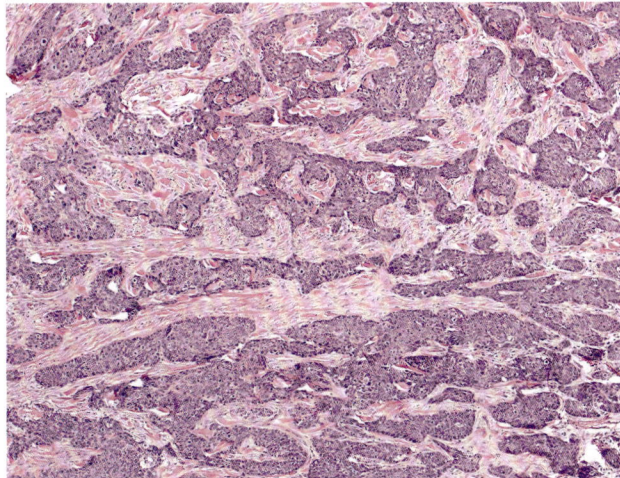

Figure 5.148. Invasive basaloid squamous cell carcinomas are high-grade undifferentiated neoplasms with a dark blue appearance at low power.

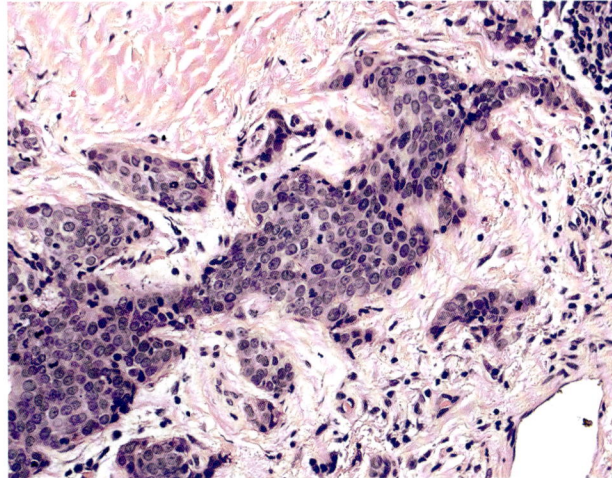

Figure 5.149. Basaloid cytology includes scant cytoplasm with enlarged nuclei, leading to a deeply basophilic appearance. Nuclear features include vesicular and clumped chromatin.

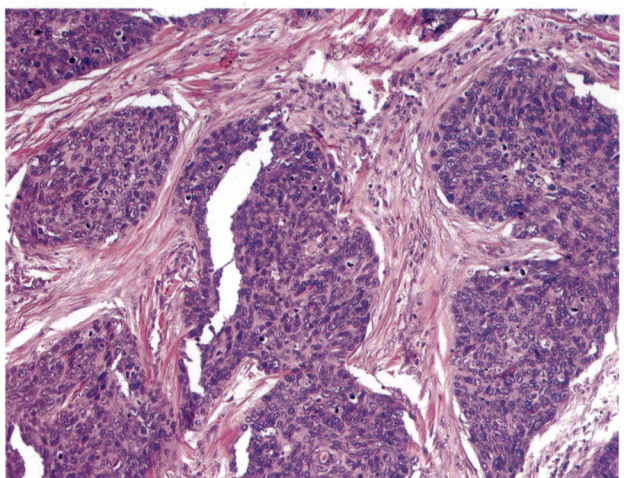

Figure 5.150. In basaloid squamous cell carcinoma, brisk mitotic activity is frequently identified along with apoptosis and karyorrhexis due to cellular turnover. The invasive nests of the tumor may also show comedo necrosis (not pictured here).

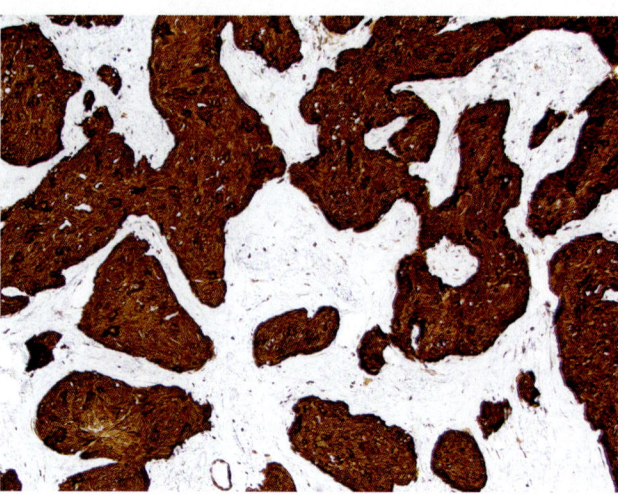

Figure 5.151. As an HPV-associated carcinoma, basaloid squamous cell carcinoma shows strong and diffuse p16 expression as demonstrated here.

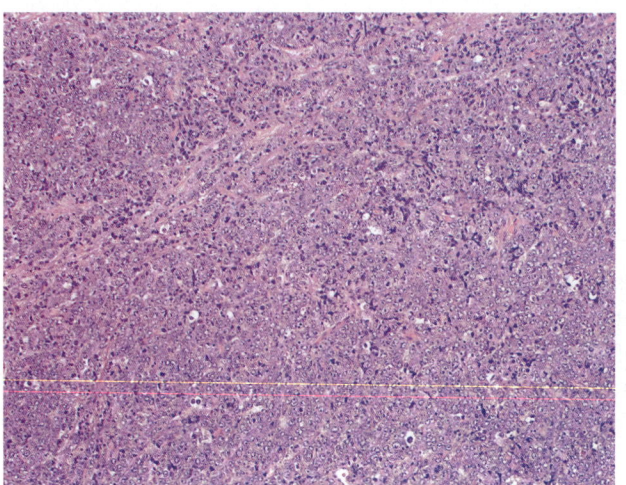

Figure 5.152. This sheet-like proliferation of high-grade undifferentiated cells leads to a broad differential diagnosis, which should include lymphoma. Most primary penile lymphomas are diffuse large B cell type, and initial immunohistochemical workup should include a CD3 and CD20.

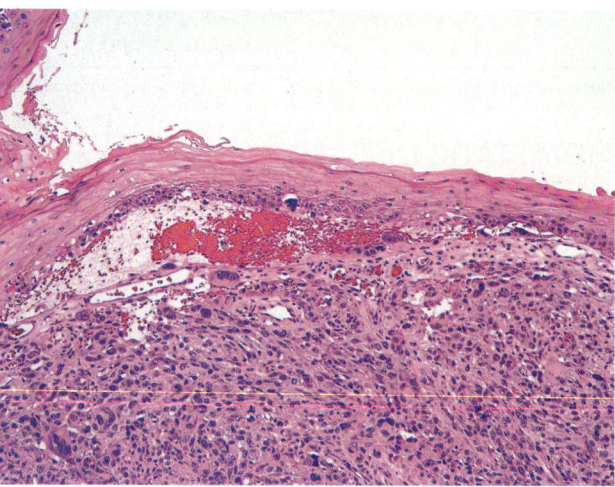

Figure 5.153. Malignant melanoma of the penis is rare but morphologically identical to melanoma in other sites. Here, a high-grade undifferentiated neoplasm is present in the subepithelial layer, and scattered atypical melanocytes are present within the epithelium, providing a hint to the diagnosis.

NEAR MISSES

A middle-age man presents with a painless scrotal mass, palpable at the head of the epididymis. The patient says the mass has been growing and, given concern for a possible malignancy, undergoes surgical scrotal exploration. A frozen section is performed, which comprises largely spindle cells, and the preliminary diagnosis is given as "Spindle cell proliferation, cannot exclude malignancy." As a result, the surgeon proceeds with radical orchiectomy. On gross examination, the mass appears centered in the epididymis with no involvement of the testicular parenchyma. The cut section shows a poorly circumscribed gray-white nodule. On permanent histologic review, the mass demonstrates the predominant spindle cell pattern seen on the frozen section; however, small tubules are identified

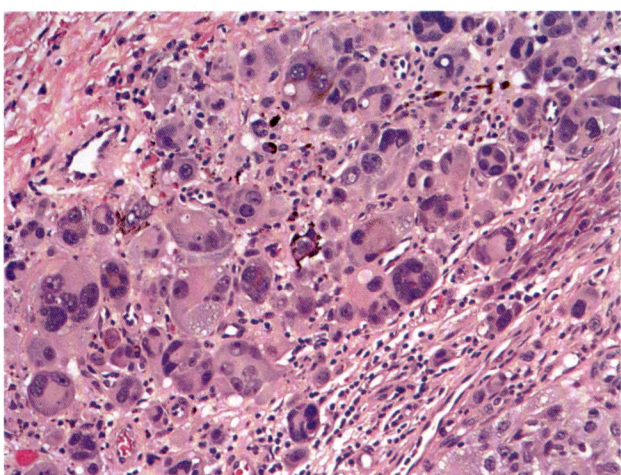

Figure 5.154. When present, the finding of intracytoplasmic melanin is also highly suggestive of malignant melanoma. Cytologic features of melanoma include extreme nuclear pleomorphism, prominent nucleoli, intranuclear inclusions, and bi- and multinucleation.

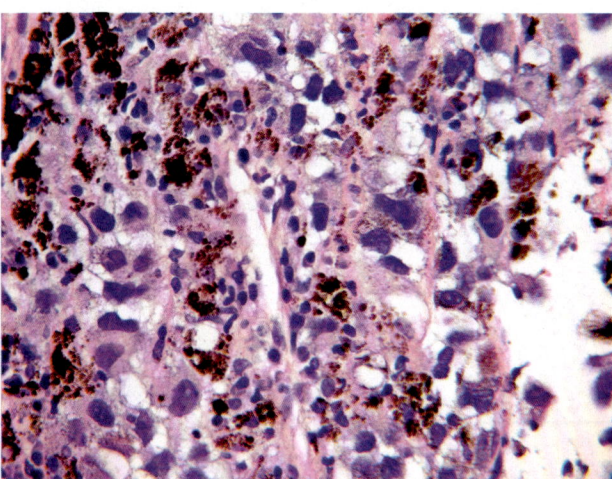

Figure 5.155. Coarse intracytoplasmic melanin is present in abundance in this example of malignant melanoma. Note that the malignant cells have cleared out cytoplasm, one of many unusual appearances of melanoma that may confuse the diagnosis.

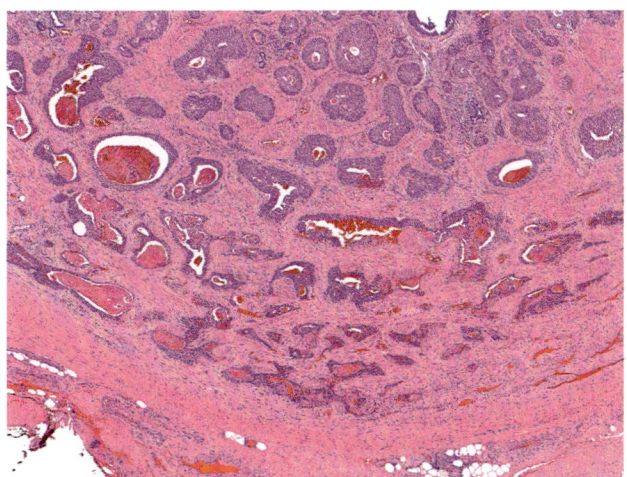

Figure 5.156. Metastatic urothelial carcinoma diffusely involving the vascular spaces of the penis. With this degree of involvement of the corporal vascular tissue, it is understandable why priapism is a presenting symptom.

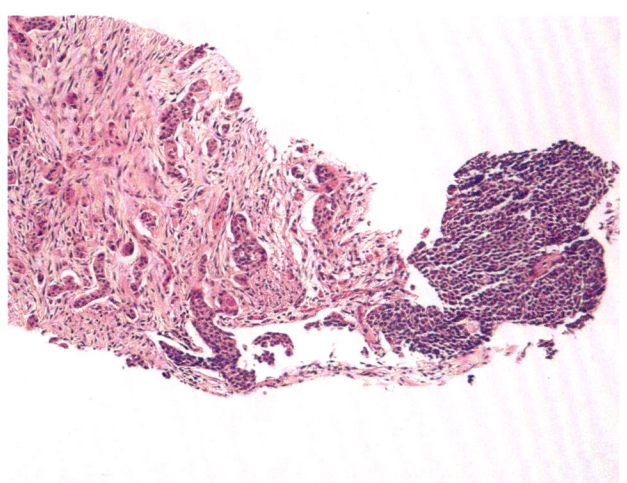

Figure 5.157. This penis biopsy demonstrates a solid nest of infiltrating tumor and adjacent small, irregular nests, some of which may represent lymphovascular invasion. Metastatic disease to the penis is rare, but the most common tumors to involve the penis are urothelial and prostate.

scattered throughout the tumor. The spaces are lined by flattened eosinophilic cells with minimal atypia. No mitotic figures or necrosis are appreciated (Figures 5.159 and 5.160).

Given the microscopic appearance and location, adenomatoid tumor with smooth muscle predominance is the number one entity in the differential diagnosis. Although the tubular component is somewhat obscured by the smooth muscle hyperplasia, it is the most helpful feature for diagnosis adenomatoid tumor. An immunohistochemical panel to include WT-1 and calretinin will help identify the lining cells as mesothelial in origin. However, caution should be taken in using just a smooth muscle marker such as SMA, as the smooth muscle component will be diffusely positive and may lead to incorrect diagnosis a leiomyoma or leiomyosarcoma. It is critical to recognize the embedded tubules and mesothelial markers can help highlight them when scarce.

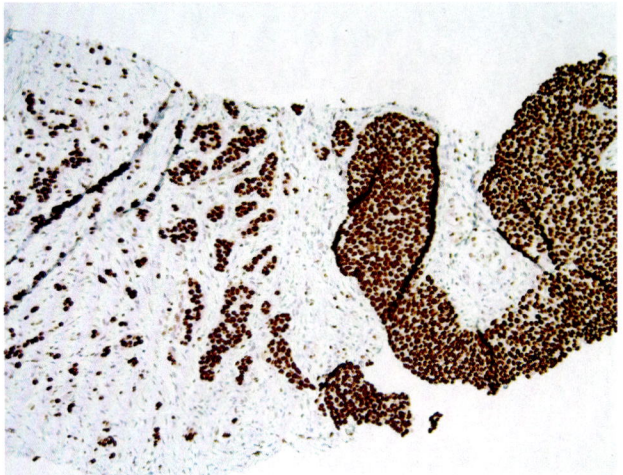

Figure 5.158. GATA3 shows strong and diffuse nuclear positivity in this metastatic lesion, consistent with involvement by urothelial carcinoma.

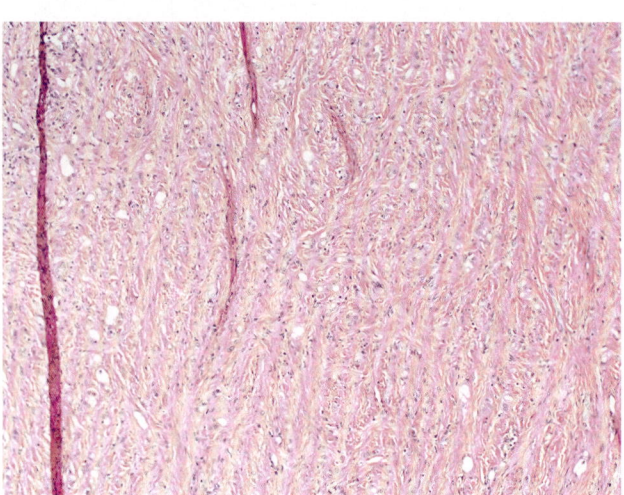

Figure 5.159. Adenomatoid tumors can have variable amounts of smooth muscle that can mimic a spindle cell neoplasm. A close search for the mesothelial tubules will usually yield the correct diagnosis.

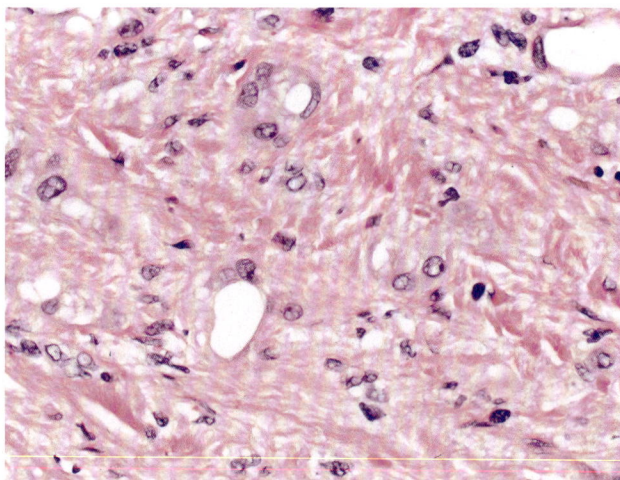

Figure 5.160. At high power, scattered tubules are present in this adenomatoid tumor along with rare vacuolated cells that resemble signet ring cells. The finding of an infiltrative tubular/glandular growth pattern can mimic an adenocarcinoma. Immunohistochemical markers such as calretinin and D2-40 will confirm the mesothelial origin.

References

1. Lane ZL, Epstein JI. Small blue cells mimicking small cell carcinoma in spermatocele and hydrocele specimens: a report of 5 cases. *Hum Pathol.* 2010;41(1):88-93. doi:10.1016/j.humpath.2009.06.018.

2. Goldman RL, Azzopardi JG. Benign neural invasion in vasitis nodosa. *Histopathology.* 1982;6(3):309-315. doi:10.1111/j.1365-2559.1982.tb02725.x.

3. Kezlarian BE, Cheng L, Gupta NS, Williamson SR. Vasitis nodosa and related lesions: a modern immunohistochemical staining profile with special emphasis on novel diagnostic dilemmas. *Hum Pathol.* 2018;73:164-170. doi:10.1016/j.humpath.2017.12.001.

4. Hes O, Perez-Montiel DM, Cabrero IA, et al. Thread-like bridging strands: a morphologic feature present in all adenomatoid tumors. *Ann Diagn Pathol.* 2003;7(5):273-277. doi:10.1016/S1092-9134(03)00085-6.

5. Schwartz EJ, Longacre TA. Adenomatoid tumors of the female and male genital tracts express WT1. *Int J Gynecol Pathol.* 2004;23(2):123-128. doi:10.1097/00004347-200404000-00006.

6. Amin W, Parwani AV. Adenomatoid tumor of testis. *Clin Med Pathol*. 2009;2009(2):17-22. doi:10.4137/cpath.s3091.

7. Skinnider BF, Young RH. Infarcted adenomatoid tumor: a report of five cases of a facet of a benign neoplasm that may cause diagnostic difficulty. *Am J Surg Pathol*. 2004;28(1):77-83. doi:10.1097/00000478-200401000-00008.

8. Algaba F, Mikuz G, Boccon-Gibod L, et al. Pseudoneoplastic lesions of the testis and paratesticular structures. *Virchows Arch*. 2007;451(6):987-997. doi:10.1007/s00428-007-0502-8.

9. Ulbright TM, Gersell DJ. Rete testis hyperplasia with hyaline globule formation: a lesion simulating yolk sac tumor. *Am J Surg Pathol*. 1991;15(1):66-74. doi:10.1097/00000478-199101000-00008.

10. Al-Obaidy KI, Idrees MT, Grignon DJ, Ulbright TM. Adenocarcinoma of the rete testis: clinico-pathologic and immunohistochemical characterization of 6 cases and review of the literature. *Am J Surg Pathol*. 2019;43(5):670-681. doi:10.1097/PAS.0000000000001219.

11. Amin MB. Selected other problematic testicular and paratesticular lesions: rete testis neoplasms and pseudotumors, mesothelial lesions and secondary tumors. *Mod Pathol*. 2005;18(suppl 2):S131-S145. doi:10.1038/modpathol.3800314.

12. Jones MA, Young RH, Scully RE. Adenocarcinoma of the epididymis: a report of four cases and review of the literature. *Am J Surg Pathol*. 1997;21(12):1474-1480. doi:10.1097/00000478-199712000-00010.

13. Ulbright TM, Young RH. *AFIP atlas of tumor pathology*. In: *Fourth Series, Fascicle 18*. Washington, DC: American Registry of Pathology; 2013.

14. Mrinakova B, Kajo K, Ondrusova M, Simo J, Ondrus D. Malignant mesothelioma of the tunica vaginalis testis. A clinicopathologic analysis of two cases with a review of the literature. *Klin Onkol*. 2016;29(5):369-374. doi:10.14735/amko2016369.

15. Chekol SS, Sun CC. Malignant mesothelioma of the tunica vaginalis testis: diagnostic studies and differential. *Arch Pathol Lab Med*. 2012;136(1):113-117. doi:10.5858/arpa.2010-0550-RS.

16. Gilcrease MZ, Schmidt L, Zbar B, Truong L, Rutledge M, Wheeler TM. Somatic von hippel-lindau mutation in clear cell papillary cystadenoma of the epididymis. *Hum Pathol*. 1995;26(12):1341-1346. doi:10.1016/0046-8177(95)90299-6.

17. Odrzywolski KJ, Mukhopadhyay S. Papillary cystadenoma of the epididymis. *Arch Pathol Lab Med*. 2010;134(4):630-633. doi:10.12771/emj.1980.3.2.87.

18. Cox R, Vang R, Epstein JI. Papillary cystadenoma of the epididymis and broad ligament: morpho-logic and immunohistochemical overlap with clear cell papillary renal cell carcinoma. *Am J Surg Pathol*. 2014;38(5):713-718. doi:10.1097/PAS.0000000000000152.

19. Xiao S-Y, Rizzo P, Carbone M. Benign papillary mesothelioma of the tunica vaginalis testis. *Arch Pathol Lab Med*. 2000;124(1):143-147.

20. Brimo F, Illei PB, Epstein JI. Mesothelioma of the tunica vaginalis: a series of eight cases with uncer-tain malignant potential. *Mod Pathol*. 2010;23(8):1165-1172. doi:10.1038/modpathol.2010.113.

21. Bürger T, Schildhaus HU, Inniger R, et al. Ovarian-type epithelial tumours of the testis: immuno-histochemical and molecular analysis of two serous borderline tumours of the testis. *Diagn Pathol*. 2015;10(1):118. doi:10.1186/s13000-015-0342-9.

22. Michal M, Kazakov DV, Kacerovska D, et al. Paratesticular cystadenomas with ovarian stroma, metaplastic serous müllerian epithelium, and male adnexal tumor of probable wolffian origin: a series of 5 hitherto poorly recognized testicular tumors. *Ann Diagn Pathol*. 2013;17(2):151-158. doi:10.1016/j.anndiagpath.2012.09.002.

23. McClure RF, Keeney GL, Sebo TJ, Cheville JC. Serous borderline tumor of the paratestis: a report of seven cases. *Am J Surg Pathol*. 2001;25(3):373-378. doi:10.1097/00000478-200103000-00012.

24. Ulbright TM, Young RH. Primary mucinous tumors of the testis and paratestis: a report of nine cases. *Am J Surg Pathol*. 2003;27(9):1221-1228. doi:10.1097/00000478-200309000-00005.

25. Clay MR, Martinez AP, Weiss SW, Edgar MA. MDM2 amplification in problematic lipomatous tumors: analysis of FISH testing criteria. *Am J Surg Pathol*. 2015;39(10):1433-1439. doi:10.1097/PAS.0000000000000468.

26. Miyamoto H, Montgomery EA, Epstein JI. Paratesticular fibrous pseudotumor: a morphologic and immunohistochemical study of 13 cases. *Am J Surg Pathol*. 2010;34(4):569-574. doi:10.1097/PAS.0b013e3181d438cb.

27. Alruwaii F, Grignon DJ, Idrees MT. Smooth muscle hyperplasia of the testicular adnexa: a clinicopathologic study of 12 cases. *Hum Pathol*. 2020;99:27-35. doi:10.1016/j.humpath.2020.03.003.

28. Barton JH, Davis CJ, Sesterhenn IA, Mostofi FK. Smooth muscle hyperplasia of the testicular adnexa clinically mimicking neoplasia: clinicopathologic study of sixteen cases. *Am J Surg Pathol.* 1999;23(8):903-909. doi:10.1097/00000478-199908000-00007.

29. Fisher C, Goldblum JR, Epstein JI, Montgomery E. Leiomyosarcoma of the parastesticular region. A clinicopathologic study. *Am J Surg Pathol.* 2001;25(9):1143-1149. doi:10.1097/00000478-200109000-00004.

30. Leuschner I, Newton WA, Schmidt D, et al. Spindle cell variants of embryonal rhabdomyosarcoma in the paratesticular region: a report of the intergroup rhabdomyosarcoma study. *Am J Surg Pathol.* 1993;17(3):221-230. doi:10.1097/00000478-199303000-00002.

31. Priemer DS, Trevino K, Chen S, Ulbright TM, Idrees MT. Paratesticular soft-tissue masses in orchiectomy specimens: a 17-year survey of primary and incidental cases from one institution. *Int J Surg Pathol.* 2017;25(6):480-487. doi:10.1177/1066896917707040.

32. Epstein J, Cubilla A, Humphrey P; American Registry of Pathology, Armed Forces Institute of Pathology (US). *Tumors of the prostate gland, seminal vesicles, penis, and scrotum.* In: *AFIP Atlas of Tumor Pathology ; 4th Ser. Fasc. 14.* Washington, DC: American Registry of Pathology in collaboration with the Armed Forces Institute of Pathology; 2011:675.

33. Shah V, Shet T. Scrotal calcinosis results from calcification of cysts derived from hair follicles: a series of 20 cases evaluating the spectrum of changes resulting in scrotal calcinosis. *Am J Dermatopathol.* 2007;29(2):172-175. doi:10.1097/01.dad.0000246465.25986.68.

34. Velazquez EF, Cubilla AL. Lichen sclerosus in 68 patients with squamous cell carcinoma of the penis: frequent atypias and correlation with special carcinoma variants suggests a precancerous role. *Am J Surg Pathol.* 2003;27(11):1448-1453. doi:10.1097/00000478-200311000-00007.

35. Oertell J, Caballero C, Iglesias M, et al. Differentiated precursor lesions and low-grade variants of squamous cell carcinomas are frequent findings in foreskins of patients from a region of high penile cancer incidence. *Histopathology.* 2011;58(6):925-933. doi:10.1111/j.1365-2559.2011.03816.x.

36. Nasca MR, Innocenzi D, Micali G. Penile cancer among patients with genital lichen sclerosus. *J Am Acad Dermatol.* 1999;41(6):911-914. doi:10.1016/S0190-9622(99)70245-8.

37. Weyers W, Ende Y, Schalla W, Diaz-Cascajo C. Balanitis of Zoon: a clinicopathologic study of 45 cases. *Am J Dermatopathol.* 2002;24(6):459-467. doi:10.1097/00000372-200212000-00001.

38. Lezcano C, Chaux A, Velazquez EF, Cubilla AL. Clinicopathological features and histogenesis of penile cysts. *Semin Diagn Pathol.* 2015;32(3):245-248. doi:10.1053/j.semdp.2014.12.014.

39. Suwa M, Takeda M, Bilim V, Takahashi K. Epidermoid cyst of the penis: a case report and review of the literature. *Int J Urol.* 2000;7(11):431-433. doi:10.1046/j.1442-2042.2000.00219.x.

40. Cole LA, Helwig EB. Mucoid cysts of the penile skin. *J Urol.* 1976;115(4):397-400. doi:10.1016/S0022-5347(17)59215-0.

41. Tomasini C, Aloi A, Puiatti P, Caliendo V. Dermoid cyst of the penis. *Dermatology.* 1997;194(2):188-190. doi:10.1159/000246096.

42. Brooks SG, Williams RED. Lymphatic cyst of the penis. *Br J Urol.* 1989;63(3):329-330. doi:10.1111/j.1464-410X.1989.tb05206.x.

43. Mulhall JP, Creech SD, Boorjian SA, et al. Subjective and objective analysis of the prevalence of Peyronie's disease in a population of men presenting for prostate cancer screening. *J Urol.* 2004;171(6 pt 1):2350-2353. doi:10.1097/01.ju.0000127744.18878.f1.

44. Hatfield BS, King CR, Udager AM, et al. Peyronie disease: clinicopathologic study of 71 cases with emphasis on histopathologic patterns and prevalent metaplastic ossification. *Hum Pathol.* July 2020. In press. doi:10.1016/j.humpath.2020.07.013.

45. Davis CJ. The microscopic pathology of Peyronie's disease. *J Urol.* 1997;157(1):282-284. http://www.ncbi.nlm.nih.gov/pubmed/8976280. Accessed April 30, 2020.

46. Farshid G, Weiss SW. Massive localized lymphedema in the morbidly obese: a histologically distinct reactive lesion simulating liposarcoma. *Am J Surg Pathol.* 1998;22(10):1277-1283. doi:10.1097/00000478-199810000-00013.

47. Lee S, Han JS, Ross HM, Epstein JI. Massive localized lymphedema of the male external genitalia: a clinicopathologic study of 6 cases. *Hum Pathol.* 2013;44(2):277-281. doi:10.1016/j.humpath.2012.05.023.

48. Oertel YC, Johnson FB. Sclerosing lipogranuloma of male genitalia. Review of 23 cases. *Arch Pathol Lab Med.* 1977;101(6):321-326. http://www.ncbi.nlm.nih.gov/pubmed/577132. Accessed June 20, 2020.

49. Bjurlin MA, Carlsen J, Grevious M, et al. Mineral oil-induced sclerosing lipogranuloma of the penis. *J Clin Aesthet Dermatol*. 2010;3(9):41-44. http://www.ncbi.nlm.nih.gov/pubmed/20877525. Accessed June 20, 2020.

50. Nucci MR, Granter SR, Fletcher CDM. Cellular angiofibroma: a benign neoplasm distinct from angiomyofibroblastoma and spindle cell lipoma. *Am J Surg Pathol*. 1997;21(6):636-644. doi:10.1097/00000478-199706000-00002.

51. Iwasa Y, Fletcher CDM. Cellular angiofibroma: clinicopathologic and immunohistochemical analysis of 51 cases. *Am J Surg Pathol*. 2004;28(11):1426-1435. doi:10.1097/01.pas.0000138002.46650.95.

52. Tsang WY, Chan JK, Lee KC, Fisher C, Fletcher CD. Aggressive angiomyxoma. A report of four cases occurring in men. *Am J Surg Pathol*. 1992;16(11):1059-1065.

53. Matoso A, Chen S, Plaza JA, Osunkoya AO, Epstein JI. Symplastic leiomyomas of the scrotum: a comparative study to usual leiomyomas and leiomyosarcomas. *Am J Surg Pathol*. 2014;38(10):1410-1417. doi:10.1097/PAS.0000000000000228.

54. McKenney JK, Collins MH, Carretero AP, Boyd TK, Redman JF, Parham DM. Penile myointimoma in children and adolescents: a clinicopathologic study of 5 cases supporting a distinct entity. *Am J Surg Pathol*. 2007;31(10):1622-1626. doi:10.1097/PAS.0b013e31804ea443.

55. Fetsch JF, Brinsko RW, Davis CJ, Mostofi FK, Sesterhenn IA. A distinctive myointimal proliferation ("myointimoma") involving the corpus spongiosum of the glans penis: a clinicopathologic and immunohistochemical analysis of 10 cases. *Am J Surg Pathol*. 2000;24(11):1524-1530. doi:10.1097/00000478-200011000-00008.

56. Velazquez EF, Melamed J, Barreto JE, Aguero F, Cubilla AL. Sarcomatoid carcinoma of the penis. *Am J Surg Pathol*. 2005;29(9):1152-1158. doi:10.1097/01.pas.0000160440.46394.a8.

57. Turgut M, Yenilmez A, Can C, Bildirici K, Erkul A, Özyürek Y. Fibroepithelial polyp of glans penis. *Urology*. 2005;65(3):593. doi:10.1016/j.urology.2004.09.071.

58. Yan H, Treacy A, Yousef G, Stewart R. Giant fibroepithelial polyp of the glans penis not associated with condom-catheter use: a case report and literature review. *J Can Urol Assoc*. 2013;7(9-10):E621-E624. doi:10.5489/cuaj.506.

59. Schiller PI, Itin PH. Angiokeratomas: an update. *Dermatology*. 1996;193(4):275-282. doi:10.1159/000246270.

60. Fabry H. Angiokeratoma corporis diffusum - fabry disease: historical review from the original description to the introduction of enzyme replacement therapy. *Acta Paediatr*. 2007;91(439):3-5. doi:10.1111/j.1651-2227.2002.tb03102.x.

61. Bai H, Cviko A, Granter S, Yuan L, Betensky RA, Crum CP. Immunophenotypic and viral (human papillomavirus) correlates of vulvar seborrheic keratosis. *Hum Pathol*. 2003;34(6):559-564. doi:10.1016/S0046-8177(03)00184-9.

62. Talia KL, McCluggage WG. Seborrheic keratosis-like lesions of the cervix and vagina: report of a new entity possibly related to low-risk human papillomavirus infection. *Am J Surg Pathol*. 2017;41(4):517-524. doi:10.1097/PAS.0000000000000762.

63. Chan MP. Verruciform and condyloma-like squamous proliferations in the Anogenital Region. *Arch Pathol Lab Med*. 2019;143(7):821-831. doi:10.5858/arpa.2018-0039-RA.

64. Patterson JW, Kao GF, Graham JH, Helwig EB. Bowenoid papulosis: a clinicopathologic study with ultrastructural observations. *Cancer*. 1986;57(4):823-836. doi:10.1002/1097-0142(19860215)57:4<823::AID-CNCR2820570424>3.0.CO;2-3.

65. Cubilla AL, Meijer CJLM, Young RH. Morphological features of epithelial abnormalities and precancerous lesions of the penis. *Scand J Urol Nephrol*. 2000;34:215-219. doi:10.1080/003655900750016652.

66. Liu H, Urabe K, Moroi Y, et al. Expression of p16 and hTERT protein is associated with the presence of high-risk human papillomavirus in Bowenoid papulosis. *J Cutan Pathol*. 2006;33(8):551-558. doi:10.1111/j.1600-0560.2006.00438.x.

67. Moch H, Cubilla AL, Humphrey PA, Reuter VE, Ulbright TM. The 2016 WHO classification of tumours of the urinary system and male genital organs—Part A: renal, penile, and testicular tumours. *Eur Urol*. 2016;70(1):93-105. doi:10.1016/j.eururo.2016.02.029.

68. Masih AS, Stoler MH, Farrow GM, Wooldridge TN, Johansson SL. Penile verrucous carcinoma: a clinicopathologic, human papillomavirus typing and flow cytometric analysis. *Mod Pathol*. 1992;5(1):48-55.

69. Del Pino M, Bleeker MCG, Quint WG, Snijders PJF, Meijer CJLM, Steenbergen RDM. Comprehensive analysis of human papillomavirus prevalence and the potential role of low-risk types in verrucous carcinoma. *Mod Pathol*. 2012;25(10):1354-1363. doi:10.1038/modpathol.2012.91.

70. Zidar N, Langner C, Odar K, et al. Anal verrucous carcinoma is not related to infection with human papillomaviruses and should be distinguished from giant condyloma (Buschke–Löwenstein tumour). *Histopathology*. 2017;70(6):938-945. doi:10.1111/his.13158.

71. Chaux A, Reuter V, Lezcano C, Velazquez EF, Torres J, Cubilla AL. Comparison of morphologic features and outcome of resected recurrent and nonrecurrent squamous cell carcinoma of the penis: a study of 81 cases. *Am J Surg Pathol*. 2009;33(9):1299-1306. doi:10.1097/PAS.0b013e3181a418ae.

72. Chaux A, Soares F, Rodríguez I, et al. Papillary squamous cell carcinoma, Not Otherwise Specified (NOS) of the penis: clinicopathologic features, differential diagnosis, and outcome of 35 cases. *Am J Surg Pathol*. 2010;34(2):223-230. doi:10.1097/PAS.0b013e3181c7666e.

73. Chaux A, Tamboli P, Ayala A, et al. Warty-basaloid carcinoma: clinicopathological features of a distinctive penile neoplasm. Report of 45 cases. *Mod Pathol*. 2010;23(6):896-904. doi:10.1038/modpathol.2010.69.

74. Cubilla AL, Lloveras B, Alemany L, et al. Basaloid squamous cell carcinoma of the penis with papillary features: a clinicopathologic study of 12 cases. *Am J Surg Pathol*. 2012;36(6):869-875. doi:10.1097/PAS.0b013e318249c6f3.

75. Cubilla AL, Lloveras B, Alejo M, et al. The basaloid cell is the best tissue marker for human papillomavirus in invasive penile squamous cell carcinoma: a study of 202 cases from Paraguay. *Am J Surg Pathol*. 2010;34(1):104-114. doi:10.1097/PAS.0b013e3181c76a49.

76. Chaux A, Pfannl R, Lloveras B, et al. Distinctive association of p16INK4a overexpression with penile intraepithelial neoplasia depicting warty and/or basaloid features: a study of 141 cases evaluating a new nomenclature. *Am J Surg Pathol*. 2010;34(3):385-392. doi:10.1097/PAS.0b013e3181cdad23.

77. Chaux A, Pfannl R, Rodríguez IM, et al. Distinctive immunohistochemical profile of penile intraepithelial lesions: a study of 74 cases. *Am J Surg Pathol*. 2011;35(4):553-562. doi:10.1097/PAS.0b013e3182113402.

78. Kuan SF, Montag AG, Hart J, Krausz T, Recant W. Differential expression of mucin genes in mammary and extramammary Paget's disease. *Am J Surg Pathol*. 2001;25(12):1469-1477. doi:10.1097/00000478-200112000-00001.

79. Liegl B, Leibl S, Gogg-Kamerer M, Tessaro B, Horn L-C, Moinfar F. Mammary and extramammary Paget's disease: an immunohistochemical study of 83 cases. *Histopathology*. 2007;50(4):439-447. doi:10.1111/j.1365-2559.2007.02633.x.

80. Zhao M, Zhou L, Sun L, et al. GATA3 is a sensitive marker for primary genital extramammary paget disease: an immunohistochemical study of 72 cases with comparison to gross cystic disease fluid protein 15. *Diagn Pathol*. 2017;12(1). doi:10.1186/s13000-017-0638-z.

81. Nowak MA, Guerriere-Kovach P, Pathan A, Campbell TE, Deppisch LM. Perianal Paget's disease: distinguishing primary and secondary lesions using immunohistochemical studies including gross cystic disease fluid protein-15 and cytokeratin 20 expression. *Arch Pathol Lab Med*. 1998;122(12):1077-1081. http://www.ncbi.nlm.nih.gov/pubmed/9870855. Accessed June 21, 2020.

82. Moch H, Humphrey PA, Ulbright T, Reuter VE. *WHO Classification of Tumours of the Urinary System and Male Genital Organs*. 4th ed.. Lyon, France: International Agency for Research on Cancer; 2016.

83. Cubilla AL, Lloveras B, Alejo M, et al. Value of p16INK4a in the pathology of invasive penile Squamous cell carcinomas: a report of 202 cases. *Am J Surg Pathol*. 2011;35(2):253-261. doi:10.1097/PAS.0b013e318203cdba.

84. Matoso A, Ross HM, Chen S, Allbritton J, Epstein JI. Squamous neoplasia of the scrotum: a series of 29 cases. *Am J Surg Pathol*. 2014;38(7):973-981. doi:10.1097/PAS.0000000000000192.

85. Matoso A, Fabre V, Quddus MR, et al. Prevalence and distribution of 15 high-risk human papillomavirus types in squamous cell carcinoma of the scrotum. *Hum Pathol*. 2016;53:130-136. doi:10.1016/j.humpath.2016.02.013.

86. Amin MB, Edge SB, Greene FL, et al, eds. *AJCC Cancer Staging Manual*. 8th ed.. New York, NY: Springer; 2017.

87. Cubilla AL, Reuter VE, Gregoire L, et al. Basaloid squamous cell carcinoma: a distinctive human papilloma virus- related penile neoplasm. A report of 20 cases. *Am J Surg Pathol*. 1998;22(6):755-761. doi:10.1097/00000478-199806000-00014.

88. Alvarado-Cabrero I, Sanchez DF, Piedras D, et al. The variable morphological spectrum of penile basaloid carcinomas: differential diagnosis, prognostic factors and outcome report in 27 cases classified as classic and mixed variants. *Appl Cancer Res.* 2017;37(1):3. doi:10.1186/s41241-017-0010-3.

89. McGregor DH, Tanimura A, Eigel JW. Basal cell carcinoma of penis. *Urology.* 1982;20(3):320-323. doi:10.1016/0090-4295(82)90653-7.

90. Haque S, Noble J, Wotherspoon A, Woodhouse C, Cunningham D. MALT lymphoma of the foreskin. *Leuk Lymphoma.* 2004;45(8):1699-1701. doi:10.1080/10428190410001683813.

91. Chaux A, Amin M, Cubilla AL, Young RH. Metastatic tumors to the penis: a report of 17 cases and review of the literature. *Int J Surg Pathol.* 2011;19(5):597-606. doi:10.1177/1066896909350468.

92. Teichman JMH, Mannas M, Elston DM. Noninfectious penile lesions. *Am Fam Physician.* 2018;97(2):102-110.

CHAPTER 1 PROSTATE

1-1. **Which of the following constitutes extraprostatic extension?**

    A. Prostatic adenocarcinoma within skeletal muscle.

    B. Prostatic adenocarcinoma within the intraprostatic ejaculatory duct.

    C. Prostatic adenocarcinoma in the "bladder neck" sections adjacent to normal benign prostatic glands present.

    D. Prostatic adenocarcinoma into the plane of fat but not touching fat cells.

1-2. **Select the correct statement:**

    A. A single-color method of multiplex antibody stain for evaluating small foci of prostatic adenocarcinoma is inferior and should be avoided.

    B. Negative ERG immunohistochemistry argues against a diagnosis of prostatic adenocarcinoma in a biopsy specimen.

    C. Absence of basal cells and positive AMACR staining is not entirely specific for prostatic adenocarcinoma.

    D. Many prostate cancers have aberrant immunohistochemical positivity for both p63 and high-molecular-weight cytokeratin.

1-3. **Which of the following is true of adenosis (atypical adenomatous hyperplasia)?**

    A. It is considered a precursor of prostatic adenocarcinoma.

    B. It typically occurs in the transition zone.

    C. The basal cell layer should be intact and continuous.

    D. It should not contain luminal crystalloids.

1-4. **Which of the following is true of partial atrophy?**

    A. Basal cells are consistently present.

    B. The cytoplasm is often barely taller than the nucleus and wide laterally.

    C. The glandular contour is angulated or tufted.

    D. *ERG* rearrangements are often present, overlapping with prostatic adenocarcinoma.

1-5. **Which of the following immunohistochemical markers is most helpful in diagnosis of nephrogenic adenoma involving the prostatic urethra?**

    A. PAX8.

    B. AMACR.

    C. p63.

    D. High-molecular-weight cytokeratin.

1-6. **Which of the following is considered pathognomonic of prostatic adenocarcinoma?**

    A. Glomeruloid structures/glomerulations.

    B. Nucleoli.

    C. Amphophilic cytoplasm.

    D. Small, round gland pattern.

1-7. **Which of the following is incorrectly matched with its grade pattern?**

    A. Separate, well-formed, round glands = pattern 3.

    B. Poorly formed glands = pattern 4.

    C. Cribriform glands = pattern 4.

    D. Ductal variant = pattern 5.

1-8. **Which of the following is true regarding prostatic adenocarcinoma with comedonecrosis?**

    A. Typically present in invasive cancer only.

    B. Eosinophilic material in the glandular lumen is sufficient for diagnosis.

    C. Frequently associated with low-grade invasive cancer.

    D. When associated with intraductal carcinoma, prognostic significance is unclear.

1-9. **Which of the following patterns is unlikely to be mimicked by prostate cancer with treatment effect (radiation or androgen deprivation therapy)?**

    A. Poorly formed glands.

    B. Single cells.

    C. Atrophy-like cancer.

    D. Large cribriform cancer.

1-10. **You reported a prostatic adenocarcinoma specimen with typical morphology, Gleason score 4 + 4 = 8 (Grade Group 4). In view of widespread metastases, the oncologist requested neuroendocrine markers to be performed, which show focal, patchy staining in the cancer. The best approach is to**

    A. Amend the diagnosis to small cell neuroendocrine carcinoma.

    B. Amend the diagnosis to large cell neuroendocrine carcinoma.

    C. Report patchy staining but not meeting criteria for neuroendocrine carcinoma.

    D. Add to the report "prostatic adenocarcinoma with neuroendocrine features."

CHAPTER 2 BLADDER

2-1. **Select the correct statement:**

    A. Staging of urothelial carcinomas is based on tumor size.

    B. Staging of urothelial carcinomas includes tumor grade.

    C. There is no difference in staging for papillary and flat tumors.

    D. Staging of urothelial carcinomas is based on extent of invasion.

2-2. **Select the correct statement:**

    A. CK20 staining limited to the umbrella cell layer supports a diagnosis of CIS.

    B. Ki-67 index is only increased in neoplastic processes such as CIS.

    C. Full-thickness staining with CD44 supports a reactive/nonneoplastic process.

    D. Wild-type p53 (heterogeneous) staining is diagnostic of CIS.

2-3. **Which of the following entities involving the muscularis propria should be considered malignant?**

    A. Urachal remnant.

    B. Mullerianosis.

    C. Nephrogenic adenoma.

    D. Bland nests of urothelium.

2-4. True/False: GATA3 is useful to distinguish urothelial carcinoma from paraganglioma.

2-5. True/False: Identification of fat within a transurethral resection of the bladder specimen should prompt an immediate call to the clinician due to risk of bladder perforation.

2-6. Select the incorrect statement:

    A. Retraction artifact surrounding tumor cells is a helpful feature of early lamina propria invasion.

    B. Inverted pattern of growth is only seen in invasive urothelial tumors.

    C. Tumor cells showing more abundant eosinophilic cytoplasm and mature features when compared to the overlying surface tumor is indicative of "paradoxical maturation" and a feature of invasion.

    D. The degree of lamina propria invasion "focal" versus "nonfocal" has prognostic significance and should be commented on in the report.

2-7. True/False: The recognition and reporting of histologic variants of urothelial carcinoma is critical for accurate diagnosis, prognosis, and treatment planning.

2-8. Lynch syndrome is associated with which of the following (choose all that apply)?

    A. Mismatch repair deficiency.

    B. Upper tract and bladder urothelial carcinoma.

    C. Decreased risk of multiple types of malignancy.

    D. Inverted growth pattern.

2-9. Which of the following immunohistochemical panels is best for distinguishing prostate from bladder origin?

    A. AE1/3, CK7, and CK20.

    B. NKX3.1, PSA, GATA3, and p40.

    C. INSM1, chromogranin, synaptophysin, and CD56.

    D. MOC31 and BerEp4.

2-10. Which of these features is incompatible with the diagnosis of benign inverted urothelial papilloma?

    A. Peripheral palisading of urothelial cells.

    B. Eosinophilic material within microcysts.

    C. Multiple well-formed exophytic papillary fronds.

    D. Jigsaw pattern of interlocking cords of urothelial cells.

CHAPTER 3 KIDNEY

3-1. Which of the following is true of normal renal anatomy/histology?

    A. Vein branches consistently include thick bundles of smooth muscle.

    B. Four to six cell nuclei per mesangial glomerular area is normal.

    C. The renal sinus is the loose fibrous and adipose tissue at the renal hilum.

    D. Distal renal tubules are strongly positive for AMACR and more eosinophilic than proximal tubules.

3-2. A metastatic bone biopsy in a 65-year-old woman shows a tumor compatible with RCC and imaging identifies a large renal mass. The immunohistochemistry shows PAX8+, cytokeratin 7 negative, AMACR weak, and carbonic anhydrase IX negative. Which conclusion is most accurate?

    A. This phenotype is strongly supportive of papillary RCC.

    B. This phenotype argues for an unrelated cancer of gynecologic origin.

    C. Although carbonic anhydrase IX is negative, clear cell RCC remains a consideration.

    D. A syndromic RCC type should be strongly considered.

3-3. Which combination of findings is most in keeping with clear cell RCC?

    A. Cytokeratin 7 minimal/negative, AMACR moderate, KIT negative, *VHL* mutated.

    B. Cytokeratin 7 diffuse positive, KIT positive, chromosome 3p25 normal.

    C. Cytokeratin 7 minimal/negative, carbonic anhydrase IX negative, *FH* mutated.

    D. AMACR negative, KIT negative, trisomy of chromosome 7 and 17.

3-4. You encounter a renal tumor that resembles type 1 papillary RCC with papillary structures and foamy macrophages, but areas of clear cytoplasm are also present. Immunohistochemistry shows diffuse cytokeratin 7, strong AMACR, and negative carbonic anhydrase IX. Fluorescence in situ hybridization is negative for *TFE3/TFEB* translocation. Which statement is most accurate?

    A. The diagnosis should be clear cell papillary RCC based on the clear cytoplasm and papillary architecture.

    B. The diagnosis should be unclassified RCC due to the mixed clear cell and papillary features.

    C. This is a morphologic variation of papillary RCC and can be reported as type 1 papillary RCC.

    D. The diagnosis should be Xp11.2 RCC based on the overlapping features of clear cell and papillary RCC.

3-5. You encounter a renal mass biopsy with suspected chromophobe RCC. Which of the following would be supportive of the diagnosis?

    A. Positive vimentin immunohistochemistry.

    B. Positive KIT (CD117) immunohistochemistry.

    C. Negative cytokeratin 7 immunohistochemistry.

    D. Negative colloidal iron special stain.

3-6. Which of the following would be in favor of a diagnosis of clear cell papillary RCC?

    A. High-molecular-weight cytokeratin negative.

    B. Tumor necrosis.

    C. Prominent branched glandular formation.

    D. Size >10 cm.

3-7. True/False: A tumor shows striking features suggestive of MITF family translocation RCC; however, break-apart fluorescence in situ hybridization tests for *TFE3* and *TFEB* are both reported as negative. A diagnosis of MITF family translocation RCC is still possible.

3-8. A renal neoplasm specimen shows spindle cell morphology with some mildly atypical cells having clear cytoplasm. You suspect angiomyolipoma. Immunohistochemistry shows substantial staining for smooth muscle actin, negative cytokeratin, and negative PAX8. Melanocytic markers are largely negative with exception of rare scattered cells positive for both. The best interpretation would be:

    A. Angiomyolipoma, because even rare cells positive for melanocytic markers would support the diagnosis.

    B. Leiomyoma, because there is smooth muscle marker positivity but extremely minimal melanocytic marker positivity.

    C. Sarcomatoid RCC, because epithelial marker staining can be decreased or absent.

    D. Leiomyosarcoma, because it is a smooth muscle neoplasm with atypia.

3-9. Which of the following is most specific for FH-deficient RCC/hereditary leiomyomatosis and RCC syndrome?

    A. Prominent nucleoli.

    B. History of uterine leiomyomas.

    C. Negative (loss of) FH immunohistochemistry.

    D. Sarcomatoid dedifferentiation.

3-10. Which of these features would be most supportive of oncocytoma diagnosis?

    A. Cytokeratin 7 staining in rare single cells making up <1% of the tumor.

    B. Negative immunohistochemical staining for KIT.

    C. Negative immunohistochemical staining for succinate dehydrogenase B.

    D. Strong cytoplasmic colloidal iron staining.

CHAPTER 4 TESTIS

4-1. Select the correct statement:

    A. Segmental infarcts of the testis are most commonly associated with torsion.

    B. Ghost tubules are seen only in segmental infarcts.

    C. Polyarteritis nodosa (PAN)-like vasculitis is the most common cause of testicular vasculitis.

    D. Isolated vasculitis of the testis is more common than systemic vasculitis involving the testis.

4-2. Select the incorrect statement:

    A. Spermatocytic tumors are GCNIS-associated tumors.

    B. Postpubertal teratomas are GCNIS-associated tumors.

    C. Isochromosome 12p is identified frequently in tumors arising from germ cell neoplasia in situ.

    D. Dermoid and epidermoid cysts are not associated with germ cell neoplasia in situ.

4-3. True/False: Granulomatous inflammation is only associated with infectious processes in the testis.

4-4. Select the correct statement:

    A. Yolk sac tumor has a single classic architectural pattern.

    B. Sarcomatoid differentiation is frequently identified in metastatic yolk sac tumor, leading to diagnostic difficulty.

    C. Call-Exner bodies are a helpful diagnostic feature of yolk sac tumor.

    D. GATA3 is a useful immunohistochemical marker for yolk sac tumor.

4-5. True/False: The identification of Leydig cells within the spermatic cord soft tissue supports a diagnosis of malignant Leydig cell tumor.

4-6. Select the incorrect statement:

A. Germ cell neoplasia in situ (GCNIS) is an intratubular growth pattern of malignant germ cells.

B. GCNIS has the same immunoprofile as seminoma.

C. GCNIS cells are distributed in a patchy manner along the basal aspect of the tubules.

D. GCNIS is never identified in spermatic tubules that contain mature spermatids.

4-7. True/False: Involvement of the paratesticular soft tissue at the base of the spermatic cord/epididymis is staged as pT3.

4-8. Specific histologic features in the diagnosis of regressed germ cell tumor include (choose all that apply):

A. Germ cell neoplasia in situ (GCNIS).

B. Scar.

C. Coarse intratubular calcifications.

D. Leydig cell hyperplasia.

4-9. Which of the following immunohistochemical panels is best for distinguishing seminoma from embryonal carcinoma?

A. SF1, inhibin, and calretinin.

B. GATA3, hCG, AFP, and glypican 3.

C. D2-40, CD117, CD30, and AE1/3.

D. MOC31 and BerEp4.

4-10. Which of these findings is not associated with cryptorchid testis?

A. Sertoli cell nodules.

B. Infertility.

C. Tubular hyperplasia with increased tubular diameter.

D. Hemosiderin deposition.

CHAPTER 5 PARATESTIS AND EXTERNAL GENITALIA

5-1. A paratesticular cyst with mesothelial hyperplasia is usually best classified as:

A. Spermatocele.

B. Hydrocele.

C. Varicocele.

D. Hematocele.

5-2. Select the correct statement:

A. Adenomatoid tumor should be negative for mesothelial markers, contrasting to mesothelioma.

B. Hyaline globules favor a diagnosis of yolk sac tumor over hyperplasia of the rete testis.

C. Restriction of mesothelial proliferation to a band-like zone favors hyperplasia over mesothelioma.

D. Papillary cystadenoma of the epididymis is negative for carbonic anhydrase IX (CA-IX), contrasting to metastatic clear cell renal cell carcinoma.

5-3. Which of the following is most accurate concerning soft tissue tumors of the paratestis?

A. A 3-cm "cord lipoma" with no appreciable atypia should be evaluated with immunohistochemistry for *MDM2* to rule out atypical lipomatous tumor/well-differentiated liposarcoma.

B. A 15-cm "cord lipoma" should be evaluated similarly to a retroperitoneal lipomatous neoplasm.

C. Fibrous pseudotumors are usually positive for ALK immunohistochemistry, suggesting they are inflammatory myofibroblastic tumors.

D. A smooth muscle proliferation with bland cytology "cuffing" around the ductules of the epididymis is most likely to be leiomyosarcoma.

5-4. True/False: Scrotal calcinosis is thought to be associated with systemic hypercalcemia.

5-5. Which of the following statements is most accurate concerning inflammatory processes of the male external genital tract?

A. A dense lichenoid inflammatory pattern with numerous plasma cells is highly specific for Zoon balanitis.

B. Balanitis xerotica obliterans is synonymous with lichen sclerosus et atrophicus.

C. Negative immunohistochemistry for treponemal organisms in a tissue section rules out a diagnosis of syphilis.

D. Lichen sclerosus has no appreciable association with penile cancer.

5-6. Which statement is most accurate regarding spindle cell lesions of the penis and scrotum?

A. Peyronie disease is often highly cellular, mimicking a sarcoma.

B. A large scrotal lesion histologically resembling liposarcoma in a morbidly obese patient may represent massive localized lymphedema.

C. Sclerosing lipogranuloma is an idiopathic process affecting the male external genital sites.

D. Myointimoma is a unique lesion that has been only described to occur on the scrotum.

5-7. Which statement is most accurate regarding papillary proliferations of the penis?

A. Angiokeratoma of the scrotum raises suspicion for Fabry disease.

B. Seborrheic keratosis of genital sites has a similar pathogenesis to that of other skin sites.

C. Warty-basaloid PeIN is associated with HPV.

D. Verrucous carcinoma is associated with HPV.

5-8. Which of the following is true regarding extramammary Paget disease of the penis/scrotum?

A. GATA3 positivity suggests secondary spread of urothelial carcinoma.

B. Cells are typically negative for cytokeratin 7 in primary disease.

C. Cells are typically positive for p63 in primary disease.

D. NKX3.1 positivity suggests secondary spread of prostatic adenocarcinoma.

5-9. **Which statement most accurately reflects the eighth edition AJCC staging of penile cancer?**

    A. Involvement of the urethra is pT3 disease.

    B. Tumors that are pT1a invade the lamina propria with or without lymphovascular invasion, high-grade cytology, or perineural invasion.

    C. Involvement of the prostate is pT3.

    D. Tumor extension to the corpus spongiosum and cavernosum is now staged differently.

5-10. **True/False: Priapism is a presenting feature of metastatic carcinoma to the penis.**

SELF-ASSESSMENT ANSWERS

CHAPTER 1 PROSTATE

1-1. Answer – D. Skeletal muscle commonly intermingles with the prostate at the apex and anterior, so involvement of skeletal muscle is not necessarily extraprostatic extension. Likewise, involvement of the ejaculatory duct is still within the prostate, although such a tumor would be of higher risk for seminal vesicle invasion. Although invasion of bladder neck muscle constitutes pT3a in the current staging system, this is restricted to involvement of large muscle bundles different from the confluent muscle of the prostate stroma. If normal benign glands are present adjacent to the cancer in the bladder neck sections, this is usually an argument against bladder neck invasion. Carcinoma at the level of fat almost always indicates extraprostatic extension, even if the tumor cells are not directly touching adipocytes.

1-2. Answer – C. There are various potential formulations for immunohistochemistry to evaluate atypical glands in prostate biopsies. Although dual-color stains are typically easy to interpret, single-color assays, such as p63 and AMACR with a brown chromogen, are also reasonable and technically easier to perform in some laboratories. Single antibodies alone (p63 only or high-molecular-weight cytokeratin only) may be more challenging to interpret without the positive component of AMACR staining. *ERG* rearrangements are present in only 40% to 50% of prostatic adenocarcinomas, and therefore, a negative result does not argue against prostatic adenocarcinoma; however, a positive result for ERG is highly suggestive of carcinoma. Absence of basal cells and AMACR staining should not be interpreted in isolation as definitive of malignancy, as some mimics, such as atypical adenomatous hyperplasia (adenosis), benign colorectal tissue, or partial atrophy, can have patchy or absent basal cells and increased AMACR. Although rare prostatic adenocarcinomas can have aberrant positivity for p63 or high-molecular-weight cytokeratin, fortunately this is rare and especially so for both markers to be positive in the same cancer.

1-3. Answer – B. Adenosis is a mimic of prostatic adenocarcinoma. Although it shares some features with adenocarcinoma, such as partial absence of basal cells, variable AMACR positivity, and small gland pattern, it is currently not thought to confer any increased risk of cancer. It does typically occur in the transition zone as a part of nodular hyperplasia. Although it should have some basal cells, the basal cell layer is often patchy and discontinuous, with some glands appearing to entirely lack basal cells. It can contain crystalloids, again mimicking cancer.

1-4. Answer – B. Partial atrophy is a mimic of prostatic adenocarcinoma. Like other mimics, basal cells may be patchy and appear absent in a subset of the glands. Typically, the cytoplasm is barely taller than the nucleus, although there may be substantial lateral cytoplasm before the next nucleus is visualized. Partial atrophy often forms small round glands, mimicking cancer, in contrast to normal benign glands (tufted) or simple atrophy (angulated). Using immunohistochemistry, benign mimics like partial atrophy have been found to be negative for ERG protein.

1-5. Answer – A. Nephrogenic adenoma is thought to be derived from shed renal tubular cells from the kidney that implant into the urinary tract mucosa and proliferate. Therefore, these lesions are consistently positive for PAX8. AMACR positivity may be deceptive, as both benign renal tubules and prostatic adenocarcinoma are positive for this marker. High-molecular-weight cytokeratin and p63 will not show a basal cell layer, again overlapping with prostatic adenocarcinoma. However, sometimes the glandular cells will be positive for high-molecular-weight cytokeratin, which can be a clue to the distinction from prostate cancer if a multiplex antibody stain is used.

1-6. Answer – A. All of these features are found in prostate cancer; however, other than glomerulations, all of these can also be observed in benign mimics. True glomeruloid structures with a cribriform tuft in the lumen of a round gland is considered diagnostic of prostatic adenocarcinoma (and Gleason pattern 4). Perineural invasion and mucinous fibroplasia/collagenous micronodules are the other features that are considered pathognomonic of cancer.

1-7. Answer – D. Ductal variant prostatic adenocarcinoma is considered inherently pattern 4. A possible exception to this is high-grade prostatic intraepithelial neoplasia (PIN)-like cancer, composed of small tufted glands resembling PIN. This can be interpreted as pattern 3. Some authors would consider this a form of ductal cancer, whereas others would regard it separately as PIN-like cancer.

1-8. Answer – D. Recent evidence shows that comedonecrosis in prostatic adenocarcinoma is enriched in intraductal carcinoma. This is frequently associated with high-grade invasive cancer. Granular eosinophilic debris in the lumen with an interface of karyorrhectic debris is usually required for diagnosis. Although there is now considerable debate as to whether it is necessary to evaluate foci of comedonecrosis with immunohistochemistry to prove or refute intraductal carcinoma, there are no data convincingly showing that intraductal carcinoma with comedonecrosis is more favorable than invasive cancer with comedonecrosis. However, this is an area of exploration.

1-9. Answer – D. Prostatic adenocarcinoma with radiation or androgen deprivation therapy effect often forms atrophic glands with scant cytoplasm, often poorly formed glands or single cells. Nuclei vary from those of typical prostatic adenocarcinoma to very small nuclei, mimicking histiocytic cells. These patterns should not be graded, as the cancer has had at least partial response to therapy. Large cribriform growth is not a known pattern of cancer with treatment effect and, if present, could be reported that there is minimal or limited evidence of treatment effect.

1-10. Answer – C. It is not unusual to find focal or patchy neuroendocrine marker staining in conventional prostatic adenocarcinoma. Currently, the significance of this is uncertain. It is not recommended to use a diagnosis of small cell or large cell neuroendocrine carcinoma based only on immunohistochemistry, unless the tumor shows overt neuroendocrine features histologically. This often includes a high proliferative rate, negative prostatic markers, and sometimes TTF1 positivity.

CHAPTER 2 BLADDER

2-1. Answer – D. Urothelial carcinomas are staged based on the extent of invasion. Noninvasive tumors are staged differently depending on their architectural growth pattern. Noninvasive papillary tumors are staged as pTa, whereas noninvasive flat tumors, or CIS, is staged as pTis. Invasion into the lamina propria is considered pT1 regardless of growth pattern. Involvement of the muscularis propria is staged as pT2, also regardless of growth pattern. In a TURBT, there is no subdivision of pT2 disease; however, in a cystectomy involvement of the inner muscularis propria is pT2a and outer muscle involvement is pT2b. Extravesical fat involvement constitutes pT3 disease. Tumor size and tumor grade are not considered in the determination of stage.

2-2. Answer – C. The usual staining pattern of CD44 in normal/reactive urothelium is full thickness. When possible, the diagnosis of CIS should be based on H&E morphology. Hyperchromasia, nuclear pleomorphism with nuclei 4-5× the size of a resting lymphocyte, architectural disorganization and frequent mitotic figures are features of CIS. When the H&E findings are not entirely diagnostic of CIS,

IHC may provide useful information to support reactive urothelium versus CIS. Full-thickness CK20 staining lends support to CIS, and loss of full-thickness CD44 staining supports CIS. Wild-type p53 staining is seen in normal urothelium, and the expected pattern for CIS is either strong, diffuse nuclear staining (most common), or, less commonly, the null/negative p53 pattern. Ki-67 should be used with caution in assessing CIS, as reactive urothelium frequently has an increased proliferation index.

2-3. Answer – D. Bland nests of urothelium should never be present within muscularis propria. Numerous benign glandular lesions may involve the muscularis propria of the bladder, including urachal remnants, mullerianosis, and nephrogenic adenoma. However, there is no benign urothelial lesion that can occur in the muscularis propria. If bland nests of urothelium are identified in the muscularis propria, the diagnosis is invasive urothelial carcinoma and it likely represents the nested variant, which is cytologically bland. Close inspection for mild atypia, rare mitotic figures, and other features of invasion will help to prove the malignant nature of the lesion.

2-4. Answer – False. GATA3 is positive in both paraganglioma and urothelial carcinoma and should not be used to distinguish the two entities. An immunohistochemical panel should include a pan-keratin, p40, synaptophysin, and chromogranin. In urothelial carcinoma, pan-keratin and p40 should be positive, whereas they are negative in paraganglioma. In paraganglioma, the opposite immunoprofile is seen with synaptophysin and chromogranin positive and pan-keratin and p40 negative. Both of these entities may be present in the muscularis propria with significant morphologic overlap; therefore, it is important to recognize the morphologic and immunophenotypic characteristics.

2-5. Answer – False. Fat can be identified at any level of the bladder, including all the way up to the lamina propria. Identifying fat in a TURBT specimen does not warrant a call to the clinician or even acknowledgment in the report. Unlike fat in a colon or endometrial biopsy, it is an acceptable finding.

2-6. Answer – B. Inverted growth pattern is commonly identified in benign entities (benign inverted urothelial papilloma) and urothelial carcinomas. Recognition that downward, bulging growth may represent inverted growth is important to avoid overdiagnosis of invasion. Smooth contours and large size of the nests of tumor favor a noninvasive, inverted growth pattern. Conversely, features of invasion include single cells or small nests, retraction artifact, paradoxical maturation and desmoplastic stromal response. When lamina propria invasion is definitively identified, a comment as to the extent of invasion should be given in the form of "focal" versus "nonfocal."

2-7. Answer – True. Histologic variants of urothelial carcinoma include 10 different patterns of urothelial carcinoma that often co-occur with usual urothelial carcinoma, but have sufficiently different morphologies that they may cause diagnostic confusion. It is essential to be familiar with the variant histologies so that the overall diagnosis of a urothelial carcinoma is rendered, followed by a description of any variant histology in the report. Some variant histologies are associated with worse prognostic outcomes, and outlining these findings can help guide treatment decisions for the clinician.

2-8. Answer – A, B, and D. Lynch syndrome is a mismatch repair deficiency leading to an increased risk for multiple malignancies, including upper tract urothelial carcinoma (the third most common tumor type in Lynch syndrome) and bladder urothelial carcinoma. Upper tract tumors commonly show inverted growth pattern as well as a brisk lymphocytic infiltrate.

2-9. Answer – B. A limited immunopanel for the differentiation of prostate from bladder should include at least NKX3.1 and GATA3. NKX3.1 is a highly sensitive and specific marker for prostate cancer. PSA is less sensitive in poorly differentiated tumors but still a helpful marker when positive. GATA3 is the most specific marker for urothelial origin and p40/p63 may also be useful to support a bladder primary. When a poorly differentiated tumor is arising in the bladder neck/prostate and no obvious morphologic features of one tumor type are present (surface urothelial component or obvious acinar or cribriform pattern with classic cytology for prostate), a limited immunopanel should be employed.

2-10. **Answer – C.** Well-formed papillary cores are not acceptable in a benign urothelial papilloma. Benign inverted urothelial papillomas demonstrate predominantly inverted growth pattern with interlocking cords of urothelium with peripheral palisading. Microcysts containing eosinophilic material are frequently present. While a rare papillary frond may be identified, a well-formed exophytic component is not compatible with this diagnosis and favors either a benign papilloma or a papillary urothelial carcinoma depending on the cytologic features.

CHAPTER 3 KIDNEY

3-1. **Answer – C.** Renal vein branches are sometimes small with inconspicuous smooth muscle in their walls. Recognition of the paired artery can be a clue to locate small vein branches, which can be important for cancer staging. More than four nuclei in a mesangial area is abnormal and may be due to glomerulonephritis or diabetic nephropathy. The renal sinus is the loose tissue and adipose tissue that envelops the renal vasculature and renal pelvis. This is also a key area for renal cancer staging. Proximal renal tubules are strongly positive for AMACR and more eosinophilic than their distal counterparts.

3-2. **Answer – C.** The weak AMACR staining in this case does not lend strong support to papillary RCC, nor does the negative cytokeratin 7, although cytokeratin 7 may be minimally positive or negative in eosinophilic papillary tumors. Given the history of a large renal mass, metastatic RCC is likely, so there is no reason to suspect an alternate primary cancer based on the provided information. Although carbonic anhydrase IX is negative, clear cell RCC always remains a consideration, as it is the most common subtype of renal cancer and otherwise the immunohistochemical results would be compatible with this diagnosis. Sometimes carbonic anhydrase IX staining can be decreased in areas of poorly differentiated or high-grade clear cell RCC. No reason to strongly suspect a hereditary syndrome is given for this case, as the patient's age is not unusual for renal cancer and findings such as multiplicity or family history are not provided.

3-3. **Answer – A.** Clear cell RCC usually has negative or minimal cytokeratin 7 staining (although exceptions occur with more extensive staining and do not exclude the diagnosis), variable AMACR staining ranging from negative to strong, negative KIT (contrasting to oncocytoma or chromophobe RCC), diffuse membranous carbonic anhydrase IX staining, and mutation of *VHL*/loss of chromosome 3p25. Mutation of *FH* is associated with hereditary leiomyomatosis and renal cell carcinoma syndrome, and trisomy of 7/17 is associated with type 1 papillary RCC.

3-4. **Answer – C.** Clear cytoplasmic changes are known to occur in type 1 papillary RCC. Clear cell papillary RCC, in contrast, is a defined entity with a specific constellation of morphologic and immunohistochemical features that has a favorable prognosis (carbonic anhydrase IX positive, AMACR negative/minimal, cytokeratin 7 diffuse positive, CD10 usually negative, GATA3/high-molecular-weight cytokeratin often positive). Clear cell papillary RCC typically does not contain prominent foamy macrophages. The negative fluorescence in situ hybridization studies do not lend support to translocation RCC (Xp11.2 translocation involving *TFE3*). A diagnosis of unclassified RCC probably should be avoided in this case, as this may give a clinical impression of an aggressive neoplasm and otherwise the features are in keeping with papillary RCC.

3-5. **Answer – B.** Although special stains and immunohistochemistry are not always perfect, positive KIT is common in both oncocytoma and chromophobe RCC, which may help in distinguishing these from clear cell or other RCC types. Vimentin is typically negative in both oncocytoma and chromophobe, with exception of "central scar" areas, especially in oncocytoma. Cytokeratin 7 may vary, especially in eosinophilic chromophobe RCC, but diffuse staining for cytokeratin 7 is the prototypical pattern of classic chromophobe. Colloidal iron can be technically challenging to perform, but the classic finding is diffuse cytoplasmic staining in chromophobe RCC.

3-6. Answer – C. Clear cell papillary RCC is typically nonaggressive and may be considered for reclassification as a low malignant potential tumor in future schemes. The vast majority are under 4 cm (pT1a) and tumor necrosis is very rare. High-molecular-weight cytokeratin is often positive, as are carbonic anhydrase IX, cytokeratin 7, and sometimes GATA3, whereas AMACR and CD10 are typically negative/minimal. Branched glands rather than round nests may be a clue to the diagnosis.

3-7. Answer – True. Several *TFE3* fusions have been recently found to result from chromosomal inversions within the X chromosome, so that fluorescence in situ hybridization may appear subtly positive or false-negative due to the close proximity of the two genes on the same chromosome. In these cases, other molecular techniques may detect the fusion, despite a negative fluorescence in situ hybridization result. Also, very rare tumors have been recently noted to have rearrangement of *MITF* rather than *TFE3* or *TFEB*.

3-8. Answer – A. Angiomyolipoma is a relatively common spindle cell neoplasm of the kidney. Substantial smooth muscle marker staining with scattered cells positive for melanocytic markers is not unusual. In contrast to melanocytic markers, cathepsin K typically shows diffuse strong staining. Focal melanocytic marker staining should not be ignored when attempting to distinguish a smooth muscle neoplasm from angiomyolipoma. Rare leiomyomas of the kidney do occur, typically in women, and these are usually positive for estrogen receptor and progesterone receptor. Leiomyosarcoma can occur around the kidney, especially in association with the renal vein or vena cava. Interpretation of an angiomyolipoma as leiomyosarcoma could lead to a serious error in treatment; therefore, angiomyolipoma should usually be considered in the differential diagnosis of spindle cell tumors of the kidney.

3-9. Answer – C. All these findings can occur with FH-deficient RCC/hereditary leiomyomatosis and RCC syndrome; however, abnormal negative FH immunohistochemistry (sometimes referred to as "loss") is highly specific for FH-deficient renal cancer. Of note, occasional mutated tumors may have normal staining, likely due to a dysfunctional protein that remains recognizable by the antibody. Therefore, a normal result does not always exclude the syndrome. Prominent nucleoli are present in many RCC types. Very prominent nucleoli with perinucleolar clearing was prototypically described in these tumors; however, this finding alone is not highly specific. Likewise, uterine leiomyomas are common. If a patient develops leiomyomas at an exceptionally young age, it may suggest the syndrome, but a precise age cutoff is not well established. Similarly, sarcomatoid dedifferentiation can occur in multiple RCC types.

3-10. Answer – A. Renal oncocytoma characteristically shows only scattered rare cells positive for cytokeratin 7, which some authors may occasionally refer to as negative. An exception to this is the central scar area of the tumor, in which the amount of staining is often increased. KIT is commonly positive, which may aid in distinguishing from clear cell or other RCC types (but not from chromophobe RCC, which is also KIT positive). Negative staining for succinate dehydrogenase B (abnormal lack of the protein/"loss") would suggest succinate dehydrogenase-deficient RCC, which is now recognized as a distinct tumor type. Colloidal iron staining is typically negative in oncocytoma, in contrast to chromophobe RCC, although this can be technically challenging in some laboratories.

CHAPTER 4 TESTIS

4-1. Answer – C. The most common cause of testicular vasculitis is PAN-like systemic vasculitis that also involves the testicular vessels. All infarcts, both segmental and global, eventually lead to necrotic "ghost tubules" of the remnant spermatic tubules. Global infarct involving the entire testis are the classic finding following testicular torsion. If a testicle is only torsed for a short period of time, blood flow may be restored prior to tubular necrosis and diffuse hemorrhage with vascular congestion may be the predominant pattern.

4-2. Answer – A. Spermatocytic tumors do not arise from germ cell neoplasia in situ (GCNIS). These tumors originate from nontransformed germ cells, possibly differentiated spermatogonia. As a result, the finding of GCNIS is not compatible with a diagnosis of spermatocytic seminoma. Postpubertal teratomas are derived from GCNIS-derived malignant germ cell tumors, even in their pure form. More commonly, they are found in mixed germ cell tumors and the diagnosis is apparent. In the pure form, the identification of isochromosome 12p in a teratoma supports its postpubertal, malignant nature. Alternatively, dermoid and epidermoid cysts of the testis are also not derived from germ cell neoplasia and would not demonstrate isochromosome 12p.

4-3. Answer – False. The finding of histiocyte-rich granulomatous inflammation in the testis should prompt thorough evaluation for the presence of seminoma. Seminomas may have such brisk granulomatous responses that the actual malignant cells comprise the minority of cells and can be missed. Other features that support a malignant process would be the identification of germ cell neoplasia in situ and OCT4, CD117, or D2-40 labeling of atypical cells. In the absence of a seminoma, granulomatous inflammation may occur in response to fungus, tuberculosis, sarcoidosis, vasculitis, malakoplakia, or sperm granuloma.

4-4. Answer – B. Sarcomatoid differentiation is frequently identified in metastatic yolk sac tumor and can lead to diagnostic difficulty. A sarcomatoid yolk sac tumor should be considered in the setting of spindle cell neoplasm of unknown origin in a patient at risk for, or with history of, germ cell tumor, and expression of AE1/3 and glypican 3 in the spindle cells would support a diagnosis of yolk sac tumor. Yolk sac tumor has myriad architectural patterns and accurate diagnosis requires recognition of its many appearances. The presence of Schiller-Duval bodies is helpful for the diagnosis of yolk sac tumor; call-Exner bodies are associated with granulosa cell tumors. GATA3 infrequently marks yolk sac tumor weakly but may be useful in the diagnosis of other germ cell tumors.

4-5. Answer – False. Benign Leydig cells may be identified in the spermatic cord soft tissue, commonly located adjacent to nerves. Testicular mediastinum, tunica albuginea, and the epididymis may also contain benign Leydig cells. The only definitive diagnostic feature for determining malignancy in Leydig cell tumors (and all sex cord stromal tumors) is metastasis. However, several features worrisome for malignancy have been proposed, including large size (>5 cm), infiltrative margins, extratesticular extension (minus the above mentioned sites), cytologic atypia, increased or atypical mitotic figures, lymphovascular invasion, necrosis, and increased Ki-67 proliferation index.

4-6. Answer – D. Germ cell neoplasia in situ (GCNIS) is a proliferation of malignant germ cells within seminiferous tubules in the spermatogonial niche (along the basement membrane). The immunohistochemical profile is similar to that of seminoma. Although GCNIS usually is present in tubules with impaired spermatogenesis (such tubules would be the best place to search for GCNIS), it is possible to occasionally encounter it in tubules with spermatogenesis. This is thought to occur when GCNIS spreads into normal tubules in a retrograde fashion.

4-7. Answer – True. Pathologic stage 3 testicular tumors directly invade the spermatic cord soft tissue. This includes the base of the spermatic cord where it meets the epididymis. Gross examination and sectioning should specifically comment on this region of the testis and sample it adequately. However, it should be noted that the finding of lymphovascular invasion in the spermatic cord, in the absence of soft tissue invasion, does not count as pT3 disease.

4-8. Answer – A and C. Spontaneous regression of germ cell tumors may occur in any germ cell tumor but is most commonly associated with seminoma. The clinical scenario often involves primary presentation of metastatic germ cell tumor without an obvious testicular mass. In the orchiectomy specimen, there may be a testicular scar, which is nonspecific for regression and may occur in other settings. The most specific features for regressed germ cell tumor are the findings of GCNIS in the surrounding tubules and intratubular coarse calcifications.

4-9. Answer – C. A panel of AE1/3, CD30, CD117, and D2-40 would be useful, with embryonal carcinoma expressing AE1/3 and CD30 and lacking CD117 and D2-40 expression. Seminoma has the opposite immunoprofile with CD117 and D2-40 positivity, with negative or minimal CD30 and AE1/3. SF1, inhibin, and calretinin are useful markers for sex cord stromal tumors, but do not play a role in the distinction of germ cell tumors. GATA3, HCG, AFP, and glypican would be a helpful immunopanel for identifying choriocarcinoma (GATA3 and HCG positive) and yolk sac tumor (AFP and glypican positive). MOC31 and BerEp4 are generic carcinoma markers and do not play a specific role in any germ cell tumor workup.

4-10. Answer – C. Tubular atrophy with decreased tubular diameter is associated with cryptorchidism, not tubular hyperplasia. Sertoli cell nodules, hemosiderin deposition, and association with infertility are all findings in cryptorchidism. Additional findings include intratubular microlithiasis, peritubular fibrosis with prominent Leydig cells and possible mixed pattern of maturation arrest, Sertoli only syndrome, and hypospermatogenesis.

CHAPTER 5 PARATESTIS AND EXTERNAL GENITALIA

5-1. Answer – B. Hydroceles are fluid accumulations in the mesothelial-lined space between the testis and the scrotal wall. The wall may contain skeletal muscle. Mesothelial hyperplasia is more typically found in hydrocele specimens. Spermatocele, in contrast, is a dilation of ejaculatory structures, especially the ductules of the epididymis. Distinction between hydrocele and spermatocele can be difficult, because the lining of spermatocele is often flattened, mimicking mesothelium; however, findings that would favor spermatocele include sperm in the lumen, presence of epididymal structures, or columnar lining cells. A varicocele is a dilated vein, and a hematocele is accumulation of blood in the scrotum.

5-2. Answer – C. A mesothelial proliferation that respects an "imaginary line," that is, restricted to a superficial, band-like zone, favors a diagnosis of mesothelial hyperplasia over mesothelioma. Also, mesothelial hyperplasia should typically not form a gross mass and should lack stromal invasion, cytologic atypia, desmoplasia, and necrosis. Adenomatoid tumor is a benign mesothelial proliferation, and therefore, mesothelial markers do not distinguish it from mesothelioma. Rather, the morphologic pattern of gland-like structures with bridging luminal strands is diagnostic of adenomatoid tumor. Hyaline globules are present in both adenomatous hyperplasia of the rete testis and yolk sac tumor. Therefore, invasion of embryonal carcinoma into the rete testis with associated rete hyperplasia could lead to misdiagnosis of mixed embryonal carcinoma and yolk sac tumor. (Clear cell) papillary cystadenoma of the epididymis is, for unknown reasons, almost identical to clear cell papillary renal cell carcinoma, including immunohistochemical positivity for carbonic anhydrase IX and cytokeratin 7, with negative results for CD10 and AMACR. Clear cell papillary renal cell carcinoma is nonaggressive, so it is unlikely to metastasize; however, metastatic conventional clear cell renal cell carcinoma can often be recognized by cytologic atypia and positivity for CD10 or RCC antigen. Clear cell renal cell carcinoma typically lacks papillary formation, is positive for CA-IX, and has minimal or no cytokeratin 7 labeling; however, exceptions occur.

5-3. Answer – B. Large lipomatous tumors from the spermatic cord (>10 cm) are technically retroperitoneal and raise concern for atypical lipomatous tumor/well-differentiated liposarcoma. Immunohistochemistry or FISH for *MDM2* may be necessary before making a benign diagnosis. Small "cord lipomas," in contrast, may not be true lipomatous neoplasms but rather nonspecific tracking of adipose tissue along the spermatic cord or inguinal canal. Therefore, extensive evaluation for small specimens without atypia is probably unnecessary in most cases, especially if the gross appearance is not that of a round or ovoid mass. Fibrous pseudotumor of the paratestis (nodular periorchitis, proliferative funiculitis, other terms) has been typically found to be negative for ALK immunohistochemistry, suggesting it is distinct from inflammatory myofibroblastic tumor. A bland smooth muscle proliferation encircling ducts of the epididymis is one of the typical patterns of smooth muscle hyperplasia of the testicular adnexa, which is a benign process of unknown etiology. Leiomyosarcoma, in contrast, is quite rare as a paratesticular lesion. Even for myoid-appearing spindle cell lesions with atypia, it may be warranted to evaluate the possibility of dedifferentiated liposarcoma before rendering a diagnosis of paratesticular leiomyosarcoma.

5-4. Answer – False. Scrotal calcinosis is thought to potentially originate from rupture and calcification of epidermal inclusions cysts, although it is unknown why this pattern of predominantly calcified nodules is common in the scrotum and uncommon in other sites where epidermal cysts occur.

5-5. Answer – B. Balanitis xerotica obliterans is an equivalent term to lichen sclerosus et atrophicus, which is better known for its gynecologic counterpart. It is associated with differentiated-type penile intraepithelial neoplasia (PeIN) and non-HPV related invasive squamous cell carcinoma (similar to the etiology of differentiated vulvar squamous cell carcinomas). Although a dense plasma cell–rich inflammatory infiltrate may represent plasma cell balanitis (Zoon balanitis), syphilis should always be a consideration, even if special stains or immunohistochemistry are negative for organisms, as these are less sensitive than serologic tests.

5-6. Answer – B. Peyronie disease is usually hypocellular, composed of collagen and spindle-shaped fibroblastic cells, sometimes with prominent ossification. It is considered a member of the group of superficial fibromatoses (including palmar and plantar fibromatoses), although it is typically less cellular than these and rarely if ever mimics a sarcoma. Massive localized lymphedema is an unusual process that forms a mass-like lesion in dependent skin sites, typically in patients with morbid obesity or other potential causes of lymphatic obstruction. These lesions can mimic liposarcoma due to large size and mildly atypical cells amidst fat and loose connective tissue; however, awareness of the history of obesity and lack of fully malignant hyperchromatic cells of liposarcoma can aid in recognition of this entity. Sclerosing lipogranuloma is not idiopathic but rather occurs as a reaction to injection of exogenous materials in the genitals, such as oil, paraffin, or silicone. Myointimoma has only been reported to occur in the penis, not the scrotum, although it bears similarity to intravascular fasciitis and may be related.

5-7. Answer – C. Warty-basaloid PeIN and other penile cancer types that have a basaloid pattern are typically associated with HPV. In contrast, verrucous carcinoma and differentiated penile cancer types are usually not associated with HPV. Although diffuse angiokeratomas are associated with Fabry disease, those localized to the scrotum are typically not regarded as suggesting the disease. Lesions that resemble seborrheic keratosis of the genitals are often HPV associated, and therefore, these may be better regarded as condylomas in most cases.

5-8. Answer – D. NKX3.1 positivity would suggest secondary spread of prostatic adenocarcinoma. Although GATA3 is a marker of urothelial carcinoma, it is also positive in almost all primary extramammary Paget disease lesions and, therefore, is not helpful alone in distinguishing these two considerations. Positivity for p63 would suggest pagetoid spread of squamous cell carcinoma rather than primary disease, which is thought to originate from skin adnexal glands. Cytokeratin 7 is typically positive in primary extramammary Paget disease.

5-9. Answer – D. The eighth edition AJCC staging of penile cancer introduced several changes. Involvement of the corpus spongiosum and cavernosum were previously both the same stage in the seventh edition; however, these are now split in the eighth edition (spongiosum pT2, cavernosum pT3). Involvement of the urethra previously dictated pT3; however, this is now compatible with either pT2 or pT3, likely because involvement of the urethral meatus is more common and less severe than invasion through the shaft into the urethra. Involvement of the prostate (adjacent organ) is pT4.

5-10. Answer – True. Prostatic adenocarcinoma and urothelial carcinoma are among the most common tumors to metastasize to the penis. Priapism can occur as a presenting finding, likely due to occlusion of the erectile tissue by tumor emboli.

Note: Page numbers followed by "f" indicate figures, "t" indicate tables and "b" indicate boxes.